Hematopoietic Cell Transplants

Concepts, Controversies, and Future Directions

Hematopoietic Cell Transplants

Concepts, Controversies, and Future Directions

Edited by

Editor-in-Chief

Hillard M. Lazarus, MD, FACP

Co-Editors

Robert Peter Gale, MD, PhD

Armand Keating, MD, FRCPC

Andrea Bacigalupo, MD

Reinhold Munker, MD

Kerry Atkinson MBBS, MD, DTM&H, FRCP, FRACP

Deputy Editor

Syed Ali Abutalib, MD

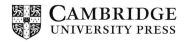

CAMBRIDGE
UNIVERSITY PRESS

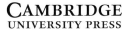

University Printing House, Cambridge CB2 8BS, United Kingdom

Cambridge University Press is part of the University of Cambridge.

It furthers the University's mission by disseminating knowledge in the pursuit of education, learning and research at the highest international levels of excellence.

www.cambridge.org
Information on this title: www.cambridge.org/9781316606698

© Cambridge University Press 2017

First published 2017

Printed in the United Kingdom by Clays St lves plc

A catalogue record for this publication is available from the British Library

Library of Congress Cataloging-in-Publication Data
Names: Lazarus, Hillard M., editor.
Title: Hematopoietic cell transplants : concepts, controversies and future directions / edited by editor-in-chief, Hillard M. Lazarus ; co-editors, Robert Peter Gale, Armand Keating, Andrea Bacigalupo, Reinhold Munker, Kerry Atkinson ; deputy editor, Syed Ali Abutalib.
Description: Cambridge, United Kingdom ; New York : Cambridge University Press, 2016. | Includes bibliographical references and index.
Identifiers: LCCN 2016008140 | ISBN 9781107115248 (hardback) | ISBN 9781316606698 (mixed media) | ISBN 9781316335727 (Cambridge books online)
Subjects: | MESH: Hematopoietic Stem Cell Transplantation | Donor Selection | Postoperative Complications–prevention & control | Leukemia–therapy | Lymphoma–therapy
Classification: LCC QH588.S83 | NLM WH 380 | DDC 616.02/774–dc23
LC record available at https://lccn.loc.gov/2016008140

9781316606698 (Mixed Media)
9781107115248 (Hardback)
9781316335727 (Cambridge Books Online)

Dedications

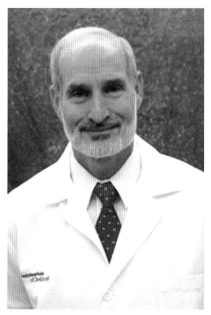

Hillard M. Lazarus, MD, FACP

Professor Lazarus dedicates this textbook to Joan, his loving and supportive wife of nearly 40 years.

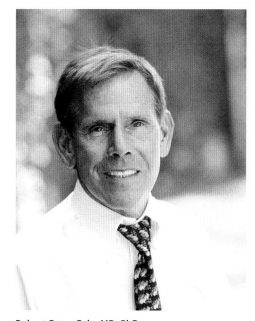

Robert Peter Gale, MD, PhD

Dedicated to my wife Laura Jane Gale and Sabine Jacob who helped immensely.

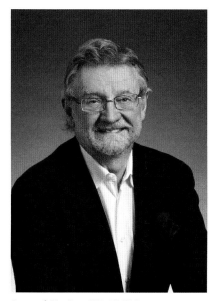

Armand Keating, MD, FRCPC

To our many, many residents and fellows and our future leaders.

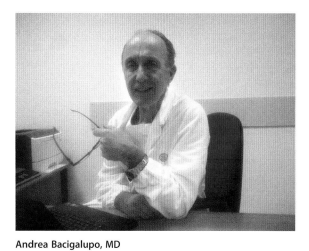

Andrea Bacigalupo, MD

To my mentor, Professor Alberto Marmont – a great scientist and a teacher

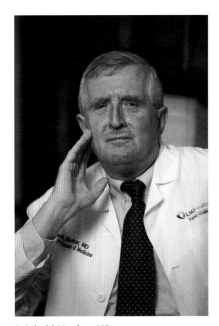

Reinhold Munker, MD

For the benefit of humanity and science.

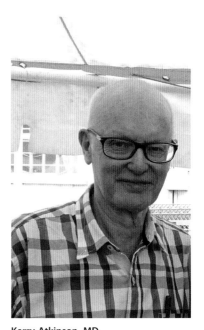

Kerry Atkinson, MD

For Virginia and Ilmar, Simon and Joanne, Sally and Jim, and Scott and Louise.

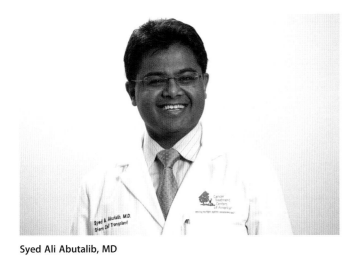

Syed Ali Abutalib, MD

To my everlasting thirst for acquiring medical knowledge, my valued patients, mentors, and to my family, most especially my daughter, Sakeena Ali.

Contents

The Editors

Editor-in-Chief:

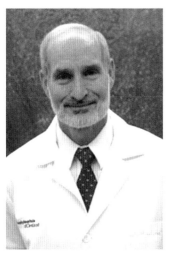

Hillard M. Lazarus, MD, FACP
Professor of Medicine, Case Comprehensive Cancer Center, Case Western Reserve University, University Hospitals Case Medical Center, Cleveland, OH, USA

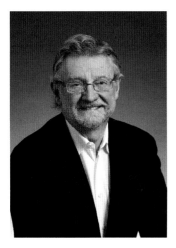

Armand Keating, MD, FRCPC
Professor of Medicine and of Biomedical Engineering, University of Toronto; Director, Cell Therapy Program, Princess Margaret Cancer Centre, Toronto, ON, Canada

Co-Editors:

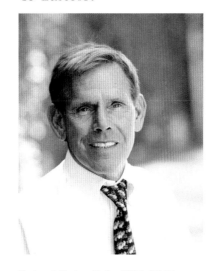

Robert Peter Gale, MD, PhD
Haematology Research Centre, Division of Experimental Medicine, Department of Medicine, Imperial College London, London, UK

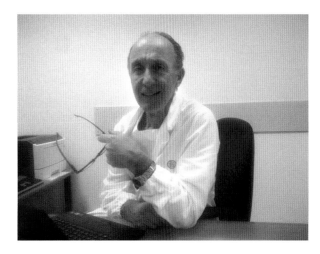

Andrea Bacigalupo, MD
Cattedra Ematologia, Universita' Cattolica del Sacro Cuore, Fondazione Policlinico, Unviersitario A Gemelli, Roma, Italia

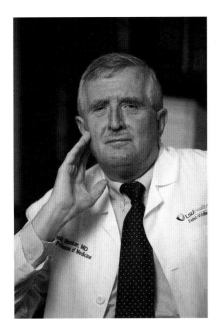

Reinhold Munker, MD
Professor of Medicine, Louisiana State University,
Shreveport, LA, USA

Deputy Editor:

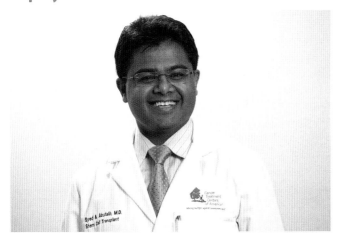

Syed Ali Abutalib, MD
Assistant Director, Hematology & Bone Marrow Transplant
Program, Cancer Treatment Centers of America, Zion,
IL, USA

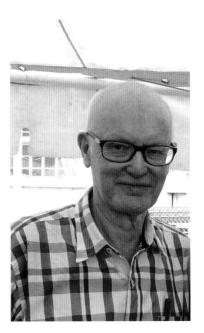

Kerry Atkinson, MBBS, MD, DTM&H, FRCP, FRACP
Adjunct Professor, University of Queensland Centre for
Clinical Research; Adjunct Professor, Stem Cell Laboratories,
Queensland University of Technology at the Translational
Research Institute; and Specialist in General Medicine,
Salisbury Medical Centre, Brisbane, QLD, Australia

List of Contributors

Edwin P. Alyea
Dana-Farber Cancer Institute, USA

Jane F. Apperley
Centre for Haematology, Faculty of Medicine, Imperial College London, Hammersmith Hospital, UK and Department of Clinical Haematology, Imperial College Healthcare NHS Trust, Hammersmith Hospital, UK

James O. Armitage
University of Nebraska Medical Center, Department of Internal Medicine, Division of Hematology-Oncology, USA

L.C.M. Arruda
Center for Cell-Based Therapy, São Paulo Research Foundation (FAPESP), Brazil and Department of Biochemistry and Immunology, Ribeirão Preto Medical School, University of São Paulo, Ribeirão Preto, Brazil

Andrew S. Artz
University of Chicago, USA

Franco Aversa
Division of Hematology and Transplant Unit, Department of Clinical and Experimental Medicine, University of Parma, Italy

Veronika Bachanova
University of Minnesota Blood and Marrow Transplant Program, Department of Medicine, Division of Hematology and Oncology, USA

Karen K. Ballen
Stem Cell Transplant Program, University of Virginia Health Center, USA

A. John Barrett
Chief Stem Cell Allotransplantation Section, Hematology Branch, National Heart. Lung and Blood Institute, National Institutes of Health, USA

Asad Bashey
The Blood and Marrow Transplant Group, Northside Hospital, Atlanta, GA, USA

Vijaya R. Bhatt
University of Nebraska Medical Center, Department of Internal Medicine, Division of Hematology-Oncology, USA

Joan Bladé
Hospital Clínic i Provincial de Barcelona, Institut d'Investigacions Biomédiques August Pi I Sunyer (IDIBAPS), Barcelona, Spain

R. Gregory Bociek
University of Nebraska Medical Center, Department of Internal Medicine, Division of Hematology-Oncology, USA

Catherine M. Bollard
Program for Cell Enhancement and Technologies for Immunotherapy, Sheikh Zayed Institute for Pediatric Surgical Innovation, and Center for Cancer and Immunology Research, Children's National Health System, USA

Renier J. Brentjens
Department of Medicine, Center for Cell Engineering, and Molecular Pharmacology and Chemistry Program, Memorial Sloan Kettering Cancer Center, USA

Sarah A. Buckley
Fred Hutchinson Cancer Research Center, University of Washington, Seattle, WA, USA

Linda J. Burns
Department of Medicine, Division of Hematology and Oncology, University of Minnesota Blood and Marrow Transplant Program, USA

Paolo F. Caimi
Department of Medicine, Division of Hematology and Oncology, Case Western Reserve University, and Case Comprehensive Cancer Center, USA

Bruce Camitta
Pediatric Hematology/Oncology, Medical College of Wisconsin/Children's Research Institute of the Children's Hospital of Wisconsin, USA

Enric Carreras
Hematology Department, Hospital Clinic Barcelona, Spain

Nelson J. Chao
Division of Hematologic Malignancies and Cellular Therapy, Department of Internal Medicine, Duke University Medical Center, Durham, NC, USA

Andy I. Chen
Center for Hematologic Malignancies, Knight Cancer Institute, Oregon Health & Science University, USA

Stefan O. Ciurea
Department of Stem Cell Transplantation and Cellular Therapy, The University of Texas, MD Anderson Cancer Center, USA

R. Coleman Lindsley
Harvard University, USA

Robert Frank Cornell
Vanderbilt University Medical Center, Nashville, TN, USA

Charles Craddock
Centre for Clinical Haematology, Queen Elizabeth Hospital, Birmingham, UK

Conrad Russell Y. Cruz
Program for Cell Enhancement and Technologies for Immunotherapy, Sheikh Zayed Institute for Pediatric Surgical Innovation, and Center for Cancer and Immunology Research, Children's National Health System, USA

Francesco d'Amore
Aarhus University, Denmark

Francesco Dazzi
King's College London, UK

Marcos de Lima
Division of Hematology and Oncology, University Hospitals Seidman Cancer Center, Case Western Reserve University, USA

Binod Dhakal
Division of Hematology/Oncology, Medical College of Wisconsin, Milwaukee, WI, USA

Elizabeth C. DiMaggio
Blood and Marrow Transplantation, Moffitt Cancer Center, USA

John F. DiPersio
University of Washington, St. Louis, MO, USA

Sarah Dobrozsi
Pediatric Hematology/Oncology, Medical College of Wisconsin/Children's Research Institute of the Children's Hospital of Wisconsin, USA

Anita D'Souza
Center for International Blood and Marrow Transplant Research (CIBMTR) and the Medical College of Wisconsin, Milwaukee, USA

Carlo Dufour
Clinical and Experimental Hematology Unit, G. Gaslini Children's Hospital, Italy

Mary Eapen
Division of Hematology and Oncology, Department of Medicine, Medical College of Wisconsin, USA

Stephane Eeckhoudt
Cliniques universitaires Saint Luc, Belgium

Lawrence Einhorn
Distinguished Professor of Medicine, Livestrong Foundation Professor of Oncology, Department of Medicine, Indiana University, Indianapolis, IN, USA

Fredrik Ellin
Department of Internal Medicine , Kalmar County Hospital, Kalmar, Sweden

Mahmoud Elsawy
Clinical Research Division, Fred Hutchinson Cancer Research Center, USA and Department of Medical Oncology, National Cancer Institute, Cairo University, Egypt

D. Farge
Unité Clinique de Médecine Interne et Pathologie Vasculaire, Hôpital Saint-Louis, Paris, France

Timothy S. Fenske
Division of Hematology & Oncology, Medical College of Wisconsin, USA

Marcelo A. Fernández-Viña
Department of Pathology, Stanford University School of Medicine, Palo Alto, CA, USA

Jürgen Finke
Hematology, Oncology, and Stem Cell Transplantation, Freiburg University Medical Center, Germany

A. Fischer
Université Paris and Institut Universitaire de France, France

Courtney D. Fitzhugh
Sickle Cell Disease Branch, National Heart, Lung, and Blood Institute, National Institutes of Health, Bethesda, MD, USA

Hua Fung
Case Western Reserve University and University Hospital of Cleveland, Cleveland, OH, USA

Javid Gaziev
International Centre for Transplantation in Thalassemia and Sickle Cell Anemia, Mediterranean Institute of Hematology, Italy

Adrian P. Gee
GMP Facilities Center for Cell & Gene Therapy, Baylor College of Medicine, Houston, TX, USA

Stanton L. Gerson
Case Western Reserve University and University Hospital of Cleveland, Cleveland, OH, USA

Morie A. Gertz
Department of Medicine, Mayo Clinic Rochester, MN, USA

Thomas Giever
Medical College of Wisconsin, Milwaukee, WI, USA

Sergio A. Giralt
Melvin Berlin Family Chair in Myeloma Research, Weill Cornell Medical College, USA

Corrado Girmenia
Dipartimento di Ematologia, Oncologia, Anatomia Patologica e Medicina Rigenerativa, Azienda Policlinico Umberto I, Italy

E. Gluckman
Eurocord, Hôpital Saint Louis, Paris, France

Dennis Goldfinger
Department of Laboratory Medicine and Pathology, David Geffen School of Medicine at UCLA, USA

Michael Green
Division of Hematologic Malignancies and Cellular Therapy, Department of Internal Medicine, Duke University Medical Center, USA

Gregory A. Hale
All Children's Hospital, USA

Parameswaran Hari
Medical College of Wisconsin, USA

Alex F. Herrera
Department of Hematology/Hematopoietic Cell Transplantation, City of Hope Medical Center, USA

Ernest Holler
Department of Internal Medicine 3 (Hematology, Oncology, and Stem Cell Transplantation), University Medical Center, Germany

Sarah A. Holstein
Division of Oncology and Hematology, Department of Internal Medicine, University of Nebraska Medical Center, USA

Netanel A. Horowitz
Department of Hematology and Bone Marrow Transplantation, Rambam Health Care Campus, and Bruce Rappaport Faculty of Medicine, Technion, Israel Institute of Technology, Israel

Christopher S. Hourigan
Myeloid Malignancies Section, Hematology Branch, National Heart, Lung and Blood Institute, National Institutes of Health, USA

Andrew J. Innes
Centre for Haematology, Faculty of Medicine, Imperial College London, Hammersmith Hospital, UK

Esa Jantunen
Department of Medicine, Kuopio University Hospital, Finland

Kimberley A. Kasow
University of North Carolina-Chapel Hill, NC, USA

Lakshmikanth Katragadda
Division of Hematology & Oncology, University of Florida, USA

Partow Kebriaei
University of Texas, MD Anderson Cancer Center, USA

Natasha Kekre
Dana Faber Cancer Institute, USA

Michael D. Keller
Program for Cell Enhancement and Technologies for Immunotherapy, Sheikh Zayed Institute for Pediatric Surgical Innovation, and Center for Cancer and Immunology Research, Children's National Health System, USA

Nandita Khera
Blood and Marrow Transplant Program, Mayo Clinic Arizona, USA

Christian Kollmannsberger
BC Cancer Centre, Canada

John Koreth
Dana-Farber Cancer Institute, USA

Amrita Krishnan
City of Hope, USA

Nicolaus Kröger
University Medical Center Hamburg-Eppendorf, Hamburg, Germany

Juan J. Lahuerta
Hospital Universitario, Madrid, Spain

Grete F. Lauritzsen
Department of Oncology, Oslo University Hospital, Oslo, Norway

Helen Leather
Division of Hematology/Oncology, College of Medicine, University of Florida, USA

Dean A. Lee
Division of Hematology, Oncology, and BMT, Nationwide Children's Hospital, Columbus, OH, USA

Michelle Limei Poon
National University Hospital Singapore, Department of Hematology Oncology, Singapore

Mark Litzow
Mayo Clinic College of Medicine Rochester, USA

Per Ljungman
Department of Hematology, Karolinska University Hospital, Division of Hematology, Department of Medicine Huddinge, Karolinska Institute, Sweden

Guido Lucarelli
International Centre for Transplantation in Thalassemia and Sickle Cell Anemia, Mediterranean Institute of Hematology, Italy

Alejandro Madrigal
Anthony Nolan Research Institute and University College London, UK

Navneet S. Majhail
Blood & Marrow Transplant Program, Cleveland Clinic, USA

K.C.R. Malmegrim
Center for Cell-Based Therapy, São Paulo Research Foundation (FAPESP), Brazil and Department of Clinical, Toxicological, and Bromatological Analysis, School of Pharmaceutical Sciences of Ribeirão Preto, University of São Paulo, Ribeirão Preto, Brazil

Susanna Mannisto
Department of Oncology, Helsinki University Central Hospital, Helsinki, Finland

Judith C.W. Marsh
Department of Haematological Medicine, King's College Hospital, London, UK

María Victoria Mateos
Hospital Universitario de Salamanca-IBSAL, IBMCC-CSIC, Spain

Sebastian Mayer
Division of Hematology/Oncology, Weill Cornell Medical College/New York Presbyterian Hospital, USA

Richard T. Maziarz
Center for Hematologic Malignancies, Knight Cancer Institute, Oregon Health & Science University, USA

Shaun McCann
St James' Hospital and Trinity College Dublin, Ireland

Philip L. McCarthy
Roswell Park Cancer Institute, USA

Jeffrey McCullough
Department of Laboratory Medicine and Pathology, University of Minnesota, USA

Donal P. McLornan
King's College London, UK

Rohtesh S. Mehta,
Department of Stem Cell Transplantation and Cellular Therapy, UT MD Anderson Cancer Center, USA

Roland Mertelsmann
Department of Internal Medicine I, Hematology, Oncology, and Stem Cell Transplantation, Freiburg University Medical Center, Germany

Peter Meyer
Hematology Oncology Unit, Stavanger University Hospital, Stavanger, Norway

Maurizio Miano
Clinical and Experimental Hematology Unit, G. Gaslini Children's Hospital, Italy

Shanna Morgan
Department of Laboratory Medicine and Pathology, University of Minnesota, USA

Lori S. Muffly
Colorado Blood Cancer Institute, Denver, CO, USA

Craig Nichols
Virginia Mason Medical Center, Seattle, WA, USA

Rebecca L. Olin
University of California San Francisco, San Francisco, CA, USA

M.C. Oliveira
Center for Cell-Based Therapy, São Paulo Research Foundation (FAPESP), Brazil and Division of Clinical Immunology, Department of Internal Medicine, Ribeirão Preto Medical School, University of São Paulo, Ribeirão Preto, Brazil

John M. Pagel
Fred Hutchinson Cancer Research Center, University of Washington, Seattle, WA, USA

Elisabeth Paietta
Montefiore Medical Center, Albert Einstein College of Medicine, Bronx, NY, USA

Soo J. Park
University of Washington, St. Louis, MO, USA

Marcelo Pasquini
Center for International Blood and Marrow Transplant Research (CIBMTR) and the Medical College of Wisconsin, Milwaukee, USA

Jakob R. Passweg
Hematology Division, Basel University Hospital, Basel, Switzerland

Steven Z. Pavletic
Experimental Transplantation and Immunology Branch, National Cancer Institute, Bethesda, MD, USA

Martin Bjerregård Pedersen
Department of Hematology, Aarhus University Hospital, Aarhus, Denmark

Régis Peffault de Latour
Hôpital Saint-Louis, Hôpitaux de Paris, France

Miguel-Angel Perales
Adult Bone Marrow Transplantation Service, Memorial Sloan Kettering Cancer Center, Weill Cornell Medical College, NY, USA

Sai Ravi Pingali
Houston Methodist Cancer Center, Weill Cornell Medical College, Cornell University, Houston, TX, USA

Victoria T. Potter
King's College London, UK

Iskra Pusic
Division of Oncology, Department of Internal Medicine, Washington University School of Medicine, USA

Sarwish Rafiq
Department of Medicine, Memorial Sloan Kettering Cancer Center, New York, NY, USA

Thomas Relander
Department of Oncology, Skane University Hospital, Lund, Sweden

Katayoun Rezvani
Department of Stem Cell Transplantation and Cellular Therapy, UT MD Anderson Cancer Center, USA

Marcie L. Riches
Division of Hematology/Oncology, Department of Medicine, The University of North Carolina at Chapel Hill, Chapel Hill, NC, USA

J. Douglas Rizzo
Center for International Blood and Marrow Transplant Research (CIBMTR) and the Medical College of Wisconsin, Milwaukee, USA

Laura Rosiñol
Hospital Clínic i Provincial de Barcelona, Institut d'Investigacions Biomédiques August Pi I Sunyer (IDIBAPS), Barcelona, Spain

Jacob M. Rowe
Department of Hematology and Bone Marrow Transplantation, Rambam Health Care Campus, Israel and Department of Hematology, Shaare Zedek Medical Center, and Bruce Rappaport Faculty of Medicine, Technion, Israel Institute of Technology, Israel

Jesus F. San Miguel
Clínica Universidad de Navarra/Centro de Investigación Médica Aplicada (CIMA), Spain

Aurore Saudemont
Anthony Nolan Research Institute and University College London, UK

Mark A. Schroeder
University of Washington, St. Louis, MO, USA

Bronwen E. Shaw
Center for International Blood and Marrow Transplant Research (CIBMTR) and the Medical College of Wisconsin, Milwaukee, WI, USA

Taimur Sher
Mayo Clinic Florida, USA

Elizabeth J. Shpall
Department of Stem Cell Transplantation and Cellular Therapy, UT MD Anderson Cancer Center, USA

Melody Smith
Adult Bone Marrow Transplantation Service, Memorial Sloan Kettering Cancer Center, Weill Cornell Medical College, New York, USA

Sonali M. Smith
Department of Medicine, The University of Chicago, USA

Robert J. Soiffer
Dana-Farber Cancer Institute, Brigham and Women's Hospital, Harvard Medical School, Boston, MA, USA

Mohamed L. Sorror
Clinical Research Division, Fred Hutchinson Cancer Research Center, USA and Division of Medical Oncology, Department of Medicine, University of Washington School of Medicine, USA

Stephen Spellman
Immunobiology and Observational Research Center for International Blood and Marrow Transplant Research (CIBMTR), Minneapolis, USA

Lode J. Swinnen
Department of Oncology, Division of Hematologic Malignancies, Johns Hopkins University, Baltimore, MD, USA

Julie-An Talano
Children's Hospital of Wisconsin, Milwaukee, WI, USA

Martin S. Tallman
Leukemia Service, Memorial Sloan Kettering Cancer Center, Weill Cornell Medical College, USA

Michael T. Tees
Colorado Blood Cancer Institute, Denver, CO, USA

John F. Tisdale
Molecular and Clinical Hematology Branch, USA

Helle Toldbod
Department of Hematology, Aarhus University Hospital, Aarhus, Denmark

Masumi Ueda
Division of Hematology and Oncology, Department of Medicine, University Hospitals Case Medical Center, Case Western Reserve University, USA

Koen van Besien
Division of Hematology/Oncology, Weill Cornell Medical College/New York Presbyterian Hospital, USA

Claudio Viscoli
Dipartimento di Malattie Infettive, IRCCS S. Martino University Hospital – IST, Italy

Zhiwei Wang
Center for International Blood and Marrow Transplant Research (CIBMTR) and the Medical College of Wisconsin, Milwaukee, USA

Dawn Ward
Department of Laboratory Medicine and Pathology, David Geffen School of Medicine at UCLA, Los Angeles, CA, USA

R. Patrick Weitzel
Molecular and Clinical Hematology Branch, USA

Basem M. William
Division of Hematology and Oncology, Stem Cell Transplantation Program, University Hospitals Seidman Cancer Center, Case Western Reserve University, USA

John R. Wingard
Division of Hematology/Oncology, University of Florida College of Medicine, USA

Preface

Hematopoietic cell transplantation is rapidly changing into directions entirely unpredictable even a decade ago. For example, in the first 40 years the focus of donor selection was on finding the *best* donor for everyone who *needed* a transplant. This strategy involved developing sophisticated techniques to unravel complexities of HLA, the major human histocompatibility complex. Today, with the use of HLA-haplotype-matched related donors, umbilical cord blood units, and more than 27 million adult unrelated donors from which to choose, we say everyone who *needs* a transplant can have one. In some sense we have moved away from selecting to de-selecting donors. But do we really know precisely who *needs* a transplant? We are less certain about this than we were 40 years ago.

Concepts underlying the pre-transplant *conditioning* also have changed dramatically. For many years the focus was on developing increasingly intensive regimens to eradicate disease. As a result of elegant pre-clinical studies that were moved into the clinical arena, this focus has shifted to decreasing the intensity of pre-transplant conditioning, relying more on immune-mediated mechanisms to prevent disease recurrence. And we have largely abandoned the notion there is a *best* donor for everyone: some people at high-risk of disease recurrence need a donor likely to cause some degree of graft-*versus*-host disease (G*v*HD) with its attendant anti-cancer efficacy but unavoidable adverse consequences. Other persons at low risk of disease recurrence might be better off receiving a transplant from a donor are less likely to cause G*v*HD. Are the trends we discuss above evidence-based? Sometimes, but often not.

Our field faces many other controversies. One *versus* two umbilical cord blood cell units? Graft-engineering *versus* use of post-transplant cyclophosphamide? Bone marrow *versus* mobilized blood cell grafts? And so on. The problem is the complexity, expense and requisite time to perform and follow the results of transplants often preclude doing appropriate clinical trials to resolve these issues. Further, at this time some problems defy resolution or may not be resolvable. Often our colleagues vote with their feet rather than their decisions being data-driven. We are no worse in this setting than our colleagues in other high technology medical fields, but we are not better either.

The situation we describe demands a different type of *textbook*. A textbook not a textbook. Not a door-stop but a living resource focused on controversies. One able to adapt rapidly by constant up-dating, linking to on-line versions and the like. We tried to develop such a resource with the help of over 150 thoughtful co-authors and over 170 lively chapters. We hope *Hematopoietic Cell Transplants: Concepts, Controversies, and Future Directions* accomplishes this goal and helps our readers appreciate what is known but especially what is unknown in our rapidly evolving field. In planning this book we were inspired by a quote from Voltaire: *Judge a man by questions rather than his answers.* We hope you agree.

Hillard M. Lazarus MD, FACP
Robert Peter Gale MD, PhD, DSc(hc), FACP, FRSM
(for The Editors)

A Brief History of Hematopoietic Cell Transplantation

Robert Peter Gale and Shaun McCann

The thing that has been is the thing that shall be; and the thing that is done is that which shall be done: There is nothing new under the sun.

Ecclesiastes

The history of bone marrow transplantation has been told by many colleagues in great detail, including some of the players. The reader is referred to these accounts for details, which are often personal views (see Suggested Reading). Our aim is to briefly summarize how bone marrow transplants developed and continue to develop. Details of most recent progress are covered in the chapters that follow. As such we see our target audience as younger colleagues who may not know some or any of this extraordinary history.

Where to begin? The *Táin Bó Cúailgne* (The Cattle Raid of Cooley), written in about 100 CE, describes Cethern, a seriously wounded warrior who in about 500 BCE was advised by Fingin, a healer, to bathe in a vessel of bone marrow (apparently stealing cattle is not taken lightly in Ireland; Figure 1.1). He was miraculously healed and returned to avenge his enemies.[1] Naturally, Fingin claimed success (or at least *proof-of-concept*), setting a continuing precedent for claiming efficacy based on a dubious study design and brief follow-up. On a cautionary note, Cethern killed 49 physicians who advised other therapies before he decided on a bone marrow cure.

Another example of bone marrow transplantation (perhaps better termed ingestion) existed among some tribes in New

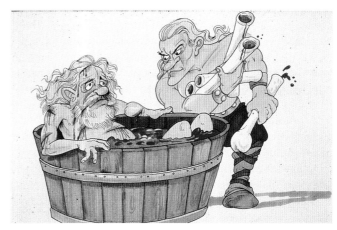

Figure 1.1. Cethern in the tub of marrow mash. With kind permission of James Cogan.

Guinea where women were expected to eat the bone marrow of decreased relatives to ensure passage into the ancestral world and continuation of their patriarchal lineage. Skip forward to the 19th century when the French physician Charles-Édouard Brown-Séquard described giving calves' bone marrow to women with chlorosis[2] or *green sickness* (hypochromic anemia), seen in languid women and virgins (brings to mind Botticelli's *Birth of Venus*; Figure 1.2). Brown-Séquard dissolved the bone marrow in glycerol (killing any living cells) and gave it to Parisian women by mouth. Not unexpectedly some of these women recovered given the considerable

---

[1] "Thereupon Fingin the prophetic leech asked of Cuchulain a vat of marrow wherewith to heal and to cure Cethern son of Fintan. Cuchulain proceeded to the camp and entrenchment of the men of Erin, and whatsoever he found of herds and flocks and droves there he took away with him. And he made a marrow-mash of their flesh and their bones and their skins; and Cethern son of Fintan was placed in the marrow-bath till the end of three days and three nights. And his flesh began to drink in the marrow-bath about him and the marrow-bath entered in within his stabs and his cuts, his sores and his many wounds. Thereafter he arose from the marrow-bath at the end of three days and three nights, [1]and he slept a day and a night after taking in the marrow." From The Ancient Irish Epic Tale *Táin Bó Cúalnge*, Author unknown, translated by Joseph Dunn. Gutenberg Project. 2005. EBook #16464.

[2] In 1554, German physician Johannes Lange described the condition as "peculiar to virgins." He prescribed sufferers should "live with men and copulate. If they conceive, they will recover." The name "chlorosis" was coined in 1615 by Montpellier professor of medicine Jean Varandal from the word "chloris" (Greek: χλωρις) meaning "greenish-yellow," "pale green," "pale," "pallid," or "fresh." Both Lange and Varande claimed Hippocrates as a reference.

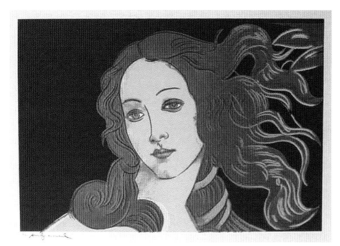

Figure 1.2. Andy Warhol. Details of Renaissance Paintings (Sando Botticelli, Birth of Venus, 1482), 1984.

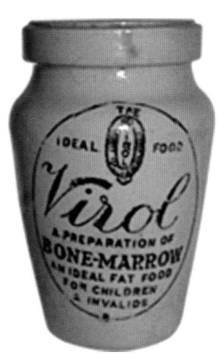

Figure 1.3. Apothecary jar for bone marrow.

amount of iron in the bone marrow extract. Brown-Séquard rightly claimed success but his explanation of how his elixir worked may have been a bit off and his cure rate may not have been more effective than that recommended by Dr. Johannes Lange in 1554 who prescribed that sufferers should "live with men and copulate. If they conceive, they will recover." Brown-Séquard was a controversial, eccentric figure known for self-reporting rejuvenated sexual prowess after eating extracts of monkey testes. Although his improvement was thought to be a placebo effect (the authors admit no personal experience), it was apparently sufficiently convincing to start the field of endocrinology. We return to hormones and hematopoiesis later. These are not isolated examples. For many centuries physicians and apothecaries gave bone marrow extracts from various creatures to treat diverse illnesses and complaints, often with remarkable success (Figure 1.3). And who can dispute the attractiveness of bone marrow on toast on a cold winter's day (a good fino sherry helps).

The development of modern bone marrow transplantation hinged on a convergence of diverse forces. This is so of many modern advances. Consider the city of Chicago. The Great Chicago Fire of 1871, caused by Ms. O'Leary's errant cow, burned the city to the ground (the Irish again). Rebuilding was needed but, with Lake Michigan on one side, it was clear the plan had to be largely vertical. The striking architecture we see today is the result of the convergence of three technologies: (1) development of steel beams, which allowed building to a greater height than possible with masonry-based structures; (2) development of elevators allowing people to ascend to high floors; and (3) harnessing electricity, which meant floor plates could be larger since not every working or living area had to be near a window.

What were the convergent forces at play in the evolution of bone marrow transplants? One was the Second World War and development of nuclear weapons and nuclear energy. Some readers will know of a letter from Albert Einstein to President Roosevelt in 1939 warning of German

efforts to develop an atomic bomb.[3] As a result, the US Government recruited scientists at the National Institutes of Health and the University of Chicago (where Enrico Fermi developed the first controlled nuclear chain reaction) to work on ways to counter the effects of radiation on humans, especially bone marrow failure.[4] Although this story is too complex for our chapter we should recall the first description of the effects of radiation on hematopoiesis which dates from 1903. Radiobiologists and physicians including Eugene Cronkite at the Brookhaven national laboratory, Arthur Compton at Washington University, Theodore Fliedner at the University of Ulm, Stafford Warren at UCLA and others from the National Cancer Institute (NCI), University of Chicago, UCLA, and Harrell in the UK and elsewhere played key roles in the field of radiation biology and radiation protection. Several led key sections of the Manhattan Project in Los Alamos.

In 1950, Leon Jacobsen and colleagues at the University of Chicago reported that shielding of the tibia or spleen and later intraperitoneal injection of spleen or bone marrow cells could *protect* an irradiated mouse from death.[5] The hypothesis was that *factors* released by the spleen or from spleen cells stimulated recovery of the irradiated bone marrow. The hypothesis (like that of Brown-Séquard and the monkey testes) was

---

[3] German plans for developing a nuclear weapon are nicely portrayed in the play *Copenhagen* of a 1941 meeting between Niels Bohr and Werner Heisenberg.

[4] Fermi fled to the USA from Italy to escape fascist race discrimination laws which would have affected his wife Laura.

[5] He was knighted for his work by King Olav of Norway and was a member of the North Dakota Rough Riders.

incorrect but eventually led Alan Erslev, John Adamson, Eugene Goldwasser, and others to isolate erythropoietin some years later. In 1952, Egon Lorenz, George Cogden, and Delta Uphoff reported that infusing spleen, or later bone marrow cells, could also rescue lethally irradiated mice and guinea pigs.

While on a holiday at Lake Windermere in the Lake District in England, Lorenz wrote to Uphoff:[6] "After talking with many people (I) am beginning to get convinced that we should not only try transfusions in mice at different intervals after irradiation but also injection (intravenous) of normal bone marrow suspension at different times after irradiation with the idea of repopulation (of) the destroyed bone marrow. As to technique, it should not be too difficult to get some bone marrow out as only (a) little may be necessary to produce the effect." And the rest is history as they say.

One interesting approach which arose from this research relates to doing bone marrow transplants in the battlefield. The idea (courtesy of Marvin Tyan) was that an enemy might use a tactical nuclear weapon; many soldiers would be irradiated and at risk of dying from bone marrow failure. Medics would roll up, extract some blood or bone marrow from a volunteer, mix it with an aliquot of the radiation victim's blood and add concanavallin-A. The donor immune cells would proliferate and commit "suicide" obviating the need for HLA-matching and preventing graft-versus-host disease (GvHD). This led George Santos to the idea, once widely used, of giving persons with aplastic anemia a unit of donor blood followed by cyclophosphamide just prior to an allo-transplant. If this sounds like using cyclophosphamide after an HLA-haplotype-matched transplant you are on the right track.

The discovery of GvHD is another interesting story. Irradiated mice receiving spleen or bone marrow cells typically died within 2 weeks. This phenomenon was termed *primary disease* (namely, death from bone marrow failure). To save monies, experiments were usually terminated at about this time point. However, on one occasion Lorenz went on vacation to Switzerland and a cage of transplanted mice was lost for another 2 weeks. When the cage was recovered by Delta Uphoff she noted that the mice had ratty fur (excuse the pun), inflamed footpads, and diarrhea. No one knew what was causing this and so (as we do today) it was termed *secondary disease* (or runt disease). It was not until 1962 when David Barnes and John Loutit showed that transplanting parental cells into an F1 hybrid recipient but not the reverse resulted in secondary disease that the pathophysiology of GvHD was understood. It was named GvHD by Morten Simonson in 1965. We recently wrote on the risk of naming diseases (such as *autologous GvHD, engraftment syndrome*)

implying an unproved etiology. *Secondary disease* (secondary to what?) is a good example.

Another technology contributing to this convergence was the development of genetically defined inbred mouse strains led mostly by George Snell at the Bar Harbor Laboratories.[7] In 1952, Joan Main and Richmond Prehn showed that a chimeric mouse would accept a skin graft from the bone marrow donor, and Ford used cytogenetics to prove that hematopoietic recovery was derived from donor bone marrow cells rather than recovery of the recipient's bone marrow.

A third enabling technology was defining the genetic loci controlling transplant acceptance and rejection, first in mice (H2), later in dogs (DLA) and subhuman primates (RhLA). In the late 1950s and early 1960s, Dausset, Benacerraf, Jan van Rood, Rose Payne, Felix Rapaport, Walter Bodmer, and others began to define the HLA system in humans by noting that the sera of some people, particularly parous women, reacted with the white blood cells (WBCs) of others. The story began when van Rood saw a parous woman in Leiden with a nonhemolytic transfusion reaction. It was previously thought that only persons receiving red blood cell (RBC) transfusions had these reactions. He realized that whereas RBC transfusion recipients could be immunized to many donors, a parous female could be immunized only to antigens from her husband. He and George Eernisse performed skin grafts between healthy volunteers. (Try this today and you will soon be at Rikers Island or HMP Wormwood Scrubs.) Their experiments led to the discovery of human leukocyte antigens or HLAs, eventuating in the first World Health Organization (WHO) conference on HLA Nomenclature in 1968. Hans Balmer in Rijswik and Rainer Storb and colleagues in Seattle then showed matching for comparable genetic loci in controlled graft rejection in monkeys and dogs. Progress in defining the HLA system allowed physicians to choose from among possible bone marrow donors.[8]

A fourth convergent technology was the development of methods to viably freeze bone marrow mononuclear cells, an advance which enabled clinicians to consider autotransplants. John Farrant, Stanley Liebo, Peter Mazur, and Seymour Perry were the scientists responsible for developing these methods later improved on by C. Dean Buckner, Roy Weiner, John Goldman, and others.

A fifth enabling technology was the development of techniques to obtain large numbers of blood cells by

---

[6] Egon Lorenz to Delta Uphoff, Aug 6, 1950, RCUT, C. C. Congdon Collection/MS838 Box 2, Folder 4.

[7] For which he received the Nobel Prize in Physiology or Medicine (with Jean Dausset and Baruj Benacerraf) in 1980.

[8] Interestingly, Dausset escaped from Vichy France to Tunisia where he joined the ambulance corps and was responsible for giving RBC transfusions, the beginning of his interest in histocompatibility testing. He also worked in Paris after the war developing exchange transfusions with Marcel Bessis at Hospital St. Louis. Meanwhile, Jon von Rood spent his nights in a secret basement in occupied Holland hiding from the Nazis whilst attending medical school during the day.

continuous flow centrifugation. Initially this approach, pioneered by Emil Freireich, Jean Hester, and A. Reginald Clift was used to collect granulocytes to transfuse into persons with granulocytopenia and infection. As readers know this approach fizzled but blood cell separators are now used to collect mononuclear cells (MNC) for auto- and allo-transplants.

Several clinical scientists seized on this convergence of technologies to move towards treating humans with life-threatening diseases. In 1956, E. Donnell Thomas (recipient of the 1990 Nobel Prize in Physiology or Medicine) performed a bone marrow transplant between genetically identical twins. In 1958, Georges Mathé, Henri Jammet, Léon Schwatzenberg, and colleagues transplanted bone marrow from several relatives to each of five workers exposed to ionizing radiations from a nuclear reactor accident in Vinca, Yugoslavia. Their reason for choosing several related donors was the notion that the *best* bone marrow would win. If this sounds like the current practice of giving two umbilical cord blood cell units to transplant recipients (and let the best man win) you are not far off.[9] We would be remiss not to mention Louis Hemplemann who directed medical research for the Manhattan Project at Los Alamos and who, in 1946, treated the first victims of an uncontrolled fission reaction or criticality called *Ticking the Dragon's Tail*.[10]

Special mention must be made of the extraordinary productivity (especially on a per capita basis; 1960 population 11.5 million) of the Radiobiological Institute TNO Rijswijk led by Dirk van Bekkum and his many talented collaborators and students including Marc de Vries, Karel Dicke (the first person to see a *stem cell*, whatever it is), Bob Lowenberg, Anton Hagenbeek, and others who developed mouse models of transplants which formed the bases for some of the early transplants in humans. The Dutch government had advance notice of the A-bombings and gave considerable support to van Bekkum to develop the TNO.

An understanding of the HLA system paved the way for selecting the best donor. In 1968, Robert Good, Richard Gatti, and colleagues reported the first successful allo-transplant from an HLA-identical sibling to a child with severe combined immune deficiency (SCID), and Fritz Bach, Mortimer Bortin, and colleagues reported similar success in a child with Wiskott–Aldrich syndrome. The irony is that after several decades of trying to find the *best* donor we are now in a situation where results of transplants from *bad* donors (HLA-haplotype-matched relatives which is also HLA-haplotype-mismatched donors) are claimed by some to have outcomes similar to those from HLA-identical siblings (don't believe it).

Another critical development was of an international system of collaboration reporting bone marrow transplant outcomes. Mortimer Bortin at Mount Sinai Hospital in Milwaukee (with help from his wife Barbara or "Babs") collected data on 203 transplants done between 1939 and 1969, "for my own edification." Because transplants were so rarely done, this compilation allowed colleagues to better evaluate outcomes. The data were not encouraging – there were only three survivors. Somewhat amusingly, our surgery colleagues, noting the word "transplant," invited Mort to undertake this activity on behalf of the American College of Surgeons. A few years later a light bulb went off and we were kicked out. This early effort led to creation of the International Bone Marrow Transplant Registry (IBMTR) and later the Autologous Bone Marrow Transplant Registry (ABMTR), the Center for International Blood and Marrow Research (CIBMTR; under Mary Horowitz) and the European Bone Marrow Transplant Group (EBMT). The CIBMTR now has data on >400 000 transplants from >450 centers worldwide and the EBMT has similar data. Many chapters in this book cite data and reports from the CIBMTR and EBMT, which have become the definitive source for analyzing transplant outcomes. These are a brilliant example of what can be achieved by international collaboration.

Meanwhile, in the preclinical and clinical arenas there was also considerable progress. Although it is impossible (and dangerous) to try to cite every contribution, a few areas deserve mention. For example, Rainer Storb, Ted Graham, and colleagues at Seattle were able to work out many important transplant-related issues in dogs. Our use of post-transplant methotrexate (later with cyclosporine) results from their efforts. George Santos, Peter Tutschka, and colleagues in Baltimore experimented using cyclophosphamide and busulfan in a rat model, which is the basis of this commonly used conditioning regimen. Bruno Speck,[11] Alois Gratwohl, and colleagues in Basel explored the efficacy of antithymocyte and antilymphocyte globulins mostly kindly provided by a Swiss horse (named Caesar) and a warren of unnamed rabbits. Many people subsequently worked on approaches to T-cell-depletion, including Herman Waldmann, Steven Cobbold and colleagues at Oxford, Yair Reisner, Richard O'Reilly and colleagues in New York and Rehovot, Paul Martin at Seattle, and others. There are many more important early contributors including (in alphabetical order): Frederick Appelbaum, Jane Apperley, James Armitage, Andrea Bacigalupo, A. John Barrett (Austin we believe), Karl Blume, Hal Broxmeyer, Rebecca Buckley, Reginald Clift, Martin Cline, Max Cooper, Hans-Joachim Deeg, John Fahey, Joseph Fay, Alex Fefer, Joseph Ferrebee, Steven Forman, Eliane Gluckman, John Goldman, Anthony Goldstone, Ted Gordon-Smith (another Edward escapee), Claude Gorin, John Hansen, Geoffrey and Roger Herzig, Richard Hong,

---

9 Mathé joined the French resistance, was captured by the Nazis and scheduled for execution just as the war ended. He was liberated and never mentioned this experience to his colleagues.

10 Played by one of the authors in the movie *Fat Man and Little Boy*, 1989.

11 Speck worked with van Rood at Leiden at an early stage.

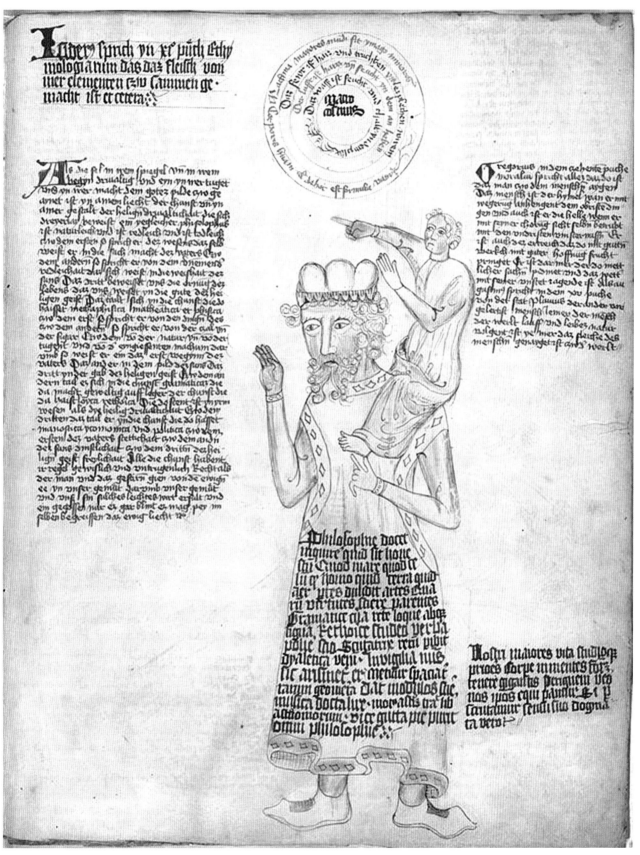

Figure 1.4. The blind giant Orion carrying his servant Cedalion on his shoulders.

Mary Horowitz, Humphrey Kay, Armand Keating, John Kersey, Hans-Joachim Kolb, Alberto Marmont, Timothy McElwain, Hilaire Meuwissen, Paul Neiman, Hans Ochs, Gordon Phillips, Raymond Powles, Alfred Rimm, Olle Ringden, Jean Sanders, Stefan Thierfelder, Robert Truitt, Huib Vriesendorp, Paul Weiden, Axel Zander, and many, many more. Each made a unique and important contribution to progress in bone marrow transplantation. This list must, unavoidably and unintentionally, omit important contributors. If you were left out it is likely because we consider you a rising star, albeit potentially with benign prostatic hypertrophy. (Or, if you have died, you might not mind. At least you won't be sending us an angry letter.)

What do we see as the major progress and setbacks of the last 40 years? First, different pretransplant conditioning regimens result in reasonably similar outcomes when compared in large randomized trials. Second, is the extension of transplants to persons lacking an HLA-identical sibling donor using HLA-matched unrelated persons, umbilical cord blood cell grafts, and HLA-haplotype-matched relatives. Third, is the good and bad impact of reduced intensity conditioning (RIC) transplants. Transplants can now be extended to older, frail persons (like the authors) but, after adjusting for confounding variables, RIC regimen transplants do not convincingly decrease transplant-related mortality (TRM) or improve outcome. They do get people out of the hospital quicker and alive, which makes everyone happy. Fourth, is the ongoing dilemma of defining graft-*versus*-cancer. We all agree that there is an anticancer effect associated with GvHD but we lack convincing evidence of a cancer-specific immune-mediated effect. Does it exist and can we harness it? Hans Kolb and Shimon Slavin think so but we are not convinced. With >5500 reports of graft-*versus*-leukemia (GvL) etc. in PubMed, perhaps we will publish it to death before we answer the question. Fifth, is the slow but steady progress in decreasing TRM using more effective diagnosis of infection and better antibacterial, antiviral and antifungal drugs, more precise dosing of drugs used for conditioning, and other factors. Most of the increasingly better outcomes of transplants come from decreases in TRM rather than fewer cancer recurrences. Sixth, is the switch from bone marrow to blood cells grafts, shifting responsibility from the transplant physician to the blood bank and freeing up time for tennis. Whether this is a leap forward, sideways, or backwards is debatable (see below). There are, of course, many other successes and failures detailed in the chapters which follow.

And so who really performed the first bone marrow transplant and does it really matter? Was it Cú Chulainn, people from New Guinea, medieval apothecaries, Brown-Séquard, E. Donnall Thomas in genetically identical twins, Georges Mathé in the Vinca victims, or someone else we don't know

of because they couldn't get their papyrus, parchment, manuscript, or typescript accepted for publication?

Many chapters which follow ours detail progress since these early days. The evolution of bone marrow transplants from mice to humans, from the Second World War until today is a remarkable story illustrating the principle of unintended consequences. It shows how developing weapons of mass destruction led to a technology which has saved many lives. Over 1 million bone marrow transplants have been done and countless lives saved. Please keep these early days in mind when you read what follows. Roy Weiner compared this chapter to the Haggadah, the story of the exodus of the Jews from Egypt, which is recited on Passover each year to remind us of history.

One is, of course, tempted to ask what lessons we have learned from the past bearing in mind the admonition of George Santayana: "Those who do not remember the past are condemned to repeat it." There are many important positive lessons from the history of bone marrow transplants but there are also some cautions. The most important, we think, is the rapid, wide adoption of unproved interventions simply because an idea sounds good. In 1967, van Bekkum and de Vries suggested that the reason some clinical transplant approaches fail is, "mainly because the clinical applications were undertaken too soon, most of them before even the minimum of basic knowledge required to bridge the gap between mouse and patient had been obtained." Our laboratory is now humans but the problem persists. Consider the leaps to T-cell-depletion in the 1980s, the use of autotransplants in women with breast cancer, and the rush to use blood cells rather than bone marrow cells in every transplant setting. We need solid clinical data, preferably results of randomized clinical trials, before adopting a new technology. But overall, and even with these missteps, there has been substantial progress.

In closing, we are reminded of a quote from Bernard of Chartres from the 12th century (*nanos gigantum humeris insidentes*), later echoed by Sir Isaac Newton: "We are like dwarfs on the shoulders of giants, so that we can see more than they, and things at a greater distance, not by virtue of any sharpness of sight on our part, or any physical distinction, but because we are carried high and raised up by their giant size" (Figure 1.4).

Acknowledgments

Professors Hillard Lazarus, Dirk van Bekkum, Jon van Rood, and Jane Apperley kindly reviewed the chapter. Professor Brown-Séquard also sent helpful comments via a medium as did Cethern, and Fingin. RPG acknowledges support from the NIHR Biomedical Research Centre funding scheme.

Suggested Reading

Ballen KK, Gluckman E, Broxmeyer HE. Umbilical cord transplantation: the first 25 years and beyond. *Blood* 2013; 122:491–8.

Little M-T, Storb R. History of haematopoietic stem-cell transplantation. *Nat Rev Cancer* 2002;2: 231–8.

Thomas ED. Bone marrow transplantation from the personal viewpoint. *Int J Hematol* 2005;81:89–93.

Thomas ED. A history of haematopoietic cell transplantation *Br J Haematol* 1999;105:330–9.

Thomas, ED, Blume KG. Historical markers in the development of allogeneic hematopoietic cell transplantation. *Biol Blood Marrow Transplant* 1999;5:341–6.

van Bekkum DW, de Vries MJ. 1967. *Radiation Chimeras.* London: Logos Press; New York and London: Academic Press.

Current Use and Trends in Hematopoietic Cell Transplantation

Anita D'Souza, Marcelo Pasquini, Zhiwei Wang, and J. Douglas Rizzo

Introduction

Hematopoietic cell transplantation (HCT) is an established curative treatment for a number of conditions including malignant hematologic diseases and nonmalignant congenital and acquired diseases involving the hematopoietic system. Over a million HCTs have been reported worldwide in the last 6 decades[1]. In this chapter, current trends and outcomes of HCT as reported to the Center for International Blood and Marrow Transplant Research (CIBMTR) are described and further discussed. The CIBMTR is a research collaboration between the National Marrow Donor Program® (NMDP)/Be The Match® and the Medical College of Wisconsin, Milwaukee and administers a clinical database of more than 370000 HCT recipients from a large network of voluntary transplant centers (Figure 2.1). Outcome data are prospectively maintained. Charts with total transplant numbers are estimates based on data reported to CIBMTR, adjusted to transplant type. Overall survival probabilities are presented according to disease, disease status, donor type, year of transplant, and conditioning regimen intensities. Comparisons across survival curves are univariate and are not adjusted for potentially important contributing factors. The CIBMTR classifies acute myeloid leukemia (AML), acute lymphocytic leukemia (ALL), and chronic myelogenous leukemia (CML) as early phase (first complete remission or first chronic phase), intermediate phase (second or subsequent complete remission or chronic phase or

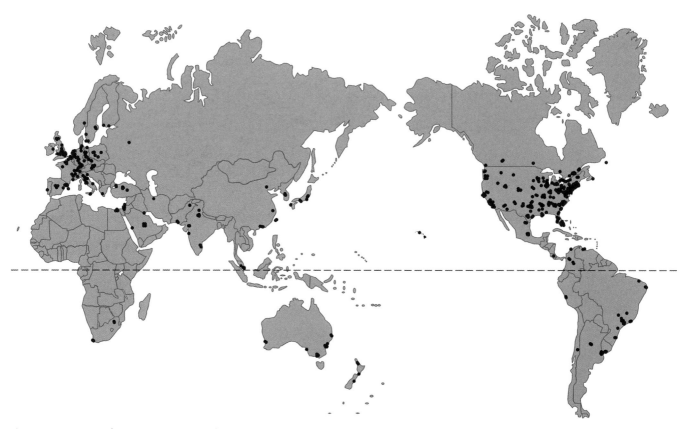

Figure 2.1. Location of centers participating in the CIBMTR.

accelerated phase), or advanced phase (primary induction failure, active disease, or blastic phase) disease. Myelodysplastic syndrome (MDS) is divided into early (refractory anemia or refractory anemia with ringed sideroblasts) and advanced (refractory anemia with excess blasts or chronic myelomonocytic leukemia) disease. Lymphoma is classified according to sensitivity to prior chemotherapy (chemosensitive or chemoresistant). These disease classifications are used throughout this chapter. The survival data reported in this chapter were compiled using transplants registered with the CIBMTR from 2001 to 2011[2].

Transplant Activity in the United States

Figure 2.2 shows the estimated annual numbers of transplants in the United States. The number of autologous HCTs in the United States has steadily increased since 2000, mainly for the treatment of plasma cell and lymphoproliferative disorders. Allogeneic HCTs from unrelated donors have steadily increased in frequency, and their annual use has surpassed related donor allogeneic HCTs since 2006. The major contributing factors to this trend were the growth of unrelated donor registries and cord blood inventories, improvement in unrelated donor transplant outcomes, and increases in the numbers of allogeneic HCT performed in patients older than 60 years with reduced intensity conditioning.

Figure 2.3 shows the indications for HCT in the United States in 2011. Multiple myeloma and lymphoma account for 58% of all HCTs. Multiple myeloma is the most common indication for autologous and AML for allogeneic HCT in the United States. Lymphoma and solid tumors are common indications for autologous transplants. In the pediatric population, allogeneic HCT is used more commonly than autologous HCT. In children, the most common indication for allogeneic HCT was acute leukemia followed by nonmalignant indications; lymphoma and solid tumors were the most common indications for autologous HCT. In adults under age 50 years, allogeneic HCT is more commonly utilized than autologous HCT. This reverses after age 50 to more autologous than allogeneic HCT. Multiple myeloma and non-Hodgkin

lymphoma account for the majority of autologous and acute leukemia for allogeneic HCT in adults. The proportion of HCT for various diseases has remained fairly stable over the last 10 years in the pediatric and adult population.

Trends in Distribution of Graft Sources for Allogeneic HCT

The annual number of unrelated donor transplants has increased in the last two decades. Among the pediatric population, in 2011, 43% of all unrelated donor HCTs utilized umbilical cord blood grafts compared to 28% in 2001. Among unrelated HCTs, bone marrow as a graft source decreased in favor of peripheral blood over the period 2001–2011. The opposite trend was seen with the related HCTs. While the number of related HCTs declined from 2001 to 2011, the proportion of bone marrow over peripheral blood as the graft source increased during this time period. Figure 2.4 shows these trends of pediatric graft sources over time.

Among adults, the number of unrelated donor transplants has surpassed the number of related donor transplants since the late 1990s. Peripheral blood remains the most common source for unrelated donor transplants in adults since 2001. The number of unrelated peripheral blood HCTs in adults has

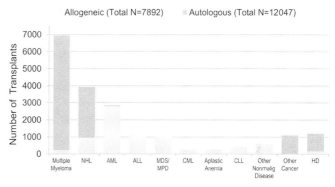

Figure 2.3. Indications for transplant. NHL, non-Hodgkin lymphoma; AML, acute myeloid leukemia; ALL, acute lymphoblastic leukemia; MDS/MPD, myelodysplastic syndrome/myeloproliferative neoplasm; CML, chronic myelogenous leukemia; CLL, chronic lymphocytic leukemia; HD, Hodgkin lymphoma.

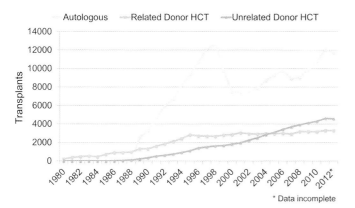

Figure 2.2. Transplant activity in the United States of America.

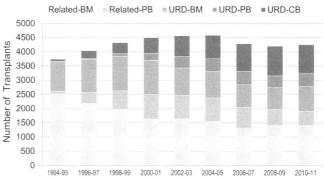

Figure 2.4. Trends in pediatric allogeneic HCTs by time and graft source. BM, bone marrow; PB, peripheral blood; CB, cord blood.

increased consistently and comprises 43% of all adult HCTs in 2011 compared to 9% in 2001. In 2011, umbilical cord blood and bone marrow grafts accounted for 12% and 13% compared to 5% and 50% in 2001 of unrelated donor transplants respectively.

Within the last few years, a trend towards alternate donor graft sources has been noted. Since 2010, 26% of grafts have been from alternate donors including mismatched unrelated, haploidentical, single and double umbilical cord graft sources. Alternate graft sources are of particular importance in non-Caucasians. Among African-Americans, haploidentical and umbilical cord HCT accounted for 18% and 19% of all HCTs in 2013. While it is too early to show these trends, alternate graft sources are anticipated to continue to increase in the next several years.

Age Trends among HCT Recipients

The number of autologous and allogeneic transplants for treatment of malignant diseases in older patients continues to increase. This change is even better demonstrated going back a

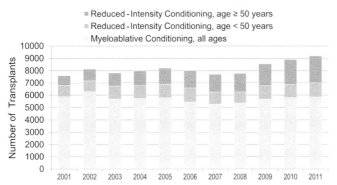

Figure 2.5. Trends in proportion of reduced intensity conditioned allogeneic HCT.

decade. Between 1991 and 1997, 7% of allogeneic HCTs occurred in patients 50 years or older; between 2005 and 2011, this increased to 38%. In 2011, 20% of all allogeneic HCT recipients were 60 years or older, up from 5% in 2001. Nearly 38% of all autologous HCT recipients are 60 years or older. Improvements in techniques leading to better patient and donor selection, the use of reduced intensity conditioning regimens, and improvements in supportive care for these patients are likely contributors to this trend.

Trends in Utilization of Pretransplant Conditioning Regimens

The CIBMTR operational definition of the intensity of conditioning regimens has been previously published[2]. The number of HCTs using reduced intensity conditioning has increased steadily in the last decade, particularly in patients aged 50 years and older (Figure 2.5). In 2011, 66% of all reduced intensity conditioned HCTs occurred in this age group compared to 44% in 2001. Among patients less than 50 years, the proportion of reduced intensity conditioned HCTs has also increased slightly from 2001 to 2011. Additionally, among transplants with reduced intensity conditioning, the use of alternate donors has increased with increasing proportion of umbilical cord transplants (Figure 2.6A). The utilization of reduced intensity conditioning varies according to the indication of transplant (Figure 2.5B). Myeloablative conditioning is still used in the majority of acute leukemias and MDS; however a trend is seen towards increased use of reduced intensity conditioning in the last 10 years reflecting an increase in HCT recipient ages (Figure 2.5B). For example, in 2011, 33% of AML transplants used reduced intensity conditioning compared to 18% in 2001.

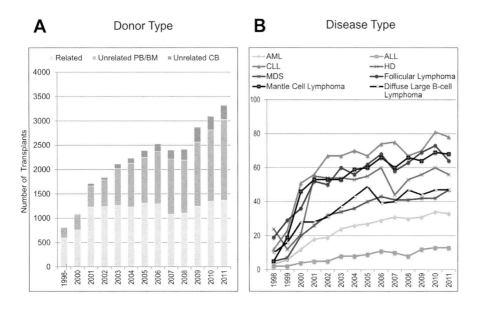

Figure 2.6. Trends in reduced intensity conditioned allogeneic HCT. (**A**) Donor source; (**B**) disease indication.

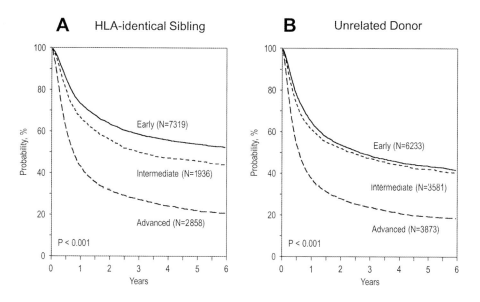

Figure 2.7. HCT in AML. (A) HLA-identical sibling HCT. (B) Unrelated donor HCT.

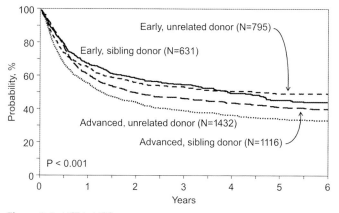

Figure 2.8. HCT in MDS.

Transplant Outcomes among Various Disease Types, 2001—2011

Acute Myeloid Leukemia (AML)

Among 25 800 patients receiving an HLA-identical sibling (n=12 113) or unrelated donor (n=13 687) transplant for AML between 2001 and 2011, disease status at transplant and the donor type predicted post-transplant survival (Figure 2.7A and B). The 3-year probabilities of survival after HLA-matched sibling transplant in this cohort were 58% ± 1%, 49% ± 1%, and 26% ± 1% for patients with early, intermediate, and advanced disease, respectively. The probabilities of survival after an unrelated donor transplant were 48% ± 1%, 46% ± 1%, and 26% ± 1% for patients with early, intermediate, and advanced disease, respectively.

Myelodysplastic Syndromes (MDS)

Among 3924 patients receiving an allogeneic transplant for MDS between 2001 and 2011, disease status at the time of transplant and donor type are predictors of survival (Figure 2.8). The 3-year probabilities of survival were 53% ± 2% and 52% ± 2% for recipients of sibling and unrelated donor transplants for early MDS, respectively. Among patients with advanced MDS, corresponding probabilities were 45% ± 2% and 38% ± 2%.

Acute Lymphoblastic Leukemia (ALL)

Among young patients with ALL, for whom traditional chemotherapy has a high success rate, allogeneic transplantation is generally reserved for patients with high-risk disease (i.e., high leukocyte count at diagnosis and the presence of poor-risk cytogenetic markers), who fail to achieve remission or who relapse after chemotherapy. Among the 2188 patients younger than 20 receiving an HLA-matched sibling transplant for ALL between 2001 and 2011, the 3-year probabilities of survival were 67% ± 2%, 55% ± 2 %, and 26% ± 3% for patients with early, intermediate, and advanced disease, respectively (Figure 2.9A). The corresponding probabilities of survival among the 3271 recipients of an unrelated donor transplant were 64% ± 2%, 47% ± 1%, and 31% ± 3% (Figure 2.9B). Older age at disease onset is a high-risk feature in ALL. Consequently, a larger proportion of ALL patients 20 years of age or older undergo allogeneic HCT for early disease. Among 3592 patients ≥20 years of age receiving HLA-matched sibling HCT for ALL between 2001 and 2011, the 3-year survival probabilities were 53% ± 1%, 32% ± 2%, and 23% ± 2% for patients with early, intermediate, and advanced disease, respectively (Figure 2.9C). Corresponding probabilities among the 3929 recipients of unrelated donor HCT were 50% ± 1%, 34% ± 2%, and 18% ± 2% (Figure 2.9D).

Chronic Myelogenous Leukemia (CML)

Chronic myeloid leukemia is no longer the most common indication for allogeneic HCTs. However, this still remains a

11

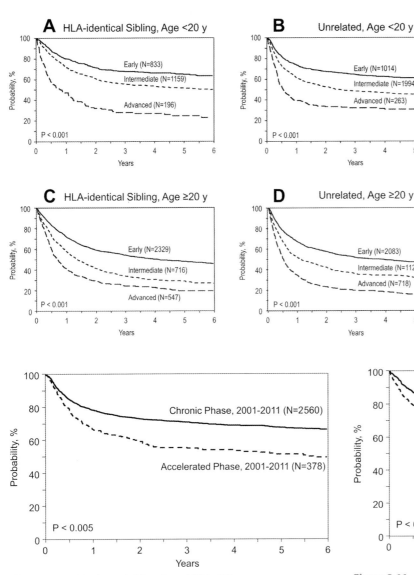

Figure 2.9. HCT in ALL. (**A**) Age <20 years, HLA-identical sibling donor. (**B**) Age <20 years, unrelated donor. (**C**) Age ≥20 years, HLA-identical donor. (**D**) Age ≥20 years, unrelated donor.

Figure 2.10. HLA-identical sibling donor HCT in CML.

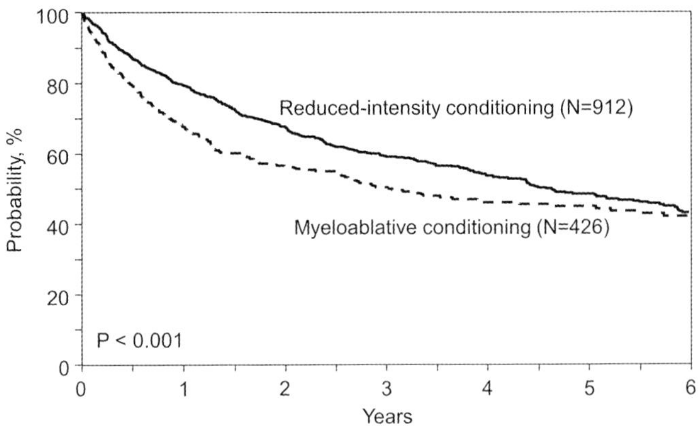

Figure 2.11. HLA-identical sibling donor HCT in CLL.

curative option for patients in whom tyrosine kinase inhibitors have failed or are poorly tolerated. The CIBMTR has data for 2938 HLA-matched sibling donor allotransplants for CML between 2001 and 2011. The 3-year probabilities of survival were 71% ± 1% and 54% ± 3% for patients in chronic phase (CP) and in accelerated phase (AP), respectively (Figure 2.10).

Chronic Lymphocytic Leukemia (CLL)

Allogeneic transplants are the main transplant modality for treatment of chronic lymphocytic leukemia (CLL) patients in whom standard chemotherapy fails or who have high-risk features (e.g., cytogenetic abnormalities, short remission intervals, purine-analog-resistant disease). The use of reduced intensity conditioning regimens for allogeneic transplant continues to increase in this population. Among the 1338 patients who underwent transplantation for CLL, the 3-year probabilities of

survival were 50% ± 3% and 58% ± 2% after myeloablative and reduced intensity conditioning regimens, respectively (Figure 2.11).

Severe Aplastic Anemia (SAA)

Allogeneic HCT is the treatment of choice for young patients with severe aplastic anemia and an available HLA-matched sibling donor. Among the 2763 patients receiving HLA-matched sibling donor HCT for severe aplastic anemia between 2001 and 2011, the 3-year probabilities of survival were 88% ± 1% for those younger than 20 years and 76% ± 1% for those 20 years of age or older. Among the 1407 recipients of unrelated donor HCT, the corresponding probabilities of survival were 70% ± 2% and 63% ± 2% (Figure 2.12).

Lymphomas

Hodgkin Lymphoma (HL)

Transplantation for HL is indicated in patients who have failed initial chemotherapy or radiation therapy. Survival after HCT for HL depends on disease response to previous salvage therapy. Among the 8343 patients receiving autotransplants for HL between 2001 and 2011, the 3-year probabilities of survival were 85% ± 1%, 74% ± 1%, and 58% ± 2% for patients in complete remission, with chemosensitive (but not CR) and with chemoresistant disease, respectively. Allogeneic HCT for HL is generally performed in patients who experience disease relapse after receiving multiple lines of therapy including autotransplant or who have refractory disease and an available HLA-matched donor. Among 545 patients receiving allotransplants for HD between 2001 and 2011, the 3-year probabilities

of survival were 48% ± 3% and 41% ± 4% after sibling and unrelated donor transplants, respectively (Figure 2.13A)

Follicular Lymphoma (FL)

Transplantation for FL is generally reserved for patients with recurrent or aggressive disease. Autotransplantation is the most common transplant approach in this disease. Among the 2927 patients receiving an autotransplant for FL between 2001 and 2011 most had chemosensitive disease. The 3-year probabilities of survival were 75% + 1% and 62% + 3% for patients with chemosensitive and chemoresistant disease, respectively. Similar to HL, allogeneic transplant for FL is performed in patients who experience disease relapse after multiple lines of therapy or who have refractory disease and an available HLA-match donor. Among 1045 patients receiving HLA-matched sibling donor transplants for FL between 2001 and 2011, the 3-year probabilities of survival were 70% ± 2% and 59% ± 4% for patients with chemosensitive and chemoresistant disease, respectively (Figure 2.13B).

Diffuse Large B-Cell Lymphoma (DLBCL)

Autotransplants are an accepted treatment indication for DLBCL and, similar to FL, most autotransplants are performed in patients with relapsed chemosensitive disease. Among the 10490 patients who received an autotransplant for DLBCL between 2001 and 2011, the 3-year probabilities of survival were 62% ± 1% and 40% ± 2% for patients with chemosensitive and chemoresistant disease, respectively. Allogeneic HCT for treatment of DLBCL is performed less frequently than for FL and is generally used only in patients with aggressive disease that has been resistant to previous therapies, including autotransplants. Among the 699 patients who

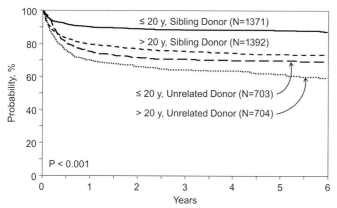

Figure 2.12. HCT in severe aplastic anemia.

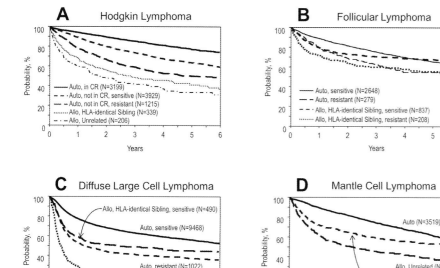

Figure 2.13. HCT in Lymphoma. (A) Hodgkin lymphoma; (B) follicular lymphoma; (C) diffuse large cell lymphoma; (D) mantle cell lymphoma. Auto, autologous HCT; Allo, allogeneic; sensitive, chemosensitive; resistant, chemoresistant.

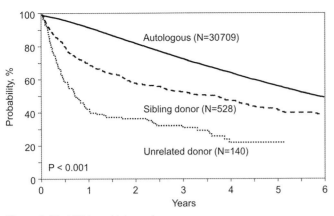

Figure 2.14. HCT in multiple myeloma.

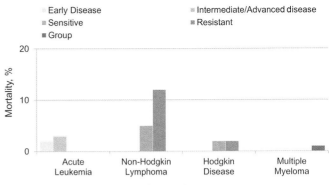

Figure 2.15. 100 day mortality after autologous HCT.

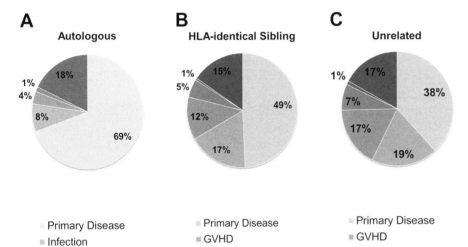

Figure 2.16. Cause of death after HCT. (A) Autologous; (B) HLA-identical sibling; (C) unrelated.

underwent an HLA-matched sibling HCT for DLBCL from 2001 to 2011, the 3-year probabilities of survival were 48% ± 3% and 17% ± 4% for patients with chemosensitive and chemoresistant disease, respectively (Figure 2.13C).

Mantle Cell Lymphoma (MCL)

The optimal timing of HCT for MCL is not well defined. As with other mature B-cell lymphoproliferative disorders, autotransplantation is the most common transplant approach. Among the 3519 patients who received an autotransplant for MCL between 2001 and 2011, the 3-year probability of survival was 74% ± 1%. Among 943 patients who underwent an allogeneic transplantation for MCL during the same period, the 3-year probabilities of survival were 59% ± 2% and 45% ± 3% for sibling and unrelated donor transplants, respectively (Figure 2.13D).

Plasma Cell Disorders

Multiple myeloma (MM) is the most common indication for autologous HCT. Among 30709 patients who received an

autologous HCT for MM between 2001 and 2011, the 3-year probability of survival was 72% ± 1%. Allogeneic transplantation for MM is reserved for patients with high-risk disease and the majority are performed after an autologous HCT with reduced intensity or nonmyeloablative conditioning regimens. Among the 668 patients who received an allogeneic HCT from 2001 to 2011, the 3-year probabilities of survival were 52% ± 2% and 31% ± 4% for recipients of HLA-matched sibling and unrelated donor grafts, respectively (Figure 2.14). Light chain amyloidosis is the other plasma cell neoplasm where autologous transplant is utilized and 1396 patients received autologous HCTs for amyloidosis between 2001 and 2011.

Trends in Mortality

The 100-day mortality rate after autologous HCT calculated for the 2010–2011 period is shown in Figure 2.15. Early mortality ranges between 1–12% with the lowest mortality seen after autologous transplant for multiple myeloma and the highest in chemotherapy-resistant non-Hodgkin lymphoma.

These rates have improved significantly from 7–22% in the period 2007–2008[3]. The most commonly reported causes of death after an autologous HCT is primary disease (69%), followed by infection (8%), organ failure (4%), secondary malignancy (1%), and others (18%)(Figure 2.16A).

Among allogeneic HCT recipients, the most common cause of death is primary disease. Graft-*versus*-host disease accounted for 17% of deaths after HLA-identical sibling transplants and 19% after unrelated donor HCT in 2010–2011 (Figure 2.16B and C). Other causes of death included infection (12% in HLA-identical sibling and 17% in unrelated HCT), organ failure (5% in HLA-identical sibling and 7% in unrelated HCT), and second malignancy in 1% in both groups. The 100-day mortality after HLA-identical sibling HCT is 7–9% for patients with AML in remission as compared to 22% for patients with active leukemia at the time of transplantation. This number is even higher at 11–13% compared to 27% respectively among unrelated donor HCT.

Overall, 1-year survival rates after allogeneic transplantation for AML, CML, or MDS have generally improved in the last 2 decades. Outcomes of unrelated donor HCT are approaching those seen with related donors. While outcomes are better for recipients under age 50 years, these trends are being observed in patients younger and older than 50 years (Figure 2.17). Among recipients under 50 years of age, 1-year survival after HLA-identical HCT improved from 72% to 78% and among unrelated donor HCT from 54% to 70% in 2011 and 2011, respectively. In adults aged 50 years and older, 1-year survival after HLA-identical HCT improved from 60% to 64% and among unrelated donor HCT from 40% to 58% in 2011 and 2011, respectively. Improvements in donor selection, HLA-matching techniques, better patient selection for transplantation, and improvements in supportive care likely contributed to these improved trends.

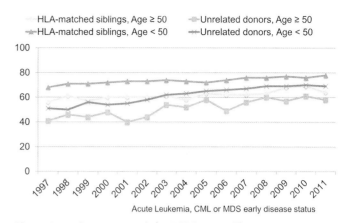

Figure 2.17. One-year survival after HCT. Footnote: The recipients represent patients with acute leukemia, chronic myelogenous leukemia, and myelodysplastic disease, early disease.

Conclusions

The numbers of HCTs performed annually continue to increase. We highlight trends showing an increasing proportion of matched unrelated donor compared to HLA-identical sibling HCT, increase in alternate donor sources, increasing utilization of HCT in older adults, and improving 100-day and 1-year survival.

Acknowledgments

The authors acknowledge Ms. Renee Dunn for assistance in developing figures. The CIBMTR is supported by the National Institutes of Health (NIH) grants # U24CA076518 and # HL069294, Health Resources and Service Administration (HRSA) contract # HHSH250201200016C.

References

1. Gratwohl A, Pasquini MC, Aljurf MD, Confer DL, Baldomero H, Bouzas LF *et al.* Global hematopoietic stem cell transplantation (HSCT) at one million: an achievement of pioneers and foreseeable challenges for the next decade. a report from the worldwide network for blood and marrow transplantation (WBMT). *Blood* 2013; 122(21): 2133.

2. Pasquini MC, Wang Z. Current use and outcome of hematopoietic stem cell transplantation: CIBMTR Summary Slides, 2013. Available at http://www.cibmtr.org.

3. Bacigalupo A, Ballen K, Rizzo D, Giralt S, Lazarus H, Ho V *et al.* Defining the intensity of conditioning regimens: working definitions. *Biol Blood Marrow Transplant* 2009; 15(12): 1628–1633. doi: 10.1016/j.bbmt.2009.07.004

Chapter 3

Biology: Critical Components of Hematopoietic Cell Transplantation

Sergio A. Giralt

Introduction

The use of high-dose chemoradiotherapy as treatment for refractory hematologic malignancies traces its origins to the 1940s when it was observed that lethal marrow aplasia would result from high-dose radiation exposure. The possibility that this potent agent could be used to eradicate resistant leukemic cells and that animals exposed to supra-lethal doses of radiation could be successfully rescued by transfusing marrow or spleen cellular extracts provided the preclinical rationale to allow initial explorations in humans[1,2].

However, the initial experience with allogeneic hematopoietic cell transplant (allo-HCT) was dismal, with less than a handful of survivors [3]. The discovery of human leukocyte antigens (HLA) and advances in supportive care allowed the modern era of allo-HCT for malignant disorders to begin in the late 1970s with the seminal article by Thomas *et al.* demonstrating the curative potential of HLA-matched allogeneic bone marrow transplants in patients with refractory acute leukemia[4].

In 1978, investigators from the National Cancer Institute were the first to report the use of high-dose chemotherapy followed by autologous BMT for patients with relapsed lymphoma [5]. These results were followed by subsequent randomized trials in chemosensitive relapsed lymphoma and multiple myeloma resulting in the clinical evidence that led to the widespread application of autologous HCT (reviewed in [6]). HCT is now an established medical procedure with more than 10000 procedures performed yearly in the United States[6]. In this chapter, we will review the different elements of the HCT procedure as well as describe ongoing controversies in the field.

The Hematopoietic Cell Transplant Procedure

HCT is a complex procedure in which an individual receives a combination of chemical and physical agents to eliminate a malignant disorder or a poorly functioning bone marrow supported by reinfusion of hematopoietic progenitor cells (HPCs) from the patient or a third-party donor. Intense and timely supportive care is required as patients recover from the effects of the conditioning regimen and throughout the period of profound immune suppression that occurs while the transplanted HPCs mature and recover normal function.

HCT Recipient

Who benefits from HCT remains one of the most common and challenging questions in clinical practice. In general, indications for HCT can be divided into malignant and nonmalignant disorders, which are summarized in Table 3.1. However, not all patients who have a condition that could be amenable to treatment with HCT are actually "transplant eligible." Transplant eligibility requires certain levels of organ function and psychosocial support to determine what the risk–benefit ratio of HCT is compared to other alternative treatment approaches and whether a specific type of HCT may be more appropriate than another in an individual patient. Table 3.2 summarizes tests and parameters currently used to determine HCT eligibility[7–10].

Table 3.1 Most common indications for hematopoietic cell transplantation

Autologous hematopoietic cell transplantation		Allogeneic hematopoietic cell transplantation	
Neoplastic disorder	No. of procedures performed in USA in 2009		No. of procedures performed in USA in 2009
Myeloma	4700	Acute myeloid leukemia	2500
Non-Hodgkin lymphoma	2800	Acute lymphoblastic leukemia	1100
Hodgkin lymphoma	1250	Myelodysplastic syndrome	1000
Non-neoplastic disorders			
Autoimmune diseases	NR	Severe aplastic anemia	

Table 3.2 Commonly used eligibility criteria for hematopoietic cell transplantation

Eligibility criteria	Test	Transplant eligible	Comments
Patient performance status	History and physical exam	Usually ECOG 2 or less Karnofsky performance status of >70	Transplant-related mortality is related to pre-HCT performance status Patients with poor performance status are generally not considered candidates for HCT unless chances for long-term cure are high if HCT is successful
Disease and disease status	Multiple	Depending on disease status at the time of HCT Patients with high-risk chemorefractory disease are not considered eligible if expected 2-year disease-free survival rate is less than 10%	Armand *et al.* recently proposed a disease and disease status risk classification for hematopoietic cell transplantation[8]
Infectious disease markers	Serologies for Hepatitis A, B, and C PCR for viral copies HIV, HTLV-1 CMV, EBV, toxoplasmosis	Generally patients should not have active viral replication	Guidelines are evolving with the advent of effective antiviral therapy
Cardiac function	Echocardiogram Nuclear medicine testing	Ejection fraction greater than 40% prior to MAC regimen Compensated cardiac disease/condition	Patients with cardiac history require more extensive pretransplant evaluation including referral to Cardiology for stress testing or Holter monitoring
Pulmonary function	Pulmonary function testing	DLCO >40% prior to MAC regimen Absence of severe symptomatic pulmonary disease	In some series, most important predictor of outcome if DLCO less than 40%
Renal function	Creatinine and creatinine clearance	Usually creatinine clearance over 40mL/min	Patients with poor renal function (including patients with ESRD) can be considered for HCT on individual basis. Auto-HCT is routinely performed in patients with multiple myeloma on dialysis
Hepatic function	Liver function tests	Bilirubin less than 2–3 × ULN unless history of Gilbert's disease	
Comorbidity scoring	HCT-CI	No cut-off determined	Comorbidity scoring more useful to decide regimen intensity. HCT-CI most commonly used scoring system[9]
Psychosocial evaluation [10]	HED PACT	Varies with institutional guidelines	Essential to determine risk of noncompliance as well as caregiver availability and social support needed throughout the transplant process

Adapted from ref [7].
MAC, myeloablative conditioning regimen.

Hematopoietic Progenitor Cell Source

HCTs have been classified according to the source of stem cells as either autologous or allogeneic, and according to where they were obtained from (i.e., marrow, peripheral blood, or cord blood):

- **Autologous HCT**. Involves using HPCs obtained from the recipient. The stem cells can be obtained directly from the recipient's marrow or through mobilization of stem cells from the marrow into the peripheral blood using G-CSF and the CXCR4 antagonist, plerixafor. Currently,

the majority (>95%) of all autologous HCTs performed in North America are using G-CSF mobilized peripheral blood HPCs[6,11].

- **Allogeneic HCT**. Involves using HPCs obtained from a third party which can be a related or unrelated donor. Unrelated donor HPCs can be obtained by live volunteer donors or from previously banked cord blood units[12]. Allogeneic HPCs from volunteer related or unrelated donors can be obtained through multiple bone marrow aspirations or through mobilization of HPCs into the

Table 3.3 Advantages and disadvantages of different hematopoietic cell sources

Hematopoietic cell source	Advantages	Disadvantages
Autologous HCT		
Bone marrow[14,15]	HPC readily available	Painful
		Limited HPC cell dose since there is a limit to the amount of marrow that can be collected at one time
		Slower neutrophil and platelet recovery which result in higher rates of infection and nonrelapse mortality
		Rarely performed replaced by peripheral blood (PB) HPCs
Peripheral blood[12]	Preferred product for autologous HCT Faster neutrophil and platelet recovery resulting in fewer infections and less morbidity and mortality	Cost
	Better tolerated for patients	5–20% mobilization failure depending on method used
Allogeneic HCT		
Bone marrow	HPC readily available	Associated with more donor complications than peripheral blood collections
	Less chronic GvHD	Requires OR time and resources
	Preferred product for low-risk disease (i.e., acute leukemias in CR1 or chronic myelogenous leukemia in chronic phase)	HPC cell dose limited by the amount of donor marrow that can be collected during one procedure. This is relevant when recipient is much larger than the donor
	Preferred product for mismatched related and unrelated donor transplants using post-transplant cyclophosphamide as GvHD prophylaxis[12]	Slower neutrophil and platelet recovery
Peripheral blood	Faster neutrophil and platelet recovery. However faster engraftment has not translated into improved survival Preferred product for CD34 selection[17]	More chronic GvHD without decrease in relapses in patients with low-risk acute leukemias or CML in chronic phase
	HPC collection procedure better tolerated by donors	
Cord blood [18]	Allows HLA disparities without severe GvHD. Improve minority access to HCT	Slower neutrophil, platelet, and immune recovery which may result in increased risks of infection and nonrelapse mortality
	Cells can be obtained quickly	Cost

peripheral blood and collection through apheresis techniques. Allogeneic peripheral blood HCT is associated with faster neutrophil and platelet recovery when compared to bone marrow, but also with higher rates of chronic graft-*versus*-host disease (GvHD) without significant survival benefits[13]. Table 3.3 summarizes the advantages and disadvantages of the different HPC sources available today[12–18].

Conditioning Regimens

The conditioning or preparative regimen is the combination of chemical and physical agents given prior to HCT. The high-dose conditioning regimen ("myeloablative") is given to eradicate the malignancy exploiting the dose-response effect. In the setting of allo-HCT the conditioning regimen should serve to

suppress recipient immune response precluding graft failure. Conditioning regimen intensity has been classified according to their myelotoxic effects into myeloablative, reduced intensity, and nonmyeloablative as summarized in Table 3.4. Table 3.5 lists the most commonly used conditioning regimens today[19].

The combination of cyclophosphamide and total body irradiation (CyTBI) was the first conditioning regimen that achieved widespread applicability[4]. Santos *et al.* substituted high-dose busulfan for total body irradiation (TBI). The BuCy conditioning regimen was rapidly adopted and in multiple randomized trials as well as meta-analysis has been shown to be as effective as TBI-containing regimens for myeloid leukemias[20]. For patients with ALL, TBI-containing regimens may be slightly superior. More recently intravenous busulfan has been shown to result in more predictable delivery of

Table 3.4 Definition of conditioning regimens according to their intensity

Intensity of preparative regimen	Definition
Myeloablative conditioning regimen (MAC regimen)	A regimen that destroys the hematopoietic cells in the bone marrow with resultant long-lasting pancytopenia usually irreversible, and in most instances fatal, unless hematopoiesis is restored by infusion of HPCs
Reduced intensity conditioning (RIC)	Regimens that are an intermediate category between MAC regimen and NMA. They do not fit the definition of MAC regimen or NMA but they result in cytopenias, which may be prolonged and require HPC rescue
Nonmyeloablative (NMA)	A regimen that results in minimal cytopenias but significant lymphopenia and does not require HPC rescue

Table 3.5 Commonly used conditioning regimens

Allogeneic HCT

Myeloablative conditioning

CyTBI	Cyclophosphamide 120 mg/kg + TBI 8–12 Gy*
BuCy	Cyclophosphamide 120 mg/kg + busulfan 16 mg/kg PO or IV equivalent
FluBu	Fludarabine 120–150 mg/m² + busulfan 16 mg/kg PO or IV equivalent

Reduced intensity conditioning

Flu Mel	Fludarabine + melphalan 140 mg/m²
Flu Bu	Fludarabine + busulfan 8 mg/kg PO or IV equivalent

Nonmyeloablative conditioning

Flu TBI	Fludarabine + TBI 2 Gy
Flu Cy	Fludarabine + cyclophosphamide 60 mg/kg
Cy ATG	Cyclophosphamide 4 gm/m² + ATG†

Common autologous HCT conditioning regimens

Lymphoma

BEAM	BCNU + etoposide + cytarabine + melphalan
BEAC	BCNU + etoposide + cytarabine + cyclophosphamide
CBV	Cyclophosphamide + BCNU + etoposide

Myeloma

High-dose melphalan	Melphalan 200 mg/m²

Abbreviation: TBI, total body irradiation; BCNU, carmustine.

busulfan and has been combined with fludarabine. The fludarabine/busulfan (FluBu) combinations have become increasingly more utilized since cyclophosphamide and its metabolites have been implicated in the development of veno-occlusive disease (VOD)[21].

The extramedullary toxicity of myeloablative conditioning regimens limited their use to patients under the age of 60 years who had a good performance status and minimal comorbidities. With the demonstration that engraftment could be achieved with reduced intensity conditioning (RIC) regimens, the age barrier to HCT was lifted, particularly for patients between 60 and 70 years of age. RIC regimens are generally associated with lower nonhematologic toxicities. Operationally, RIC regimens have been defined by the following doses of commonly administered agents: melphalan less than 150 mg/m²; busulfan less than 9 mg/kg of the oral equivalent; thiotepa less than 10 mg/kg and TBI less than 500 cGy single fraction or 800 cGy fractionated.

Retrospective comparisons suggest similar outcomes with RIC regimens when compared to myeloablative conditioning regimens. However, results of a prospective randomized trial comparing RIC *versus* myeloablative conditioning regimens in AML and MDS will soon be available[22].

Supportive Care during HCT Procedure

The HCT procedure can be viewed as five time-dependent phases:

Phase I: chemotherapy phase (usually day −7 to day 0): This is the phase in which the conditioning regimen is administered. Phase I finishes with the infusion of the graft.

Phase II: cytopenic phase (usually day +1 to day +10 through +21): The effects of the conditioning regimen are made evident during the period. In the case of myeloablative conditioning regimens, severe myelosuppression is universal moderate to severe, and gastrointestinal toxicity manifested as stomatitis and diarrhea occurs frequently.

Phase III: early recovery phase (usually day +10 through day +28): Traditionally with bone marrow grafts the neutrophil engraftment defined as an absolute neutrophil count of 500 per microliter or greater for 3 consecutive days occurs between days 21 and 28 after transplant. With filgrastim mobilized peripheral HPCs the neutrophil recovery happens usually within 9 to 12 days of infusion. Engraftment kinetics of cord blood grafts are much slower with median time to neutrophil engraftment of 24 days for children and 14 days for adults. Double cord blood grafts in adults have been associated with faster neutrophil recovery in adults but not in children. During this initial phase of neutrophil recovery patients can develop a syndrome

Table 3.6 Common complications post-HCT and current treatment and prevention strategies[23–29]

Complications	Timing post-HCT	Cause	Prevention & treatment
Gastrointestinal:			
Nausea/Vomiting Anorexia	During conditioning and immediate post-HCT	Direct side effect of conditioning regimen	5HT3 antagonists Steroids Antiemetics
Diarrhea	Immediate post-HCT	Direct side effect of conditioning regimen	Symptomatic treatment
	Postengraftment	In allo setting need to rule out GvHD *versus* Infection *versus* delayed GI recovery. Engraftment syndrome less common compared to auto-setting In auto setting infection *versus* delayed GI recovery *versus* engraftment syndrome	Treat underlying cause if documented Symptomatic treatment in addition to work-up including radiologic and endoscopic evaluation as needed
Mucositis/stomatitis	Days post-HCT usually peaks around day 10	Direct side effect of conditioning regimen	Palifermin and cryotherapy . Optimize oral hygiene and health Treatment is symptomatic pain control and hydration
Myelosuppression	Days post-HCT	Direct side effect of conditioning regimen	Growth factors and supportive care (transfusions)
Infections			
Herpes simplex virus	Immediate post-HCT	Immunedeficiency	Acyclovir or equivalents
Cytomegalovirus reactivation	After engraftment	Immunedeficiency post-HCT rare post-auto HCT	PCR monitoring with preemptive therapy
Bacterial infections	Early and at any time	Neutropenia with gastrointestinal mucosa destruction Indwelling catheters (CVC)	Antibiotic prophylaxis and treatment of breakthrough fevers or infections
Fungal infections	Early thrush Late-fungal pneumonias or invasive fungal infections	Neutropenia and immunedeficiency. Fungal overgrowth due to antibacterials	Antifungals for prevention and treatment
Acute graft-*versus*-host disease	After engraftment	HLA disparities between donor and recipient	Prevention Calcineurin inhibitors and methotrexate Post-transplant cyclophosphamide CD34 selection Treatment: steroids +/− other agents
Chronic graft-*versus*-host disease	3 months or later as immunosuppression is being tapered	HLA disparities between donor and recipient	Prevention Post-transplant cyclophosphamide CD34 selection Treatment: steroids +/− others

Adapted from ref [7].

characterized by fever, rash, and pulmonary infiltrates known as the "engraftment syndrome," which when identified should be treated promptly with steroids and G-CSF should be discontinued. This period also marks the most common time when graft-*versus*-host disease (GvHD) can begin to manifest itself in the allograft setting.

Phase IV: early convalescence phase (usually day +28 through day +180 for autografts and day +360 for allografts): This period is characterized by continued immune suppression despite normal peripheral blood cell counts. Patients remain at risk of serious life-threatening opportunistic infections that require antibiotic, antiviral, and antifungal prophylaxis as well as close monitoring by the transplant team.

Phase V: late convalescence: This final phase is characterized by the almost full recovery of the immune system and by the potential of late complications such as organ dysfunction or recurrence of the original malignancy.

Table 3.6 summarizes the most common complications that happen during HCT and the strategies used to prevent or treat them.

Table 3.7 General controversies in HCT procedure"

Selected controversies in HCT procedure	Ongoing trial and/or suggestions to tackle the controversies
Autologous HCT-related controversies	
1. Use of post-SCT maintenance using disease-specific drugs in the auto-HCT setting	Lenalidomide maintenance for myeloma Brentuximab vedotin maintenance for Hodgkin disease Randomized trials performed, follow-up studies in planning
2. Timing of auto HCT in different disorders	Upfront *versus* salvage in both myeloma and lymphoma Multiple randomized trials either planned or ongoing
3. Post-auto HCT immunotherapy using checkpoint blockade or vaccines	Phase 1/2 trials ongoing of PD1 blockade post-autograft as well as CD19 CAR T-cells Randomized phase 2 trial of myeloma/dendritic cell fusion vaccine to be performed by the BMT CTN
Mobilization-related controversies	
1. Optimal mobilization in the auto-HCT setting	G+plerixafor *versus* chemo *versus* chemo-plerixafor
2. G-Mobilized marrow *versus* PB	Randomized Canadian study ongoing
3. Optimal stem cell dose	
Graft selection-related controversies	
1. Optimal alternative donor source (cord blood *versus* haplo *versus* mismatched unrelated)	BMT CTN 1102 Trial
2. HLA-matching *versus* timing of HCT	None ongoing
3. PB *versus* bone marrow in high-risk disease	None ongoing
4. KIR advantageous donor	One prospective trial ongoing, one planned
Early and late HCT-associated complication related controversies	
1. Optimal GvHD prevention strategy for ablative regimens	BMT CTN Progress II Trial
2. Optimal GvHD prevention strategy for nonablative regimen	BMT CTN Progress I Trial
3. Preemptive strategies for reduced NRM (i.e., difibrotide)	No trials ongoing
4. Use of biomarkers to predict events (i.e., GvHD)	Part of correlative trials

Summary and Current Controversies in HCT

High-dose therapy with hematopoietic progenitor cell support either autologous or allogeneic has become established curative treatment for a variety of malignant and nonmalignant disorders. It is a complex procedure that in the hands of well-trained multidisciplinary teams following appropriate guidelines for supportive care is associated with long-term disease control in a substantial number of patients.

Transplant outcomes have improved significantly over the last 4 decades primarily due to decreases in nonrelapse mortality (NRM) rates, and not due to reductions in the risk of post-HCT relapses. However, the advent of new chemotherapy agents targeting specific antigens (new monoclonal antibodies) and new small molecules (targeting disease-specific pathways) have opened a new era in HCT research, focusing on improving patients' disease status prior to HCT as well as potentially reducing the risks of relapse post-HCT through post-HCT therapies. Likewise access to HCT has increased with the advent of new less toxic conditioning regimens that can be safely delivered to older patients and new alternative donor sources for patients who lack a fully matched donor within their family or the volunteer donor registries.

Results of ongoing prospective trials may change the way HCTs are performed in the near future. Table 3.7 summarizes some of the most salient controversial issues in HCT today.

References

1. Thomas ED, Lochte HL Jr, Cannon JH, Sahler OD, Ferrebee JW. Supralethal whole body irradiation and isologous marrow transplantation in man. *J Clin Invest* 1959; 38:1709–16.

2. Appelbaum F. Hematopoietic stem cell transplantation at 50. *N Engl J Med* 2007;357(15):1472–5.

3. Bortin MM. A compendium of reported human bone marrow transplants. *Transplantation* 1970;9(6):571–87.

4. Thomas ED, Buckner CD, Clift RA, *et al.* Marrow transplantation for acute

nonlymphoblastic leukemia in first remission. *N Engl J Med* 1979;301:597–9.

5. Applebaum F, Herzig G, Ziegler J, *et al.* Successful engraftment of cryopreserved autologous bone marrow in patients with malignant lymphoma. *Blood* 1978;52;85–95.

6. Pasquini MC, Wang Z. Current use and outcome of hematopoietic stem cell transplantation: CIBMTR Summary Slides, 2013. Available at: http://www.cibmtr.org

7. Giralt S, Radich J. Clinical bone marrow and stem cell transplantation. In *American Society of Hematology – Self Assessment Program (ASH-SAP),* 5th edition; Chapter 14.

8. Armand P, Gibson C, Cutler C, *et al.* A disease risk index for patients undergoing allogeneic stem cell transplantation. *Blood* 2012;120:905–13.

9. Sorror ML, Maris MB, Storb R, *et al.* Hematopoietic cell transplantation (HCT)-specific comorbidity index: a new tool for risk assessment before allogeneic HCT. *Blood* 2005;106:2912–19.

10. Foster LW, McLellan L, Rybicki L, *et al.* Utility of the psychosocial assessment of candidates for transplantation (PACT) scale in allogeneic BMT. *Bone Marrow Transplant* 2009;44;375–80.

11. Gyurcokza B, Sandmaier B. Conditioning regimens for hematopoietic cell transplantation: one size does not fit all. *Blood* 2014;124(3):344–53.

12. Ballen KK, Koreth J, Chen YB, Dey BR, Spitzer TR. Selection of optimal alternative graft source: mismatched unrelated donor, umbilical cord blood, or haploidentical transplant. *Blood* 2012;119:1972–80.

13. Stem Cell Transplant Trialist Group. Allogeneic peripheral blood stem-cell compared with bone marrow transplantation in the management of hematologic malignancies: an individual patient data meta-analysis of nine randomized trials. *J Clin Oncol* 2005; 23:5074–87.

14. Thomas E.D and Storb R. Technique for human marrow grafting. *Blood* 1970;36:507–515.

15. Luznik L, O'Donnell PV, Symons HJ, *et al.* HLA-haploidentical bone marrow transplantation for hematologic malignancies using nonmyeloablative conditioning and high-dose, posttransplantation cyclophosphamide. *Biol Blood Marrow Transplant* 2008;14(6):641–50.

16. Aversa F, Terenzi A, Tabilio A. *et al.* Full haplotype-mismatched hematopoietic stem-cell transplantation: a phase II study in patients with acute leukemia at high-risk of relapse. *J Clin Oncol* 2005;23;3447–34.

17. Laughlin MJ, Barker J, Bambach B, *et al.* Hematopoietic engraftment and survival in adult recipients of umbilical-cord blood from unrelated donors. *N Engl J Med* 2001;344:1815–22.

18. Sheppard D, Bredeson C, Allan D, Tay J. Systematic review of randomized controlled trials of hematopoietic stem cell mobilization strategies for autologous transplantation for hematologic malignancies. *Biol Blood Marrow Transplant* 2012;18:1191–203.

19. Santos GW, Tutschka PJ, Brookmeyer R, *et al.* Marrow transplantation for acute non lymphocytic leukemia after treatment with busulfan and cyclophosphamide. *N Engl J Med* 1983;309(22):1347–53.

20. Tutschka PJ, Copelan EA, Klein JP. Bone marrow transplantation for leukemia following a new busulfan and cyclophosphamide regimen.*Blood* 1987;70(5):1382–88.

21. Bacigalupo A, Ballen K, Rizzo D, *et al.* Defining the intensity of conditioning regimens: working definitions. *Biol Blood Marrow Transplant* 2009;15:1628–33.

22. Luger S, Ringden O, Zhang MJ *et al.* Similar outcomes using myeloablative versus reduced intensity regimens for allogeneic transplants for AML or MDS. *Bone Marrow Transplant* 2012;47:203–11.

23. Tomblyn M, Chiller T, Einsele H, *et al.* Guidelines for preventing infectious complications among hematopoietic cell transplant recipients: a global perspective. *Biol Blood Marrow Transplant* 2009;15:1143-238. Important consensus statement.

24. Tuncer HD, Rana N, Milani C, Darko A, Al-Hasmi S. Gastrointestinal and hepatic complications of hematopoietic stem cell transplantation. *World J Gastroenterol* 2012;18:1851–60.

25. Ferrara JL, Levine JE, Reddy P, Holler E. Graft-vs-host-disease. *Lancet* 2009;373:1550–61.

26. Filipovich AH. Diagnosis and manifestations of chronic graft-*versus*-host disease. *Best Pract Res Clin Haematol* 2008;21:251–7.

27. Joseph RW, Couriel DR, Komanduri KV. Chronic graft-*versus*-host disease after allogeneic stem cell transplantation: challenges in prevention, science, and supportive care. *J Support Oncol* 2008;6:361–72.

28. Rizzo JD, Wingard JR, Tichelli A, *et al.* Recommended screening and preventive practices for long-term survivors after hematopoietic cell transplantation: joint recommendations of the European Group for Blood and Marrow Transplantation, the Center for International Blood and Marrow Transplant Research, and the American Society of Blood and Marrow Transplantation. *Biol Blood Marrow Transplant.* 2006;12:138–51.

29. Tichelli A, Rovó A, Gratwohl A. Late pulmonary, cardiovascular, and renal complications after hematopoietic stem cell transplantation and recommended screening practices. *Hemat Am Soc Hematol Educ Program* 2008:125–33.

Chapter 4

Assessment of Comorbidities for Hematopoietic Cell Transplants: Achievements and Controversies

Mahmoud Elsawy and Mohamed L. Sorror

Introduction

Allogeneic conventional HCT (hematopoietic cell transplantation) is a potentially curative therapy for many patients with hematologic malignant or nonmalignant diseases. Historically, conditioning regimens for conventional HCT have been intensified to the limits of organ tolerance in order to optimize cancer eradication. Consequently, serious toxicities to organs, such as gut, lung, kidney, heart, and liver, have been observed which, additionally, have limited the ability to deliver adequate doses of postgrafting immunosuppression needed for control of graft-*versus*-host disease (GvHD). Until recently, these regimen-related toxicities associated with high-dose myeloablative conditioning have limited allogeneic HCT to patients without significant comorbidities who are less than 55 to 60 years of age. This age restriction has been unfortunate since the median ages of patients with most blood cancers have ranged from 65 to 70 years. Also, in many cases, medical comorbidities precluded treatment with allogeneic HCT even in younger patients[1,2]. In an effort to expand treatment options for patients with hematologic malignancies, several HCT regimens have been developed that have reduced the intensity of the conditioning therapy, thereby minimizing toxicities. The regimens rely in part or almost entirely on graft-*versus*-leukemia effects for tumor cell kill. The use of reduced intensity regimens has expanded the use of HCT to include elderly and comorbid patients with various hematologic malignancies. Therefore, it has become important to comprehensively study differences in comorbidities among patient groups, to investigate the impacts of comorbidities on HCT outcomes and quality of life, and to standardize comorbidity assessment for future clinical trials.

Comorbidities are likely the main factor behind morbidity and mortality after treatment of older patients with cancer for the following reasons. First, in a "typical" geriatric series, individuals who are 65 years of age and older suffer on average from three different diseases[3]. Second, previous research has demonstrated that severity of a given comorbidity could significantly alter the type of initial anticancer treatment. For example, Van Spronsen *et al.* determined that 50% and 15% less chemotherapy was administered to older patients with Hodgkin and non-Hodgkin lymphomas and comorbidities, respectively, when compared to those without

comorbidities[4]. In addition, comorbidities have been identified as one of the prognostic factors for long-term quality of life (QoL) of cancer patients[5–9]. Comorbidity was found to have an independent impact from (or regardless of) functional status and, therefore, could provide additional prognostic information in older cancer patients[10]. Nevertheless, patients with comorbidities have often been excluded from clinical trials, and there has been little information on how to translate results from cooperative studies to given patients with comorbidities. Likewise, the impact of different comorbidities on treatment compliance, toxicity, eligibility for HCT, and the eventual outcomes of patients with blood cancers is unknown.

Achievements

Introducing the Use of Comorbidity Indices in Comparative Effectiveness Research of Allogeneic HCT

The interactions between the primary disease and different comorbidities could vary based on the type and degree of organ involvement. In addition, comorbidities are so diverse that systematic accounts of every possible diagnosis and degree of severity would create an unmanageable amount of information, especially when these data have been gathered for clinical studies or prognostic purposes. As a result, several indices have been introduced as a way to rate the impacts of different comorbidities on the primary disease. The Charlson comorbidity index (CCI)[11] has been the most widely used comorbidity index in predicting mortality risks in various solid malignancies. The 19 comorbidities included in the index have been selected and weighted on the basis of their strengths of associations with 1-year mortality in a cohort of 559 patients admitted to a general medical center. A summary score based on the sum of the weights was then validated in a cohort of breast cancer patients by evaluating the ability of scores to predict mortality.

Up until 2004, there has been almost no effort to evaluate the distribution of comorbidities among HCT recipients, to investigate their impacts on HCT outcomes, or to include them in designing clinical trials. The first study on the impact

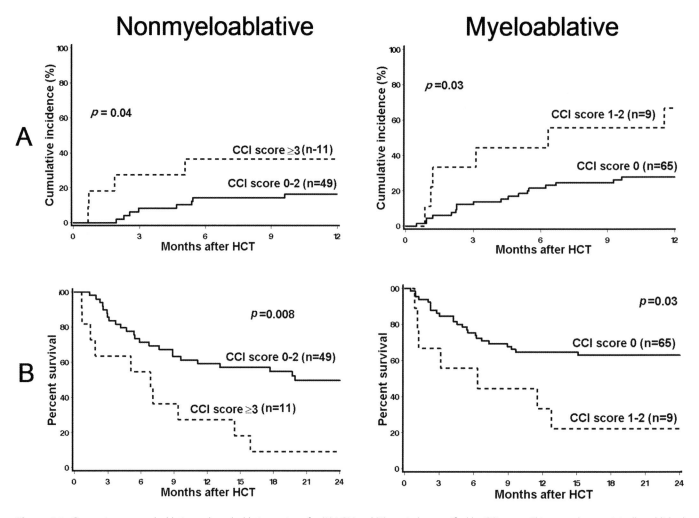

Figure 4.1. Comparing nonmyeloablative and myeloablative patients for (A) NRM and (B) survival as stratified by CCI scores. This research was originally published in *Blood*. Sorror ML, Maris MB, Storer B, Sandmaier BM, Diaconescu R, Flowers C, *et al*. Comparing morbidity and mortality of HLA-matched unrelated donor hematopoietic cell transplantation after nonmyeloablative and myeloablative conditioning: influence of pretransplant comorbidities. *Blood* 104(4): 961-8, 2004. © the American Society of Hematology.

of comorbidity indices on HCT outcomes utilized the CCI. The study assessed the pretransplant clinical differences among recipients of nonmyeloablative and high-dose conditioning followed by HLA-matched unrelated grafts to determine the differences in outcomes between the two cohorts of patients. To that end, associations between the CCI, as a measure of comorbidities, and other known risk factors with post-HCT nonrelapse mortality (NRM) and survival were evaluated. In that study, the lessened cumulative incidences of 1-year (20% *versus* 32%, P=1.4) NRM among nonmyeloablative patients did not reach statistical significance. After adjustment for pretransplant differences, including CCI scores, statistically significant lower hazard ratios (HRs) for 1-year (0.3, P=0.04) NRM were found for nonmyeloablative patients (Figure 4.1), confirming the importance of a single scoring system for comorbidities. In multivariate analyses of risk factors for outcomes, comorbidities as scored by the CCI, proved to be the only independent factor for predicting overall grade IV toxicity and NRM[12].

Development of the HCT-Specific Comorbidity Index (HCT-CI)

The CCI had two major limitations among HCT recipients. First, some of the comorbidities described by Charlson were rarely encountered due either to existing exclusion criteria, for example for hepatic comorbidities, or lack of inclusion of laboratory data, for example for pulmonary comorbidities. Second, the CCI did not capture some of the comorbidities that were frequently seen among transplanted patients, such as infections and psychiatric problems. As a result, the CCI identified comorbidities in only 35% of all patients and 12% of recipients of high-dose HCT[12]. To address these limitations, the CCI was modified in a way that better detected comorbidities among HCT recipients[13]. First, the definitions of several comorbidities were modified by adding progressive impairments of diffusion capacity of carbon monoxide (DLCO) and/or forced expiratory volume in 1-second (FEV1), left ventricular ejection fraction (LVEF) of ≤50%,

Table 4.1 Comparing definitions of comorbidities between CCI and HCT-CI

Comorbidity	CCI definition	New definition, from HCT-CI
Mild pulmonary	Dyspnea on moderate activity	Dyspnea on moderate activity or DLco and/or FEV1 81–90%
Moderate pulmonary	Dyspnea on slight activity	Dyspnea on slight activity or DLco and/or FEV1 66–80%
Severe pulmonary	Dyspnea at rest or requires oxygen	Dyspnea at rest or requires oxygen or DLco and/or FEV1$\leq$65%
Cardiac	Congestive heart failure (symptomatic and requiring treatment) and myocardial infarction were included as independent comorbidities, each acquiring a score of 1	Includes coronary artery disease,*congestive heart failure, myocardial infarction, or ejection fraction <50%: one or more acquiring a score of 1
Mild hepatic	Chronic hepatitis or cirrhosis Chronic hepatitis	bilirubin > ULN to 1.5 × ULN, or AST/ALT > ULN to 2.5 × ULN
Moderate–severe hepatic	Cirrhosis with portal hypertension ± bleeding varices	Cirrhosis, fibrosis, bilirubin >1.5 × ULN, or AST/ALT >2.5 × ULN
Mild renal	Serum creatinine 2–3 mg/dL	Creatinine 1.2–2 mg/dL
Moderate–severe renal	Creatinine >3 mg/dL, renal dialysis, or renal transplant	Creatinine >2 mg/dL, renal dialysis, or renal transplant
Prior solid tumor	Initially treated in the last 5 years	Treated at any time point in the patient's past history, excluding nonmelanoma skin cancer

* One or more vessel-coronary artery stenosis requiring medical treatment, stent, or bypass graft.
Abbreviations: DLco = diffusion capacity of carbon monoxide; FEV1 = forced expiratory volume in one second; ULN = upper limit of normal; AST = aspartate aminotransferase; ALT = alanine aminotransferase.

and progressive elevations of levels of bilirubin and hepatic transaminases to the clinical definitions of pulmonary, cardiac, and hepatic comorbidities, respectively (Table 4.1). In addition, new cut-offs for serum creatinine levels were set to better define renal comorbidity. Second, all comorbidities encountered in transplanted patients were included in the risk assessment analysis.

The study included 1055 patients with different hematologic diseases who were given allogeneic HCT after nonmyeloablative (n=294) or myeloablative (n=761) conditioning. Two-thirds of the patients were randomly assigned to a training set and one-third to a validation set. Integer weights of comorbidities were calculated based on adjusted HRs from Cox proportional hazard models of 2-year NRM. The new HCT-CI included 17 comorbidities acquiring scores from 1 to 3 (Table 4.2). In the validation set, HCT-CI scores showed higher sensitivity than the CCI scores in capturing comorbidities. HCT-CI scores of 1–2 and $\geq$3 were found in 34% and 28% of patients, while only 10% and 3% of patients had CCI scores of 1 and $\geq$2, respectively. The HCT-CI scores of 0, 1–2, and $\geq$3 showed good discrimination of NRM (14%, 21%, and 41%) and survival (71%, 60%, and 34%), respectively (Figure 4.2). The HCT-CI scores showed higher discriminative power than the CCI scores both for NRM (c-statistic estimate of 0.692 *versus* 0.546, P <0.001) and survival (c-statistic estimate of 0.661 *versus* 0.561, P < 0.001).

Use of the HCT-CI for Comparative Effectiveness of Different Conditioning Regimens and Intensities

The HCT-CI could be used to optimize treatment selections for a given hematologic malignancy.

Acute Myeloid Leukemia (AML)/Myelodysplastic Syndromes (MDS)

Multiple retrospective studies have shown similar rates of overall mortality among patients with AML and MDS after high-dose compared to nonmyeloablative conditioning regimens. Whether comorbidities could refine risk stratification was an important question. One study analyzed outcomes among patients with AML (n=391) or MDS (n=186) given either nonmyeloablative (n=125) or high-dose conditioning (n=452). Multivariate analyses of risk factors among all patients showed that high HCT-CI scores and high disease risk were the most significant factors predicting NRM (P < 0.0001 and P=0.004), overall survival (OS, P < 0.0001 and P < 0.0001), and relapse-free survival (RFS, P < 0.0001 and P <0.0001), respectively. Therefore, all patients were stratified into four risk groups incorporating the impacts of both comorbidities and disease risk (Table 4.3). Rates of 2-year OS were 70% and 78% among AML/MDS patients with HCT-CI scores of 0–2 and low-risk diseases following nonmyeloablative and high-dose HCT, respectively, and they were 57% and 51%, respectively, if patients had high-risk AML/MDS[14]. The results suggested that AML/MDS patients with low

Table 4.2 Definitions of comorbidities included in the HCT-CI and HCT-CI scores as compared to CCI scores

Comorbidity	Definitions of comorbidities included in the new HCT-CI	HCT-CI weighted scores	Original CCI scores
Arrhythmia	Atrial fibrillation or flutter, sick sinus syndrome, or ventricular arrhythmias	1	0
Cardiac[b]	Coronary artery disease,[c] congestive heart failure, myocardial infarction, or EF $\leq$ 50%	1	1
Inflammatory bowel disease	Crohn disease or ulcerative colitis	1	0
Diabetes	Requiring treatment with insulin or oral hypoglycemics but not diet alone	1	1
Cerebrovascular disease	Transient ischemic attack or cerebrovascular accident	1	1
Psychiatric disturbance[a]	Depression or anxiety requiring psychiatric consult or treatment	1	Not included
Hepatic, mild[b]	Chronic hepatitis, bilirubin > ULN to 1.5 × ULN, or AST/ALT> ULN to 2.5 × ULN	1	1
Obesity[a]	Patients with a body mass index >35 kg/m^2	1	Not included
Infection[a]	Requiring continuation of antimicrobial treatment after day 0	1	Not included
Rheumatologic	SLE, RA, polymyositis, mixed CTD, or polymyalgia rheumatica	2	1
Peptic ulcer	Requiring treatment	2	1
Moderate/severe renal[b]	Serum creatinine >2 mg/dL, on dialysis, or prior renal transplantation	2	2
Moderate pulmonary[b]	DLco and/or FEV1 66–80% or dyspnea on slight activity	2	1
Prior solid tumor[b]	Treated at any time point in the patient's past history, excluding nonmelanoma skin cancer	3	2
Heart valve disease	Except mitral valve prolapse	3	0
Severe pulmonary[b]	DLco and/or FEV1 $\leq$65% or dyspnea at rest or requiring oxygen	3	1
Moderate/severe hepatic[b]	Liver cirrhosis, bilirubin >1.5 × ULN, or AST/ALT >2.5 × ULN	3	3

[a] Newly investigated comorbidities.
[b] Comorbidities with modified definitions compared with the original CCI.
[c] One or more vessel-coronary artery stenosis requiring medical treatment, stent, or bypass graft.
Abbreviations: EF = ejection fraction; ULN = upper limit of normal; SLE = systemic lupus erythmatosis; RA = rheumatoid arthritis; CTD = connective tissue disease; DLco = diffusion capacity of carbon monoxide.

comorbidity burden are candidates for prospective randomized studies to determine the role of conditioning intensity. Unsurprisingly, patients with higher HCT-CI scores ($\geq$3) overall had relatively inferior survivals, in particular those with high-risk AML/MDS (OS of 29% and 24%, respectively). The poor survival rates were due to more relapses (49%) among nonmyeloablative recipients and more frequent NRM (46%) among high-dose recipients (Figure 4.3). Another study reported similar results with an OS rate of 32% among 128 patients with AML/MDS and HCT-CI scores of $\geq$3 after alemtuzumab-based reduced intensity conditioning (RIC) HCT[15]. Patients with scores of 0 and 1–2 had survival rates of 69% and 39%, respectively. The European Group of Blood and Marrow Transplantation (EBMT) reported 2-year NRM incidences of 9%, 15%, 18%, and 31%, respectively, in patients with scores of 0, 1, 2, and $\geq$3, who were treated with RIC HCT

for AML in first complete remission (CR)[16]. The HCT-CI was also found to provide strong stratification of survival rates among patients with chronic myelomonocytic leukemia, who were treated mostly with conventional allo-HCT. Rates were 15% *versus* 54% among those with scores of $\geq$3 *versus* 0–2, respectively[17]. Studies suggest that patients with high HCT-CI scores could benefit from novel conditioning regimens that target leukemia while avoiding the lethal toxicities.

Chronic Lymphocytic Leukemia (CLL), Lymphoma, or Multiple Myeloma

A large proportion of patients offered allo-HCT for CLL, lymphoma, or myeloma are older than 60 years, and heavily pretreated with multiple lines of chemotherapy which often includes an autologous HCT. One study comparing outcomes

Table 4.3 Two-year NRM, relapse, OS, and RFS incidences among nonmyeloablative compared to myeloablative patients as stratified into four risk groups based on HCT-CI scores and disease status

Risk groups	Patients	NRM (%)	Relapse (%)	OS (%)	RFS (%)
Group I (HCT-CI scores 0–2 and low-risk diseases)	Myeloablative (n=138)	11	14	78	75
	Nonmyeloablative (n=28)	4	33	70	63
Group II (HCT-CI scores 0–2 and intermediate and high-risk diseases)	Myeloablative (n=176)	24	34	51	43
	Nonmyeloablative (n=34)	3	42	57	56
Group III (HCT-CI scores ≥3 and low-risk diseases)	Myeloablative (n=52)	32	27	45	41
	Nonmyeloablative (n=19)	27	37	41	36
Group IV (HCT-CI scores ≥3 and intermediate and high-risk diseases)	Myeloablative (n=86)	46	34	24	20
	Nonmyeloablative (n=44)	29	49	29	23

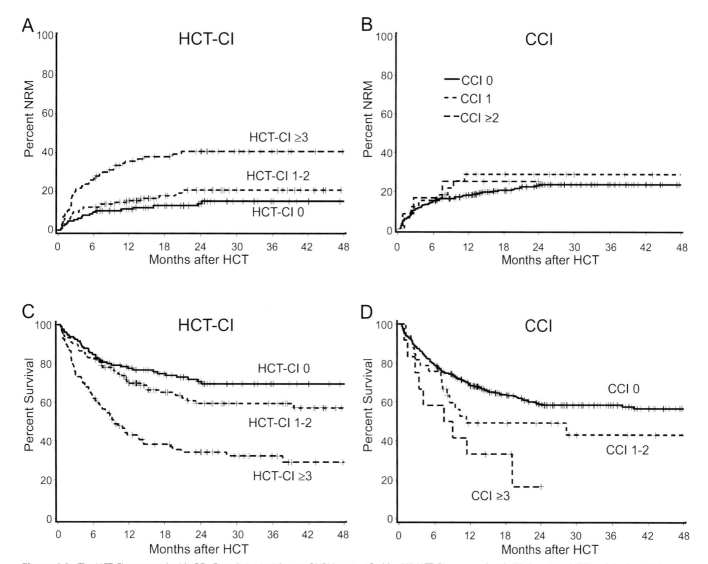

Figure 4.2. The HCT-CI compared with CCI. Cumulative incidence of NRM as stratified by (**A**) HCT-CI compared with (**B**) the original CCI and Kaplan–Meier estimates of survival as stratified by (**C**) the HCT-CI compared with (**D**) the original CCI. This research was originally published in *Blood*. Sorror ML, Maris MB, Storb R, Baron F, Sandmaier BM, Maloney DG, *et al*. Hematopoietic cell transplantation (HCT)-specific comorbidity index: a new tool for risk assessment before allogeneic HCT. *Blood* 106(8): 2912–9, 2005. © the American Society of Hematology.

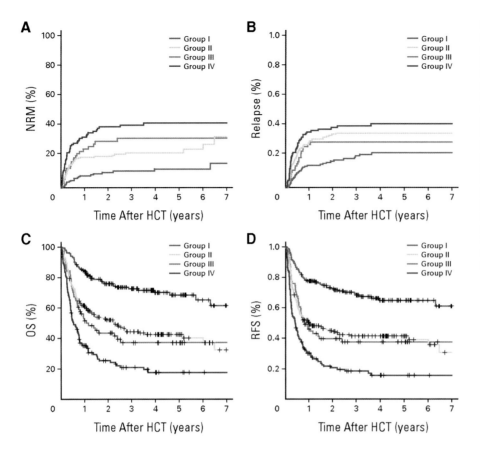

Figure 4.3. Risk stratification of patients with acute myeloid leukemia/myelodysplasia and receiving allogeneic hematopoietic cell transplant (HCT). Group I (gray) included HCT-specific comorbidity index (CI) scores 0 to 2 plus low disease risk; group II (yellow) included HCT-CI scores 0 to 2 plus intermediate and high disease risks; group III (blue) included HCT-CI scores ≥3 plus low disease risks; and group IV (red) included HCT-CI scores ≥3 plus intermediate and high disease risks. NRM, nonrelapse mortality; OS, overall survival; RFS, relapse-free survival. From Sorror ML, Sandmaier BM, Storer BE, Maris MB, Baron F, Maloney DG, *et al.* Comorbidity and disease status-based risk stratification of outcomes among patients with acute myeloid leukemia or myelodysplasia receiving allogeneic hematopoietic cell transplantation. *J Clin Oncol* 25(27): 4246–54, 2007 14. Reprinted with permission. © 2007 American Society of Clinical Oncology. All rights reserved.

among patients with lymphoma or CLL given either nonmyeloablative (n=152) or high-dose (n=68) conditioning found that conditioning intensity and HCT-CI scores were the two major predictive factors for NRM and OS. Patients with no comorbidities had 3-year NRM rates of 18% and 15% and overall survival rates of 68% and 60% following nonmyeloablative and high-dose regimens, respectively. These differences were not statistically significant. There were also no differences in mean number of hospitalization or outpatient follow-up days. Alternatively, patients with scores ≥1 had significantly lower rates of NRM, 28% *versus* 50%, and better OS rates, 47% *versus* 35%, following nonmyeloablative *versus* high-dose HCT [18]. Overall, there was no evidence for a role of conditioning intensity to reduce relapse in both cohorts. While prospective randomized studies are needed for patients with no comorbidities, nonmyeloablative HCT should be preferred to those with comorbidities.

Another study of outcomes among 203 patients with NHL, Hodgkin lymphoma (HL), and MM given RIC allo-HCT showed 2-year survival rates of 87%, 51%, and 49%, respectively, in those with scores of 0, 1–2, and ≥3 (Figure 4.4)[19]. When 63 lymphoma patients were conditioned with fludarabine and cyclophosphamide regimen followed by allo-HCT, those with scores of 0–2 had NRM of 13.6% *versus* 36.8% among those with scores of ≥3[20]. In 84 patients with CLL, the combination of the HCT-CI with an adverse disease-feature, namely lymph node size of ≥5cm, could stratify

patients into four risk groups. Patients with or without comorbidities who had lymph node size under 5 cm achieved 5-year overall survival of 60% and 78%, respectively, while those with lymph node size of ≥5cm had overall survival of 27% and 43%, respectively (Figure 4.5)[21].

Chronic Myeloid Leukemia (CML)

Among 271 patients diagnosed with imatinib-resistant CML and treated with allogeneic high-dose HCT, those with an HCT-CI score of 0 had 5-year NRM and survival of 5.3% and 69.6% compared to 18.5% and 55.5%, respectively, among those with comorbidities. In that study, an inflammatory biomarker, C-reactive protein (CRP), also had independent prognostic impacts on HCT outcomes. Those with CRP of ≤9 mL/L had 5-year survival of about 70% compared to 40% among those with higher values. The study suggested that patients with no comorbidities and low CRP values are good candidates for early allogeneic HCT after failing treatment with first-generation tyrosine kinase inhibitors[22].

Use of the HCT-CI to Compare Outcomes at Two Different Institutions

The HCT-CI was used to compare outcomes among two cohorts of patients diagnosed with a single disease entity, acute myeloid leukemia in first CR, transplanted at two different institutions, the Fred Hutchinson Cancer Research Center

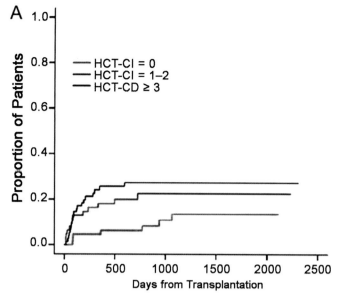

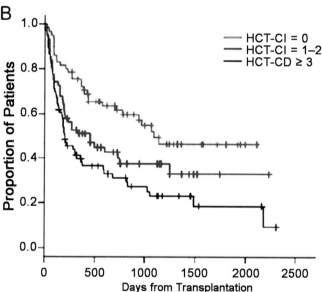

Figure 4.4. (A) Cumulative incidence of nonrelapse mortality (P≤0.04) and (B) progression-free survival (P≤0.001) as stratified by pretransplant HCT-CI among patients with lymphoma, CLL, and multiple myeloma. Reprinted by permission from Farina L, Bruno B, Patriarca F, Spina F, Sorasio R, Morelli M, et al. The hematopoietic cell transplantation comorbidity index (HCT-CI) predicts clinical outcomes in lymphoma and myeloma patients after reduced-intensity or nonmyeloablative allogeneic stem cell transplantation. *Leukemia* 23(6): 1131–8, 2009. Copyright 2009.

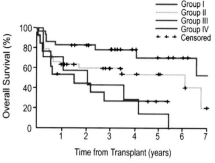

Figure 4.5. Kaplan–Meier probabilities of survival among patients with advanced CLL who were treated with allo-NMA-HCT as stratified into four risk groups on the basis of consolidated HCT-CI scores and lymph node diameter. Group I included patients who had no comorbidities and who had lymphadenopathy of ≤5cm ; group II, patients with comorbidities only; group III, patients with lymphadenopathy of ≥5cm only; and group IV, patients with both comorbidities and lymphadenopathy of ≥5cm . Five-year survival rates were 78%, 60%, 43%, and 27% for risk groups I, II, III, and IV, respectively. From Sorror ML, Storer BE, Sandmaier BM, Maris M, Shizuru J, Maziarz R, et al. Five-year follow-up of patients with advanced chronic lymphocytic leukemia treated with allogeneic hematopoietic cell transplantation after nonmyeloablative conditioning. *J Clin Oncol* 26(30): 4912-20, 2008. Reprinted with permission. © 2008 American Society of Clinical Oncology. All rights reserved.

was detected (HR: 0.98, *P*=0.94), highlighting the importance of the HCT-CI in comparing trial results at different institutions[23].

Use of the HCT-CI in Combination with Other Models to Improve Risk Assessment (Table 4.4)

The HCT-CI and Performance Status (PS)

Comorbidity indices and PS scales independently predict cancer treatment outcomes[10]. However, the greatest benefit of PS scales appears to result when they are combined with a comorbidity index[24,25].The integration of PS with the HCT-CI allowed better outcome stratification among recipients of nonmyeloablative conditioning followed by allogeneic HCT[26]. A refined risk-stratification model was proposed by consolidating the HCT-CI and Karnofsky PS resulting in four risk groups for NRM and survival (Figure 4.6).

The HCT-CI and the EBMT Risk Score

The EBMT risk score was originally developed in patients with chronic myeloid leukemia but later validated among other hematologic malignancies[27]. It comprises five risk factors: age, donor type, time from diagnosis to HCT, disease stage, and donor/recipient gender combinations[28]. In a recent study of a cohort of 1616 recipients of allogeneic HCT from various high-dose and RIC/nonmyeloablative conditioning regimens, the HCT-CI and the EBMT risk scores were consolidated resulting in six risk groups for outcomes (Figure 4.7). The combined model had a better c-statistic estimate of 0.630 for OS compared to the HCT-CI (0.613) and the EBMT (0.558) alone[29].

(FHCRC) and MD Anderson Cancer Center (MDACC). HCT-CI scores of 0, 1–2, and ≥3 predicted comparable NRM (7% *versus* 7%, 19% *versus* 21%, and 37% *versus* 27%) among FHCRC *versus* MDACC patients, respectively. In multivariate models, HCT-CI scores were associated with the highest HRs for NRM and survival among each cohort. The 2-year survival rates among FHCRC and MDACC patients were 71% *versus* 56%, respectively. After adjustment for risk factors, including HCT-CI scores, no difference in survival

Table 4.4 Combining the HCT-CI with other models to improve risk assessment

Composite model	Risk groups		Outcomes at 2 years		Outcomes at 4 or 5 years	
	HCT-CI	KPS	NRM (%)	OS (%)	NRM (%)	OS (%)
Comorbidity / PS[26]	0–2	>80%	16	68		
	0–2	≤80%	17	58		
	≥3	>80%	30	41		
	≥3	≤80%	39	32		
	HCT-CI/age					
Comorbidity/age score [31] (nonmyeloablative *versus* RIC)	0		5–12	81–87		
	1–2		9–18	66–67		
	3–4		17–36	47–54		
	≥5		35–41	34–35		
Comorbidity/relapse score [34]	HCT-CI	Relapse risk score				
	0	Low				69
	0	Standard				45
	0	High				41
	1–2	Low				56
	1–2	Standard				44
	1–2	High				15
	≥3	Low				56
	≥3	Standard				23
	≥3	High				23
Comorbidity/Biomarkers[37] (HCT-CI + ferritin, albumin, and platelets): *Each of the three biomarkers acquire a weight of 1 to be added to the HCT-CI score*	Augmented HCT-CI					
	0–1		8	79		
	2		16	64		
	3		22	52		
	4		31	47		
	≥5		42	30		
HCT-CI/EBMT[29]	HCT-CI	EBMT				
	0	<4			11	72
	0	≥4			19	61
	1–2	<4			16	63
	1–2	≥4			28	48
	≥3	<4			31	40
	≥3	≥4			41	30
HCT-CI/IADL[40] *HCT-CI score of ≥3 or IADL score < 14 acquire a score of 1. Both abnormalities get a score of 2*	Scores					
	0			62		
	1			44		
	2			13		

From Hematology Am Soc Hematol Educ Program. 2014;2014(1):21–33. doi: 10.1182/asheducation-2014.1.21 [Epub Nov 18 2014].
Abbreviations: EBMT, European bone marrow transplant; HCT-CI, hematopoietic cell transplantation comorbidity index; IADL, instrumental activities of daily living; KPS, Karnofsky performance scores; NRM, nonrelapse mortality; OS, overall survival; PS, performance status; RIC, reduced intensity conditioning.

The HCT-CI and Age

Age, *per se*, was shown to be a poor prognostic factor for allo-HCT. Nevertheless, it is true that up until now assignment of patients to allo-HCT is based to a great extent on age. Usage of age alone as a selection criterion could be responsible for significant loss of life and/or resources. However, incorporation of age into the HCT-CI gives a better understanding of the (often small) effect of age in a given patient, an important consideration given that pretransplant assessment has been greatly biased against older patients[30]. Age was added to

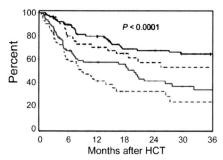

Figure 4.6. Kaplan–Meier probabilities of survival among patients with hematologic malignancies treated with allo-NMA-HCT as stratified into four risk groups based on a consolidated HCT-CI and KPS scale. Group I (solid black line) includes patients with HCT-CI scores of 0 to 2 and a KPS of >80%; group II (dotted black line) includes patients with HCT-CI scores of 0 to 2 and a KPS of ≤80%; group III (solid blue line) includes patients with HCT-CI scores of ≥3 and a KPS of >80%; group IV (dotted blue line) includes patients with HCT-CI scores of ≥3 and a KPS of ≤80%. Survival rates at 2 years were 68%, 58%, 41%, and 32% for risk groups I, II, III, and IV, respectively. From Sorror M, Storer B, Sandmaier BM, Maloney DG, Chauncey TR, Langston A, *et al.* Hematopoietic cell transplantation-comorbidity index and Karnofsky performance status are independent predictors of morbidity and mortality after allogeneic nonmyeloablative hematopoietic cell transplantation. *Cancer* 112: 1992–2001, 2008. Reprinted with permission. © 2008, John Wiley and Sons.

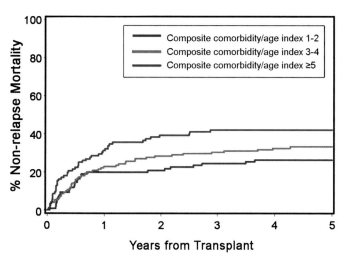

Figure 4.8. Stratification of the probabilities of nonrelapse mortality among patients (n=387) who were 60 years or older using the composite comorbidity/age scores. From Sorror *et al. J Clin Oncol* 2014;32:8153–8157. Reprinted with permission. © 2014 American Society of Clinical Oncology. All rights reserved.

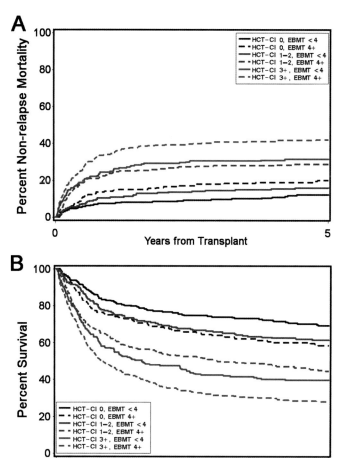

Figure 4.7. Probabilities of (A) nonrelapse mortality and (B) Kaplan–Meier estimates of overall survival as stratified by a combined model comprising the hematopoietic cell transplantation comorbidity index (HCT-CI) and the European Group for Blood and Marrow Transplantation (EBMT). Reprinted from *Biology of Blood and Marrow Transplantation*, in press, Elsawy M, Storer BE, Sorror ML. "To combine or not to combine": Optimizing risk assessment before allogeneic hematopoietic cell transplantation (Letter). *Biol Blood Marrow Transplant* [Epub ahead of print May 7 2014]. doi: 10.1016/j.bbmt.2014.05.005. Copyright 2014 with permission from Elsevier.

the HCT-CI as an additional variable, acquiring a weight of 1 for patients aged ≥40 years with proven risk stratification capacity[31] (Figure 4.8).

A significant change in the practice of referral to allo-HCT is expected where age is not to be considered solely for protocol criteria or treatment selection. Instead, all patients should be evaluated with the composite comorbidity/age score, summating the impact of comorbidities and age, as well as appropriate features of their primary disease for selection of the most beneficial transplant strategy. Regardless of age, patients with low scores should be considered for randomized clinical trials or offered higher intensity regimens. An exclusion would be

patients older than 65 years as there are limited data on usage of high-dose regimens in that group. Likewise, regardless of age, patients with higher scores would be more suitable candidates for lesser intensity regimens. This information would improve future knowledge of physicians and patients in regards to effectiveness of medical interventions with the ultimate goal of improving outcomes and quality, and reducing costs[32].

The HCT-CI and The Relapse Risk Score

A relapse risk score that was specifically developed for recipients of nonmyeloablative HCT[33] was integrated with the HCT-CI to enhance prediction of OS among patients of ≥60 years. The combined comorbidity/relapse score stratified older patients into nine risk groups, with 5-year OS rates ranging from 69% in those with an HCT-CI score of 0 and AML in first CR to 23% in those with HCT-CI scores of ≥3 and advanced or secondary AML[34].

The HCT-CI and Biomarkers

The integration of biomarkers into current health measures could refine decision-making. Additionally, they could serve as potential targets for future interventions. As mentioned earlier, the HCT-CI could be complemented by CRP, an inflammatory biomarker thought to aid in host defense, to risk-stratify patients diagnosed with TKI-failed CML before allogeneic HCT. Serum albumin concentration can serve as a marker of inflammation and predicts cardiovascular and all-cause mortality[35]. High serum ferritin can indicate iron overload or acute inflammation and is thought to predict morbidity and mortality after HCT[36]. Low blood counts may indicate progressive malignancy, extensive prior cytotoxic treatment, or stromal damage. Since these particular biomarkers are closely tied to medical comorbidities, their independent roles from the HCT-CI were evaluated in a relatively large study. Each biomarker value acquired a weight of 1 that could be added to the HCT-CI scores to yield an augmented model. The augmented index had a statistically significantly higher c-statistic estimate (0.61) for NRM prognostication in comparison to the HCT-CI alone (0.58) (P=0.0007)[37]. Table 4.5 summarizes definitions and scoring guidelines of the augmeted HCT-CI.

The HCT-CI and Instrumental Activities of Daily Living

Functional status is considered as a component of geriatric assessment (GA) for older patients. Prior to HCT, functional status has been mostly evaluated using PS scales. Those scales provide limited information compared to measures of basic (BADL) and instrumental (IADL) activities of daily living [38,39]. A recent study in a group of recipients of allogeneic HCT with a median age of 58 (range 50–73) years showed independent impacts of IADL and HCT-CI on overall morality. The authors assigned a single point to either of HCT-CI score of ≥ 3 or IADL score of < 14 to have a combined model of either 0, 1, or 2 points[40]. Patients with 0,1, and 2 points had 2-year survival rates of 62%, 44%, and 13%, respectively. All patients older than 60 years with a combined score of 2 had less than 2 years of survival.

Associations between the HCT-CI and Post-HCT Morbidities

The biology underlying the associations between comorbidities and post-HCT mortality has not been, so far, extensively evaluated. One recent study comprising data from 2985 recipients of allogeneic HCT treated at five institutions evaluated the associations between the HCT-CI scores and development and fate of acute GvHD[41]. Increasing HCT-CI scores, as a continuous variable, was associated with the risks for grades II–IV (HR=1.03, P=0.04) and more strongly with those for grades III–IV acute GvHD (HR=1.12, P<0.0001). Patients with scores of 0, 1–4, and ≥ 5 had 120-day rates of grades III–IV acute GvHD of 13%, 18%, and 24%, respectively. These associations were persistently significant among recipients of high-dose, RIC, and nonmyeloablative conditioning regimens.

Additional analyses revealed that 9 out of the 17 comorbidities of the HCT-CI were associated with severe acute GvHD; the majority of those comorbidities had underlying inflammatory pathology. While increasing comorbidity scores were associated with increasing age, age *per se* had no statistically significant association with development of acute GvHD. Finally, increasing HCT-CI scores predicted survival following diagnosis of acute GvHD. Both pretransplant comorbidities and development of acute grades II–IV GvHD had additive effects on subsequent mortality[41]. Findings set the stage for targeting specific comorbidities to alleviate post-HCT complications. In another recent study, while an increasing HCT-CI score was not predictive of chronic GvHD development, the index has been shown to correlate with higher risk of NRM (HR=1.29, P<0.0001) and overall mortality (HR=1.25, P<0.001) following the diagnosis of chronic GvHD. This correlation was independent of donor type and stem cell source. Hence, prospective clinical trials targeting treatment of chronic GvHD could utilize the HCT-CI score in their design (https://www.ncbi.nlm.nih.gov/pubmed/26194447).

Another study evaluated the impacts of comorbidities on long-term QoL among a group of 1775 adult survivors 3–18 years after HCT. Those survivors were surveyed prospectively using the Short-Form Health Survey (SF-36), Fatigue Symptom Inventory (FSI), Symptom Check List-90-Revised (SCL-90-R) for depression, Cancer and Treatment Distress (CTXD) scale, ENRICHD Social Support Instrument (ESSI), Social Activity Log (SAL), and self-reported comorbidity index (SR-CI) for general health. Comorbidities were coded retrospectively. Increasing pretransplant HCT-CI scores independently resulted in impaired physical health, increased depression, increased distress, diminished social support, and increased comorbidity burden among long-term survivors[42].

Controversies and Solutions

Validity of the HCT-CI in Single and Multiple Center Experiences

Validity of the HCT-CI as a prognostic model for transplant outcomes has been under some debate. Given the proven value of comorbidity assessment before allo-HCT, it is of prime importance to validate the performance of the index in adequately sampled, well-designed, and appropriately analyzed retrospective and prospective studies. We have performed an online search using PubMed as well as blood journal websites to identify studies that used the HCT-CI to study allo-HCT outcomes. No exclusions were made based on number of patients, direction of the results, or characteristics of study populations. Studies including recipients of autologous HCT or conventional chemotherapy for any type of hematologic malignancies were excluded as we intended to focus on performance of the index in recipients of allo-HCT. Thirty-three studies were identified. Details on numbers of patients, types of donors and regimens, outcomes predicted or not predicted by

Table 4.5 Definitions of comorbidities included in the HCT-CI and the augmented HCT-CI and their corresponding scores

The HCT-CI

Comorbidity	Definition	Score
Arrhythmia	Any type of arrhythmia that has necessitated the delivery of a specific anti-arrhythmia treatment at any time point in the patient's past medical history.	1
Cardiac	Coronary artery disease,§ congestive heart failure, myocardial infarction, or EF ≤50%	1
Inflammatory bowel disease	Crohn's disease or ulcerative colitis requiring treatment at any time point in patient's past medical history.	1
Diabetes	Requiring treatment with insulin or oral hypoglycemic agents continuously for 4 weeks before start of conditioning	1
Cerebrovascular disease	Transient ischemic attack or cerebrovascular accident	1
Psychiatric disturbance	Any disorder requiring continuous treatments for 4 weeks before start of conditioning	1
Hepatic, mild	Chronic hepatitis, bilirubin > ULN to 1.5 × ULN, or AST/ALT> ULN to 2.5 × ULN; at least two values of each within 2 or 4 weeks before start of conditioning.	1
Obesity	Patients with a body mass index >35 kg/m^2 for patients older than 18 years or a BMI-for-age of ≥95th percentile for patients of ≤18 years of age	1
Infection	Requiring antimicrobial treatment starting from before conditioning and continued beyond day 0	1
Rheumatologic	Requiring specific treatment at any time point in the patient's past medical history	2
Peptic ulcer	Based on prior endoscopic or radiologic diagnosis	2
Moderate/severe renal	Serum creatinine >2mg/dL (at least two values of each within 2 or 4 weeks before start of conditioning), on dialysis, or prior renal transplantation	2
Moderate pulmonary	Corrected DLco (via Dinakara equation) and/or FEV1 of 66–80% or dyspnea on slight activity	2
Prior malignancy	Treated at any time point in the patient's past history, excluding non-melanoma skin cancer	3
Heart valve disease	Of at least moderate severity, prosthetic valve, or symptomatic mitral valve prolapse as detected by echocardiogram	3
Severe pulmonary	Corrected DLco (via Dinakara equation) and/or FEV1 ≤ 65% or dyspnea at rest or requiring oxygen	3
Moderate/severe hepatic	Liver cirrhosis, bilirubin >1.5 × ULN, or AST/ALT >2.5 × ULN; at least two values of each within 2 or 4 weeks before start of conditioning	3
Augmented HCT-CI: all of the above +		
High ferritin	Values of ≥2500 as measured the closest prior to start of conditioning	1
Mild Hypoalbuminemia	Values of <3.5-3.0 as measured the closest prior to start of conditioning	1
Thrombocytopenia	Values of <100,000 as measured the closest prior to start of conditioning	1
Moderate Hypoalbuminemia	Values of <3.0 as measured the closest prior to start of conditioning	2

Abbreviations: EF = ejection fraction; ULN= upper limit of normal; DLco= diffusion capacity of carbon monoxide: FEV1= forced expiratory volume in 1 second. §One or more vessel-coronary artery stenosis requiring medical treatment, stent, or bypass graft.

the HCT-CI, and the methods used for assessing index performance are described in Table 4.6. The majority of these studies focused on NRM and OS as the outcomes of interest, while few analyzed, in addition, progression-free survival. The most commonly used statistical methods were cumulative incidence estimates for NRM; Kaplan–Meier rates for survivals; and hazard ratios, confidence interval, and *P*-values from regression models. Only seven studies utilized c-statistic estimates to validate findings. This raises concerns about the adequacy of some of the studies since concordance probability estimates (such as c-statistic) are the most appropriate methods to evaluate model performance as they are not influenced by sample size or scale marker.

Overall, 25 of the 33 studies have shown statistically significant associations between the HCT-CI scores and some or all of the evaluated outcomes[43–49]. Some of the 25 studies were performed in disease-specific cohorts of patients [14,15,17–19,23,46,47,50], while others were done in patients

Table 4.6 Performance of the HCT-CI as a prognostic factor in single and multicenter retrospective and prospective studies

Study	No. of patients	Types of donors	Types of conditioning intensity	Outcomes Predicted by the HCT-CI	Outcomes Not predicted by the HCT-CI	Comments	Statistical methods used for validation Rates	Multivariate HRs	c-Statistic estimates
Kerbauy et al., 2005 [17]	43	HLA-matched (n=35) HLA-MM (n=8)	MA (n=37) NMA (n=6)	4-year NRM and OS	—	Small sample size Diagnoses: chronic myelomonocytic leukemia	✓	—	—
Maruyama et al., 2007 [51]	132	Related (n=70) Unrelated (n=62)	MA (n=52) RIC (n=80)	2-year NRM and OS in MA patients	2-year NRM and OS on RIC patients	Diagnoses: leukemia/lymphoma in nonremission	✓	✓	—
Kerbauy et al., 2007 [50]	104	Related (n=58) Unrelated (n=45)	MA (n=95) NMA (n=9)	5-year NRM and OS	—	Diagnoses: idiopathic myelofibrosis, advanced polycythemia vera, and essential thrombocythemia	✓	✓	—
Sorror et al., 2007 [23]	244	HLA-matched (n=220) HLA-MM (n=24)	MA (n=202) NMA (n=18) RIC (n=24)	2-year NRM and OS	—	Diagnoses: AML in 1st complete remission	✓	✓	✓
Sorror et al., 2007 [14]	577	HLA-matched (n=523) HLA-MM (n=54)	MA (n=425) NMA (n=125)	2-year NRM and OS	—	Adding disease status improved prediction Diagnoses: AML/MDS	✓	✓	—
Sorror et al., 2008 [26]	341	Related (n=160) Unrelated (n=181)	NMA (n=341)	2-year NRM and OS	—	Adding KPS improved prediction Diagnoses: malignant and nonmalignant hematologic disorders	✓	✓	—
Artz et al., 2008[52]	112	HLA-matched (n=103) HLA-MM (n=9)	RIC	1-year OS	1-year NRM	Small sample size Diagnoses: malignant and nonmalignant hematologic disorders	✓	✓	—
Sorror et al., 2008 [18]	220	HLA-matched (n=205) HLA-MM (n=15)	MA (n=68) NMA (n=152)	3-year NRM and OS	—	Diagnoses: chronic lymphocytic leukemia and lymphoma	✓	✓	—
Xhaard et al., 2008 [64]	286	Related (n=149) Unrelated (n=63) Other (n=74)	MA (n=167) NMA (n=119)	—	2-year NRM and OS	Lack of information on PFT Diagnoses: malignant and nonmalignant hematologic disorders	✓	✓	✓

Reference	n	HLA match	Conditioning	Endpoints (overall cohort)	Endpoints (subgroup)	Comments			
Majhail et al., 2008 [53]	373	HLA-matched (n=184) UCB (=189)	MA (n=150) NMA (n=223)	2-year NRM and OS in overall cohort	2-year NRM and OS in subgroup analysis	Small number of patients in subgroups Diagnoses: malignant and nonmalignant hematologic disorders	✓	✓	—
Farina et al., 2009 [19]	203	Related (n=121) Unrelated (n=82)	RIC (n=154) NMA (n=49)	2-year NRM, OS, and PFS	—	Lymphoma and myeloma	✓	✓	—
Guilfoyle et al., 2009 [65]	187	Related (n=138) Unrelated (n=49)	MA (n=177) NMA (n=10)	—	2-year NRM and OS	1. High incidence of pulmonary comorbidities; 2. small sample size; 3. data collected from 1990–2005 (significant heterogeneity in treatment protocols and supportive care). Diagnoses: malignant and nonmalignant hematologic disorders	✓	✓	—
Kataoka et al., 2010 [54]	187	HLA-matched (n=143) HLA-MM (n=44)	MA (n=170) NMA (n=17)	1. 3-year NRM and OS; 2. OS in low-risk disease subgroup	OS in high-risk disease subgroup	Small number of patients in subgroups Diagnoses: malignant and nonmalignant hematologic disorders	✓	✓	—
Lim et al., 2010[15]	128	HLA-matched (n=94) HLA-MM (n=34)	RIC	3-year NRM, OS, and DFS	—	Diagnoses: AML/MDS	✓	✓	—
Barba et al., 2010[55]	194	Related (n=153) Unrelated or MM (n=41)	RIC	2-year NRM and OS	—	Diagnoses: malignant and nonmalignant hematologic disorders	✓	✓	✓
Terwey et al., 2010 [63]	151	HLA-matched (n=134) HLA-MM (n=17)	MA (n=138) RIC (n=13)	—	2-year NRM and OS	High frequency of intermediate and high-risk patients (71%) Diagnoses: ALL	✓	✓	—
DeFor et al., 2010 [61]	444	HLA-matched (n=211) UCB (n=233)	MA (n=169) NMA (n=275)	—	2-year NRM and OS	Diagnoses: malignant and nonmalignant hematologic disorders	✓	✓	✓
Birninger et al., 2011 [62]	340	Related (n=116) Other (n=224)	MA (n=133) NMA (n=207)	—	3-year NRM and OS	1. Unbalanced score categories 2. Possible overscoring of some comorbidities Diagnoses: high-risk AML	✓	✓	—
Smith et al., 2011 [45]	252	HLA-matched (n=149) HLA-MM (n=55) UCB (n=48)	MA (n=189) RIC/NMA (n=61) None (n=2)	1-year NRM and OS	—	Pediatric population-based study Diagnoses: malignant and nonmalignant hematologic disorders	✓	✓	—

Table 4.6 (cont.)

Study	No. of patients	Types of donors	Types of conditioning intensity	Outcomes Predicted by the HCT-CI	Outcomes Not predicted by the HCT-CI	Comments	Statistical methods used for validation Rates	Multivariate HRs	c-Statistic estimates
Castagna et al., 2011 [66]	63	HLA-matched (n=59) HLA-MM (n=2) UCB (n=2)	RIC	—	1-year TRM and 2-year OS	Small sample size Diagnoses: malignant and nonmalignant hematologic disorders	✓	—	—
Williams et al., 2012 [67]	96	Related (n=34) Unrelated (n=62)	MA (n=33) RIC (n=63)	—	1-year NRM and OS	Small sized heterogeneous sample Diagnoses: malignant and nonmalignant hematologic disorders	✓	✓	—
Bokhari et al., 2012 [47]	121	Related (n=57) Unrelated (n=64)	RIC	2-year NRM and OS when combined with age and disease status	2-year NRM and OS	Diagnoses: AML/MDS	✓	✓	—
Raimondi et al., 2012 [56]	1937	Related (n=958) Unrelated (n=979)	MA (n=1083) RIC (n=854)	2-year NRM and OS	—	A large multicenter prospective study Diagnoses: malignant and nonmalignant hematologic disorders	✓	✓	✓
Mo et al., 2013 [58]	526	HLA-MM related	MA	2-year NRM, OS, and relapse risk	—	Diagnoses: malignant and nonmalignant hematologic disorders	✓	✓	—
Le et al., 2013 [48]	79	HLA-matched	MA	5-year NRM and OS	—	Diagnoses: malignant and nonmalignant hematologic disorders	✓	✓	—
Ratan el al., 2013 [46]	218	HLA-matched	MA	5-year NRM, OS, and RFS	—	Diagnoses: AML/MDS	✓	✓	—
Hashmi et al., 2013 [57]	103	Related (n=45) Unrelated (n=58)	RIC	1-year OS	—	Diagnoses: malignant and nonmalignant hematologic disorders	✓	✓	—
Bayraktar et al., 2013 [59]	377	HLA-matched (n=277) HLA-MM (n=100)	MA (n=199) NMA (n=178)	Mortality and 1-year OS in patients admitted to ICU	—	Diagnoses: Overall recipients of allo-HCT who were admitted to the ICU	✓	✓	—

Study	N	Donor	Conditioning	Outcome	Outcome	Notes			
Chemnitz et al., 2014 [60]	245	Related (n=87) Unrelated (n=158)	MA/RIC (n=167) NMA (n=35) Other (n=43)	5-year NRM and OS	—	Diagnoses: malignant and nonmalignant hematologic disorders	✓	✓	—
Nakaya et al.,2014 [76]	243	Related (n=68) Unrelated (n=175)	MA (n=166) RIC (n=77)	—	2-year NRM and OS	A multi-center prospective study Diagnosis: malignant and benign hematological disorders HCT-CI was predictive of 2-year NRM and OS using new cut-offs for risk groups (low risk for scores of 0-3 and high risk for scores ≥4)	✓	✓	—
Elsawy et al., 2014 [77]	492	HLA-MM (n=254) UCB (n=238)	MA (n=308) NMA/RIC (n=184)	2-year NRM and OS	—	The HCT-CI scores could be used to optimize graft source selection for patients with no suitable matched donors. Diagnosis: malignant and benign hematological disorders	✓	✓	✓
Sorror et al., 2015 [78]	19767	Related (19%) Unrelated (23%) Autologous (58%)—	MA (67%) NMA/RIC (33%)—	1- and 3-year NRM and OS3-year TRM and OS	—	A large multicenter prospective study Diagnoses: malignant and nonmalignant hematologic disorders	✓	✓	—
Elsawy et al., 2015 [79]	2523	Related (56%) Unrelated (44%)	MA (62%) RIC (18%) NMA (20%)	2-year NRM and OS	—	Diagnoses: malignant and nonmalignant hematologic disorders	✓	✓	✓

Abbreviations: ALL = acute lymphoblastic leukemia; AML = acute myeloid leukemia; DFS = disease-free-survival; HCT-CI = hematopoietic cell transplantation comorbidity index; HLA = human leukocyte antigen; HCT = hematopoietic cell transplantation; HRs = hazard ratios; ICU = intensive care unit; KPS = Karnofsky performance status; MA = myeloablative; MDS =myelodysplastic syndromes; MM = mismatched; NMA = nonmyeloablative; NRM = non relapse mortality; OS = overall survival; PFS = progression-free survival; PFTs = pulmonary function test; RFS = relapse-free survival; RIC = reduced intensity conditioning regimen; TCD = T-cell depleted; TRM = transplant-related mortality; UCB = umbilical cord blood.

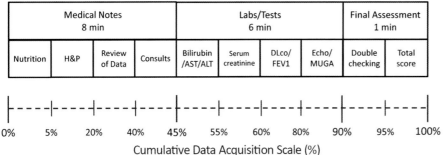

Three-Step Process (15 minutes)

Medical Notes 8 min				Labs/Tests 6 min				Final Assessment 1 min	
Nutrition	H&P	Review of Data	Consults	Bilirubin /AST/ALT	Serum creatinine	DLco/ FEV1	Echo/ MUGA	Double checking	Total score

0%   5%   20%   40%   45%   55%   60%   80%   90%   95%   100%

Cumulative Data Acquisition Scale (%)

Figure 4.9. Three-step methodology for comorbidity coding. This research was originally published in *Blood*. Sorror M. How I assess comorbidities prior to hematopoietic cell transplantation. *Blood* 121(15): 2854–63, 2013. © the American Society of Hematology.

with various hematologic malignancies[26,43–45,48,51–60]. Eight studies reported lack of associations between the HCT-CI and any of the reported outcomes[61–68]. The majority of those studies were done outside the United States[63–65,67]. Limited sample size of patients and/or limited number of events have probably been responsible for lack of statistical significance in the majority of the seven studies. In fact, a recent study has shown that an overall sample size of at least 200 patients is required to achieve convincing levels of power and statistical significance to detect differences between subgroups conditional on a roughly equally sized distribution of patients among the subgroups[31,69]. In the former study, when the performance of the HCT-CI was validated simultaneously in five collaborating institutions, the index was associated in all but a single site, with less than 200 overall patient samples, with statistically significant HRs for NRM and survival[44,69]. Other problems that affected the seven studies included lack of essential comorbidity data elements[64] or unbalanced distribution of patients within the subgroups of comorbidity scores[63,65]. Limited ability to accurately assign comorbidity scores could have led to an over- or underscoring of some comorbidities[62], which is another concern that will be addressed below in the section on "Reliability of the HCT-CI".

It is important to note that all the adequately sampled multicenter studies[43–45,56], particularly those with a prospective design[43,56], have proven the validity of the HCT-CI in providing prognostic information about NRM and survivals following allogeneic HCT.

Reliability of the HCT-CI

Poor agreement on interpretation of comorbidity definitions has been reported for some comorbidity indices[70] and it could constitute an obstacle against worldwide use of an index. A study from the FHCRC showed that the use of the HCT-CI to score comorbidities by four novice evaluators without instructive guidelines resulted in only fair inter-rater agreement as measured by weighted kappa statistic (Kw) values of 0.433−0.585 where 1 indicates excellent agreement and 0, no agreement at all[71]. This is not surprising since the HCT-CI is a newly introduced tool in the field of pretransplant assessment. Similar findings were reported by the Center of

International Blood and Marrow Transplantation Research (CIBMTR). IRR were evaluated among data managers from three participating institutions *versus* their respective investigators. Kw statistic estimates were 0.54, 0.81, and 0.47, respectively, indicating fair−moderate agreement rate among evaluators[43].

To address this issue, a brief training program was developed, consisting of systematic methodology for data acquisition (Figure 4.9) and consistent guidelines for comorbidity coding that were summarized in a Web-based calculator (www.hctci.org). The methodology and the guidelines were delivered in a document format to four different evaluators as a brief training program on comorbidity coding. Data from 98 randomly selected patients were used for assessment of comorbidities independently by four novice evaluators as well as by the developer of the training program. Comparisons of the Kw values across all five evaluators showed marked improvement in the magnitude of the inter-evaluator agreement on assigning HCT-CI scores to an excellent rate with weighted k values in the range of 0.89 to 0.97[71]. Fleiss' kappa statistic estimates also improved from 0.380 (during the initial assessment phase) to 0.800 during validation of the training program. Of note, none of the four evaluators had prior experience in comorbidity coding suggesting utility of this training program in preparing a wide variety of individuals with variable qualifications, ranging from study coordinators and data managers to experienced transplant physicians, for comorbidity coding. The new methodology, guidelines, and Web-based application constituted a major step in worldwide applicability of the HCT-CI in clinical practice and comparative effectiveness research of HCT.

Summary and Future Directions

Comorbidity assessment has become a critical component of risk assessment before allo-HCT. The HCT-CI was developed to capture organ comorbidities and to provide prognostic information specifically about allo-HCT outcomes. Studies have demonstrated that the index could provide information to decide which older patients are medically fit to tolerate high-dose conditioning regimens with resultant better OS, and which are less fit and might have longer OS and better quality of life with RIC/nonmyeloablative conditioning regimens.

While results of allogeneic HCT following RIC/nonmyeloablative conditioning regimens suggest tolerance of some older patients to these regimens, it is not clear how to translate these results to the general population of older patients since selection criteria might have excluded patients with greater comorbidity burdens. Lack of prospective randomized studies and the suspicion of inherent selection bias have failed to generate definitive evidence for a role of HCT in older patients. However, only 12% and 6% of patients who are ≥ 60 or ≥ 65 years old are treated with HCT and these proportions have not changed substantially for years[72–74]. Ongoing efforts focus on understanding the role of comorbidities assessed at the time of diagnosis of a blood cancer in determining feasibility of transplant and comparing the value of transplant *versus* nontransplant conventional therapies (NCT01929408).

The HCT-CI was found to be a key factor in comparing trial results across institutions. It can be used in adjusting regression analyses for the confounding effects of comorbidities and in ensuring balanced distribution of patients among treatment groups in randomized prospective studies (NCT00322101). It is important to note that comorbidity assessment is only a single component of the pretransplant evaluations. The impact of other patient-specific risk factors, such as PS[26] or age[31], should be taken into account. Although evaluation of comorbidities and performance status is important, they can be complemented by other domains of GA evaluating physical, cognitive, affective, social, financial, and other factors that could affect the health of an older adult. Prospective studies with multicenter design are needed to study the integration of measures of frailty, physical functions like IADL, cognition, nutrition, gait speed, and other components of GA into models used for decision-making about the choice of transplant for an older patient. Likewise, gaining further knowledge about the most important markers of single nucleotide polymorphisms (SNPs) that affect HCT outcomes could enhance our ability for prognostication prior to transplant. These studies are underway[75]. Physicians and investigators should also weigh the information about comorbidity and other patient-risk factors carefully against the burden and biologic behavior of the primary disease. The inclusion of a model that captures variable disease features[39,76,77] and/or the use of a composite HCT-CI/EBMT model is desirable in risk assessment before HCT[29].

A fair number of studies have dealt with validation of the HCT-CI. Clearly, appropriate sample size of patients (at least 200), roughly equal stratification of patients into comorbidity risk groups, and the inclusion of possible confounders in the analyses would be critical for such studies. Current evidence from large multicenter and prospective studies reveals the validity of the HCT-CI to guide decision-making about transplant *versus* no transplant and the decision about the most suitable intensity of conditioning regimens. Enhancing IRR by the newly developed training guidelines and the establishment of an online website for assigning comorbidity scores (www.hctci.org) are critical steps to ensure excellent agreement on comorbidity evaluation at different institutions. These efforts will lead to consistent inclusion of comorbidity assessment in daily practice. Current evidence suggests the need for having a preclinical model to study the biology behind the association between comorbidities and post-HCT morbidity and mortality[41]. These studies could set the stage for future intervention studies to alleviate the burden of comorbidities and hence improve HCT outcomes.

Acknowledgments

The authors are grateful for the help of Bonnie Larson and Helen Crawford in manuscript preparation. They are also grateful for research support by grant HL08802 from the National Heart Lung Blood Institute, National Institute of Health; Research Scholar Grant #RSG-13-084-01-CPHPS from the American Cancer Society; a Patient-Centered Outcome Research Institute contract #CE-1304–7451 (M.L.S.); and for grant JS2865 from the Egyptian Ministry of Higher Education (M.E.).

References

1. Thomas ED, Blume KG, Forman SJ, eds. *Hematopoietic Cell Transplantation*. 2nd edition. Blackwell Science, Inc., Boston, MA: 1999

2. Atkinson K, ed. *Clinical Bone Marrow and Blood Stem Cell Transplantation*. 2nd edition. Cambridge University Press, Cambridge, UK: 2000

3. Fried LP, Bandeen-Roche K, Kasper JD, Guralnik JM. Association of comorbidity with disability in older women: the Women's Health and Aging Study. *J Clin Epidemiol* 52(1): 27–37, 1999

4. van Spronsen DJ, Janssen-Heijnen ML, Breed WP, Coebergh JW. Prevalence of co-morbidity and its relationship to treatment among unselected patients with Hodgkin's disease and non-Hodgkin's lymphoma, 1993–1996. *Ann Hematol* 78(7): 315–9, 1999

5. Greimel ER, Padilla GV, Grant MM. Physical and psychosocial outcomes in cancer patients: a comparison of different age groups. *Br J Cancer* 76(2): 251–5, 1997

6. Kurtz ME, Kurtz JC, Stommel M, Given CW, Given B. The influence of symptoms, age, comorbidity and cancer site on physical functioning and mental health of geriatric women patients. *Women Health* 29(3): 1–12, 1999

7. Given CW, Given B, Azzouz F, Stommel M, Kozachik S. Comparison of changes in physical functioning of elderly patients with new diagnoses of cancer. *Med Care* 38(5): 482–93, 2000

8. Pinto A, Zagonel V, Ferrara F. Acute myeloid leukemia in the elderly: biology and therapeutic strategies (Review). *Crit Rev Oncol Hematol* 39(3): 275–87, 2001

9. van Spronsen DJ, Janssen-Heijnen ML, Lemmens VE, Peters WG, Coebergh JW. Independent prognostic effect of co-morbidity in lymphoma patients: results of the population-based

Eindhoven Cancer Registry. *Eur J Cancer* 41(7): 1051–7, 2005

10. Extermann M, Overcash J, Lyman GH, Parr J, Balducci L. Comorbidity and functional status are independent in older cancer patients. *J Clin Oncol* 16(4): 1582–7, 1998

11. Charlson ME, Pompei P, Ales KL, MacKenzie CR. A new method of classifying prognostic comorbidity in longitudinal studies: development and validation. *J Chronic Dis* 40(5): 373–83, 1987

12. Sorror ML, Maris MB, Storer B, Sandmaier BM, Diaconescu R, Flowers C, *et al.* Comparing morbidity and mortality of HLA-matched unrelated donor hematopoietic cell transplantation after nonmyeloablative and myeloablative conditioning: influence of pretransplant comorbidities. *Blood* 104(4): 961–8, 2004

13. Sorror ML, Maris MB, Storb R, Baron F, Sandmaier BM, Maloney DG, *et al.* Hematopoietic cell transplantation (HCT)-specific comorbidity index: a new tool for risk assessment before allogeneic HCT. *Blood* 106(8): 2912–9, 2005

14. Sorror ML, Sandmaier BM, Storer BE, Maris MB, Baron F, Maloney DG, *et al.* Comorbidity and disease status-based risk stratification of outcomes among patients with acute myeloid leukemia or myelodysplasia receiving allogeneic hematopoietic cell transplantation. *J Clin Oncol* 25(27): 4246–54, 2007

15. Lim ZY, Ingram W, Brand R, Ho A, Kenyon M, Devereux S, *et al.* Impact of pretransplant comorbidities on alemtuzumab-based reduced-intensity conditioning allogeneic hematopoietic SCT for patients with high-risk myelodysplastic syndrome and AML. *Bone Marrow Transplant* 45(4): 633–9, 2010

16. Mohty M, Labopin M, Basara N, Cornelissen JJ, Tabrizi R, Malm C, *et al.* Association between the Hematopoietic Cell Transplantation-Specific Comorbidity Index (CI) and non-relapse mortality (NRM) after reduced intensity conditioning (RIC) allogeneic stem cell transplantation (allo-SCT) for acute myeloid leukemia (AML) in first complete remission (CR1). [Abstract] *Blood* 114(22): 270, #650,2009

17. Kerbauy DMB, Chyou F, Gooley T, Sorror ML, Scott B, Pagel JM, *et al.* Allogeneic hematopoietic cell transplantation for chronic myelomonocytic leukemia. *Biol Blood Marrow Transplant* 11: 713–20, 2005

18. Sorror ML, Storer BE, Maloney DG, Sandmaier BM, Martin PJ, Storb R. Outcomes after allogeneic hematopoietic cell transplantation with nonmyeloablative or myeloablative regimens for treatment of lymphoma and chronic lymphocytic leukemia. *Blood* 111(1): 446–52, 2008

19. Farina L, Bruno B, Patriarca F, Spina F, Sorasio R, Morelli M, *et al.* The hematopoietic cell transplantation comorbidity index (HCT-CI) predicts clinical outcomes in lymphoma and myeloma patients after reduced-intensity or non-myeloablative allogeneic stem cell transplantation. *Leukemia* 23(6): 1131–8, 2009

20. Pollack SM, Steinberg SM, Odom J, Dean RM, Fowler DH, Bishop MR. Assessment of the hematopoietic cell transplantation comorbidity index in non-Hodgkin lymphoma patients receiving reduced-intensity allogeneic hematopoietic stem cell transplantation. *Biol Blood Marrow Transplant* 15(2): 223–30, 2009

21. Sorror ML, Storer BE, Sandmaier BM, Maris M, Shizuru J, Maziarz R, *et al.* Five-year follow-up of patients with advanced chronic lymphocytic leukemia treated with allogeneic hematopoietic cell transplantation after nonmyeloablative conditioning. *J Clin Oncol* 26(30): 4912–20, 2008

22. Pavlu J, Kew AK, Taylor-Roberts B, Auner HW, Marin D, Olavarria E, *et al.* Optimizing patient selection for myeloablative allogeneic hematopoietic cell transplantation in chronic myeloid leukemia in chronic phase. *Blood* 115(20): 4018–20, 2010

23. Sorror ML, Giralt S, Sandmaier BM, de Lima M, Shahjahan M, Maloney DG, *et al.* Hematopoietic cell transplantation-specific comorbidity index as an outcome predictor for patients with acute myeloid leukemia in first remission: Combined FHCRC and MDACC experiences. *Blood* 110(13): 4608–13, 2007

24. Appelbaum FR, Gundacker H, Head DR, Slovak ML, Willman CL, Godwin JE, *et al.* Age and acute myeloid leukemia. *Blood* 107(9): 3481–5, 2006

25. Artz AS, Pollyea DA, Kocherginsky M, Stock W, Rich E, Odenike O, *et al.* Performance status and comorbidity predict transplant-related mortality after allogeneic hematopoietic cell transplantation. *Biol Blood Marrow Transplant* 12(9): 954–64, 2006

26. Sorror M, Storer B, Sandmaier BM, Maloney DG, Chauncey TR, Langston A, *et al.* Hematopoietic cell transplantation-comorbidity index and Karnofsky performance status are independent predictors of morbidity and mortality after allogeneic nonmyeloablative hematopoietic cell transplantation. *Cancer* 112: 1992–2001, 2008

27. Gratwohl A, Stern M, Brand R, Apperley J, Baldomero H, de Witte T, *et al.* Risk score for outcome after allogeneic hematopoietic stem cell transplantation: a retrospective analysis. *Cancer* 115(20): 4715–26, 2009

28. Gratwohl A, Hermans J, Goldman JM, Arcese W, Carreras E, Devergie A, *et al.* Risk assessment for patients with chronic myeloid leukaemia before allogeneic blood or marrow transplantation. *Lancet* 352(9134): 1087–92, 1998

29. Elsawy M, Storer BE, Sorror ML. "To combine or not to combine": Optimizing risk assessment before allogeneic hematopoietic cell transplantation (Letter). *Biol Blood Marrow Transplant* 20(9):1455–6, 2014

30. Appelbaum FR. Preparative regimens and ageism. *Biol Blood Marrow Transplant* 17(10): 1419–20, 2011

31. Sorror ML, Storb R, Sandmaier BM, Maziarz RT, Pulsipher MA, Maris MB, *et al.* Comorbidity-age index: a clinical measure of biological age prior to allogeneic hematopoietic cell transplantation. *J Clin Oncol* 32(29):3249–56, 2014

32. Orszag PR, Emanuel EJ. Health care reform and cost control. *N Engl J Med* 363(7): 601–3, 2010

33. Kahl C, Storer BE, Sandmaier BM, Mielcarek M, Maris MB, Blume KG, *et al.* Relapse risk among patients with malignant diseases given allogeneic hematopoietic cell transplantation after nonmyeloablative conditioning. *Blood* 110(7): 2744–8, 2007

34. Sorror ML, Sandmaier BM, Storer BE, Franke GN, Laport GG, Chauncey TR, *et al.* Long-term outcomes among older patients following nonmyeloablative conditioning and allogeneic

hematopoietic cell transplantation for advanced hematologic malignancies. *JAMA* 306(17): 1874–83, 2011

35. Djousse L, Rothman KJ, Cupples LA, Levy D, Ellison RC. Serum albumin and risk of myocardial infarction and all-cause mortality in the Framingham Offspring Study. *Circulation* 106(23): 2919–24, 2002

36. Deeg HJ, Spaulding E, Shulman HM. Iron overload, hematopoietic cell transplantation, and graft-*versus*-host disease. *Leuk Lymphoma* 50(10): 1566–72, 2009

37. Sorror ML, Storer BE, Schoch G, Sandmaier BM, Martin PJ, Scott BL, *et al*. Low albumin, high ferritin, and thrombocytopenia before transplant predict non-relapse mortality (NRM) independent of the hematopoietic cell transplantation comorbidity index (HCT-CI). [Abstract] *Blood* 114(22): 271, #651,2009. https://www.ncbi.nlm.nih.gov/pubmed/25862589

38. Sherman AE, Motyckova G, Fega KR, DeAngelo DJ, Abel GA, Steensma D, *et al*. Geriatric assessment in older patients with acute myeloid leukemia: a retrospective study of associated treatment and outcomes. *Leuk Res* 37(9): 998-1003, 2013

39. Deschler B, Ihorst G, Platzbecker U, Germing U, Marz E, de Figuerido M, *et al*. Parameters detected by geriatric and quality of life assessment in 195 older patients with myelodysplastic syndromes and acute myeloid leukemia are highly predictive for outcome. *Haematologica* 98(2): 208–16, 2013

40. Muffly LS, Kocherginsky M, Stock W, Chu Q, Bishop MR, Godley LA, *et al*. Geriatric assessment to predict survival in older allogeneic hematopoietic cell transplantation recipients. *Haematologica*;99(8):1373–9, 2014

41. Sorror ML, Martin PJ, Storb R, Bhatia S, Maziarz RT, Pulsipher MA, *et al*. Pretransplant comorbidities predict severity of acute graft-*versus*-host disease and subsequent mortality. *Blood* 124(2): 287–95, 2014

42. Sorror ML, Yi JC, Storer BE, Rock EE, Artherholt SB, Storb R, *et al*. Association of pre-transplant comorbidities with long-term quality of life (QOL) among survivors after allogeneic hematopoietic cell transplantation (HCT). [Abstract] *Biol*

Blood Marrow Transplant 19(2): S153, 2013

43. Sorror ML, Logan BR, Zhu X, Rizzo JD, Cooke KR, McCarthy PL, *et al*. Prospective validation of the predictive power of the hematopoietic cell transplantation comorbidity index: a Center for International Blood and Marrow Transplant Research study. *Biol Blood Marrow Transplant* 21(8): 1479–87, 2015

44. Sorror ML, Ostronoff F, Storb R, Bhatia S, Maziarz RT, Pulsipher MA, *et al*. Multi-institutional validation of the predictive power of the hematopoietic cell transplantation comorbidity index (HCT-CI) for HCT outcomes. [Abstract] *Blood* 118(21): #145, 2011

45. Smith AR, Majhail NS, MacMillan ML, Defor TE, Jodele S, Lehmann LE, *et al*. Hematopoietic cell transplantation comorbidity index predicts transplantation outcomes in pediatric patients. *Blood* 117(9): 2728–34, 2011

46. Ratan R, Ceberio I, Hilden P, Devlin SM, Malloy MA, Barker JN, *et al*. The Hematopoietic Cell Transplant-Co-Morbidity Index (HCT-CI) predicts outcomes after T cell depleted (TCD) allogeneic HCT for AML and MDS. [Abstract] *Blood* 122(21): 2045, 2013

47. Bokhari SW, Watson L, Nagra S, Cook M, Byrne JL, Craddock C, *et al*. Role of HCT-comorbidity index, age and disease status at transplantation in predicting survival and non-relapse mortality in patients with myelodysplasia and leukemia undergoing reduced-intensity-conditioning hemopoietic progenitor cell transplantation. *Bone Marrow Transplant* 47(4): 528–34, 2012

48. Le RQ, Jain NA, Tian X, Ito S, Lu K, Haggerty J, *et al*. Comorbidity measures in ex vivo T cell depleted allogeneic hematopoietic stem cell transplantation (HCT). [Abstract] *Blood* 122(21), 2013

49. Sorror ML. Comorbidities and hematopoietic cell transplantation outcomes. pp. 237–47. In Gewirtz AM, Mikhael JR, Schwartz BS, Crowther MA, editors. *Hematology 2010: American Society of Hematology Education Program Book*. American Society of Hematology, Washington, DC: 2010

50. Kerbauy DMB, Gooley TA, Sale GE, Flowers MED, Doney KC, Georges GE, *et al*. Hematopoietic cell transplantation as curative therapy for idiopathic

myelofibrosis, advanced polycythemia vera, and essential thrombocythemia. *Biol Blood Marrow Transplant* 13(3): 355–65, 2007

51. Maruyama D, Fukuda T, Kato R, Yamasaki S, Usui E, Morita-Hoshi Y, *et al*. Comparable antileukemia/lymphoma effects in nonremission patients undergoing allogeneic hematopoietic cell transplantation with a conventional cytoreductive or reduced-intensity regimen. *Biol Blood Marrow Transplant* 13(8): 932–41, 2007

52. Artz AS, Wickrema A, Dinner S, Godley LA, Kocherginsky M, Odenike O, *et al*. Pretreatment C-reactive protein is a predictor for outcomes after reduced-intensity allogeneic hematopoietic cell transplantation. *Biol Blood Marrow Transplant* 14(11): 1209–16, 2008

53. Majhail NS, Brunstein CG, McAvoy S, Defor TE, Al-Hazzouri A, Setubal D, *et al*. Does the hematopoietic cell transplantation specific comorbidity index predict transplant outcomes? A validation study in a large cohort of umbilical cord blood and matched related donor transplants. *Biol Blood Marrow Transplant* 14(9): 985–92, 2008

54. Kataoka K, Nannya Y, Ueda K, Kumano K, Takahashi T, Kurokawa M. Differential prognostic impact of pretransplant comorbidity on transplant outcomes by disease status and time from transplant: a single Japanese transplant centre study. *Bone Marrow Transplant* 45(3): 513–20, 2010

55. Barba P, Piñana JL, Martino R, Valcárcel D, Amorós A, Sureda A, *et al*. Comparison of two pretransplant predictive models and a flexible HCT-CI using different cut points to determine low-, intermediate-, and high-risk groups: the flexible HCT-CI is the best predictor of NRM and OS in a population of patients undergoing allo-RIC. *Biol Blood Marrow Transplant* 16(3): 413–20, 2010

56. Raimondi R, Tosetto A, Oneto R, Cavazzina R, Rodeghiero F, Bacigalupo A, *et al*. Validation of the Hematopoietic Cell Transplantation-Specific Comorbidity Index: a prospective, multicenter GITMO study. *Blood* 120(6): 1327–33, 2012

57. Hashmi S, Oliva JL, Liesveld JL, Phillips GL, Milner L, Becker MW. The hematopoietic cell transplantation specific comorbidity index and survival

after extracorporeal photopheresis, pentostatin, and reduced dose total body irradiation conditioning prior to allogeneic stem cell transplantation. *Leuk Res* 37(9): 1052–6, 2013

58. Mo XD, Xu LP, Liu DH, Zhang XH, Chen H, Chen YH, *et al.* The hematopoietic cell transplantation-specific comorbidity index (HCT-CI) is an outcome predictor for partially matched related donor transplantation. *Am J Hematol* 88(6): 497–502, 2013

59. Bayraktar UD, Shpall EJ, Liu P, Ciurea SO, Rondon G, de LM, *et al.* Hematopoietic cell transplantation-specific comorbidity index predicts inpatient mortality and survival in patients who received allogeneic transplantation admitted to the intensive care unit. *J Clin Oncol* 31(33): 4207–14, 2013

60. Chemnitz JM, Chakupurakal G, Basler M, Holtick U, Theurich S, Shimabukuro-Vornhagen A, *et al.* Pretransplant comorbidities maintain their impact on allogeneic stem cell transplantation outcome 5 years posttransplant: a retrospective study in a single German institution. *ISRN Hematology*: Article ID 853435, 2014

61. DeFor TE, Majhail NS, Weisdorf DJ, Brunstein CG, McAvoy S, Arora M, *et al.* A modified comorbidity index for hematopoietic cell transplantation. *Bone Marrow Transplant* 45(5): 933–8, 2010

62. Birninger N, Bornhäuser M, Schaich M, Ehninger G, Schetelig J. The hematopoietic cell transplantation-specific comorbidity index fails to predict outcomes in high-risk AML patients undergoing allogeneic transplantation: investigation of potential limitations of the index. *Biol Blood Marrow Transplant* 17(12): 1822–32, 2011

63. Terwey TH, Hemmati PG, Martus P, Dietz E, Vuong LG, Massenkeil G, *et al.* A modifed EBMT risk score and the hematopoietic cell transplantation-specific comorbidity index for pre-transplant risk assessment in adult acute lymphoblastic leukemia. *Haematologica* 95(5): 810–8, 2010

64. Xhaard A, Porcher R, Chien JW, de Latour RP, Robin M, Ribaud P, *et al.* Impact of comorbidity indexes on non-relapse mortality. *Leukemia* 22(11): 2062–9, 2008

65. Guilfoyle R, Demers A, Bredeson C, Richardson E, Rubinger M, Szwajcer D, *et al.* Performance status, but not the hematopoietic cell transplantation comorbidity index (HCT-CI), predicts mortality at a Canadian transplant center. *Bone Marrow Transplant* 43(2): 133–9, 2009

66. Castagna L, Furst S, Marchetti N, El CJ, Faucher C, Mohty M, *et al.* Retrospective analysis of common scoring systems and outcome in patients older than 60 years treated with reduced-intensity conditioning regimen and alloSCT. *Bone Marrow Transplant* 46(7): 1000–5, 2011

67. Williams M, Murray J, Kulkarni S, Bloor A. HCT-CI correlates poorly with outcome following allogeneic stem cell transplant: impact of underlying diagnosis, patient selection and assessment of organ function. 38th Annual Meeting of the European Group for Blood and Marrow Transplantation. [Abstract] *Bone Marrow Transplant* 47(1): S205–S206, #646, 2012

68. Nakaya A, Mori T, Tanaka M, Tomita N, Nakaseko C, Yano S, *et al.* Does the hematopoietic cell transplantation specific comorbidity index predict transplantation outcomes? *Biol Blood Marrow Transplant* 20(10):1553–9, 2014

69. Elsawy M, Storer BE, Pulsipher MA, Maziarz RT, Bhatia S, Maris MB, *et al.* Multi-centre validation of the prognostic value of the haematopoietic cell transplantation-specific comorbidity index among recipient of allogenic haematopoietic cell transplantation. *Br J Haematol.* 2015;170(4):574–83

70. Imamura K, McKinnon M, Middleton R, Black N. Reliability of a comorbidity measure: the Index of Co-Existent Disease (ICED). *J Clin Epidemiol* 50(9): 1011–6, 1997

71. Sorror M. How I assess comorbidities prior to hematopoietic cell transplantation. *Blood* 121(15): 2854–63, 2013

72. Pasquini MC, Griffith LM, Arnold DL, Atkins HL, Bowen JD, Chen JT, *et al.* Hematopoietic stem cell transplantation for multiple scerosis: collaboration of the CIBMTR and EBMT to facilitate international clinical studies. *Biol Blood Marrow Transplant* 16(8): 1076–83, 2010

73. Bentley TS, Hanson SG. U.S. organ and tissue transplant cost estimates and discussion. Milliman Research Report. Available at http://publications.milliman.com/research/health-rr/pdfs/2011-us-organ-tissue.pdf, 2011

74. Ortner NJ. U.S. organ and tissue transplant cost estimates and discussion. Milliman Research Report, Available at: http://publications .milliman.com/research/health-rr/pdfs/US-Organ-Tissue-Transplant-2005-RR06-01–05.pdf, 2005

75. Comorbidity and Regimen Related Toxicity (RRT) Committee Report. Improving prognostic assessment for patients 60 years and older undergoing allogeneic HCT. BMT CTN State of the Science Symposium, Feb 24–25, 2014. Available at http://www.cvent.com/events/bmt-ctn-state-of-the-science-symposium/custom-17-d54c4d401ae642c4b2f549b39e52c539.aspx, 2014

76. Armand P, Gibson CJ, Cutler C, Ho VT, Koreth J, Alyea EP, *et al.* A disease risk index for patients undergoing allogeneic stem cell transplantation. *Blood* 120(4): 905–13, 2012

77. Deeg HJ, Scott BL, Fang M, Shulman HM, Gyurkocza B, Myerson D, *et al.* Five-group cytogenetic risk classification, monosomal karyotype, and outcome after hematopoietic cell transplantation for MDS or acute leukemia evolving from MDS. *Blood* 120(7): 1398–408, 201

78. Elsawy M, Storer BE, Sandmaier B, Delaney C, Appelbaum F, Woolfrey AE, *et al.* Role of comorbidities in prognostic evaluation of outcomes following allogeneic hematopoietic cell transplantation from HLA-mismatched and umbilical cord blood donor grafts. *Blood* 124:2583, 2014

79. Sorror ML, Logan BR, Zhu X, Rizzo JD, Cooke KR, McCarthy PL, *et al.* Prospective validation of the predictive power of the hematopoietic cell transplantation comorbidity index. *Biol Blood Marrow Transplant* 21(8):1479–87, 2015

Chapter

5

Michael T. Tees and Marcie L. Riches

Infectious Diseases: Evaluation and Implications of Results in Hematopoietic Cell Transplants

Introduction

Infections have a significant impact on morbidity and mortality in the peri- and post-hematopoietic cell transplant (HCT) setting; therefore, pre-HCT assessment of risk is necessary. Excluding patients with certain hemoglobinopathies, all patients proceeding to HCT have impaired immunity due to the primary disease, initial myelosuppressive therapies, and previous infections[1]. A myriad of factors must be considered and placed in the context of an individual patient's risk.

Indeed, a thorough evaluation could affect the selection of the conditioning regimen and even the donor source, but will also provide an opportunity to plan appropriate interventions, such as adjusting common peri-HCT antimicrobial prophylaxis (see Chapters 23–25). A thorough infectious disease evaluation is easily incorporated into a patient's general risk assessment. A conceptual framework of the factors under consideration is illustrated in Figure 5.1. Obtaining a complete medical history, physical examination, and appropriate

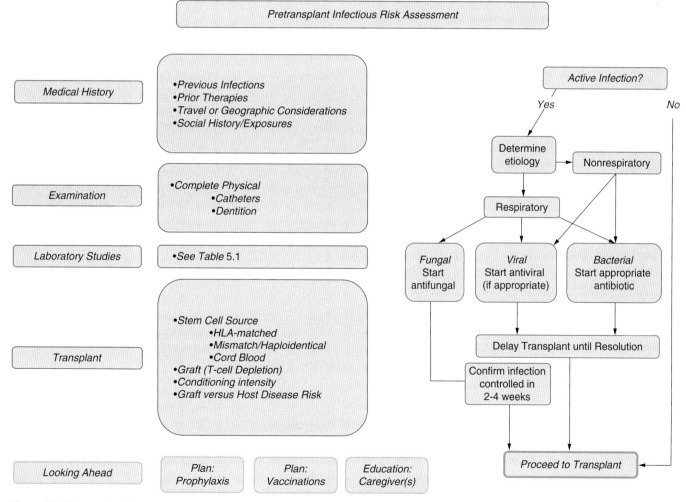

Figure 5.1. Pretransplant risk assessment.

laboratory studies is fundamental, but acknowledgment of the conditioning intensity and hematopoietic cell source is necessary for a cohesive assessment of a patient's risk.

Pretransplant Infectious Disease Work-Up

The HCT comorbidity index (HCT-CI) administers one point if a patient meets one of the following criteria: active/documented infection requiring continuation of antimicrobial treatment beyond day 0, fever of unknown origin, pulmonary nodules suspicious for fungal pneumonia, or a positive purified protein derivative (PPD) screen requiring prophylaxis against tuberculosis (see Chapter 16) [2,3]. While the HCT-CI is an indispensable tool (see Chapter 4), it cannot factor unique infectious disease history and potential risks, and certain consideration should occur in the pre-HCT assessment to identify these risks. Focused questioning and discussion should inquire about previous serious infections/complications, as well as chronic issues, such as the need for multiple dental procedures or known diagnoses of viral infections.

Previous Therapies

History of prior anticancer therapy is important to assess the potential immune status of the patient proceeding with HCT. Previous therapies and duration of neutropenia frequently correlate with infection history and serve as a starting point in the risk assessment. Immunosuppressive agents, such as fludarabine or alemtuzumab, also have implications in the peri- and post-HCT setting. Realistically, all regimens contribute to a variably weakened immune system.

Previous Infections

Fungal

A history of prior invasive fungal infection increases the risk of fungal infection recurrence [4,5]. Clearance of this infection may be incomplete by the time of HCT, and thus, it is important to obtain CT imaging of the chest in search of residual disease. Despite apparent clinical clearance of disease, these patients still have an increased risk of reinfection. Patients often continue antifungal therapy through conditioning, peri-HCT, and engraftment; alternatively prophylaxis with a second-generation triazole may be advised (see Chapter 18).

Bacterial

Prior bacterial infections can increase the risk of peri-HCT infections, notably *Clostridium difficile*. Often with reinfection of *C. difficile*, the symptoms are milder and occur early in the peri-HCT period, raising the possibility of misdiagnosis [6]. Acknowledging a previous infection may reduce the time to diagnosis and institution of appropriate isolation precautions [7]. Other prior infections that may impact patient care decisions include *S. pneumoniae* and those from the viridans streptococcal group [8]. Patients with prior invasive pneumococcal infection may theoretically have an increased risk of

reinfection due to one of three possible scenarios: the patient has not received a multivalent conjugated vaccination, the patient has received a vaccination but was unable to develop central memory formation, or the patient was exposed to a strain not covered by multivalent vaccines. In patients with a history of viridans group infections, taking note of the dentition on physical examination is necessary. Previous infections with fluoroquinolone-resistant organisms are important to note as it impacts the choice of antimicrobial prophylaxis and the acute management of peri-HCT neutropenic fever [9,10] (see Chapter 16).

Viral

While the history or presence of a chronic viral infection will be confirmed by laboratory studies, this must be addressed with the patient as well (see Chapter 17). Screening positive for HBcAb and/or HBsAg necessitates testing for hepatitis B virus (HBV)-DNA viral load. In recipients with a positive HBV-DNA viral load, obtaining a liver biopsy may be indicated, as assessment of liver injury would alter decisions in conditioning regimens. Initiation of treatment is advised, and should continue through transplantation. In recipients with HBcAb with or without a positive HBsAb but a negative HBV-DNA viral load, the risk of reactivation is present, albeit low. Risk increases if the development of graft-versus-host disease (GvHD) necessitates steroid use, and therefore prophylaxis with lamivudine or entecavir (see Chapter 17) should be considered with routine monitoring of HBV-DNA [11]. In patients with hepatitis C virus (HCV), historical data note an increased risk of nonrelapse mortality and shortened overall survival, as well as a faster progression to cirrhosis compared to nontransplant HCV patients [12,13]. However, a more contemporary study did not identify inferior outcomes in patients receiving related donor transplants [14]. A liver biopsy is advised to assess for degree of hepatic injury for patients with either a history of infection >10 years, unknown duration of infection with elevated viral load, iron overload, excess alcohol use, or clinical evidence of liver disease. In the presence of persistently elevated transaminases or early fibrosis on liver biopsy, the clinician should avoid conditioning with cyclophosphamide or total body irradiation (TBI) [15]. Treatment of HCV in the immediate pre- or peri-HCT period has not been studied and is not advised at this time. The prevalence of patients with hematologic malignancies and HIV continues to increase; at present, the data suggest that these patients fare quite well with autologous HCT [16,17]. In some individuals receiving allogeneic HCT for other indications, HIV has been eradicated [18]. Additional data in this population are needed so enrollment of the patient in a clinical trial is advised (see Chapter 58). Involvement of an infectious disease specialist is necessary to develop an appropriate treatment plan, as almost all antiretrovirals have drug interactions with either conditioning agents and/or GvHD prophylactic agents [19].

Table 5.1 Laboratory studies in pretransplant risk assessment

Study	Recipient	Donor
Cytomegalovirus IgM/IgG	Yes	Yes
Epstein–Barr virus IgG/PCR	Yes	Yes
Hepatitis B virus core Ab, surface Ag (HBcAb, HBsAg)	Yes	Yes
Hepatitis C virus PCR	Yes	Yes
Herpes simplex virus 1/2 IgG	Yes	Yes
Human immunodeficiency virus 1/2 PCR	Yes	Yes
Human T-lymphotrophic virus 1/2 IgG[a]	Yes	Assess risk
Varicella-zoster virus IgG/PCR	Yes	Yes
Treponema pallidum RPR (FTA-ABS for confirmation)	Yes	Yes
Toxoplasmosis gondii IgG	Yes	Assess risk
Aspergillosis galactomannan Ag[b]	Yes	No
TB screening test (PPD or interferon-gamma release assay)[a]	Assess risk	Assess risk
Others[a]	Assess risk	Assess risk

[a] A clinician should assess the risk and necessity for certain studies in both the recipient and donor.
[b] A meta-analysis demonstrated a 71% sensitivity and 89% specificity of detecting a proven invasive aspergillosis (IA) infection, and in proven or probable IA infections, a 61% sensitivity with 93% specificity. A large heterogeneity between the studies was noted, suggested to be secondary to antifungal prophylaxis, which decreases the sensitivity of the test [31].

Geographic and Social Influences

Patient assessment should include consideration of primary residence and recent travel to areas with vector-borne illnesses. There are rare circumstances when augmentation of the pre-HCT laboratory studies is necessary and should be guided by clinical signs or symptoms. In regions where infections with *Plasmodium* spp., *Trypanosoma cruzi*, or others are of higher prevalence, infection should be ruled out if clinically indicated [20–22]. Furthermore, infection with tick-borne illnesses including *Borrelia burgdorferi*, *Babesia* spp, *Anaplasma* spp., *Histoplasmosis*, and *Coccidioides* spp. may need consideration [23]. Occupational exposures may necessitate consideration of *Coxiella* spp. or tuberculosis. Testing for tuberculosis may also be indicated in patients from regions with a high prevalence, those with a known contact, recent incarceration, or other identifiable risk factors [15]. Identification of previous infections with any of the above is useful for an appropriate differential diagnosis in the peri-HCT period. Helpful resources include national centers of disease epidemiology, such as the US Centers for Disease Control and Prevention (wwwnc.cdc.gov/travel/page/clinician-information-center).

Physical Examination

A complete physical examination is a critical component of the pre-HCT work-up to identify active or potential sources of infection. This includes a thorough examination of a patient's oral cavity, as periodontal disease and caries may be a potential source of infection in the peri-HCT period. Many transplant centers require a dental evaluation prior to proceeding to transplant, which may necessitate extraction or adjustment of prosthetic dental devices [24,25]. A decision analysis determined that patients without dental evaluation had a slightly higher risk of death due to dental associated infections (1.8/ 1000 patients) compared to those with pre-HCT dental clearance [26]. While this probability is low, it is an opportunity to decrease a potential risk of morbidity and mortality associated with transplant. If a dental procedure is necessary, allowing 10–14 days for healing is recommended prior to proceeding to HCT.

Assessment of the head, ears, eyes, nose, and throat are important, in particular if a patient has had recent or sustained periods of neutropenia. Auscultation of the lungs should not be replaced by a pulmonary function test, as any abnormalities may warrant a baseline noncontrast CT. A genitourinary and perianal inspection may detect potential infectious sources, such as a perianal abscess. A full dermatologic evaluation is also advised to assess for areas of injury and to identify indwelling lines.

Laboratory Studies of Recipient and Donor

Table 5.1 lists both the recipient and donor laboratory studies recommended. Donor evaluation essentially mirrors that of the recipient, and implications of positive results are discussed in this section.

Cytomegalovirus (CMV) serostatus is a necessary component of a work-up, as CMV reactivation or infection is a major complication affecting allogeneic HCT recipients. CMV sero-negative autologous or allogeneic recipients with a CMV seronegative donor must receive CMV-negative products. If an allogeneic recipient is CMV seropositive regardless of donor serostatus, diligent surveillance and either prophylactic or preemptive therapy is necessary (see Chapter 17) [27,28]. In the event that a recipient is seronegative but a donor is seropositive, any blood products the patient receives up until transplant must be from a seronegative donor. It is rare to identify an acute EBV infection or presence of viral replication at the pre-HCT evaluation, but serology indicating prior exposure should be assessed given the risk of reactivation after HCT. In fact, EBV reactivation is also associated with CMV reactivation in the allogeneic HCT recipient [29].

Positive herpes simplex virus (HSV), Varicella-zoster virus (VZV), or *Toxoplasmosis gondii* IgG titer in a recipient does not result in adjustment of the treatment plan, although the potential for reactivation must be acknowledged. A positive study for *T. palladium* should warrant treatment, which can be initiated at the time of evaluation for either the donor or recipient. If there is suspicion of active *T gondii* infection in the recipient or donor, treatment and clearance of this infection is indicated prior to conditioning regimen and/or hematopoietic cell collection. It is important to note that prophylactic therapy with a sulfa-based agent may also require desensitization in a sulfa-allergic patient. Seropositivity of HTLV-1/2 may be present in a recipient from an endemic region, or in a patient being considered for transplant for adult T-cell leukemia/lymphoma (ATLL). If a potential donor comes from a region where HTLV 1/2 is prevalent, he/she may be screened. If a carrier, he/she should be excluded from consideration. Even in the setting of a sibling donor transplant for adult T-cell leukemia/lymphoma, limited data suggest that these patients have inferior outcomes from donors with HTLV 1/2 seropositivity [30]. Evidence of HIV 1/2 should exclude donors as well. Obtaining a serum aspergillosis galactomannam antigen from a recipient is controversial in that its sensitivity is variable, and more likely than not, historical and clinical findings would be available indicating the possibility of active fungal infection [31]. If TB screening is indicated, there remains considerable question on the most appropriate study, such as the PPD skin test or the interferon-gamma release assay, as well as when prophylaxis is indicated [32–34]. In general, patients with latent TB or close exposure to someone with active TB should receive prophylaxis with isoniazid and pyridoxine, although location-based and institutional guidelines should dictate the approach. Other geographic considerations are previously discussed and are equally applicable in the donor infectious disease evaluation.

The status of HBV or HCV in either the recipient or donor requires consideration and planning for appropriate management. The management of recipients who screen positive for HBV or HCV are discussed in the Previous Infections section above. In the event a recipient is negative for HBcAb and HBsAg, assessment of the donor's HBV status is critical. Screening positive for HBcAb and/or HBsAg necessitates testing for HBV-DNA viral load. If a donor has HBV-DNA

active replication, a dual approach is advised. The donor should initiate therapy with entecavir for approximately 1 month prior to hematopoietic cell collection, and viral load should be measured at the time of collection as presumably, there is a greater risk of viral transmission if virus is detected in the stem cell product. Consider a minimum CD34+ dose without increasing the risk of primary graft failure. The recipient should begin immunizations prior to transplant; however, this may be ineffective in decreasing infection from the donor given the difficulty in completing the series in a limited time frame before HCT and the high likelihood of vaccination failure in an immunocompromised patient. The recipient HBsAb titer should be checked prior to transplant, and in the event that a patient has HBsAb titers <10IU/L, the recipient should receive HBIG 0.016mL/kg prior to the hematopoietic cell infusion and resume immunizations between 6 and 12 months post-HCT as recommended by international guidelines [15,35]. Prophylaxis with lamivudine starting at day 0 through at least 6 months beyond discontinuation of immunosuppressive agents is advised [15,36,37]. It is important to note that HBV infection of either the donor or recipient is not associated with increased mortality; however, this is based on retrospective analyses [14,38]. HCV infection status is determined by PCR and discussed previously in the Previous Infections section above. Similar to HBV, the risk of recipient infection from a positive donor appears dependent upon the viral load at the time of donation. Clearance of HCV from the donor is ideal prior to donation; however, realistically, this is almost never possible with current commonly available therapies. The recipient should be informed of the risk of HCV infection from the donor, and its potential short- and long-term implications[39].

Infectious disease screening is often performed by a national registry, such as the National Marrow Donor Program (NMDP). Potential donors may be deemed "ineligible" due to donor travel outside of his/her home country within the past 12 months. However, it is also important to note that collaboration between international registries is increasing, and therefore, the clinician should not necessarily exclude "ineligible" donors. Most importantly, explanation of the risks and complications of transmissibility of known or unknown diseases must be discussed with the recipient, and informed consent is obligatory.

Pre-HCT imaging is not supported by robust evidence, although institutional and clinician preferences may dictate otherwise. Clinician assessment based on the history and physical should guide a decision to obtain further studies, in particular whether the results of the imaging would change the pre- and peri-HCT management.

Type of HCT and Relationship to Infection

Consideration of the hematopoietic cell source and conditioning regimen planned is important to identify the relative risk to the recipient. Allogeneic HCT recipients receiving an

HLA-matched sibling or unrelated hematopoietic cell source have a relatively comparable risk of nonrelapse mortality [40,41]. Moving beyond HLA-matched adult sources, the use of HLA-mismatched or haploidentical sources require an intensification of conditioning regimens to decrease the risk of rejection and GvHD, thus increasing the risk of infection and mortality [42–44]. One method employed is to decrease the number of T-cells via antithymocyte globulin (ATG), alemtuzumab, or ex-vivo T-cell depletion of the graft [45]. Patients receiving cord blood transplants have a longer time to neutrophil engraftment, and a longer time to complete immune reconstitution, and the clinician must anticipate intensive monitoring post-HCT [46].

Active Infection at Time of HCT

A patient who presents for initiation of conditioning therapy with a fever or symptoms of infection should have a full evaluation. Examination may reveal the likely etiology, such as a recent central venous catheter placement as central venous catheters are a common source of infection [47]. Bacterial infections should prompt initiation of therapy and appropriate interventions, and the HCT would proceed after resolution of the acute illness. Some clinicians may opt to continue antimicrobial coverage through conditioning therapy to decrease a potential risk of recurrence. While no evidence suggests this decreases the risk of reinfection, often art overcomes science. In the setting of a new diagnosis of a fungal infection, therapy should be initiated and HCT may proceed with the continuation of the antifungal therapy.

If a respiratory viral infection is diagnosed, it is advised to delay HCT until resolution of symptoms. The broader adoption of respiratory panels by PCR has allowed easier detection and more rapid diagnosis. Treatment of parainfluenza, metapneumovirus, adenovirus, and respiratory synctial viruses with ribavirin may be applicable although the utility of this agent could be debated. Influenza treatment with osletamivir would be advised. It is important to note that all of the above viral illnesses are associated with increased mortality when patients are infected in the peri-HCT setting, so proceeding with an active respiratory viral infection is ill-advised [48–51]. In theory, coronavirus and rhinovirus, usually associated with the common cold may be safer; however, coronavirus in the post-HCT setting has long-term mortality rates comparable to other flu-like viruses in a recent analysis [51]. Recently, a retrospective study demonstrated no increased risk of proceeding to HCT with an active rhinovirus infection [52]. However, at present, data are limited and risks must be discussed with the patient.

Planning Ahead

The pre-HCT infectious disease evaluation is an opportune time to address several issues and discuss post-HCT prevention strategies. In the pre-HCT period, it is advised that caregivers and close friends/family obtain the 7-valent pneumococcal vaccine (PCV7), which has demonstrated better efficacy compared to the 23-valent vaccine in the HCT population [53]. Caregivers and close friends/family should also receive the seasonal influenza vaccine, avoiding the live intranasal preparation. In the event that a recent contact develops influenza, the patient should be instructed to contact his/her provider as starting prophylactic treatment is indicated. Other recommendations include administration of only inactivated vaccines, when possible, to children who may be in contact with the patient in the peri HCT period. If the measles, mumps, and rubella (MMR), varicella, or rotavirus vaccines are administered, the child should avoid contact with the immunocompromised person for at least 7 days to allow adequate time for viral shedding to cease. Varicella revaccination or obtaining zoster vaccination in either the recipient or caregiver is not advised in the pre- or peri-HCT period. Caregivers and close contacts who do get vaccinated and subsequently develop rash or cutaneous manifestation should cover the lesions and avoid the patient and the transplant center. Educating the patient and caregiver to discourage visits from those with symptoms of upper respiratory infections is necessary. Recipients should also be made aware of the need of reimmunization in the post-HCT setting (see Chapters 23–25).

A comprehensive education program for patients and caregivers to address the many aspects of the HCT process is important. Disease prevention by avoidance of certain foods and consumption of water that is safe from *Crytosporidium* should be advised. Protected sex and avoidance of others' bodily fluids and feces after HCT should be recommended. Even in situations of monogamous relationships, discordant HBV, HCV, or CMV status could theoretically increase risk to the HCT recipient.

Controversies

Considering a patient with HIV for HCT was only recently considered noncontroversial. This may have stemmed from the few patients who presented for HCT and the unclear outcomes in a new population with a baseline immunodeficiency. However, as more clinicians and institutions have transplanted patients with HIV, there is little controversy that these patients appear to have comparable outcomes following autologous HCT, and in fact, allogeneic HCT may be an avenue to therapy of the underlying infection (see Chapter 58). Enrollment in a clinical trial is advised.

Also controversial is the declination of seasonal influenza vaccinations by healthcare workers, as vaccination contributes considerably towards preventing transmission of a potentially deadly disease to an immunocompromised patient. Excluding those who have allergies, all workers in a transplant unit or clinic should receive an annual vaccination. The risk to patients far outweighs the negligible personal risk of vaccination, and it is recommended that institutions develop policies to address these situations.

Summary

The pre-HCT infectious disease work-up allows an assessment of potential risk factors in the recipient, including the extent and type of previous infections associated with prior therapy, chronic viral infections such as HBV, HCV, and HIV, and geographic considerations. Assessment of infectious exposures in the donor as well as acknowledging the planned conditioning regimen and HCT are also critical for appropriate pre- and peri-HCT management decisions. The pre-HCT infectious disease assessment also provides an opportunity for educating the patient, caregiver(s), and family members on prevention strategies to decrease the recipient risks of exposure and infection throughout the entire transplant period.

References

1. Myers LA, Patel DD, Puck JM, Buckley RH. Hematopoietic stem cell transplantation for severe combined immunodeficiency in the neonatal period leads to superior thymic output and improved survival. *Blood.* 2002;99(3):872–8.

2. Sorror ML, Maris MB, Storb R, Baron F, Sandmaier BM, Maloney DG, *et al.* Hematopoietic cell transplantation (HCT)-specific comorbidity index: a new tool for risk assessment before allogeneic HCT. *Blood.* 2005;106(8):2912–9.

3. Sorror ML. How I assess comorbidities before hematopoietic cell transplantation. *Blood.* 2013;121(15):2854–63.

4. Zhang P, Song A, Wang Z, Feng S, Qiu L, Han M. Hematopoietic SCT in patients with a history of invasive fungal infection. *Bone Marrow Transplant.* 2009;43(7):533–7.

5. Georgiadou SP, Lewis RE, Best L, Torres HA, Champlin RE, Kontoyiannis DP. The impact of prior invasive mold infections in leukemia patients who undergo allo-SCT in the era of triazole-based secondary prophylaxis. *Bone Marrow Transplant.* 2013;48(1):141–3.

6. Kinnebrew MA, Lee YJ, Jenq RR, Lipuma L, Littmann ER, Gobourne A, *et al.* Early Clostridium difficile infection during allogeneic hematopoietic stem cell transplantation. *PLoS one.* 2014;9(3):e90158.

7. Zacharioudakis IM, Ziakas PD, Mylonakis E. Clostridium difficile infection in the hematopoietic unit: a meta-analysis of published studies. *Biol Blood Marrow Transplant.* 2014.[Epub ahead of print].

8. Kumar D, Humar A, Plevneshi A, Siegal D, Franke N, Green K, *et al.* Invasive pneumococcal disease in adult hematopoietic stem cell transplant recipients: a decade of prospective population-based surveillance. *Bone Marrow Transplant.* 2008;41(8):743–7.

9. Prabhu RM, Piper KE, Litzow MR, Steckelberg JM, Patel R. Emergence of quinolone resistance among viridans group streptococci isolated from the oropharynx of neutropenic peripheral blood stem cell transplant patients receiving quinolone antimicrobial prophylaxis. *Eur J Clin Microbiol Infect Dis.* 2005;24(12):832–8.

10. Guthrie KA, Yong M, Frieze D, Corey L, Fredricks DN. The impact of a change in antibacterial prophylaxis from ceftazidime to levofloxacin in allogeneic hematopoietic cell transplantation. *Bone Marrow Transplant.* 2010;45(4):675–81.

11. Giaccone L, Festuccia M, Marengo A, Resta I, Sorasio R, Pittaluga F, *et al.* Hepatitis B virus reactivation and efficacy of prophylaxis with lamivudine in patients undergoing allogeneic stem cell transplantation. *Biol Blood Marrow Transplant.* 2010;16(6):809–17.

12. Peffault de Latour R, Lévy V, Asselah T, Marcellin P, Scieux C, Adès L, *et al.* Long-term outcome of hepatitis C infection after bone marrow transplantation. *Blood.* 2003;103(5):1618–24.

13. Nakasone H, Kurosawa S, Yakushijin K, Taniguchi S, Murata M, Ikegame K, *et al.* Impact of hepatitis C virus infection on clinical outcome in recipients after allogeneic hematopoietic cell transplantation. *Am J Hematol.* 2013;88(6):477–84.

14. Tomblyn M, Chen M, Kukreja M, Aljurf MD, Al Mohareb F, Bolwell BJ, *et al.* No increased mortality from donor or recipient hepatitis B- and/or hepatitis C-positive serostatus after related-donor allogeneic hematopoietic cell transplantation. *Transpl Infect Dis.* 2012;14(5):468–78.

15. Tomblyn M, Chiller T, Einsele H, Gress R, Sepkowitz K, Storek J, *et al.* Guidelines for preventing infectious complications among hematopoietic cell transplantation recipients: a global perspective. *Biol Blood Marrow Transplant.* 2009;15(10):1143–238.

16. Re A, Michieli M, Casari S, Allione B, Cattaneo C, Rupolo M, *et al.* High-dose therapy and autologous peripheral blood stem cell transplantation as salvage treatment for AIDS-related lymphoma: long-term results of the Italian Cooperative Group on AIDS and Tumors (GICAT) study with analysis of prognostic factors. *Blood.* 2009;114(7):1306–13.

17. Krishnan A, Palmer JM, Zaia JA, Tsai NC, Alvarnas J, Forman SJ. HIV status does not affect the outcome of autologous stem cell transplantation (ASCT) for non-Hodgkin lymphoma (NHL). *Biol Blood Marrow Transplant.* 2010;16(9):1302–8.

18. Durand CM, Ambinder RF. Hematopoietic stem cell transplantation in HIV-1-infected individuals: clinical challenges and the potential for viral eradication. *Curr Opin Oncol.* 2013;25(2):180–6.

19. Hutter G, Zaia JA. Allogeneic haematopoietic stem cell transplantation in patients with human immunodeficiency virus: the experiences of more than 25 years. *Clin Exp Immunol.* 2011;163(3):284–95.

20. Dictar M, Sinagra A, Veron MT, Luna C, Dengra C, De Rissio A, *et al.* Recipients and donors of bone marrow transplants suffering from Chagas' disease: management and preemptive therapy of parasitemia. *Bone Marrow Transplant.* 1998;21(4):391–3.

21. Villeneuve L, Cassaing S, Magnaval JF, Boisseau M, Huynh A, Demur C, *et al.* Plasmodium falciparum infection following allogeneic bone-marrow transplantation. *Ann Trop Med Parasitol.* 1999;93(5):533–5.

22. Mejia R, Booth GS, Fedorko DP, Hsieh MM, Khuu HM, Klein HG, *et al.* Peripheral blood stem cell transplant-related Plasmodium falciparum infection in a patient with sickle cell

disease. *Transfusion.* 2012;52(12):2677–82.

23. Klein MB, Miller JS, Nelson CM, Goodman JL. Primary bone marrow progenitors of both granulocytic and monocytic lineages are susceptible to infection with the agent of human granulocytic ehrlichiosis. *J Infect Dis.* 1997;176(5):1405–9.

24. Goldman KE. Dental management of patients with bone marrow and solid organ transplantation. *Dent Clin North Am.* 2006;50(4):659–76, viii.

25. Yamagata K, Onizawa K, Yanagawa T, Hasegawa Y, Kojima H, Nagasawa T, *et al.* A prospective study to evaluate a new dental management protocol before hematopoietic stem cell transplantation. *Bone Marrow Transplant.* 2006;38(3):237–42.

26. Elad S, Thierer T, Bitan M, Shapira MY, Meyerowitz C. A decision analysis: the dental management of patients prior to hematology cytotoxic therapy or hematopoietic stem cell transplantation. *Oral Oncol.* 2008;44(1):37–42.

27. George B, Pati N, Gilroy N, Ratnamohan M, Huang G, Kerridge I, *et al.* Pre-transplant cytomegalovirus (CMV) serostatus remains the most important determinant of CMV reactivation after allogeneic hematopoietic stem cell transplantation in the era of surveillance and preemptive therapy. *Transpl Infect Dis.* 2010;12(4):322–9.

28. Chemaly RF, Ullmann AJ, Stoelben S, Richard MP, Bornhauser M, Groth C, *et al.* Letermovir for cytomegalovirus prophylaxis in hematopoietic-cell transplantation. *N Engl J Med.* 2014;370(19):1781–9.

29. Zallio F, Primon V, Tamiazzo S, Pini M, Baraldi A, Corsetti MT, *et al.* Epstein–Barr virus reactivation in allogeneic stem cell transplantation is highly related to cytomegalovirus reactivation. *Clin Transplant.* 2013;27(4):E491–7.

30. Kato K, Kanda Y, Eto T, Muta T, Gondo H, Taniguchi S, *et al.* Allogeneic bone marrow transplantation from unrelated human T-cell leukemia virus-I-negative donors for adult T-cell leukemia/lymphoma: retrospective analysis of data from the Japan Marrow Donor Program. *Biol Blood Marrow Transplant.* 2007;13(1):90–9.

31. Pfeiffer CD, Fine JP, Safdar N. diagnosis of invasive aspergillosis using a galactomannan assay: a meta-analysis. *Clin Infect Dis.* 2006;42(10):1417–727.

32. Lee J, Lee MH, Kim WS, Kim K, Park SH, Lee SH, *et al.* Tuberculosis in hematopoietic stem cell transplant recipients in Korea. *Int J Hematol.* 2004;79(2):185–8.

33. Kobashi Y, Mouri K, Obase Y, Fukuda M, Miyashita N, Oka M. Clinical evaluation of QuantiFERON TB-2G test for immunocompromised patients. *Eur Respir J.* 2007;30(5):945–50.

34. Moon SM, Lee SO, Choi SH, Kim YS, Woo JH, Yoon DH, *et al.* Comparison of the QuantiFERON-TB Gold In-Tube test with the tuberculin skin test for detecting latent tuberculosis infection prior to hematopoietic stem cell transplantation. *Transpl Infect Dis.* 2013;15(1):104–9.

35. Onozawa M, Hashino S, Darmanin S, Okada K, Morita R, Takahata M, *et al.* HB vaccination in the prevention of viral reactivation in allogeneic hematopoietic stem cell transplantation recipients with previous HBV infection. *Biol Blood Marrow Transplant.* 2008;14(11):1226–30.

36. Hsiao LT, Chiou TJ, Liu JH, Chu CJ, Lin YC, Chao TC, *et al.* Extended lamivudine therapy against hepatitis B virus infection in hematopoietic stem cell transplant recipients. *Biol Blood Marrow Transplant.* 2006;12(1):84–94.

37. Lin PC, Poh SB, Lee MY, Hsiao LT, Chen PM, Chiou TJ. Fatal fulminant hepatitis B after withdrawal of prophylactic lamivudine in hematopoietic stem cell transplantation patients. *Int J Hematol.* 2005;81(4):349–51.

38. Ramos CA, Saliba RM, de Padua Silva L, Khorshid O, Shpall EJ, Giralt S, *et al.* Resolved hepatitis B virus infection is not associated with worse outcome after allogeneic hematopoietic stem cell transplantation. *Biol Blood Marrow Transplant.* 2010;16(5):686–94.

39. Shuhart MC, Myerson D, Childs BH, Fingeroth JD, Perry JJ, Snyder DS, *et al.* Marrow transplantation from hepatitis C virus seropositive donors: transmission rate and clinical course. *Blood.* 1994;84(9):3229–35.

40. Ho VT, Kim HT, Aldridge J, Liney D, Kao G, Armand P, *et al.* Use of matched unrelated donors compared with matched related donors is associated with lower relapse and superior progression-free survival after reduced-intensity conditioning hematopoietic stem cell transplantation. *Biol Blood Marrow Transplant.* 2011;17(8):1196–204.

41. Peffault de Latour R, Brunstein CG, Porcher R, Chevallier P, Robin M, Warlick E, *et al.* Similar overall survival using sibling, unrelated donor, and cord blood grafts after reduced-intensity conditioning for older patients with acute myelogenous leukemia. *Biol Blood Marrow Transplant.* 2013;19(9):1355–60.

42. Bachanova V, Brunstein CG, Burns LJ, Miller JS, Luo X, Defor T, *et al.* Fewer infections and lower infection-related mortality following non-myeloablative *versus* myeloablative conditioning for allotransplantation of patients with lymphoma. *Bone Marrow Transplant.* 2009;43(3):237–44.

43. Deeg HJ, Sandmaier BM. Who is fit for allogeneic transplantation? *Blood.* 2010;116(23):4762–70.

44. Xuan L, Huang F, Fan Z, Zhou H, Zhang X, Yu G, *et al.* Effects of intensified conditioning on Epstein–Barr virus and cytomegalovirus infections in allogeneic hematopoietic stem cell transplantation for hematological malignancies. *J Hematol Oncol.* 2012;5:46.

45. Roux E, Helg C, Chapuis B, Jeannet M, Roosnek E. T-cell repertoire complexity after allogeneic bone marrow transplantation. *Hum Immunol.* 1996;48(1–2):135–8.

46. Komanduri KV, St John LS, de Lima M, McMannis J, Rosinski S, McNiece I, *et al.* Delayed immune reconstitution after cord blood transplantation is characterized by impaired thymopoiesis and late memory T-cell skewing. *Blood.* 2007;110(13):4543–51.

47. Lukenbill J, Rybicki L, Sekeres MA, Zaman MO, Copelan A, Haddad H, *et al.* Defining incidence, risk factors, and impact on survival of central line-associated blood stream infections following hematopoietic cell transplantation in acute myeloid leukemia and myelodysplastic syndrome. *Biol Blood Marrow Transplant.* 2013;19(5):720–4.

48. Renaud C, Xie H, Seo S, Kuypers J, Cent A, Corey L, *et al.* Mortality rates of human metapneumovirus and respiratory syncytial virus lower respiratory tract infections in

hematopoietic cell transplantation recipients. *Biol Blood Marrow Transplant.* 2013;19(8):1220–6.

49. Kim YJ, Guthrie KA, Waghmare A, Walsh EE, Falsey AR, Kuypers J, *et al.* Respiratory syncytial virus in hematopoietic cell transplant recipients: factors determining progression to lower respiratory tract disease. *J Infect Dis.* 2014;209(8):1195–204.

50. Seo S, Xie H, Campbell AP, Kuypers JM, Leisenring WM, Englund JA, *et al.* Parainfluenza virus lower respiratory tract disease after hematopoietic cell transplant: viral detection in the lung predicts outcome. *Clin Infect Dis.* 2014;58(10):1357–68.

51. Wolfromm A, Porcher R, Legoff J, de Latour RP, Xhaard A, de Fontbrune FS, *et al.* Viral respiratory infections diagnosed by multiplex PCR after allogeneic hematopoietic stem cell transplantation: long-term incidence and outcome. *Biol Blood Marrow Transplant.* 2014. [Epub ahead of print].

52. Abandeh FI, Lustberg M, Devine S, Elder P, Andritsos L, Martin SI. Outcomes of hematopoietic SCT recipients with rhinovirus infection: a matched, case-control study. *Bone Marrow Transplant.* 2013;48(12):1554–7.

53. Kumar D, Chen MH, Welsh B, Siegal D, Cobos I, Messner HA, *et al.* A randomized, double-blind trial of pneumococcal vaccination in adult allogeneic stem cell transplant donors and recipients. *Clin Infect Dis.* 2007;45(12):1576–82.

6

Hematopoietic Cell Transplantation: Is There Any Age Limit?

Andrew S. Artz and Rebecca L. Olin

Epidemiology

The percentage of hematopoietic cell transplants being performed for older patients has steadily increased over the years, as evidenced by Center for International Blood and Marrow Transplant Research (CIBMTR) data[1]. In the 1990s, fewer than 10% of transplants were performed for older patients (≥50 years for allogeneic, ≥60 years for autologous). This is in sharp contrast to the most recent reporting period 2005–2011, when older patients comprised close to 40% of transplant recipients.

Table 6.1 displays preliminary data examining the age composition of allogeneic transplant recipients 50 years of age or above at first transplant registered with the CIBMTR. There has been a marked increase in the relative percentage of such transplants performed for recipients over 60 years old. Transplant for patients over 70 years old, while uncommon, has seen the most striking growth.

Many factors underlie greater hematapoietic cell transplantation (HCT) utilization in older patients[2] (Table 6.2). Of note, while reduced intensity or nonmyeloablative conditioning has been widely credited, the rise in allogeneic transplant mirrors the rise in autologous transplant for older adults, which employs ablative regimens. Improvements in supportive care, including infectious disease monitoring, prophylaxis, and treatment, have played a key role in expanding the use of both allogeneic and autologous transplants. Finally, demographic trends have resulted in an increase in the number of older adults nationwide, who also suffer a disproportionate burden of the incidence and mortality related to most hematologic malignancies.

Despite the increased ability to safely transplant older adults with hematologic malignancies, only a small fraction of older patients with transplant-eligible diseases receive a transplant. Estimates of the percentage of older patients diagnosed with acute myeloid leukemia (AML) who ultimately undergo allogeneic transplant range from 0.8 to 6%[3,4]. Although some patients may not be eligible due to lack of disease control and/or health impairments, undoubtedly under-referral, donor availability, and patient and physician preference all contribute.

Allogeneic Transplant

Controversy: Should an Older Sibling Be Preferred over a Younger Unrelated Donor?

For younger adults, a matched sibling donor will be the preferred option for similar to better outcomes, but also for ready

Table 6.1 Number of first allogeneic HCT recipients 50 years of age and older registered with CIBMTR by centers worldwide from 2000 through 2013*, by year of transplant and age group

	All Years	2000–2001	2002–2003	2004–2005	2006–2007	2008–2009	2010–2011	2012–2013
Total N	40319	3238	3887	4599	5282	6494	7924	8895
Age group, N (%)								
50–59	24365 (60)	2567 (79)	2883 (74)	3186 (69)	3339 (63)	3759 (58)	4347 (55)	4284 (48)
60–69	14601 (36)	639 (20)	949 (24)	1342 (29)	1824 (35)	2548 (39)	3240 (41)	4059 (46)
70–74	1240 (3)	24 (1)	50 (1)	68 (1)	103 (2)	178 (3)	316 (4)	501 (6)
75–79	101 (<1)	4 (<1)	4 (<1)	2 (<1)	15 (<1)	8 (<1)	20 (<1)	48 (1)
80+	12 (<1)	4 (<1)	1 (<1)	1 (<1)	1 (<1)	1 (<1)	1 (<1)	3 (<1)
Age group, N (%)								
50–69	38966 (97)	3206 (99)	3832 (99)	4528 (98)	5163 (98)	6307 (97)	7587 (96)	8343 (94)
70+	1353 (3)	32 (1)	55 (1)	71 (2)	119 (2)	187 (3)	337 (4)	552 (6)

* Registration of allogeneic transplant with CIBMTR is voluntary for non-US centers and was voluntary for US centers through 2007; US centers have been required to register all allogeneic transplants with CIBMTR since 2008. The data presented here are preliminary and were obtained from the Statistical Center of the Center for International Blood and Marrow Transplant Research. The analysis has not been reviewed or approved by the Advisory or Scientific Committees of the CIBMTR.

Table 6.2 Trends promoting hematopoietic cell transplant (HCT) for older adults

Characteristic	Example
Reduced intensity conditioning[a]	Fewer acute regimen-related toxicities
Peripheral blood hematopoietic cells	Reduces time to neutrophil engraftment Easier collection of hematopoietic cells for patients and older donors
Supportive care	
Infectious disease	Better infectious disease monitoring (e.g. CMV detection) and better treatments for opportunistic infections
Growth factors	Facilitate stem cell collection and reduce neutropenia phase post-HCT
Immunosuppression[a]	More tolerable immunosuppression reducing toxicity
Human leukocyte antigen (HLA) Matching[a]	Better HLA-matching reduces post-HCT complications
Donor registries [a]	Merging of registry databases electronically facilitates unrelated donor identification. Cord blood banks provide resource for unrelated cord blood
Patient health	Older adults have fewer disabilities and longer life expectancy allowing more intensive treatment
Societal attitudes	Patient and physician attitudes have shifted to expect life-prolonging treatment for older adults
Availability	More transplant centers and insurance coverage for older adults

[a] Restricted to Allogeneic HCT.
Adapted from Artz A, Ershler W. Hematopoietic cell transplantation in older adults. In Hurria A, Cohen HJ, editors. *Practical geriatric oncology.* Cambridge, New York: Cambridge University Press; 2010, p. 282.]

availability and flexibility to manipulate the product and/or give post-transplant cellular therapy. Health conditions and concern about hematopoietic health of the harvest may raise concerns for older donors. Older age is associated with mobilizing fewer CD34+ progenitor cells after G-CSF[5]. Comorbid conditions do not appear to impede ability to mobilize CD34+ cells, although lower donor performance score may. In general, a medically cleared donor aged 50–70 will likely have an adequate collection; there are little data on donors >70 years of age.

We advocate an older healthy matched sibling donor for an older patient over a younger unrelated donor. A large CIBMTR analysis of 2172 recipients aged ≥50 years compared grafts from matched siblings 50 years or above compared to unrelated

donors under 50 years of age[6]. Rates of both acute and chronic graft-*versus*-host disease (GvHD) were higher after an unrelated allograft. For older patients with preserved performance status (KPS of 90% or more), survival was best after sibling allografts. However, for recipients with Karnofsky performance score (KPS) ≤80, there was no difference in outcomes between sibling and unrelated donor sources. Limitations of this analysis include limited numbers of both recipients and donors aged >70. Smaller series generally show at least equivalent outcomes using sibling *versus* unrelated donors, with one exception[7–9]. Therefore, we recommend the use of a medically eligible older sibling donor up to the age of 70, and do not perform an unrelated donor search when one is available. Donors 70 and older are acceptable but require careful clearance and may justify cryopreservation of the graft prior to patient conditioning to ensure an adequate yield. A parallel unrelated donor search is prudent should the sibling donor not clear.

In the absence of a matched sibling or readily available matched unrelated donor, older patients may still be considered for alternative graft source such as umbilical cord blood or haploidentical donors. In the case of umbilical cord blood grafts, emerging evidence supports outcomes equivalent to sibling/unrelated donors[10].

Effect of Increasing Age on Transplant Outcome

Older age has historically prohibited transplant. Modern evidence still supports worse outcomes in the older *versus* younger transplant recipients, though the gap may be narrowing. CIBMTR data demonstrate that 1-year overall survival is still better for transplant recipients <50 years *versus* ≥50 years, though the difference is 10% or less depending on whether the donor used is related or unrelated[1]. An analysis of 1853 patients aged 0.1–75 years and transplanted from 2000 to 2006 showed that risk of non-relapse mortality (NRM) still increases with increasing age. Using age groups of 20-year increments with the 0- to 19-year-old group as a reference point, NRM became significantly worse once over age 40[11].

Several retrospective studies have evaluated the effect of increasing recipient age, within an older patient population, on transplant outcomes[8,12–16] (Table 6.3). There has generally been no demonstration of worsening NRM or overall survival (OS) with increasing age, and no clear effect on acute or chronic GvHD. However, studies comparing younger to older patients provide limited insight into the benefits of transplant for older patients.

Transplant *versus* Nontransplant Therapy

In older patients, prospective studies comparing allogeneic transplant to other therapies (i.e., donor *versus* nondonor biologic assignment) do not exist. Therefore, data regarding the efficacy of transplant for this population have been derived from retrospective and case–control analyses, and have been largely limited to AML.

Table 6.3 Studies evaluating effect of age on allogeneic transplant outcomes

Study	Population	NRM	GvHD	OS
Koreth *et al.*, 2010[12]	n=158, aged 60–71, mixed indications	No effect	Lower risk of cGvHD in age >65 *versus* 60–65	No effect
Sorror *et al.*, 2011[8]	n=372, aged 60–75, mixed indications	No effect	No effect	No effect
Chevallier *et al.*, 2012[13]	n=600, aged 60–71, mixed indications	No effect	No effect	No effect
McClune *et al.*, 2010[14]	n=1080, aged 40–79, AML CR1 or MDS	No effect	Borderline higher risk of cGvHD in age >65	No effect
McClune *et al.*, 2014[16]	n=1248, aged 40–75, NHL	Worse NRM for age ≥55	No effect	Worse OS in age ≥55
Lim *et al.*, 2010[15]	n=1333, aged 50–74, MDS	No effect	NR	No effect

cGvHD, chronic graft-*versus*-host disease; NHL, non-Hodgkin lymphoma; MDS, myelodysplastic syndrome; NRM, nonrelapse mortality; OS, overall survival; NR, not reported.

Estey *et al.* studied consecutive AML patients >50 years of age seen at MD Anderson Cancer Center, and performed a case–control study comparing the outcomes of transplanted patients *versus* those who received chemotherapy[17]. The analysis demonstrated longer relapse-free survival in the transplanted patients, with limitations including selection bias and small sample size. Farag *et al.* compared the outcomes of patients aged 60–70 with AML in first remission receiving RIC regimen transplants reported to the CIBMTR with outcomes of patients receiving induction and consolidation chemotherapy on CALGB cooperative group trials (n=94 *versus* n=96, respectively)[18]. Allogeneic transplant was associated with a lower risk of relapse, higher NRM, longer leukemia-free survival, but only a borderline difference in overall survival that was not statistically significant. Kurosawa *et al.* reported a retrospective study of patients aged 50–70 with AML in first remission, using a Japanese national registry data, comparing transplanted *versus* nontransplanted patients (n=152 *versus* 884, respectively)[19]. Transplant was associated with lower relapse risk and longer relapse-free and overall survival. In subgroup analysis, transplant was associated with improved overall survival among patients with an eligible sibling donor, but not among patients with only an unrelated donor.

One prospective multicenter study of allogeneic transplant in older patients exists, conducted through the Alliance cooperative group and the Blood and Marrow Transplant Clinical Trials Network (BMT CTN) (CALGB 100103/BMT CTN 0502)[20]. Patients with AML in first remission aged 60–74 underwent sibling or unrelated RIC regimen transplant including T-cell depletion from 2004–2011. The trial enrolled 123 patients with a median age of 64. At 2 years, DFS and OS were 39% and 46%, respectively, with transplant-related mortality (TRM) 14%. Acute severe GvHD at 100 days was 3% and chronic GvHD at 2 years was 26% (similar to a large study of nonmyeloablative transplant reported by Sorror and colleagues in patients 60 years and older[8]). These studies demonstrate

that reduced intensity conditioning (RIC) regimen allogeneic transplant in the older patient population is feasible and outcomes are reasonable. A prospective donor-*versus*-no-donor comparison trial is clearly warranted, but is not yet underway.

Decision analysis has been a particularly informative approach in understanding the role of allogeneic transplant for older patients with myelodyplastic syndrome (MDS). Koreth *et al.* used Markov modeling to compare reduced intensity transplant *versus* nontransplant strategies for patients aged 60–70[21]. For patients with low/intermediate-1 MDS, nontransplant therapies remain the favored approach, but for patients with intermediate-2/high-risk MDS, allogeneic transplant improves both life expectancy and quality-adjusted life expectancy.

Controversy: Which Older Patient Is a Candidate for Allogeneic Transplant?

A common statement posed from observational studies has been "older age is not a barrier to transplant" based on reasonable survival for hematologic malignancies after allogeneic HCT. The questions remain, from a practical perspective, how to evaluate an older patient's candidacy for transplant and how old is too old? We recommend candidacy be determined based on assessment of disease relapse risk and transplant tolerance (Figure 6.1):

1. **Disease risk.** Disease relapse remains the most common cause of transplant failure, and poorly controlled disease precludes HCT in a large number if not the majority of older patients. Common transplant indications of AML, ALL, and MDS have lower rates and durations of remission in older patients. Poor disease-free survival without transplant will generally spur consideration of HCT. We recommend prognostic disease-based models either including age (e.g., age-adjusted Revised International Prognostic Scoring System (IPSS)) or using studies derived from older adults. For example, patients 60 and older fare

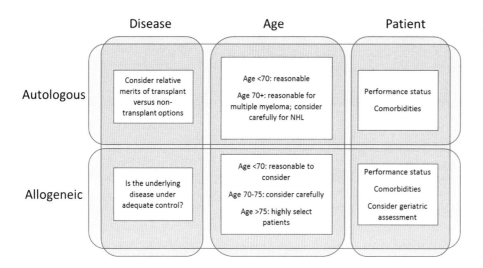

Figure 6.1. Evaluation of autologous or allogeneic transplant candidacy in older patients including disease-specific and patient-specific factors.

considerably worse after standard induction and consolidation relative to younger patients for the same cytogenetic and molecular markers[22]. We strongly advocate early consideration of transplant to account for shortened remission duration.

2. **Transplant tolerance.** For older adults, impaired transplant tolerance measured by risks of nonrelapse mortality relative to younger adults complicate disease risk-based decisions to pursue transplant. While transplant morbidity and impaired quality of life are of central importance, death without relapse (nonrelapse mortality or transplant-related mortality) is the best studied marker of tolerance. We use the following criteria to assess transplant tolerance:

    a. Age. Chronologic age remains important. Older age is associated with higher TRM even when adjusted for other health parameters below[11,23]. We are quite cautious in patients 70 years and older and consider only the most robust adults 75 years of age or greater for allogeneic HCT. A protocol is highly preferred. Determination of a patient's "physiologic age" complements chronologic age. Below we discuss both traditional and novel prognostic factors we consider.

    b. Performance status. Physician-rated performance status, most commonly measured using the Karnofsky index (KPS), is the easiest prognostic factor to assess. The majority of older adults undergoing allogeneic transplant have a high KPS of $\geq$80%, making performance status a relatively coarse measure. Performance status has been associated with TRM and overall survival after allogeneic transplant; specifically KPS $\leq$80 was associated with decreased overall survival in a large CIBMTR analysis of AML patients[6]. Most older patients with KPS less than 80% are not good candidates. Patients with an intercurrent event or recent treatment may recover KPS but loss of performance status may still be a marker of impairment.

    c. Comorbidity. We recommend measuring comorbidity by the Hematopoietic Cell Transplantation Comorbidity Index (HCT-CI)[24]. The HCT-CI has been validated and shown to be predictive of treatment-related mortality and overall survival in a wide variety of patient populations and transplant settings[25,26]. The HCT-CI can predict TRM in all age groups, including older patients specifically, and is a stronger predictor of TRM than age[8,11]. Sorror et al. recently published the composite Comorbidity–Age Index, which can risk-stratify patients based on the combination of these two variables[11].

    It is important to assess the HCT-CI correctly, which includes pulmonary function testing; since forced expiratory volume in 1 second (FEV1) and diffusion capacity of carbon monoxide (DLCO) abnormalities are heavily weighted in the HCT-CI index, omission of pulmonary function tests (PFTs) may result in falsely low comorbidity scores. Higher comorbidity, such as HCT-CI of 3 and particularly 4 or more, is linked to very high TRM. We caution against decisions based on the score alone and advise clinical interpretation for severity. For example, an HCT-CI score of 3 will be obtained from either a low Gleason score prostate cancer remotely resected or locally advanced lung cancer after chemoradiation, though only the latter would markedly impair transplant tolerance. Also, comorbid conditions not scored by the HCT-CI are often relevant, such as other concurrent hematologic malignancies or thromboembolic disease.

    Of note, outcomes for nontransplant therapy will also suffer in the presence of higher comorbidity [27,28]. Therefore, the decision of whether to avoid transplant based solely on high comorbidity is complex.

    d. Geriatric assessment (GA). GA is a comprehensive health assessment designed to measure a wide variety of health domains, frequently including functional status, comorbidity, cognition, nutritional status/weight loss, social support, psychologic health, polypharmacy, frailty, and others. Brief cancer-specific geriatric assessments have been developed and shown to predict chemotherapy-related toxicity in older solid tumor patients, as well as survival in older AML patients [29,30]. Recent evidence suggests that GA is feasible in the older stem cell transplant population, and can uncover significant vulnerabilities not captured by more traditional measures such as performance status. In a study of 166 allogeneic transplant recipients aged 50–73 who were clinically deemed fit for transplant, 51% were found to be pre-frail and 25% were frail, using the widely accepted Fried Frailty Index[31]. Forty percent had limitations in their Instrumental Activities of Daily Living (IADL), a measure of functional status; among patients with an Eastern Cooperative Oncology Group (ECOG) performance status of 0, 28% were still limited in IADL.

Many of the limitations identified by GA adversely affect transplant outcomes. In a larger sample of 203 older patients, the presence of IADL limitation, slow walk speed, and poor mental health were each independently associated with reduced overall survival, even when adjusted for traditional prognostic factors such as age, comorbidity, and active disease[23]. Using a simple risk score with 1 point each for IADL impairment and HCT-CI score ≥ 3, 2-year overall survival was 63%, 29%, and 0% for 0, 1, and 2 points, respectively, among the cohort 60 years and older.

Other measures such as social support, emotional health, nutrition, and polypharmacy are standard tools in GA and may uncover important vulnerabilities (e.g., health impairment of sole caregiver). We believe that GA supplements other prognostic tools and either an informal or formal evaluation be pursued. GA-guided interventions may also be used to mitigate transplant-related complications such as exercise programs for those with reduced function.

e. Biomarkers. High levels of clinically available biomarkers of c-reactive protein and serum ferritin

track with worse outcomes. We do not believe these should influence candidacy until validated studies show an independent influence from the factors described above.

Autologous Transplant

Multiple Myeloma

Effect of Increasing Age on Transplant Outcomes

For autologous transplant to be feasible, adequate numbers of hematopoietic stem cells must be obtainable. Older patients with multiple myeloma may have more difficulty mobilizing adequate CD34+ progenitor cells than younger patients. A large cohort study of myeloma patients did demonstrate an inverse correlation of age with CD34+ cell collection; however, 92% of older patients were able to collect adequate stem cells for a single autologous transplant[32]. The advent of plerixafor has improved rates of successful mobilization even further[33].

Historically, in the era of TBI-based autologous transplants and bone marrow hematopoietic cell grafts, the rate of TRM for older patients was 25–35%. In the modern era, using a melphalan-based preparative regimen, peripheral blood hematopoietic cells, and better supportive care, tolerability and TRM have been greatly improved. As a result, the definition of "older" for patients with multiple myeloma has shifted somewhat from the definition for other diseases, as patients in their 50s and early 60s generally have excellent transplant tolerance using melphalan-based conditioning. Modern studies investigating the safety and efficacy of patients ≥ 65 or ≥ 70 years with multiple myeloma reflect excellent tolerance with TRM in the 0–5% range. Several retrospective studies have examined the effect of increasing age on transplant outcome, with variable results[34–37] (Table 6.4).

Bashir et al. recently published the largest series to date of 84 patients ≥ 70 years with multiple myeloma receiving a melphalan-based autologous transplant (65% received 200 mg/m^2)[38]. There was no comparator group of younger patients; however, results were impressive with an 85% overall

Table 6.4 Studies evaluating effect of increasing age on autologous transplant outcomes for multiple myeloma

Study	Population	ORR	TRM	TTP	OS
Jantunen et al., 2006[34] (Finland)	n=22 $\geq$65 n=79 <65	No effect (94% ORR)	No effect (0%)	No effect (median 23 months PFS)	No effect (median 57 months OS)
Lenhoff et al., 2006[35] (Nordic)	n=120 60–64 n=294 <60	No effect (90% ORR)	No effect (1%)	Worse EFS in 60–64 (19% at 4 years)	Worse OS in 60–64 (50% at 4 years)
Kumar et al., 2008[36] (Mayo)	n=33 >70 n=60 <65 (matched controls)	No effect (97% ORR)	No effect (3%)	No effect (median 28.5 months TTP)	No effect (median not reached)
El-Cheikh et al., 2011[37] (France)	n=82 >65 n=104 60–65	–	No effect (3.7)	Worse PFS in >65	No effect (32% at 10 years)

ORR, overall response rate; TRM, treatment-related mortality; TTP, time to progression; PFS, progression-free survival; EFS, event-free survival; OS, overall survival.

Table 6.5 Studies evaluating effect of increasing age on autologous transplant outcomes for NHL

Study	Population	NRM	PFS	OS
Jantunen *et al.*, 2008[41] DLBCL	n=463 ≥60 n=2149 <60	Worse (4.4%)	Worse (51% at 3 years)	Worse (60% at 3 years)
Lazarus *et al.*, 2008[42] NHL indolent	n=173 ≥55 n=615 <55	No effect (7% at 5 years)	Worse (29% at 5 years)	Worse (54% at 5 years)
Lazarus *et al.*, 2008[42] NHL aggressive	n=632 ≥55 n=1334 <55	Worse (15% at 5 years)	Worse (19% at 5 years)	Worse (30% at 5 years)
Wildes *et al.*, 2008[43] NHL	n=59 ≥60 n=93 <60	No effect (8.5%)	No effect (median 22 months)	No effect (median 48 months)
Jantunen *et al.*, 2012[44] MCL	n=79 ≥65 n=633 <65	No effect (3.8%)	No effect (29% at 5 years)	No effect (61% at 5 years)

NRM, nonrelapse mortality; PFS, progression-free survival; OS, overall survival; DLBCL, diffuse large B-cell lymphoma; NHL, non-Hodgkin lymphoma; MCL, mantle cell lymphoma.

response rate, 3% TRM, a time to progression of 27% at 5 years, and an overall survival of 67% at 5 years.

Transplant *versus* Other Therapy

Three studies have examined the effectiveness of autologous transplant relative to nontransplant therapies in older adults with multiple myeloma. Lenhoff *et al.* demonstrated using a retrospective registry study that adults aged 60–64 who received autologous transplant had better overall survival compared to those who received conventional chemotherapy[35]. On the other hand, Offidani *et al.* compared outcomes of adults ≥65 who received chemotherapy followed by transplant if eligible, *versus* chemotherapy alone if ineligible for transplant; there was no difference in progression-free survival (PFS) or OS[39]. Finally, Facon *et al.* reported results of a trial randomizing older patients aged 65–75 to receive melphalan-prednisone chemotherapy, MP with addition of thalidomide, or MP followed by transplant (melphalan $100\,mg/m^2$)[40]. The winning arm was the thalidomide-containing regimen, and there was no survival benefit of chemotherapy plus transplant *versus* chemotherapy alone. While the relative benefit and morbidity of transplant for older patients with myeloma in the era of novel therapeutics is unclear, autologous HCT in select older patients has quite low transplant-related mortality.

Non-Hodgkin Lymphoma

Effect of Increasing Age on Transplant Outcomes

Several studies, including some very large international database studies, have compared the toxicity and efficacy of transplant in older patients with non-Hodgkin lymphoma (NHL) (indolent, aggressive and mantle cell)[41–44] (Table 6.5) Although the smaller studies have tended to show no difference in NRM, PFS, or OS, the larger studies have shown worse PFS and OS in older patients.

Nevertheless, there is evidence from small series of selected patients with lymphoma that autologous transplant is feasible even in patients over the age of 70. Elstrom *et al.* published

results on 21 patients aged 69–86[45]. NRM at 100 days was 19%. Age ≥75 was associated with worse PFS and borderline worse OS in a small number of patients. High comorbidity scores by HCT-CI predicted worse outcome. Andorsky *et al.* published results on 17 patients ≥70; NRM was 18% at 100 days and 35% at 1 year[46]. Compared to 39 patients aged 65–69, relapse mortality and overall survival were both worse in the older cohort. In this series, a history of falls (which may be a marker of frailty) was associated with worse outcomes.

Controversy: Which Older Patient Should Be Considered for Autologous HCT?

We believe that older adults who are fit and have reasonable nondisease-related survival are candidates for autologous transplant (Figure 6.1). Most patients with KPS of 80% or more and controlled comorbidity under the age of 75 years of age will be expected to have reasonable nondisease-related survival (and therefore may live long enough to realize the benefits of transplant), though more formal estimates can be derived by consulting with the patient's primary care provider or by using a comprehensive geriatric assessment (CGA) and/or online calculator (e.g., eprognosis.ucsf.edu). Higher HCT-CI has a statistically significant but clinically small effect on rates of TRM and OS after autologous HCT[47]. As before, higher comorbidity also tracks with worse survival without transplant.

The rapid evolution of nontransplant therapies for multiple myeloma and lymphoma, the main autologous transplant indications, present challenges in quantifying the benefits of transplant for young and old alike. Tolerance in general for adults even into their early 70s for melphalan conditioning and autologous transplant are quite good; patients >75 should be evaluated on a case by case basis. For diffuse large B-cell lymphoma (DLBCL), older patients can tolerate transplant, although they may have a greater chance of toxicity and worse PFS/OS relative to younger adults. Autologous transplant should be reserved for the highly selected patient >70 with NHL.

References

1. Pasquini M, Wang Z. Current use and outcome of hematopoietic stem cell transplantation: CIBMTR Summary Slides. 2013.

2. Artz A, Ershler W. Hematopoietic cell transplantation in older adults. In Hurria A, Cohen HJ, editors. *Practical geriatric oncology.* Cambridge, New York: Cambridge University Press; 2010. p. 1 online resource (x, 435 p.).

3. Ustun C, Lazarus HM, Weisdorf D. To transplant or not: a dilemma for treatment of elderly AML patients in the twenty-first century. *Bone Marrow Transplant.* 2013;48(12):1497–505.

4. Oran B, Weisdorf DJ. Survival for older patients with acute myeloid leukemia: a population-based study. *Haematologica.* 2012;97(12):1916–24.

5. Richa E, Papari M, Allen J, Martinez G, Wickrema A, Anastasi J, *et al.* Older age but not donor health impairs allogeneic granulocyte colony-stimulating factor (G-CSF) peripheral blood stem cell mobilization. *Biol Blood Marrow Transplant.* 2009;15(11):1394–9.

6. Alousi AM, Le-Rademacher J, Saliba RM, Appelbaum FR, Artz A, Benjamin J, *et al.* Who is the better donor for older hematopoietic transplant recipients: an older-aged sibling or a young, matched unrelated volunteer? *Blood.* 2013;121(13):2567–73.

7. De Latour RP, Labopin M, Cornelissen J, Vindelov L, Blaise D, Milpied N, *et al.* Equivalent outcome between older siblings and unrelated donors after reduced intensity allogeneic hematopoietic stem cell transplantation for patients older than 50 years with acute myeloid leukemia in first complete remission: A report from the ALWP of EBMT. *Blood* 2012;120: Abstract 961.

8. Sorror ML, Sandmaier BM, Storer BE, Franke GN, Laport GG, Chauncey TR, *et al.* Long-term outcomes among older patients following nonmyeloablative conditioning and allogeneic hematopoietic cell transplantation for advanced hematologic malignancies. *JAMA : The Journal of the American Medical Association.* 2011;306(17):1874–83.

9. Kroger N, Zabelina T, de Wreede L, Berger J, Alchalby H, van Biezen A, *et al.* Allogeneic stem cell transplantation for older advanced MDS patients: improved survival with young unrelated donor in comparison with HLA-identical siblings. *Leukemia.* 2013;27(3):604–9.

10. Peffault de Latour R, Brunstein CG, Porcher R, Chevallier P, Robin M, Warlick E, *et al.* Similar overall survival using sibling, unrelated donor, and cord blood grafts after reduced-intensity conditioning for older patients with acute myelogenous leukemia. *Biol Blood Marrow Transplant* 2013;19(9):1355–60.

11. Sorror ML, Storb RF, Sandmaier BM, Maziarz RT, Pulsipher MA, Maris MB, *et al.* Comorbidity-age index: a clinical measure of biologic age before allogeneic hematopoietic cell transplantation. *J Clin Oncol.* 2014.

12. Koreth J, Aldridge J, Kim HT, Alyea EP, 3rd, Cutler C, Armand P, *et al.* Reduced-intensity conditioning hematopoietic stem cell transplantation in patients over 60 years: hematologic malignancy outcomes are not impaired in advanced age. *Biol Blood Marrow Transplant.* 2010;16(6):792–800.

13. Chevallier P, Szydlo RM, Blaise D, Tabrizi R, Michallet M, Uzunov M, *et al.* Reduced-intensity conditioning before allogeneic hematopoietic stem cell transplantation in patients over 60 years: a report from the SFGM-TC. *Biol Blood Marrow Transplant.* 2012;18(2):289–94.

14. McClune BL, Weisdorf DJ, Pedersen TL, Tunes da Silva G, Tallman MS, Sierra J, *et al.* Effect of age on outcome of reduced-intensity hematopoietic cell transplantation for older patients with acute myeloid leukemia in first complete remission or with myelodysplastic syndrome. *J Clin Oncol.* 2010;28(11):1878–87.

15. Lim Z, Brand R, Martino R, van Biezen A, Finke J, Bacigalupo A, *et al.* Allogeneic hematopoietic stem-cell transplantation for patients 50 years or older with myelodysplastic syndromes or secondary acute myeloid leukemia. *J Clin Oncol.* 2010;28(3):405–11.

16. McClune BL, Ahn KW, Wang HL, Antin JH, Artz AS, Cahn JY, *et al.* Allotransplantation for patients age ≥40 years with non-Hodgkin lymphoma: encouraging progression-free survival. *Biol Blood Marrow Transplant.* 2014;20(7):960–8.

17. Estey E, de Lima M, Tibes R, Pierce S, Kantarjian H, Champlin R, *et al.* Prospective feasibility analysis of reduced-intensity conditioning (RIC) regimens for hematopoietic stem cell transplantation (HSCT) in elderly patients with acute myeloid leukemia (AML) and high-risk myelodysplastic syndrome (MDS). *Blood.* 2007;109(4):1395–400.

18. Farag SS, Maharry K, Zhang MJ, Perez WS, George SL, Mrozek K, *et al.* Comparison of reduced-intensity hematopoietic cell transplantation with chemotherapy in patients age 60–70 years with acute myelogenous leukemia in first remission. *Biol Blood Marrow Transplant.* 2011;17(12):1796–803.

19. Kurosawa S, Yamaguchi T, Uchida N, Miyawaki S, Usuki K, Watanabe M, *et al.* Comparison of allogeneic hematopoietic cell transplantation and chemotherapy in elderly patients with non-M3 acute myelogenous leukemia in first complete remission. *Biol Blood Marrow Transplant.* 2011;17(3):401–11.

20. Devine S, Owzar K, Blum W, DeAngelo D, Stone R, Hsu J, *et al.* A Phase II study of allogeneic transplantation for older patients with AML in first complete remission using a reduced intensity conditioning regimen: results from CALGB 100103/BMT CTN 0502. *Blood.* 2012;120:Abstract 230.

21. Koreth J, Pidala J, Perez WS, Deeg HJ, Garcia-Manero G, Malcovati L, *et al.* Role of reduced-intensity conditioning allogeneic hematopoietic stem-cell transplantation in older patients with de novo myelodysplastic syndromes: an international collaborative decision analysis. *J Clin Oncol.* 2013;31(21):2662–70.

22. Buchner T, Berdel WE, Haferlach C, Haferlach T, Schnittger S, Muller-Tidow C, *et al.* Age-related risk profile and chemotherapy dose response in acute myeloid leukemia: a study by the German Acute Myeloid Leukemia Cooperative Group. *J Clin Oncol.* 2009;27(1):61–9.

23. Muffly LS, Kocherginsky M, Stock W, Chu Q, Bishop MR, Godley LA, *et al.* Geriatric assessment to predict survival in older allogeneic hematopoietic cell transplantation recipients. *Haematologica.* 2014;99(8):1373–9.

24. Sorror ML, Maris MB, Storb R, Baron F, Sandmaier BM, Maloney DG, *et al.* Hematopoietic cell transplantation (HCT)-specific comorbidity index: a new tool for risk assessment before

allogeneic HCT. *Blood.* 2005;106(8):2912–9.

25. Sorror M. Impacts of pretransplant comorbidities on allogeneic hematopoietic cell transplantation (HCT) outcomes. *Biol Blood Marrow Transplant.* 2009;15(1 Suppl):149–53.

26. Raimondi R, Tosetto A, Oneto R, Cavazzina R, Rodeghiero F, Bacigalupo A, et al. Validation of the Hematopoietic Cell Transplantation-Specific Comorbidity Index: a prospective, multicenter GITMO study. *Blood.* 2012;120(6):1327–33.

27. Giles FJ, Borthakur G, Ravandi F, Faderl S, Verstovsek S, Thomas D, et al. The haematopoietic cell transplantation comorbidity index score is predictive of early death and survival in patients over 60 years of age receiving induction therapy for acute myeloid leukaemia. *Br J Haematol.* 2007;136(4):624–7.

28. Sperr WR, Wimazal F, Kundi M, Baumgartner C, Nosslinger T, Makrai A, et al. Comorbidity as prognostic variable in MDS: comparative evaluation of the HCT-CI and CCI in a core dataset of 419 patients of the Austrian MDS Study Group. *Ann Oncol.* 2010;21(1):114–9.

29. Hurria A, Togawa K, Mohile SG, Owusu C, Klepin HD, Gross CP, et al. Predicting chemotherapy toxicity in older adults with cancer: a prospective multicenter study. *J Clin Oncol.* 2011;29(25):3457–65.

30. Klepin HD, Geiger AM, Tooze JA, Kritchevsky SB, Williamson JD, Pardee TS, et al. Geriatric assessment predicts survival for older adults receiving induction chemotherapy for acute myelogenous leukemia. *Blood.* 2013; 121(21):4287–94.

31. Muffly LS, Boulukos M, Swanson K, Kocherginsky M, Cerro PD, Schroeder L, et al. Pilot Study of Comprehensive Geriatric Assessment (CGA) in Allogeneic Transplant: CGA Captures a High Prevalence of Vulnerabilities in Older Transplant Recipients. *Biol Blood Marrow Transplant.* 2013;19(3):429–34.

32. Morris CL, Siegel E, Barlogie B, Cottler-Fox M, Lin P, Fassas A, et al. Mobilization of CD34+ cells in elderly patients (>/=70 years) with multiple myeloma: influence of age, prior therapy, platelet count and mobilization regimen. *Br J Haematol.* 2003;120(3):413–23.

33. Micallef IN, Stiff PJ, Stadtmauer EA, Bolwell BJ, Nademanee AP, Maziarz RT, et al. Safety and efficacy of upfront plerixafor + G-CSF versus placebo + G-CSF for mobilization of CD34(+) hematopoietic progenitor cells in patients >/=60 and <60 years of age with non-Hodgkin's lymphoma or multiple myeloma. *Am J Hematol.* 2013;88(12):1017–23.

34. Jantunen E, Kuittinen T, Penttila K, Lehtonen P, Mahlamaki E, Nousiainen T. High-dose melphalan (200 mg/m^2) supported by autologous stem cell transplantation is safe and effective in elderly (>or=65 years) myeloma patients: comparison with younger patients treated on the same protocol. *Bone Marrow Transplant.* 2006;37(10):917–22.

35. Lenhoff S, Hjorth M, Westin J, Brinch L, Backstrom B, Carlson K, et al. Impact of age on survival after intensive therapy for multiple myeloma: a population-based study by the Nordic Myeloma Study Group. *Br J Haematol.* 2006;133(4):389–96.

36. Kumar SK, Dingli D, Lacy MQ, Dispenzieri A, Hayman SR, Buadi FK, et al. Autologous stem cell transplantation in patients of 70 years and older with multiple myeloma: Results from a matched pair analysis. *Am J Hematol.* 2008;83(8):614–7.

37. El-Cheikh J, Kfoury E, Calmels B, Lemarie C, Stoppa AM, Bouabdallah R, et al. Age at transplantation and outcome after autologous stem cell transplantation in elderly patients with multiple myeloma. *Hematol Oncol Stem Cell Ther.* 2011;4(1):30–6.

38. Bashir Q, Shah N, Parmar S, Wei W, Rondon G, Weber DM, et al. Feasibility of autologous hematopoietic stem cell transplant in patients aged >/=70 years with multiple myeloma. *Leuk Lymphoma.* 2012;53(1):118–22.

39. Offidani M, Leoni P, Corvatta L, Polloni C, Gentili S, Savini A, et al. ThaDD plus high-dose therapy and autologous stem cell transplantation does not appear superior to ThaDD plus maintenance in elderly patients with de novo multiple myeloma. *Eur J Haematol.* 2010;84(6):474–83.

40. Facon T, Mary JY, Hulin C, Benboubker L, Attal M, Pegourie B, et al. Melphalan and prednisone plus thalidomide versus melphalan and prednisone alone or reduced-intensity autologous stem cell transplantation in elderly patients with multiple myeloma (IFM 99-06): a randomised trial. *Lancet.* 2007;370(9594):1209–18.

41. Jantunen E, Canals C, Rambaldi A, Ossenkoppele G, Allione B, Blaise D, et al. Autologous stem cell transplantation in elderly patients (> or =60 years) with diffuse large B-cell lymphoma: an analysis based on data in the European Blood and Marrow Transplantation registry. *Haematologica.* 2008;93(12):1837–42.

42. Lazarus HM, Carreras J, Boudreau C, Loberiza FR, Jr., Armitage JO, Bolwell BJ, et al. Influence of age and histology on outcome in adult non-Hodgkin lymphoma patients undergoing autologous hematopoietic cell transplantation (HCT): a report from the Center For International Blood & Marrow Transplant Research (CIBMTR). *Biol Blood Marrow Transplant.* 2008;14(12):1323–33.

43. Wildes TM, Augustin KM, Sempek D, Zhang QJ, Vij R, Dipersio JF, et al. Comorbidities, not age, impact outcomes in autologous stem cell transplant for relapsed non-Hodgkin lymphoma. *Biol Blood Marrow Transplant.* 2008;14(7):840–6.

44. Jantunen E, Canals C, Attal M, Thomson K, Milpied N, Buzyn A, et al. Autologous stem-cell transplantation in patients with mantle cell lymphoma beyond 65 years of age: a study from the European Group for Blood and Marrow Transplantation (EBMT). *Ann Oncol.* 2012;23(1):166–71.

45. Elstrom RL, Martin P, Hurtado Rua S, Shore TB, Furman RR, Ruan J, et al. Autologous stem cell transplant is feasible in very elderly patients with lymphoma and limited comorbidity. *Am J Hematol.* 2012;87(4):433–5.

46. Andorsky DJ, Cohen M, Naeim A, Pinter-Brown L. Outcomes of auto-SCT for lymphoma in subjects aged 70 years and over. *Bone Marrow Transplant.* 2011;46(9):1219–25.

47. Pasquini M, Logan B, Ho V, McCarthy Jr. P, Cooke K, Rizzo J, et al. Comorbidity Index (CI) in autologous hematopoietic cell transplantation (HCT) for malignant diseases: validation of the HCT-CI. *Blood.* 2012: Abstract 814.

Chapter

7

Selecting the Best Donor for an Allogeneic Hematopoietic Cell Transplant

Mary Eapen

Introduction

There are several potential donor sources for allogeneic transplants including HLA-matched siblings, HLA-mismatched relatives, and HLA-matched or -mismatched unrelated donors. HLA-matched siblings and HLA-partially or HLA-completely matched unrelated donors are the most widely used. Recently, increasing numbers of HLA-mismatched related donor transplants are being done. Concurrently, *peripheral blood* grafts have largely replaced *bone marrow* in the setting of HLA-matched sibling and HLA-matched or -mismatched adult unrelated donor transplantation. Bone marrow is the predominant graft for HLA-mismatched related donor transplantation. Umbilical cord blood grafts are also increasingly used for both children and adults. The proportion of umbilical cord blood transplantation relative to unrelated adult donor transplantation is higher in children. In this chapter I discuss types of donors for allotransplants, types of grafts, donor safety, and regulations affecting use of donors and grafts.

HLA-Identical Siblings *versus* HLA-Matched Unrelated Donors

Transplants from an HLA-matched sibling are considered to have the best outcomes. However, there was debate whether an older HLA-identical is better than a younger HLA-matched unrelated donor. A recent study by the Center for International Blood and Marrow Transplant (CIBMTR) addressed this question. Transplants for persons 50 years or older with leukemia or lymphoma were analyzed to compare outcomes between recipients of HLA-identical sibling donors aged $\geq$50 years (n=1415) *versus* HLA-matched unrelated donors aged <50 years (n=757). Risks of acute graft-*versus*-host disease (GvHD) grade 2–4 (hazard ratio [HR] 1.63, 95% CI 1.48−2.01; P<0.001), grade 3–4 (HR 1.85, 95% CI 1.54−2.23; P<0.001), and chronic GvHD (HR 1.48, 95% CI 1.29−1.70; P<0.001) were higher after HLA-matched unrelated donor transplantation. The effect of donor type on nonrelapse mortality (NRM), relapse, and survival was confounded by performance score. In subjects with performance scores of 90 or 100%, risks of NRM (HR 1.42, 95% CI 1.15−1.74; P=0.001), relapse (HR 1.57, 95% CI 1.29−1.91; P<0.001), and death (HR 1.66, 95% CI 1.45−1.91; P=0.001) were higher after unrelated donor transplantation compared to

HLA-identical sibling transplantation. However, with performance scores less than 90%, NRM (HR 0.96, 95% CI 0.74−1.24; P=0.76), relapse (HR 0.86, 95% CI 0.66−1.12; P=0.25), and death (HR 0.90, 95% CI 0.75−1.09; P=0.29) were similar after HLA-matched sibling and HLA-matched unrelated donor transplants[1]. Considering acute and chronic GvHD risks and survival, the data support the notion that an HLA-matched sibling is the preferred donor even when the subject is >50 years old.

Peripheral Blood Cell Grafts *versus* Bone Marrow Grafts

Peripheral blood cell grafts have largely replaced *bone marrow* grafts for HLA-matched sibling donor transplants in adults, primarily attributed to ease of collection. This shift is supported by data from several clinical trials reporting comparable survivals in adults after both types of grafts[2]. However, in persons with chronic-phase chronic myeloid leukemia, *bone marrow* grafts are preferred because of less chronic GvHD[3] (see Chapter 38).

HLA Haplotype-Identical Donors

Most potential transplant recipients have one or more relatives who share an HLA haplotype. These donors are termed HLA-haplotype-matched or HLA-haplotype-mismatched causing considerable confusion. This confusion and preference for terms is caused by variability in numbers of HLA antigens matched or mismatched on the second HLA haplotype. For example, two people can share an HLA haplotype as well as one or more HLA antigens on the second haplotype. In this section I use the term HLA-haplotype-matched for these transplants.

There are several potential advantages of using this type of donor including immediate availability, flexibility in obtaining a graft, avoidance of an unrelated donor search (cost and time), and donor availability for repeated graft collections such as for therapy of relapse post-transplant (see Chapters 59 and 61). Early studies of HLA haplotype-identical transplants reported high rates of NRM, graft failure, and GvHD associated with increasing HLA disparity between donor and recipient[4,5]. Recently, several groups report improved outcomes after HLA haplotype-identical transplants. These studies used diverse strategies to overcome these problems by focusing on graft engineering. These can be fundamentally divided into those which manipulate the graft *in-vitro* pretransplant (Chapter 59) and those which give cyclophosphamide post-transplant. In one study, Aversa and colleagues selectively depleted T-cells in the graft with low rates of GvHD but substantial NRM[6]. In a recent report they combined this approach with infusion of T-cells and natural killer (NK) cells thought to increase antivirus immunity[7]. Although this approach seems effective, it is rarely used by others due to reasons discussed in subsequent text. In this study, and most others I discuss, there is no control cohort to prove the interventions being done are effective; most comparisons are to historical controls and are fraught with biases such as subject selection and small sample sizes. Others have reported results of *bone marrow* transplants followed by post-transplant cyclophosphamide after conventional or reduced intensity (RIC) pretransplant conditioning[8,9]. The NRM, graft failure, and GvHD rates are low. However, there is concern that relapse rates may be higher than compared to HLA-matched unrelated donor transplantation, a concern that can only be addressed with longer follow-up. Two recent reports on haploidentical donor transplantation also report favorable outcomes[10,11]. One study used high-dose post-transplant cyclophosphamide, cyclosporine, and mycophenolate after conventional conditioning [10]. Another used a complex GvHD prophylaxis regimen after conventional or RIC regimen[11]. The former report that employed post-transplant cyclophosphamide demonstrated adequate recovery of immune reconstitution as evidenced by CD4+ lymphocyte recovery at day +100 and +150 post-transplantation (see Chapter 22). Data on immune reconstitution are lacking for the later report. To date, the effect of HLA mismatching appears to be negligible[12,13]. It is possible that the augmented or selective elimination of T-cell alloreactivity (post-transplant cyclophosphamide) GvHD prophylaxis regimen may have mitigated the negative impact of HLA disparity to the point that outcomes of such transplants are comparable to outcomes after HLA-identical related and unrelated donor transplants[9].

HLA-Matched Unrelated Donors

Most data suggest a direct association between number of donor−recipient HLA-matches and transplant outcomes with the best outcomes when donor and recipient are matched at the allele-level at HLA-A, HLA-B, HLA-C, and HLA-DRB1 loci[14–16] (also see Chapter 8). Some data suggest a further benefit from matching at the HLA-DQ locus. However, >95% of donor−recipient pairs matched at the allele-level at HLA-A, HLA-B, HLA-C, and HLA-DRB1 are also matched at HLA-DQ. Also, an isolated mismatch at the HLA-DQ locus has no detectable adverse impact on survival[16,17].

The above conclusions are based on pooling data from *peripheral blood* and *bone marrow* grafts. However, *peripheral blood*-based grafts differ from *bone marrow* grafts because

they contain substantially more CD3+ and CD34+ cells. This difference might influence the impact of different degrees of HLA-matching. In a report limited to *peripheral blood* transplantation from unrelated donors, transplants mismatched at 1 HLA-locus for HLA-A, -B, -C, or -DRB1 was associated with higher mortality compared with transplants matched at HLA-A, -B, -C, and -DRB1[18]. These data suggest the effects of HLA mismatching on survival after unrelated donor transplantation are consistent regardless of graft type (see Chapters 8 and 9).

It is also important to know if the impact of HLA-matching on outcomes of conventional transplants also operates after RIC regimen transplants. A recent study reported results of matching at HLA-A, -B, -C, and -DRB1 in 2500 donor−recipient pairs receiving RIC regimen transplants. Most of these transplants were HLA-matched; only one-fifth were mismatched at ≥1 HLA-locus and there was no matching for HLA-DQ. Despite these limitations a 1 locus HLA mismatch was associated with higher mortality risks[19].

Practice Points

In summary, most data indicate an important role for HLA-matching on transplant outcomes after *unrelated* donor transplants using *peripheral blood* or *bone marrow* grafts following conventional "myeloablative" conditioning and RIC regimen (Figure 7.1).

Is Matching for HLA-DPB1 and Other Lesser Expressed (Low-Expression) HLA Alleles Important for Improved Outcomes after Allografts?

HLA-A, -B, -C, and -DRB1 are the *high-expression* HLA alleles. However, there are several *low-expression* HLA alleles. Matching between unrelated donors and recipients does not routinely consider these *low-expression* alleles. Three recent reports explored the effects of matching at these *low-expression* HLA alleles (see Chapter 8). Fleischauer and colleagues considered the impact of matching at HLA-DPB1 on transplant outcomes. Donor−recipient pairs were grouped as matched, permissive-, or nonpermissive mismatch based on T-cell epitope matching[20]. HLA-matched was defined as donor−recipient pairs matched at the allele-level at HLA-A, -B, -C, -DRB1, and -DQB1. There were no significant differences in mortality risks between HLA-matched transplants and transplants with a permissive mismatch at HLA-DPB1 locus. In contrast, nonpermissive mismatch at HLA-DPB1 locus was associated with a higher mortality risk for matched and 1 HLA-locus mismatched transplants. Interestingly, permissive mismatch at HLA-DPB1 locus was well tolerated with no significant differences in mortality risks between HLA-matched transplantations and single HLA-locus mismatched transplantations. These data support avoiding a nonpermissive mismatch at the HLA-DPB1 locus (see Figure 7.1). The report

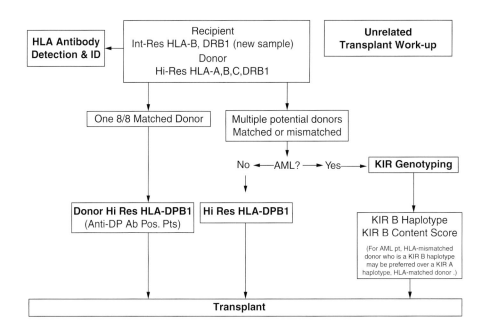

Figure 7.1. Recipient/sibling donor work-up.

by Pidala and colleagues also supports higher mortality after isolated nonpermissive HLA-DPB1 mismatched transplantations that are HLA-matched at HLA-A, -B, -C, and -DRB1[17].

Fernández-Viña et al. adopted a slightly different approach in that they explored the effects of multiple mismatches at HLA-DP, -DQ, and -DRB3/4/5[21]. Their results suggest that matching at *low-expression* HLA alleles can be ignored when donors and recipients are matched at the high-expression HLA alleles, i.e., matched at HLA-A, -B, -C, and -DRB1. However, single mismatch at any of the *high-expression* HLA alleles plus ≥3 mismatches (in the direction of graft-*versus*-host) at *low-expression* HLA alleles is associated with a higher mortality. Consequently, if there is 7/8 HLA-matched *unrelated* donor it is important to consider HLA-matching status at HLA-DP, DQ, and DRB3/4/5. In the absence of direct comparative studies after HLA-mismatched (7/8 matched) *unrelated* donor transplantations including three or more mismatches at the *low-expressing* HLA alleles it is impossible to offer definitive recommendations on the merits of selecting such an HLA-mismatched (7/8 HLA-matched) unrelated donor *versus* an alternative such as HLA-haploidentical donor or unrelated umbilical cord blood.

Availability of HLA-Matched Unrelated Donors

The huge polymorphism of HLA genes and allelic variation is population-specific. Consequently, sometimes an HLA-matched unrelated donor cannot be found even with large registries most of whose participants are persons of predominately European descent[22,23]. The Bioinformatics Division of the National Marrow Donor Program (NMDP) recently developed mathematical models to predict likelihood of identifying an HLA-matched unrelated donor for persons in the United States likely to benefit from a transplant[24]. Not surprisingly, the ethnic and racial group of a person influences the likelihood of finding a suitable donor. An HLA-matched unrelated donor can be easily identified for persons with common HLA genotypes. About 75% of persons of European descent will have an HLA-matched donor at the *high-expressing* alleles (HLA-A, -B, -C, -DRB1) and 25% will have a donor mismatched at one of the *high-expressing* HLA loci. For persons of other races and/or ethnicities, the likelihood of finding a completely HLA-matched donor is substantially lower (15–50%) but most non-Caucasians will have a donor mismatched at a single *high-expressing* locus. The model did not consider matching at the *low-expression* HLA alleles so the likelihood of finding an appropriate donor may be less than estimated.

Unrelated Cord Blood Grafts

Umbilical cord blood cells are increasingly used as a source of HLA-matched unrelated donors (see Chapters 60 and 66). Most cord blood transplants are done in children and adolescents. However, increasing numbers are being done in adults. Cord blood units are readily available and require less-stringent HLA-matching than unrelated adult donors. Several reports from observation databases that compared transplant outcomes in adults after HLA-matched *unrelated* donor and cord blood transplantation confirm similar rates of leukemia-free and overall survival except in selected populations such as first complete remission acute myeloid leukemia that showed an advantage for transplantation of grafts from an HLA-matched adult unrelated donor[25–28]. However, it should be noted that NRM rates are high after umbilical cord blood transplantation. This is in part being addressed by infusing relatively high cell doses by infusing two *unmanipulated* cord blood units, an *ex-vivo* expanded cord blood unit and an unmanipulated cord blood unit or combining one cord blood unit with CD34-selected *bone marrow* cells from a HLA-haplotype-matched relative[29–34]. All of these strategies support faster hematopoietic recovery but there are no published reports that support better leukemia-free or overall survival after transplantation of an *ex-vivo* expanded cord blood unit and an unmanipulated cord blood unit or combining a one cord blood unit with CD34-selected *bone marrow* cells from an HLA-haplotype-matched relative compared to that after transplantation of two unmanipulated cord blood cell units (see Chapter 66).

An important difference in selecting HLA-matched unrelated *peripheral blood* or *bone marrow* donors and a cord blood cell unit is criteria for HLA-matching. Unrelated blood cell and bone marrow are selected based on closeness of high-resolution HLA-matching[14–16]. In contrast, umbilical cord blood units are selected using low-resolution HLA typing (antigen-level) for HLA-A and -B and at the allele-level for HLA-DRB1. Matching for HLA-C is not typically considered in cord blood selection (see Chapter 60). However, two recent reports support allele-level HLA-matching including matching for HLA-C results in better hematopoietic recovery and less NRM in the setting of *single* umbilical cord blood transplantation for hematologic malignancy[35,36]. The effects of better HLA-matching, if any, in the setting of double cord blood transplantation is not known.

Controversies and Limitations in Selecting Donors When an HLA-Identical Sibling Is Not Available

When an HLA-matched sibling is not available most but not all would initiate a search for a suitably HLA-matched adult unrelated donor. Others, although a minority, would argue a mismatched related donor such as a haploidentical donor or unrelated cord blood graft are acceptable alternatives to matched sibling donor transplantation. The concept of prospectively randomizing subjects to an HLA-matched unrelated *versus* a mismatched related or umbilical cord blood is difficult for physician and patients alike. Therefore studies on transplantation outcomes with different types of donors have utilized data collected in large observational databases. Several of these studies that compared outcome after HLA-matched unrelated adult donor transplantation to that after mismatched umbilical cord blood transplantation are described above. Transplantation of grafts from an HLA-mismatched relative has been adopted only recently and there is a paucity of data comparing outcomes after this transplantation to others such as umbilical cord blood or HLA-matched unrelated donor. In the United States, there is a phase 3 clinical trial of the Blood and Marrow Transplant Clinical Trials Network (BMT CTN 1101) that randomizes subjects with acute leukemias or non-Hodgkin lymphomas to receive a transplant from an HLA-haplotype-matched relative or an HLA-mismatched transplant of two cord blood cell units. The trial, which opened late 2011, is expected to accrue over 4–4.5 years and the primary outcome is 2-year disease-free survival (see Chapter 61).

An often unaddressed issue is the time it takes between searching for a suitable *unrelated* adult donor and procuring the graft for transplantation. The average time needed to find an HLA-matched unrelated donor is about 7 weeks, which may be too long for a patient with acute leukemia in second remission. Another issue is donor attrition from unrelated donor registries. Attrition rates vary; higher attrition rates are associated with large-volume donor centers, donors in high-population, urban areas with large minority representation, and with less stable populations[37]. Commitment to donate, realistic expectations, few medical concerns, and frequent contact with the donor center are associated with less potential donor attrition[38]. These issues do not affect related donors, who are highly motivated, or umbilical cord blood units that are banked making them potentially attractive alternatives even when a suitable HLA-matched unrelated adult donor is available. However, the absence of published data prevents one from offering definitive recommendations on donor choice when a HLA-matched sibling is not available. Published reports suggest transplantation of grafts from a suitably HLA-matched unrelated donor, haploidentical relative, and umbilical cord blood are all acceptable and extends hematopoietic cell transplantation as a treatment option for everyone who may benefit from this treatment procedure

Safety, Regulations, and Registries

The rather large body of published work confirms transplantation from unrelated adult donor and banked unrelated umbilical cord blood is a safe procedure for patients and the transplantation of umbilical cord blood either as a single unit or two units to augment cell dose delivered has increased access to transplantation. With the exception of bone marrow, the Food and Drug Administration (FDA) has jurisdiction over all human and cellular-based products in the United States. Unlike accreditation which is voluntary, regulation is mandated by the governing body and provides a minimum set of standards to be able to provide a product, in this case, hematopoietic cells, within the regulated jurisdiction. In the United States, the majority of adult unrelated donor transplantations are facilitated by the NMDP. The NMDP maintains a donor registry, facilitates donor recruitment, and provides oversight and advocacy for its volunteer unrelated donors including their safety. The Center for Biologics, Evaluation, and Research (CBER) within the FDA has oversight of cord blood banking. CBER regulations require registration and listing of establishments that manufacture publically available cord blood units, established standards for donor eligibility (focus on safety and prevention of communicable diseases), application of current good tissue practice to cord blood banking (21 CFR 1271), and licensure (cord blood banks intending to sell units in the United States for clinical use hold a biologics license). Recognizing that the majority of units are stored in the United States and the fact that several hundred units annually are shipped from cord blood banks outside the United States, the FDA also issued guidance for creation of an Investigational New Drug (IND) application under which unlicensed cord blood units could still be used. The FDA guidance does not apply to autologous products or products intended for use in first or secondary relatives. Consequently, cord blood units stored for autologous use or for relatives need not be licensed and may be used for the treatment of diseases not specified for licensed unit use. A unique difference between the volunteer adult donor and banked unrelated umbilical cord blood is that the former may be contacted by the donor registry for subsequent donations for a patient whereas umbilical cord blood donation is "one-time only" and donor identity is protected with no subsequent contact with the donor or his/her family.

Practice Points for Selecting the Best Donor for Allograft

Most data support using an HLA-identical sibling donor if available. If not, several steps, not mutually exclusive, can be done including: (1) HLA typing of relatives to identify an HLA-haplotype-matched person(s); (2) searching large donor registries for a suitable HLA-matched unrelated donor; and (3) searching cord blood cell registries for a suitable unit(s). Results of these searches form the calculus for deciding on the *best* donor. An HLA-matched unrelated donor is typically the first choice in the absence of an HLA-matched sibling donor. If such a donor is not found one can consider an HLA-mismatched unrelated donor (7/8 HLA-matched), an HLA-haplotype-matched relative, or HLA-matched umbilical cord blood cells (Figure 7.1; implications of *KIR genotyping* in acute myelogenous leukemia are discussed elsewhere in this book). There are no data from randomized trials comparing these approaches and the imperfect data from controlled and uncontrolled trials suggest roughly comparable outcomes. Obviously only well-designed clinical trials can determine which approach, if any, is better.

References

1. Alousi AM, Le-Rademacher J, Saliba RM, *et al.* Who is the better donor for older hematopoietic transplant recipients: an older-aged sibling or a young, matched unrelated volunteer? *Blood.* 2013;121(13):2567–2773.

2. Stem Cell Trialists' Collaborative Group. Allogeneic peripheral blood stem-cell compared with bone marrow in the management of hematologic malignancies: an individual patient data meta-analysis of nine randomized trials. *J Clin Oncol.* 2005;23(22):5074–5087.

3. Schmitz N, Eapen M, Horowitz MM, *et al.* Long-term outcome of patients transplanted with mobilized blood or bone marrow: a report from the International Bone Marrow Transplant Registry and the European Group for Blood and Marrow Transplantation. *Blood.* 2006;108:4288–4290.

4. Anasetti C, Beatty PG, Storb R, *et al.* Effect of HLA incompatibility on graft-*versus*-host disease, relapse, and survival after marrow transplantation for patients with leukemia or lymphoma. *Hum Immunol.* 1990;29(2):79–91.

5. Szydlo R, Goldman JM, Klein JP, *et al.* Results of allogeneic bone marrow transplants for leukemia using donors other than HLA-identical siblings. *J Clin Oncol.* 1997;15(5):1767–1777.

6. Aversa F, Tabilio A, Velardi A, *et al.* Treatment of high risk acute leukemia with T-cell depleted stem cells from related donors with one fully mismatched haplotype. *N Eng J Med.* 1998;339(17):1186–1193.

7. Ruggeri L, Capanni M, Urbani E, Perruccio K, Shlomchik WD. Effectiveness of donor natural killer cell alloreactivity in mismatched hematopoietic transplants. *Science.* 2002;295(5562):2097–2100.

8. Luznik L, O'Donnell PV, Symons HJ, *et al.* HLA-haploidentical bone marrow transplantation for hematologic malignancies using nonmyeloablative conditioning and high-dose, posttransplantation cyclophosphamide. *Biol Blood Marrow Transplant.* 2008;14(6):641–650.

9. Bashey A, Zhang X, Sizemore CA, *et al.* T-Cell replete HLA-haploidentical hematopoietic transplantation for hematologic malignancies using post-transplantation cyclophosphamide results in outcomes equivalent to those of contemporaneous HLA-matched related and unrelated donor transplantation. *J Clin Oncol.* 2013;31(10):1310–1316.

10. Raiola AM, Dominietto A, Ghiso A, *et al.* Unmanipulated haploidentical bone marrow transplantation and posttransplant cyclophosphamide for hematologic malignancies after myeloablative conditioning. *Biol Blood Marrow Transplant.* 2013;19(1):117–122.

11. Di Bartolomeo P, Santarone S, De Angelis G, *et al.* Haploidentical unmanipulated GCSF primed bone marrow transplantation for patients with high-risk hematologic malignancies. *Blood.* 2013;121(5):849–857.

12. Kasamon YL, Luznik L, Leffell MS, *et al.* Nonmyeloablative HLA-haploidentical BMT with high-dose post-transplantation cyclophosphamide: effect of HLA disparity on outcome. *Biol Blood Marrow Transplant.* 2010;16(4):482–489.

13. Huo MR, Xu L, Li D, *et al.* The effect of HLA disparity on clinical outcome after HLA-haploidentical blood and marrow transplantation. *Clin Transplant.* 2012;26(2):284–291.

14. Morishima Y, Sasazuki T, Inoko H, *et al.* The clinical significance of human leukocyte antigen (HLA) allele compatibility in patients receiving a marrow transplant from serologically HLA-A, HLA-B and HLA-DR matched unrelated donors. *Blood.* 2002;99(11):4200–4206.

15. Flomenberg N, Baxter-Lowe LA, Confer D, *et al.* Impact of HLA class I and class II high-resolution matching on outcomes of unrelated donor bone marrow transplantation: HLA-C mismatching is associated with a strong adverse effect on transplantation outcome. *Blood.* 2004;104(7):1923–1930.

16. Lee SJ, Klein J, Haagenson M, *et al.* High-resolution donor-recipient HLA matching contributes to the success of unrelated donor marrow transplantation. *Blood.* 2007;110(13):4576–4583.

17. Pidala J, Lee SJ, Ahn KW, *et al.* Non-permissive HLA-DPB1 mismatch increases mortality after myeloablative unrelated allogeneic hematopoietic cell transplantation. *Blood.* 2014;124(16):2596–2606.

18. Woolfrey A, Klein JP, Haagenson M, *et al.* HLA-C antigen mismatch is associated with worse outcome in unrelated donor peripheral blood stem cell transplantation. *Biol Blood Marrow Transplant.* 2011;17(6):885–892.

19. Koreth J, Ahn KW, Pidala J, *et al.* HLA-mismatch is associated with worse outcomes after unrelated donor reduced intensity hematopoietic cell transplantation: a CIBMTR analysis. *Blood.* 2013;122:547a.

20. Fleischhauer K, Shaw BE, Gooley T, *et al.* Effect of T-cell-epitope matching at HLA-DPB1 in recipients of unrelated donor haematopoietic cell transplantation: a retrospective study. *Lancet Oncol.* 2012;13(4):366–374.

21. Fernández-Viña MA, Klein JP, Haagenson M, *et al.* Multiple mismatches at the low expression HLA loci DP, DQ, and DR3/4/5 associate with adverse outcomes in hematopoietic stem cell transplantation. *Blood.* 2013;121(22):4603–4610.

22. Beatty PG, Mori M, Milford E. Impact of racial genetic polymorphism on the probability of finding an HLA-matched donor. *Transplantation.* 1995;60(8):778–783.

23. Kollman C, Maiers M, Gragert L, *et al.* Estimation of HLA-A, -B, -DRB1 haplotype frequencies using mixed resolution data from a national registry with selective retyping of volunteers. *Hum Immunol.* 2007;68(12):950–958.

24. Garget L, Eapen M, Williams E, *et al.* HLA match likelihoods for unrelated donor grafts in the U.S. registry. *N Engl J Med.* 2014;371(4):339–348.

25. Eapen M, Rocha V, Sanz G, *et al.* Effect of graft source on unrelated donor haematopoietic stem-cell transplantation in adults with acute leukaemia: a retrospective analysis. *Lancet Oncol.* 2010;11(7):653–660.

26. Brunstein CG, Gutman JA, Weisdorf DJ, *et al.* Allogeneic hematopoietic cell transplantation for hematologic malignancy: relative risk and benefits of double umbilical cord blood. *Blood.* 2010;116(22):4693–4699.

27. Brunstein CG, Eapen M, Ahn KW, *et al.* Reduced-intensity conditioning transplantation in acute leukemia: the effect of source of unrelated donor stem cells on outcomes. *Blood.* 2012;119(23):5591–5598.

28. Weisdorf D, Eapen M, Ruggeri A, *et al.* Alternative donor hematopoietic transplantation for older patients with AML in first complete remission: a center for international blood and marrow transplant research-eurocord analysis. *Biol Blood Marrow Transplant.* 2014;20(6):816–822.

29. Brunstein CG, Barker JN, Weisdorf DJ, *et al.* Umbilical cord blood transplantation after nonmyeloablative conditioning: impact on transplantation outcomes in 110 adults with hematologic disease. *Blood.* 2007;110(8):3064–3070.

30. Scaradavou A, Brunstein CG, Eapen M, *et al.* Double unit grafts successfully extend the application of umbilical cord blood transplantation in adults with acute leukemia. *Blood.* 2013;121(5):752–758.

31. van Besien K, Liu H, Jain N, Stock W, Artz A. Umbilical cord blood transplantation supported by third-party donor cells: rationale, results and applications. *Biol Blood Marrow Transplant.* 2013;19(5):682–691.

32. Liu H, Rich ES, Godley L, *et al.* Reduced-intensity conditioning with combined haploidentical and cord blood transplantation results in rapid engraftment, low GvHD and durable remission. *Blood.* 2011;118(24):6438–6445.

33. Delaney C, Heimfeld S, Brashem-Stein C, Voorhies H, Manger RL, Bernstein ID. Notch-mediated expansion of human cord blood progenitor cells capable of rapid myeloid reconstitution. *Nat Med.* 2010;16(20):232–236.

34. de Lima M, McNiece I, Robinson SN, *et al.* Cord-blood engraftment with ex vivo mesenchymal-cell coculture. *N Engl J Med.* 2012;367(24):2305–2315.

35. Eapen M, Klein JP, Sanz GF, *et al.* Effect of donor-recipient HLA matching at HLAA, B, C and DRB1 on outcomes after umbilical-cord blood transplantation for leukaemia and myelodysplastic syndrome: a retrospective analysis. *Lancet Oncol.* 2011;12(13):1214–1221.

36. Eapen M, Klein JP, Ruggeri A, *et al.* Impact of allele-level HLA matching on outcomes after myeloablative single unit umbilical cord blood transplantation for hematologic malignancy. *Blood.* 2014;123(1):133–140.

37. Myaskovsky L, Switzer GE, Dew MA, Goycoolea JM, Confer DL, Abress L. The association of donor center characteristics with attrition from the National Marrow Donor Registry. *Transplantation.* 2004;77(6):874–880.

38. Switzer GE, Dew MA, Goycoolea JM, Myaskovsky L, Abress L, Confer DL. Attrition of potential bone marrow donors at two key decision points leading to donation. *Transplantation.* 2004;77(10):1529–1534.

Chapter

8

Unrelated Donor Selection: Human Leukocyte Antigen Testing and Matching – Permissive and Non–permissive Matches

Stephen Spellman and Bronwen E. Shaw

Introduction

Allogeneic hematopoietic cell transplant (HCT) offers the opportunity for a durable cure for a myriad of malignant and nonmalignant diseases. The optimal allogeneic donor choice is an HLA-identical sibling donor; however, the majority of patients (~70%) will not have a suitable match within their family. Patients without an optimal related donor can turn to alternative sources of allogeneic grafts including volunteer unrelated donors and cryopreserved umbilical cord blood units (UCB). Unrelated donor and UCB selection has evolved over time with the advent of more advanced high-resolution HLA testing technologies and observational studies that have demonstrated the importance of specific HLA loci and donor demographics for optimal HCT outcomes. This chapter provides an evidence-based review of the literature to define the state of the art requirements for HLA typing and matching for unrelated graft sources. In addition, the chapter includes a discussion of efforts to identify permissive and non-permissive mismatches to optimize graft selection for patients unable to identify an optimally HLA-matched unrelated graft source.

Current Standard for HLA Testing and Matching

HLA testing technologies and matching strategies have evolved significantly since the first use of unrelated donors in the late 1980s[1]. The advent of DNA-based typing technologies and enhanced databases of well characterized HLA allele sequences have increased the precision and accuracy of typing leading to improved matching. Current National Marrow Donor Program/Be The Match guidelines recommend that potential unrelated donor candidates undergo complete HLA-A, -B, -C, -DRB1/3/4/5, -DQB1, and -DPB1 high-resolution DNA-based testing to select the best HLA match[2]. High-resolution matching is defined as identical HLA DNA sequences between the donor and recipient across the antigen-binding domain, i.e., exons 2 and 3 for HLA class I (HLA-A, -B, and -C) and exon 2 for HLA class II (HLA-DRB1)[3]. Multiple methodologies exist to generate HLA typing at the high-resolution level, e.g., high-definition sequence-specific oligonucleotide probe-based, traditional Sanger sequencing and next generation sequencing techniques (Table 8.1). The specific methodology employed to generate an HLA typing is not critical. The critical element is having the support from an American Society of Histocompatibility and Immunogenetics (ASHI) or European Federation for Immunogenetics (EFI) accredited laboratory with guidance from an accredited histocompatibility and immunogenetics laboratory director to assist the clinical team with interpretation of the typing results and match assessment between the prospective donor(s) and patient.

Along with the evolution of typing techniques, the definition of an optimal HLA-match has changed over time. The current National Marrow Donor Program (NMDP)/Center for International Blood and Marrow Transplant Research (CIBMTR)[2]and Blood and Marrow Transplant Clinical Trials Network[4] standard for an optimal match is a high-resolution match at HLA-A, -B, -C, and -DRB1 (8/8 match). The 8/8 match standard is supported by multiple large studies that have found strong associations with matching at HLA-A, -B, -C, and -DRB1 and overall survival[5–8]. The optimal match definition can also be augmented by applying various *tie-breaker criteria* among donors equivalently matched at HLA-A, -B, -C, and -DRB1. For example, donor-specific anti-HLA antibodies are a potent barrier to engraftment and have been demonstrated to target most HLA loci including the *low-expression* loci (HLA-DQB1 and DPB1)[9,10] (see Chapter 9). Patient HLA sensitivities should be evaluated and mismatches avoided in the selected donor, if possible. An unrelated donor selection hierarchy is illustrated in Figure 8.1 and incorporates additional tie-breaker criteria that will be discussed further in the chapter.

Unfortunately, not all searching patients will find an optimal match and they will have to pursue a HLA-mismatched donor. The likelihood of finding a suitably HLA-matched unrelated donor or umbilical cord blood unit varies significantly due to the racial and ethnic background of the patient (see also Chapter 7). A recent study from the NMDP led by Gragert *et al.* evaluated the likelihood of finding a match among 21 distinct racial/ethnic subgroups defined within the United States population (Figure 8.2)[11]. The likelihood of finding an optimally matched (8/8 match at HLA-A, -B, -C, and -DRB1) ranged from 75% for patients of European descent down to 16% for black people of South or Central American descent. With other suitably matched donors (7/8 match) or

Table 8.1 HLA typing techniques and resulting resolution

Methodology	Approach	Interpretation	Resolution	Application	Results
Serology	Cellular assay based on complement fixation by HLA-specific antibodies	Cell death – yes/no	Low	Family screening Null allele confirmation	A2, A24
Sequence-specific primers (PCR-SSP)	HLA sequence-specific PCR primers	Amplification – yes/no	Low to high, dependent on DNA sequence coverage	Family screening Verification typing	Low — A*02:XX, A*24:XX or A*02AB, A*24:BC High – A*0201g, A*24:02g
Sequence-specific oligonucleotide probes (PCR-SSOP)	HLA sequence-specific oligonucleotide probes that bind to polymorphic sequences of amplified DNA	Probe binding – yes/no	Low to high depending on DNA sequence coverage	Family screening Verification typing	Low — A*02:XX, A*24:XX or A*02AB, A*24:BC High – A*02:01G, A*24:02G
Sanger sequence-based typing (SBT)	HLA amplicon sequencing using base termination	Base pair reads and consensus alignment	High to allele-level depending on coverage	All	High – A*02:01G, A*24:02G Allele – A*02:01:01:03, A*24:02:01:01
Next generation sequencing (NGS)	Multiple platforms, based on massive parallel sequencing reactions	Base pair calling and consensus alignment	High to allele-level depending on coverage	All	High – A*02:01G, A*24:02G Allele – A*02:01:01:03, A*24:02:01:01

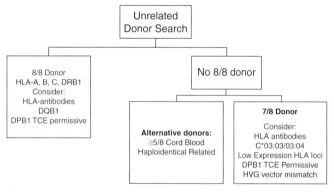

Figure 8.1. Diagram illustrating the HLA-matching factors that should be considered in the selection of unrelated donors. TCE, T-cell epitope; low-expression HLA loci — HLA-DP, DQ, and DRB 3,4,5; HVG, host-*versus*-graft.

umbilical cord blood units (≥4/6 match), the likelihoods increase to over 90% for adult (>20 years old) and over 95% for pediatric (<20 years old) patients.

How Should HLA-Mismatched Donors Be Prioritized?

Many studies have attempted to define permissive and nonpermissive HLA mismatches. The following section will describe various approaches and the relative utility of each, and summarize the negative and positive findings with recommendations for incorporation into donor prioritization in the HLA-mismatched setting.

HLA Mismatch Prioritization Algorithms and Strategies

Various investigators have attempted to develop algorithms to stratify HLA mismatch risk. These approaches varied from serologic cross-reactivity to complex models based on the structure and function of HLA molecules and their interactions with the T-cell receptor (Table 8.2).

Cross-Reactive Groups (CREGs)

Wade *et al.* investigated the benefit of matching for HLA alleles that belonged to serologic cross-reactive groups (CREGs), the rationale being that alleles that generated cross-reactive HLA antibodies would be structurally similar and therefore less likely to generate an alloreactive response. A cohort of 2709 cases was scored for CREG mismatches at HLA-A or -B according to the Rodey *et al.* scheme. HLA-A or -B mismatches within CREG groups were coded as a minor mismatch and those outside CREG groups as major mismatches. When compared to fully HLA-matched cases, CREG matched donors and recipients had similar outcomes to pairs mismatched for alleles outside of CREG groups[12].

HLA Matchmaker

The HLA Matchmaker algorithm, developed by Rene Duquesnoy et al., proved effective at predicting kidney graft survival in the HLA-mismatched setting[13]. The algorithm considers short sequences of polymorphic amino acid residues in the mismatched HLA molecule as key elements of immunogenic

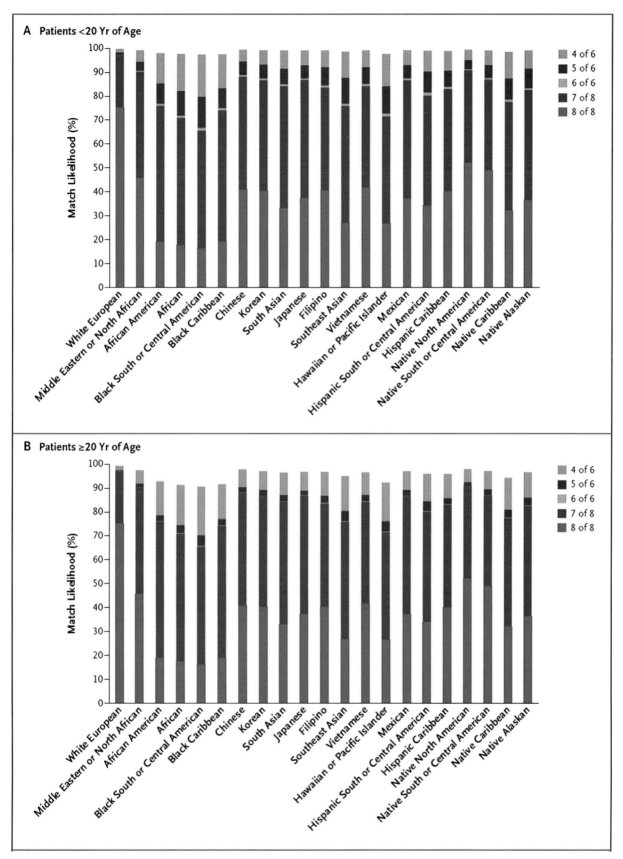

Figure 8.2. HLA-match likelihoods according to racial/ethnic group and age. Likelihood of finding a suitable HLA match (defined as an 8/8 or 7/8 adult unrelated donor or ≥4/6 single or double umbilical cord blood unit(s) with a minimum cell dose of 2.5 x 10⁷/kg) for (A) a pediatric patient (<20 years of age) and (B) an adult patient (>20 year of age), respectively.

Table 8.2 Failed HLA mismatch prioritization algorithms

Algorithm	Studies	Approach	Results
Cross-reactive groups (CREGs)	Wade et al. 2007[12]	Scoring based on HLA mismatch sharing of CREGs	No benefit of selecting HLA mismatches within CREGs
HLA Matchmaker	Duquesnoy et al. 2008[14]	Mismatch scoring based on structural epitope sharing between HLA molecules	No association between epitope sharing and clinical outcome
HistoCheck	Shaw et al. 2004[17], Askar et al. 2011[18], Spellman et al. 2012[19]	Mismatch scoring based on HLA molecular similarity	No association between HistoCheck score and clinical outcome

epitopes. Duquesnoy et al. hypothesized that the allogenicity predicted by HLA Matchmaker may also be applicable to the mismatched unrelated donor transplant setting. They evaluated a cohort of 744 unrelated HCT cases with 1 HLA-A, -B, or -C mismatch and 1690 fully HLA-A, -B, -C, -DR, or -DQ allele-matched cases. In multivariate models adjusting for other significant clinical risk factors, the degree of triplet mismatching did not significantly correlate with any outcomes[14].

HistoCheck

Elsner and Blasczyk hypothesized that a rating system based on the structure of HLA class I molecules might be used to identify acceptable mismatches[15]. They developed the HistoCheck algorithm that scored HLA mismatches based on the functional similarity of amino acids using a distance matrix developed by Risler et al.[16] and assigned importance based on the position of the disparity in the HLA molecule (i.e., location in the peptide binding or T-cell receptor recognition site). Shaw et al. used HistoCheck to score 26 single HLA-A allele mismatched recipients and nine single HLA-B mismatches in the Anthony Nolan clinical database [17]. No associations were observed between the HistoCheck scores and neutrophil engraftment, acute or chronic graft-versus-host disease (GvHD), relapse, or survival in this small study. Askar et al.[18] evaluated the correlation between HistoCheck score and high-risk HLA allele mismatch combinations previously described by Kawase et al. They found that HistoCheck score distribution was no different between high- and low-risk allele combinations, and did not correlate with mismatch risk stratification in the Japanese population. The CIBMTR evaluated the HistoCheck algorithm in a cohort of 744 cases of single HLA class I mismatched transplants. HistoCheck scores were tested as a categorical variable by quartiles and also as a continuous variable. The analysis found no differences among the quartiles and no association between increasing scores and worse outcomes [19]. The findings suggested that the HistoCheck scoring system for HLA class I mismatches was not predictive of transplant outcomes as measured by survival, GvHD, relapse, or engraftment and were consistent with the prior studies from Shaw and Askar.

Evaluation of Amino Acid Substitutions and Positions

Multiple studies have attempted to evaluate the impact of mismatching at specific amino acid (AA) positions. A study by Ferrara et al. was the first to describe a high-risk/non-permissive AA position. They found that AA116 in HLA class I was associated with increased risk for acute GvHD and treatment-related mortality (TRM)[20]. The acute GvHD risk finding was validated and refined in a recent study by Pidala et al. The group demonstrated that an HLA-C mismatch at AA116 conferred increased risk for severe acute GvHD above risk imposed by other mismatches[21]. Additional studies have attempted to classify specific AA mismatches as high risk or protective and are summarized in Table 8.3.

Identification of Permissive HLA Mismatches

HLA Mismatch Direction

HLA mismatches can be characterized by directionality based on the presence of an alloreactive target within the host or graft. Host-versus-graft (HvG) only vector mismatches occur when the recipient is homozygous (HLA-A*02:01/02:01) and the donor heterozygous (HLA*02:01/24:01) for the mismatched locus. Graft-versus-host (GvH) only vector mismatches can occur when the donor is homozygous (HLA-A*02:01/02:01) and the recipient heterozygous (HLA*02:01/24:01). Bidirectional mismatches occur when both the donor (HLA-A*02:01/24:01) and recipient (HLA-A*01:01/24:01) carry an alloreactive target. Two recent studies have evaluated the impact of unidirectional mismatching in unrelated donor HCT. Hurley et al. assessed the impact of HLA homozygosity at mismatched loci in a cohort of 2687 myeloablative unrelated donor HCT for malignant disease based on 8/8, 7/8 HvG only, 7/8 GvH only, and 7/8 bidirectional mismatches[25]. HvG mismatches lead to lower levels of aGvHD compared to GvH only or bidirectional mismatches and were not significantly different than the 8/8 group. All the 7/8 groups were associated with worse overall survival compared to the fully matched group. Kanda et al. evaluated a cohort of 3756 unrelated donor HCT cases for hematologic malignancy. The group observed that bidirectional HLA mismatches were associated with increased risk of aGvHD and worse OS and TRM

Table 8.3 Summary of some of the studies that have attempted to identify high-risk amino acid or allele combinations

Study	Locus/gene	Numbers	Patient and transplant characteristics	Era	Outcomes
Ferrara et al., 2001[20]	Amino acid	100	CML and other leukemia MA TC-replete marrow	1994–1999	Non-permissive amino acid MM: MM at position 116 in HLA class I associated with increased risk of aGvHD and TRM.
Kawase et al., 2007[22]	Allele combinations	5210	Various diseases MA/RIC TC-replete marrow, <10% ATG	1993–2006	Non-permissive HLA MM: Identified 16 high-risk HLA allele combinations associated with aGvHD grades III–IV (4 – HLA-A, 1 – HLA-B, 7 – HLA-C, 1 – HLA-DRB1, 2 – HLA-DPB1 and 1 – HLA-DRB1-DQB1 combination). Non-permissive amino acid MM: Identified 6 HLA class I amino acid MM associated with aGvHD grades III–IV
Kawase et al., 2009[23]	Amino acid	4643	ALL, AML, CML, malignant lymphoma, MM TC-replete marrow, <10% ATG	1993–2005	Relapse protection MM: 4 – HLA-C and 6 – HLA-DPB1 MM combinations associated with a decreased risk of relapse and better OS than fully matched pairs. Specific amino acid MM in HLA-C, but not HLA-DPB1 associated with less relapse
Marino et al., 2012[24]	Amino acid	2107	ALL, AML, CML and MDS MA TC-replete	1988–2004	31 AAS associated with increased risk of day 100 mortality
Pidala et al., 2013[21]	Amino acid	7313	ALL, AML, CML and MDS MA/RIC TC-replete/TCD	1988–2009	Non-permissive amino acid MM: HLA-C AAS 99 associated with increased TRM. HLA-C AAS 116 associated with increased aGvHD III–IV. HLA-B AAS 9 associated with increased cGvHD

compared to fully HLA-matched donor and recipients[26]. GvH only mismatches were associated with increased aGvHD risk, but did not differ from the fully matched group for OS and TRM. HvG only mismatches did not differ from the fully HLA-matched group for any outcomes. These results differed from the Hurley et al. findings suggesting that the limited numbers of unidirectional mismatches in each study may have led to some instability in the models. The consistent finding that HvG only mismatches associated with lower rates of acute GvHD appears to make the most biologic sense and could be applied to 7/8 HLA-mismatched donor prioritization.

HLA Expression Level Effects

Not all HLA molecules are expressed at the same level on the cell surface leading some investigators to believe that some loci or alleles may be more immunogenic than others. HLA-A, -B, and -DRB1 are considered high-expression loci (HEL) with all allotypes constitutively expressed. HLA-C and -DPB1 alleles vary in expression level due to polymorphisms in the promoter regions upstream of the loci[27]. Petersdorf et al. evaluated the association between the HLA-C allotype expression levels and mismatching. Using a cohort of 1975 HLA-C mismatched unrelated donor HCT for various diseases, they found that recipient HLA-C expression levels associated with an increased

risk of acute GvHD and mortality and mismatches with low-expression alleles were well tolerated[28]. Petersdorf et al. demonstrated lower expression levels of HLA-DPB1 in individuals carrying a genetic marker for a low-expression variant. Following assessment of expression variant linkage to single mismatched HLA-DPB1 alleles in a cohort of 1441 HLA-A, -B, -C, -DRB1, and -DQB1 matched unrelated donor HCT for ALL, AML, CML, and MDS, they found that the risk of acute GvHD was higher for high-expression recipients receiving grafts from low-expression donors[29]. HLA-DRB3/4/5, -DQA1, -DQB1, and -DPA1 are also expressed at lower levels on the cell surface. Single mismatches at HLA-DRB3/4/5, -DQ, or -DP have not been demonstrated to associate with a decrease in OS. However, a recent study by Fernández-Viña et al. found that in the 7/8 matched setting minimizing the cumulative total of mismatches of HLA-DP, -DQ, and -DRB3/4/5 to <3 resulted in improved survival[30] (see Chapter 7).

Permissive HLA-C Mismatch: HLA-C*03:03/*03:04

An interesting finding from the Lee et al. Blood 2007 study was that HLA-C allele-level mismatches did not appear to correlate with worse outcomes, while outcomes for all other loci (HLA-A, -B, and -DRB1) were demonstrated to not differ between allele versus antigen mismatches. Fernández-Viña and colleagues hypothesized that this difference at the HLA-C locus

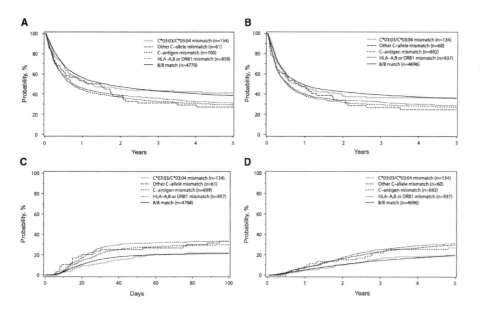

Figure 8.3. Adjusted probabilities of (**A**) overall survival, (**B**) disease-free survival, (**C**) grade III–IV acute GvHD, and (**D**) transplant-related mortality in patients presenting no mismatch (8/8), HLA-C*03:03/C*03:04 mismatch, other HLA-C allele mismatch, HLA-C antigen mismatch, or one mismatch in either HLA-A, B or DRB1 loci.

may be due to the permissivity of a specific mismatch, HLA-C*03:03 *versus* *03:04. This particular mismatch is quite common in the US Caucasian population and accounted for 69% of the HLA-C allele-level mismatches in the Lee *et al.* cohort. Prior *in-vitro* analyses by Oudshoorn *et al.* demonstrated that mixed lymphocyte cultures mismatched for only HLA-C*03:03/03:04 failed to generate a cytotoxic T-cell response[31]. This was surprising as the alleles C*03:03/C*03:04 type distinctly by serology as HLA-Cw9 and Cw10, respectively. HLA-C*03:03 and C*03:04 differ by a single amino acid substitution that is located outside the antigen-recognition site, so it is likely that this difference does not impact peptide binding or the T-cell receptor interaction domain. Fernandez-Viña *et al.* evaluated a cohort of 6633 cases and found that the C*03:03/C*03:04 mismatched and the 8/8 matched groups had virtually identical outcomes. In contrast, all other 7/8 matched cases were associated with worse OS (Figure 8.3)[32].

Permissive HLA-DPB1 Mismatch: T-Cell Epitope Groups

HLA-DPB1 is difficult to match in unrelated donors due to the poor linkage disequilibrium with other HLA loci. HLA-DPB1 allele mismatching consistently associates with increased risks of acute GvHD and TRM with a corresponding benefit of lower relapse, but varies in associations with OS[5–8]. Zino *et al.* observed that certain combinations of HLA-DPB1 mismatches elicited varying degrees of cytotoxic T-cell responses *in-vitro* and developed a classification scheme that defined permissive and non-permissive mismatches[33]. Several large retrospective studies have shown that the T-cell epitope (TCE) algorithm can be used to classify HLA-DPB1 mismatched HCT pairs into permissive and non-permissive mismatched groups that associate with OS (Figure 8.4)[34,5]. The majority of searching patients (>70%) should be able to identify a

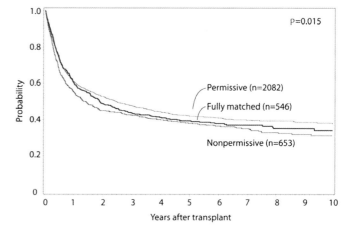

Figure 8.4. Adjusted OS curves for HLA-DPB1 matched, permissive mismatch, and non-permissive mismatch cases.

matched or permissive HLA-DPB1 mismatched donor, which is significant improvement over the ~20% that find an HLA allele-level match (Figure 8.4).

Controversies and Future Directions

HLA mismatches are associated with bad outcomes with very few exceptions as discussed. Many investigators have attempted to define a continuum of risk associated with various HLA mismatches at the molecular, antibody epitope, and allele level with limited success. What is clear is that the HLA-peptide-T-cell receptor interaction is a highly specific, sensitive, and complex system that can detect minute changes in structure and expression levels resulting in a robust alloreactive response in the unrelated HCT setting. Even perfectly HLA-matched transplants (matched sibling donor) experience aGvHD and TRM rates that are undesirable. The impact of minor histocompatibility antigens cannot be overlooked. New strategies to suppress or abrogate the alloreactive immune response while preserving the graft-*versus*-cancer effect required to cure hematologic malignancy are desperately needed. However, there may be hope in the form of 1950s technology. Post-transplant high-dose cyclophosphamide G*v*HD prophylaxis strategies employed successfully in HLA haplotype mismatched HCT[35,36] may be extensible to the mismatched unrelated donor setting. This would permit all patients in need to receive a suitable graft with the best HLA match available without fear of a strong alloreactive response and prolonged immune suppression. The suitability of the post-transplant cyclophosphamide approach in unrelated donors remains to be seen and trials are warranted.

References

1. Spellman S, Setterholm M, Maiers M, Noreen H, Oudshoorn M, Fernandez-Viña M *et al*. Advances in the selection of HLA-compatible donors: refinements in HLA typing and matching over the first 20 years of the National Marrow Donor Program Registry. *Biol Blood Marrow Transplant*. 2008;14(9 Suppl):37–44. doi: 10.1016/j.bbmt.2008.05.001. Epub 2008 Jun 20 (Review).

2. Spellman SR, Eapen M, Logan BR, Mueller C, Rubinstein P, Setterholm MI *et al*.; National Marrow Donor Program; Center for International Blood and Marrow Transplant Research. A perspective on the selection of unrelated donors and cord blood units for transplantation. *Blood*. 2012;120 (2):259–65. doi: 10.1182/blood-2012-03-379032. Epub 2012 May 17.

3. Nunes E, Heslop H, Fernandez-Vina M, Taves C, Wagenknecht DR, Eisenbrey AB *et al*. Definitions of histocompatibility typing terms. *Blood*. 2011;118(23):e180–3. doi:10.1182/ blood-2011-05-353490. Epub 2011 Oct 14.

4. Howard CA, Fernandez-Vina MA, Appelbaum FR, Confer DL, Devine SM, Horowitz MM *et al*. Recommendations for donor human leukocyte antigen assessment and matching for allogeneic stem cell transplantation: consensus opinion of the Blood and Marrow Transplant Clinical Trials Network (BMT CTN). *Biol Blood Marrow Transplant*. 2015;21(1):4–7. doi: 10.1016/j.bbmt.2014.09.017. Epub 2014 Sep 30.

5. Pidala J, Lee SJ, Ahn KW, Spellman S, Wang HL, Aljurf M *et al*. Nonpermissive HLA-DPB1 mismatch increases mortality after myeloablative unrelated allogeneic hematopoietic cell transplantation. *Blood*. 2014;124 (16):2596–606. doi: 10.1182/blood-2014-05-576041. Epub 2014 Aug 26.

6. Lee SJ, Klein J, Haagenson M, Baxter-Lowe LA, Confer DL, Eapen M *et al*. High-resolution donor-recipient HLA matching contributes to the success of unrelated donor marrow transplantation. *Blood*. 2007;110(13):4576–83. Epub 2007 Sep 4.

7. Verneris MR, Lee SJ, Ahn KW, Wang HL, Battiwalla M, Inamoto Y *et al*. HLA mismatch is associated with worse outcomes after unrelated donor reduced-intensity conditioning hematopoietic cell transplantation: an analysis from the Center for International Blood and Marrow Transplant Research. *Biol Blood Marrow Transplant*. 2015 Jun 6. pii: S1083-8791(15)00389-4. doi: 10.1016/j. bbmt.2015.05.028 Epub ahead of print.

8. Fürst D, Müller C, Vucinic V, Bunjes D, Herr W, Gramatzki M *et al*. High-resolution HLA matching in hematopoietic stem cell transplantation: a retrospective collaborative analysis. *Blood*. 2013;122(18):3220–9. doi: 10.1182/blood-2013-02-482547. Epub 2013 Sep 17. [Erratum in: Blood. 2014 Mar 13;123(11):1768.]

9. Spellman S, Bray R, Rosen-Bronson S, Haagenson M, Klein J, Flesch S *et al*. The detection of donor-directed, HLA-specific alloantibodies in recipients of unrelated hematopoietic cell transplantation is predictive of graft failure. *Blood*. 2010;115(13):2704–8. doi:10.1182/blood-2009-09-244525. Epub 2010 Jan 20.

10. Ciurea SO, Thall PF, Wang X, Wang SA, Hu Y, Cano P *et al*. Donor-specific anti-HLA Abs and graft failure in matched unrelated donor hematopoietic stem cell transplantation. *Blood*. 2011;118(22):5957–64. doi: 10.1182/blood-2011-06-362111. Epub 2011 Oct 3.

11. Gragert L, Eapen M, Williams E, Freeman J, Spellman S, Baitty R *et al*. HLA match likelihoods for hematopoietic stem-cell grafts in the U.S. registry. *N Engl J Med*. 2014;371 (4):339–48. doi: 10.1056/ NEJMsa1311707.

12. Wade JA, Hurley CK, Takemoto SK, Thompson J, Davies SM, Fuller TC *et al*. HLA mismatching within or outside of cross-reactive groups (CREGs) is associated with similar outcomes after unrelated hematopoietic stem cell transplantation. *Blood*. 2007;109(9):4064–70. Epub 2007 Jan 3.

13. Duquesnoy RJ, Takemoto S, de Lange P, Doxiadis II, Schreuder GM, Persijn GG *et al*. HLA matchmaker: a molecularly based algorithm for histocompatibility determination. III. Effect of matching at the HLA-A,B amino acid triplet level on kidney transplant survival. *Transplantation*. 2003;75(6):884–9.

14. Duquesnoy R, Spellman S, Haagenson M, Wang T, Horowitz MM, Oudshoorn M. HLA matchmaker-defined triplet matching is not associated with better survival rates of patients with class I HLA allele mismatched hematopoietic cell transplants from unrelated donors. *Biol Blood Marrow Transplant*. 2008;14 (9):1064–71. doi: 10.1016/j. bbmt.2008.07.001.

15. Elsner H, Blasczyk R. Sequence similarity matching: proposal of a structure-based rating system for bone marrow transplantation. *Eur J Immunogenet*. 2002;29:229–36.

16. Risler JL, Delorme MO, Delacroix H, Henaut A. Amino acid substitutions in structurally related proteins: A pattern recognition approach. Determination of a new and efficient scoring matrix. *J Mol Biol*. 1988; 204(4):1019–29.

17. Shaw BE, Barber LD, Madrigal JA, Cleaver S, Marsh SG. Scoring for HLA matching? A clinical test of HistoCheck. *Bone Marrow Transplant*. 2004; 34 (4):367–8.

18. Askar M, Sobecks R, Morishima Y, Kawase T, Nowacki A, Makishima H *et al*. Predictions in the face of clinical reality: HistoCheck versus high-risk HLA allele mismatch combinations responsible for severe acute graft-versus-host disease. *Biol Blood Marrow Transplant*. 2011;17(9):1409–15.

19. Spellman S, Klein J, Haagenson M, Askar M, Baxter-Lowe LA, He J et al. Scoring HLA class I mismatches by HistoCheck does not predict clinical outcome in unrelated hematopoietic stem cell transplantation. *Biol Blood Marrow Transplant*. 2012;18(5):739–46. doi: 10.1016/j.bbmt.2011.09.008. Epub 2011 Sep 29.

20. Ferrara GB, Bacigalupo A, Lamparelli T, Lanino E, Delfino L, Morabito A et al. Bone marrow transplantation from unrelated donors: the impact of mismatches with subsitutions at position 116 of the human leukocyte antigen class I heavy chain. *Blood*. 2001; 98(10):3150–5.

21. Pidala J, Wang T, Haagenson M, Spellman SR, Askar M, Battiwalla M et al. Amino acid substitution at peptide-binding pockets of HLA class I molecules increases risk of severe acute GVHD and mortality. *Blood*. 2013;122(22):3651–8. doi: 10.1182/blood-2013-05-501510. Epub 2013 Aug 27.

22. Kawase T, Morishima Y, Matsuo K, Kashiwase K, Inoko H, Saji H et al.; Japan Marrow Donor Program. High-risk HLA allele mismatch combinations responsible for severe acute graft-*versus*-host disease and implication for its molecular mechanism. *Blood*. 2007;110(7):2235–41. Epub 2007 Jun 6.

23. Kawase T, Matsuo K, Kashiwase K, Inoko H, Saji H, Ogawa S et al.; Japan Marrow Donor Program. HLA mismatch combinations associated with decreased risk of relapse: implications for the molecular mechanism. *Blood*. 2009;113(12):2851–8. doi: 10.1182/blood-2008-08-171934. Epub 2008 Nov 7.

24. Marino SR, Lin S, Maiers M, Haagenson M, Spellman S, Klein JP et al. Identification by random forest method of HLA class I amino acid substitutions associated with lower survival at day 100 in unrelated donor hematopoietic cell transplantation. *Bone Marrow Transplant*. 2012;47 (2):217–26. doi: 10.1038/bmt.2011.56. Epub 2011 Mar 28.

25. Hurley CK, Woolfrey A, Wang T, Haagenson M, Umejiego J, Aljurf M et al. The impact of HLA unidirectional mismatches on the outcome of myeloablative hematopoietic stem cell transplantation with unrelated donors. *Blood*. 2013;121(23):4800–6. doi: 10.1182/blood-2013-01-480343. Epub 2013 May 1.

26. Kanda J, Ichinohe T, Fuji S, Maeda Y, Ohashi K, Fukuda T et al.; HLA Working Group of the Japan Society for Hematopoietic Cell Transplantation. Impact of HLA mismatch direction on the outcome of unrelated bone marrow transplantation: a retrospective analysis from the Japan Society for Hematopoietic Cell Transplantation. *Biol Blood Marrow Transplant*. 2015;21 (2):305–11. doi: 10.1016/j.bbmt.2014.10.015. Epub 2014 Oct 18.

27. Thomas R, Thio CL, Apps R, Qi Y, Gao X, Marti D et al. A novel variant marking HLA-DP expression levels predicts recovery from hepatitis B virus infection. *J Virol*. 2012;86(12):6979–85. doi: 10.1128/JVI.00406-12. Epub 2012 Apr 11. PubMed PMID: 22496224; PubMed Central PMCID: PMC3393572.

28. Petersdorf EW, Gooley TA, Malkki M, Bacigalupo AP, Cesbron A, Du Toit E et al; International Histocompatibility Working Group in Hematopoietic Cell Transplantation. HLA-C expression levels define permissible mismatches in hematopoietic cell transplantation. *Blood*. 2014;124(26):3996–4003. doi:10.1182/blood-2014-09-599969. Epub 2014 Oct 16.

29. Petersdorf EW, Malkki M, O'hUigin C, Carrington M, Gooley T, Haagenson MD et al. High HLA-DP expression and graft-versus-host disease. *N Engl J Med*. 2015;373(7):599–609. doi:10.1056/NEJMoa1500140. PubMed PMID: 26267621.

30. Fernández-Viña MA, Klein JP, Haagenson M, Spellman SR, Anasetti C, Noreen H et al. Multiple mismatches at the low expression HLA loci DP, DQ, and DRB3/4/5 associate with adverse outcomes in hematopoietic stem cell

transplantation. *Blood*. 2013;121 (22):4603–10. doi: 10.1182/blood-2013-02-481945. Epub 2013 Apr 17.

31. Oudshoorn M, Doxiadis II, van den Berg-Loonen PM, Voorter CE, Verduyn W, Claas FH. Functional *versus* structural matching: can the CTLp test be replaced by HLA allele typing? *Hum Immunol*. 2002;63(3):176–84.

32. Fernandez-Viña MA, Wang T, Lee SJ, Haagenson M, Aljurf M, Askar M et al. Identification of a permissible HLA mismatch in hematopoietic stem cell transplantation. *Blood*. 2014;123(8):1270–8. doi:10.1182/blood-2013-10-532671. Epub 2014 Jan 9.

33. Zino E, Frumento G, Marktel S, Sormani MP, Ficara F, Di Terlizzi S et al. A T-cell epitope encoded by a subset of HLA-DPB1 alleles determines nonpermissive mismatches for hematologic stem cell transplantation. *Blood*. 2004;103(4):1417–24. Epub 2003 Oct 23.

34. Fleischhauer K, Shaw BE, Gooley T, Malkki M, Bardy P, Bignon JD et al; International Histocompatibility Working Group in Hematopoietic Cell Transplantation. Effect of T-cell-epitope matching at HLA-DPB1 in recipients of unrelated-donor haemopoietic-cell transplantation: a retrospective study. *Lancet Oncol*. 2012;13(4):366–74. doi:10.1016/S1470-2045(12)70004-9. Epub 2012 Feb 15. Erratum in: Lancet Oncol. 2012;13(4):e134-5.

35. Fuchs EJ. HLA-haploidentical blood or marrow transplantation with high-dose, post-transplantation cyclophosphamide. *Bone Marrow Transplant*. 2015;50(Suppl 2):S31–6. doi: 10.1038/bmt.2015.92.

36. Bashey A, Solomon SR. T-cell replete haploidentical donor transplantation using post-transplant CY: an emerging standard-of-care option for patients who lack an HLA-identical sibling donor. *Bone Marrow Transplant*. 2014;49(8):999–1008. doi: 10.1038/bmt.2014.62. Epub 2014 May 19 (Review).

Chapter

9

Donor-Specific Anti-Human Leukocyte Antigen Antibodies and Risk of Graft Failure after Hematopoietic Cell Transplants

Marcelo A. Fernández-Viña and Stefan O. Ciurea

Introduction

Transplantation of allogeneic hematopoietic cells (allo-HCT) is an effective treatment for a broad range of both malignant and nonmalignant hematologic diseases[1–3]. Approximately 30% of the patients will have an HLA-matched related donor; for the remaining patients, HLA-matched unrelated donors (MUDs), cord blood units (CBUs), and related donors mismatched in one HLA haplotype (HaploD) serve as a vital alternative donor graft source[4,5].

With the exception of transplants using donor grafts obtained from HLA-identical siblings, most allogeneic hematopoietic cell transplants (allo-HCT) include donors who are mismatched at one or several HLA loci compared to the recipient. Early engraftment is crucial for achieving optimal transplant outcomes. Primary graft failure (PGF) associates with HLA mismatch[6], thus is more frequently observed in transplants with use of alternative mismatched grafts (Table 9.1). The incidence of PGF varies from 3% in MUD-HCT to 20% in HCT using CBU or T-cell-depleted HaploD grafts[7–11]. Despite advances in HLA-matching and supportive care, PGF remains an important problem because of the high morbidity and treatment-related mortality (TRM) that results from this event. More than 90% of the patients will succumb primarily to TRM related to opportunistic infections in the setting of prolonged neutropenia or relapse due to absence of the

graft-*versus*-tumor effect of the graft. Several factors appear to affect engraftment in which T-cell-mediated and antibody-mediated effects are the primary causative factors of PGF (Table 9.1). T-cell-mediated graft destruction is more prevalent as it may happen in HLA-matched transplants; clinically it is difficult to anticipate or to document this cause. Presence of donor specific antibodies (DSA) in the patient sera can cause PGF in approximately 25–35% of cases with HLA mismatched donor when examined retrospectively.

The lessons learned from the findings and observations of graft rejection in solid organ transplantation are quite instructive. The presence of anti-HLA antibodies in the patient are associated with graft rejection, organ dysfunction, and patient survival[12–18]. The pioneering work by Anasetti and colleagues[19] performed more than two decades ago showed that PGF was more likely in the presence of a positive cross-match for detection of anti-donor lymphocytotoxic antibodies than in patients not alloimmunized against the donor (relative risk [RR] 2.3, CI 1.8–2.8, $P=0.0038$)[19]. However, the same group identified residual host lymphocytes in 11 of 14 patients with graft failure and suggested that the mechanism of PGF could be host-mediated immune rejection. The association between a positive cross-match and PGF in allo-HCT has been confirmed by other investigators as well[20]. A direct causative role of DSAs and PGF, however, has remained controversial

Table 9.1 Causes of primary graft failure in allo-HCT

Mechanism	Cause	Prevention
B-cell-mediated rejection	Donor-specific anti-HLA antibodies	Screen recipient sera for DSA and modify graft selection Preemptive therapy before transplant[a]
T-cell-mediated rejection	Persistence of recipient T-cells	Enhance anti T-cell therapy (addition of low-dose TBI, or thiotepa to conditioning)
Myelosuppressive drugs	Trimethoprim-sulfamethoxazole, linezolid, ganciclovir	Avoid/remove offending agent
Opportunistic infections	Viral – HHV6, CMV Bacterial sepsis	Monitoring for viral reactivation Early treatment and/or prophylaxis
Other	T-cell depletion Nonmyeloablative conditioning	Use of a T-cell-replete graft Use of a higher intensity conditioning regimen

[a] Pretransplant treatment to decrease antibody levels

Table 9.2 Comparison between direct (complement-dependent cytotoxicity [CDC], flow cytometric cross-match [FXM]), and virtual cross-match (solid phase [SPA], single, and phenotype) assays for presence or absence of anti-HLA antibodies in the patient's sera

Method	Direct cross-match assays (CDC, FXM)	Virtual cross-match assays (SPA)
Patient's serum needed	Yes	Yes
Donor's viable lymphocytes needed	Yes	No
Interference by biologic antibodies (i.e., anti-CD20, anti-CD52, etc.)	Yes Increase false-positive results	No
Interference with IVIG	Yes Increase false-positive results (avoid IVIG infusion 1–2 weeks prior to testing)	Yes Increase false-positive results (avoid IVIG infusion 1–2 weeks prior to testing)
Ease of testing	Cumbersome with requirement of donor's lymphocytes	Simpler and faster
Retesting	New collection of viable T-cells from the donor	Stored DNA from previous samples from the donor (in the event HLA-specific antibodies were present previously)
Specificity	Low (interferences by other methods)	High (single antigen SPA) (method used in our centers) Intermediate (phenotype SPA)
Sensitivity	Low (CDC) High (FXM)	High (single antigen SPA) (method used in our centers) Intermediate (phenotype SPA)

SPA: solid phase assays, IVIG: intravenous immunoglobulin, CDC: complement dependent cytotoxicity, FXM: flow cytometric cross-match.

until recently. Better techniques to detect the antibodies (Table 9.2) have been developed and facilitated understanding the relationship between DSA and PGF.

Methods to Identify DSA?

In-vitro assays for the detection of anti-HLA-DSA in the patient's serum pretransplant provide significant information to predict graft failure and allow for PGF risk assessment. The detection of these antibodies against donor antigens can be performed by direct cross-matches using several methods. The patient's serum can be reacted with a sample of prospective donor cells. Alternatively, a "virtual cross-match" can be undertaken in which the patient's serum is assayed for the specific anti-HLA antibody reactivity against the donor mismatched antigens (Table 9.2)[18,21,22].

The direct cross-match testing involves patient's serum with donor viable lymphocytes and can be performed by complement-dependent cytotoxicity (CDC) or by flow cytometric cross-matches (FXM). These tests require the collection of viable donor lymphocytes. When the selected donor becomes unavailable, the required collection of cells from the new selected donor may add additional delays if the DSA assessment is performed by direct cross-matching.

The cross-match assays present limitations in their specificity as different types of antibodies (autoreactive or therapeutic antibodies like rituximab) may cause positive cross-match results (clinically irrelevant with regard to graft rejection) via reactivity of non-HLA antibodies (Table 9.2). Pretransplant

some patients may undergo treatment with agents such as antithymocyte globulin or humanized monoclonal antibodies (e.g., rituximab, alemtuzumab), which may affect the viability of patients' lymphocytes and interfere with the cross-match testing. Therefore, results of CDC or FXM may become difficult to interpret[9,22].

In contrast to the physical (CDC and FXM) cross-matches, the "virtual cross-match" only requires *in-vitro* screening of the patient's serum[12,23]. The assessment of humoral compatibility can be accomplished rapidly when the patient, the selected donor, and a few alternative potential candidates are pretyped for all relevant HLA loci. The HLA mismatches that can serve as targets of recognition by patient's alloantibodies or allo-reactive T-cells are evaluated to assess (unwanted reactivity against allograft) risk for rejection. The host-*versus*-graft (HvG) direction mismatch implies HLA antigen present in the donor but absent in the patient. The recipient's immune recognition of HvG mismatches remains a barrier for successful engraftment

Historically, the HLA specificities present in a serum specimen are assigned by making inferences through correlation analyses of reactivity against lymphocytes from a panel of HLA-typed subjects. The positive and negative reactions were correlated with each of the specificities present in the various phenotypes of the panel members. The determination of reactivity through this process was difficult and often the assigned specificity was not precise or some specificities were not detected. Because the products of various loci (e.g., *A*, *B*, and *C*) are expressed simultaneously and because many individuals carry two alleles per locus, the panel design was crucial in order to provide the discernment of possible specificities; in some situations because some alleles of different loci associate tightly, the assignment of some specificities could not be achieved. Improvement in anti-HLA antibody detection using preparations of single HLA antigen allows precise detection and quantification of DSA, and has provided new insights into methods of graft rejection

HLA Typing and Solid-Phase Assays for Detection of DSA

The novel solid-phase immunoassays utilize purified preparations of HLA molecules corresponding to a single HLA antigen and allow accurate identification of HLA antibody specificities. The information gained from the application of these sensitive technologies can be used to predict *cross-match* results in solid organ transplantation; however, the accuracy of these predictions may be suboptimal when HLA typing of the donor is incomplete (i.e., HLA typing not beyond A, B, C, and HLA-DRB1). Therefore, the use of solid-phase immunoassays with fluorescent beads coated with single HLA antigens should be paired with high resolution and typing of **all** HLA loci (including HLA-DP) in the patient and the eligible donor to achieve an assessment of humoral compatibility with high precision.

Histocompatibility laboratories have designed multistep tiered testing processes for rapid/low-cost initial assessment of HLA reactivity utilizing fluorescent beads, each one coated with HLA molecules extracted from cells from a single or multiple volunteer donors. The patient's sera that show reactivity with the mixed HLA antigen preparations are further tested (this requires actual transplant donor lymphocytes) against panels of fluorescent beads, each one coated with a preparation from a single antigen. In this manner the specific reactivity of the patient's serum is directly assessed and is not just inferred through correlation analysis of reactivity patterns. The two-step testing process may present the limitation that the initial screening may have limited sensitivity resulting in false-negative detection of alloantibodies in the patient's serum. To decrease the chances of having false-negative detection of alloantibodies, some transplant centers and histocompatibility laboratories have adopted testing protocols in which there is a single step testing only for DSA with single antigen preparations.

Assignment of DSA

The HLA class I molecules are heterodimers in which one subunit (alpha, HLA encoded) is highly polymorphic while the second subunit (beta-2 microglobulin, encoded in chromosome 15) is nonpolymorphic. Therefore, all variations and immunogenicity defined by mismatches in the class I molecules (A, B, and C) is determined by the variable alpha subunit. Similarly, DR molecules are heterodimers in which one subunit presents extensive allelic and isotypic variability (DR-beta subunit) while the second subunit (DR-alpha) is not variable. In contrast, the DQ and DP molecules are made of

two polymorphic subunits[24]. The analysis of antibody reactivity (present in a patient's serum; DSA) is relatively simple for mismatches in alleles of the HLA class I or DRB loci. In contrast, the determination of DSA against DQ or DP mismatches must involve a thorough analysis of the allele composition of the alpha and beta subunits of heterodimers with one or both alleles mismatched. Many serologic allo-epitopes of the DQ (and possibly DP) molecules are defined by the combination of both subunits; these combinatorial epitopes may be immunogenic in spite of one of the subunits being matched between the patient and donor. It should be noted that the pairing between DQA1 and DQB1 encoded subunits presents restrictions in pairing; these phenomena were well described by Kwok et al.[25] who identified that the alleles of the DQA1*01 groups can only pair with alleles of the DQB1*05 and DQB1*06 groups; in contrast, it is thought that other DQA1 and DQB1 groups can pair with each other but not with DQA1*01, DQB1*05, and DQB1*06. It appears that there are no restrictions in pairing between DPA1 and DPB1 encoded subunits.

The evaluation of potential DSA against HLA class I and DRB mismatched alleles in the HvG direction is simple and the analysis should focus in the antigen preparations corresponding to the mismatched allele or if not represented in the panel of alleles corresponding to the same serotype. In contrast, the evaluation of DSA against mismatches in DQA1, DQB1, DPA1, and DPB1 requires the examination of all possible heterodimers that may be formed and may be present in the donor and absent in the recipient following the reactivity of the serum against heterodimers containing the donor's mismatched alleles.

It should be noted that the panels of single antigen preparations may not include the mismatched donor alleles or antigens; in these cases a thorough antibody analysis can lead to identification of amino acid sequence motifs or combinations of amino acid replacements in alleles reactive with the patient's serum that may define the putative epitopes recognized by the patient's serum[26–29]. If the antigen mismatched in the donor (e.g., DPB1*03:01 or DPB1(11:01)) bears the sequence motif likely to determine the putative epitope recognized by the patient's serum, then this donor should be considered incompatible according to anti-HLA antibody reactivity. Once the putative epitope is identified, one may query if the mismatched allele may present the same amino acid substitutions that most likely define the recognized epitope. There is a significant amount of work in the definition of serologic epitopes that may be shared by more than one allele or antigen group.

Controversies and Areas of Investigation
Controversy #1: Do Both T-cells and DSAs Contribute to Allograft Rejection?

Preclinical animal model studies in the 1970s demonstrated the role of T-cells as mediators for allograft rejection;

engraftment was enhanced by greater numbers of donor T-cells; use of increased immunosuppression post-transplant; and the empiric addition of anti-T-cell therapy, like antithymocyte globulin[30,31]. T-cell-mediated graft rejection can be mechanistic in HLA-matched and HLA-mismatched transplantation; however, humoral mediated rejection (anti-HLA antibodies [DSA]) appears to be more prevalent in HCT with HLA-mismatched grafts including "matched" unrelated donor (MUD) HCT, as 75% of MUD transplants are mismatched in at least one HLA-DP locus[10,11]. The main mechanism of allosensitization appears to be pregnancy[11]; previously pregnant females' recipient of haplotype matched related graft may be at higher risk for rejecting the graft from her children. It is likely that with worldwide expansion of mismatched related (haplotype matched) donors, the role of DSA and its link to PGF will be further elucidated.

Controversy #2: Does Complement Pathway Play a Role in Allograft Failure?

Yes. Large registry studies suggest that DSA are an important cause of engraftment failure in HCT especially recipients of HLA-mismatched allografts. In solid organ transplantation, the data suggest an important role for complement-binding DSA[32] in graft failure[33]. Data on allo-HCT from the MD Anderson Cancer Center clearly show that patients with high DSA levels are more likely to have complement-binding DSA; these patients are at higher risk for allograft rejection[34]. Future research will elucidate the exact role of complement pathway in this setting.

Controversy #3: Is There a Defined DSA Threshold Level Beyond Which Allograft Rejection Is Evident?

No. The serum antibody concentrations are interpreted as normalized MFI, as defined by the manufacturer of the kit, against the donor's HLA-mismatched locus. In general, DSA levels higher than 1000 MFI are considered positive. It is generally agreed that there is higher risk for PGF with higher MFI DSA or if multiple DSA are detected in the patient's serum. The risk in this setting of DSA depends not only on absolute MFI levels but many other factors are important as well. These include graft source, graft cell dose, method of graft manipulation (if done), patient's conditioning and immunosuppressive regimens, type of disease, etc. As such, it is difficult to define actionable MFI values. Although precise DSA MFI cut-offs for considering high-risk for PGF are not clearly defined yet, several centers (for whatever reason "center preference") consider DSA levels >3000 MFI as a contraindication to allo-HCT. In this circumstance, selection of an alternative DSA negative donor or, if no alternative donor is available in a timely fashion, a decision to apply a therapy to reduce the DSA levels in the recipient is suggested. Finally, in addition to DSA evaluation, testing for complement-binding DSA (C1q) appears to be important and may be available in the future[33–35].

Controversy #4: Can Treatment of Patients with Positive DSA Mitigate the Risk of Allograft Failure?

Probably yes. Early studies on a smaller number of patients suggest that treatment of patients with positive DSA before allo-HCT can decrease the risk or eliminate the risk of engraftment failure at least in the haplotype-matched transplant setting[9,35]. However, solid organ transplantation, although applied widely for allosensitized patients, has produced mixed results[36].

Controversy #5: How Best to Eliminate DSA from the Recipient of an Allograft?

A multimodality treatment for allosensitized recipients is borrowed from treatment of solid organ transplant recipients and has been implemented in at least two transplant centers in the United States (MD Anderson Cancer Center and Johns Hopkins Sidney Kimmel Comprehensive Cancer Center). The treatment is usually administered for 1–3 weeks prior to conditioning regimen with the goal to neutralize and/or prevent further generation of DSA. The approach uses plasma exchange, intravenous immunoglobulin, and rituximab (elimination of B-cells), or bortezomib ("elimination" of plasma cells). A novel approach explored by the MD Anderson group employs an irradiated buffy coat prepared from the donor cells (using donor HLA antigens). This product is infused 1 day before allograft infusion (day 0) in order to neutralize or "block" the circulating antibodies and/or exhaust complement, thereby sparing allograft the injury[34]. This strategy may offer a fast, cheap, and easy way to clear the DSA, at least in the haplotype matched transplant setting. Anti-complement therapy (anti-C5 [eculizumab], anti-C1q) may also represent a possible therapeutic approach and will be investigated in the future.

Conclusions

DSAs in the recipient are associated with primary graft failure in all forms of allogeneic hematopoietic cell transplant. While the exact DSA levels above which the risk is much higher and treatment needs to be initiated or the donor changed are less well described, transplant centers have their own methods to tackle this unwanted situation. It is likely that future research will answer many questions that currently remain unanswered.

References

1. Beatty PG, Clift RA, Mickelson EM, Nisperos BB, Flournoy N, Martin PJ, *et al.* Marrow transplantation from related donors other than HLA-identical siblings. *N Engl J Med.* 1985;313(13):765–71.

2. Saber W, Opie S, Rizzo JD, Zhang MJ, Horowitz MM, Schriber J. Outcomes after matched unrelated donor *versus* identical sibling hematopoietic cell

transplantation in adults with acute myelogenous leukemia. *Blood.* 2012;119(17):3908–16.

3. Arora M, Weisdorf DJ, Spellman SR, Haagenson MD, Klein JP, Hurley CK, *et al.* HLA-identical sibling compared with 8/8 matched and mismatched unrelated donor bone marrow transplant for chronic phase chronic myeloid leukemia. *J Clin Oncol.* 2009;27(10):1644–52.

4. Foeken LM, Green A, Hurley CK, Marry E, Wiegand T, Oudshoorn M. Donor Registries Working Group of the World Marrow Donor Association (WMDA). Monitoring the international use of unrelated donors for transplantation: the WMDA annual reports. *Bone Marrow Transplant.* 2010;45(5):811–8.

5. Petz LD, Spellman SS, Gragert L. The underutilization of cord blood transplantation: extent of the problem, causes, and methods improvement. In Broxmeyer HE, ed. *Cord Blood: Biology, Transplantation, Banking, and Regulation.* Bethesda, MD: AABB Press; 2011: 557–84.

6. Flomenberg N, Baxter-Lowe LA, Confer D, Fernandez-Vina M, Filipovich A, Horowitz M, *et al.* Impact of HLA class I and class II high-resolution matching on outcomes of unrelated donor bone marrow transplantation: HLA-C mismatching is associated with a strong adverse effect on transplantation outcome. *Blood.* 2004;104(7):1923–30.

7. Cutler C, Kim HT, Sun L, Sese D, Glotzbecker B, Armand P, *et al.* Donor-specific anti-HLA antibodies predict outcome in double umbilical cord blood transplantation. *Blood.* 2011;118(25):6691–7.

8. Takanashi M, Atsuta Y, Fujiwara K, Kodo H, Kai S, Sato H, *et al.* The impact of anti-HLA antibodies on unrelated cord blood transplantations. *Blood.* 2010;116(15):2839–46.

9. Ciurea SO, de Lima M, Cano P, Korbling M, Giralt S, Shpall EJ, *et al.* High risk of graft failure in patients with anti-HLA antibodies undergoing haploidentical stem-cell transplantation. *Transplantation.* 2009;88(8):1019–24.

10. Spellman S, Bray R, Rosen-Bronson S, Haagenson M, Klein J, Flesch S, *et al.* The detection of donor-directed, HLA-specific alloantibodies in recipients of

unrelated hematopoietic cell transplantation is predictive of graft failure. *Blood.* 2010;115(13):2704–8.

11. Ciurea SO, Thall PF, Wang X, Wang SA, Hu Y, Cano P, *et al.* Donor-specific anti-HLA Abs and graft failure in matched unrelated donor hematopoietic stem cell transplantation. *Blood.* 2011;118(22):5957–64.

12. Patel R, Terasaki PI. Significance of the positive crossmatch test in kidney transplantation. *N Engl J Med.* 1969;280(14):735–9.

13. Held PJ, Kahan BD, Hunsicker LG, Liska D, Wolfe RA, Port FK, *et al.* The impact of HLA mismatches on the survival of first cadaveric kidney transplants. *N Engl J Med.* 1994;331(12):765–70.

14. Suciu-Foca N, Reed E, Marboe C, Harris P, Yu PX, Sun YK, *et al.* The role of anti-HLA antibodies in heart transplantation. *Transplantation.* 1991;51(3):716–24.

15. Terasaki PI, Ozawa M. Predicting kidney graft failure by HLA antibodies: a prospective trial. *Am J Transplant.* 2004;4(3):438–43.

16. Mao Q, Terasaki PI, Cai J, Briley K, Catrou P, Haisch C, Rebellato L. Extremely high association between appearance of HLA antibodies and failure of kidney grafts in a five-year longitudinal study. *Am J Transplant.* 2007;7(4):864–71.

17. McKenna RM, Takemoto SK, Terasaki PI. Anti-HLA antibodies after solid organ transplantation. *Transplantation.* 2000;69(3):319–26.

18. Bray RA, Nolen JD, Larsen C, Pearson T, Newell KA, Kokko K, *et al.* Transplanting the highly sensitized patient: The Emory algorithm. *Am J Transplant.* 2006;6(10):2307–15.

19. Anasetti C, Amos D, Beatty PG, Appelbaum FR, Bensinger W, Buckner CD, *et al.* Effect of HLA compatibility on engraftment of bone marrow transplants in patients with leukemia or lymphoma. *N Engl J Med.* 1989;320(4):197–204.

20. Ottinger HD, Rebmann V, Pfeiffer KA, Beelen DW, Kremens B, Runde V, *et al.* Positive serum crossmatch as predictor for graft failure in HLA-mismatched allogeneic blood stem cell transplantation. *Transplantation.* 2002;73(8):1280–5.

21. Pei R, Lee JH, Shih NJ, Chen M, Terasaki PI. Single human leukocyte antigen flow cytometry beads for accurate identification of human leukocyte antigen antibody specificities. *Transplantation.* 2003;75(1):43–9.

22. Zachary AA, Leffell MS. Detecting and monitoring human leukocyte antigen-specific antibodies. *Hum Immunol.* 2008;69(10):591–604.

23. Gebel HM, Liwski RS, Bray RA. Technical aspects of HLA antibody testing. *Curr Opin Organ Transplant.* 2013;18(4):455–62.

24. Mignot E, Thorsby E. Narcolepsy and the HLA system. *N Engl J Med.* 2001;344(9):692.

25. Kwok WW, Kovats S, Thurtle P, Nepom GT. HLA-DQ allelic polymorphisms constrain patterns of class II heterodimer formation. *J Immunol.* 1993;150(6):2263–72.

26. Bodmer J, Bodmer W, Heyes J, So A, Tonks S, Trowsdale J, Young J. Identification of HLA-DP polymorphism with DP alpha and DP beta probes and monoclonal antibodies: correlation with primed lymphocyte typing. *Proc Natl Acad Sci U S A.* 1987;84(13):4596–600.

27. Klohe E, Pistillo MP, Ferrara GB, Goeken NE, Greazel NS, Karr RW. Critical role of HLA-DR beta 1 residue 58 in multiple polymorphic epitopes recognized by xenogeneic and allogeneic antibodies. *Hum Immunol.* 1992;35(1):18–28.

28. Cano P, Fernández-Viña M. Two sequence dimorphisms of DPB1 define the immunodominant serologic epitopes of HLA-DP. *Hum Immunol.* 2009;70(10):836–43.

29. El-Awar N, Lee JH, Tarsitani C, Terasaki PI. HLA class I epitopes: recognition of binding sites by mAbs or eluted alloantibody confirmed with single recombinant antigens. *Hum Immunol.* 2007;68(3):170–80.

30. Deeg HJ, Storb R, Weiden PL, Shulman HM, Graham TC, Torok-Storb BJ, Thomas ED. Abrogation of resistance to and enhancement of DLA-nonidentical unrelated marrow grafts in lethally irradiated dogs by thoracic duct lymphocytes. *Blood.* 1979;53(4):552–7.

31. Ciurea SO, Saliba RM, Hamerschlak N, Karduss Aurueta AJ, Bassett R, Fernandez-Vina M, *et al.* Fludarabine, melphalan, thiotepa and anti-thymocyte

globulin conditioning for unrelated cord blood transplant. *Leuk Lymphoma.* 2012;53(5):901–6.

32. Chen G, Tyan DB. C1q assay for the detection of complement fixing antibody to HLA antigens. *Methods Mol Biol.* 2013;1034:305–11.

33. Loupy A, Lefaucheur C, Vernerey D, Prugger C, Duong van Huyen JP, Mooney N, *et al.* Complement-binding anti-HLA antibodies and kidney-allograft survival. *N Engl J Med.* 2013;369(13):1215–26.

34. Ciurea SO, Thall PF Milton DR, *et al.* Complement-binding donor-specific anti-HLA antibodies and risk of primary graft failure in hematopoietic stem cell transplantation. *Biol Blood Marrow Transplant.* 2015;21(8):1392–8.

35. Leffell MS, Jones RJ, Gladstone DE. Donor HLA-specific Abs: to BMT or not to BMT? *Bone Marrow Transplant.* 2015 Feb 23. doi: 10.1038/bmt.2014.331. [Epub ahead of print].

36. Marfo K, Lu A, Ling M, Akalin E. Desensitization protocols and their outcome. *Clin J Am Soc Nephrol.* 2011;6(4):922–36.

Chapter

10

CD34+ Cell Mobilization in Autologous and Allogeneic Hematopoietic Cell Transplants

Soo J. Park, Mark A. Schroeder, and John F. DiPersio

Introduction

Hematopoietic cell transplantation (HCT) remains a potentially curative treatment for patients with a variety of hematologic malignancies and select solid tumors treated with high-dose chemotherapy. Peripheral blood hematopoietic cells (PBHCs) have essentially replaced bone marrow as the graft source for both autologous and allogeneic HCT worldwide. Mobilized PBHCs have the advantages of more rapid engraftment, reduced infectious complications, and enhanced immune reconstitution[1–4]. Current methods to optimize peripheralization of hematopoietic stem cells (HSCs) are based on the use of cytokines and/or cytotoxic agents to disrupt stromal adhesion or induce marrow aplasia, respectively.

Successful HCT requires the collection of an adequate number of CD34+ cells, a surrogate marker of hematopoietic stem cells, capable of consistent trilineage engraftment for sustained hematopoietic recovery. Clinical studies suggest that a minimum CD34+ cell dose of 2×10^6 cells/kg is necessary to ensure successful hematopoietic reconstitution for autologous hematopoietic cell transplant[5–8]. Larger doses of CD34+ cells have resulted in more rapid and consistent platelet recovery[9–12]. A CD34+ cell dose threshold of ≥ 4.2–4.5×10^6 cells/kg has been associated with improved overall survival for recipients of matched unrelated donor allogeneic hematopoietic cell transplantation (SCT) though larger doses in this setting have been linked to an increased risk for graft-*versus*-host disease[13,14]. No such dose effect has ever been demonstrated for autologous hematopoietic cell transplant. Although no true optimal cell dose for mobilization has been defined for either autologous or allogeneic transplantation, consensus lower limit for both procedures is $>2 \times 10^6$ CD34+ cells/kg with optimal target yields $>5 \times 10^6$ CD34+ cells/kg[9–12].

Unfortunately, a significant number of patients, especially those with non-Hodgkin lymphoma and Hodgkin disease, mobilized with conventional regimens respond poorly and fail to collect the minimum CD34+ cell dose[9,15,16]. Failure to successfully mobilize on initial attempt results in increased morbidity and healthcare utilization. Those patients who undergo remobilization do so with a higher likelihood of failing remobilization[17]. The causes of mobilization failure remain unknown though numerous risk factors have been associated with an increased tendency for inadequate mobilization. Recent studies have shown that direct alteration of the hematopoietic niche, such as that which occurs in diabetic patients and those with impaired glucose tolerance, has been independently associated with poor mobilization[18–20]. It remains difficult to predict which patients will be poor mobilizers though new strategies are currently being evaluated for the purpose of optimizing HSC mobilization.

The growing understanding of the mechanisms involved in PBHC mobilization and the dynamic forces that define the HSC niche have allowed the identification of critical pathways involved in the trafficking and homing of HSCs to their niches. These critical pathways have given researchers new pharmacologic targets for mobilization. This chapter will discuss the standard approaches to HSC mobilization for autologous and allogeneic transplantation and explore the use of novel agents for mobilization. We will first define the bone marrow niche in order to fully appreciate the biology of mobilization. The critical axes of mobilization will be reviewed to provide a greater understanding of the mechanisms of action underlying these new agents.

The Bone Marrow Niche

Bone Marrow Niche

The bone marrow niche is an *in-vivo* microenvironment that is capable of indefinitely maintaining and regulating the self-renewal and differentiation of HSCs[21]. This niche is composed of a diverse stromal network supported by a self-secreting extracellular matrix[22]. The bone marrow niche is strategically organized in this fashion to provide optimal support for stem cell homeostasis and production. The marrow environment is classically divided into two separate niches based on anatomic location and function, the endosteal niche and the perivascular niche[22]. The components and roles of each niche will be discussed in greater detail below and are represented schematically in **Figure 10.1**.

The Endosteal Niche

The endosteal niche is termed so for its proximity to trabecular bone[22]. It is primarily comprised of osteolineage cells with

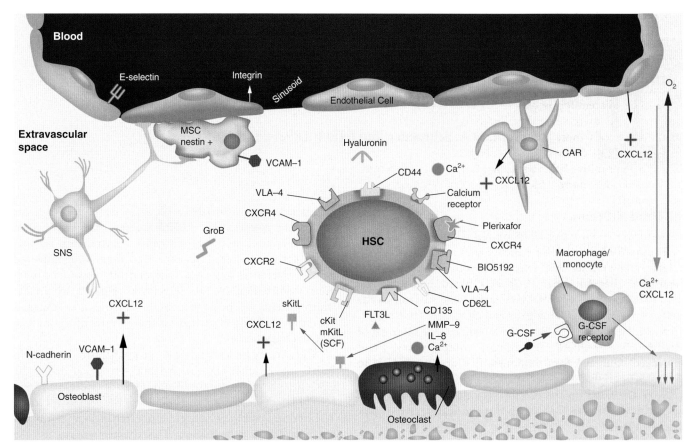

Figure 10.1. Model of the bone marrow niche and hematopoietic stem cell mobilization. Models of HSC mobilization by (**a**) G-CSF, decreased CXCL12 expression via osteoblast suppression; (**b**) GM-CSF, possible alterations in adhesion molecules on HSC surface, not pictured; (**c**) stem cell factor (SCF), disruption of the interaction between m-KitL and c-Kit to inactivate downstream signals mediating HSC adhesion; (**d**) CXCR4 inhibitors, disruption of the CXCL12/CXCR4 axis to induce rapid mobilization, plerixafor; (**e**) VLA-4 inhibitors, disruption of the VCAM-1/VLA-4 axis to induce rapid mobilization, BIO5192; (**f**) Groβ_{Δ4}, truncated CXCR2 ligand; (**g**) FLT3L, truncated CD135 ligand that is structurally homologous to SCF, CDX-301. BIO5192, VLA-4 inhibitor; Ca^{2+}, calcium; c-Kit, receptor tyrosine kinase; CAR, CXCL12 abundant reticular cell; FLT3L, FMS-related tyrosine kinase 3 ligand; G-CSF, granulocyte-colony stimulating factor; Groβ_{Δ4}, truncated XXX; IL-8, interleukin-8; HSC, hematopoietic stem cell; MMP-9, matrix metalloproteinase-9; m-KitL, membrane-bound Kit ligand; MSC, mesenchymal stem cell; sKitL, soluble Kit ligand; SDF-1, stromal derived factor-1; SNS, sympathetic nervous system; VCAM-1, vascular cell adhesion molecule-1; VLA-4, very late antigen-4.

most of the attention centered on osteoblasts. Although this niche had previously been thought to be responsible for the direct regulation of HSCs, recent studies have called the role and importance of this niche into question[23].

Historical data describing the use of osteoblastic cytokines to support primitive HSCs in culture have suggested a large endosteal niche component[24]. These *in-vitro* observations gave way for *in-vivo* studies that utilized specific gene promoters to encourage bone formation[25–27]. The finding of increasing numbers of both osteoblasts and HSCs provided solid evidence for some type of endosteal regulating effect on the bone marrow[23]. However, localization studies performed during bone marrow mapping have placed HSCs adjacent to vasculature, thus conflicting with the idea of a singular endosteal niche[28,29].

Though initial studies centered around osteoblastic effects on HSC regulation, several studies soon followed that sought to determine the exact nature of this effect. Such studies found that neither changes in sheer osteoblastic cell numbers nor

genetic modification of these cells had any significant effect on HSC proliferation[29–32]. It now appeared that the relationship between osteoblasts and HSCs was indeed indirect. Osteoblastic cells were previously thought to regulate HSC numbers via an N-cadherin-mediated mechanism though studies employing *Cdh2* gene deletion have shown no effect on the bone marrow niche[33–35].

Current data do not minimize the role of osteoblasts in HSC regulation but clarifies the specific pathways and exact mechanisms by which they regulate the endosteal niche. Preventing proper osteoblastic differentiation through conditional gene deletion of *Sp7* has resulted in the near complete absence of hematopoiesis[36]. Other bone-forming progenitor cells that reside within the endosteal niche have been capable of creating sufficient bone scaffolds to support HSCs and their associated anatomic elements[37,38]. We emphasize these collective findings to relay the overall importance of the endosteal niche as a regulatory region upon which osteoblasts play a supporting role.

The Perivascular Niche

Akin to the terminology applied for the endosteal niche, the perivascular niche is named for its proximity to the vascular endothelium[22]. The concept of a perivascular niche is supported by early mapping studies discovering the propensity for HSCs to be adjacent to vasculature[28,39]. Stained HSCs have been observed to preferentially localize in juxtaposition to sinusoidal vessels more so than their other hematopoietic counterparts[29]. Studies utilizing high-resolution imaging have shown primitive HSCs trafficking towards specific microdomains of bone marrow blood vessels where they later proliferate[40,41].

Within the perivascular niche, HSCs have been found to localize adjacent to *Nestin*+ mesenchymal stromal cells (MSCs) located around blood vessels throughout the bone marrow [42]. The high expression of stem cell factor (SCF) and stromal cell-derived factor 1 (SDF-1) by these MSCs was found to promote HSC maintenance. Endothelial cells join alongside MSCs to affect HSC quiescence and localization[28]. Loss of function within the CD130 (IL-6 receptor β subunit) receptor complex on endothelial cells as well as faulty angiogenesis leading to impaired sinusoidal regeneration have both been found to result in decreased hematopoiesis[43,44].

Further studies to elucidate the relationship between HSCs and the cells of the perivascular niche emphasized the importance of niche factors, specifically SCF and SDF-1. Conditional gene deletion of *Scf* from MSCs was shown to result in HSC depletion[45]. Normal hematopoiesis was observed to take effect only in the presence of membrane-bound SCF[46]. SDF-1 demonstrated similar effects as shown by gene deletion of the chemokine itself or its receptor, CXCR4, causing HSC depletion in certain strains of transgenic mice[39,47,48].

Cells are not the only regulators of the perivascular niche. The sympathetic nervous system (SNS) has interestingly been shown to have a critical role in HSC mobilization[49,50]. Preclinical studies using mice deficient in key enzymes needed for proper myelin sheath production have shown nearly absent mobilization when treated with G-CSF[51]. These mice suffer from decreased adrenergic tone and osteolineage cell dysfunction. Ablative studies reveal these pathologic findings to be driven by poor norepinephrine signaling. It appears the SNS harbors an important role in regulating HSC retention and egress.

Novel Factors and Signaling Pathways in Niche Regulation

Reviewing the two anatomic bone marrow niches shows us the diversity of cells and factors involved in HSC regulation. There may also be many other unknown factors and signaling mechanisms by which the bone marrow niche is maintained. The observation that HSCs cannot be sustainably expanded in culture has led to speculation surrounding the existence of unidentified growth factors required to preserve the bone marrow microenvironment. Recent work to uncover these niche factors has highlighted the role of pleiotrophin (PTN), a heparin-binding growth factor produced by sinusoidal endothelial cells, in promoting HSC renewal and retention. The addition of PTN to both mice and human cord blood HSCs resulted in a marked increase in long-term repopulating HSC counts in culture[52]. Irradiated mice were able to mount a pronounced HSC expansile response after receiving systemic PTN. *Ptn* knockout mice were shown to display significantly decreased HSC content and impaired hematopoietic regeneration after myelosuppression. Along similar lines, mice receiving anti-PTN antibody demonstrate impaired HSC homing and retention[53]. These collective findings identify PTN as a regulator of both HSC expansion and regeneration in the perivascular niche.

Recent evidence has also shown proinflammatory cytokines to promote short-term hematopoiesis via niche regulation led by resident macrophages[54]. Type I and II interferons, tumor necrosis factor (TNF), and lipopolysaccharide (LPS) have all been demonstrated to influence HSC proliferation and differentiation as a means to increase the granulopoiesis response in times of physiologic stress. In contrast, it appears that chronic inflammatory signaling can lead to HSC exhaustion and subsequent bone marrow failure. Studies utilizing mice HSCs deficient in proinflammatory cytokines have found a repopulating advantage and propose that inflammatory signaling may play a regulatory role in HSC proliferation. These findings may expound upon the mechanisms underlying poor mobilization in conditions marked by chronic inflammation such as diabetes mellitus. Studies to identify the signals by which bone marrow macrophages regulate the niche are ongoing.

Additional factors have been reported to influence HSC numbers in the bone marrow though further characterization is needed to properly define their role with respect to the niche [55–58].

Niche Perspectives

Research over the past 10 years has corroborated the niche concept and shed light on the molecular and cellular elements that comprise the bone marrow niche. With the development of more sophisticated molecular and imaging techniques, it is becoming possible to measure hematopoiesis in real-time to study the intricacies of niche physiology. A better understanding of niche physiology will allow us to elucidate the mechanisms responsible for normal hematopoiesis, as well as altered hematopoiesis and leukemogenesis. Continued efforts to unravel the cellular complexities of the bone marrow niche heralds new therapeutic approaches for both malignant hematology and HSC mobilization.

Standard Approaches to CD34+ Cell Mobilization

The current agents used for HSC mobilization are summarized in Table 10.1 and below.

Table 10.1 Approved agents for hematopoietic stem cell mobilization

Drug	Mechanism of action	Name	Clinical trial status
G-CSF	Down-regulation of CXCL12 in bone marrow osteoblasts; release of proteases	Filgrastim Neupogen	Approved for HSC mobilization
Pegylated G-CSF	Same mechanism as G-CSF but prolonged	Pegfilgrastim Neulasta	Not approved for HSC mobilization
GM-CSF	Possible alterations of adhesion molecules on HSC surface	Sargramostim Leukine	Approved for HSC mobilization
G/C	Induction of marrow aplasia		Approved for HSC mobilization
Plerixafor	CXCR4 antagonist	Mozobil	Approved for HSC mobilization in combination with G-CSF in lymphoma and multiple myeloma
Stem cell factor	Down-regulation of c-Kit	Ancestim Stemgen	Approved for use in Canada and New Zealand but not currently available in the United States

Abbreviations: G-CSF, granulocyte-colony stimulating factor; G/C, G-CSF plus chemotherapy; GM-CSF, granulocyte-macrophage colony-stimulating factor; HSC, hematopoietic stem cell.

Granulocyte Colony-Stimulating Factor (G-CSF)

The optimal regimen for PBHC mobilization has yet to be defined though a number of different approaches have been used. Granulocyte colony-stimulating factor (G-CSF, filgrastim, Neupogen, Amgen, Thousand Oaks, CA, USA) continues to be the most commonly used agent for inducing egress of HSCs. G-CSF is a recombinant cytokine that functions as a myeloid growth factor whose mechanism of action has not been fully understood. It is known that G-CSF down-regulates CXCL12 and activates CD26 protease, thereby causing integrin-β1 dysfunction and ultimately disruption of HSC niche interaction[54]. Additional work with transgenic and wild-type mice has suggested a mechanistic role for bone marrow monocytic cells in G-CSF-induced HSC mobilization. Putative trophic factors produced by the monocytic cell lineage are thought to promote osteoblast maintenance and HSC retention. G-CSF receptor (G-CSFR) signaling within these cells inhibits trophic factor production and decreases CXCL12 expression via osteoblast suppression to ultimately induce HSC mobilization[59,60]. Further characterization of the monocytic cell population and identification of these factors remain active areas of investigation.

G-CSF is usually given by subcutaneous injection at a standard dose of 10 μg/kg per day followed by daily apheresis from day 5 until the minimum CD34+ cell dose has been collected. G-CSF is well tolerated with the most frequently observed adverse effects being skeletal pain, fatigue, nausea, and headache[61,62]. Of note, there have been rare reports of thrombosis-mediated deaths and splenic rupture though universal splenic enlargement has been observed with G-CSF administration and shown to regress once G-CSF is stopped [63–65].

The use of G-CSF for PBHC mobilization remains the standard for autologous hematopoietic cell transplant (auto-HCT) in the United States while chemomobilization is largely favored in Europe[66]. Cytokine mobilized PBHCs are now the preferred graft source and have virtually replaced bone marrow in this role. More rapid hematopoietic reconstitution and lower transplant-related mortality have also extended this transplant paradigm into the allogeneic setting[1,67–69]. Additionally, the harvest of mobilized PBHCs is a relatively indolent procedure that typically does not require hospitalization or general anesthesia.

While the use of G-CSF alone usually results in successful PSBC mobilization for the majority of patients, a significant number of patients fail to mobilize adequately[9,15,16]. Nearly 20% of patients with non-Hodgkin lymphoma (NHL), multiple myeloma (MM), or Hodgkin disease (HD) mobilized with G-CSF alone required remobilization to obtain the minimal CD34+ cell dose necessary for transplantation[17]. Strategies to manage mobilization failure have included dose escalation of G-CSF, which has been shown in several small studies to improve mobilization and allow for adequate PBHC collection [70]. The presumed synergistic effect provided by the addition of chemotherapy is another remobilization strategy that will be discussed later in further detail. However, patients who require remobilization tend to fail regardless of the regimen used[17].

Pegylated G-CSF (Pegfilgrastim)

Pegfilgrastim (Neulasta, Amgen, Thousand Oaks, CA, USA) is the pegylated form of G-CSF that confers reduced renal excretion to allow elevated G-CSF serum levels for up to 14 days after a single injection[71]. Pegfilgrastim was first considered a potential mobilizing agent after it was observed to have equivalent effects to daily administration of G-CSF for neutropenic prophylaxis after cytotoxic chemotherapy[72]. While G-CSF remains the current gold standard mobilizing regimen, interest in pegfilgrastim as a mobilizing agent continues to grow in response to concerns regarding patient compliance and unpredictable pharmacokinetics.

There remains a paucity of studies reporting the efficacy of pegfilgrastim in HSC mobilization though published studies to date tend to view pegfilgrastim as an equally effective mobilizing agent relative to G-CSF. Two published studies of pegfilgrastim for cytokine mobilization in the autologous setting have demonstrated equivalence to filgrastim though the earlier study was not truly comparative and far too small to generate any statistical comparison[72]. Evidence for the use of pegfilgrastim in the allogeneic setting is much more substantial with two studies reporting the majority of donors achieving target stem cell yields in one apheresis[72].

Some of these studies have suggested the functional properties and subset composition of a pegfilgrastim mobilized product differ when compared to those mobilized by G-CSF. Gene expression analysis revealed higher expression levels in genes indicative of early hematopoiesis and cell cycle promotion[73]. These findings have clinically translated into more rapid neutrophil and platelet recovery when compared to subjects who had received a G-CSF mobilized graft[74]. It was thought that these biologic and functional differences were secondary to continuous receptor stimulation mediated by pegfilgrastim though pharmacologic studies have shown ligand trafficking dynamics to play a major role in regulating drug potency[74,75].

Immunologic studies have also shown interesting differences conferred by G-CSF pegylation. Modulation of the original G-CSF molecule through pegylation enhances expansion of invariant natural killer T-cells to augment CD8+ T-cell mediated toxicity, in turn mediating a graft-*versus*-leukemia (G*v*L) effect[76]. Although the most recent studies comparing pegfilgrastim and G-CSF have shown pegfilgrastim to be an equivalent mobilizing agent in both the autologous and allogeneic setting[72], these immunologic graft differences require further studies to better define the role of pegfilgrastim in PBHC transplantation. The use of pegfilgrastim in HSC mobilization may theoretically help retain G*v*L effects, thus making it a useful mobilizing agent for those patients who are at higher risk for relapse or have persistent disease[76].

Pegfilgrastim is currently only approved for the prophylaxis of chemotherapy-induced neutropenia. It has not gained approval for HSC mobilization.

Granulocyte-Macrophage Colony-Stimulating Factor (GM-CSF)

Granuloctye-macrophage colony-stimulating factor (GM-CSF, sargramostim, Leukine, Sanofi, Bridgewater, NJ, USA) is another recombinant cytokine that functions to mobilize HSCs into the periphery. This agent has been shown to have a high incidence of mobilization failure relative to G-CSF and has subsequently fallen out of favor[77–79]. The higher doses of GM-CSF required to mobilize an adequate number of CD34+ cells cause considerable toxicity. However, one study did report a lower than expected incidence of acute graft-*versus*-host disease (G*v*HD) in recipients of sibling donor allogeneic

hematopoietic cell transplant recipients mobilized solely with GM-SCF[80]. Regardless, other larger studies do not support this observation and evidence suggesting this correlation remains limited. Accordingly, the use of GM-CSF as a single agent for mobilization is comparatively rare.

GM-CSF does yield lower numbers of CD34+ cells but is able to mobilize a higher percentage of myeloid-derived suppressor cells and CD4+ and CD25+ regulatory T-cells[81,82]. Studies in mice have shown enhanced CD34+ HSC mobilization when GM-CSF is synergistically combined with plerixafor [82]. These observations lead us to speculate about the potential for a fully mobilized product capable of reducing rates of post-transplant G*v*HD. Such studies have preliminarily demonstrated adequate mobilization using a combined GM-CSF and plerixafor regimen with ongoing phenotypic and functional assessments of cellular graft contents[82]. These findings suggest an intriguing possibility of combining GM-CSF with plerixafor as a mobilizing approach, especially in the allogeneic setting.

G-CSF plus Chemotherapy (G/C)

The use of chemotherapy to augment mobilization was based on the observation that cytotoxic chemotherapy induces marrow aplasia thereby stimulating hematopoietic recovery. The addition of chemotherapy to G-CSF is presumed to produce a synergistic effect on protease release that results in enhanced mobilization relative to G-CSF alone[83]. With newer mobilizing agents on the horizon, the role and benefit of G/C for HSC mobilization has been scrutinized.

A large retrospective analysis of 1040 patients with NHL, MM, or HD who had one prior mobilization with either G-CSF alone or G/C revealed similar failure rates of 18% based on a target threshold of 2×10^6 CD34+ cells/kg[17]. A higher percentage of patients who had received G/C were able to collect a defined optimal yield of 5×10^6 cells/kg compared to patients who had received G-CSF alone[17]. Failure rates remained similar across disease groups regardless of the mobilizing regimen[17]. More patients treated with G/C were able to collect the optimal target yield across all diseases though patients with MM had the highest total CD34+ cell count regardless of the mobilizing regimen[17]. Both mobilizing regimens reported about 75% of patients who were able to collect the minimum cell dose of 2×10^6 cells/kg within the first 2 apheresis days[17]. MM patients who were mobilized with G/C had a significantly higher percentage of patients reaching the minimum cell dose on the first apheresis day [17]. This singularity of MM is thought to be attributed to the less toxic regimens these patients undergo compared to the high-dose chemotherapy regimens many NHL and HD patients undergo[17,84].

Remobilization analysis was performed with the entire database of 269 patients with the disease subtypes listed above. Only 62% of patients were able to achieve the minimum cell dose with remobilization. Failure rates for remobilization were statistically significant and highest for patients treated with G-CSF ± GM-CSF and G/C and lowest for those treated with G-CSF and Plerixafor (G/P) though they were largely similar between G-CSF ± GM-CSF and G/C[17]. Surprisingly, G/C had the highest pooled failure rate when compared to G-CSF ± GM-CSF and G/P[17]. Remobilization with G/P had the lowest pooled failure rate[17].

Toxicity, immunosuppression, and increased resource utilization continue to be major concerns surrounding chemomobilization[85–88]. These findings urge one to consider whether the mobilizing effects of chemotherapy outweigh the risks of adverse cytotoxic effects if no discernible benefit can be seen. It is apparent from the study above that mobilization with G/C does not significantly impact the ability to collect the minimum cell dose needed to proceed to autologous SCT. While mobilization with G/C does increase the frequency of obtaining optimal cell yields, failure rates remain the same. No remobilization advantage is seen when G/C is used. G/C use may be considered appropriate and preferable in MM patients in preparation for tandem autologous SCT and heavily pretreated patients who have been identified as poor mobilizers[17,84]. However, the arrival of new mobilizing agents with greater efficacy and an improved side-effect profile begs us to re-evaluate the role of chemotherapy in HSC mobilization.

Stem Cell Factor (SCF)

Stem cell factor (SCF), also known as steel factor or c-Kit ligand, is a hematopoietic growth factor that is primarily produced by endothelial cells and *Lepr*-expressing perivascular stromal cells of the vascular niche[89]. SCF exists in two forms, soluble (s-KitL) and membrane-bound (m-KitL)[90]. SCF is critical to the maintenance and engraftment of HSCs. The ligand−receptor complex between m-KitL and the c-Kit receptor serves to maintain HSC retention within the bone marrow microenvironment via very late antigen-4 (VLA-4) mediated adhesion[91,92]. HSC egress is facilitated by cytokine induction of matrix metalloproteinase-9 (MMP-9) to sever m-KitL binding within the osteoblastic niche [22]. Blocking the complex between m-KitL/c-Kit and promoting MMP-9 production are two potential mechanisms that may be investigated for pharmacologic mobilization.

Recombinant human SCF (Ancestim, Stemgen, Amgen, Thousand Oaks, CA, USA) in combination with G-CSF has been used to enhance HSC mobilization in patients who had failed a prior mobilization regimen. Study results are conflicting as one phase 2 study did not find any increase in the stem cell yield with the addition of Ancestim while another study reported nearly a 50% increase in successful mobilization [93,94]. A retrospective analysis of a large French cohort consisting of 513 patients who had failed prior mobilization with G-CSF or G/C reported approximately one-third of patients who received Ancestim were able to attain a target cell dose threshold of 2×10^6 cells/kg[95]. SCF activates mast cells and has been known to produce serious side effects though this has been managed with appropriate premedication

across many of the Ancestim trials[89]. Unfortunately, this has limited the use of Ancestim as a mobilizing adjunct to the regions of Canada and New Zealand. It is not available in the United States.

Plerixafor

Plerixafor (AMD3100, Mozobil, Sanofi, Bridgewater, NJ, USA), a small molecule antagonist of the CXCR4, has rapidly become an exciting new agent in HSC mobilization. This bicyclam derivative was first tested as a potential antiviral agent for HIV but was incidentally noted to cause a dose-dependent CD34+ leukocytosis during clinical studies[96,97]. Phase 1 studies soon found this dose-dependent mobilizing effect to be statistically significant and associated with a minimal side effect profile[98]. Plerixafor was able to elicit a maximum six-fold increase in circulating CD34+ cells in patients with NHL and MM[98].

Phase 2 studies of plerixafor demonstrated its mobilization superiority when combined with G-CSF relative to G-CSF alone. Patients with NHL or MM treated with G/P were able to mobilize more CD34+ cells per apheresis session, required fewer sessions to reach target yields, and had higher total CD34+ cell yields[99]. Slightly over one-half of the patients were able to mobilize the minimum cell dose after one apheresis session with all of the patients attaining this goal after two sessions. Those who failed to adequately mobilize with G-CSF alone were rescued with the use of plerixafor.

Plerixafor has also shown efficacy in patients who have previously failed other mobilization regimens. A cohort of 115 patients with NHL, MM, and HD under the Compassionate Use Protocol were remobilized with G/P for autologous SCT and demonstrated high success rates with durable engraftment[94]. Akin to poor mobilizers, patients with NHL, MM, and HD who had been heavily pretreated with chemotherapy had similar successful results[101–103]. Few studies assessing plerixafor in combination with G/C have shown increasing rates of higher stem cell yields though an adequate yield of HSCs can also be collected with G/P alone, thus bypassing the need for cytotoxic chemotherapy exposure[104].

Two large phase 3 trials echoed similar findings to those seen in phase 2 studies[105,106]. A total of 298 NHL patients and 302 MM patients were randomized to either mobilization with G/P or G-CSF alone in preparation for autologous SCT. Patients treated with G/P in both disease groups experienced statistically significant results favoring the addition of plerixafor to reach the primary and secondary target CD34+ cell yields. Those patients unable to collect cells to meet the secondary endpoint of 2×10^6 cells/kg were eligible for rescue mobilization with plerixafor. Mobilization failure was primarily seen in the placebo arm. Autologous SCT with G/P-mobilized HSCs was found to be rapid and durable. Completion of these phase 3 trials led to plerixafor's Food and Drug Administration (FDA) approval in December 2008.

Based upon these favorable findings, the use of plerixafor has been extended to the allogeneic setting where clinical studies remain ongoing and so far have shown a reduction in the time needed for PBHC mobilization and procurement [107]. Interestingly, a higher percentage of CD34^{dim} cells were found to be mobilized by plerixafor and thus may reduce the relative risk of acute GvHD, an important consideration for allogeneic mobilization[108]. Currently, plerixafor is only approved to be used in combination with G-CSF for HSC mobilization in patients with lymphoma and myeloma[89]. Unfortunately, the high cost of plerixafor and its administration have largely prohibited its widespread use, of which it has been the subject of great debate.

The emergence of plerixafor represents significant advancement in the world of mobilization though its use as a single agent has been limited by high rates of mobilization failure in healthy donors[108]. To this end, the pharmacologic industry has been seeking efforts to develop more potent inhibitors against the CXCL12/CXCR4 axis. These lead compounds are in various stages of clinical research and have shown promising results as will be discussed later.

Clinical Controversies of Hematopoietic Stem Cell Mobilization

Chemotherapy *versus* Plerixafor with G-CSF

Regardless of the chosen mobilizing regimen, the main goal of HSC mobilization has always been to collect a sufficient number of CD34+ cells for successful transplantation. Ideally, this would occur in the first mobilization attempt with a minimum number of apheresis sessions. Although G-CSF continues to remain the gold standard agent for mobilization, a large retrospective study of 1834 patients with NHL, HD, and MM reported mobilization failure rates up to 27% with G-CSF alone[17]. G/C is another mobilizing regimen frequently used by many institutions both in the United States and in Europe. The addition of chemotherapy to G-CSF has been shown to be more effective in mobilizing HSCs than G-CSF alone though one randomized study was unable to detect any significant differences between the two regimens[84]. However, the latter study did suggest G/C may aid certain subsets of patients in achieving successful mobilization.

The development of plerixafor has marked a significant step forward in HSC mobilization. Mobilization with G-CSF and Plerixafor (G/P) in autologous SCT reduces the mobilization failure rate and confers benefits of a higher HSC yield and fewer apheresis procedures[105]. Several compassionate use studies have shown that plerixafor will facilitate, when given with G-CSF, successful remobilization in patients who had failed previous mobilization attempts[100]]. Patients who have been heavily pretreated with chemotherapy represent a special cohort given their higher risk of mobilization failure[103]. A study of 28 patients who had been treated with multiple cycles of chemotherapy and/or radiotherapy reported similar increases in circulating CD34+ cells as those who were considered minimally pretreated after treatment with G/P[103].

Controversy exists in regards to the use of plerixafor to replace chemomobilization. Two retrospective analyses have compared G/P with G/C and found similar and adequate HSC harvests with both regimens being superior to G-CSF alone [109,110]. The smaller study did emphasize that plerixafor's predictable kinetics, fewer days of G-CSF and apheresis, and less treatment-related toxicity may help tip the balance in its favor and away from G/C[110]. Data from a large retrospective analysis showed that remobilization with G/C had the highest pooled failure rate while remobilization with G/P had the lowest failure rate[17]. In addition, the more primitive HSCs mobilized by plerixafor may confer G/P a greater reconstituting capacity relative to a G/C mobilized product, thus having important implications in post-transplant outcomes and costs[111].

The success of plerixafor has addressed many of the limitations involved with the use of G-CSF alone and G/C in HSC mobilization. Based on the current literature, we expect plerixafor to become the adjunctive agent of choice for HSC mobilization though G/C may still be preferable in heavily pretreated patients where this regimen has a significantly higher probability of successful mobilization. "Just-in-time" approaches dictating plerixafor use to rescue patients with a poor mobilization response have now begun to emerge as a successful mobilization and remobilization strategy for patients failing or likely to fail standard mobilization with G-CSF alone or G/C[112–114]. This approach has allowed poor mobilizers to timely advance towards transplant while avoiding remobilization with its increased costs and treatment delays[115,116]. Collectively, plerixafor has proven itself to be an effective agent for adequate upfront mobilization when part of a cytokine-based regimen.

G-CSF in the Allogeneic Setting

Although many other cytokines have been investigated for autologous use, G-CSF continues to be the predominant cytokine used for allogeneic PBHC mobilization. It remains the most extensively studied mobilizing agent in this setting. Though the mobilizing efficacy of G-CSF has been consistently demonstrated in patients and normal donors, concerns continue to surround the use of G-CSF in healthy individuals as they relate to mobilization success, donor morbidity, and transplant outcomes.

The success of stem cell mobilization is largely dependent on the CD34+ cell dose. Multiple risk factors have been identified to predict the likelihood of achieving target cell yields for autologous donors though no such concrete data are present for allogeneic donors. Significant inter-donor variability exists in the ability to mobilize PBHCs[117]. Retrospective analyses performed in studies of normal donors who were stimulated with G-CSF have identified several clinical and demographic factors as predictors of successful PBHC mobilization[118–120]. Studies are ongoing to determine the effect of donor comorbidities on allogeneic stem cell mobilization and whether the presence of comorbidities favors use of one mobilizing agent over another. Recently, conditions related to lower steady-state CD34+ cell levels and neuronal alteration of the bone marrow niche have been associated with poor PBHC mobilization, as seen in patients with diabetes mellitus[25,26].

G-CSF is generally well tolerated but is not without its share of adverse effects, some of which harbor serious health consequences. By virtue of extramedullary myelopoiesis, numerous reports have documented the development of transient splenomegaly in response to G-CSF administration. Though this finding normally regresses after completion of apheresis, several healthy donors have been reported to suffer from spontaneous splenic rupture necessitating surgical repair [121–122]. Thrombosis-related events also represent a potentially serious toxicity likely related to the procoagulant effects of G-CSF[65]. Furthermore, G-CSF use has been associated with disease exacerbation in potential donors who suffer from autoimmune disease and is not recommended[123–127].

Currently, G-CSF and GM-CSF are the only cytokines that are approved for HSC mobilization in the United States for both autologous and allogeneic transplants. The use of plerixafor is only approved in combination with G-CSF for HSC mobilization in patients with lymphoma or multiple myeloma. All three agents have been used for allogeneic mobilization with varying rates of success. Numerous studies have assessed the graft composition unique to each mobilizing agent and/or regimen to determine the impact on engraftment and HSC function. While randomized studies have demonstrated that the combination of G-CSF and GM-CSF is not more effective than G-CSF or GM-CSF alone, differences in graft content have suggested that GM-CSF and Plerixafor may be preferred for allogeneic mobilization due to their protective effects against GvHD[82,128,129]. It is important to note that such studies were not statistically powered to detect GvHD differences and thus the rates of GvHD could very well be similar [82]. Larger studies are needed for more appropriate, informative analyses.

Plerixafor in the Allogeneic Setting

Plerixafor has also been studied for use in HSC mobilization for allogeneic SCT. A phase 1 and 2 study in 25 normal sibling donors who were treated with a single subcutaneous injection of plerixafor followed by leukapheresis 4 hours later showed that about two-thirds of the donors were able to mobilize the "minimum" cell dose of 2×10^6 cells/kg after a single 20-L apheresis with all donors reaching this number after a second collection[107]. Transplantation with this plerixafor-only mobilized product resulted in complete and durable engraftment with grade II–IV acute GvHD occurring in 35% of the patients.

A phase 1 trial in 21 healthy donors who were mobilized with increasing doses of intravenous plerixafor demonstrated a

similar time to reach peak numbers of peripheral CD34+ cells with near equivalent potency when compared to the subcutaneous formulation[130]. A clear dose–response relationship was evident with a maximum eight-fold increase in circulating CD34+ cells occurring after treatment with 320 μg/kg of intravenous plerixafor. Prolonged mobilization was associated with higher drug doses and did not seem to confer any additional benefit.

Based on the pharmacokinetic data gathered from phase 1 trials, phase 2 studies commenced in which 28 healthy sibling donors were treated with 320 μg/kg of intravenous plerixafor though only 23 of these donors were evaluable[131]. Six donors were unable to collect the minimum cell dose after a single 20-L apheresis resulting in a failure rate similar to that which was seen with subcutaneous plerixafor. Four of these donors were able to collect the minimum cell dose after a second day of mobilization and collection. Mobilization failure rates after two doses of plerixafor and 2 days of mobilization and collection were similar between the subcutaneous and intravenous formulations of plerixafor.

Plerixafor Cost

The high cost of plerixafor has limited its use to those patients who are at high-risk for mobilization failure. Although it has been difficult to determine which patients will ultimately be poor mobilizers, a predetermined peripheral blood CD34+ cell count has been used as a surrogate marker for mobilization success and failure[17].

Institutions have since been using risk-adapted algorithms to financially optimize plerixafor use. "Just-in-time" approaches, the preemptive administration of plerixafor, has been shown to timely rescue failed mobilization, thus avoiding the morbidity and costs associated with repeated plerixafor mobilization[112–114]. This approach relies on the circulating CD34+ cell count as a surrogate marker of peak mobilization response to determine eligibility for plerixafor administration. Patients who fail to reach the target circulating CD34+ cell count after 4 days of G-CSF administration are given plerixafor on the fifth day to augment mobilization[112,115]. Variants of these protocols allow for peak mobilization synergy to patients who have declared themselves as poor mobilizers. Patients who are also predicted to be poor mobilizers on the basis of known clinical factors that impair HSC mobilization may benefit from plerixafor as first-line treatment to help avoid the potential need for repeat mobilization.

A cost-utility evaluation of G/P compared to G-CSF alone for HSC mobilization in 20 patients with relapsed diffuse large B-cell lymphoma (DLBCL) did report increased costs associated with plerixafor use though a beneficial incremental cost-utility ratio of $14574 per quality-adjusted life-year was calculated[133]. The use of plerixafor met accepted standards for cost-effectiveness primarily due to its superior efficacy as a mobilizing agent. Results were robust even in the face of unaccounted indirect costs and differences in DLBCL

Table 10.2 Novel agents currently being tested for hematopoietic stem cell mobilization

Drugs/Pathways	Mechanism of action	Specific agents	Clinical trial status
CXCL12/CXCR4 modulators	CXCR4 antagonists	POL 6326	Phase 1, 2 ongoing
	Neutralization of CXCL12	BKT-140	Phase 1/2a completed
	Inhibition of CXCL12-mediated Ca flux	NOX-A12	Phase 1 completed
		TG-0054	Phase 1, 2 completed
		MDX-1338	Phase 1/1b ongoing
		PZ-218/PZ-305/PZ-210	Preclinical studies
		ALX-0651	Phase 1 terminated
		GSK812397	No studies available
		KRH-3955	No studies available
		FC131	No studies available
		MSX-122	Phase 1 suspended
VCAM/VLA-4 inhibitors	Inhibition of VLA-4 mediated HSC adhesion to VCAM-1 within the bone marrow stroma	BIO5192	Development terminated
Groβ$_{\Delta 4}$/CXCL2	Release of proteases that alter HSC adhesion to the bone marrow niche	SB-251353	Preclinical studies
FLT3 ligand	CD135 agonist	CXD-301	Phase 1 completed

Abbreviations: Ca, calcium; HSC, hematopoietic stem cell; VCAM-1, vascular cell adhesion molecule-1; VLA-4, very late antigen-4.

treatment. Larger economic analyses are needed to fully justify the costs of plerixafor to the public though this study has laid the foundation for using rigorous economic methods to evaluate healthcare interventions.

Future Directions of Novel Mobilizing Agents

A number of newer drugs have been designed to exploit pathways critical for stem cell mobilization and are now in clinical development. These are summarized below and in Table 10.2.

Inhibitors of CXCL12/CXCR4

CXCL12, also known as SDF-1, is a chemokine that is primarily produced by stromal cells of the bone marrow niche, namely osteoblasts, endothelial cells, Nestin$^+$ MSCs, and CXCL12-abundant reticular (CAR) cells[22,25,134–137]. This chemokine is strongly chemotactic for lymphocytes and stem cells and has been shown to regulate HSC migration and angiogenesis[22,39,138,139]. Studies using genetically modified mice have highlighted the importance of signaling via the CXCL12/CXCR4 axis to promote HSC quiescence and retention[48,140–143].

The quest to seek alternative drugs targeting the CXCL12/CXCR4 axis has been led by the development of POL6326 (Polyphor, Allschwil, Switzerland). POL6326, a synthetic cyclic peptide, is a selective and reversible CXCR4 inhibitor that has a 50- to 100-fold better affinity for CXCR4 when compared to

plerixafor[144]. Mice have shown an 11- to 12-fold increase in peripheral HSCs after a single injection of POL6326. A phase 1 trial in 74 healthy volunteers confirmed POL6326 was safe and effective. Recently, a phase 2a, proof-of-concept study, was recently completed in patients with primary multiple myeloma though results are pending[145]. Currently, a phase 2 study to determine the number of allogeneic donors who require a second leukapheresis for sibling donor HSC procurement in patients with advanced hematologic malignancies is ongoing.

Many other lead drug candidates targeting the CXCL12/CXCR4 axis are currently being studied in phase 1 and 2 trials for HSC mobilization.

Targeting the VCAM/VLA-4 Axis

Numerous adhesion molecules involved in HSC homing and mobilization are expressed on the surface of endothelial cells within the perivascular niche. VLA-4, a $\alpha_4\beta_3$ integrin heterodimer on HSCs, binds to its receptor vascular cell adhesion molecule-1 (VCAM-1), to facilitate HSC retention in the bone marrow microenvironment[146]. Conditional ablation of the VLA-4 α_4 subunit in mice models has resulted in enhanced HSC peripheralization[147]. Other transplant studies have shown impaired homing and similar peripheralization in α_4-deficient bone marrow cells[147–149]. These observations suggest that expression of the $\alpha_4\beta_3$ integrin plays an important role in HSC retention.

Natalizumab, a humanized monoclonal antibody against the $\alpha_4\beta_3$ integrin, is currently used as an immunomodulatory agent for multiple sclerosis and Crohn's disease. This drug is believed to exert its therapeutic effects by preventing the adhesion and migration of immune cells to their target organs. Patients under active treatment with natalizumab were observed to have elevated circulating HSC levels[150,151]. However, this increase was found to be quite modest when compared to current mobilizing agents. Furthermore, natalizumab's mobilizing effects seemed to be restricted by a tachyphylactic phenomenon. Phenotyping studies performed on the mobilized product revealed an abundance of quiescent HSCs destined for the erythrocytic lineage[150,151].

The potential for natalizumab as a mobilizing agent has been met with modest to negligible enthusiasm given its limited mobilizing potential and prolonged immunosuppressive effects. A significant number of patients treated with natalizumab for multiple sclerosis have developed progressive multifocal leukoencephalopathy (PML) in a dose-dependent fashion, rendering the drug a black box warning[152, 153].

In response to the observation that blockade of the $\alpha_4\beta_3$ integrin with natalizumab results in clinically significant mobilization, many small molecule α_4 integrin antagonists have been developed by industry[154–156]. Unfortunately, further development of these early compounds was hampered by poor bioavailability and short half-lives. New-generation antagonists have exhibited a more favorable pharmacologic profile though these agents are currently being studied in clinical trials for the treatment of autoimmune diseases[157–159]. As such, their ability to enhance CD34+ cell peripheralization has not been evaluated.

In preclinical studies, BIO5192, another α_4 integrin antagonist, was shown to significantly enhance HSC mobilization and confer durable engraftment[160]. Combining BIO5192 with plerixafor demonstrated an additive mobilizing effect in the order of three-fold compared to plerixafor alone. Similar results were seen when BIO5192 was combined with G-CSF and G/P, five-fold and 17-fold, respectively[160]. These studies provide evidence for the utility of targeting the α_4 integrin for HSC mobilization though such findings have yet to be reproduced in human subjects. Unfortunately, the clinical development of BIO5192 has been terminated. However, similar mobilization results were obtained with firategrast, a small molecule VLA-4 antagonist developed for the treatment of multiple sclerosis[108]. Firategrast is currently undergoing phase 1 and 2 studies to determine its safety and efficacy in reducing leukocyte migration into the central nervous system.

Groβ$_{\Delta 4}$/CXCR2

Groβ is a chemokine belonging to the CXC chemokine family that serves as a selective ligand for the CXC receptor 2 (CXCR2). The truncated form of Groβ (Groβ$_{\Delta 4}$), the N-terminal peptidase-processed variant, is significantly more potent than the full length protein in HSC mobilization[161].

Studies in murine models have shown this chemokine to provide an equivalent mobilizing effect when compared to G-CSF. Mobilization synergy has been observed when Groβ$_{\Delta 4}$ and G-CSF are used in combination[162,163]. Mice receiving Groβ$_{\Delta 4}$ mobilized graft products have been shown to engender more rapid neutrophil and platelet engraftment[161]. These studies have suggested the utility of Groβ$_{\Delta 4}$ as a rapid and effective HSC mobilizer with enhanced long-term repopulating capacity. Of particular importance is that Groβ$_{\Delta 4}$, like CXCR4 inhibitors and small molecule VLA-4 antagonists, is a very rapid stem cell mobilizing agent inducing its maximum effects in minutes[161].

Although extensive work in mobilization has highlighted the importance of HSC cell dose for hematopoietic recovery, preclinical studies on Groβ$_{\Delta 4}$-mobilized blood suggest hematopoietic recovery is associated with an increased percentage of more primitive long-term repopulating Sca-1$^+$-c-Kit$^+$lineage$^-$ (SKL) cells and CD34$^-$-SKL cells relative to G-CSF alone[164–166]. Numerous studies have cited the importance of primitive HSCs in mediating rapid marrow recovery and the early phase of engraftment. The graft product of Groβ$_{\Delta 4}$ plus G-CSF demonstrated greater engraftment and repopulating capacity likely by virtue of more primitive HSCs[166]. Decreased rates of apoptosis of SKL (primitive murine HSCs) cells are also thought to contribute to accelerated engraftment[167].

Although numerous studies to understand the bone marrow microenvironment have implicated the CXCL12/CXCR4 axis in homing and engraftment, studies of Groβ$_{\Delta 4}$-mobilized cells question the importance of this axis. It appears that the enhanced adhesion of Groβ$_{\Delta 4}$-mobilized SKL cells to VCAM-1-expressing endothelial cells is elevated relative to G-CSF mobilized cells and perhaps responsible for the enhanced homing properties seen with Groβ$_{\Delta 4}$[167,168]. Homing remained unaffected in the presence of plerixafor and CD26 antagonists. Groβ$_{\Delta 4}$ may thus play a potential role in HSC mobilization though future studies are needed to determine its safety and efficacy in humans[167].

FMS-Related Tyrosine Kinase 3 Ligand (FLT3L)

FLT3L is a hematopoietic cytokine that is structurally homologous to SCF. FLT3L binds to its receptor CD135 expressed on HSCs to promote proliferation and normal differentiation [169]. Recent studies utilizing FLT3L and truncated FLT3L to mobilize murine HSCs demonstrate their promise as adjunctive mobilizing agents in mouse and man[170]. These preclinical studies assessed the number and phenotype of HSCs mobilized with FLT3L relative to G-CSF alone and G-CSF combined with plerixafor (G/P). FLT3L synergized with plerixafor (F/P) was found to result in a six-fold increase in frequency and 12-fold increase in absolute number of mobilized Lin$^-$Sca-1$^+$c-Kit$^+$ (LSK) cells (mouse HSCs). Moreover, lethally irradiated syngeneic mice were only able to be hematopoietically rescued by using PBHC grafts mobilized by F/P

[170]. Transplanting these mice with grafts mobilized with G-CSF or G/P resulted in engraftment failure and death.

F/P-mobilized PBHC grafts were also shown to promote improved survival and less GvHD compared to G-CSF mobilized grafts after allogeneic SCT[170]. This observation has been attributed to the greater number of myeloid dendritic cells that are mobilized by a FLT3L-based regimen. In addition, greater numbers of natural killer cells and regulatory T-cells were also seen in FLT3L mobilized PBHC products[170–172]. All of these cell types in donor grafts have been demonstrated to generate protective effects against acute GvHD and thus improve survival post-allogeneic SCT in mouse models.

A phase 1 trial of CDX-301, a recombinant human truncated FLT3L, is currently underway, and phenotypic and functional assessments of cellular graft contents are ongoing[173].

Physical Exercise

Endothelial progenitor cells (EPCs) and circulating progenitor cells (CPCs) play an important role in the processes of neo-vascularization and endothelial repair due to their pluripotent nature[174]. They constitute an extremely small fraction of the circulating cells in the peripheral blood[175]. Physical exercise has been known to promote the release of bone marrow EPCs in cardiac patients by virtue of vascular endothelial growth factor (VEGF) release[174]. A systematic review analyzing the effect of different types of exercise on EPC mobilization has shown conflicting results though some generalized points can be made as detailed below[176].

Both endurance and maximal exercise can influence the numbers of HSCs, CPCs, and EPCs in healthy subjects. It appears that endurance exercise is dependent on a hypoxic environment for these mobilizing effects. Endurance exercise mimics physiologic ischemia to promote stabilization of hypoxic inducible factor-1, thus stimulating gene expression of VEGF[177–179]. The presence of VEGF activates endothelial nitric oxide synthase (eNOS) and increases NO bioavailability, in turn mobilizing EPCs from the bone marrow[180]. On the other hand, maximal exercise relies on the shear stress activation of protein kinase 3 to activate eNOS, along with reduced NADPH expression, to increase NO bioavailability and EPC mobilization[181].

EPC and CPC mobilization appear to be more prominent in endurance exercise and is correlated with VEGF plasma levels[176,182]. VEGF does not seem to play a role in EPC mobilization with maximal exercise[176]. EPC release in maximal exercise is driven by the bioavailability of NO with a longer exercise duration correlated with greater EPC release [180,183]. Both pathways utilize NO to mobilize EPCs thus identifying a potential lifestyle and therapeutic adjunct to optimize HSC mobilization[176].

Conclusions

Although significant advances in our understanding of the hematopoietic niche and stem cell trafficking have been made over the past 15 years, there have been few novel approaches for stem cell mobilization in the clinic. G-CSF and G/C continue to remain the gold standards of mobilization. The development of novel CXCR4 antagonists, FDA approval of plerixafor, and the preclinical and early clinical development of other rapid and robust stem cell mobilizing agents such as VLA-4 inhibitors and $Gro\beta_{\Delta4}$, as well as novel cytokines such as pegfilgrastim and FLT3L, continues to provide hope for the future. Additional basic science insights into the architecture and key tethers that comprise the hematopoietic niche as well as those pathways involved in stem cell trafficking and retention will likely lead to new clues and approaches that can be validated in both preclinical models and in early clinical trials.

References

1. Bensinger WI, Martin PJ, Storer B, Clift R, Forman SJ, Negrin R, et al. Transplantation of bone marrow as compared with peripheral-blood cells from HLA-identical relatives in patients with hematologic cancers. *N Engl J Med*. 2001; 344(3):175–81.

2. Beyer J, Schwella N, Zingsem J, Strohscheer I, Schwaner I, Oettle H, et al. Hematopoietic rescue after high-dose chemotherapy using autologous peripheral-blood progenitor cells or bone marrow: a randomized comparison. *J Clin Oncol*. 1995; 13 (6):1328–35.

3. Hartmann O, Le Corroller AG, Blaise D, Michon J, Phillip I, Norol F, et al. Peripheral blood stem cell and bone marrow transplantation for solid tumors and lymphomas: hematologic recovery and costs. A randomized, controlled trial. *Ann Intern Med*. 1997; 126(8):600–7.

4. Schmitz N, Linch DC, Dreger P, Goldstone AH, Boogaerts MA, Ferrant A, et al. Randomised trial of filgrastim-mobilised peripheral blood progenitor cell transplantation *versus* autologous bone-marrow transplantation in lymphoma patients. *Lancet*. 1996; 347 (8998):353–7.

5. Bender JG, To LB, Williams S, Schwartzberg LS. Defining a therapeutic dose of peripheral blood stem cells. *J Hematother*. 1992; 1(4):329–41.

6. Passos-Coelho JL, Braine HG, Davis JM, Huelskamp AM, Schepers KG, Ohly K, et al. Predictive factors for peripheral-blood progenitor-cell collections using a single large-volume leukapheresis after cyclophosphamide and granulocyte-macrophage colony-stimulating factor mobilization. *J Clin Oncol*. 1995; 13(3):705–14.

7. Gandhi MK, Jestice K, Scott MA, Bloxham D, Bass G, Marcus RE. The minimum CD34 threshold depends on prior chemotherapy in autologous peripheral blood stem cell recipients. *Bone Marrow Transplant*. 1999; 23(1):9–13.

8. Montgomery M, Cottler-Fox M. Mobilization and collection of autologous hematopoietic progenitor/stem cells. *Clin Adv Hematol Oncol*. 2007; 5(2):127–36.

9. Weaver CH, Hazelton B, Birch R, Palmer P, Allen C, Schwartzberg L, et al. An analysis of engraftment

kinetics as a function of the CD34 content of peripheral blood progenitor cell collections in 692 patients after the administration of myeloablative chemotherapy. *Blood.* 1995; 86(10):3961–9.

10. Beguin Y, Baudoux E, Sautois B, Fraipont V, Schaaf-Lafontaine N, Pereira M, *et al.* Hematopoietic recovery in cancer patients after transplantation of autologous peripheral blood CD34+ cells or unmanipulated peripheral blood stem and progenitor cells. *Transfusion.* 1998; 38(2):199–208.

11. Reiffers J, Faberes C, Boiron JM, Marit G, Foures C, Ferrer AM, *et al.* Peripheral blood progenitor cell transplantation in 118 patients with hematological malignancies: analysis of factors affecting the rate of engraftment. *J Hematother.* 1994; 3(3):185–91.

12. Bolwell BJ, Pohlman B, Rybicki L, Sobecks R, Dean R, Curtis J, *et al.* Patients mobilizing large numbers of CD34+ cells ('super mobilizers') have improved survival in autologous stem cell transplantation for lymphoid malignancies. *Bone Marrow Transplant.* 2007; 40(5):437–41.

13. Pulsipher MA, Chitphakdithai P, Logan BR, Leitman SF, Anderlini P, Klein JP, *et al.* Donor, recipient, and transplant characteristics as risk factors after unrelated donor PBSC transplantation: beneficial effects of higher CD34+ cell dose. *Blood.* 2009; 114(13):2606–16.

14. Baron F, Maris MB, Storer BE, Sandmaier BM, Panse JP, Chauncey TR, *et al.* High doses of transplanted CD34+ cells are associated with rapid T-cell engraftment and lessened risk of graft-*versus*-host disease after nonmyeloablative conditioning and unrelated hematopoietic cell transplantation. *Leukemia.* 2005; 19(5):822–8.

15. Dreger P, Kloss M, Petersen B, Haferlach T, Loffler H, Loeffler M, *et al.* Autologous progenitor cell transplantation: prior exposure to stem cell-toxic drugs determines yield and engraftment of peripheral blood progenitor cell but not of bone marrow grafts. *Blood.* 1995; 86(10):3970–8.

16. Tarella C, Di Nicola M, Caracciolo D, Zallio F, Cuttica A, Omede P. High-dose ara-C with autologous peripheral blood progenitor cell support induces a

marked progenitor cell mobilization: an indication for patients at risk for low mobilization. *Bone Marrow Transplant.* 2002; 30(11):725–32.

17. Pusic I, Jiang SY, Landua S, Uy GL, Rettig MP, Cashen AF, *et al.* Impact of mobilization and remobilization strategies on achieving sufficient stem cell yields for autologous transplantation. *Biol Blood Marrow Transplant.* 2008; 14(9): 1045–56.

18. Fadini GP, Pucci L, Vanacore R, Baesso I, Penno G, Balbarini A, *et al.* Glucose tolerance is negatively associated with circulating progenitor cell levels. *Diabetologia.* 2007; 50(10):2156–63.

19. Fadini GP, Boscaro E, de Kreutzenberg S, Agostini C, Seeger F, Dimmeler S, *et al.* Time course and mechanisms of circulating progenitor cell reduction in the natural history of type 2 diabetes. *Diabetes Care.* 2010; 33(5):1097–102.

20. Ferraro F, Lymperi S, Mendez-Ferrer S, Saez B, Spencer JA, Yeap BY, *et al.* Diabetes impairs hematopoietic stem cell mobilization through alteration of niche function. *Sci Transl Med.* 2011; 3(104):104ra101.

21. Heazlewood SY, Oteiza A, Cao H, Nilsson SK. Analyzing hematopoietic stem cell homing, lodgment and engraftment to better understand the bone marrow niche. *Ann N Y Acad Sci.* 2014; 1310:119–28.

22. Rettig MP, Schroeder MA, DiPersio JF. Marrow microenvironment and biology of mobilization of stem cells. In: Appelbaum FR, Forman SJ, Negrin RS, Blume KG, editors. *Thomas' Hematopoietic Cell Transplantation,* 5th edition. New Jersey: Wiley-Blackwell; 2013.

23. Morrison SJ, Scadden DT. The bone marrow niche for haematopoietic stem cells. *Nature.* 2014; 505(7483):327–34.

24. Taichman RS, Emerson SG. Human osteoblasts support hematopoiesis through the production of granulocyte colony-stimulating factor. *J Exp Med.* 1994; 179(5):1677–82.

25. Calvi LM, Adams GB, Weibrecht KW, Weber JM, Olson DP, Knight MC, *et al.* Osteoblastic cells regulate the haematopoietic stem cell niche. *Nature.* 2003; 425:841–6.

26. Park D, Spencer JA, Koh BI, Kobayashi T, Fujisaki J, Clemens TL, *et al.* Endogenous bone marrow MSCs are dynamic, fate-restricted participants in

bone maintenance and regeneration. *Cell Stem Cell.* 2012; 10(3):259–72.

27. Zhang J, Niu C, Ye L, Huang H, He X, Tong WG, *et al.* Identification of the haematopoietic stem cell niche and control of the niche size. *Nature.* 2003; 425(6960):836–41.

28. Kiel MJ, Yilmaz OH, Iwashita T, Yilmaz OH, Terhorst C, Morrison SJ. SLAM family receptors distinguish hematopoietic stem and progenitor cells and reveal endothelial niches for stem cells. *Cell.* 2005; 121(7):1109–21.

29. Kiel MJ, Radice GL, Morrison SJ. Lack of evidence that hematopoietic stem cells depend on N-cadherin-mediated adhesion to osteoblasts for their maintenance. *Cell Stem Cell.* 2007; 1(2):204–17.

30. Visnjic D, Kalajzic Z, Rowe DW, Katavic V, Lorenzo J, Aquila HL. Hematopoiesis is severely altered in mice with an induced osteoblast deficiency. *Blood.* 2004; 103(9):3258–64.

31. Zhu J, Garrett R, Jung Y, Zhang Y, Kim N, Wang J, *et al.* Osteoblasts support B-lymphocyte commitment and differentiation from hematopoietic stem cells. *Blood.* 2007; 109(9):3706–12.

32. Raaijmakers MH, Mukherjee S, Guo S, Zhang S, Kobayashi T, Schoonmaker JA, *et al.* Bone progenitor dysfunction induces myelodysplasia and secondary leukemia. *Nature.* 2010; 464(7290):852–7.

33. Kiel MJ, Acar M, Radice GL, Morrison SJ. Hematopoietic stem cells do not depend on N-cadherin to regulate their maintenance. *Cell Stem Cell.* 2009; 4(2):170–9.

34. Greenbaum AM, Revollo LD, Woloszynek JR, Civitelli R, Link DC. N-cadherin in osteolineage cells is not required for maintenance of hematopoietic stem cells. *Blood.* 2012; 120(2):295–302.

35. Bromberg O, Frisch BJ, Weber JM, Porter RL, Civitelli R, Calvi LM. Osteoblastic N-cadherin is not required for microenvironmental support and regulation of hematopoietic stem and progenitor cells. *Blood.* 2012; 120(2):303–13.

36. Zhou X, Zhang Z, Feng JQ, Dusevich VM, Sinha K, Zhang H, *et al.* Multiple functions of Osterix are required for bone growth and homeostasis in postnatal mice. *Proc Natl Acad Sci USA.* 2010; 107(29):12919–24.

37. Chan CK, Chen CC, Luppen CA, Kim JB, DeBoer AT, Wei K, et al. Endochondral ossification is required for haematopoietic stem-cell niche formation. *Nature.* 2009; 457:490–4.

38. Sacchetti B, Funari A, Michienzi S, Di Cesare S, Piersanti S, Saggio I, et al. Self-renewing osteoprogenitors in bone marrow sinusoids can organize a hematopoietic microenvironment. *Cell.* 2007; 131(2):324–36.

39. Sugiyama T, Kohara H, Noda M, Nagasawa T. Maintenance of the hematopoietic stem cell pool by CXCL12-CXCR4 chemokine signaling in bone marrow stromal cell niches. *Immunity.* 2006; 25(6):977–88.

40. Lo CC, Fleming HE, Wu JW, Zhao CX, Miake-Lye S, Fujisaki J, et al. Live-animal trafficking of individual haematopoietic stem/progenitor cells in their niche. *Nature.* 2009; 457(7225):92–6.

41. Sipkins DA, Wei X, Wu JW, Runnels JM, Cote D, Means TK, et al. In vivo imaging of specialized bone marrow endothelial microdomains for tumour engraftment. *Nature.* 2005; 435(7044):969–73.

42. Mendez-Ferrer S, Michurina TV, Ferraro F, Mazloom AR, MacArthur BD, Lira SA, et al. Mesenchymal and haematopoietic stem cells form a unique bone marrow niche. *Nature.* 2010; 466:829–34.

43. Yao L, Yokota T, Xia L, Kincade PW, McEver RP. Bone marrow dysfunction in mice lacking the cytokine receptor gp130 in endothelial cells. *Blood.* 2005; 106(13):4093–101.

44. Hooper AT, Butler JM, Nolan DJ, Kranz A, Iida K, Kobayashi M, et al. Engraftment and reconstitution of hematopoiesis is dependent on VEGFR2-mediated regeneration of sinusoidal endothelial cells. *Cell Stem Cell.* 2009; 4(3):263–74.

45. Oguro H, Ding L, Morrison SJ. SLAM family markers resolve functionally distinct subpopulations of hematopoietic stem cells and multipotent progenitors. *Cell Stem Cell.* 2013; 13(1):102–16.

46. Barker JE. Early transplantation to a normal microenvironment prevents the development of Steel hematopoietic stem cell defects. *Exp Hematol.* 1997; 25(6):542–7.

47. Tzeng YS, Li H, Kang YL, Chen WC, Cheng WC, Lai DM. Loss of Cxcl12/Sdf-1 in adult mice decreases the quiescent state of hematopoietic stem/progenitor cells and alters the pattern of hematopoietic regeneration after myelosuppression. *Blood.* 2011; 117(2):429–39.

48. Zou YR, Kottmann AH, Kuroda M, Taniuchi I, Littman DR. Function of the chemokine receptor CXCR4 in haematopoiesis and in cerebellar development. *Nature.* 1998; 393(6685):595–9.

49. Katayama Y, Battista M, Kao WM, Hidalgo A, Peired AJ, Thomas SA, et al. Signals from the sympathetic nervous system regulate hematopoietic stem cell egress from bone marrow. *Cell.* 2006; 124(2):407–21.

50. Mendez-Ferrer S, Lucas D, Battista M, Frenette PS. Haematopoietic stem cell release is regulated by circadian oscillations. *Nature.* 2008; 452(7186):442–7.

51. Katayama Y, Battista M, Kao WM, Hidalgo A, Peired AJ, Thomas SA, et al. Signals from the sympathetic nervous system regulate hematopoietic stem cell egress from bone marrow. *Cell.* 2006; 124(2):407–21.

52. Himburg HA, Muramoto GG, Daher P, Meadows SK, Russell JL, Doan P, et al. Pleiotrophin regulates the expansion and regeneration of hematopoietic stem cells. *Nat Med.* 2010; 16(4):475–82.

53. Himburg HA, Harris JR, Ito T, Daher P, Russell JL, Quarmyne M, et al. Pleiotrophin regulates the retention and self-renewal of hematopoietic stem cells in the bone marrow vascular niche. *Cell Rep.* 2012; 2(4):964–75.

54. Petit I, Szyper-Kravitz M, Nagler A, Lahav M, Peled A, Habler L, et al. G-CSF induces stem cell mobilization by decreasing bone marrow SDF-1 and up-regulating CXCR4. *Nat Immunol.* 2002; 3(7):687–94.

55. Nakamura-Ishizu A, Okuno Y, Omatsu Y, Okabe K, Morimoto J, Uede T, et al. Extracellular matrix protein tenascin-C is required in the bone marrow microenvironment primed for hematopoietic regeneration. *Blood.* 2012; 119(23):5429–37.

56. Stier S, Ko Y, Forkert R, Lutz C, Neuhaus T, Grunewald E, et al. Osteopontin is a hematopoietic stem cell niche component that negatively

regulates stem cell pool size. *J Exp Med.* 2005; 201(11):1781–91.

57. Nilsson SK, Johnston HM, Whitty GA, Williams B, Webb RJ, Denhardt DT, et al. Osteopontin, a key component of the hematopoietic stem cell niche and regulator of primitive hematopoietic progenitor cells. *Blood.* 2005; 106(4):1232–9.

58. Sugimura R, He XC, Venkatraman A, Arai F, Box A, Semerad C, et al. Noncanonical Wnt signaling maintains hematopoietic stem cells in the niche. *Cell.* 2012; 150(2):351–65.

59. Christopher MJ, Rao M, Liu F, Woloszynek JR, Link DC. Expression of the G-CSF receptor in monocytic cells is sufficient to mediate hematopoietic progenitor mobilization by G-CSF in mice. *J Exp Med.* 2011; 208(2):251–60.

60. Liu F, Poursine-Laurent J, Link DC. Expression of the G-CSF receptor on hematopoietic progenitor cells is not required for their mobilization by G-CSF. *Blood.* 2000; 95(10):3025–31.

61. Anderlini P, Przepiorka D, Seong D, Miller P, Sundberg J, Lichtiger B, et al. Clinical toxicity and laboratory effects of granulocyte-colony-stimulating factor (filgrastim) mobilization and blood stem cell apheresis from normal donors, and analysis of chargers for the procedures. *Transfusion.* 1996; 36(7):590–5.

62. Stroncek DF, Clay ME, Petzoldt ML, Smith J, Jaszcz W, Oldham FB, et al. Treatment of normal individuals with granulocyte-colony-stimulating factor: donor experiences and the effects on peripheral blood CD34+ cell counts and on the collection of peripheral blood stem cells. *Transfusion.* 1996; 36(7):601–10.

63. Becker PS, Wagle M, Matous S, Swanson RS, Pihan G, Lowry PA, et al. Spontaneous splenic rupture following administration of granulocyte colony-stimulating factor (G-CSF): occurrence in an allogeneic donor of peripheral blood stem cells. *Biol Blood Marrow Transplant.* 1997; 3(1):45–9.

64. Stroncek D, Shawker T, Follmann D, Leitman SF. G-CSF-induced spleen size changes in peripheral blood progenitor cell donors. *Transfusion.* 2003; 43(5):609–13.

65. Rothe L, Collin-Osdoby P, Chen Y, Sunyer T, Chaudhary L, Tsay A, et al. Human osteoclasts and osteoclast-like

cells synthesize and release high basal and inflammatory stimulated levels of the potent chemokine interleukin-8. *Endocrinology.* 1998; 139(10):4353–63.

66. Korbling M, Fliender TM. History of blood stem cell transplants. Blood stem cell transplants. In: Gale RP, Juttner CA, Henon P, editors. *Peripheral blood stem cell autographs.* New York: Cambridge University Press; 1994:9.

67. Blaise D, Kuentz M, Fortanier C, Bourhis JH, Milpied N, Sutton L, *et al.* Randomized trial of bone marrow *versus* lenograstim-primed blood cell allogeneic transplantation in patients with early-stage leukemia: a report from the Societe Francaise de Greffe de Moelle. *J Clin Oncol.* 2000; 18(3):537–46.

68. Couban S, Simpson DR, Barnett MJ, Bredeson C, Hubesch L, Howson-Jan K, *et al.* A randomized multicenter comparison of bone marrow and peripheral blood in recipients of matched sibling allogeneic transplants for myeloid malignancies. *Blood.* 2002; 100(5):1525–31.

69. Schmitz N, Beksac M, Hasenclever D, Bacigalupo A, Ruutu T, Nagler A, *et al.* Transplantation of mobilized peripheral blood cells to HLA-identical siblings with standard-risk leukemia. *Blood.* 2002; 100(3):761–7.

70. Goterris R, Hernandez-Boluda JC, Teruel A, Gomez C, Lis MJ, Terol MJ, *et al.* Impact of different strategies of second-line stem cell harvest on the outcome of autologous transplantation in poor peripheral blood stem cell mobilizers. *Bone Marrow Transplant.* 2005; 36(10):847–53.

71. Costa LJ, Kramer C, Hogan KR, Butcher CD, Littleton AL, Shoptaw KB, *et al.* Pegfilgrastim-*versus* filgrastim-based autologous hematopoietic stem cell mobilization in the setting of preemptive use of plerixafor: efficacy and cost analysis. *Transfusion.* 2012; 52(11):2375–81.

72. Herbert KE, Gambell P, Link EK, Mouminoglu A, Wall DM, Harrison SJ, *et al.* Pegfilgrastim compared with filgrastim for cytokine-alone mobilization of autologous haematopoietic stem and progenitor cells. *Bone Marrow Transplant.* 2013; 48(3):351–6.

73. Bruns I, Steidl U, Fischer JC, Raschke S, Kobbe G, Fenk R, *et al.* Pegylated

G-CSF mobilizes CD34+ cells with different stem and progenitor cell subsets and distinct functional properties in comparison with unconjugated G-CSF. *Blood* (ASH Annual Meeting Abstracts). 2006; 108: Abstract 3382.

74. Kobbe G, Bruns I, Fenk R, Czibere A, Haas R. Pegfilgrastim for PBSC mobilization and autologous haematopoietic SCT. *Bone Marrow Transplant.* 2009; 43(9):669–77.

75. Sarkar CA, Lowenhaupt K, Wang PJ, Horan T, Lauffenburger DA. Parsing the effects of binding, signaling, and trafficking on the mitogenic potencies of granulocyte colony-stimulating factor analogues. *Biotechnol Prog.* 2003; 19(3):955–64.

76. Morris ES, MacDonald KP, Hill GR. Stem cell mobilization with G-CSF analogs: a rational approach to separate GVHD and GVL? *Blood.* 2006; 107(9):3430–5.

77. Brown RA, Adkins D, Khoury H, Vij R, Goodnough LT, Shenoy S, *et al.* Long-term follow-up of high-risk allogeneic peripheral-blood stem-cell transplant recipients: graft-*versus*-host disease and transplant-related mortality. *J Clin Oncol.* 1999; 17(3):806–12.

78. Lane TA, Law P, Maruyama M, Young D, Burgess J, Mullen M, *et al.* Harvesting and enrichment of hematopoietic progenitor cells mobilized into the peripheral blood of normal donors by granulocyte-macrophage colony-stimulating factor (GM-CSF) or G-CSF: potential role in allogeneic marrow transplantation. *Blood.* 1995; 85(1):275–82.

79. Gazitt Y, Shaughnessy P, Liu Q. Differential mobilization of CD34+ cells and lymphoma cells in non-Hodgkin's lymphoma patients mobilized with different growth factors. *J Hematother Stem Cell Res.* 2001; 10(1):167–76.

80. Devine SM, Brown RA, Mathews V, Trinkaus K, Khoury H, Adkins D, *et al.* Reduced risk of acute GvHD following mobilization of HLA-identical sibling donors with GM-CSF alone. *Bone Marrow Transplant.* 2005; 36(6):531–8.

81. Gazitt Y, Shaughnessy P, Devore P. Mobilization of dendritic cells and NK cells in non-Hodgkin's lymphoma patients mobilized with different growth factors. *J Hematother Stem Cell Res.* 2001; 10(1):177–86.

82. Schroeder MA, Merida S, Schwab D, Rettig MP, Meier S, Lopez S, *et al.* Sargramostim (GM-CSF) combined with IV Plerixafor to mobilize peripheral blood stem cells (PBSC) from normal HLA-matched allogeneic sibling donors. BMT Tandem "Scientific" Meeting, March, 2014; Session N(Abstract 32):Abstract 32.

83. Ford CD, Greenwood J, Anderson J, Snow G, Petersen FB. CD34+ cell adhesion molecule profiles differ between patients mobilized with granulocyte-colony-stimulating factor alone and chemotherapy followed by granulocyte-colony-stimulating factor. *Transfusion.* 2006; 46(2):193–8.

84. Milone G, Leotta S, Indelicato F, Mercurio S, Moschetti G, Di Raimondo F, *et al.* G-CSF alone vs cyclophosphamide plus G-CSF in PBPC mobilization of patients with lymphoma: results depend on degree of previous treatment. *Bone Marrow Transplant.* 2003; 31(9):747–54.

85. Krishnan A, Bhatia S, Slovak ML, Arber DA, Niland JC, Nademanee A, *et al.* Predictors of therapy-related leukemia and myelodysplasia following autologous transplantation for lymphoma: an assessment of risk factors. *Blood.* 2000; 95(5):1588–93.

86. Desikan KR, Barlogie B, Jagannath S, Vesole DH, Siegel D, Fassas A, *et al.* Comparable engraftment kinetics following peripheral-blood stem-cell infusion mobilized with granulocyte colony-stimulating factor with or without cyclophosphamide in multiple myeloma. *J Clin Oncol.* 1998; 16(4):1547–53.

87. Koc ON, Gerson SL, Cooper BW, Laughlin M, Meyerson H, Kutteh L, *et al.* Randomized cross-over trial of progenitor-cell mobilization: high-dose cyclophosphamide plus granulocyte colony-stimulating factor (G-CSF) *versus* granulocyte-macrophage colony-stimulating factor plus G-CSF. *J Clin Oncol.* 2000; 18(9):1824–30.

88. Gupta S, Zhou P, Hassoun H, Kewalramani T, Reich L, Costello S, *et al.* Hematopoietic stem cell mobilization with intravenous melphalan and G-CSF in patients with chemoresponsive multiple myeloma: report of a phase II trial. *Bone Marrow Transplant.* 2005; 35(5):441–7.

89. Hopman RK, DiPersio JF. Advances in stem cell mobilization. *Blood Rev.* 2014; 28(1):31–40.

90. Ding L, Saunders TL, Enikolopov G, Morrison SJ. Endothelial and perivascular cells maintain haematopoietic stem cells. *Nature.* 2012; 481(7382):457–62.

91. Broudy VC. Stem cell factor and hematopoiesis. *Blood.* 1997; 90(4):1345–64.

92. Levesque JP, Leavesley DI, Niutta S, Vadas M, Simmons PJ. Cytokines increase human hematopoietic cell adhesiveness by activation of very late antigen (VLA)-4 and VLA-5 integrins. *J Exp Med.* 1995; 181(5):1805–15.

93. da Silva MG, Pimentel P, Carvalhais A, Barbosa I, Machado A, Campilho F, *et al.* Ancestim (recombinant human stem cell factor, SCF) in association with filgrastim does not enhance chemotherapy and/or growth factor-induced peripheral blood progenitor cell (PBPC) mobilization in patients with a prior insufficient PBPC collection. *Bone Marrow Transplant.* 2004; 34(8):683–91.

94. To LB, Bashford J, Durrant S, MacMillan J, Schwarer AP, Prince HM, *et al.* Successful mobilization of peripheral blood stem cells after addition of ancestim (stem cell factor) in patients who had failed a prior mobilization with filgrastim (granulocyte colony-stimulating factor) alone or with chemotherapy plus filgrastim. *Bone Marrow Transplant.* 2003; 31(5):371–8.

95. Lapierre V, Rossi JF, Heshmati F, Azar N, Vekhof A, Makowski C, *et al.* Ancestim (r-metHuSCF) plus filgrastim and/or chemotherapy for mobilization of blood progenitors in 513 poorly mobilizing cancer patients: the French compassionate experience. *Bone Marrow Transplant.* 2011; 46(7):936–42.

96. De Clercq E. The bicyclam AMD3100 story. *Nat Rev Drug Discov.* 2003; 2(7):581–7.

97. Donzella GA, Schols D, Lin SW, Este JA, Nagashima KA, Maddon PJ, *et al.* AMD3100, a small molecule inhibitor of HIV-1 entry via the CXCR4 co-receptor. *Nat Med.* 1998; 4(1):72–7.

98. Devine SM, Flomenberg N, Vesole DH, Liesveld J, Weisdorf D, Badel K, *et al.* Rapid mobilization of CD34+ cells following administration of the CXCR4 antagonist AMD3100 to patients with multiple myeloma and non-Hodgkin's lymphoma. *J Clin Oncol.* 2004; 22(6):1095–102.

99. Flomenberg N, Devine SM, DiPersio JF, Liesveld JL, McCarty JM, Rowley SD, *et al.* The use of AMD3100 plus G-CSF for autologous hematopoietic progenitor cell mobilization is superior to G-CSF alone. *Blood.* 2005; 106(5):1867–74.

100. Calandra G, McCarty J, McGuirk J, Tricot G, Crocker SA, Badel K, *et al.* AMD3100 plus G-CSF can successful mobilize CD34+ cells from non-Hodgkin's lymphoma, Hodgkin's disease and multiple myeloma patients previously failing mobilization with chemotherapy and/or cytokine treatment: compassionate use data. *Bone Marrow Transplant.* 2008; 41(4):331–8.

101. Cashen A, Lopez S, Gao F, Calandra G, MacFarland R, Badel K, *et al.* A phase II study of plerixafor (AMD3100) plus G-CSF for autologous hematopoietic progenitor cell mobilization in patients with Hodgkin lymphoma. *Biol Blood Marrow Transplant.* 2008; 14(11):1253–61.

102. Fowler CJ, Dunn A, Hayes-Lattin B, Hansen K, Hansen L, Lanier K, *et al.* Rescue from failed growth factor and/or chemotherapy HSC mobilization with G-CSF and plerixafor (AMD3100): an institutional experience. *Bone Marrow Transplant.* 209; 43(12):9–17.

103. Stiff P, Micallef I, McCarthy P, Magalhaes-Silverman M, Weisdorf D, Territo M, *et al.* Treatment with plerixafor in non-Hodgkin's lymphoma and multiple myeloma patients to increase the number of peripheral blood stem cells when given a mobilizing regimen of G-CSF: implications for the heavily pretreated patient. *Biol Blood Marrow Transplant.* 2009; 15(2):249–56.

104. Dugan MJ, Maziarz RT, Bensinger WI, Nademanee A, Liesveld J, Badel K, *et al.* Safety and preliminary efficacy of plerixafor (Mozobil) in combination with chemotherapy and G-CSF: an open-label, multicenter, exploratory trial in patients with multiple myeloma and non-Hodgkin's lymphoma undergoing stem cell mobilization. *Bone Marrow Transplant.* 2010; 45(1):39–47.

105. DiPersio JF, Micallef IN, Stiff PJ, Bolwell BJ, Maziarz RT, Jacobsen E, *et al.* Phase III prospective randomized double-blind placebo-controlled trial of plerixafor plus granulocyte colony-stimulating factor compared with placebo plus granulocyte colony-stimulating factor for autologous stem-cell mobilization and transplantation for patients with non-Hodgkin's lymphoma. *J Clin Oncol.* 2009; 27(28):4767–73.

106. DiPersio JF, Stadtmauer EA, Nademanee A, Micallef IN, Stiff PJ, Kaufman JL, *et al.* Plerixafor and G-CSF *versus* placebo and G-CSF to mobilize hematopoietic stem cells for autologous stem cell transplantation in patients with multiple myeloma. *Blood.* 2009; 113(23):5720–6.

107. Devine SM, Vij R, Rettig M, Todt L, McGlauchlen K, Fisher N, *et al.* Rapid mobilization of functional donor hematopoietic cells without G-CSF using AMD3100, an antagonist of the CXCR4/SDF-1 interaction. *Blood.* 2008; 112(4):990–8.

108. Rettig MP, Ansstas G, DiPersio JF. Mobilization of hematopoietic stem and progenitor cells using inhibitors of CXCR4 and VLA-4. *Leukemia.* 2012; 26(1):34–53.

109. Nazha A, Cook R, Vogl DT, Mangan PA, Hummel K, Cunningham K, *et al.* Plerixafor and G-CSF *versus* cyclophosphamide and G-CSF for stem cell mobilization in patients with multiple myeloma. *Blood (ASH Annual Meeting Abstracts).* 2009 Dec; 114: Abstract 2146.

110. Shaughnessy P, Islas-Ohlmayer M, Murphy J, Hougham M, MacPherson J, Winkler K, *et al.* Plerixafor plus G-CSF compared to chemotherapy plus G-CSF for mobilization of autologous CD34+ cells resulted in similar cost but more predictable days of apheresis and less hospitalization. *Blood (ASH Annual Meeting Abstracts).* 2009; 114:Abstract 2277.

111. Fruehauf S, Veldwijk MR, Seeger T, Schubert M, Laufs S, Topaly J, *et al.* A combination of granulocyte-colony-stimulating factor (G-CSF) and plerixafor mobilizes more primitive peripheral blood progenitor cells than G-CSF alone: results of a European phase II study. *Cytotherapy.* 2009; 11(8):992–1001.

112. Costa LJ, Alexander ET, Hogan KR, Schaub C, Fouts TV, Stuart RK. Development and validation of a decision-making algorithm to guide the use of plerixafor for autologous hematopoietic stem cell mobilization. *Bone Marrow Transplant.* 2011; 46(1):64–9.

113. Smith VR, Popat U, Ciurea S, Nieto Y, Anderlini P, Rondon G, et al. Just-in-time rescue plerixafor in combination with chemotherapy and granulocyte-colony stimulating factor for peripheral blood progenitor cell mobilization. *Am J Hematol.* 2013; 88(9):754–7.

114. Farina L, Spina F, Guidetti A, Longoni P, Ravagnani F, Dodero A, et al. Peripheral blood CD34+ cell monitoring after cyclophosphamide and granulocyte-colony-stimulating factor: an algorithm for the preemptive use of plerixafor. *Leuk Lymphoma.* 2014; 55(2):331–6.

115. Basak GW, Mikala G, Koristek Z, Jaksic O, Basic-Kinda S, Cegledi A, et al. Plerixafor to rescue failing chemotherapy-based stem cell mobilization: it's not too late. *Leuk Lymphoma.* 2011; 52(9):1711–9.

116. Vishnu P, Roy V, Paulsen A, Zubair AC. Efficacy and cost-benefit analysis of risk-adaptive use of plerixafor for autologous hematopoietic progenitor cell mobilization. *Transfusion.* 2012; 52(1):55–62.

117. Li J, Hamilton E, Vaughn L, Graiser M, Renfroe H, Lechowicz MJ, et al. Effectiveness and cost analysis of "just-in-time" salvage plerixafor administration in autologous transplant patients with poor stem cell mobilization kinetics. *Transfusion.* 2011; 51(10):2175–82.

118. Cashen AF, Lazarus HM, Devine SM. Mobilizing stem cells from normal donors: is it possible to improve upon G-CSF? *Bone Marrow Transplant.* 2007; 39(10):577–88.

119. Anderlini P, Przepiorka D, Seong C, Smith TL, Huh YO, Lauppe J, et al. Factors affecting mobilization of CD34+ cells in normal donors treated with filgrastim. *Transfusion.* 1997; 37(5):507–12.

120. Grigg AP, Roberts AW, Raunow H, Houghton S, Layton JE, Boyd AW, et al. Optimizing dose and scheduling of filgrastim (granulocyte colony-stimulating factor) for mobilization and collection of peripheral blood progenitor cells in normal volunteers. *Blood.* 1995; 86(12):4437–45.

121. Holm M. Not all healthy donors mobilize hematopoietic progenitor cells sufficiently after G-CSF administration to allow for subsequent CD34 purification of the leukapheresis product. *J Hematother.* 1998; 7(2):111–3.

122. Platzbecker U, Prange-Krex G, Bornhauser M, Koch R, Soucek S, Aikele P, et al. Spleen enlargement in healthy donors during G-CSF mobilization of PBPCs. *Transfusion.* 2001; 41(2):184–9.

123. Stroncek DF, Dittmar K, Shawker T, Heatherman A, Leitman SF. Transient spleen enlargement in peripheral blood progenitor cell donors given G-CSF. *J Transl Med.* 2004; 2:25.

124. Horowitz MM, Confer DL. Evaluation of hematopoietic stem cell donors. *Hematology Am Soc Hematol Educ Program.* 2005:469–75.

125. Nash RA, Bowen JD, McSweeney PA, Pavletic SZ, Maravilla KR, Park MS, et al. High-dose immunosuppressive therapy and autologous peripheral blood stem cell transplantation for severe multiple sclerosis. *Blood.* 2003; 102(7):2364–72.

126. Stricker RB, Goldberg B. G-CSF and exacerbation of rheumatoid arthritis. *Am J Med.* 1996; 100(6):665–6.

127. Burt RK, Fassas A, Snowden J, van Laar JM, Kozak T, Wulffraat NM, et al. Collection of hematopoietic stem cells from patients with autoimmune diseases. *Bone Marrow Transplant.* 2001; 28(1):1–12.

128. Gottenberg JE, Roux S, Desmoulins F, Clerc D, Mariette X. Granulocyte colony-stimulating factor therapy resulting in a flare of systemic lupus erythematosus: comment on the article by Yang and Hamilton. *Arthritis Rheum.* 2001; 44(10):2458–60.

129. Spitzer G, Adkins D, Mathews M, Velasquez W, Bowers C, Dunphy F, et al. Randomized comparison of G-CSF + GM-CSF vs G-CSF alone for mobilization of peripheral blood stem cells: effects on hematopoietic recovery after high-dose chemotherapy. *Bone Marrow Transplant.* 1997; 20(11):921–30.

130. Gazitt Y. Comparison between granulocyte colony-stimulating factor and granulocyte-macrophage colony-stimulating factor in the mobilization of peripheral blood stem cells. *Curr Opin Hematol.* 2002; 9(3):190–8.

131. Rettig MP, Shannon WD, Ritchey J, Holt M, McFarland K, Lopez S, et al. Characterization of human CD34+ hematopoietic stem cells following administration of G-CSF or plerixafor. *Blood* (ASH Annual Meeting Abstracts). 2008 Dec; 112:Abstract 3476.

132. Rettig MP, Lopez S, McFarland K, DiPersio JF. Rapid and prolonged mobilization of human CD34+ hematopoietic stem cells following intravenous (IV) administration of plerixafor. *Blood* (ASH Annual Meeting Abstracts). 2010 Dec; 116:Abstract 2261.

133. Kymes SM, Pusic I, Lambert DL, Gregory M, Carson KR, DiPersio JF. Economic evaluation of Plerixafor for stem cell mobilization. *Am J Manag Care.* 2012; 18(1):33–41.

134. Dar A, Goichberg P, Shinder V, Kalinkovich A, Kollet O, Netzer N, et al. Chemokine receptor CXCR4-dependent internalization and resecretion of functional chemokine SDF-1 by bone marrow endothelial and stromal cells. *Nat Immunol.* 2005; 6(10):1038–46.

135. Imai K, Kobayashi M, Wang J, Shinobu N, Yoshida H, Hamada J, et al. Selective secretion of chemoattractants for haemopoietic progenitor cells by bone marrow endothelial cells: a possible role in homing of haemopoietic progenitor cells to bone marrow. *Br J Haematol.* 1999; 106(4):905–11.

136. Jung Y, Wang J, Schneider A, Sun YX, Koh-Paige AJ, Osman NI, et al. Regulation of SDF-1 (CXCL12) production by osteoblasts; a possible mechanism for stem cell homing. *Bone.* 2006; 38(4):497–508.

137. Ponomaryov T, Peled A, Petit I, Taichman RS, Habler L, Sandbank J, et al. Induction of the chemokine stromal-derived factor-1 following DNA damage improves human stem cell function. *J Clin Invest.* 2000; 106(11):1331–9.

138. Watt SM, Forde SP. The central role of the chemokine receptor, CXC4R, in haemopoietic stem cell transplantation: will CXCR4 antagonists contribute to the treatment of blood disorders? *Vox Sang.* 2008; 94(1):18–32.

139. Peled A, Petit I, Kollet O, Magid M, Ponomaryov T, Byk T, et al. Dependence of human stem cell engraftment and repopulation on NOD/SCID mice on CXCR4. Science. 1999; 283(5403):845–8.

140. Nagasawa T, Hirota S, Tachibana K, Takakura N, Nishikawa S, Kitamura Y, et al. Defects of B-cell lymphopoiesis and bone-marrow myelopoiesis in mice lacking the CXC chemokine PBSF/SDF-1. Nature. 1996; 382(6592):635–8.

141. Tachibana K, Hirota S, Iizasa H, Yoshida H, Kawabata K, Kataoka Y, et al. The chemokine receptor CXCR4 is essential for vascularization of the gastrointestinal tract. Nature. 1999; 393(6685):591–4.

142. Ma Q, Jones D, Borghesani PR, Segal RA, Nagasawa T, Kishimoto T, et al. Impaired B-lymphopoiesis, myelopoiesis, and derailed cerebellar neuron migration in CXCR4-and SDF-1-deficient mice. Proc Natl Acad Sci USA. 1998; 95(16):9448–53.

143. Ma Q, Jones D, Springer TA. The chemokine receptor CXCR4 is required for the retention of B lineage and granulocytic precursors within the bone marrow microenvironment. Immunity. 1999; 10(4):463–71.

144. Robinson JA, Demarco S, Gombert F, Moehle K, Obrecht D. The design, structures and therapeutic potential of protein epitope mimetics. Drug Discov Today. 2008; 13(21–22):944–51.

145. Schmitt S, Weinhold N, Dembowsky K, Neben K, Witzens-Harig M, Braun M, et al. First results of a phase-II study with the new CXCR4 antagonist POL6326 to mobilize hematopoietic stem cells (HSC) in multiple myeloma (MM). Blood (ASH Annual Meeting Abstracts). 2010 Dec; 116:Abstract 824.

146. Elices MJ, Osborn L, Takada Y, Crouse C, Luhowskyj S, Hemler ME, et al. VCAM-1 on activated endothelium interacts with the leukocyte integrin VLA-4 at a site distinct from the VLA-4/fibronection binding site. Cell. 1990; 60(4):577–84.

147. Scott LM, Priestley GV, Papayannopoulou T. Deletion of alpha4 integrins from adult hematopoietic cells reveals roles in homeostasis, regeneration, and homing. Mol Cell Biol. 2003; 23(24):9349–60.

148. Priestley GV, Ulyanova T, Papayannopoulou T. Sustained alterations in biodistribution of stem/progenitor cells in Tie2Cre+ alpha4(f/f) mice are hematopoietic cell autonomous. Blood. 2007; 109(1):109–11.

149. Priestley GV, Scott LM, Ulyanova T, Papayannopoulou T. Lack of alpha4 integrin expression in stem cells restricts competitive function and self-renewal activity. Blood. 2006; 107(7):2959–67.

150. Jing D, Oelschlaegel U, Ordemann R, Holig K, Ehninger G, Reichmann H, et al. CD49d blockade by natalizumab in patients with multiple sclerosis affects steady-state hematopoiesis and mobilizes progenitors with a distinct phenotype and function. Bone Marrow Transplant. 2010; 45(10):1489–96.

151. Zohren F, Toutzaris D, Klarner V, Hartung HP, Kieseier B, Haas R. The monoclonal anti-VLA-4 antibody natalizumab mobilizes CD34+ hematopoietic progenitor cells in humans. Blood. 2008; 111(7):3893–5.

152. Foley J. Recommendations for the selection, treatment, and management of patients utilizing natalizumab therapy for multiple sclerosis. Am J Manag Care. 2010; 16(6 Suppl): S178–83.

153. Ransohoff RM. Natalizumab for multiple sclerosis. N Engl J Med. 2007; 356(25):2622–9.

154. Davenport RJ, Munday JR. Alpha4-integrin antagonism – an effective approach for the treatment of inflammatory diseases? Drug Discov Today. 2007; 12(13–14):569–76.

155. Jackson DY. Alpha 4 integrin antagonists. Curr Pharm Des. 2002; 8(14):1229–53.

156. Yang GX, Hagmann WK. VLA-4 antagonists: potent inhibitors of lymphocyte migration. Med Res Rev. 2003; 23(3):369–92.

157. Ghosh S, Panaccione R. Anti-adhesion molecule therapy for inflammatory bowel disease. Therap Adv Gastroenterol. 2010; 3(4):239–58.

158. Takazoe M, Watanabe M, Kawaguchi T, Matsumoto T, Oshitani N, Hiwatashi N, et al. Oral alpha-4 integrin inhibitor (AJM300) in patients with active Crohn's disease – a randomized, double-blind, placebo-controlled trial. Gastroenterology. 2009; 136(5 Suppl 1): A-181

159. Muro F, Iimura S, Sugimoto Y, Yoneda Y, Chiba J, Watanabe T, et al. Discovery of trans-4-[1-[[2,5-Dichloro-4-(1-methyl-3-indolylcarboxamido)phenyl]acetyl]-(4S)-methoxy-(2S)-pyrrolidinylmethoxy] cyclohexanecarboxylic acid: an orally active, selective very late antigen-4 antagonist. J Med Chem. 2009; 52(24):7974–92.

160. Ramirez P, Rettig MP, Uy GL, Deych E, Holt MS, Ritchey JK, et al. BIO5192, a small molecule inhibitor of VLA-4, mobilizes hematopoietic stem and progenitor cells. Blood. 2009; 114(7):1340–3.

161. King AG, Johanson K, Frey CL, DeMarsh PL, White JR, McDevitt P, et al. Identification of unique truncated KC/GROβ chemokines with potent hematopoietic and anti-infective activities. J Immunol. 2000; 164(7):3774–82.

162. King AG, Horowitz D, Dillon SB, Levin R, Farese AM, MacVittie TJ, et al. Rapid mobilization of murine hematopoietic stem cells with enhanced engraftment properties and evaluation of hematopoietic progenitor cell mobilization in rhesus monkeys by a single injection of SB-251353, a specific truncated form of the human CXC chemokine GROβ. Blood. 2001; 97(6):1534–42.

163. Pelus LM, Bian H, King AG, Fukuda S. Neutrophil-derived MMP-9 mediates synergistic mobilization of hematopoietic stem and progenitor cells by the combination of G-CSF and the chemokines GROβ/CXCL2 and GROβT/CXCL2Δ4. Blood. 2004; 103(1):110–9.

164. Pelus LM, Fukuda S. Peripheral blood stem cell mobilization: the CXCR2 ligand GROβ rapidly mobilizes hematopoietic stem cells with enhanced engraftment properties. Exp Hematol. 2006; 34(8):1010–20.

165. Osawa M, Hanada K, Hamada H, Nakauchi H. Long-term lymphohematopoietic reconstitution by a single CD34-low/negative hematopoietic stem cell. Science. 1996; 273(5272):242–5.

166. Matsuzaki Y, Kinjo K, Mulligan RC, Okano H. Unexpectedly efficient homing capacity of purified murine hematopoietic stem cells. Immunity. 2004; 20(1):87–93.

167. Fukuda S, Bian H, King AG, Pelus LM. The chemokine GROβ mobilizes early hematopoietic stem cells characterized by enhanced homing and engraftment. *Blood*. 2007; 110(3):860–9.

168. Sackstein R. The lymphocyte homing receptors: gatekeepers of the multistep paradigm. *Curr Opin Hematol*. 2005; 12(6):444–50.

169. Wodnar-Filipowicz A. Flt3 ligand: role in control of hematopoietic and immune functions of the bone marrow. *News Physiol Sci*. 2003; 18:247–51.

170. He S, Chu J, Vasu S, Deng Y, Yuan S, Zhang J, et al. FLT3L and Plerixafor combination increases hematopoietic stem cell mobilization and leads to improved transplantation outcome. *Biol Blood Marrow Transplant*. 2014; 20(3):309–13.

171. Olson JA, Leveson-Gower DB, Gill S, Baker J, Beilhack A, Negrin RS. NK cells mediate reduction of GVHD by inhibiting activated, alloreactive T cells while retaining GVT effects. *Blood*. 2010; 115(21):4293–301.

172. Rezvani K, Mielke S, Ahmadzadeh M, Kilical Y, Savani BN, Zeilah J, et al. High donor FOXP3-positive regulatory T-cell (Treg) content is associated with a low risk of GVHD following HLA-matched allogeneic SCT. *Blood*. 2006; 108(4):1291–7.

173. Anandasabapathy N, Hurley A, Breton G, Caskey M, Trumpfheller C, Sarma P, et al. A phase 1 trial of the hematopoietic growth factor CDX-301 (rhuFlt3L) in healthy volunteers. *Biol Blood Marrow Transplant*. 2013; 19(2 Suppl):S112–S113.

174. Hill JM, Zalos G, Halcox JP, Schenke WH, Waclawiw MA, Quyyumi AA, et al. Circulating endothelial progenitor cells, vascular function, and cardiovascular risk. *N Engl J Med*. 2003; 348(7):593–600.

175. Khan SS, Solomon MA, McCoy JP Jr. Detection of circulating endothelial cells and endothelial progenitor cells by flow cytometry. *Cytometry B Clin Cytom*. 2005; 64(1):1–8.

176. Wojakowski W, Landmesser U, Bachowski R, Jadczyk T, Tendera M. Mobilization of stem and progenitor cells in cardiovascular diseases. *Leukemia*. 2012; 26(1):23–33.

177. Asahara T, Takahashi T, Masuda H, Kalka C, Chen D, Iwaguro H, et al. VEGF contributes to postnatal neovascularization by mobilizing bone marrow-derived endothelial progenitor cells. *EMBO J*. 1999; 18(14):3964–72.

178. Schroder K, Kohnen A, Aicher A, Liehn EA, Buchse T, Stein S, et al. NADPH oxidase Nox2 is required for hypoxia-induced mobilization of endothelial progenitor cells. *Circ Res*. 2009; 105(6):537–44.

179. Lundby C, Gassmann M, Pilegaard H. Regular endurance training reduces the exercise induced HIF-1α and HIF-2α mRNA expression in human skeletal muscle in normoxic conditions. *Eur J Appl Physiol*. 2006; 96(4):363–9.

180. Cubbon RM, Murgatroyd SR, Ferguson C, Bowen TS, Rakobowchuk M, Baliga V, et al. Human exercise-induced circulating progenitor cell mobilization is nitric oxide-dependent and is blunted in South Asian men. *Arterioscler Thromb Vasc Biol*. 2010; 30(4):878–84.

181. Hambrecht R, Adams V, Erbs S, Linke A, Krankel N, Shu Y, et al. Regular physical activity improves endothelial function in patients with coronary artery disease by increasing phosphorylation of endothelial nitric oxide synthase. *Circulation*. 2003; 107(25):3152–8.

182. Bonsignore MR, Morici G, Riccioni R, Huertas A, Petrucci E, Veca M, et al. Hemopoietic and angiogenetic progenitors in healthy athletes: different responses to endurance and maximal exercise. *J Appl Physiol (1985)*. 2010; 109(1):60–7.

183. Jenkins NT, Witkowski S, Spangenburg EE, Hagberg JM. Effects of acute and chronic endurance exercise on intracellular nitric oxide in putative endothelial progenitor cells: role of NADPH oxidase. *Am J Physiol Heart Circ Physiol*. 2009; 297(5):H1798–805.

Chapter

11

New Perspectives in Manufacturing Hematopoietic Cells

Adrian P. Gee

Introduction

The rapid growth in cell therapies over the last few years has outpaced development of new technologies for manufacturing cellular products. In parallel, manufacturers have been faced with an evolving regulatory strategy making it somewhat difficult to anticipate requirements. To some extent this situation has improved in that the Food and Drug Administration (FDA or Agency) has settled on a risk-based strategy for regulating these products[1]. Essentially, this consists of two pathways[2], one for cells that are minimally manipulated *ex-vivo* and are intended to be used to provide their normal function (homologous use); and the second for more-than-minimally manipulated products (e.g., that have been cultured ex-vivo, activated, transduced, etc.) and/or are to be used to provide therapeutic effects beyond their normal function (e.g., marrow cells used in cardiac regenerative therapy). The latter are regulated as biologic pharmaceuticals under current Good Manufacturing Practices (cGMP) and clinical trials must be performed under the Investigational New Drug (IND) regulations. Minimally manipulated cells are regulated under the newer current good tissue practice (cGTP) regulations, which resemble less-stringent cGMP regulations, and do not require an IND for their clinical use.

In both cases, however, the FDA has expectations when it comes to the manufacturing of the cells. These are intended to ensure that the products are not contaminated or cross-contaminated, that they meet specifications in terms of safety and purity, and that the manufacturing procedures are consistent and under quality review.

This chapter describes the origin of the most common manufacturing methods and indicates improvements that are in process or required for cellular therapies to advance.

Original Methods

Many cellular therapies can trace their origins to bone marrow transplantation. Developed in the 1950s[3], this treatment required the collection of bone marrow from an individual and its subsequent transfer to a cancer patient. This required the development of harvesting and testing procedures, but little *ex-vivo* manipulation was used in its initial application.

As the importance of HLA-matching to avoid severe or fatal graft-*versus*-host disease (GvHD) was realized, it became apparent that HLA-identical donors were in short supply. This in turn prompted the development of registries for unrelated HLA-typed donors and of methods to try to remove the cells that were thought to mediate GvHD – T-lymphocytes [4]. T-cell depletion was one of the first methods used to manufacture a cell therapy *ex-vivo* to achieve a desired effect *in-vivo*. A variety of T-cell depletion technologies were developed (Figure 11.1), some of which would now provoke an adverse reaction from the FDA, e.g., removal of T-cells by rosetting with sheep erythrocytes. These approaches were, however, clinically effective and as knowledge of the identity of the T-cells mediating GvHD increased, methods for their removal became more selective, involving the use of monoclonal antibodies (MAbs) to identify the effector cells and to mediate their removal, by attachment to a solid matrix, e.g., magnetic and nonmagnetic particles.

In parallel, autologous transplantation was growing. This avoided the risk of GvHD by harvesting the patient's own marrow, cryopreserving it, and returning it after high-dose therapy. This required the development of methods for freezing the cells[5], resulting in the use of dimethyl sulfoxide as the cryoprotectant and controlled rate freezers, followed by storage in liquid nitrogen. These technologies have remained largely unchanged, although nitrogen vapor phase storage has replaced immersion of the products, to avoid potential cross-contamination. A potential risk from the use of autologous grafts was the possibility of contamination of the harvested marrow by occult tumor cells that would be returned to the patient. This stimulated the field of removal or purging of tumor cells from autologous grafts *ex-vivo*[6]. As with T-cell removal from allogeneic grafts, this required a method to identify the tumor cells and a way to remove them. Pharmacologic purging was used, but sometimes resulted in delayed engraftment due to toxicity towards the normal stem cells. Monoclonal antibodies provided a more selective method and, as described earlier, could also be used to effect cell removal. One of the most popular methods was to coat the tumor cells with a panel of tumor-directed MAbs and capture the cells by coating with anti-immunoglobulin-coated magnetic beads and passage through a magnetic field – immunomagnetic

Evolution of T-Cell Manipulation

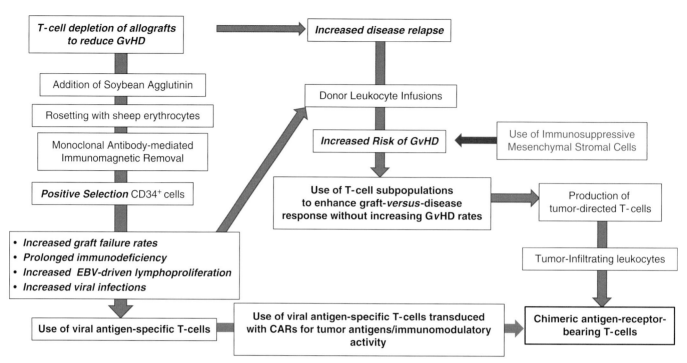

Figure 11.1. Evolution of T-cell depletion. Shown at the top left are methods that were originally used to deplete T-cells from allogeneic hematopoietic grafts to prevent graft-*versus*-host disease. As the figure moves towards the bottom left the development of hematopoietic progenitor cells is shown as an alternative strategy. To the right are methods used to combat the increased incidence of graft-*versus*-host disease associated with T-cell depletion, resulting in the development of T-cells bearing chimeric antigen receptors. Boxes with italicized text show the clinical consequences of using manipulated grafts.

purging. A device was developed for this purpose by Baxter but did not achieve widespread clinical application.

The removal of a subset of cells, be they tumor or T-cells (negative selection), was thought to be less effective than positive selection or enrichment of hematopoietic progenitor cells; development of this approach was hampered by the fact that these cells could not easily be identified. Discovery of the CD34 antigen present on hematopoietic progenitors resulted in the production of an anti-CD34 monoclonal antibody that could effect their enrichment[7]. The risk was that this approach might deplete cells that were needed for engraftment. Devices were developed to achieve CD34+ cell separation, e.g., the CellPro device (that used MAbs linked to Sepharose beads to collect the cells and physical disruption to detach them) and the Isolex and CliniMACS devices that use linkage to magnetic materials (beads and magnetic colloids, respectively) to collect the cells and a competitive peptide or removal of the magnetic field (respectively) to harvest the cells. These devices marked the first real automation of complex cell processing with their functionally closed disposables and programmed washing and cell collection technologies.

As predicted, use of purified CD34+ cells was not the universal panacea. Pan T-cell depletion resulted in delayed engraftment and results from T-cell-depleted allografts had indicated higher incidences of disease relapse (see Chapter 29),

suggesting that some T-cells may have a beneficial GvHD effect. Nonetheless, CD34+ enrichment is still used in transplants where there is a high risk of severe GvHD (see Chapters 12, 30, 59, and 61). There is no doubt, however, that the benefits of "engineering" the graft were becoming apparent, and as knowledge of the effects of various cell populations has increased, interest in manufacturing therapeutic cells with a range of specific effects has developed beyond applications in bone marrow transplantation.

Current and New Methods for Manufacturing Therapeutic Cells

Newer cellular therapies are based on the use of specific cell populations to effect killing of diseased cells, to enhance engraftment of transplanted cells and organs, to replace or regenerate tissues and organs damaged by disease, and to act as delivery vehicles for various therapeutic agents[8]. Potential and current applications are too numerous to review, however, there are certain manufacturing requirements that are common to all cell therapy products.

A primary concern for the FDA is the possibility of contamination of the product. This starts with potentially transmissible infectious agents being present in the cells collected from the donor. For this reason the donor is required to

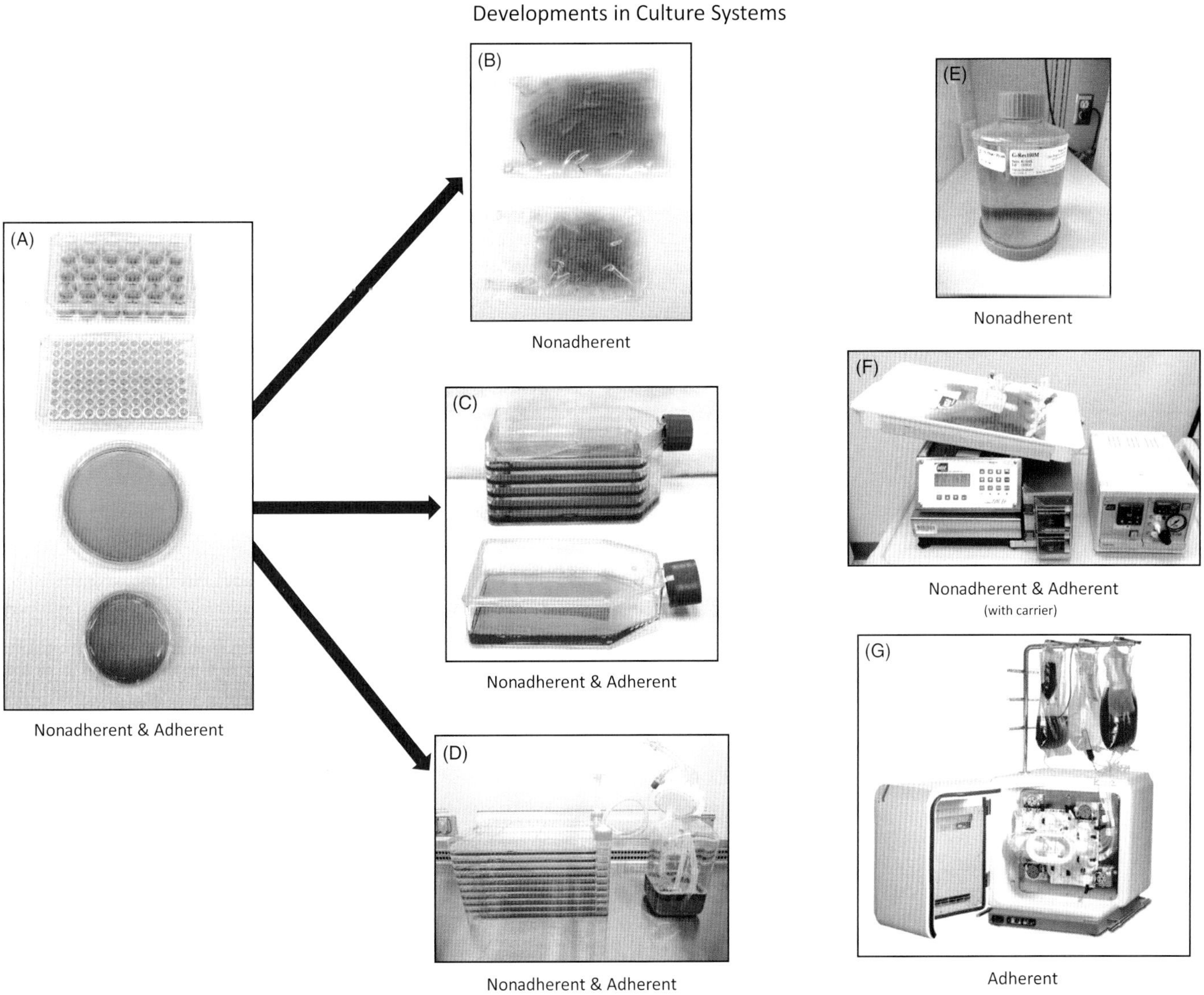

Developments in Culture Systems

Figure 11.2. Developments in culture systems. (**A**) Open culture systems for adherent and nonadherent cells. (**B**) Gas-permeable bags for culture of nonadherent cells. (**C**) Single layer and multilayer T flasks for nonadherent and adherent cell culture. (**D**) Cell Factories – large-scale multilayer flasks for culture of adherent and nonadherent cells. (**E**) The G-Rex bioreactor for nonadherent cells. (**F**) The Wave Bioreactor system for culture of nonadherent cells and for adherent cells attached to carrier substrates. (**G**) The Terumo Quantum hollow fiber bioreactor for culture of adherent cells.

undergo an assessment of eligibility[2]. This involves testing for a panel of infectious diseases, completion of a questionnaire to assess potential risks for infection, and a medical examination. It is very likely that additional infectious disease tests will be added to the current panel, and that testing procedures will become more rapid, sensitive, and inexpensive.

Starting cells were initially collected predominantly from bone marrow or peripheral blood, but now the sources are numerous, including adipose tissue, cord and menstrual blood, organs, and tissues, etc. In all cases functionally closed collection systems are preferred to avoid risk of contamination during harvesting. This has been facilitated by the development of specific devices for cell collection, e.g., the apheresis systems for blood stem cells, the Cytori device for harvesting adipose tissue, etc. As ideal sources for particular applications

are determined, it is likely that more automated collection systems will be produced.

Manufacturing usually requires expansion of the cells *invitro*. The initial collection volume and cell numbers will determine the expansion options available. Small cell numbers do not lend themselves well to closed or automated culture systems. They often need specific cell densities to grow well and have to be nursed through a series of culture vessels to get to the numbers that can grow in "devices." The initial culture vessels are open systems (Figure 11.2A, B, and D) and present a high-risk for contamination and cross-contamination. They are frequently labor intensive and would not lend themselves well to manufacturing of a commercial alternative. At present there do not seem to be any commercially available functionally closed systems for expanding small numbers of cells.

One of the most promising devices for larger cell numbers is the G-Rex device manufactured by Wilson Wolfe (Figure 11.2E)[9]. This is a small bioreactor in which the cells are suspended on a gas-permeable membrane with nutrient medium above and air below. This allows static culture without frequent feeding, but with excellent gas exchange. The cells can be harvested automatically using a harvest device. The G-Rex has produced impressive and predictable expansion of nonadherent cells with minimal technician intervention. Growth is monitored by lactose production or glucose consumption, measured by sampling the medium.

For large-scale expansion there is a wider choice of commercial systems. For nonadherent cells gas-permeable bags have been used (Figure 11.2B)[10]. These require ongoing attention as the cells expand and can be difficult to handle when volumes become large. An alternative is the Wave Bioreactor from General Electric (Figure 11.2F)[11]. This device consists of a culture bag connected to medium delivery and monitoring systems. This greatly automates cell expansion and the device has been widely used in phase 1 studies. The Wave system can also be used to culture adherent cells by the introduction of a solid-phase matrix into the bag. The cells attach to the matrix particles and can be recovered using recombinant trypsin equivalents.

Other methods for growing adherent cells range from cluster plates where the cells are grown in wells, through a variety of sizes of T flasks, up to various designs of cell factories, which consist of stacks of culture plates contained in an outer vessel (Figure 11.2C). Smaller devices are essentially open, whereas there are mechanisms available to functionally close the larger systems. Recently automated devices have become available for expanding adherent cell populations, e.g., the Quantum system from Terumo (Figure 11.2G)[12] and the PRIMER HF reactor from Biovest International[13].

Cells in the Quantum are grown on microfibers contained within a sterile disposable cartridge. This fits into a device that can be programmed to allow cell attachment, feeding, and harvesting. Growth is assessed by measuring lactate production, and when predetermined levels are reached, the flow of medium through the cartridge is increased by the user. The development of such systems is likely to be spurred on by identification of clinically effective cellular therapies in widely occurring diseases. At present the market is not well established and until it is, biotech companies are reluctant to develop equipment that may never find widespread use.

Media

For the approval of a cellular therapy product the FDA would prefer that the cells are grown in chemically defined medium that is protein free and contains only essential well-characterized supplements, e.g., X-VIVO 15 (Lonza). Unfortunately this is often not possible, but the recommendations should be borne in mind. Serum-free defined media are becoming commercially available and should always be the first choice for evaluation. The user needs to understand the formulations and determine whether supplements will be required. For cells that require serum the two main choices are fetal bovine and human AB serum[14], both available from many sources. A prerequisite for bovine serum is that it is obtained from herds from countries where bovine spongiform encephalitis is not endemic – this usually means Australia, New Zealand, and the United States. This must be documented on the certificate of analysis (CofA) from the distributer, together with all other testing that has been performed on the material. Human AB serum must be obtained from donors who have undergone eligibility screening (2), which includes testing for infectious diseases, assessment of risk behaviors, and a medical examination. Commercial lots are pooled from multiple donors and certification that they were all screened should be obtained from the manufacturer.

Supplements, such as cytokines, should be of GMP or clinical grade wherever possible. These are becoming increasingly available, e.g., from GellGenix, Totipotent SC, and Humanzyme, but where they are not, the purest form should be sourced, a CofA obtained, and the information submitted to the FDA, who will determine if additional testing is required before use. Supplements should always be kept to the minimum number required to achieve satisfactory cell growth. Regulatory authorities may question the purpose of each, and justification for its inclusion[15]. Hopefully the future will bring a wider range of approved media that can be used for cell culture and that may also be suitable as the excipient used to administer the cells.

Cryopreservation and Storage of Hematopoietic Cells

Cryopreservation of cells has become a routine manufacturing step, since the product is readily available when required, it provides a method to hold the cells to allow full testing before release, it facilitates shipment, and it allows multiple treatments from the same lot. The development of new methods for cryopreservation has been rather neglected by the cell therapy community. This is because the standardized method, which uses a final concentration of 10% dimethyl sulfoxide and controlled rate freezing followed by storage in liquid nitrogen fluid or vapor, has generally produced good results[16]. Recently there have been reports, e.g., for NK cells and hematopoietic "stem" cells, that while this approach may maintain cell viability, the functionality upon thawing may be compromised[17–19]. If this proves to be a widespread finding, it may require that cells be cultured for a period before administration, or that fresh cultures are formulated at the receiving institution. Both options would pose an impediment to commercialization, since they are logistically complex. A clearer understanding of the factors that are producing this effect may result in changes to the cryoprotectant and the methods for freezing and thawing that would overcome this effect.

Storage methods for frozen cells still predominantly use liquid nitrogen. A cell therapy manufacturing facility typically can be identified by the presence of a number of these "banks." Outwardly they have looked much the same over the years, but storage by immersion in liquid nitrogen has largely been replaced by keeping the cells in the vapor phase, thereby reducing the likelihood of cross-contamination between products. Vapor phase temperatures are achieved by maintaining a fixed amount of liquid nitrogen at the bottom of the storage bank, or by absorbing it into the walls of the vessel, the latter providing a more uniform temperature distribution. We are likely to see dramatic improvements in the inventory systems used to locate products within the banks. At present, the physical location is recorded at the time of freezing and retrieval is based on this information. In future radiofrequency tagging of products[20] will provide real-time location information, reducing the chance for errors.

Shipping methods for cryopreserved cells have become standardized, in that they generally use a dry shipper, in which liquid nitrogen is absorbed into the lining of the shipping vessel. The shippers contain a temperature-monitoring device and are usually transported by air. This method has been demonstrated to be efficient and safe[21], and there are unlikely to be major changes to it. In contrast, there is ample opportunity to improve procedures and equipment for transporting fresh cells. At present these predominantly consist of packaging cells in bags or flasks into a sturdy container[22]. In some cases, the shipping procedure becomes part of the manufacturing procedure[23], in that cells continue to expand during transportation. Although there are a variety of outer containers available, there is no integrated system specifically designed for shipment of cell cultures under defined conditions. Depending on a better understanding of the potential adverse effects of cryopreservation[17–19], this could be become a commercial opportunity.

Hematopoietic Product Testing

A panel of release tests is usually completed before a product can be released and distributed for clinical use. Traditionally these tests must address product purity, identity, and potency. Over the years the regulatory authorities have approved a number of specific tests to measure these parameters. These are listed in the *Code of Federal Regulations* and the FDA has published a number of Guidances as to their use. The trend has been to improve turnaround time for these assays thereby accelerating product release. Implementation of these faster methods may require a formal validation of the method against the approved test. This can be complex, lengthy, and expensive. Gradually some of the faster tests are achieving regulatory approval and the FDA has encouraged the development of new methods to improve sensitivity and turnaround times. Part of this is to permit full testing of products that are to be administered fresh. This requires a very short turnaround time that is not possible with some of the approved test methods. In the case of sterility testing, fresh products can

only be released using a Gram stain, which is recognized as insensitive and inconsistent. The requirement, therefore, is to perform 14-day sterility tests in addition to the Gram stain. These may be supplemented by testing sterility in process. Gradually some rapid methods have appeared, e.g., endotoxin assays using the approved Endosafe device. Others are available, e.g., *Mycoplasma* testing using the MycoAlert system, but are not yet fully approved, and the end-user may be required to perform a formal validation. There is definitely a move towards development of rapid test systems that should eventually result in completion of all release testing prior to the administration of noncryopreserved cells.

"Off-the-Shelf" Cell Therapy

As was discussed earlier, the development of cellular therapies was impacted by the importance of HLA-matching of the cells and the recipients. For many cell products this meant that allogeneic products were essentially tailor-made for an individual recipient. This boutique type of therapy was of considerably less interest for commercialization, where the model was to produce a universal pharmaceutical. For many years biotechnology companies struggled with the business model for cellular therapies. Should it be product or service based? Some service-based companies have taken off, but widespread commercialization will be stimulated if cellular therapy products can be manufactured, easily stored, and provided to a wide range of patients. We are starting to see this happen. For example, mesenchymal stromal cells (see Chapter 68) and multipotent adult progenitor cells lack HLA class II antigens and have been administered across histocompatibility barriers to provide immunosuppression in transplant recipients[24], and for regenerative medicine applications. Large banks of these cells could be manufactured, tested, and made available to a wide variety of patients.

Similarly allogeneic virus-directed T-cells (see Chapter 64) were developed initially as a single patient product; however, in recent years it has been shown that these cells can be administered to partially HLA-matched individuals without risk of GvHD (see Chapter 58)[25]. As a result a small number of banks of these cells representing major HLA types can be prepared, and can cover the greater part of the HLA spectrum.

Controversies and Future Directions

As our understanding of the factors modulating immune responses and our ability to engineer cells to provide specific properties develop, it is likely that cellular therapies will begin to more closely resemble small molecule drugs (Figure 11.3) in that they will be "off-the-shelf" and designed to treat a wider range of patients. When this is achieved cell therapy will have crossed a very important barrier to its widespread commercial development.

Perhaps the main controversy is whether the current strategy of regulating these products as pharmaceuticals is appropriate. We have already seen a few cellular therapy products reach licensure, e.g., cord blood in the United States, a process

Developments in Manufacturing of Cellular Therapy Products

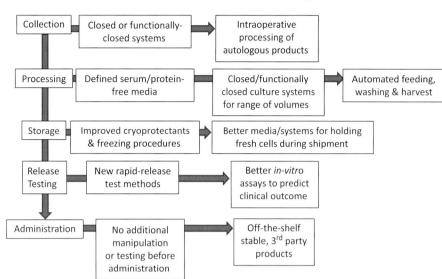

Figure 11.3. Developments in manufacturing of cellular therapy products. This figure shows on the left the major steps in the manufacturing of cellular therapy products. To the right of each box are shown the advances in each step that have been made or need to be made to optimize each step.

that has involved considerable expense for the banks. In contrast, bone marrow transplantation remains largely unregulated and allogeneic peripheral blood progenitor cell transplantation remains somewhere in between, but is probably heading towards licensure. This is the approach that the cellular therapy community originally proposed to the FDA as an alternative to regulation using the blood banking model. Whether this was the correct decision remains to be established as more products move towards licensure.

Acknowledgments

This work was supported in part by contract # HHSN268201000007C Production Assistance for Cellular Therapy (PACT) contract from NIH/NHLBI and Grant RP130256 TACCT Texas Assistance for Cancer Cell Therapy (TACCT) from the Cancer Prevention and Research Institute of Texas. The author thanks Sara Richman for her assistance in the preparation of the manuscript.

References

1. Halme DG, Kessler DA. FDA regulation of stem cell based therapies. *N Engl J Med.* 2006;355(16):1730–5.

2. The Code of Federal Regulations. Human cells, tissues and cellular and tissue-based products. 2014; Part 1271.

3. Eapen M, O'Donnell P, Brunstein CG, Wu J, Barowski K, Mendizibal A et al. Mismatched related and unrelated donors for allogeneic hematopoietic cell transplantation for adults with hematologic malignancies. *Biol Blood Marrow Transplant.* 2014;20(10):1485–92.

4. Mielke S, McIver ZA, Shenoy, Fellowes V, Khuu H, Stroncek DF et al. Selectively T cell depleted allografts from HLA-matched sibling donors followed by low-dose posttransplantation immunosuppression to improve transplantation outcome in patients with hematologic malignancies. *Biol Blood Marrow Transplant.* 2011;17(12):1855–61.

5. Berz D, McCormack EM, Winer ES, Colvin GA, Quesenberry PJ. Cryopreservation of hematopoietic stem cells. *Am J Hematol.* 2007;82(6):463–72.

6. Melillo L, Cascavilla N, Lerma E, Corsetti MT, Carella AM. The significance of minimal residual disease in stem cell grafts and the role of purging: is it better to purge in vivo or in vitro? *Acta Haematol* 2005;114(4):206–13.

7. Sidney LE, Branch MJ, Dunphy SE, Dua HS, Hopkinson A. Concise review: evidence for CD34 as a common marker for diverse progenitors. *Stem Cells.* 2014;32(6):1380–9.

8. Basel MT, Shrestha TB, Bossmann SH, Troyer DL. Cells as delivery vehicles for cancer therapeutics. *Ther Deliv.* 2014;5(5):555–67.

9. Lapteva N, Vera JF. Optimization manufacture of virus and tumor-specific T cells. *Stem Cells Int.* 2011;2011:434392. doi: 10.4061/2011/434392. Epub 2011 Sep 11.

10. Gulen D, Abe F, Maas S, Reed E, Cowan K, Pirruccello S et al. Closing the manufacturing process of dendritic cell vaccines transduced with adenovirus vectors. *Int Immunopharmacol.* 2008;8(13–14):1728–36.

11. Donia M, Larsen SM, Met O, Svane IM. Simplified protocol for clinical grade tumor-infiltrating lymphocyte manufacturing with use of the Wave bioreactor. *Cytotherapy.* 2014;16(8):1117–20.

12. Hanley PJ, Mei Z, Durett AG, de Graca Cabreira-Harrison M, Klis M, Li W et al. Efficient manufacturing of therapeutic mesenchymal stromal cells with the use of the Quantum cell expansion system. *Cytotherapy.* 2014;16(8):1048–58.

13. Tapia F, Vogel T, Genzel Y, Behrendt I, Hirschel M, Gangemi JD et al. Production of high-titer influenza A virus with adherent and suspension MDCK cells cultured in a single use hollow fiber bioreactor. *Vaccine.* 2014;32(8):1003–11.

14. Canovas D, Bird N. Human AB serum as an alternative to fetal bovine serum for endothelial and cancer cell culture. *ALTEX* 2012;29(4):426–8.

15. Read E. Ancillary materials for cell and tissue-based products. US Pharmacopeia. Available from: http://c.ymcdn.com/sites/www .celltherapysociety.org/resource/resmgr/ uploads/files/Cell Therapy Liaison Meetings/November 2011/2. CTLM_ Read_29MOV2011.pdf

16. Winter JM, Jacobson P, Bullough B, Christensen AP, Boyer M, Reems JA. Long-term effects of cryopreservation on clinically prepared hematopoietic progenitor cell products. *Cytotherapy.* 2014;16(7):965–75.

17. Miller JS, Rooney CM, Curtsinger J, McElmurry R, McCullar V, Verneris MR *et al.* Expansion and homing of adoptively transferred human natural killer cells in immunodeficient mice varies with product preparation and *in vivo* cytokine administration: implications for clinical therapy. *Biol Blood Marrow*

Transplant. 2014;20(8):1252–7. doi: 10.1016/j.bbmt.2014.05.004. Epub 2014 May 9.

18. Lapteva N, Szmania SM, van Rhee F, Rooney CM. Clinical grade purification and expansion of natural killer cells. *Crit Rev Oncol.* 2014:19(1–2):121–32.

19. Shu Z, Heimfeld S, Gao D. Hematopoietic SCT with cryopreserved grafts: adverse reactions after transplantation and cryoprotectant removal before infusion. *Bone Marrow Transplant.* 2014;49(4):469–76.

20. Kozma N, Speletz H, Reiter U, Lanzer G, Wagner T. Impact of 13.56-MHz radiofrequency identification systems on the quality of stored red blood cells. *Transfusion.* 2011;51(11):2384–90.

21. Bielanski A. Non-transmission of bacterial and viral microbes to embryos and semen stored in vapour phase of liquid nitrogen dry shippers. *Cryobiology.* 2005;50(2):206–10.

22. Veronesi E, Murgia A, Caselli A, Grisendi G, Picinno MS, Rasini V *et al.* Transportation conditions for prompt

use of ex vivo expanded and freshly harvested clinical-grade bone marrow mesenchymal stromal/stem cells for bone regeneration. *Tissue Eng Part C Methods.* 2014;20(3):239–51.

23. Klingemann H, Grodman C, Cutler E, Duque M, Kadidlo D, Klein AK *et al.* Autologous stem cells transplant recipients tolerate haploidentical related-donor natural killer cell-enriched infusion. *Transfusion.* 2013;53(2):412–8.

24. Eggenhofer E, Popp FC, Mendicino M, Silber P, Van't Hof W, Renner P *et al.* Heart grafts tolerized through third-party multipotent cells can be retransplanted to secondary hosts with no immunosuppression. *Stem Cells Transl Med.* 2013;2(8):595–606.

25. Leen AM, Bollard CM, Mendizabal AM, Shpall EJ, Szabolics P, Antin JH *et al.* Multicenter study of banked third-party virus-specific T cells to treat severe viral infections after hematopoietic stem cell transplantation. *Blood.* 2013;121(26):5113–23.

Prevention of Acute Graft-*versus*-Host Disease — One Size Fits All?

Chapter 12

Nelson J. Chao and Michael Green

Introduction

Allogeneic hematopoietic cell transplant (allo-HCT) is a therapy capable of curing patients with various hematologic malignancies. Graft-*versus*-host disease (GvHD) is the immune response of donor T-lymphocytes responding to the recipient"s alloantigens and is a complication of allo-HCT associated with significant morbidity and mortality[1]. GvHD can manifest early (approximately 100 days) or later (greater than 100 days) after stem cell transplantation. Acute graft-*versus*-host disease (aGvHD) is a T-cell-mediated disorder that classically presents in the early post-transplantation period and causes injury to host skin, intestines, and liver[2, 3]. There has been much research focused on the prevention and treatment of GvHD over several decades, however our current management practices have not changed significantly[4]. Despite the use of pharmacologic GvHD prophylaxis the rate of grade II–IV aGvHD ranges from 35 to 50% in matched related donor transplants and up to 70% in those from unrelated donors [5]. New insights into the pathophysiology[6], prevention, and treatment of GvHD offer a promising landscape for the future study and management of allo-HCT.

Prophylaxis of aGvHD centers on immunosuppression of the donor T-cells, either pharmacologically or via T-cell depletion[1,7]. A recent survey involving 79 centers from the European Group for Blood and Marrow Transplantation (EBMT) highlighted that there is no currently agreed upon standard regimen, and clinical practice varies by institution [8]. Methotrexate combined with a calcineurin inhibitor (cyclosporine or tacrolimus) is the most common GvHD prophylaxis used in myeloablative conditioning allo-HCT, while mycophenolate mofetil (MMF) combined with a calcineurin inhibitor is frequently used in nonmyeloablative conditioned or umbilical cord transplants. The graft-*versus*-tumor response is a valuable treatment consideration when pursuing an allo-HCT and T-cells also mediate this process in a similar manner to GvHD. There is much interest in identifying therapeutic approaches to decrease GvHD without abrogating the graft-*versus*-tumor effect[3].

The pathophysiology for aGvHD has been characterized over many years (Figure 12.1). In a recent review, Sung and Chao[6] examined the pathophysiology behind aGvHD. They characterized the five steps involved in the development of aGvHD

which include: (1) chemotherapy\radiation causing tissue damage leading to production of proinflammatory cytokines resulting in (2) T-cell activation through antigen-presenting cell T-cell interaction leading to (3) T-cell differentiation and expansion, (4) T-cell trafficking, and finally (5) T-cell recruitment and tissue destruction. This review will attempt to explore the most significant recent developments in the prevention of aGvHD categorized by effect on the underlying pathophysiologic step leading to disease.

T-Cell Depletion

Alemtuzumab

Alemtuzumab is a monoclonal antibody directed at CD52 with activity against T-cells both *in-vivo* and *ex-vivo*. Many reports have been published using alemtuzumab for GvHD prophylaxis in patients with aplastic anemia. One recent Canadian series examined the effect of the addition of intermediate dose alemtuzumab (50–60 mg) to either a cyclophosphamide-based or fludarabine-based conditioning regimen with additional GvHD prophylaxis with cyclosporine. Forty-one patients with aplastic anemia received allo-HCT after conditioning. No patients in this series developed grades III–IV aGvHD or severe chronic GvHD. A large number of viral infections with CMV, HSV, VZV, and BK virus were seen[9].

Researchers from Duke University performed a comparative study of 124 patients with a variety of hematologic malignancies who underwent reduced intensity conditioning (fludarabine, melphalan or busulfan, and alemtuzumab followed by transplant [either matched related donor (MRD), matched unrelated donor (MUD), or haplotype matched]). In this study, the cumulative incidence of grade III–IV aGvHD was 3% for MRDs, 11% for MUDs, and 27% for patients who had undergone haplotype matched transplants. There was no significant difference in relapse rates among the groups but the 2 year overall survival was much less in those who underwent matched unrelated (22%) and haplotype matched (23%) transplantation (compared to those with MRD transplants 51%). There was a high incidence of graft failure that was likely related to the use of busulfan in the conditioning regimen[10].

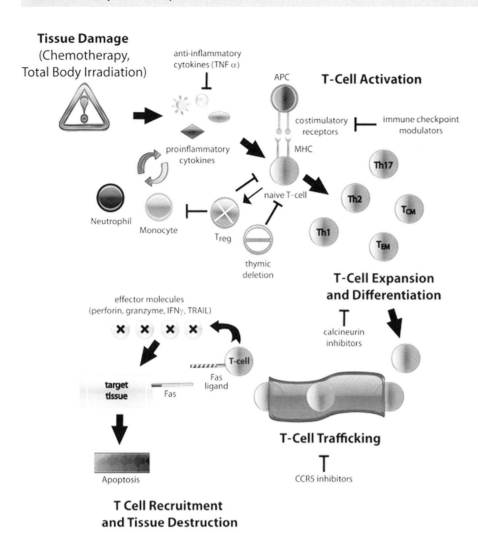

Tissue Damage
(Chemotherapy,
Total Body Irradiation)

anti-inflammatory
cytokines (TNF α)

APC

T-Cell Activation

costimulatory
receptors

immune checkpoint
modulators

MHC

proinflammatory
cytokines

Th17

naive T-cell

Th2

TCM

Neutrophil

Monocyte

Treg

Th1

thymic
deletion

TEM

effector molecules
(perforin, granzyme, IFNγ, TRAIL)

**T-Cell Expansion
and Differentiation**

calcineurin
inhibitors

T-cell

Fas
ligand

target
tissue

Fas

Apoptosis

T-Cell Trafficking

CCR5 inhibitors

**T Cell Recruitment
and Tissue Destruction**

Figure 12.1. Pathophysiology of acute GvHD. Chemotherapy and radiation cause tissue damage, producing proinflammatory cytokines, resulting in T-cell activation through APC-T-cell interaction via MHC-T-cell receptor binding and costimulatory signals. This leads to T-cell expansion and differentiation into various subtypes, which traffic through blood vessels to target organs, where they cause tissue destruction and recruitment of other inflammatory cells through pathways such as perforin/granzyme and cytokine release. These inflammatory cells and cytokines can further propagate the cycle of GvHD. This process is internally regulated by Treg cells as well as thymic deletion of alloreactive T-cells. Exogenous means of treating GvHD include inhibitors of inflammation and cytokines, immune checkpoint modulators, calcineurin inhibitors, and CCR5 inhibitors. Abbreviations: APC, antigen-presenting cell; CCR5, chemokine receptor type 5; IFN-γ, interferon-γ; MHC, major histocompatibility complex; TCM, central memory T-cell; TEM, effector memory T-cell; Treg, regulatory T-cell; TNF-α, tumor necrosis factor-α; TRAIL, TNF-related apoptosis-inducing ligand. Reprinted from Sung AD, Chao NJ. Acute graft-*versus*-host disease: are we close to bringing the bench to the bedside? *Best Pract Res Clin Haematol.* 2013;26(3):285–92., Copyright (2013), with permission from Elsevier.

Antithymocyte Globulin

Antithymocyte globulin (ATG) is a polyclonal immunoglobulin directed against human T-lymphocytes and is used in autologous hematopoietic cell transplant (auto-HCT) for prophylaxis of GvHD which, as previously discussed, is T-cell mediated[11]. Prospective and retrospective studies have had mixed results regarding the efficacy and safety of various ATG preparations for the prevention of GvHD[12–14].

An Italian group performed two consecutive trials in which 109 patients with varying hematologic malignancies were randomized to receive either rabbit ATG (two different doses 7.5 mg/kg and 15°mg/kg) *versus* no ATG as part of the conditioning regimen (total body irradiation and cyclophosphamide) prior to unrelated donor allo-HCT. They demonstrated that patients whose conditioning regimen included 15 mg/kg of rabbit ATG had reduced severe acute GvHD (11% *versus* 50%); however there was no reduction in transplant-related mortality (49% *versus* 47%) because this population was at increased risk for developing severe\fatal infections. They also found that time to platelet engraftment was longer in patients receiving ATG (38 *versus* 23 days; *P*=0.02)[12].

A related German study randomly assigned 202 patients with varying hematologic malignancies undergoing allo-HCT from MUDs to receive GvHD prophylaxis (cyclosporine plus methotrexate), with or without rabbit ATG. Severe aGvHD (grade III–IV) was no different between the ATG group and control group. However, the cumulative incidence of aGvHD (grade II–IV) was reduced in the ATG group *versus* the control group (33% *versus* 51%). They also found that extensive chronic GvHD was greatly decreased in the ATG group as well (12.2% *versus* 42.6%). There were no differences between relapse, nonrelapse mortality, overall survival, and mortality from infectious causes[13].

Researchers from Dana-Farber performed a retrospective analysis of 1676 adult patients with hematologic malignancies who underwent reduced intensity allo-HCT and compared patients who underwent *in-vivo* T-cell depletion with ATG (n=584) or alemtuzumab (n=213) with those patients who did not undergo T-cell depletion (n=879). When compared to T-cell-replete transplants those patients who received ATG had similar rates of aGvHD (38% *versus* 40%) but lower rates of chronic GvHD and lower disease-free and overall survival[14].

A Cochrane review was performed on six randomized controlled trials involving a total of 568 patients who underwent auto-HCT to investigate the utility of the addition of ATG for GvHD prophylaxis. This meta-analysis found that severe aGvHD (grade II–IV) was significantly lower in patients who received ATG (RR 0.68, NNT 8); however, there was no impact of the addition of ATG to overall survival or incidence of relapse[15].

One can infer from the totality of these studies that the addition of ATG is effective in decreasing the rate of aGvHD in allo-HCT recipients without significant impact on survival. The data from the German study with the suggestion of lower chronic GvHD are currently being studied in a prospective randomized trial (NCT01295710).

Cyclophosphamide

The alkylating agent cyclophosphamide has varying utilities in the treatment of hematologic and nonhematologic conditions with much of its efficacy secondary to its immunomodulatory effects. Preclinical studies in murine models demonstrated that high doses of cyclophosphamide after auto-HCT target proliferating alloreactive T-cells and prevent GvHD[16]. This led researchers at Johns Hopkins to perform a phase I/II study utilizing single-agent high-dose cyclophosphamide for GvHD prophylaxis after myeloablative condition and HLA-matched allo-HCT. One hundred and seventeen patients with various hematologic malignancies received myeloablation with busulfan and cyclophosphamide followed by T-cell-replete bone marrow; they received 50 mg/kg per day of cyclophosphamide on days 3 and 4 after transplantation. The incidence of acute GvHD grades II–IV and III–IV was 43% and 10%, respectively. The nonrelapse mortality (NRM) at day 100 and 2 years after transplantation was 9% and 17%, respectively. At the median follow-up of 26 months the cumulative incidence of chronic GvHD was 10%.

While reasonable efficacy was seen in the myeloablative setting its utility after reduced intensity conditioning and non-myeloablative conditioning regimens was less remarkable[17]. More studies are needed before any meaningful conclusions can be presented.

T-Cell Migration
Maraviroc

Recruitment of lymphocytes into tissues is involved in the pathophysiology of GvHD. Manipulation of T-cell trafficking using a first in class small molecule chemokine receptor 5 antagonist, maraviroc, was studied in a phase I/II trial at the University of Pennsylvania[18]. Thirty-eight patients with a variety of hematologic malignancies received a matched related or unrelated allo-HCT after reduced intensity conditioning; they then received maraviroc along with tacrolimus and methotrexate afterwards. Day 100 and day 180 grades II–IV aGvHD were 14.7% and 23.6, respectively, with low rates involving the gut (8.8%) or liver (2.9%). At day 180 the cumulative incidence of aGvHD (grade III–IV) was 5.9%. The cumulative incidence of moderate to severe chronic GvHD was 23.6% at 1 year. This study demonstrates that inhibition of lymphocyte trafficking is a potentially effective approach to abate visceral GvHD.

Sirolimus

Sirolimus is a lipophilic macrocyclic lactone (mTOR inhibitor) that is presumed to inhibit cytotoxic T-cells while leaving Tregs intact[19]. It also demonstrates inhibition of antigen presentation and dendritic cell maturation. A recent phase III multicenter trial conducted by the Bone Marrow Transplant Clinical Trials Network examined whether the combination of tacrolimus and sirolimus was more effective than tacrolimus and methotrexate in patients undergoing matched related donor allo-HCT after myeloablative conditioning (total body irradiation(TBI) with cyclophosphamide or etoposide). Three hundred and four patients with a variety of hematologic conditions were randomly assigned to the two groups. At day 114 grade II–IV aGvHD rates for the tacrolimus\sirolimus group compared to the tacrolimus\methotrexate group were 67% and 62%, respectively. There was also a trend for an increased cumulative incidence of chronic GvHD at 2 years from transplantation in the tacrolimus\sirolimus arm. However, more rapid engraftment was seen in the tacrolimus\sirolimus group. Previous studies demonstrated that the use of sirolimus was associated with increased rates of sinusoidal obstruction syndrome. Although not identified formally in the above study, moving forward it should be a big consideration. The researchers above did find that tacrolimus with sirolimus led to more rapid engraftment.

Ctyokine Secretion
Bortezomib

Bortezomib is a proteasome inhibitor and has immunomodulatory properties with the ability to selectively deplete proliferating alloreactive T-lymphocytes, reduce T-helper type 1 cytokines, block antigen-presenting cell activation, and potentially spare regulatory T-cells[20]. The addition of bortezomib to standard prophylaxis with methotrexate and tacrolimus was examined in a study by researchers at Dana-Farber Cancer Institute. Forty-five patients receiving mismatched auto-HCT after reduced intensity conditioning were included in this phase I/II study and given a short course of bortezomib administered on days +1, +4, and +7. The cumulative incidence of aGvHD at 180 days was 22%. The 1-year cumulative incidence of chronic GvHD was 29%. These data suggest that even in a high-risk population of mismatched patients bortezomib had some impact on control of GvHD, and like other early phase studies these data must be expanded before any broad application can be made. It must also be stated that bortezomib itself has potential activity against some hematologic malignancies and this in itself may reduce the incidence of relapse.

Pentostatin

Pentostatin is a purine-analog that inhibits adenosine deaminase, leading to increased lymphocyte apoptosis and decreased interleukin 2-production[21] and leads to functional impairment of T-lymphocytes while sparing natural killer and humoral responses. This ability of pentostatin led researchers at M.D. Anderson to perform a phase I/II study examining its impact when added to GvHD prophylaxis with methotrexate and tacrolimus in mismatched related (n=10) or unrelated (n=137) allo-HCT. Pentostatin was given intravenously on days +8, +15, +22, and +30 following transplantation. One hundred and forty-seven patients with various hematologic malignancies and conditioning protocols were randomly assigned to five treatment groups (control, 0.5, 1.0, 1.5, and 2.0 mg/m^2 pentostatin). Patients receiving the 1.0 and 1.5 mg/m^2 dose had the most success with grade II–IV aGvHD of 41.1% and 35.7%, when compared to the control group (55.6%). No grades III–IV aGvHD occurred in 11 HLA-mismatched recipients in the 1.5 mg/m^2 group[22].

Vorinostat

Inhibitors of histone deacetylases (HDAC) have antitumor effects, modify gene expression, and reduce production of inflammatory cytokines[23]. Vorinostat (an HDAC inhibitor) was recently studied in a phase I/II trial at the University of Michigan and Washington University. Fifty adult patients with various hematologic malignancies underwent reduced intensity conditioning (fludarabine and melphalan) prior to related donor allo-HCT, and then received verinostat along with tacrolimus and MMF[24]. Mean rates of day 100 and day 180 aGvHD (grades II–IV) were 22% and 28%, respectively. The authors found no cases of primary or secondary graft failure. The cumulative incidence of moderate to severe cGvHD at 1 year was 45%. The incidence of relapse was 16% at both 1 and 2 years. All-cause nonrelapse mortality and GvHD-related (acute and chronic) nonrelapse mortality were 10% and 6%, respectively. These results suggest that vorinostat in combination with standard GvHD prophylaxis after related donor reduced intensity conditioning had reasonable control of aGvHD, but as this was a single-center study more data are needed before the true impact of this addition is determined.

Statin Therapy

Statins are lipid-lowering drugs that reduce cholesterol production by inhibiting HMG-CoA reductase. Besides lowering of cholesterol, statins have also demonstrated immunomodulatory effects[25]. Researchers from West Virginia University have studied the addition of atorvastatin to GvHD prophylaxis in matched related allogeneic transplant recipients[26]. A total of 30 patients with various hematologic malignancies were

recruited into this phase II trial and given 40 mg of atorvastatin in conjunction with tacrolimus and short course methotrexate and underwent MRD transplantation. Cumulative incidence rates of aGvHD (grades II–IV) at days 100 and 180 were 3.3% (95% CI, 0.2% to 14.8%) and 11.1% (95% CI, 2.7% to 26.4%), respectively. These researchers are currently in the process of recruiting patients to their study (NCT01665677).

T-Cell Subset Manipulation
Total Lymphoid Irradiation

Preclinical studies using murine models have demonstrated that host natural killer T-lymphocytes and donor T-regulatory lymphocytes regulate aGvHD[27]. These regulatory T-cells inhibit the proliferation and cytokine secretion by donor T-cells implicated in the injury of the skin, intestines, and liver associated with acute GvHD. However, the impact on the graft-*versus*-tumor is maintained. Adaptation of this study led researchers at Stanford University to perform a study of 37 patients with various hematologic malignancies using reduced intensity conditioning with total lymphoid irradiation and ATG (15 mg/kg) in addition to cyclosporine and mycophenolate mofetil followed by matched auto-HCT [28]. Total lymphoid irradiation was administered starting at day 11 to a total dose of 800 cGy in 10 fractions. The radiation field consisted of a supradiaphragmatic mantle field, a subdiaphragmatic field that included an inverted Y, and splenic ports encompassing all major lymphoid organs including the thymus, spleen, and lymph nodes, mirroring protocols used in the treatment of Hodgkin disease. The incidence of acute GvHD (grades II–IV) was 3% (1 of 37 patients); this is especially remarkable as 14 patients received transplants from unrelated donors. They also noted that 12 of 16 patients who entered the study in partial remission were in complete remission after day +100, which suggests that the graft-*versus*-tumor effect is not negatively impacted by this treatment regimen. At a median follow-up of 425 days 73% of patients were still alive (27 out of 37). Expansion of this study to 111 patients reported cumulative probability of acute GvHD (grades II–IV) by day 100 was 2% among related donor transplants and 10% among unrelated donor transplant recipients. Nonrelapse mortality at 1 year was less than 4% and there was no increase in disease relapse[29].

A multicenter trial using this same protocol of total lymphoid irradiation and ATG was performed by an Italian team [30]. Forty-five heavily pretreated patients with lymphoid and myeloid malignancies were enrolled at nine centers. These patients underwent this study protocol followed by matched (related or unrelated) or one antigen mismatched (unrelated) allo-HCT. Donor engraftment was reached in 95% of patients. Rates of acute and chronic GvHD were 13.3% and 35.8%, respectively. One-year nonrelapse mortality was 9.1%. After a median follow-up of 28 months (range, 3–57 months) median overall survival was not reached.

These results are quite encouraging and offer a novel approach to greatly reduce the incidence of acute graft-*versus*-host disease following reduced intensity conditioning allo-HCT without abrogating the graft-*versus*-tumor effect.

Controversies

Controversy #1: Is T-Cell Depletion a Viable Strategy to Prevent Acute Graft-*versus*-Host Disease

Yes. T-cell depletion has reduced the incidence of acute and chronic GvHD in a variety of trials[31–34]. ATG is effective in decreasing rates of acute and chronic GvHD and its varied efficacy is likely related to the intensity of the conditioning regimen employed. In general ATG has shown promise in both unrelated and haploidentical donor transplantation with myeloablative and reduced intensity conditioning. Other methods of T-cell depletion have also been associated with less GvHD.

No. T-cell depletion has been associated with increases in graft failure, disease relapse, delayed immune reconstitution, and post-transplant lymphoproliferative disorder. While there may be less GvHD, there is higher treatment-related mortality especially from infections and a higher relapse rate; thus there is no improvement in overall survival.

Which of these would one pick? One way to finesse this would be to use T-cell depletion for patients in first remission or those without malignant disease. There the need for GvL is lower or not necessary and the consequences of GvHD are much higher. Ultimately, the best option would be to selectively deplete only those cells that cause GvHD, allowing the rest of the T-cells to exert their important biologic function.

Controversy#2: Is Methotrexate a Necessary Component of GvHD Prophylaxis Regimens?

Yes. Methotrexate remains the backbone of all drug prophylaxis regimens. It is tried and true and results in significant prevention of GvHD with known and expected results. The major drawback of methotrexate is its toxicity especially the associated mucosits, delay in hematopoietic engraftment, and potential hepatic toxicity. However, with better chemotherapy drug dosing such as using busulfan levels and better supportive care, the risks are small.

No. There is no reason to expose patients to the toxicity of methotrexate. A recent open-label phase 3 study assessed the combination of tacrolimus and sirolimus compared to methotrexate and tacrolimus after matched related donor peripheral blood transplantation.[35]. The combination of tacrolimus and sirolimus had equivalent efficacy with regards to GvHD but showed marked improvement in engraftment. There was some concern for a trend towards increased rates of sinusoidal obstruction syndrome in the sirolimus-containing regimen; however, it was not statistically significant and did not appear to impact mortality.

Which would one pick? The good news is that there are choices. If your patient is at high risk for mucositis (say prior radiation to the GI mucosa) or there are concerns around delays in engraftment, then a non-methotrexate regimen would be useful. If there were concerns around VOD, then it would probably be best to avoid sirolimus although with possible prophylaxis against VOD, the risk of this side effect could be lessened.

Conclusion and Future Directions

Graft-*versus*-host disease is a serious and complex disease following allo-HCT. It is an orchestra of events that culminates in the destruction of both healthy and cancerous tissues. It would be hard to imagine that the "one size fits all" approach would effectively impact this disease. Many interventions, even those reviewed above, are directed at individual instruments in the orchestra; while this may work to mute or dampen the song the remaining sections will still play on. The goal for prevention of GvHD is to target the conductor. The likely strategy to prevent aGvHD will be based on the established therapeutic backbone with additional targeted therapies individualized to take into account patient comorbidities, conditioning regimen, and underlying disease.

References

1. Barrett AJ, Le Blanc K. Prophylaxis of acute GVHD: manipulate the graft or the environment? *Best Practice & Research Clinical Haematology.* 2008;21(2):165–76.

2. Wysocki CA, Panoskaltsis-Mortari A, Blazar BR, Serody JS. Leukocyte migration and graft-*versus*-host disease. *Blood.* 2005;105(11): 4191–9.

3. Goker H, Haznedaroglu IC, Chao NJ. Acute graft-vs-host disease: pathobiology and management. *Experimental Hematology.* 2001;29(3):259–77.

4. Alousi AM, Bolanos-Meade J, Lee SJ. Graft-*versus*-host disease: state of the science. *Biology of Blood and Marrow Transplantation: Journal of the American Society for Blood and Marrow Transplantation.* 2013;19(1 Suppl): S102–8.

5. Al-Kadhimi Z, Gul Z, Chen W, Smith D, Abidi M, Deol A, *et al.* High incidence of severe acute graft-*versus*-host disease with tacrolimus and mycophenolate mofetil in a large cohort of related and unrelated allogeneic transplantation patients. *Biology of Blood and Marrow Transplantation: Journal of the American Society for Blood and Marrow Transplantation.* 2014;20(7):979–85.

6. Sung AD, Chao NJ. Acute graft-*versus*-host disease: are we close to bringing the bench to the bedside? *Best Practice & Research Clinical Haematology.* 2013;26(3):285–92.

7. Ferrara JL, Levine JE, Reddy P, Holler E. Graft-*versus*-host disease. *Lancet.* 2009;373(9674):1550–61.

8. Ruutu T, van Biezen A, Hertenstein B, Henseler A, Garderet L, Passweg J, *et al.*

Prophylaxis and treatment of GVHD after allogeneic haematopoietic SCT: a survey of centre strategies by the European Group for Blood and Marrow Transplantation. *Bone Marrow Transplantation*. 2012;47(11):1459–64.

9. Hamad N, Del Bel R, Messner HA, Kim D, Kuruvilla J, Lipton JH, *et al*. Outcomes of hematopoietic cell transplantation in adult patients with acquired aplastic anemia using intermediate dose alemtuzumab-based conditioning. *Biology of Blood and Marrow Transplantation: Journal of the American Society for Blood and Marrow Transplantation*. 2014;20(11):1722–8.

10. Kanda J, Long GD, Gasparetto C, Horwitz ME, Sullivan KM, Chute JP, *et al*. Reduced-intensity allogeneic transplantation using alemtuzumab from HLA-matched related, unrelated, or haploidentical related donors for patients with hematologic malignancies. *Biology of Blood and Marrow Transplantation: Journal of the American Society for Blood and Marrow Transplantation*. 2014;20(2):257–63.

11. Grullich C, Ziegler C, Finke J. Rabbit anti T-lymphocyte globulin induces apoptosis in peripheral blood mononuclear cell compartments and leukemia cells, while hematopoetic stem cells are apoptosis resistant. *Biology of Blood and Marrow Transplantation: Journal of the American Society for Blood and Marrow Transplantation*. 2009;15(2):173–82.

12. Bacigalupo A, Lamparelli T, Bruzzi P, Guidi S, Alessandrino PE, di Bartolomeo P, *et al*. Antithymocyte globulin for graft-*versus*-host disease prophylaxis in transplants from unrelated donors: 2 randomized studies from Gruppo Italiano Trapianti Midollo Osseo (GITMO). *Blood*. 2001;98(10):2942–7.

13. Finke J, Bethge WA, Schmoor C, Ottinger HD, Stelljes M, Zander AR, *et al*. Standard graft-*versus*-host disease prophylaxis with or without anti-T-cell globulin in haematopoietic cell transplantation from matched unrelated donors: a randomised, open-label, multicentre phase 3 trial. *The Lancet Oncology*. 2009;10(9):855–64.

14. Soiffer RJ, Lerademacher J, Ho V, Kan F, Artz A, Champlin RE, *et al*. Impact of immune modulation with anti-T-cell antibodies on the outcome of reduced-intensity allogeneic hematopoietic stem cell transplantation for hematologic malignancies. *Blood*. 2011;117(25):6963–70.

15. Theurich S, Fischmann H, Shimabukuro-Vornhagen A, Chemnitz JM, Holtick U, Scheid C, *et al*. Polyclonal anti-thymocyte globulins for the prophylaxis of graft-*versus*-host disease after allogeneic stem cell or bone marrow transplantation in adults. *The Cochrane Database of Systematic Reviews*. 2012;9:CD009159.

16. Luznik L, Bolanos-Meade J, Zahurak M, Chen AR, Smith BD, Brodsky R, *et al*. High-dose cyclophosphamide as single-agent, short-course prophylaxis of graft-*versus*-host disease. *Blood*. 2010;115(16):3224–30.

17. Luznik L, O'Donnell PV, Symons HJ, Chen AR, Leffell MS, Zahurak M, *et al*. HLA-haploidentical bone marrow transplantation for hematologic malignancies using nonmyeloablative conditioning and high-dose, posttransplantation cyclophosphamide. *Biology of Blood and Marrow Transplantation: Journal of the American Society for Blood and Marrow Transplantation*. 2008;14(6):641–50.

18. Reshef R, Luger SM, Hexner EO, Loren AW, Frey NV, Nasta SD, *et al*. Blockade of lymphocyte chemotaxis in visceral graft-*versus*-host disease. *The New England Journal of Medicine*. 2012;367(2):135–45.

19. Ram R, Storb R. Pharmacologic prophylaxis regimens for acute graft-*versus*-host disease: past, present and future. *Leukemia & Lymphoma*. 2013;54(8):1591–601.

20. Koreth J, Stevenson KE, Kim HT, McDonough SM, Bindra B, Armand P, *et al*. Bortezomib-based graft-*versus*-host disease prophylaxis in HLA-mismatched unrelated donor transplantation. *Journal of Clinical Oncology: Official Journal of the American Society of Clinical Oncology*. 2012;30(26):3202–8.

21. Kraut EH, Neff JC, Bouroncle BA, Gochnour D, Grever MR. Immunosuppressive effects of pentostatin. *Journal of Clinical Oncology: Official Journal of the American Society of Clinical Oncology*. 1990;8(5):848–55.

22. Parmar S, Andersson BS, Couriel D, Munsell MF, Fernandez-Vina M, Jones RB, *et al*. Prophylaxis of graft-*versus*-host disease in unrelated donor transplantation with pentostatin, tacrolimus, and mini-methotrexate: a phase I/II controlled, adaptively randomized study. *Journal of Clinical Oncology: Official Journal of the American Society of Clinical Oncology*. 2011;29(3):294–302.

23. Dinarello CA, Fossati G, Mascagni P. Histone deacetylase inhibitors for treating a spectrum of diseases not related to cancer. *Molecular Medicine*. 2011;17(5–6):333–52.

24. Choi SW, Braun T, Chang L, Ferrara JL, Pawarode A, Magenau JM, *et al*. Vorinostat plus tacrolimus and mycophenolate to prevent graft-*versus*-host disease after related-donor reduced-intensity conditioning allogeneic haemopoietic stem-cell transplantation: a phase 1/2 trial. *The Lancet Oncology*. 2014;15(1):87–95.

25. Zeiser R, Youssef S, Baker J, Kambham N, Steinman L, Negrin RS. Preemptive HMG-CoA reductase inhibition provides graft-*versus*-host disease protection by Th-2 polarization while sparing graft-*versus*-leukemia activity. *Blood*. 2007;110(13):4588–98.

26. Hamadani M, Gibson LF, Remick SC, Wen S, Petros W, Tse W, *et al*. Sibling donor and recipient immune modulation with atorvastatin for the prophylaxis of acute graft-*versus*-host disease. *Journal of Clinical Oncology: Official Journal of the American Society of Clinical Oncology*. 2013;31(35):4416–23.

27. Pillai AB, George TI, Dutt S, Strober S. Host natural killer T cells induce an interleukin-4-dependent expansion of donor CD4+CD25+Foxp3+ T regulatory cells that protects against graft-*versus*-host disease. *Blood*. 2009;113(18):4458–67.

28. Lowsky R, Takahashi T, Liu YP, Dejbakhsh-Jones S, Grumet FC, Shizuru JA, *et al*. Protective conditioning for acute graft-*versus*-host disease. *The New England Journal of Medicine*. 2005;353(13):1321–31.

29. Kohrt HE, Turnbull BB, Heydari K, Shizuru JA, Laport GG, Miklos DB, *et al*. TLI and ATG conditioning with low risk of graft-*versus*-host disease retains antitumor reactions after allogeneic hematopoietic cell transplantation from related and unrelated donors. *Blood*. 2009;114(5):1099–109.

30. Messina G, Giaccone L, Festuccia M, Irrera G, Scortechini I, Sorasio R, *et al*. Multicenter experience using total lymphoid irradiation and antithymocyte globulin as conditioning for allografting in hematological malignancies. *Biology of Blood and Marrow Transplantation: Journal of the American Society for Blood and Marrow Transplantation*. 2012;18(10):1600–7.

31. Ringden O, Pihlstedt P, Markling L, Aschan J, Baryd I, Ljungman P, *et al*. Prevention of graft-*versus*-host disease with T-cell depletion or cyclosporin and methotrexate. A randomized trial in adult leukemic marrow recipients. *Bone Marrow Transplantation*. 1991;7(3):221–6.

32. Wagner JE, Thompson JS, Carter SL, Kernan NA, members of the Unrelated Donor Marrow Transplantation Trial. Effect of graft-*versus*-host disease prophylaxis on 3-year disease-free survival in recipients of unrelated donor bone marrow (T-cell Depletion Trial): a multi-centre, randomised phase II-III trial. *Lancet*. 2005;366(9487):733–41.

33. Pavletic SZ, Carter SL, Kernan NA, Henslee-Downey J, Mendizabal AM, Papadopoulos E, *et al*. Influence of T-cell depletion on chronic graft-*versus*-host disease: results of a multicenter randomized trial in unrelated marrow donor transplantation. *Blood*. 2005;106(9):3308–13.

34. Pasquini MC, Devine S, Mendizabal A, Baden LR, Wingard JR, Lazarus HM, *et al*. Comparative outcomes of donor graft CD34+ selection and immune suppressive therapy as graft-*versus*-host disease prophylaxis for patients with acute myeloid leukemia in complete remission undergoing HLA-matched sibling allogeneic hematopoietic cell transplantation. *Journal of Clinical Oncology: Official Journal of the American Society of Clinical Oncology*. 2012;30(26):3194–201.

35. Cutler C, Logan B, Nakamura R, Johnston L, Choi S, Porter D, *et al*. Tacrolimus/sirolimus versus tacrolimus/methotrexate as GVHD prophylaxis after matched, related donor allogeneic hematopoietic cell transplantation. *Blood*. 2014;124(8):1372–7.

Progress Treating Acute Graft-*versus*-Host Disease?

Ernest Holler

Introduction

Although numerous new approaches to prevent acute graft-*versus*-host disease (aGvHD) following allogeneic hematopoietic cell transplant (allo-HCT) including exploitation of post-transplantation cyclophosphamide[1]] have been developed, there is so far little progress in treatment of aGvHD once clinical symptoms require systemic treatment. However, deeper understanding of the pathophysiology and pathophysiology-based approaches of predicting outcome may translate into substantial progress in the near future.

The actual situation in the treatment of aGvHD has been summarized in recommendations by expert panels in recent years[2,3]. No drug or approach has been shown to be superior to the use of corticosteroids in combination with calcineurin inhibitors (Table 13.1). Topical treatment can be considered for skin disease in the early stages, and lower doses of systemic corticosteroids may be used in upper gastrointestinal aGvHD together with nonabsorbable oral corticosteroids. There is no standard for second-line treatment, and expert panels recommend that specific agents are chosen based on individual clinical characteristics of the patient. In a review by Martin *et al.* on behalf of the American Society of Blood and Marrow Transplantation (ASBMT)[2], the frequently neglected impact of number of patients included in individual trials on confidence intervals for response is nicely demonstrated and convincingly explains failure of superiority or inferiority for almost all of the alternative agents tested so far in second-line settings. In a recent survey from the Swiss−Austrian−German GvHD consortium, the heterogeneity of second-line approaches used in different centers

reflects this lack of standardization, and mycophenolate mofetil as well as extracorporeal photopheresis (ECP) were the most widely used approaches[4].

The paucity of well-controlled data on treatment of GvHD is highlighted by the 2010 Cochrane database analysis on the use of corticosteroids in aGvHD. Even for the most widely used drug, there were only four acceptable trials to be included in the analysis, which at least argued against the use of higher doses of more than 2 mg/kg per day of methylprednisolone (MP) as initial treatment (Table 13.1)[5].

Progress with Standard Immunosuppression

First-Line Treatment

Owing to its favorable effects in the Clinical Trials Network (CTN) phase 2 trial comparing four agents as potential partners of corticosteroids[6], mycophenolate mofetil (MMF) was chosen for a subsequent randomized phase 3 trial comparing corticosteroids *versus* corticosteroids plus MMF as initial treatment. The trial was recently closed due to the lack of superiority of the combined approach (BMT CTN Protocol 0802). Even in subgroups of more severe aGvHD there was no evidence of superiority of a combined approach[7] thus confirming once again that corticosteroid results are hard to improve if all patients requiring treatment are included and assessed. Tumor necrosis factor (TNF)-blocking agents seemed promising candidates; however, when added to corticosteroids, they did not show additional beneficial effect, neither in the CTN phase 2 trial using etanercept nor in a randomized study using infliximab[8].

Table 13.1 Treatment of acute GvHD: current approaches

First-line treatment	Grade II–IV	Methylprednisolone 2 mg/kg per day
	Grade I, upper GI	Methylprednisolone 1 mg/kg/day + topical steroid
Second-line treatment	Pharmacologic	MMF, mTOR inhibitors (sirolimus, everolimus[a])
	Cytokine blocking	Anti-CD25, TNF-antibodies and etanercept, agents anti-IL6[a]
	T-cell antibodies	alemtuzumab, ATGs
	Immunomodulation	Extracorporeal photopheresis

[a] Early stage.

A few studies have so far addressed the question of whether milder manifestations of aGvHD can be treated less aggressively: TNF-blocking agents might substitute for some of the corticosteroid effects, and therefore, a phase 2 trial addressed the use of etanercept and topical steroids in grade I GvHD. Although long-term results looked promising and a lower proportion of patients seemed to progress to more severe aGvHD as compared to contemporary controls, the study was terminated due to poor accrual of patients[9]. An alternative approach to reduce systemic steroid dose is achieved by the use of oral beclomethasone in upper GI aGvHD. Although a first randomized trial showed promising results and several centers introduced this approach, confirmation in further cohorts is pending. Single-center phase 2 trials continuously confirm some efficacy with regard to progress of aGvHD[10]. Considering the numerous and severe side effects of long-term use of systemic corticosteroids, especially in older patients as included in reduced intensity transplants, further efforts to reduce cumulative systemic steroid dose are urgently needed.

Second-Line Treatment

For second-line treatment, reliable randomized trials are missing. Most of the candidates tested for improving outcome of first-line treatment have shown some efficacy; however, none of the drugs used gave uniform reproducible results underlining the urgent need for standardizations of definition of steroid refractoriness and indications for second-line treatment. A well-known approach of intra-arterial application of corticosteroids in gastrointestinal refractory aGvHD has regained interest, and several reports indicate success in about 60% of several small series of 2 to 11 patients[11,12], both in pediatric and adult patients, without substantial side effects. Intra-arterial application can be considered as a "special form of topical treatment." In patients with refractory skin aGvHD, topical application of ultraviolet (UV) as UVA or narrow band UVB should be considered[13].

As in prophylaxis, mTOR inhibitors with a potential positive expansion of regulatory T-cells have gained interest in pharmacologic suppression of steroid-refractory GvHD (Table 13.2). Sirolimus has been applied in >60 patients with resistant or steroid-dependent GvHD and resulted in response rates of >60%. Toxicities may be of concern such as cytopenias and, if combined with calcineurin inhibitors, a high rate of thrombotic microangiopathy (TMA)[14]. The toxicity profile of everolimus, another mTOR inhibitor with shorter half-life, may be favorable with similar positive outcome, as is suggested by recent application in chronic GvHD[15].

Anticytokine treatment has been widely discussed and applied as a second-line option; CD25 blockade which has failed in first-line treatment still seems to give a favorable outcome in second-line treatment; inolinomab gave a response rate of 42% in a large series of 92 patients from Spain[16]; similarly, basiliximab was reported to have activity >70% in refractory GvHD outside the GI tract but only 39% in GI

Table 13.2 Treatment of acute GvHD: new approaches

Cellular Immunomodulation	Mesenchymal stem cells (donor/3rd party) Regulatory T-cells (donor)[a] Apoptotic T-cells (donor)[a]
Drugs restoring epithelial immunoregulation approaches	HDAC inhibitors[a] alpha1-antitrypsin[b] Induction of IDO: ßHCG[a], tryptophane metabolites[b]
Nondrug restoring epithelial immunoregulation approaches	Microbiome modulation (probiotics, prebiotics[a]) Induction of innate lymphoid cells[b]
Steroid saving agents	JAK-1/2 inhibitors, i.e., ruxolitinib[a] Proteasome inhibitors, i.e., bortezomib[a]
Risk stratification at onset or pre-	Biomarker development: plasmabiomarkers (sTNFR, emptive treatment Reg3alpha, ST2 and others)[a], urinary proteomics[a]

[a] Early stage.
[b] Experimental only.

GvHD[17]. Besides the confusing and controversial question of how interleukin-2 receptor blockade interferes with reconstitution of regulatory T-cells, a common concern of blocking antibodies refers to the fact that they show only transient responses as they tend to suppress rather than eliminate alloreactive T-cells. This is supported by long-term results of the basiliximab study, but is also suggested by a more recent analysis by the Paris group, who report a 2-year survival of only 30% although patients initially responded to either inolimomab or the TNF-blocking agent, etanercept[18]. Tocilizumab, an antagonist of interleukin-6 as a further cytokine involved in aGvHD, may end with the same long-term results although initial responses again are promising with 67% partial response and complete responses[19].

Alemtuzumab, a pan T-cell antibody directed against CD52, may act differently and eliminate GvHD reactive T-cells. At least three reports in a substantial number of patients show response rates >60%, and one report suggests that the high rate of infectious complications may be lower if alemtuzumab is applied in reduced weekly doses[20–22].

Progress with Extracorporeal Photopheresis

Among the nonpharmacologic approaches, ECP has become the most widely used approach although true randomized trials are lacking (Table 13.1). In a recent review of published trials on ECP in 323 patients with acute and chronic GvHD, response rates were 84% (95% CI 75–92) for cutaneous and still 65% (95% CI 52–78) for gastrointestinal GvHD[23]. In line with this, several national societies recommend ECP as a treatment for steroid-dependent or refractory GvHD[24,25]. Recently, ECP was compared with anticytokine therapy in a standardized approach for patients developing steroid-refractory aGvHD: ECP results were superior (CR and PR 66% *versus* 32%) to results of anticytokine strategies and highly improved long-term survival (HR 2.12, *P 0.015*), even after adjustment for advanced (grade III/IV) GvHD[26]. Whereas previous analyses favored modulation of regulatory T-cells by ECP, induction of myeloid-derived suppressor cells might be an additional mechanism of action[27]. Direct infusion of donor apoptotic cells has been developed as a new concept to induce tolerance; the mechanism of ECP and this new approach might be overlapping[28].

Cellular Immune Modulation

Pharmacologic immunosuppression lacks selectivity regarding elimination of alloreactive *versus* elimination of anti-infectious T-cell activity, and this partially explains the difficulties to improve results of GvHD treatment. Mimicking immunoregulation is an approach which should partially overcome this dilemma. Thus far, mesenchymal stem cells (MSCs) exerting immunomodulatory and tissue repair activity as well as regulatory T-cells (T regs) have been applied in the setting of aGvHD. MSCs, mainly from third party donors, have been used in steroid-refractory GvHD, in most studies by applying repeated infusions. The initial positive results have been confirmed with 60–70% response rates and favorable long-term results[29–31], although some studies observed an increase of infectious complications. Regulatory T-cells have been successfully used for prophylaxis of aGvHD; based on convincing experimental data now clinical trials on treatment of steroid-resistant aGvHD with donor regulatory T-cells are on the way[32].

Controversies, Major Issues Explaining Lack of Progress and Possible Solutions

While failure to achieve substantial progress in treatment of GvHD is frequently seen as a consequence of inadequate efficacy of current immunosuppressive drugs and approaches, we favor an alternative explanation: The promising results of cellular approaches as well as ECP point to one important but neglected aspect in pathophysiology and treatment of GvHD. GvHD is not only target cell destruction by alloreactive T-cells but also reflects a massive disequilibrium in tissue-specific immunoregulation which is necessary to maintain homeostasis and tolerance in epithelial targets. Our current immunosuppressive drugs eliminate both alloreactive T-cells and immunoregulatory cells and thus do not support immunoreconstitution as required. This is reflected by an ongoing diagnostic trial on biopsies from patients with gastrointestinal symptoms after allo-HCT: When biopsies were grouped according to the histologic stage of aGvHD and dosing of

corticosteroids at the time of biopsy, a reactive increase in FoxP3 regulatory T-cells was only seen in patients receiving no or low doses of prednisolone (Figure 13.1A,B). Based on these findings, currently three approaches may help to overcome the disappointing results in treatment of aGvHD as shown in Figure 13.1.

Restoration of Immunoregulation

Approaches restoring immunoregulation are urgently needed, and current experimental and clinical trials using histone deacetylase inhibitors aim at restoration of regulatory T-cells and another immunoregulatory pathway in antigen-presenting cells (APCs), the induction of indoleamine 2,3-dioxygenase (IDO)[33]. In the same direction, alpha1-antitrypsin treatment of donor cells modulates GvHD, and shifts towards regulatory T-cells have been repeatedly reported[34,35]. Although tryptophan metabolites increase in patients with GvHD indicating activation of IDO[36], this reflects an attempt of restoring immunoregulation *in-vivo*, and some new approaches therefore aim at induction of IDO, such as application of *beta*-HCG or experimental use of immunoregulatory tryptophan metabolites[37].

The importance of epithelial immunoregulation is also highlighted by the recent reports on the role of diversity of the intestinal microbiome in aGvHD and related outcome [38,39]. Loss of diversity of the intestinal microbiome may result from Paneth cell destruction in aGvHD and subsequent disturbed function of antimicrobial peptides[40]. A diverse and intact microbiome is a prerequisite not only for intestinal T reg homeostasis but also for induction of innate lymphoid cells which seem to play a role in early aGvHD, especially in epithelial protection by IL-22[41,42].

Steroid Saving Agents

Based on the broad inflammatory cytokine activation in aGvHD, approaches interfering with early activation of cytokine pathways may substitute for some of the corticosteroid effects. Among these, inhibition of JAK1/2 with ruxolitinib has shown efficacy in experimental GvHD and also in a first set of patients[43], both on the level of proinflammatory cytokines and GvHD-related symptoms. Clinical trials applying ruxolitinib in GvHD are currently starting. Bortezomib, a proteasome inhibitor, is currently tested and reported to interfere with the IL-6 pathways[44].

Biomarker Guided Individualized Treatment or Preemptive Treatment

In daily clinical practice, aGvHD grade II−IV is treated with 2mg/kg per day MP independent of clinical severity and prognostic parameters with few exceptions as discussed above. This partially reflects the lack of clinically useful parameters predicting course and outcome of aGvHD at the time of onset. Only recently, clinical factors predicting outcome and steroid

(A)

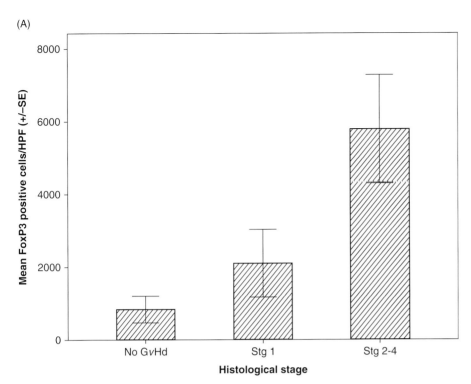

(B)

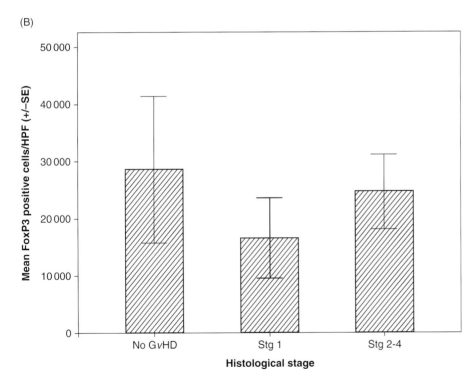

Figure 13.1. Immunohistology of FoxP3 positive cells in intestinal biopsies from patients receiving allogeneic hematopoietic cell transplantation. Patients were grouped according to histologic staging of acute GvHD and the impact of different doses of corticosteroids at the time of biopsy was analyzed. (**A**) Patients receiving <20mg/day prednisolone. Stage 0 n=22, Stage 1 n=9, Stage 2–4 n=20. Differences in FoxP3 positive cells between the histologic stages were highly significant (*P 0.003*). (**B**) Patients receiving >20mg/day prednisolone. Stage 0 n=13, Stage 1 n=18, Stage 2 n=41. No differences between the groups were detected.

refractoriness at onset have been suggested such as grade III/IV at onset, stage 2–4 gastrointestinal disease, hyperacute GvHD, and low albumin levels at onset of GvHD[45–47] but none of these criteria has so far been used to guide risk-adapted treatment. In the few last years, biomarkers have been described which associate with diagnosis and prognosis of aGvHD such as proteomics in urine samples (for early diagnosis)[48], Reg3a[49] as a biomarker of gastrointestinal disease, and ST2[50] as a marker of steroid refractoriness. If confirmed in prospective trials, these markers or combined biomarker profiles may be used for either preemptive or risk-adjusted treatment approaches allowing reduction or even avoidance of corticosteroids in low-risk and upfront intensification in high-risk aGvHD.

Selected Clinical Trials Titles and ClinicalTrials.gov Identification Number

1. Mesenchymal Stem Cell Infusion as Treatment for Steroid-Resistant Acute Graft vversus Host Disease (GvHD) or Poor Graft Function — NCT00603330
2. Mesenchymal Stem Cells for Treatment of Refractory Acute Graft-*versus*-Host Disease — NCT01765634
3. Phase 2 Study of Tocilizumab for Patients with Glucocorticoid-Refractory Acute GvHD After Allogeneic Hematopoetic Cell Transplant (allo-HCT) — NCT01757197
4. MSCs Combined with CD25 Monoclonal Antibody and Calcineurin Inhibitors for Treatment of Steroid-Resistant aGvHD — NCT02241018
5. Alpha 1 AntiTrypsin in Treating Patients with Acute Graft-*versus*-Host Disease — NCT01523821

Acknowledgments

The contribution of E. Huber, MD, Department of Pathology, University Medical Center, Regensburg is acknowledged by providing results of immunohistology of FoxP3 positive cells in intestinal biopsies.

References

1. Luznik L, O'Donnell PV, Fuchs EJ. Post-transplantation cyclophosphamide for tolerance induction in HLA-haploidentical bone marrow transplantation. *Semin Oncol.* 2012;39(6):683–93.
2. Martin PJ, Rizzo JD, Wingard JR, Ballen K, Curtin PT, Cutler C, *et al.* First-and second-line systemic treatment of acute graft-*versus*-host disease: recommendations of the American Society of Blood and Marrow Transplantation. *Biol Blood Marrow Transplant.* 2012;18(8):1150–63.
3. Ruutu T, Gratwohl A, de Witte T, Afanasyev B, Apperley J, Bacigalupo A, *et al.* Prophylaxis and treatment of GVHD: EBMT-ELN working group recommendations for a standardized practice. *Bone Marrow Transplant.* 2014;49(2):168–73
4. Wolff D, Ayuk F, Elmaagacli A, Bertz H, Lawitschka A, Schleuning M, *et al.* Current practice in diagnosis and treatment of acute graft-*versus*-host disease: results from a survey among German-Austrian-Swiss hematopoietic stem cell transplant centers. *Biol Blood Marrow Transplant.* 2013;19(5):767–76.
5. Salmasian H, Rohanizadegan M, Banihosseini S, Rahimi Darabad R, Rabbani-Anari M, Shakiba A, Ferrara JL. Corticosteroid regimens for treatment of acute and chronic graft *versus* host disease (GvHD) after allogenic stem cell transplantation. *Cochrane Database Syst Rev.* 2010;(1): CD005565.
6. Alousi AM, Weisdorf DJ, Logan BR, Bolaños-Meade J, Carter S, Difronzo N, *et al.* Blood and Marrow Transplant Clinical Trials Network. Etanercept, mycophenolate, denileukin, or pentostatin plus corticosteroids for acute graft-*versus*-host disease: a randomized phase 2 trial from the *Blood* and Marrow Transplant Clinical Trials Network. *Blood.* 2009;114(3):511–7.
7. Bolaños-Meade J, Logan BR, Alousi AM, Antin JH, Barowski K, Carter SL, *et al.* Phase 3 clinical trial of steroids/mycophenolate mofetil vs steroids/placebo as therapy for acute GVHD: BMT CTN 0802. *Blood.* 2014;124(22):3221–7.
8. Couriel DR, Saliba R, de Lima M, Giralt S, Andersson B, Khouri I, *et al.* A phase III study of infliximab and corticosteroids for the initial treatment of acute graft-*versus*-host disease. *Biol Blood Marrow Transplant.* 2009;15(12):1555–62.
9. Gatza E, Braun T, Levine JE, Ferrara JL, Zhao S, Wang T, *et al.* Etanercept plus topical corticosteroids as initial therapy for grade one acute graft-*versus*-host disease after allogeneic hematopoietic cell transplantation. *Biol Blood Marrow Transplant.* 2014;20(9):1426–34.
10. Takashima S, Eto T, Shiratsuchi M, Hidaka M, Mori Y, Kato K, *et al.* The use of oral beclomethasone dipropionate in the treatment of gastrointestinal graft-*versus*-host disease: the experience of the Fukuoka blood and marrow transplantation (BMT) group. *Intern Med.* 2014;53(12):1315–20.
11. Bürgler D, Medinger M, Passweg J, Fischmann A, Bucher C. Intra-arterial catheter guided steroid administration for the treatment of steroid-refractory intestinal GvHD. *Leuk Res.* 2014;38(2):184–7.
12. Milner LA, Becker MW, Bernstein SH, Bruckner L, Friedberg JW, Holland GA, *et al.* Intra-arterial methylprednisolone for the management of steroid-refractory acute gastrointestinal and hepatic graft *versus* host disease. *Am J Hematol.* 2011;86(8):712–4.
13. Feldstein JV, Bolaños-Meade J, Anders VL, Abuav R. Narrowband ultraviolet B phototherapy for the treatment of steroid-refractory and steroid-dependent acute graft-*versus*-host disease of the skin. *J Am Acad Dermatol.* 2011;65(4):733–8.
14. Hoda D, Pidala J, Salgado-Vila N, Kim J, Perkins J, Bookout R, *et al.* Sirolimus for treatment of steroid-refractory acute graft-*versus*-host disease. *Bone Marrow Transplant.* 2010;45(8):1347–51.
15. Mielke S, Lutz M, Schmidhuber J, Kapp M, Ditz D, Ammer J, *et al.* Salvage therapy with everolimus reduces the severity of treatment-refractory chronic GVHD without impairing disease control: A dual center retrospective analysis. *Bone Marrow Transplant.* 2014;49(11):1412–8.
16. García-Cadenas I, Valcárcel D, Martino R, Piñana JL, Novelli S, Esquirol A, *et al.* Updated experience with inolimomab as treatment for corticosteroid-refractory acute graft-*versus*-host disease. *Biol Blood Marrow Transplant.* 2013;19(3):435–9.
17. Wang JZ, Liu KY, Xu LP, Liu DH, Han W, Chen H, *et al.* Basiliximab for the treatment of steroid-refractory acute graft-*versus*-host disease after unmanipulated HLA-mismatched/haploidentical hematopoietic stem cell transplantation. *Transplant Proc.* 2011;43(5):1928–33.

18. Xhaard A, Rocha V, Bueno B, de Latour RP, Lenglet J, Petropoulou A, et al. Steroid-refractory acute GvHD: lack of long-term improved survival using new generation anticytokine treatment. *Biol Blood Marrow Transplant.* 2012;18(3):406–13.

19. Drobyski WR, Pasquini M, Kovatovic K, Palmer J, Douglas Rizzo J, Saad A, et al. Tocilizumab for the treatment of steroid refractory graft-*versus*-host disease. *Biol Blood Marrow Transplant.* 2011;17(12):1862–8.

20. Meunier M, Bulabois CE, Thiebaut-Bertrand A, Itzykson R, Carre M, Carras S, et al. Alemtuzumab for severe steroid-refractory gastrointestinal acute graft-*versus*-host disease. *Biol Blood Marrow Transplant.* 2014;20(9):1451–4.

21. Khandelwal P, Lawrence J, Filipovich AH, Davies SM, Bleesing JJ, Jordan MB, et al. The successful use of alemtuzumab for treatment of steroid-refractory acute graft-*versus*-host disease in pediatric patients. *Pediatr Transplant.* 2014;18(1):94–102.

22. Schub N, Günther A, Schrauder A, Claviez A, Ehlert C, Gramatzki M, Repp R. Therapy of steroid-refractory acute GVHD with CD52 antibody alemtuzumab is effective. *Bone Marrow Transplant.* 2011;46(1):143–7.

23. Abu-Dalle I, Reljic T, Nishihori T, Antar A, Bazarbachi A, Djulbegovic B, et al. Extracorporeal photopheresis in steroid-refractory acute or chronic graft-*versus*-host disease: results of a systematic review of prospective studies. *Biol Blood Marrow Transplant.* 2014;20(11):1677–86.

24. Das-Gupta E, Dignan F, Shaw B, Raj K, Malladi R, Gennery A, et al. Extracorporeal photopheresis for treatment of adults and children with acute GvHD: UK consensus statement and review of published literature. *Bone Marrow Transplant.* 2014;49(10):1251–8.

25. Pierelli L, Perseghin P, Marchetti M, Messina C, Perotti C, Mazzoni A, et al.; Società Italiana di Emaferesi and Manipolazione Cellulare (SIdEM); Gruppo Italiano Trapianto Midollo Osseo (GITMO). Extracorporeal photopheresis for the treatment of acute and chronic graft-*versus*-host disease in adults and children: best practice recommendations from an Italian Society of Hemapheresis and Cell Manipulation (SIdEM) and Italian Group for Bone Marrow Transplantation (GITMO) consensus process. *Transfusion.* 2013;53(10):2340–52.

26. Jagasia M, Greinix H, Robin M, Das-Gupta E, Jacobs R, Savani BN, et al. Extracorporeal photopheresis *versus* anticytokine therapy as a second-line treatment for steroid-refractory acute GVHD: a multicenter comparative analysis. *Biol Blood Marrow Transplant.* 2013;19(7):1129–33

27. Rieber N, Wecker I, Neri D, Fuchs K, Schäfer I, Brand A, et al. Extracorporeal photopheresis increases neutrophilic myeloid-derived suppressor cells in patients with GvHD. *Bone Marrow Transplant.* 2014;49(4):545–52.

28. Mevorach D, Zuckerman T, Reiner I, Shimoni A, Samuel S, Nagler A, et al. Single infusion of donor mononuclear early apoptotic cells as prophylaxis for graft-*versus*-host disease in myeloablative HLA-matched allogeneic bone marrow transplantation: a phase I/IIa clinical trial. *Biol Blood Marrow Transplant.* 2014;20(1):58–65.

29. Sánchez-Guijo F, Caballero-Velázquez T, López-Villar O, Redondo A, Parody R, Martínez C, et al. Sequential third-party mesenchymal stromal cell therapy for refractory acute graft-*versus*-host disease. *Biol Blood Marrow Transplant.* 2014;20(10):1580–5.

30. Introna M, Lucchini G, Dander E, Galimberti S, Rovelli A, Balduzzi A, et al. Treatment of graft *versus* host disease with mesenchymal stromal cells: a phase I study on 40 adult and pediatric patients. *Biol Blood Marrow Transplant.* 2014;20(3):375–81.

31. Ball LM, Bernardo ME, Roelofs H, van Tol MJ, Contoli B, Zwaginga JJ, et al. Multiple infusions of mesenchymal stromal cells induce sustained remission in children with steroid-refractory, grade III–IV acute graft-*versus*-host disease. *Br J Haematol* 2013;163(4):501–9.

32. Schneidawind D, Pierini A, Negrin RS. Regulatory T cells and natural killer T cells for modulation of GvHD following allogeneic hematopoietic cell transplantation. *Blood.* 2013;122(18):3116–21.

33. Reddy P. Targeting deacetylases to improve outcomes after allogeneic bone marrow transplantation. *Trans Am Clin Climatol Assoc.* 2013;124:152–62.

34. Marcondes AM, Li X, Tabellini L, Bartenstein M, Kabacka J, Sale GE, et al. Inhibition of IL-32 activation by α-1 antitrypsin suppresses alloreactivity and increases survival in an allogeneic murine marrow transplantation model. *Blood.* 2011;118(18):5031–9.

35. Tawara I, Sun Y, Lewis EC, Toubai T, Evers R, Nieves E, et al. Alpha-1-antitrypsin monotherapy reduces graft-*versus*-host disease after experimental allogeneic bone marrow transplantation. *Proc Natl Acad Sci U S A.* 2012;109(2):564–9.

36. Landfried K, Zhu W, Waldhier MC, Schulz U, Ammer J, Holler B, et al. Tryptophan catabolism is associated with acute GvHD after human allogeneic stem cell transplantation and indicates activation of indoleamine 2,3-dioxygenase. *Blood.* 2011;118(26):6971–4.

37. Elmaagacli AH, Ditschkowski M, Steckel NK, Gromke T, Ottinger H, Hillen U, et al. Human chorionic gonadotropin and indolamine 2,3-dioxygenase in patients with GvHD. *Bone Marrow Transplant.* 2014;49(6):800–5.

38. Holler E, Butzhammer P, Schmid K, Hundsrucker C, Koestler J, Peter K, et al. Metagenomic analysis of the stool microbiome in patients receiving allogeneic stem cell transplantation: loss of diversity is associated with use of systemic antibiotics and more pronounced in gastrointestinal graft-versus-host disease. *Biol Blood Marrow Transplant.* 2014;20(5):640–5.

39. Jenq RR, Ubeda C, Taur Y, Menezes CC, Khanin R, Dudakov JA, et al. Regulation of intestinal inflammation by microbiota following allogeneic bone marrow transplantation. *J Exp Med.* 2012;209(5):903–11.

40. Eriguchi Y, Takashima S, Oka H, Shimoji S, Nakamura K, Uryu H, et al. Graft-*versus*-host disease disrupts intestinal microbial ecology by inhibiting Paneth cell production of α-defensins. *Blood.* 2012;120(1):223–31.

41. Munneke JM, Björklund AT, Mjösberg JM, Garming-Legert K, Bernink JH, Blom B, et al. Activated innate lymphoid cells are associated with a reduced susceptibility to graft-*versus*-host disease. *Blood.* 2014;124(5):812–21.

42. Hanash AM, Dudakov JA, Hua G, O'Connor MH, Young LF, Singer NV, et al. Interleukin-22 protects intestinal

stem cells from immune-mediated tissue damage and regulates sensitivity to graft *versus* host disease. *Immunity.* 2012;37(2):339–50.

43. Spoerl S, Mathew NR, Bscheider M, Schmitt-Graeff A, Chen S, Mueller T, *et al.* Activity of therapeutic JAK 1/2 blockade in graft-*versus*-host disease. *Blood.* 2014;123(24):3832–42.

44. Pai CC, Hsiao HH, Sun K, Chen M, Hagino T, Tellez J, *et al.* Therapeutic benefit of bortezomib on acute graft-*versus*-host disease is tissue specific and is associated with interleukin-6 levels. *Biol Blood Marrow Transplant.* 2014 Jul 23. pii: S1083-8791(14)00448-0. doi: 10.1016/j.bbmt.2014.07.022. [Epub ahead of print]

45. Castilla-Llorente C, Martin PJ, McDonald GB, Storer BE, Appelbaum FR, Deeg HJ, *et al.* Prognostic factors and outcomes of severe gastrointestinal GVHD after allogeneic hematopoietic cell transplantation. *Bone Marrow Transplant.* 2014;49(7):966–71.

46. Ayuk F, Bussmann L, Zabelina T, Veit R, Alchalby H, Wolschke C, *et al.* Serum albumin level predicts survival of patients with gastrointestinal acute graft-*versus*-host disease after allogeneic stem cell transplantation. *Ann Hematol.* 2014;93(5):855–61.

47. MacMillan ML, DeFor TE, Weisdorf DJ. What predicts high risk acute graft-*versus*-host disease (G*v*HD) at onset?: identification of those at highest risk by a novel acute G*v*HD risk score. *Br J Haematol.* 2012;157(6):732–41.

48. Weissinger EM, Metzger J, Dobbelstein C, Wolff D, Schleuning M, Kuzmina Z, *et al.* Proteomic peptide profiling for preemptive diagnosis of acute graft-*versus*-host disease after allogeneic stem cell transplantation. *Leukemia.* 2014;28(4):842–52.

49. Ferrara JL, Harris AC, Greenson JK, Braun TM, Holler E, Teshima T, *et al.* Regenerating islet-derived 3-alpha is a biomarker of gastrointestinal graft-*versus*-host disease. *Blood.* 2011;118(25): 6702–8.

50. Vander Lugt MT, Braun TM, Hanash S, Ritz J, Ho VT, Antin JH, *et al.* ST2 as a marker for risk of therapy-resistant graft-*versus*-host disease and death. *N Engl J Med.* 2013;369(6):529–39.

14

Hematopoietic Growth Factors after Hematopoietic Cell Transplantation: Are They Useful?

Jürgen Finke and Roland Mertelsmann

Introduction

Since the availability of granulocyte colony-stimulating factor (G-CSF) in the early 1990s the field of autologous and allogeneic hematopoietic cell transplant (HCT) has shifted from bone marrow harvested grafts to G-CSF mobilized peripheral blood (PB) grafts collected via an apheresis procedure. Growth factors have a defined role post-transplant for reducing morbidity and mortality. The application of growth factors is based on randomized trials as well as empiric experience. This chapter covers the use of hematopoietic growths factors which influence the three main hematologic cell lineages, i.e., granulocytopoiesis, erythrocytopoiesis, and thrombocytopoiesis. Clinically available cytokines with immunomodulatory effects targeting lymphocytes such as interferon-alpha, interleukin-2 will not be dealt with in this chapter but are appropriately covered in other chapters of this book.

The Role of Granulocyte Colony-Stimulating Factors

Recombinant human G-CSF is available in several forms: filgrastim is produced in *E. coli* and lenograstim as a glycosolated G-CSF in a Chinese hamster kidney cell line. Furthermore, various generic G-CSF preparations are available as well as a pegylated form of filgrastim, allowing single-dose application.

G-CSF Following Autologous HCT: Timing and Benefits?

Early trials demonstrated a significant acceleration of neutrophil engraftment after autologous HCT with a difference of 6 to 8 days after marrow grafts and 2 to 4 days after PB grafts [1–5]. In these early trials G-CSF was given from day +1 after HCT. Later randomized trials showed that G-CSF application could safely be delayed to days +3, to +7 after PB autologous HCT with the same beneficial effect[6–9]. The use of G-CSF post-marrow grafts reduced the number of days of febrile neutropenia and intravenous antibiotics. When used after PB grafts no difference regarding antibiotic use, transfusion requirements, or platelet engraftment was described. Pegfilgrastim, given as a single fixed dose at day +1 after PB

autografts, has been compared to filgrastim, given either from day +1 or +5 post-HCT, showing equally rapid neutrophil engraftment absolute neutrophil count (ANC) >500/μL (days +10.8 to +12) without further untoward effects[10–13].

G-CSF Following Allogeneic HCT

A similar acceleration of neutrophil engraftment by 4 days as seen after autologous HCT could be observed after marrow or PB allograft, from either an HLA-matched sibling or unrelated donors[14–18]. No untoward effects were seen regarding platelet or erythrocyte engraftment, GvHD, or early mortality. Again, delayed application of G-CSF starting from days +5, +6, or +10 following allogeneic HCT resulted in similar outcome to the start on day 0[16,19].

Concerns have been raised regarding possible detrimental effects of growth factors on the immune system post-allogeneic transplant. Furthermore, the contributing role of neutrophils in acute GvHD has been elucidated recently[20]. A retrospective analysis by the Acute Leukemia Working Party of the European Bone Marrow Transplant (EBMT) showed faster neutrophil recovery and delayed platelet engraftment in 2223 patients with acute leukemia receiving either marrow or PB grafts from HLA-matched sibling donors. In the G-CSF group, they also observed an increased rate of acute GvHD grades II–IV in marrow graft recipients (50%) and 39% in the control group; $P=0.007$[21]. In the recipients of marrow allografts, the use of G-CSF was also associated with an increased risk of chronic GvHD (RR, 1.29) and an increased treatment-related mortality (RR, 1.73), and reduced overall survival (RR, 0.59) and leukemia-free survival (LFS) (RR, 0.64). This effect was not seen in recipients of PB allografts[21]. A long-term (>9 years) follow-up study from the EBMT in 1887 adult patients receiving marrow allografts for acute leukemias after "myeloablative" conditioning regimens revealed faster neutrophil and delayed platelet engraftment, and decreased GvHD-free and leukemia-free survival[22]. After HLA haplotype-mismatch transplant, the application of G-CSF delayed T-lymphocyte reconstitution and omitting G-CSF led to a more rapid increase of T-cells and an improved anti-infectious defense[23]. A meta-analysis based on 34 randomized controlled trials of prophylactic G-CSF and GM-CSF after autologous and allogeneic HCT demonstrated a reduced risk of documented infections and duration of intravenous antibiotic use but not reduction in infection-related mortality. The absolute decrease in the risk of documented infections was 8% and 13 patients were needed to be treated with G-CSFs in order to prevent one infection[24].

Practice Points

Based on the available data and in our opinion, administration of G-CSF after autologous HCT from day +7 until WBC >1000/μL is acceptable in order to decrease the risk of infections and accelerate safe discharge from hospital. We do not routinely give G-CSF after allogeneic HCT, mainly due to concern over cytokine release/engraftment syndromes (see Chapter 21; also seen in auto-HCT) and possible negative effects related to the immune system, incidence of GvHD, and overall outcome. However, we give G-CSF when ANC >500/μL is not reached by day +21, in order to decrease risk of infections. Furthermore we do see an indication for G-CSF in drug-induced neutropenia, e.g., as frequently observed during application of ganciclovir.

Erythrocyte-Stimulating Agents

Anemia is frequent prior to transplant and post-transplant; patients usually have adapted to the reduced hemoglobin levels. Previous notion of maintaining hemoglobin levels close to normal (adjusted for age and gender) is no longer true. Randomized trials have shown that transfusion strategies aiming at high hemoglobin levels can be detrimental. In our practice, individually tolerated red blood cell transfusion triggers are used and post-transplant hemoglobin levels are usually kept above 7°g/dL in asymptomatic patients. Apart from the direct toxic effects of high-dose chemotherapy, anemia post-transplant can also be caused by other clinical complications and medications, e.g., infections, inflammation, and antiviral agents; calcineurin inhibitor induced renal insufficiency post-allograft resulting in insufficient endogenous erythropoietin (EPO) levels is also not uncommon and is an indication for EPO therapy.

Erythrocyte-Stimulating Agents Following Autologous HCT

Randomized trials have shown a significant effect of EPO alone or in combination with G-CSF after autologous HCT on red cell regeneration without affecting overall outcome[25,26].

In patients with religious objection to blood products, EPO in combination with G-CSF, intravenous iron, folic acid, and aminocaproic acid has been successfully given to avoid blood transfusions, infections, and bleeding after PB autologous HCT[27].

Erythrocyte-Stimulating Agents Following Allogeneic HCT

After allograft, EPO significantly reduced red cell transfusion requirements without affecting other post-transplant parameters[28–30]. The prolonged time to red blood cell engraftment after allogeneic HCT with major ABO blood group incompatibility (see Chapter 15) can be successfully shortened with EPO[31,32].

A high creatinine level during the first month after allogeneic HCT was shown to be a risk factor for persistent anemia and inadequate EPO secretion; adminstration of EPO was successful in these patients[33]. A recently published prospective randomized trial showed that erythropoietin therapy reduces transfusion requirements after allo-HCT. In this trial, erythropoietin therapy (500 U/kg per week) hastened erythroid recovery and decreased transfusion requirements when started 1 month after allo-HCT. The proportion of complete correctors (i.e., hemoglobin $\geq$13 g/dL) before day +126 post-transplant was 8.1% in the control arm (median not reached) and 63.1% in the erythropoietin arm (median, 90 days) ($P<0.001$). Hemoglobin levels were higher and transfusion requirements decreased ($P<0.001$) in the erythropoietin arm. Of note, when erythropoietin therapy was started on day +28, only five patients had a hemoglobin level higher than 11 g/dL (mean hemoglobin approximately 9 g/dL), in keeping with current guidelines for initiation of erythrocyte-stimulating agent (ESA) therapy[34].

Practice Points

EPO after autologous HCT showed marginal benefits. However, the effect after allogeneic HCT was more prominent. Anemia associated with impaired EPO secretion after allogeneic HCT is more frequent than generally recognized and it is associated with renal insufficiency, chronic inflammation, or chronic GvHD. We do not give EPO routinely after autologous HCT. After allogeneic HCT, we give EPO in selected clinical situations: low reticulocyte counts and inadequate serum EPO levels associated with decreased renal function; major blood group differences between donor and recipient, especially in patients with high antibody titers against the donor A or B blood groups. We usually determine endogenous EPO levels prior to therapy with EPO. For practical purposes, we prefer pegylated EPO applications once weekly. Furthermore, we do not stimulate hemoglobin levels >10 g/dL for safety reasons; however, this might change due to recent prospective data described above. We consider general medical aspects, such as cardiac disease, hypertension, and history of thromboembolic events, prior to use of EPO application.

Thrombopoietic Growth Factors

Thrombopoietin (TPO) is naturally produced by the liver and serum levels are inversely correlated with platelet counts. Recombinant TPO or megakaryocyte growth factor has been shown to induce rapid platelet regeneration in clinical trials. However, due to the development of neutralizing antibodies, thrombophilia, and increase in marrow fibrosis these recombinant factors have not been licensed for clinical use in the setting of HCT[35].

Two TPO-mimetic agents are available: romiplostin is a TPO-mimetic peptide linked to human IgG fragments and is applied weekly subcutaneously for patients with immune thrombocytopenia purpura (ITP). Eltrombopag is a small molecule with TPO-mimetic effect and is taken orally for ITP as well[36–38]. Despite lack of Food and Drug Administration (FDA) induction, both drugs have been used successfully in clinical trials for the treatment of acute GvHD-associated thrombocytopenia[39] or prolonged thrombo cytopenia after HCT[40]. Eltrombopag was given with increasing doses post-transplantation without dose-limiting toxicities. One episode of pulmonary embolism was observed [40,41].

Practice Points

Although it is tempting to use these novels agents, no randomized trials endorse their application post-transplant. Since ITP is a not infrequent complication post-allogeneic HCT, either romiplostin or eltrombpag could be useful in this setting. TPO mimetics are not applied routinely. Special situations after allogeneic HCT like ITP or drug- or infection-induced marrow damage are potential indications on an individual basis. We do not use TPO mimetics after transplantation except in selected patients with refractory ITP.

References

1. Gisselbrecht C, Prentice HG, Bacigalupo A, Biron P, Milpied N, Rubie H, et al. Placebo-controlled phase III trial of lenograstim in bone-marrow transplantation. *Lancet* 1994;343(8899):696–700.

2. Stahel RA, Jost LM, Cerny T, Pichert G, Honegger H, Tobler A, et al. Randomized study of recombinant human granulocyte colony-stimulating factor after high-dose chemotherapy and autologous bone marrow transplantation for high-risk lymphoid malignancies. *J Clin Oncol* 1994;12(9):1931–8.

3. Klumpp TR, Mangan KF, Goldberg SL, Pearlman ES, Macdonald JS. Granulocyte colony-stimulating factor accelerates neutrophil engraftment following peripheral-blood stem-cell transplantation: a prospective, randomized trial. *J Clin Oncol* 1995;13(6):1323–7.

4. Schmitz N, Dreger P, Zander AR, Ehninger G, Wandt H, Fauser AA, et al. Results of a randomised, controlled, multicentre study of recombinant human granulocyte colony-stimulating factor (filgrastim) in patients with Hodgkin's disease and non-Hodgkin's lymphoma undergoing autologous bone marrow transplantation. *Bone Marrow Transplant* 1995;15(2):261–6.

5. Linch DC, Milligan DW, Winfield DA, Kelsey SM, Johnson SA, Littlewood TJ, et al. G-CSF after peripheral blood stem cell transplantation in lymphoma patients significantly accelerated neutrophil recovery and shortened time in hospital: results of a randomized BNLI trial. *Br J Haematol* 1997;99(4):933–8.

6. Faucher C, Le Corroller AG, Chabannon C, Novakovitch G, Manonni P, Moatti JP, et al. Administration of G-CSF can be delayed after transplantation of autologous G-CSF-primed blood stem cells: a randomized study. *Bone Marrow Transplant* 1996;17(4):533–6.

7. Bolwell BJ, Pohlman B, Andresen S, Kalaycio M, Goormastic M, Wise K, et al. Delayed G-CSF after autologous progenitor cell transplantation: a prospective randomized trial. *Bone Marrow Transplant* 1998;21(4):369–73.

8. Bence-Bruckler I, Bredeson C, Atkins H, McDiarmid S, Hamelin L, Hopkins H, et al. A randomized trial of granulocyte colony-stimulating factor (Neupogen) starting day 1 vs day 7 post-autologous stem cell transplantation. *Bone Marrow Transplant* 1998;22(10):965–9.

9. Piccirillo N, Sica S, Laurenti L, Chiusolo P, La Barbera EO, Sora F, et al. Optimal timing of G-CSF administration after CD34+ immunoselected peripheral blood progenitor cell transplantation. *Bone Marrow Transplant* 1999;23(12):1245–50.

10. Martino M, Pratico G, Messina G, Irrera G, Massara E, Messina G, et al. Pegfilgrastim compared with filgrastim after high-dose melphalan and autologous hematopoietic peripheral blood stem cell transplantation in multiple myeloma patients. *Eur J Haematol* 2006;77(5):410–5.

11. Rifkin R, Spitzer G, Orloff G, Mandanas R, McGaughey D, Zhan F, et al. Pegfilgrastim appears equivalent to daily dosing of filgrastim to treat neutropenia after autologous peripheral blood stem cell transplantation in patients with non-Hodgkin lymphoma. *Clin Lymphoma Myeloma Leuk* 2010;10(3):186–91.

12. Gerds A, Fox-Geiman M, Dawravoo K, Rodriguez T, Toor A, Smith S, et al. Randomized phase III trial of pegfilgrastim versus filgrastim after autologus peripheral blood stem cell transplantation. *Biol Blood Marrow Transplant* 2010;16(5):678–85.

13. Sebban C, Lefranc A, Perrier L, Moreau P, Espinouse D, Schmidt A, et al. A randomised phase II study of the efficacy, safety and cost-effectiveness of pegfilgrastim and filgrastim after autologous stem cell transplant for lymphoma and myeloma (PALM study). *Eur J Cancer* 2012;48(5):713–20.

14. Schriber JR, Chao NJ, Long GD, Negrin RS, Tierney DK, Kusnierz-Glaz C, et al. Granulocyte colony-stimulating factor after allogeneic bone marrow transplantation. *Blood* 1994;84(5):1680–4.

15. Locatelli F, Pession A, Zecca M, Bonetti F, Prete L, Carra AM, et al. Use of recombinant human granulocyte colony-stimulating factor in children given allogeneic bone marrow transplantation for acute or chronic leukemia. *Bone Marrow Transplant* 1996;17(1):31–7.

16. Hagglund H, Ringden O, Oman S, Remberger M, Carlens S, Mattsson J. A prospective randomized trial of Filgrastim (r-metHuG-CSF) given at different times after unrelated bone marrow transplantation. *Bone Marrow Transplant* 1999;24(8):831–6.

17. Bishop MR, Tarantolo SR, Geller RB, Lynch JC, Bierman PJ, Pavletic ZS, et al. A randomized, double-blind trial of filgrastim (granulocyte colony-stimulating factor) versus placebo following allogeneic blood stem cell transplantation. *Blood* 2000;96(1):80–5.

18. Przepiorka D, Smith TL, Folloder J, Anderlini P, Chan KW, Korbling M, et al. Controlled trial of filgrastim for acceleration of neutrophil recovery after allogeneic blood stem cell transplantation from human leukocyte antigen-matched related donors. *Blood* 2001;97(11):3405–10.

19. Ciernik IF, Schanz U, Gmur J. Delaying treatment with granulocyte colony-stimulating factor after allogeneic bone marrow transplantation for hematological malignancies: a prospective randomized trial. *Bone Marrow Transplant* 1999;24(2):147–51.

20. Schwab L, Goroncy L, Palaniyandi S, Gautam S, Triantafyllopoulou A, Mocsai A, et al. Neutrophil granulocytes recruited upon translocation of intestinal bacteria enhance graft-*versus*-host disease via tissue damage. *Nat Med* 2014;20(6):648–54.

21. Ringden O, Labopin M, Gorin NC, Le Blanc K, Rocha V, Gluckman E, et al. Treatment with granulocyte colony-stimulating factor after allogeneic bone marrow transplantation for acute leukemia increases the risk of graft-*versus*-host disease and death: a study from the Acute Leukemia Working Party of the European Group for Blood and Marrow Transplantation. *J Clin Oncol* 2004;22(3):416–23.

22. Ringden O, Labopin M, Gorin NC, Volin L, Torelli GF, Attal M, et al. Growth factor-associated graft-*versus*-host disease and mortality 10 years after allogeneic bone marrow transplantation. *Br J Haematol* 2012;157(2):220–9.

23. Volpi I, Perruccio K, Tosti A, Capanni M, et al. Postgrafting administration of granulocyte colony-stimulating factor impairs functional immune recovery in recipients of human leukocyte antigen haplotype-mismatched hematopoietic transplants. *Blood* 2001;97(8):2514–21.

24. Dekker A, Bulley S, Beyene J, Dupuis LL, Doyle JJ, Sung L. Meta-analysis of randomized controlled trials of prophylactic granulocyte colony-stimulating factor and granulocyte-macrophage colony-stimulating factor after autologous and allogeneic stem cell transplantation. *J Clin Oncol* 2006;24(33):5207–15.

25. Vannucchi AM, Bosi A, Ieri A, Guidi S, Saccardi R, Lombardini L, et al. Combination therapy with G-CSF and erythropoietin after autologous bone marrow transplantation for lymphoid malignancies: a randomized trial. *Bone Marrow Transplant* 1996;17(4):527–31.

26. Chao NJ, Schriber JR, Long GD, Negrin RS, Catolico M, Brown BW, et al. A randomized study of erythropoietin and granulocyte colony-stimulating factor (G-CSF) *versus* placebo and G-CSF for patients with Hodgkin's and non-Hodgkin's lymphoma undergoing autologous bone marrow transplantation. *Blood* 1994;83(10):2823–8.

27. Ballen KK, Becker PS, Yeap BY, Matthews B, Henry DH, Ford PA. Autologous stem-cell transplantation can be performed safely without the use of blood-product support. *J Clin Oncol* 2004;22(20):4087–94.

28. Klaesson S, Ringden O, Ljungman P, Lonnqvist B, Wennberg L. Reduced blood transfusions requirements after allogeneic bone marrow transplantation: results of a randomised, double-blind study with high-dose erythropoietin. *Bone Marrow Transplant* 1994;13(4):397–402.

29. Link H, Boogaerts MA, Fauser AA, Slavin S, Reiffers J, Gorin NC, et al. A controlled trial of recombinant human erythropoietin after bone marrow transplantation. *Blood* 1994;84(10):3327–35.

30. Biggs JC, Atkinson KA, Booker V, Concannon A, Dart GW, Dodds A, et al. Prospective randomised double-blind trial of the in vivo use of recombinant human erythropoietin in bone marrow transplantation from HLA-identical sibling donors. The Australian Bone Marrow Transplant Study Group. *Bone Marrow Transplant* 1995;15(1):129–34.

31. Paltiel O, Cournoyer D, Rybka W. Pure red cell aplasia following ABO-incompatible bone marrow transplantation: response to erythropoietin. *Transfusion* 1993;33(5):418–21.

32. Fujisawa S, Maruta A, Sakai R, Taguchi J, Tomita N, Ogawa K, et al. Pure red cell aplasia after major ABO-incompatible bone marrow transplantation: two case reports of treatment with recombinant human erythropoietin. *Transpl Int* 1996;9(5):506–8.

33. Gaya A, Urbano-Ispizua A, Fernandez-Aviles F, Salamero O, Roncero JM, Rovira M, et al. Anemia associated with impaired erythropoietin secretion after allogeneic stem cell transplantation: incidence, risk factors, and response to treatment. *Biol Blood Marrow Transplant* 2008;14(8):880–7.

34. Jaspers A, Baron F, Willems E, et al. Erythropoietin therapy after allogeneic hematopoietic cell transplantation: a prospective, randomized trial. *Blood*. 2014;124(1):33–41.

35. Bolwell B, Vredenburgh J, Overmoyer B, Gilbert C, Chap L, Menchaca DM, et al. Phase 1 study of pegylated recombinant human megakaryocyte growth and development factor (PEG-rHuMGDF) in breast cancer patients after autologous peripheral blood progenitor cell (PBPC) transplantation. *Bone Marrow Transplant* 2000;26(2):141–5.

36. Cheng G, Saleh MN, Marcher C, Vasey S, Mayer B, Aivado M, et al. Eltrombopag for management of chronic immune thrombocytopenia (RAISE): a 6-month, randomised, phase 3 study. *Lancet* 2011;377(9763):393–402.

37. Molineux G, Newland A. Development of romiplostim for the treatment of patients with chronic immune thrombocytopenia: from bench to bedside. *Br J Haematol* 2010;150(1):9–20.

38. Kuter DJ. New thrombopoietic growth factors. *Blood* 2007;109(11):4607–16.

39. Ruiz-Delgado GJ, Lutz-Presno J, Ruiz-Arguelles GJ. Romiplostin may revert the thrombocytopenia in graft-*versus*-host disease. *Hematology* 2011;16(2):108–9.

40. Reid R, Bennett JM, Becker M, Chen Y, Milner L, Phillips GL, et al. Use of eltrombopag, a thrombopoietin receptor agonist, in post-transplantation thrombocytopenia. *Am J Hematol* 2012;87(7):743–5.

41. Liesveld JL, Phillips GL, Becker M, Constine LS, Friedberg J, Andolina JR, et al. A phase 1 trial of eltrombopag in patients undergoing stem cell transplantation after total body irradiation. *Biol Blood Marrow Transplant* 2013;19(12):1745–52.

Chapter 15

Blood Group Incompatibilities and Transfusion Support after Hematopoietic Cell Transplant

Shanna Morgan, Dawn Ward, Dennis Goldfinger, and Jeffrey McCullough

Introduction

Allogeneic hematopoietic cell transplant (HCT) can be done successfully between donor–recipient pairs that are mismatched for RBC blood group antigens. ABO incompatibility occurs in 25–30% of transplants requiring manipulation of the graft if necessary and transfusion strategy may be complex. The indications for transfusion are no different from nonmismatched transplants, but the selection of the specific blood component must be based on the specific antigen/antibody ABO mismatch. Also the timing of appearance of a donor's RBCs – red blood cell engraftment – may be affected by the ABO mismatch.

Definitions of RBC Blood Group Incompatibilities

The two graft-related factors of importance are the RBC antigen type and RBC antibody content to determine the kind of donor–recipient mismatch. Mismatches are divided into major and minor (Table 15.1). In a major ABO mismatch, the patient has antibodies against donor RBC antigens. For instance, in mismatch of blood type A group into a blood type O recipient, the recipient would have circulating anti-A that could be expected to hemolyze the type A RBCs contained in the graft.

Table 15.1 Major and minor ABO incompatibilities

Type of mismatch	Recipient ABO	Donor ABO
Major	0	A
(antibody in the recipient's	0	B
plasma against donor RBC)	0	AB
	A	AB
	B	AB
Minor	A	0
(antibody in the donor's	B	0
plasma against recipient RBC)	AB	0
	AB	A
	AB	B
Bidirectional	A	B
	B	A

This situation can be managed by removing the anti-A from the patient (discussed later) or the RBCs from the graft. In a minor ABO mismatch, the donor has antibodies in the plasma against the recipient such as when blood type O containing anti-A is infused into a blood type A recipient (Table 15.1). The plasma in the graft could hemolyze recipient RBCs, or donor lymphocytes (passenger lymphocytes in minor ABO incompatibility discussed later) as they engraft can produce antibodies that could hemolyze residual patient RBCs. In some donor–recipient pairs, both a major and minor mismatch can occur. This is called bidirectional mismatch.

Influence of ABO Incompatibility on Neutrophil Engraftment

In general, allogeneic hematopoietic cell transplant (allo-HCT) with ABO-incompatible blood groups are regarded as safe and are not clearly linked to impaired overall survival (OS). However, two reports raise the possibility that ABO incompatibility may affect engraftment. Goldman et al. reported a retrospective cohort study evaluating OS of all bone marrow (BM) and peripheral blood (PB) hematopoietic cell allografts from related and unrelated HLA-matched donors between 1994 and 2000[1]. The study was limited to patients with acute leukemia (ALL, AML), CML, and MDS. Allo-HCT were characterized as: ABO identical, donor cell incompatible (major), and donor plasma incompatible (minor). OS was reported as 50–60% at 5 years. There was no statistically significant survival difference between two types of ABO mismatches except for a prolonged time to platelet engraftment in five ABO bidirectional incompatible patients. A second study from Remberger et al. showed that the presence of major ABO mismatch in an HLA-matched unrelated donor was indeed associated with an increased risk of graft failure[2]. However, in 224 patients with acute leukemia (n=139), chronic leukemia (n=71), or MDS (n=14) there was no statistically significant difference in graft failure among patients with mismatch for RhD, MNSs, Kidd, or with minor ABO mismatch. One hundred and fifty-two patients received BM grafts and 72 patients received PB grafts. ABO-matched grafts were used in 89 (40%) cases, ABO-mismatched in 135 (60%) of cases with 67 (29%) major, 68 (30%) minor, and bidirectional in 16 (7%) of cases. Non-ABO mismatches were RhD mismatch in 53 (24%) cases,

Table 15.2 Potential immune consequences of ABO-incompatible HCT

Major ABO incompatibility	Minor ABO incompatibility
Engraftment failure	Acute hemolysis of recipient RBCs from patient antibodies during infusion
Delay in onset of erythropoiesis	Passenger lymphocyte syndrome
Acute hemolysis of donor RBCs during infusion	
Delayed hemolysis associated with persistence of patient pretransplant RBC isohemagglutinin	
Pure red cell aplasia	

Kidd (Jka/b) mismatch in 99 (44%) of cases, and MNSs mismatch in 144 (64%) cases. The graft failure rate with major ABO match was 0.6%, with HLA allele match 2.0%, with major ABO mismatch 7.5%; with HLA allele mismatch it was 8.3% and with major ABO mismatch plus HLA allele mismatch it was 20% (see Chapter 9). Despite these data, experience supports the conclusion that antidonor isoagglutinins can delay RBC engraftment but have no clear effect on neutrophil and platelet engraftment although these cells express/absorb ABO antigens. It is generally concluded that ABO incompatibility is not a cause of primary or secondary graft failure. However, both major and minor ABO incompatibility may result in a number of other immunologic consequences, which are elaborated in Table 15.2

Major ABO Incompatibility: Complications and How Best to Avoid and Tackle Them

Peripheral Blood as Graft Source

The primary potential complications of major ABO incompatibility are immediate hemolysis of RBCs in the graft, delayed hemolysis if the recipient continues to have circulating antibodies, and pure red cell aplasia (PRCA). In the past, plasma exchange was used to reduce circulating isoagglutinin levels in the recipient, but rebounding high antibody titers and subsequent hemolysis demonstrated this to be of temporary value[3–5]. The practice was discontinued when methods became available to remove the RBCs from the graft. Antibody removal could be revisited as recent studies have shown it to be safe and avoid the need to reduce the number of RBCs in the transplant product[5,6]. Another strategy uses recipient plasma exchange (removal of antibody) coupled with transfusion of donor-type ABO plasma on day of the graft infusion (day 0) to absorb any additional circulating recipient isohemagglutinins[6].

Practice Points

Manipulation of the graft to reduce donor RBCs is the more widely used strategy, with a target of less than 10 mL RBC contamination in the infusion product. There is no general consensus about the maximum number of incompatible RBCs that may be safely infused to the recipient. Volumes ranging between 10 and 20 mL have been cited[7]. We suggest limiting the maximum infusion of RBC content to 0.3 mL per kg body weight of the recipient. While graft manipulation is more convenient than antibody removal from the recipient, this does create the possibility of inadvertently removing CD34+ cells from the product; therefore caution is advised especially if the acquired graft has the bare minimum of CD34+ cells and/or viability of the graft is compromised[8,9].

Bone Marrow and Cord Blood Units as Graft Source

Bone marrow usually contains greater numbers of RBCs making RBC reduction necessary in case of major ABO mismatch. The method involves RBC sedimentation with either 6% hydroxyethyl starch or dextran and an automated cell separation procedure. Most cord blood units are RBC-reduced prior to cryopreservation[10,11]. While there are different methods of RBC depletion or mononuclear cell concentration, engraftment rates are similar for all[11]. The residual erythrocytes lyse during cryopreservation, therefore immediate hemolysis is not a problem with cord blood transplants and further RBC depletion steps after thawing are not necessary. Because the volume of a thawed cord blood unit is usually 20–30 mL, there is no concern about transfusion of RBC antibody. However, it is important to minimize the infusion of free hemoglobin as this can cause a reaction similar to acute intravascular hemolysis[12]. This is accomplished by washing the cord blood unit after it is thawed[11].

Delay in Erythrocyte Engraftment and Pure Red Blood Cell Aplasia

In major ABO incompatibility when recipients have antibodies against the donor RBCs, delayed erythrocyte engraftment and/or PRCA may ensue. This occurs most often when group O patients receive a group A blood type, or with bidirectional ABO mismatches[13]. Antibodies against minor RBC antigens are less frequently reported, and cause less severe hemolysis[14]. Consequently, dependence on RBC transfusion is prolonged. Another complication, PRCA, results when recipient isohemagglutinins enter the marrow and destroy donor progenitor erythroid cells as they develop A or B antigen. Subsequently, reticulocytopenia ensues while the other cellular groups within the marrow engraft. The incidence of PRCA is dependent upon the conditioning regimen[13,15,16]. Anemia is usually severe and the resolution of PRCA may take several months during which transfusion of RBCs of the original recipient red cell type must be used.

Minor ABO Incompatibility: Complications and How Best to Avoid and Tackle Them

Acute Hemolysis Prevention Strategy

Minor ABO-incompatible transplant occurs when the donor's plasma is incompatible with a recipient's RBCs (Table 15.1). Thus infusion of graft with characteristics of minor ABO mismatch may result in acute hemolysis in the recipient. An attempt to avoid infusion of donor incompatible plasma is strongly preferred, but this recommendation is not evidence based. The likelihood of a hemolytic event is not always predictive with the measurement of donor mismatched isohemagglutinin titers[17]. Plasma reduction may be performed as a way to decrease the volume of incompatible plasma within the graft[7]. There are no standards or guidelines for "ideal" plasma volume or "ideal" isohemagglutinin titer. The decrease in plasma volume does not effectively reduce the number of donor lymphocytes' "passenger lymphocytes," which may still lead to immunologic consequences (Table 15.2)

Passenger Lymphocytes and Delayed Hemolysis

Infusion of donor lymphocytes in the setting of minor ABO mismatch also has potential to cause hemolysis. Since the donor lacks RBC antigens that the recipient has, i.e., minor ABO mismatch, the donor lymphocytes within the graft recognize the recipient RBCs as foreign and may produce antibody against mismatched RBC antigen. This passenger lymphocyte syndrome (PLS) usually presents 7–14 days after the transplant with the abrupt onset of hemolysis. Usually ABO or sometimes other red cell antigens mismatch may be involved. The hemolysis ranges from mild to severe, and may be intra- or extravascular, depending upon the nature of the antibody involved. PLS occurs most frequently in transplants that have a donor with group O blood type and a recipient with group A blood type[18]. Hemolysis should be suspected if the patient develops an acute drop in hemoglobin in the absence of bleeding between day +7 and day +14 after allo-HCT. Diagnosis of PLS is supported by routine hemolytic laboratory evaluation including the direct antiglobulin test (DAT) due to the transfused antibody. A positive DAT with anti-A and/or anti-B recovered in the eluate in the setting of hemolysis occurs in 10–15% of minor ABO-incompatible transplants. PLS-related hemolysis continues for 5–10 days or until the recipient RBCs are destroyed or replaced by transfused RBCs[19]. Donor-derived isohemagglutinins (antibody) remain for the duration of the lymphocyte lifespan. During this period group O RBCs are provided for management of anemia. Risk factors for PLS include the pretransplant conditioning regimen (myeloablative < non-myeloablative), group A or group AB recipient with a group B donor, HLA-mismatched donors, graft source (BM > PB), and graft manipulation (T-cell depletion < non-T-cell-depleted)[20,21].

RhD Blood Group Incompatibility in Allo-HCT

The RhD antigen is the most potent immunogen of all the non-ABO antigens. Despite this fact Rh mismatch between donor and recipient is not a deterrent. Because antibodies against the Rh group are not naturally occurring, the overall risk of hemolytic reactions is quite low to negligible[22].

RhD-Incompatible (RhD Donor$^+$/Recipient$^-$)

In RhD-negative woman with two or more RhD-positive pregnancies, there is an approximately 15–20% chance of developing anti-D antibodies; however, this is the case in situations where the immune system is intact[23]. Unlike the scenario in pregnancy, subjects on immunosuppressive therapy, AIDS patients, and cardiac and liver transplant recipients have reduced rates of anti-D formation if transfused with RhD-positive RBCs[24–27]. Cummins et al. detected anti-D in only one of 52 RhD-negative recipients of RhD-positive donor heart and/or lung grafts and two of six RhD-negative recipients who were transfused between 6 and 32 RhD-positive RBC units[26]. Similarly, Casanueva et al. reported that in a series of 17 RhD-negative liver transplant recipients that received in the range of 5–41 units of RhD-positive RBC units, alloimmunization did not appear in any of the recipients[27]. In a series of eight RhD-negative AIDS patients who received multiple RhD-positive RBC transfusions, none developed anti-D antibodies[24]. Patients on chemotherapeutic agents who receive RhD-incompatible (donor$^+$/recipient$^-$) platelet concentrates have an incidence of anti-D alloimmunization in the range of 0 to 19%[28]. Alloimmunization rate differences can be attributed to variable RBC content of platelet concentrates and also variable intensity of chemotherapy regimens.

RhD-Incompatible (RhD Donor$^-$/Recipient$^+$)

On the contrary, some RhD-positive recipients of RhD-negative blood and marrow grafts have developed anti-D since patients' RhD-positive RBCs continue to circulate for weeks after the transplant and may stimulate donor lymphocytes; hemolysis would typically not start until about 6 months post-transplantation[29–33]. These cases have shown a variable clinical prognosis and hemolysis can persist for months or years[34–36].

Controversy#1: Does RhD Incompatibility Influence Allo-HCT Outcomes?

For the majority of these cases, the hemolysis does not represent a fatality risk as that is usually from other underlying conditions such as graft-versus-host disease (GvHD) or relapse of primary disease +/− infection[37–40]. Erker et al.[41] have shown that donor–recipient Rh mismatch in 32 of 143 patients had a decreased OS, though only two of those patients developed anti-D, which lends us to believe that the anti-D was not the cause of poorer survival. There was no effect seen on neutrophil engraftment, incidence of acute or chronic GvHD, or relapse. Wirk *et al.* reported that of 258 transplants with Rh-mismatched donors, there were no significant associations to be made between OS, event-free survival, transplant-related mortality, or incidence of acute or chronic GvHD[42]. In conclusion, Rh incompatibility does not affect allo-HCT outcomes.

Controversy#2: Preformed RhD Antibody in Recipient and Rh-Positive Blood Group of the Donor: What To Do?

Presence of an anti-D antibody in the recipient does not preclude the allo-HCT of an individual with Rh-positive RBCs in the graft as the engraftment of Rh-mismatched transplants can be successful, even when RhD-positive RBC grafts are transplanted into recipients with anti-D[43,44]. Because CD34+ cells do not contain Rh antigens, the only concern is the possibility of hemolysis of Rh-positive RBCs in the graft by preformed anti-D.

Practice Points

Prior to allo-HCT, therapeutic plasma exchange and high-dose intravenous immunoglobulin may be employed in an attempt to decrease the isoagglutinin titer in the recipient to prevent the hemolysis. No standard protocols exist for how low the titer should be prior to deployment of allo-HCT and this is not routinely done[44,45]. The recommended approach is to perform red blood cell depletion on the donor product thereby removing incompatible erythrocytes to less than 10–20 mL as for ABO incompatibility (discussed above).

Transfusion Strategies in ABO and Rh-Incompatible Blood Groups

Blood transfusion supportive care is complex especially if ABO incompatibility exists. Transfusion practices are based on known pathophysiology and the desire to minimize the risk of exposure to incompatible blood products and/or hemolysis. Transfusion services should seek blood components that are compatible with the donor and recipient as early as possible in the peri-transplantation period. This typically begins when the patient receives the immunosuppressive preparative regimen. Transfusion therapy initiated prior to the transplant should continue through engraftment[22]. In the post-transplantation period, native recipient RBCs will continue to circulate and donor lymphocytes may produce RBC antibodies as discussed above.

Transfusion Strategies for ABO Blood Group Mismatch allo-HCT

When providing transfusion support, the goal in ABO mismatch allo-HCT is to provide transfusion of RBCs that are

Table 15.3 Guidelines for blood component selection

Any type of allograft							
		Product		Platelets			
Recipient ABO	Donor ABO	RBC	Plasma/ CRYO	1st	2nd	3rd	4th
O	A	O	A or AB	A	AB	B	O
	B	O	B or AB	B	AB	A	O
	AB	O	AB	AB	B	A	O
A	O	O	A or AB	A	AB	B	O
	B	O	AB	AB	B	A	O
	AB	A or O	AB	AB	A	B	O
B	O	O	B or AB	B	AB	A	O
	A	O	AB	AB	A	B	O
	AB	B or O	AB	AB	B	A	O
AB	O	O	AB	AB	B	A	O
	A	A or O	AB	AB	A	B	O
	B	B or O	AB	AB	B	A	O

compatible with both the recipient isohemagglutinins and donor isohemagglutinins and to provide transfusion of plasma or platelet products whereby the infusion does not contain isohemagglutinins that are incompatible with either the recipient or donor RBCs. Nonetheless, it is standard practice to have a transfusion strategy to minimize incompatible RBC, plasma, and platelet products (Table 15.3) to decrease complications due to ABO incompatibility. For transfusion purposes, there are four phases of the transplant process: (1) preparative regimen to transplant, (2) transplant to initial appearance of donor RBCs, (3) initial donor RBC appearance to complete RBC engraftment to new donor type, and (4) after RBC engraftment is fully established and DAT is negative. This should be established by two negative DATs along with two consecutive samples with recipient cell and serum typing demonstrating donor ABO status. Some institutions begin RBC selection (Table 15.3) at the time the preparative regimen begins while others begin RBC selection on the day of transplant. While either approach is satisfactory, we prefer to begin RBC selection at the time the preparative regimen is begun. We recommend blood component selection using the guidelines shown in Table 15.3. Other institutions provide group O RBCs to recipient–donor ABO-incompatible transplant pairs regardless of the mismatch. The change to group O RBCs may occur during transplant conditioning or within the immediate peri-transplant period. Recipients are maintained on group O or donor ABO-compatible RBCs and blood components until the recipient forward and reverse typing reflects the donor RBC type without discrepancy. Theoretically, one could continue to transfuse a recipient with group O RBCs indefinitely if unsure when to switch to donor RBC type. However, the unnecessary use of type O RBCs in not recommended because it diverts O RBCs from other patients in need.

Transfusion Strategy for Rh Blood Group Mismatch Allo-HCT

In the scenario in which an RhD-positive recipient receives an RhD-negative graft, a small potential for anti-D immunization exists[22,40,46]. It is unknown whether post-transplant avoidance of RhD-positive blood products would decrease this risk since the bulk of the RBCs are from the patient. However, we suggest the use of RhD-negative RBCs as early as possible in the post-transplant setting. The risk of alloimmunization is increased after nonmyeloablative conditioning[47,48]. RhD-negative patients receiving RhD-positive stem cells can receive RhD-positive blood components after the transplant.

In institutions that perform PB and BM transplants, large numbers of patients may be transfusion-dependent. When there is a limited supply of RhD-negative blood components, most notably platelets, it may be necessary to transfuse RhD-incompatible platelets. Though platelet apheresis products have less than 0.1 mL of RBCs per unit, the very few RBCs present still have the ability to alloimmunize. While Lichtiger et al.[49] reported that transfusion of RhD-positive platelets to Rh-negative immunosuppressed patients resulted in no cases of anti-D formation, the general consensus is that while the risk is not zero, it is very small. Asfour et al.[50] reported an incidence of RhD alloimmunization of 3 of 78 (4%) in RhD-negative patients transfused with multiple RhD-positive platelets, which is similar to that reported in the 1970s by Goldfinger and McGinniss[51]. McLeod et al. reported an alloimmune response of 3 of 16 (19%) in immunosuppressed autologous bone marrow allo-HCT patients[52]. This difference in alloimmunization rate is probably due to less transplant-related immune suppression in the autologous transplant patients and the early appearance of antibody suggesting that patients had been immunized previously.

Practice Points

In conclusion, immunosuppressed PB or BM transplant recipients are significantly less likely to mount an immunization response to the D antigen; this knowledge is beneficial for inventory management in periods of RhD-negative platelet shortages. The administration of Rh immunoglobulin can prevent the formation of anti-D if given within 72 hours of exposure to RhD-positive blood products, though this practice is not necessary in the allo-HCT setting[53]. Furthermore, RhD-positive platelets transfused into RhD-negative patients with anti-D show normal in-vivo survival times because platelets do not contain Rh antigens[54].

Rh Donor⁺/Recipient⁻: How About Fresh Frozen Plasma Transfusion?

Residual RBCs and RBC fragments in RhD-positive plasma given to an RhD-negative recipient can pose a small risk of both primary alloimmunization and a secondary response in an already immunized patient[55,56]. The freeze–thaw process

in fresh frozen plasma (FFP) hemolyzes most of the RBCs thus rendering them less immunogenic[55,57,58]. Given the risk is so low, plasma derived from RhD-positive donors may be transfused to RhD-negative recipients.

Rh Donor⁺/Recipient⁻: How About Cryoprecipitate Transfusion?

Cryoprecipitate may contain enough RhD-positive substance to stimulate an immune response but this has not been studied in HCT patients. Thus it is not necessary to select for RhD-negative units nor is the use of Rh immunoglobulin recommended.

Practice Points

The main Rh antigens are D, C, c, E, and e. Rh-positive and Rh-negative denote the presence or absence of the D antigen, which is the most immunogenic of the Rh antigens. There are no evidence-based data to support the refusal of Rh-negative blood in Rh-positive patients in order to avoid non-D (C,c,E,e) Rh alloimmunization. Several studies have shown that for transfusion purposes C+D− and D−E+ units should still be considered Rh-negative[59,60]. In the nonimmunized patient, typing for C and E antigens on the D antigen-negative units is nonefficient use of time, reagents, and money. Second, the short supply of Rh-negative blood should not be intensified by calling C+D− and D−E+ units Rh-positive. The c and e antigens are rather poor immunogens. The majority of Rh-negative blood is c+ and e+ and much Rh-positive blood is also c+ and e+. Thus, with respect to the c and e antigens (or C or E antigens), there is no reason to match patient and donor on a routine basis.

Passenger Lymphocytes in Rh Mismatch Antigen Allo-HCT

The majority of healthy donors have not been transfused and consequently do not have the alloantibodies against Rh antigens so transfusion of donor antibody is not a concern. However, as in the minor ABO-incompatible allo-HCT scenario, donor lymphocytes may produce alloantibodies against foreign RBCs, triggering hemolysis of RBCs in the recipient. This would be exacerbated by the further transfusion of Rh-incompatible RBG during the immediate post-transplant period. Formation of non-ABO (Rh+) RBC antibodies after transplantation occurs in about 2–9% of patients[29,61–65]. One series showed that 8 of 217 (3.7%) allograft recipients developed non-ABO alloantibodies after allo-HCT at a median of 23 (range 16–672) days post-allo-HCT. Conditioning regimen, GvHD prophylaxis, and graft source did not predict development of alloantibodies; however, 2 of 156 (2.1%) patients receiving ABO-compatible grafts and 5 of 62 (9.6%) of patients receiving ABO-incompatible grafts developed alloantibodies, which might suggest facilitation of antibody production in the ABO-incompatible setting.

Furthermore, four of six patients with identified antibodies had alloantibodies directed against antigens absent in both the donor and recipient signifying that alloantibody formation can occur against transfused RBCs despite profound immunosuppression[63]. Abou-Elells *et al.* reported that although seven (3.6%) of 193 patients had alloantibodies prior to transplants, only four (2.1%) developed new alloantibodies during the course of transplantation[29]. Therefore, 98% of allo-HCT patients did not form new or additional RBC alloantibodies to non-ABO or Rh antigens.

Other Types of Rh (not D) Blood Group Incompatibilities

Similar to Rh-mismatched blood group transplants, though the potential for alloimmunization exists, there are very few patients that develop clinically relevant hemolysis. Erker *et al.* described how 17 Kell-mismatched transplants (nine minor, eight major) had no effect on transfusion requirements, length of hospitalization in transplantation unit, overall survival, or incidence of acute or chronic GvHD[41]. Additionally, 23 patients with non-ABO blood group antibodies did not show significant difference in transfusion requirements, delayed engraftment, survival, or GvHD[40]. In patients in which preformed antibody is present to a known donor positive RBC antigen, it would be reasonable to follow a similar algorithm as with a major ABO-incompatible blood type allo-HCT, which should be defined by each allo-HCT. Though there is no defined safe isoagglutinin titer, a management strategy as Rowley suggests can potentially minimize the risk of acute hemolytic reactions while avoiding the major risk of loss of CD34+ cells due to unnecessary RBC depletion. Rowley [9] suggests that no avoidance strategy is necessary

when antidonor antibody titers in the recipient are $\geq$1:32 with less than 20 mL RBC in the graft or recipient antidonor titers $\leq$1:16; however, it is suggested to monitor for acute hemolytic reactions during infusion[9]. If the antidonor antibody titers in the recipient are $\geq$1:32 and with greater than or equal to 20 mL RBC in the graft, then management should include RBC depletion of donor product (the authors prefer this method) or isoagglutinin depletion of recipient (older method), as well as monitoring for acute hemolytic reactions upon infusion[9,46,66,67]. Transfusion support in RBC incompatible HPC transplants should accommodate both the recipient and donor beginning at day 0 or earlier if possible to avoid hemolysis[22].

Practice Points

RBC depletion of cord blood units: Almost all RBCs are hemolyzed during processing and freezing of cord blood units and thus RBC depletion is not necessary. However, free hemoglobin, which may cause serious reactions, remains in the cord blood units.

Converting blood type in recipient: When selecting the ABO types of RBCs for transfusion, it is possible to use type O indefinitely or switch to donor-type RBCs. We recommend converting the patient to the donor blood type once the following criteria are met: (1) 100 days without a RBC transfusion, (2) complete (100%) chimera, (3) RBC ABO type of patient is donor type, and (4) serum ABO type of patient is compatible with donor type.

Use of Rh-negative blood type components: The extent to which RhD-negative platelets are to be used, especially for women in the childbearing years, and the use of Rh immune globulin for women in the childbearing years who receive RhD-positive blood products are not generally agreed upon.

References

1. Goldman J, Liesveld J, Nichols D, *et al.* ABO incompatibility between donor and recipient and clinical outcomes in allogeneic stem cell transplantation. *Leuk Res* 2003; 27:489–91.

2. Remberger M, Watz E, Ringden O, Mattsson J, Shjanwell A, Wikman A. Major ABO blood group mismatch increases the risk for graft failure after, unrelated donor hematopoietic stem cell transplantation. *Biol Blood Marrow Transplant* 2007;13(6):675–82.

3. Buckner CD, Clift RA, Sanders JE, *et al.* ABO-incompatible marrow transplants. *Transplantation* 1978; 26:233–8.

4. Warkentin Pl, Yomtovian R, Hurd D, *et al.* Severe delayed hemolytic transfusion reaction complicating

an ABO-incompatible bone marrow transplantation. *Vox Sang* 1983; 45:40–7.

5. Klummp TR, Herman JH, Ulicny J, *et al.* Lack of effect of donor-recipient ABO mismatching outcome following allogeneic hematopoietic stem cell transplantation. *Bone Marrow Transplant* 2006; 38:615–20.

6. Curley C, Pillai E, Mudie K, *et al.* Outcomes after major or bidirectional ABO-mismatched allogeneic hematopoietic progenitor cell transplantation after pretransplant isoagglutinin reduction with donor-type secreter plasma with or without plasma exchange. *Transfusion* 2012; 52:291–7.

7. Robeck JD, Grossman BJ, Harris T, Hillyer CD. *Technical manual.* Bethesda, MD: AABB; 2011.

8. Bender JG, Bikto L, Williams S, *et al.* Defining a therapy dose of peripheral blood stem cells. *J Hematother* 1992; 1:329–41.

9. Rowley SD. Hematopoietic stem cell transplantation between red cell incompatible donor-recipient pairs. *Bone Marrow Transplant* 2001; 28(4):315–21.

10. Cohn C, Gaensler K, Nambiar A. Engraftment associated complications: Is it an allo-or an autoantibody? *Transfusion* 2010; 50(2S).

11. Akel S, Regan D, Petz L, McCullough J. Current thawing and infusion practice of cryopreserved cord blood: the impact on graft quality, recipient safety, and transplantation outcomes. *Transfusion* 2014; 54(11):2997–3009.

12. Stroncek DF, Fautsch SK, Lasky LC, Hurd DD, Ramsay NKC, McCullough

J. Adverse reactions in patients transfused with cryopreserved marrow. *Transfusion* 1991; 31:521–7.

13. Malfuson JV, Amor RB, Bonin P, Rodet M, Boccaccio C, Pautas C, et al. Impact of nonmyeloablative conditioning regimens on the occurrence of pure red cell aplasia after ABO-incompatible allogeneic haematopoietic stem cell transplantation. *Vox Sang* 2007; 92(1):85–9.

14. Petz LD. Immune hemolysis associated with transplantation. *Semin Hematol* 2005; 42(3):145–55.

15. Fleur MA, Lichtiger B, Bassett R, et al. Incidence and natural history of pure red cell aplasia in major ABO-mismatched haematopoietc cell transplantation. *Br J Haematol* 2013; 160:798–805.

16. Yazar MH, Triulzi DJ. Immune hemolysis following ABO-mismatched stem cell or solid organ transplantation. *Curr Opin Hematol* 2007; 14:664–70.

17. Karafin MS, Blagg L, Tobian AA, et al. ABO antibody titers are not predictive of hemolytic reactions due to plasma-incompatible platelet transfusions. *Transfusion* 2012; 52:2087–93.

18. Mollison P, Engelfriet C, Contreras M, editors. *ABO, lewis and P groups and l antigens.* 10th ed. Oxford, UK: Blackwell Science; 1997.

19. Petz LO. Hemolysis associated with transplantation. *Transfusion* 1998; 38:224–8.

20. Bolan CD, Childs RW, Proter JL, et al. Massive immune haemolysis after allogeneic peripheral blood stem cell transplantation with minor ABO incompatibility. *Br J Haematol* 2001; 112:787–95.

21. Daniel-Johnson J, Schwartz J. How do I approach ABO-incompatible hematopoietic progenitor cell transplantation? *Transfusion* 2011; 51:1143–9.

22. Gajewski JL, Johnson VV, Sandler SG, et al. A review of transfusion practice before, during, and after hematopoietic progenitor cell transplantation. *Blood* 2008; 112:3036–47.

23. McCullough J. *Transfusion medicine.* 3rd ed, Chapter 8. Oxford, UK: Wiley-Blackwell; 2012: 1–597.

24. Boctor FN, Ali NM, Mohandas K, et al. Absence of D-alloimmunization in AIDS patients receiving D-mismatched RBCs. *Transfusion* 2003; 43:(2):173–6.

25. Ramsey G, Hahn LF, Cornell FW, et al. Low rate of Rhesus immunization from Rh-incompatible blood transfusions during liver and heart transplant surgery. *Transplantation* 1989; 47(6):993–5.

26. Cummins D, Contreras M, Amin S, et al. Red cell alloantibody development associated with heart and lung transplantation. *Transplantation* 1995, 59:1432–5.

27. Casanueva M, Valdes MD, Ribera MC. Lack of alloimmunisation to D antigen in D-negative immunosuppressed liver transplant patients. *Transfusion* 1994; 34:570–2.

28. Menitove JE. Immunoprophylaxis for D-patients receiving platelets from D+ donors? *Transfusion* 2002; 42:136–8.

29. Abou-Elells AA, Camarillo TA, Allen BM, et al. Low incidence of red cell and HLA antibody formation by bone marrow transplant patients. *Transfusion* 1995; 35:931–5.

30. Parkman R. Immunological reconstitution following bone marrow transplantation. In *Bone marrow transplantation.* Boston, MA: Blackwell Scientific; 1994; 504–12.

31. Atkinson K. Reconstruction of the haemopoietic and immune systems after marrow transplantation. *Bone Marrow Transplant* 1990; 5(4):209–26.

32. Friedberg RC. Transfusion therapy in the patient undergoing hematopoietic stem cell transplantation. *Hematol Oncol Clin North Am* 1994; 8(6):1105–16. Review.

33. Heddle NM, Soutar RL, O'Hoski PL, et al. A prospective study to determine the frequency and clinical significance of alloimmunization post-transfusion. *Br J Haematol* 1995; 91(4):1000–5.

34. Azuma E, Nishihara H, Hanada M. Recurrent cold hemagglutinin disease following allogeneic bone marrow transplantation successfully treated with plasmapheresis, corticosteroid and cyclophosphamide. *Bone Marrow Transplant* 1996; 18(1):243–6.

35. Wennerberg A, Backman KA, Gillerlain C. Mixed erythrocyte chimerism: implications for tolerance of the donor immune system to recipient non-ABO system red cell antigens. *Bone Marrow Transplant* 1996; 18(2):433–5.

36. Sachs V. Immune haemolysis after organ transplantation. *Transf Med* 1995; 5(1):87.

37. Chen F, Owen I, Savage D, et al. Late onset haemolysis and red cell autoimmunisation after allogeneic bone marrow transplant. *Bone Marrow Transplant* 1997; 19:491–5.

38. Drobyski WR, Potluri J, Sauer D, Gottschall JL. Autoimmune hemolytic anemia following T cell-depleted allogeneic bone marrow transplantation. *Bone Marrow Transplant* 1996; 17(6):1093–9.

39. Horn B, Viele M, Mentzer W, et al. Autoimmune hemolytic anemia in patients with SCID after T cell-depleted BM and PBSC transplantation. *Bone Marrow Transplant* 1999; 24(9):1009–13.

40. Mijovic A. Alloimmunization to RhD antigen in RhD-incompatible haemopoietic cell transplants with non-myeloablative conditioning. *Vox Sang* 2002; 83:358–362.

41. Erker CG, Steins MB, Fischer RJ, et al. The influence of blood group differences in allogeneic hematopoietic peripheral blood progenitor cell transplantation. *Transfusion* 2005; 45:1382–90.

42. Wirk B, Klumpp TR, Ulicny J, et al. Lack of effect of donor-recipient Rh mismatch on outcomes after allogeneic hematopoietic stem cell transplantation. *Transfusion* 2008; 48:163–8.

43. Berkman EM, Caplan SN. Engraftment of RH-positive marrow in a recipient with RH antibody. *Transplant Proc* 1977; 9(1 Suppl 1):215–8.

44. Rigal D, Monestier M, Meyer F, Tremisi PJ, et al. Transplant of rhesus-positive bone marrow in a rhesus-negative woman having anti-rhesus D alloantibodies. *Acta Haematol* 1985; 73(3):153–6.

45. Taylor PA, Ehrhardt MJ, Roforth MM, et al. Preformed antibody, not primed T cells, is the initial and major barrier to bone marrow engraftment in allosensitized recipients. *Blood* 2007; 109:1307–15.

46. Warkentin PI, Hilden JM, Kersey JH, et al. Transplantation of major ABO-incompatible bone marrow depleted of red cells by hydroxyethyl starch. *Vox Sang* 1985; 48(2):89–104.

47. Kalacioglu M, Copelan E, Avalos B, *et al.* Survival after ABO-incompatible allogeneic bone marrow transplant after a preparative regimen of busulfan and cyclophosphamide. *Bone Marrow Transplant* 1995; 15:105–10.

48. Booth GS, Gerhie EA, Bolan CD, Savani BN. Clinical guide to ABO-incompatible allogeneic stem cell transplantation. *Biol Blood Marrow Transplant* 2013; 19:1152–8.

49. Lichtiger B, Hester JP. Transfusion of Rh-incompatible blood components to cancer patients. *Haematologia* 1986; 19:81–8.

50. Asfour M, Narvios A, Lichtiger B. Transfusion of RhD-incompatible blood components in RhD-negative blood marrow transplant recipients. *Med Gen Med* 2004; 13:22.

51. Goldfinger D, MGinniss MH. Rh-incompatible platelet transfusion: risks and consequences of sensitizing immunosuppressed patients. *N Engl J Med* 1971; 284:942.

52. McLeod BC, Piehl MR, Sassetti RJ. Alloimmunizaation to RhD by platelet transfusion in autologous bone marrow transplant recipients. *Vox Sang* 1990; 59:185–9.

53. Avache S, Herman JH. Prevention of D sensitization after mismatched transfusion of blood components: toward optimal use of RhIG. *Transfusion* 2008; 48:1990–9.

54. Pfisterer H, Thierfelder S, Kottusch H, *et al.* Examination of human thrombocytes for Rhesus antigens using decomposition studies in vivo following Cr 51 labelling. *Klin Wochenschr* 1967; 45(10):519–22.

55. Burnie KM, Barr RM. Unpublished observations cited by Mollsion PL, Engelfriet CP, Contreras M. In *Blood transfusion in clinical medicine*, 9th edition. Oxford: Blackwell; 1993: 235.

56. McBride JA, O'Hoski P, Blasjchman MA, *et al.* Rhesus alloimmunisation following intensive plasmapheresis. *Transfusion* 1978; 18:626–7.

57. O'Shaughnessy DF, Atterbury C, Bolton Maggs P, *et al.* Guidelines for the use of fresh-frozen plasma, cryoprecipitate and cryosupernatant. British Committee for Standards in Haematology, Blood Transfusion Task Force. *Br J Haematol* 2004; 126(1):11–28.

58. Barclay GR, Greiss MA, Urbaniak SJ. Adverse effect of plasma exchange on anti-D production in rhesus immunization owing to removal of inhibitory factors. *BMJ* 1980; 280(6231):1569–71.

59. Schorr JB, Schorr PT, Francis R, *et al.* *The antigenicity of C and E antigens when transfused into Rh-negative (rr) and Rh-positive recipients.* Chicago, IL: Commun Am Assoc Blood Banks; 1971.

60. Huestis DW. International forum: what constitutes adequate routine Rh typing on donors and recipients? *Vox Sang* 1971; 21:183.

61. Leo A, Mytilineos J, Voso MT, *et al.* Passenger lymphocyte syndrome with severe hemolytic anemia due to an anti-Jk(a) after allogeneic PBPC transplantation. *Transfusion* 2000; 40(6):632–6.

62. Ting A, Pun A, Dodds AJ, Atkinson K, *et al.* Red cell alloantibodies produced after bone marrow transplantation. Red cell alloantibodies produced after bone marrow transplantation. *Transfusion* 1987; 27(2):145–7.

63. de la Rubia J, Arriaga F, Andreu R, *et al.* Development of non-ABO RBC alloantibodies in patients undergoing allogeneic HPC transplantation. Is ABO incompatibility a predisposing factor? *Transfusion* 2001; 41:106–10.

64. Zupańska B, Zaucha JM, Michalewska B, *et al.* Multiple red cell alloantibodies, including anti-Dib, after allogeneic ABO-matched peripheral blood progenitor cell transplantation. *Transfusion* 2005; 45(1):16–20.

65. López A, de la Rubia J, Arriaga F, *et al.* Severe hemolytic anemia due to multiple red cell alloantibodies after an ABO-incompatible allogeneic bone marrow transplant. *Transfusion* 1998; 38(3):247–51.

66. Dinsmore RE, Reich LM, Kapoor N, *et al.* ABH incompatible bone marrow transplantation: removal of erythrocytes by starch sedimentation. *Br J Haematol* 1983; 54(3):441–9.

67. Lasky LC, Warkentin PI, Kersey JH, *et al.* Hemotherapy in patients undergoing blood group incompatible bone marrow transplantation. *Transfusion* 1983; 23(4):277–85.

Chapter

16

Prevention and Treatment of Bacterial Infections in Hematopoietic Cell Transplants

Corrado Girmenia and Claudio Viscoli

Introduction

Hematopoietic cell transplant (HCT) patients receiving cytotoxic conditioning regimens, particularly those with myeloablative activity, sufficient to determine a profound, prolonged neutropenia and adversely affect the integrity of the gastrointestinal mucosa, are at risk for endogenous origin invasive infection due to colonizing bacteria that translocate across intestinal mucosal surfaces[1–3]. Bacterial infection by exogenous origin also occurs, particularly in patients with indwelling venous devices which may be contaminated regardless of the immunologic status of the patient[4]. The risk of severe bacterial infection in the early post-transplant period is lower in autologous-HCT (auto-HCT) as compared to allogeneic HCT (allo-HCT) and in allo-HCT it is markedly reduced when nonmyeloablative conditioning is used. After engraftment, due to the delayed immunologic recovery and the prolonged immunosuppressive therapy, allo-HCT patients may continue to be at risk for severe infections, including those caused by bacterial pathogens[1].

The epidemiology of bacterial infections in immunocompromised patients, including HCT populations, is characterized by a continuous evolution represented not only by the increasing incidence of some bacterial species but also by the emergence of antimicrobial resistance, particularly against gram-negative bacteria[5]. An awareness of these epidemiologic phenomena is crucial in the definition of prevention strategies and in the choice of antibiotic protocols aimed at the targeted treatment of infections by microorganisms with reduced susceptibility, at the containment of the induction of resistance to antimicrobials, and at overall hospital infection control.

Epidemiology of Bacterial Infections in Recipients of HCT: Why Has It Changed over Time?

Continuous modification in the epidemiologic spectrum of bloodstream bacterial isolates obtained from febrile neutropenic and HCT patients has occurred over the past decades. During the 1960s and 1970s, gram-negative bacilli represented the predominant pathogens causing life-threatening infections. Then, during the 1980s and 1990s, gram-positive organisms

became more common, probably due to the increased use of venous catheters and systemic prophylaxis with fluoroquinolones which can allow colonization by and entry of gram-positive skin and intestinal flora[6–9]. Currently, coagulase-negative staphylococci continue to be the most common blood isolates; however, a new emergence of infections by enterobacteriacae (i.e., *Escherichia coli* and *Klebsiella pneumoniae*) and nonfermenting gram-negative pathogens (i.e., *Pseudomonas aeruginosa* and *Stenotrophomonas maltophilia*) has been observed in several centers[10–17]. In particular, drug-resistant gram-negative bacterial species are causing an increasing number of infections in neutropenic and nonneutropenic patients. *Klebsiella pneumoniae* and *E. coli* strains with acquired Extended-Spectrum Beta Lactamases (ESBL) genes show a broad range of beta-lactam antibiotic resistance. These ESBL producers are often only susceptible to carbapenems, antibiotics with a very broad spectrum of activity, but their use may induce the selection of bacteria with even greater resistance patterns such as *K. pneumoniae* and *P. aeruginosa* carbapenem-resistant strains. The spread of infections by multidrug-resistant (MDR) gram-negative strains may represent a devastating problem considering also that the molecules recently added to the antibacterial armamentarium are mainly oriented against gram-positive bacteria.

Despite the increasing attention given to the clinical and therapeutic aspects of infection in persons with hematologic malignancies, few data are available on the incidence, microbiologic characteristics, *in-vitro* susceptibility pattern, and clinical outcome of bacterial infections, specifically in the HCT populations. Data from studies on bacterial infections in HCT patients published in the last few years are summarized in Table 16.1[18–27]. These studies generally confirm that staphylococci still continues to be the most commonly isolated bacterial pathogen and that a variable emergence of resistance in gram-negative bacteria, in particular enterobacteria, is observed.

Quinolone Prophylaxis and Timing of Appropriate Antibiotics: Influence on Epidemiology and Outcomes?

The impact of *in-vitro* susceptibility pattern in the outcome of bacterial infections in HCT populations may be extrapolated

Table 16.1 Epidemiology of bacterial infections in HCT populations

Author, year (reference)	Type of transplant, population (no. of pts)	Period, type of study, country	Incidence of bacterial infection	% of gram-positive/gram-negative	More frequent bacterial pathogens	In-vitro susceptibility data
Busca et al., 2011[18]	Allo-HCT, adults (269)	2001–2009, retrospective, Italy	12%	60/40	Staphylococci, 53% E. coli, 23% Pseudomonas spp., 10%	Methicillin resistance: 81% of staphylococci: ESBL+: 17% of gram-negative
Mikulska et al., 2012 [19]	Allo-HCT, adults (382)	2004–2008, retrospective, Italy	34%	62/38	Enterococci, 27% Staphylococci, 22% E. coli, 19%	No detailed susceptibility data
Mendes et al., 2012 [20]	Allo- and auto-HCT, adults (429)	2001–2010, retrospective, Brazil	17%	43/57	P. aeruginosa, 22.5% Staphylococci, 20% Enterococci, 19% Acinetobacter, 15%	
Hong et al., 2013[21]	Allo-HCT, adults (59)	2002–2012, retrospective, Korea	37%	36/64	Staphylococci, 25% E. coli, 18% K. pneumoniae, Acinetobacter, Enterococcus, 11% each	MDR 44% of gram-negative: Methicillin resistant: 71% of staphylococci
	Auto-HCT, adults (75),		19%	31/69	K. pneumoniae, 37% Staphylococci, 25% E. coli, 19%	MDR 9% of gram-negative Methicillin resistant: 75% of staphylococci
Srinivasan et al., 2013 [22]	Allo-HCT, pediatric (211)	2005–2009, retrospective, United States	0–30 days post-transpl: 9% 31–100 days post-transpl: 23% 101 days–2 years post-transpl: 33%	0–30 days post-transpl: 66/33 31–100 days post-transpl: 74/26 101 days–2 years post-transpl: 76/24	Staphylococci, 31% Streptococci, 7% K. pneumoniae, 8% E. coli, 8% Clostridium difficile, 14%	No detailed susceptibility data
Kim et al., 2013[23]	Allo-HCT, adults (231)	2004–2005, retrospective, United States	23%	50/50	E. coli, 17% Enterococci, 17% K. pneumoniae, 11%	No detailed susceptibility data

Study	Population	Period, design, country	Incidence	Organisms	Susceptibility
Sarashina et al., 2013 [24]	Allo-HCT, pediatric (277)	1988–2009, retrospective, Japan	9% (6% during the pre-engraftment period and 3% after engraftment)	Staphylococci, 29% Streptococci, 25% K. pneumoniae, 13%	No detailed susceptibility data
Bock et al., 2013 [25]	Allo-HCT, adults (555)	2005–2010, retrospective, United States	51%	Staphylococci, 64% Enterococci, 28% P. aeruginosa, 5%	P. aeruginosa resistance: gentamicin (>40%), levofloxacin (>30%), ceftazidime (>30%). In the years 2009–2010, 40% and 25% of E. coli and K. pneumoniae strains, respectively, were resistant to ceftazidime (suspect of ESBL). With regard to staphylococci and enterococci 0% and 81%, respectively, were resistant to vancomycin
	Auto-HCT, adults (279)	2005–2010, retrospective, United States	24%	Staphylococci, 83% Enterococci, 6% Corynebacterium, 5%	
Pinana et al., 2014 [26]	Auto-HCT, adults (720)	1998–2003, prospective, multicenter, Spain	20%	Staphylococci, 43% E. coli, 19% Streptococci, 13% Pseudomonas, 6%	No detailed susceptibility data
Seo et al., 2014 [27]	Allo-HCT, adults (696)	2006–2011, retrospective, United States	29%	Enterococci, 30% Staphylococci, 17% E. coli, 14% K. pneumoniae, 14%	Enterococci: 34% vancomycin-resistant Enterobacteria: 10% ESBL positive, 9% carbapenem resistant, 14% multidrug resistant

Data from recently published studies.

from studies in cancer patients in which HCT patients were included. In an adult Spanish cancer center, 272 bloodstream infections documented in the period 1991–1996 (labeled as the first period) when quinolone prophylaxis was used were compared to 283 documented during the period 2006–2010 (labeled as the second period) when antibacterial prophylaxis was stopped[28]. Overall, 20% of the patients had been submitted to HCT. Gram-positive bloodstream infections were more frequent in the first period (64% *versus* 41%; $P < 0.001$), mainly due to coagulase-negative staphylococci and viridans group streptococci. In the second period gram-negative infections increased (28% *versus* 49%; $P < 0.001$), *E. coli*, *P. aeruginosa*, and *K. pneumoniae* being the most frequently isolated pathogens (51%, 23%, and 22%, respectively). Antimicrobial susceptibility testing showed a significantly lower rate of quinolone resistance among all *E. coli* strains isolated in the second period (37% *versus* 71%; $P < 0.001$), when quinolone prophylaxis was stopped. On the other hand, in the second period MDR gram-negative infections increased (1% *versus* 6%; $P < 0.001$). The resistant gram-negative bacteria isolated in the second period included ESBL-*E. coli*, MDR *P. aeruginosa* and *S. maltophilia*, and AmpC cephalosporinase hyperproducing *Enterobacter cloacae*. In a previous paper from the same group, related to the period 2006–2009, the authors compared treatment and prognostic factors of the patients with MDR *versus* no MDR gram-negative bacteremias[12]. Patients with MDR gram-negative bacteremias more frequently received inadequate initial antibiotic therapy (69% *versus* 9%; $P < 0.001$) and the mean time to adequate therapy was longer in this group (2.13 days *versus* 0.33 days; $P < 0.001$). Patients in the resistant group more frequently required intensive care unit admission (14% *versus* 5%; $P = 0.023$), had greater need for mechanical ventilation (14% *versus* 3%; $P = 0.005$), and had a higher overall case-fatality rate (41% *versus* 21%; $P = 0.003$).

What About Carbapenem-Resistant K. pneumoniae?

An emerging pathogen increasingly causing hospital acquired severe infections in the last few years is carbapenem-resistant *K. pneumoniae* (CRKp), which has been reported particularly in Italy, the United States, Israel, Greece, China, and South America[29–35]. Infections caused by CRKp isolates are associated with high morbidity and mortality rates particularly in high-risk intensive care units and solid organ transplant patients[36–38]. Infection and colonization by these multiresistant bacteria may represent a challenging problem in HCT recipients not only for the management of post-transplant complications but also for the eligibility to transplant itself when patients acquire the pathogen before the transplant procedure[17,39–41]. To assess the current epidemiology, clinical characteristics, and outcome of CRKp infection in HCT, the Gruppo Italiano Trapianto Midollo Osseo (GITMO) retrospectively collected data of patients undergoing auto- and

allo-HCT during the period 2010–2013[42]. Overall 6058 patients from 50 transplant centers and 4389 patients from 47 transplant centers received auto- and allo-HCT, respectively. They accounted for 54% of auto-HCTs and 72% of allo-HCTs performed in Italy during the study period. Overall, 25 and 87 cases of CRKp infection were reported 8 median days from auto-HCT and 15 median days from allo-HCT, respectively. The incidence of CRKp infections was 0.4% (from 0.1% in 2010 to 0.7% in 2013) in auto-HCT and 2% (from 0.4% in 2010 to 2.9% in 2013) in allo-HCT populations. A post-transplant infection occurred in about one-third of patients with a CRKp colonization documented before or after transplant. The attributable mortality rate at 3 months from the diagnosis of CRKp infection was 16% in auto-HCT and 64.4% in allo-HCT patients. The analysis of the variables of survival demonstrated the independent impact of the history of an infection documented prior to transplant (HR 0.33, 95% CI 0.15–0.74; $P = 0.007$) and of the adequacy of the first-line antimicrobial therapy (HR 2.67, 95% CI 1.43–4.99; $P = 0.002$) in the survival of the patients in allo-HCT. No survival variable was statistically significant for auto-HCT.

Practice Points

All these experiences show the increasing epidemiologic burden of severe infections by resistant gram-negative bacteria in HCT populations. A crucial problem in the management of these infections is the choice of prophylaxis and initial antibacterial therapy considering that it may dramatically affect the patient's outcome.

Prevention of Bacterial Infections in Recipients of HCT

Prolonged severe neutropenia and breaks in the mucocutaneous barrier resulting from conditioning regimens are two critical risk factors for endogenous bacterial infection during the engraftment phase in both auto- and allo-HCT recipients. After the postengraftment period, despite the recovery of the neutrophil count, recipients of allo-HCT continue to be predisposed to several infections for a prolonged period due to the defects in cell-mediated immunity and the immunosuppressive treatments. Defective reconstitution of B-cell immunity associated with serum opsonic deficiency and immunosuppressive therapy for GvHD are major factors contributing to increased infection susceptibility by encapsulated bacteria, such as *Streptococcus pneumoniae*, *H. influenzae* and *Meningococcus*, in the postengraftment transplant period between 3 months to years after allo-HCT.

Practice Points

Antibacterial agents and vaccines are the cornerstones of the prevention of bacterial diseases; however, infection control should also consider the prevention of transmission of pathogens. Healthcare workers and others in contact with HCT

Table 16.2 European Conference on Infection in Leukemia (ECIL) and Infectious Diseases Society of America (IDSA) guidelines on antibacterial prophylaxis in neutropenic hematology and hematopoietic cell transplant patients[5,47]

Guideline	Recommendation and grading
ECIL	A fluoroquinolone with systemic activity including *P. aeruginosa* should be used Levofloxacin: 500 mg od, OS (AI) Ciprofloxacin: 500 mg bid, OS (AI) Norfloxacin: 400 mg bid, OS (BI) (less effective than ciprofloxacin) Ofloxacin: 200–300 mg bid, OS (BI) (less tested than ciprofloxacin in randomized controlled trials and at variable daily doses, lower activity against *P. aeruginosa* and less effective than ciprofloxacin)
IDSA	Fluoroquinolone prophylaxis should be considered for high-risk patients with expected prolonged and profound neutropenia (ANC <100 cells/mm^3 for >7 days) (BI). Levofloxacin and ciprofloxacin have been evaluated most comprehensively and are considered to be roughly equivalent, although levofloxacin is preferred in situations with increased risk for oral mucositis-related invasive viridans group streptococcal infection. A systematic strategy for monitoring the development of fluoroquinolone resistance among gram-negative bacilli is recommended (A-II). Addition of a gram-positive active agent to fluoroquinolone prophylaxis is generally not recommended (A-I)

recipients should routinely follow appropriate hand hygiene practices to avoid exposing recipients to bacterial pathogens. Additional precautions for patients colonized with certain contagious pathogens (e.g., MRSA, VRE, resistant gram-negative, *Clostridium difficile*) and instructions with regard to visitors, pets, and plants are crucial aspects in the overall prevention of bacterial infections in HCT recipients[43–45].

Do all Persons Undergoing HCT Require the Same Antibacterial Prophylaxis during Neutropenia?

Based on evidence that antibiotic prophylaxis improves the clinical outcome, including the incidences of documented infections and all-cause mortality in patients with chemotherapy-induced neutropenia, current guidelines recommend prophylaxis with fluoroquinolones in high-risk patients who are expected to show prolonged and profound neutropenia, such as patients undergoing HCT (Table 16.2) [5,46]. The prophylaxis should be discontinued after recovery from neutropenia.

A meta-analysis based on prospective, randomized studies on systemic antibiotic prophylaxis including HCT recipient was recently performed to evaluate the impact of antibiotic prophylaxis in this population[47]. Systemic antibiotic prophylaxis was compared with placebo or no prophylaxis or with nonabsorbable antibiotics. Systemic antibiotics other than fluoroquinolones and the effect of the addition of antibiotics for gram-positive bacteria to fluoroquinolones were also evaluated. As a result, systemic antibiotic prophylaxis with fluoroquinolones reduced the incidence of febrile episodes, clinically or microbiologically documented infection, and bacteremia without significantly affecting all-cause mortality or infection-related mortality. Since there was a significant increase in adverse events in patients who received additional antibiotics for Gram-positive bacteria without clear benefit with regard to morbidity and mortality, the routine use of gram-positive prophylaxis is not advisable. In the last few years only two publications evaluated the

effect of antibacterial prophylaxis specifically in myeloablative allo-HCT[48] and auto-HCT[49] patients. In the study in allo-HCT, conducted over the period 2000–2004, 435 patients received prophylaxis with either ceftazidime or levofloxacin and there was not a placebo/no prophylaxis control arm[48]. Among recipients of levofloxacin, there was a higher probability of developing a fever, and more patients failed to respond to prophylaxis resulting in a greater likelihood of starting empiric antibiotic therapy (63 *versus* 45%). Despite these findings, patients receiving levofloxacin had lower rates of bacteremia with virulent organisms than those receiving ceftazidime (19.2 *versus* 29.6%, $P = 0.02$) with a similar spectrum of bacteria causing bacteremia. Furthermore, the cost of treatment with levofloxacin was considerably lower compared to the ceftazidime cohort. In the second study in auto-HCT recipients the combination of ciprofloxacin plus vancomycin was associated with a reduction in the incidence of neutropenic fever (71.3% in prophylaxis group *versus* 91.2% in the no prophylaxis group, $P < 0.001$), bacteremias (5.6% *versus* 35%, respectively), and overall microbiologically documented infections[49]. Of note, no gram-negative bacteremias occurred in those receiving prophylaxis. Interesting findings from this study that warrant consideration include the occurrence of gram-positive infections in the prophylaxis group, suggesting that vancomycin inclusion in the prophylaxis strategy was not associated with any advantage. Among patients developing neutropenic fever, the likelihood of success with first-line empiric antibacterials was significantly reduced among patients receiving prophylaxis (66% prophylaxis *versus* 84.1% no prophylaxis; $P=0.025$). In this study, there were no significant improvements in hospital length of stay, duration of fever, duration of antibacterial treatment, or treatment failure with prophylaxis. Therefore, the authors concluded that their results do not support the use of antibacterial prophylaxis in auto-HCT patients. Although this experience is not able to counteract the general opinion that antibacterial prophylaxis is required in auto-HCT patients, it raises the question of a revision in the antimicrobial prevention strategies at least in lower risk auto-HCT populations.

Another important issue concerning antibacterial prophylactic strategy is antibiotic resistance. An alarm over the emergence of resistant bacteria or *C. difficile* infection as a result of the expansive use of fluoroquinolones has been raised. Since only a few clinical trials fully evaluated the emergence of resistant bacteria in HCT patients, a meta-analysis on this issue was not performed. On the other hand, a systematic review of the effect of quinolone prophylaxis in neutropenic patients showed a nonsignificant increase in colonization and infection with resistant organisms[50]. In conclusion, the problem of resistance during fluoroquinolone prophylaxis in neutropenic patients and its clinical implication remains controversial.

Practice Points

Although actually the phenomenon of quinolone resistance does not seem to be a contraindication to the use of these drugs in prophylaxis during neutropenia, the possible transmission of multiclass antimicrobial resistance genes among gram-negative bacilli should be carefully monitored and the proficiency of the practice of antibacterial prophylaxis periodically re-evaluated. There is no solid evidence to point out a measure and percentage of resistance that may serve as a threshold for deciding not to use prophylaxis, although prophylaxis efficacy seems to be reduced when the prevalence of quinolone gram-negative bacillary resistance exceeds 20% [51]. This practice should be re-evaluated in institutions where a progressive and significant increase of quinolone resistance is observed, particularly when it is associated with concomitant emergence of resistance to other classes of antibiotics used in therapy.

What is Appropriate Prevention for Postengraftment Bacterial Infections?

Patients undergoing allo-HCT are at increased risk for encapsulated bacteria (*S. pneumoniae, H. influenzae*, and *Meningococcus*) sepsis from functional asplenia and impaired B-cell immunity, therefore prophylaxis against these infections is advised[43,44]. Penicillin (penicillin V or amoxicillin, adult 250–500 mg q12h – although 500 mg q24h may be more realistic if compliance is a particular problem; in penicillin allergy clarithromycin 250 mg q12h orally; reduce the dose for children) is the drug of choice. It should be initiated at 3 months after HCT and be continued until at least 1 year after transplant or until immunosuppressive therapy has been discontinued in patients with chronic graft-*versus*-host disease (GvHD). Patients should receive prophylaxis regardless of prior administration of pneumococcal vaccines.

Vaccination against *S. pneumoniae* is strongly recommended for all HCT recipients. A 13-valent pneumococcal conjugate vaccine (PCV13) should be administered to eligible pediatric and adult HCT patients. Patients should receive a dose of PCV13 beginning 3–6 months after the transplant, followed by another two doses 2 and 4 months later. Following the primary series of 3 PCV13 doses, a dose of the 23-valent pneumococcal polysaccharide vaccine (PPSV23) to broaden the immune response might be given. For patients with chronic GvHD who are likely to respond poorly to PPSV23, a fourth dose of the PCV13 should be considered instead of PPSV23.

A three-dose regimen of *H. influenzae* type B vaccine should be administered beginning 6 months after transplant; at least 1 month should separate the doses. A single dose of meningococcal conjugate vaccine at 6–12 months from HCT is sufficient in high-risk populations.

Treatment of Bacterial Infections in Recipients of HCT

The use of antibacterial therapy in HCT recipients should follow the rules defined for persons with hematologic cancers [3]. Fever in a neutropenic transplant patient should be considered a medical emergency and broad-spectrum antibacterials should be given as soon as possible (within 60 minutes of triage) and at full doses, adjusted for renal and/or hepatic function. In addition, the diagnostic evaluation should be obtained quickly. Antibiotics are usually administered empirically, but should always include appropriate coverage for suspected or known infections.

Practice Points

Even when the pathogen is known, the antibiotic regimen should provide broad-spectrum empiric coverage for the possibility of other pathogens, unlike the treatment strategy adopted in many immunocompetent hosts. In general, the following indications should be used:

- In high-risk neutropenic patients, antibiotics should generally be administered intravenously in a hospital setting.
- Initial antibiotic selection should be guided by the patient's history, allergies, symptoms, signs, recent antibiotic use and culture data, and awareness of the susceptibility patterns of institutional nosocomial pathogens.
- Empiric broad-spectrum antibacterial therapy should be initiated within 60 minutes of triage after blood cultures have been obtained and before any other investigations have been completed
- Ideally, antibiotics should be bactericidal. Monotherapy with an antipseudomonal b-lactam agent is recommended and other antimicrobials (aminoglycosides, fluoroquinolones, and/or glycopeptides) may be added to the initial regimen for management of complications (e.g., hypotension and pneumonia) or if antimicrobial resistance is suspected or proven. Glycopeptides (or other agents active against aerobic gram-positive cocci) are not recommended as a standard part of the initial antibiotic

regimen for fever and neutropenia. These agents should be considered for specific clinical indications, including suspected catheter-related infection, skin and soft-tissue infection, pneumonia, or hemodynamic instability.

- Clinical response and culture and susceptibility results should be monitored closely, and therapy should be adjusted in a timely fashion in response to this information.

Controversies and New Perspectives in the Choice of Antibacterial Therapy

The emergence of resistant gram-negative bacteria potentially unsusceptible to the conventional antibiotic treatments raises the challenging problem of the choice of empiric antibacterial therapy in post-transplant febrile neutropenia. The relatively unsatisfactory efficacy of the available antimicrobial armamentarium and the paucity of new active antibacterial drugs in the near future represent challenging issues in the management of infections by MDR pathogens. The dramatically poor outcome observed in HCT patients when affected by resistant gram-negative infections, particularly those undergoing the allo-HCT, makes the problem even more serious in this population. An Expert Panel of the 4th European Conference on Infections in Leukemia (ECIL-4) group has developed guidelines for the management of emerging resistant gram-negative pathogens in leukemic patients and HCT recipients[5]. A key issue of the treatment of infections by MDR gram-negative bacteria is represented by the need of the use of unconventional agents such as colistin/polymyxin B, tigecyclin, and fosfomycin as the only remaining treatment options. These agents should be preferably used in combination with other agents that remain active *in-vitro* (such as gentamicin or amikacin, or carbapenems if a certain, although reduced, *in-vitro* activity remains), because of suboptimal efficacy (e.g., tigecyclin) and risk of emergent resistance (e.g., fosfomycin). The use of these drugs should be limited to the situations where no alternative exists and *in-vitro* susceptibility pattern isolate should be considered for the choice of the drugs. However, considering that culture-based techniques to identify resistant bacteria lead to a 48- to 72-hour delay from blood culture collection and that the outcome of such infections may be rapidly fatal in high-risk neutropenic patients, a strategy leading to an early, empiric, tailored, unconventional antibiotic treatment before the microbiologic documentation may be considered in selected settings[45]. A strict correlation between intestinal colonization and endogenous infection by MDR gram-negative bacteria has been observed in immunocompromised patients. In particular, a high rate of severe infections (about 30%) has been reported in allo-HCT patients with a documented carbapenem-resistant *K. pneumoniae* colonization[42]. In this specific setting, the administration of a tailored, empiric therapy including the above-mentioned unconventional antibiotics and guided by the susceptibility pattern of the colonizing microorganism may be considered at the onset of febrile neutropenia. However, no recommendation can be made considering the lack of any experience on the efficacy and safety of this practice.

In the present era of growing resistance, while new antibiotic associations will be increasingly used in the HCT setting, antibacterial strategies should be managed in the context of an antimicrobial stewardship, aiming to minimize unnecessary broad-spectrum antibiotic use and further resistance selection.

References

1. Marr KA. Delayed opportunistic infections in hematopoietic stem cell transplantation patients: a surmountable challenge. *Hematology Am Soc Hematol Educ Program.* 2012;2012:265–70.

2. Hiemenz JW. Management of infections complicating allo-hematopoietic stem cell transplantation. *Semin Hematol.* 2009;46:289–312.

3. Freifeld AG, Bow EJ, Sepkowitz KA, Boeckh MJ, Ito JI, Mullen CA, *et al.* Infectious Diseases Society of America. Clinical practice guideline for the use of antimicrobial agents in neutropenic patients with cancer: 2010 update by the infectious diseases society of America. *Clin Infect Dis.* 2011;52:e56–93.

4. Martinho GH, Romanelli RM, Teixeira GM, Macedo AV, Chaia JM, Nobre V.

Infectious complications associated with the use of central venous catheters in patients undergoing hematopoietic stem cell transplantation. *Am J Infect Control.* 2013;41:642–4.

5. Averbuch D, Cordonnier C, Livermore DM, Mikulska M, Orasch C, Viscoli C, *et al.*; ECIL4, a joint venture of EBMT, EORTC, ICHS, ESGICH/ESCMID and ELN. Targeted therapy against multi-resistant bacteria in leukemic and hematopoietic stem cell transplant recipients: guidelines of the 4th European Conference on Infections in Leukemia (ECIL-4, 2011). *Haematologica.* 2013;98:1836–47.

6. Viscoli C, Bruzzi P, Castagnola E, Boni L, Calandra T, Gaya H, *et al.* Factors associated with bacteraemia in febrile, granulocytopenic cancer patients. The International Antimicrobial Therapy Cooperative Group (IATCG) of the European Organization for

Research and Treatment of Cancer (EORTC). *Eur J Cancer.* 1994;30A:430–7

7. Viscoli C; EORTC International Antimicrobial Therapy Group. Management of infection in cancer patients. studies of the EORTC International Antimicrobial Therapy Group (IATG). *Eur J Cancer.* 2002;38(Suppl 4):S82–7.

8. Zinner SH. Changing epidemiology of infections in patients with neutropenia and cancer: emphasis on Gram-positive and resistant bacteria. *Clin Infect Dis.* 1999;29:490–4.

9. Wisplinghoff H, Seifert H, Wenzel RP, Edmond MB. Current trends in the epidemiology of nosocomial bloodstream infections in patients with hematological malignancies and solid neoplasms in hospitals in the United States. *Clin Infect Dis.* 2003;36:1103–10.

10. Oliveira AL, de Souza M, Carvalho-Dias VM, Ruiz MA, Silla L, Tanaka PY, et al. Epidemiology of bacteremia and factors associated with multi-drug-resistant Gramnegative bacteremia in hematopoietic stem cell transplant recipients. *Bone Marrow Transplant.* 2007;39:775–81.

11. Weinstock DM, Conlon M, Iovino C, Aubrey T, Gudiol C, Riedel E, et al. Colonization, bloodstream infection, and mortality caused by vancomycin-resistant enterococcus early after allo-hematopoietic stem cell transplant. *Biol Blood Marrow Transplant.* 2007;13:615–21.

12. Gudiol C, Tubau F, Calatayud L, Garcia-Vidal C, Cisnal M, Sánchez-Ortega I, et al. Bacteraemia due to multidrug-resistant Gram-negative bacilli in cancer patients: risk factors, antibiotic therapy and outcomes. *J Antimicrob Chemother.* 2011;66:657–63.

13. Arnan M, Gudiol C, Calatayud L, Liñares J, Dominguez MÁ, Batlle M, et al. Risk factors for, and clinical relevance of, faecal extended-spectrum β-lactamase producing Escherichia coli (ESBL-EC) carriage in neutropenic patients with haematological malignancies. *Eur J Clin Microbiol Infect Dis.* 2011;30:355–60.

14. Gudiol C, Calatayud L, Garcia-Vidal C, Lora-Tamayo J, Cisnal M, Duarte R, et al. Bacteraemia due to extended-spectrum beta-lactamase-producing Escherichia coli (ESBL-EC) in cancer patients: clinical features, risk factors, molecular epidemiology and outcome. *J Antimicrob Chemother.* 2010;65:333–41.

15. Trecarichi EM, Tumbarello M, Spanu T, Caira M, Fianchi L, Chiusolo P, et al. Incidence and clinical impact of extended-spectrum-beta-lactamase (ESBL) production and fluoroquinolone resistance in bloodstream infections caused by Escherichia coli in patients with hematological malignancies. *J Infect.* 2009;58:299–307.

16. Trecarichi EM, Tumbarello M, Caira M, Candoni A, Cattaneo C, Pastore D, et al. Multidrug resistant Pseudomonas aeruginosa bloodstream infection in adult patients with hematologic malignancies. *Haematologica.* 2011; 96: e1–3

17. Satlin MJ, Jenkins SG, Walsh TJ. The global challenge of carbapenem-resistant Enterobacteriaceae in transplant recipients and patients with hematologic malignancies. *Clin Infect Dis.* 2014;58:1274–83.

18. Busca A, Cavecchia I, Locatelli F, D'Ardia S, De Rosa FG, Marmont F, et al. Blood stream infections after allo-stem cell transplantation: a single-center experience with the use of levofloxacin prophylaxis. *Transpl Infect Dis.* 2012;14:40–8.

19. Mikulska M, Del Bono V, Bruzzi P, Raiola AM, Gualandi F, Van Lint MT, et al. Mortality after bloodstream infections in allo-haematopoietic stem cell transplant (HSCT) recipients. *Infection.* 2012;40:271–8.

20. Mendes ET, Dulley F, Basso M, Batista MV, Coracin F, Guimarães T, et al. Healthcare-associated infection in hematopoietic stem cell transplantation patients: risk factors and impact on outcome. *Int J Infect Dis.* 2012;16: e424–8.

21. Hong J, Moon SM, Ahn HK, Sym SJ, Park YS, Park J, et al. Comparison of characteristics of bacterial bloodstream infection between adult patients with allo- and auto- hematopoietic stem cell transplantation. *Biol Blood Marrow Transplant.* 2013;19:994–9.

22. Srinivasan A, Wang C, Srivastava DK, Burnette K, Shenep JL, Leung W, et al. Timeline, epidemiology, and risk factors for bacterial, fungal, and viral infections in children and adolescents after allo- hematopoietic stem cell transplantation. *Biol Blood Marrow Transplant.* 2013;19:94–101.

23. Kim SH, Kee SY, Lee DG, Choi SM, Park SH, Kwon JC, et al. Infectious complications following allo- stem cell transplantation: reduced-intensity vs. myeloablative conditioning regimens. *Transpl Infect Dis.* 2013;15:49–59.

24. Sarashina T, Yoshida M, Iguchi A, Okubo H, Toriumi N, Suzuki D, et al. Risk factor analysis of bloodstream infection in pediatric patients after hematopoietic stem cell transplantation. *J Pediatr Hematol Oncol.* 2013;35:76–80.

25. Bock AM, Cao Q, Ferrieri P, Young JA, Weisdorf DJ. Bacteremia in blood or marrow transplantation patients: clinical risk factors for infection and emerging antibiotic resistance. *Biol Blood Marrow Transplant.* 2013;19:102–8.

26. Piñana JL, Montesinos P, Martino R, Vazquez L, Rovira M, López J, et al. Incidence, risk factors, and outcome of bacteremia following auto-hematopoietic stem cell transplantation in 720 adult patients. *Ann Hematol.* 2014;93:299–307.

27. Seo SK, Xiao K, Huang YT, Jongwutiwes U, Chung D, Maloy M, et al. Impact of peri-transplant vancomycin and fluoroquinolone administration on rates of bacteremia in allo- hematopoietic stem cell transplant (HSCT) recipients: A 12-year single institution study. *J Infect.* 2014 Jun 12. pii: S0163-4453(14)00163-7.

28. Gudiol C, Bodro M, Simonetti A, Tubau F, González-Barca E, Cisnal M, et al. Changing aetiology, clinical features, antimicrobial resistance, and outcomes of bloodstream infection in neutropenic cancer patients. *Clin Microbiol Infect.* 2013;19:474–9.

29. Munoz-Price LS, Poirel L, Bonomo RA, Schwaber MJ, Daikos GL, Cormican M, et al. Clinical epidemiology of the global expansion of Klebsiella pneumoniae carbapenemases. *Lancet Infect Dis.* 2013;13:785–96.

30. Tzouvelekis LS, Markogiannakis A, Psichogiou M, Tassios PT, Daikos GL. Carbapenemases in Klebsiella pneumoniae and other Enterobacteriaceae: an evolving crisis of global dimensions. *Clin Microbiol Rev.* 2012;25:682–707.

31. Cantón R, Akóva M, Carmeli Y, Giske CG, Glupczynski Y, Gniadkowski M, et al. Rapid evolution and spread of carbapenemases among Enterobacteriaceae in Europe. *Clin Microbiol Infect.* 2012;18:413–31.

32. Giani T, D'Andrea MM, Pecile P, Borgianni L, Nicoletti P, Tonelli F, et al. Emergence in Italy of Klebsiella pneumoniae sequence type 258 producing KPC-3 Carbapenemase. *J Clin Microbiol.* 2009;47:3793–4.

33. Fontana C, Favaro M, Sarmati L, Natoli S, Altieri A, Bossa MC, et al. Emergence of KPC-producing Klebsiella pneumoniae in Italy. *BMC Res Notes.* 2010;3:40.

34. Gaibani P, Ambretti S, Berlingeri A, Gelsomino F, Bielli A, Landini MP, et al. Rapid increase of carbapenemase-producing Klebsiella

pneumoniae strains in a large Italian hospital: surveillance period 1 March - 30 September 2010. *Euro Surveill.* 2011;16(8).

35. Giani T, Pini B, Arena F, Conte V, Bracco S, Migliavacca R; AMCLI-CRE Survey Participants, Pantosti A, Pagani L, Luzzaro F, Rossolini GM. Epidemic diffusion of KPC carbapenemase-producing Klebsiella pneumoniae in Italy: results of the first countrywide survey, 15 May to 30 June 2011. *Euro Surveill.* 2013;18(22).

36. Tumbarello M, Viale P, Viscoli C, Trecarichi EM, Tumietto F, Marchese A, *et al.* Predictors of mortality in bloodstream infections caused by Klebsiella pneumoniae carbapenemase-producing K. pneumoniae: importance of combination therapy. *Clin Infect Dis.* 2012;55:943–50.

37. Zarkotou O, Pournaras S, Tselioti P, Dragoumanos V, Pitiriga V, Ranellou K, *et al.* Predictors of mortality in patients with bloodstream infections caused by KPC-producing Klebsiella pneumoniae and impact of appropriate antimicrobial treatment. *Clin Microbiol Infect.* 2011;17:1798–803.

38. Clancy CJ, Chen L, Shields RK, Zhao Y, Cheng S, Chavda KD, *et al.* Epidemiology and molecular characterization of bacteremia due to carbapenem-resistant Klebsiella pneumoniae in transplant recipients. *Am J Transplant.* 2013;13:2619–33.

39. Gupta N, Limbago BM, Patel JB, Kallen AJ. Carbapenem-resistant Enterobacteriaceae: epidemiology and prevention. *Clin Infect Dis.* 2011;53:60–7.

40. Zuckerman T, Benyamini N, Sprecher H, Fineman R, Finkelstein R, Rowe JM, *et al.* SCT in patients with carbapenem resistant Klebsiella pneumoniae: a single center experience with oral gentamicin for the eradication of carrier state. *Bone Marrow Transplant.* 2011;46:1226–30.

41. Satlin MJ, Calfee DP, Chen L, Fauntleroy KA, Wilson SJ, Jenkins SG, *et al.* Emergence of carbapenem-resistant Enterobacteriaceae as causes of bloodstream infections in patients with hematologic malignancies. *Leuk Lymphoma.* 2013;54:799–806.

42. Girmenia C, Rossolini GM, Piciocchi A, Bertaina A , Pisapia G, Pastore D, *et al.,* for the Gruppo Italiano Trapianto Midollo Osseo (GITMO). Infections by carbapenem-resistant Klebsiella pneumoniae in stem cell transplant recipients: a nationwide retrospective survey from Italy. *Bone Marrow Transplant.* 2015;50:282–8.

43. Tomblyn M, Chiller T, Einsele H, Gress R, Sepkowitz K, Storek J, *et al.*; Center for International Blood and Marrow Research; National Marrow Donor Program; European Blood and Marrow Transplant Group; American Society of Blood and Marrow Transplantation; Canadian Blood and Marrow Transplant Group; Infectious Diseases Society of America; Society for Healthcare Epidemiology of America; Association of Medical Microbiology and Infectious Disease Canada; Centers for Disease Control and Prevention. Guidelines for preventing infectious complications among hematopoietic cell transplantation recipients: a global perspective. *Biol Blood Marrow Transplant.* 2009;15:1143–238.

44. Engelhard D, Akova M, Boeckh MJ, Freifeld A, Sepkowitz K, Viscoli C, *et al.*; Center for International Blood and Marrow Research; National Marrow Donor ProGram; European Blood and Marrow Transplant Group; American Society of Blood and Marrow Transplantation; Canadian Blood and Marrow Transplant Group; Infectious Disease Society of America; Society for Healthcare Epidemiology of America; Association of Medical Microbiology and Infectious Diseases Canada; Centers for Disease Control and Prevention. Bacterial infection prevention after hematopoietic cell transplantation. *Bone Marrow Transplant.* 2009;44:467–70.

45. Girmenia C, Viscoli C, Piciocchi A, Cudillo L, Botti S, Errico A, *et al.* Management of carbapenem resistant Klebsiella pneumoniae infections in stem cell transplant recipients: an Italian multidisciplinary consensus statement. *Haematologica.* 2015;100: c373–6.

46. Meunier F, Lukan C. The First European Conference on Infections in Leukaemia – ECIL1: a current perspective. *Eur J Cancer.* 2008;44:2112–7.

47. Kimura S, Akahoshi Y, Nakano H, Ugai T, Wada H, Yamasaki R, *et al.* Antibiotic prophylaxis in hematopoietic stem cell transplantation. A meta-analysis of randomized controlled trials. *J Infect.* 2014;69:13–25.

48. Guthrie KA, Yong M, Frieze D, Corey L, Fredricks DN. The impact of a change in antibacterial prophylaxis from ceftazidime to levofloxacin in allo-hematopoietic cell transplantation. *Bone Marrow Transplant.* 2010;45:675–81.

49. Eleutherakis-Papaiakovou E, Kostis E, Migkou M, Christoulas D, Terpos E, Gavriatopoulou M, *et al.* Prophylactic antibiotics for the prevention of neutropenic fever in patients undergoing auto- stem-cell transplantation: results of a single institution, randomized phase 2 trial. *Am J Hematol.* 2010;85:863–7.

50. Gafter-Gvili A, Paul M, Fraser A, Leibovici L. Effect of quinolone prophylaxis in afebrile neutropenic patients on microbial resistance: systematic review and meta-analysis. *J Antimicrob Chemother.* 2007;59:5–22.

51. Bow EJ. Fluoroquinolones, antimicrobial resistance and neutropenic cancer patients. *Curr Opin Infect Dis.* 2011;24(6):545–53.

17

Prevention and Treatment of Viral Infections in Hematopoietic Cell Transplants

Per Ljungman

Introduction

Viral infections have traditionally been important complications to allogeneic hematopoietic cell transplant (allo-HCT). Many advances were reached especially in early diagnosis by nucleic acid testing techniques such as polymerase chain reaction (PCR). This, however, resulted in other challenges for patient management such as the detection of multiple viruses and the clinical implication of the detection of a virus. Several viruses (Table 17.1) can cause the most common clinical syndromes (pneumonia, encephalitis, hepatitis, gastroenteritis). The introduction of new allo-HCT techniques such as cord blood and haplotype matched transplants has added to these challenges. After several years of low activity regarding development of new antivirals, several new compounds are in clinical testing against a number of the important viruses. The increase in knowledge about immune reconstitution (see Chapter 22) and control has resulted in the development of adoptive immunotherapy with single- or multispecific T-cells, but this topic will be covered in another chapter of this book (see Chapter 64).

Table 17.1 Some viruses important for different clinical syndromes in HCT patients

Pneumonia	Encephalitis	Hepatitis	Gastrointestinitis
CMV	CMV	CMV	CMV
Influenza	HHV-6	EBV	HSV
Adenovirus	Adenovirus	Adenovirus	Adenovirus
Respiratory syncytial virus (RSV)	VZV	HBV	EBV
Parainfluenza viruses	HSV	HCV	Rotaviruses
Metapneumovirus	Measles	VZV	Noroviruses
Rhinoviruses	JCV	HAV	
Coronaviruses	EBV	HCV	
EBV	Rabies	HEV	
HHV-6 (?)	West Nile virus		

CMV

Serologic Status of Patients and Donors: Does It Matter Today?

Many studies have shown worse outcome in CMV-seropositive compared to CMV-seronegative patients. Schmidt-Hieber *et al.* recently used the registry of the European Blood and Marrow Transplant (EBMT) and studied the effect of CMV serologic status in patients transplanted for acute leukemia[1]. CMV-seropositive patients had lower overall survival (OS), leukemia-free survival (LFS), and higher nonrelapse mortality (NRM) than CMV-seronegative patients receiving grafts from CMV-seronegative donors. In contrast, Mariotti *et al.* studied a group of 265 patients transplanted for B-cell lymphoma and found no effect of CMV serostatus on outcome[2] but this study was most likely too small to find the expected effect size.

CMV can be transmitted from a seropositive donor to a seronegative patient. The risk for primary infection in the patient has been reported to be approximately 20–30% and it was recognized several years ago that this negatively impacts the OS and increases the transplant-related mortality (TRM)[3]. More recently, Pergam *et al.* performed a retrospective cohort study of 447 allo-HCT patients[4]. They found a transmission rate of 19% with a median time to infection of 47 days. In multivariate analysis only higher cell count in the graft was associated with CMV infection of the recipient. The study found in contrast to previous studies no effect on the risk for gram-negative bacterial infection, fungal infection, TRM, or OS.

A study using the EBMT registry found a reduced OS, relapse-free survival, and increased TRM in CMV-seronegative patients receiving a CMV-seropositive *unrelated* donor graft and a strong trend for reduced (*P*=0.06) survival in CMV-seronegative patients receiving CMV-seropositive grafts from HLA-identical sibling donors[5]. Another study found not only a negative impact of using a CMV-seropositive donor on OS, LFS, and NRM but also on relapse incidence[1].

The impact of the donor CMV serostatus on outcome of CMV-seropositive patients has been more controversial[6,7]. A recent study revisited this issue and found that using a CMV-seronegative donor to a CMV-seropositive patient had a negative impact on OS, LFS, and NRM in patients receiving

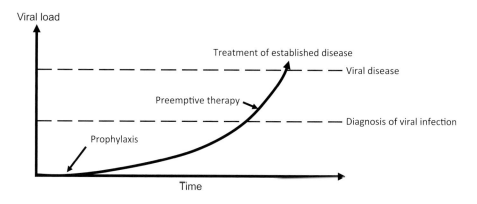

Figure 17.1. Different strategies for management of CMV infections in HCT recipients using viral load measurements.

grafts from *unrelated* donors after myeloablative conditioning regimen (MAC regimen) but not after reduced intensity conditioning (RIC) regimens[5]. However, there was no impact in patients receiving grafts from sibling donors regardless of conditioning intensity. *How can these results be explained?* CMV-seropositive patients receiving grafts from CMV-seronegative donors experience more episodes of CMV replication and have an increased risk for development of CMV disease. In patients receiving the MAC regimen, most of the existing recipient-specific T-cell immunity is depleted by the conditioning while some recipient immunity is retained in patients receiving the RIC regimen helping to protect the patient during the most vulnerable period early after allo-HCT. In summary, the use of a CMV-seropositive donor has a negative impact on survival in patients receiving unrelated but not human leukocyte antigen-identical sibling grafts. In CMV-seropositive patients, the donor serologic status influences outcome in patients receiving unrelated donor grafts after MAC but not RIC.

Prophylaxis *versus* Preemptive Therapy

For an allo-HCT patient to develop CMV disease is a failure of strategy since mortality especially from CMV pneumonia remains unacceptably high. It is therefore strongly recommended to implement a management strategy reducing the risk for CMV disease in allo-HCT centers. The two commonly used strategies are antiviral prophylaxis or preemptive therapy. The different strategies are graphically illustrated in Figure 17.1.

During the last decade, preemptive therapy has been the dominant strategy. The development of this strategy was facilitated by the rapid development of diagnostic techniques allowing quantitation of CMV load in peripheral blood. Many centers have developed their own assays and therefore there has been variability between assays. Recently a WHO standard was published to allow standardization of methods although there is a need for future development to make different methods comparable[8].

When to start preemptive therapy varies among centers and also among different patient groups at some centers[9]

(Figure 17.2). Published data suggest that preemptive therapy can safely be initiated from 100 copies/mL to 10000 copies/mL depending on the patient group[10,11].

Ganciclovir iv, valganciclovir, and foscarnet have all been shown to be effective as first-line therapy[12–14]. A common problem is what to do if the viral load continues to increase or does not decrease. In most situations, this represents "clinical resistance" and not "antiviral resistance" although mutations conferring both ganciclovir and foscarnet resistance can be found but usually not during first-line therapy. Figure 17.3 illustrates why the viral load might not decrease during the first week of therapy. However, a slow decrease in viral load was shown to be a risk factor for later development of CMV disease[15].

A common problem is repeated episodes of CMV replication. This is usually due to poor immune control by CMV-specific T-cells and is more common in high-risk patients such as patients with severe acute graft-*versus*-host disease (G*v*HD), CMV-seronegative donors to CMV-seropositive patients, and mismatched either family or unrelated donors.

The use of antiviral prophylaxis is hampered by the lack of reasonably atoxic and effective drugs. High-dose acyclovir/valacyclovir has been used for this purpose but the antiviral efficacy is quite low and ganciclovir/valganciclovir are seen as too marrow toxic for widespread use. Combination strategies with ganciclovir given before transplant followed by high-dose acyclovir, and monitoring and preemptive therapy have been studied in cord blood patients and reduced the risk for CMV replication and CMV disease compared to historical controls [16]. For the future, there might be new options with the development of new drugs and the possibility of a CMV vaccine.

Maribavir has good *in-vitro* efficacy against CMV through effects on the *UL97* kinase. It showed promising results in a phase 2 prophylactic study[17] but a large, randomized trial failed to show efficacy against the primary endpoint, CMV disease[18]. The results of the phase 3 study illustrate the problem with developing antiviral drugs against CMV.

Letermovir is a "pure" CMV antiviral having no effect against any other human virus. Phase 2 data have been

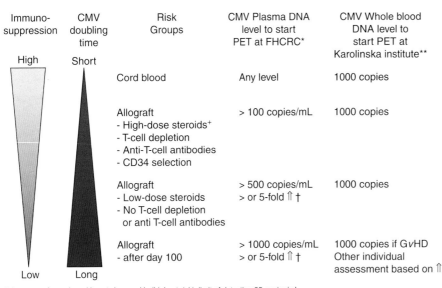

Immuno-suppression	CMV doubling time	Risk Groups	CMV Plasma DNA level to start PET at FHCRC*	CMV Whole blood DNA level to start PET at Karolinska institute**
High / Short		Cord blood	Any level	1000 copies
		Allograft - High-dose steroids+ - T-cell depletion - Anti-T-cell antibodies - CD34 selection	> 100 copies/mL	1000 copies
		Allograft - Low-dose steroids - No T-cell depletion or anti T-cell antibodies	> 500 copies/mL > or 5-fold ⇑ †	1000 copies
Low / Long		Allograft - after day 100	> 1000 copies/mL > or 5-fold ⇑ †	1000 copies if GvHD Other individual assessment based on ⇑

Figure 17.2. Management strategies for CMV infections in HCT recipients.

* Assays performed weekly or twice weekly (highest risk); limit of detection 25 copies/mL
+ 1mg per kg of prednisone or higher
† If initial level is less than threshold
** Assays performed weekly, limit of detection 50 copies

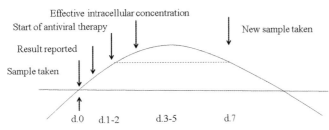

Figure 17.3. CMV replication kinetics; effects on DNA levels by antiviral therapy.

published and showed a very high efficacy in preventing CMV replication when letermovir was given in a dose of 240 mg/day with very limited toxicity[19]. Recently preliminary data from the phase III study were made public and showed a reduction in significant CMV infection in the letermovir arm.

Brincidofovir is a lipid conjugate of cidofovir that can be given orally. It has *in-vitro* efficacy against a wide range of DNA viruses including all human herpesviruses, adenovirus, polyomaviruses, and poxviruses. Phase 2 data showed good prophylactic efficacy against CMV replication when brincido-fovir was given in a dose of 100 mg twice weekly[20]. Unfortunately, the phase 3 study failed to show efficacy at 180 days (the primary endpoint). In addition, there was increased gastro-intestinal toxicy and a difficulty separating gastrointestinal acute GvHD from effects of the drug. There are also a couple of CMV vaccines in clinical trials. The currently best tested vaccine candidate in HCT patients is a DNA vaccine based on two plasmids (pp65 and glycoprotein B) and in a phase 2 trial demonstrated significantly reduced occurrence and recurrence of CMV viremia and improved the time-to-event for viremia episodes compared with placebo[21]. A phase 3 study has finalized inclusion but no results are yet available.

Difficult to Treat Patients: Other Options

Patients who experience repeated CMV reactivations and need multiple courses of antiviral therapy represent a significant management problem. These patients frequently have either renal or marrow toxicity making the use of standard agents difficult. Furthermore, among these patients "true" antiviral resistance with mutations in the *UL87* gene conferring resistance to ganciclovir and/or in the *DNA polymerase gene* conferring resistance to foscarnet are more common[22,23]. Higher doses of maribavir (300–600 mg BID) have been given to patients with resistant CMV or to those not tolerating licensed antiviral agents and showed that maribavir can be effective with limited toxicity[24]. A phase II study has been performed and a phase III is in the late planning stage. Leflunomide is an immunosuppressive drug with the indication for rheumatoid arthritis. Small case series and case reports have been published suggesting efficacy in difficult to treat CMV infections [25,26]. Artesunate is an antimalaria agent that also was reported in case reports to have some efficacy[27]. No controlled or larger study was performed and it is likely that the true efficacy of these two agents is limited. Another option is the use of CMV-specific T-cells (see Chapter 64).

What is the Role of CMV Replication in Leukemia Relapse?

More than 25 years ago, it was suggested that CMV replication could reduce the risk for relapse in acute leukemia after allo-HCT[28]. More recently, Elmaagacli *et al.* showed a reduction in the risk for acute myelogenous leukemia (AML) relapse in patients with documented CMV replication[29]. Green *et al.* confirmed this observation in a larger cohort of patients with different hematologic malignancies showing a decreased risk for relapse in patients with AML by day 100. This association was not seen in patients with acute lymphoblastic leukemia (ALL), chronic myeloid leukemia (CML), lymphoma, or myelodysplastic syndrome (MDS). The effect was seen only early after allo-HCT and was independent of CMV viral load, acute G*v*HD, or ganciclovir-associated neutropenia. Most important, there was no effect on OS. Other studies looking at different cohorts of patients have also seen effects on relapse especially in myeloid malignancies. *What is the mechanism?* There have been speculations for example regarding NK cells, γ/δ T-cells, or direct effects of CMV on leukemic blasts. Other studies analyzed CMV serologic status and found no impact on relapse risk suggesting that CMV replication itself is the important event[1,5]. In the future, we might get important information from the studies with new antiviral agents effectively suppressing CMV replication and CMV vaccines that boost CMV-specific immunity.

Epstein–Barr Virus (EBV)

EBV becomes latent after primary infection in B-cells and epithelial cells. Although detection of replicating virus is very common after HCT, direct virus-induced complications are quite rare. Instead, the important EBV-associated complication is EBV post-transplant lymphoproliferative disease (PTLD). The major risk factors for PTLD include having an unrelated or mismatched donor, T-cell depletion, EBV serologic mismatch, splenectomy, and cord blood HCT (see Chapter 20).

Monitoring: When, How, and What Method?

Several studies have shown a correlation between the presence of EBV DNAemia in peripheral blood and the development of PTLD and other EBV-associated disorders. However, it has not been a consistent finding that EBV DNAemia precedes the onset of clinical symptoms. EBV DNA levels can rise very rapidly and therefore once weekly monitoring might not be enough[30].

Should We Give Preemptive Therapy?

Despite the lack of controlled studies, many centers use rituximab as preemptive therapy based on the presence of high or increasing EBV DNA levels. Different cut-offs have been suggested in the literature for when intervention shall be considered, but currently available information does not allow the definition of a firm threshold value especially since the PCR techniques vary from center to center.

Other Approaches for Prevention or Treatment of PTLD

Currently available antiviral drugs are not effective in the prevention or treatment of EBV PTLD (see Chapter 20). Brincidofovir has antiviral activity against EBV *in-vitro* but whether prophylaxis with this drug will be able to reduce the

risk for EBV replication and possibly PTLD will require further study. Reduction/withdrawal of immunosuppression is an important strategy for treatment of PTLD after solid organ transplantation but there might be an increased risk of graft rejection or G*v*HD. Recent data show, however, that in combination with rituximab, a reduction of immunosuppression of as little as 20% of the daily dose of immunosuppressants can significantly reduce the mortality from PTLD[31]. Specific T-cells are also a management option shown to be effective against EBV PTLD.

HHV-6; One (or Two) Important Pathogen(s) in HCT Recipients?

Today HHV-6 is seen as two different viruses, HHV-6A and HHV-6B, and molecular studies show that HHV-6B reactivation is commonly detected in HCT recipients. HHV-6 can be integrated in the germ line; a property that is unique among herpesviruses. Chromosomally integrated HHV-6 (CIHHV-6) is characterized by very high HHV-6 DNA loads in blood and exists in 1–2% of the population[32,33]. An important unresolved question is whether CIHHV-6 is associated with disease.

Clinical Implications of HHV-6

HHV-6 is a common cause of viral encephalitis after allo-HCT [34]. Many case reports and small case series have been published. The majority of HHV-6 encephalitis cases occur during the first month after allo-HCT. The clinical picture of post-transplant acute limbic encephalitis (PALE) is the most common presentation. Common symptoms of PALE are short-term memory loss, confusion, disorientation, and depressed consciousness[35,36]. HHV-6 has tropism for astrocytes in the hippocampus fitting with the symptoms. In a large prospective study, Zerr *et al.* showed that patients with HHV-6 DNA in plasma were significantly more likely to present with delirium and neurocognitive decline during the first months after allo-HCT[37]. Another suggested complication of HHV-6 is the syndrome of inappropriate diuretic hormone secretion (SIADH). Risk factors for HHV-6 CNS disease are acute G*v*HD grade II–IV, the use of HLA-mismatched or unrelated donors, and CBT. A systematic review showed a risk of 8.3% in CB graft recipients compared to 0.5% in recipients of other graft sources[38]. The long-term prognosis is quite poor with significant mortality as well as a high frequency of long-term neurologic deficits[39,40].

Regarding other manifestations of HHV-6, the data are conflicting. Associations between HHV-6 reactivation and patient mortality[41], bone marrow suppression, especially delayed platelet engraftment, pneumonitis, and acute G*v*HD have been suggested on the basis of cohort studies.

Management

Assuming that HHV-6 has important effects after allo-HCT, how should patients be managed? Clinical suspicions followed by diagnostic procedures, usually PCR on CSF and MRI scans, in patients with signs of encephalitis are obvious and patients with a proven or probable infection should be treated. *In-vitro* studies suggest that HHV-6 is susceptible to foscarnet, ganciclovir, and cidofovir, and moderately susceptible to acyclovir. No controlled study has, however, been performed. Zerr *et al.* reported decreases of HHV-6 viral loads in CSF or serum during ganciclovir or foscarnet therapy[42]. Schmidt-Hieber *et al.* reported a response rate of 63% with either foscarnet or ganciclovir therapy of HHV-6 encephalitis[34]. Brincidofovir is an interesting new option but no data exist. *What about monitoring?* Quantitative PCR techniques are available in many laboratories. An important unresolved question is what to do with the results and two small studies have both found that encephalitis developed concomitantly with the detection of HHV-6 in plasma suggesting only limited effectiveness of a preemptive strategy.

Herpes Simplex Virus (HSV) and Varicella-Zoster Virus (VZV)

These infections although important as causes of morbidity rarely become serious in allo-HCT recipients. Acyclovir-resistant HSV can be documented in approximately 10% of the patients with increased risk in the more immunosuppressed recipients. Foscarnet is the current therapy of choice in this situation but brincidofovir might become an option in the future. It is important to be aware of visceral VZV disease without skin manifestations since this is a serious complication with a risk for mortality. The best management strategy is long-term antiviral prophylaxis with acyclovir or valacyclovir and that is strongly recommended in allo-HCT recipients for at least 12 months after HCT[43,44]. The benefit in autologous recipients is likely to be less. Rebound disease occurs after discontinuation.

Adenoviruses

More than 55 different adenovirus (Adv) types able to infect humans have been identified. Adv can be contracted from an outside source and outbreaks in HCT units have been reported but Adv can also be reactivated from a persistent state, especially in younger children. A main risk factor for both Adv infection and disease is *in-vivo* and *ex-vivo* T-cell depletion. Other risk factors are unrelated cord blood grafts, severe acute GvHD, and a low lymphocyte count ($<0.2 \times 10^9$/L). The common denominator for all these risk factors is the absence of Adv-specific T-cells[45–47].

Monitoring

PCR-based assays are the standard diagnostic techniques for detection of Adv. In allo-HCT patients, high levels of Adv-DNA in peripheral blood correlate with Adv-associated mortality and rising viral loads are predictive for poor outcome[48].

Should all patients be monitored by PCR for Adv? This is probably unnecessary in low-risk patients, for example in children and adults undergoing HLA-identical sibling donor HCT and in adults undergoing well-matched unrelated transplantation especially with the RIC regimen[49,50]

Treatment

Adv disease usually occurs between 2 and 3 months post-transplant[51]. Although patients with Adv viremia can remain asymptomatic and clear the virus, the viral load might increase rapidly and result in multiorgan disease with high mortality. Although no controlled trial has been performed, many centers use preemptive treatment of Adv infection with cidofovir based on the results of uncontrolled studies. These have usually shown an effect on the Adv-load in peripheral blood but the effect on mortality has been variable.

A new promising management option is brincidofovir, which is highly efficacious against Adv *in-vitro*. Brincidofovir has been studied in patients failing other therapies[52] and in a phase 2 dose-finding study of HCT patients with Adv viremia [53]. Both studies showed virologic responses and that patients who responded with a viral load decrease had a prolonged survival[52].

Respiratory Viruses

Community-acquired respiratory virus (CARV) infections include a variety of RNA- and DNA-viruses. These infections are common in the general population and the epidemiology in HCT patients commonly reflects the activity in the surrounding community. Detection of a CARV before allogeneic SCT in a symptomatic patient was reported to increase the risk for overall mortality[54]. The most studied infections are caused by respiratory syncytial virus (RSV), influenza viruses, and parainfluenza viruses (PIV), but with the availability of multiplex PCR techniques, information is rapidly emerging regarding infections with other CARVs as well. The importance of these other CARVs is still somewhat controversial as is management of most CARVs.

RSV

RSV was recognized in the early 1990s as a cause of severe disease in HCT patients. It is an important nosocomial pathogen and therefore infection control measures are very important in HCT units. Risk factors for lower respiratory tract RSV infections were analyzed in several publications. Allogeneic rather than autologous HCT recipients, low lymphocyte count, and pretransplant RSV infection are risk factors for poorer outcome. A couple of recent studies, however, have not seen a higher risk after allo-HCT[55,56]. Lymphocytopenia is probably the most important risk factor for outcome of RSV and there is a gradual risk increase for lower respiratory tract disease as the lymphocyte count at diagnosis of RSV infection decreases[56].

No controlled clinical study of sufficient size to allow conclusions regarding efficacy of any therapeutic intervention against RSV was performed. There have been several reports, mostly retrospective, on ribavirin therapy for RSV infection. The only existing controlled trial of aerosolized ribavirin in HCT recipients was able to recruit just 14 patients[57]. There was a trend for lower viral loads in the ribavirin-treated patients but no difference in outcome. A large recent study of 280 patients with upper respiratory tract infection showed that use of aerosolized ribavirin was the most important factor for reducing the risk for RSV lower respiratory tract disease, RSV associated, and for all-cause mortality[58]. In Europe, oral or intravenous ribavirin has been commonly used against RSV. The use of ribavirin by any route is supported by a systematic review showing a reduction in the risk for lower respiratory tract disease when treatment is given at the upper respiratory virus stage and an improvement in outcome of RSV pneumonia by ribavirin therapy[59]. The addition of immune globulin or pavilizumab to ribavirin is also controversial[60] but a systematic review suggested better outcome if immune globulin was given to patients with lower respiratory tract disease[59]. New treatment options such as RNA interference therapy (ALN-RSV01) and an RSV fusion inhibitor (GS-5806) are in development.

Influenza

Influenza viruses can cause severe and fatal infections in HCT recipients. New strains are a particular threat as shown by the high morbidity and significant mortality caused by the "swine flu" pandemic[61–63]. Existing evidence supports no major difference in the risk for complicated and possibly fatal infections between autologous and allogeneic recipients[64–66]. Vaccination is the recommended preventive strategy but some controversy exists as to when it is meaningful to start vaccination after transplantation and regarding its efficacy[67,68]. The vaccination response improves with time after transplant and uncontrolled data showed a reduction of influenza illness when vaccination was given 6 months after HCT[69]. The recommendations are based upon the observations that there is no risk with starting vaccination earlier, there might be some protective effect, and doses can be repeated if felt necessary.

Historical data showed a high mortality from influenza seemingly reduced with the introduction of neuramidase inhibitors, mainly oseltamivir. Treatment is therefore recommended for HCT recipients[70]. However, resistance is quite common and it was shown during the pH1N1 outbreak that the mortality was increased in patients infected with oseltamivir-resistant virus[61–63]. New neuramidase inhibitors (peramivir, laninamivir) as well as drugs with different mechanisms of action are in development as are different types of vaccines with the aim to improve the immunogenicity.

Parainfluenzaviruses (PIV)

There are four types of PIV and in HCT recipients approximately one-third of infections with PIV cause lower respiratory tract disease[71,72]. Hospital outbreaks are seen necessitating infection control strategies. PIV type 3 is the most commonly detected type. Risk factors for lower respiratory tract disease are higher corticosteroid doses, neutropenia, lymphopenia, and infection early after allo-HCT[71,73,74]. A recent study showed poorer outcome with PIV detected from the lower respiratory tract (proven/probable PIV in the lung) compared to PIV detected in the upper respiratory tract associated with new pulmonary infiltrates (possible PIV in the lung)[75].

Current treatment options are limited and current data do not support an effect by treating patients with upper respiratory tract disease. However, some centers are using ribavirin and IVIG especially in treating lower respiratory tract disease. New promising drugs are in clinical development.

Human Metapneumovirus (HMPV)

HMPV is closely related to RSV. HPMV infection in HCT patients can present with influenza-like illness. Cases of severe lower respiratory tract disease and fatal outcome have been reported and the outcome has been described as similar to that of RSV[76–78]. No recommendation for treatment can be made due to lack of data, although some centers consider treating HMPV lower respiratory tract disease with ribavirin and/or IVIG.

Rhinovirus (RhV)

RhVs are divided into three species encompassing more than 100 serotypes and are the most frequent respiratory virus infection infecting more than 20% of HCT recipients[16]. More severe presentations of lower respiratory tract disease with pneumonia and/or hypoxia seem to be quite rare. However, a recent study reported that the outcome of RhV pneumonia is not much different from pneumonia due to RSV[79].

Papovaviruses: Does Monitoring in Blood Matter for Management?

Papoviruses are DNA viruses infecting most individuals early in life. JC virus and BK virus are associated with disease after HCT while the newer respiratory papovaviruses have yet to be documented as important in this setting. JC virus can cause progressive multifocal leukoencephalopathy (PML); this complication is very difficult to manage but is rare. In several cohort studies, BK virus has been associated with hemorrhagic cystitis (HC) after HCT although there are several uncertainties regarding the pathogenesis. First, most patients excrete BK virus in urine but only a small proportion develop HC. An association with high urinary viral load exists but there are large overlaps in viral loads between patients with or without HC[80,81]. Autologous patients also commonly have BK viruria but rarely develop HC suggesting that there also might be an immunopathogenic mechanism playing a role in allo-HCT recipients. Other risk factors found in some but not all studies are MAC, acute GvHD, cord blood grafts, and the use of mismatched or unrelated donors. BK viremia is also associated with HC but again there are overlaps in viral load, although higher viral loads have been associated with more severe grades of HC[82–84].

Is it meaningful to monitor for BK viremia and intervene with preemptive therapy? Until now, no such study was reported and no ideal antiviral drug exists. Cidofovir has been used for therapy of severe HC and the results were reported in retrospective, cohort studies[85–88]. Leflunomide has also been suggested as a possible therapy[89]. Brincidofovir has effects *in-vitro* and is an interesting future option. These different options need to be evaluated in prospective, controlled studies.

Hepatitis Viruses after HCT

Many different viruses can cause liver damage with clinical signs of hepatitis including several already covered in this chapter such as VZV, adenovirus, and CMV. The hepatitis viruses (A, B, C, and E) rarely cause disease outside the liver although hepatitis C virus (HCV) has been associated with cryoglobulinemia. Hepatitis A virus can cause acute liver disease but the data in HCT patients are limited. Hepatitis E virus is increasingly recognized as a pathogen that can be transmitted by blood products and possibly by stem cell grafts, is able to become chronic, and has also been implicated in rapid development of liver fibrosis[90].

Hepatitis B Virus (HBV)

HBV infects a large proportion of the world's population early in life. Previously, transfusions were an important route of transmission but this is a rare cause today. The importance of HBV in HCT is therefore mainly in the management of chronically infected individuals. In chronic HBV infections, the initial phase with high-level HBV replication is followed by a phase of immune-system-mediated clearance followed by loss of HBeAg and development of HBe antibody resulting in an "inactive carrier" state. The inactive carrier state is characterized by minimal liver inflammation, undetectable or low serum HBV DNA, and normal liver function tests. In many patients, the inactive carrier state results in clearance of HBsAg with or without the appearance of anti-HBs antibodies. Patients who have cleared HBsAg mostly remain positive for anti-HBc. HBsAg-negative patients in whom serum HBV DNA is still detectable are defined as having an occult HBV infection. Immunosuppression, such as allo-HCT, can trigger the increase in HBV replication in patients who have previously achieved control of HBV. It was reported that 20–50% of patients with HBV infection undergoing immunosuppressive treatment develop viral reactivation possibly resulting in fulminant hepatitis. Liver damage can also develop when the immune system is reconstituted. In patients with positive HBsAg who receive allo-HCT hepatitis flares can occur in up to 50% in the absence of antiviral prophylaxis[91]. HBsAg seroreversion was found in 40% and 70% of patients at 2 and 5 years after transplantation, respectively[92]. Patients treated with B-cell targeting antibodies are at especially high-risk. HBV-infected donors for allogeneic transplants pose a risk of disease transmission to the recipient of up to 30% with some infections resulting in liver failure[93,94]. If possible, use of an HBV-infected donor should be avoided.

The European Conference on Infections in Leukemia has developed recommendations for management of HCT patients infected with HBV or having an HBV-infected donor[95]. These recommendations are as follows:

a. All HBsAg-positive patients should receive antiviral therapy starting with the chemotherapy. Any licensed antiviral drug for HBV can be used but if HBV DNA is >2000 IU/mL, entecavir or tenofovir is recommended. Treatment should continue until at least 6 months after completion of immunosuppressive therapy.

b. All HBc-positive HCT patients should receive antiviral therapy.

c. An HBsAg-negative and anti-HBc-negative recipient receiving an HBc-antibody-positive donor graft should receive antiviral therapy; adding hepatitis B immune globulin could be considered.

HCV

Short-term outcome of HCV-infected HCT recipients is comparable to noninfected although flares of liver disease and rare episodes of liver failure are described[96,97]. The risk of acute flares in patients undergoing HCT seems to be increased in patients undergoing rituximab-containing treatment regimens [96]. Therefore, chronic HCV infection is not a contraindication to HCT. Treatment regimens limiting the risk of sinusoidal obstruction syndrome should be considered. Importantly, and in contrast to HBV, patients who have successfully cleared HCV RNAemia are not at risk of reactivation[98].

An accelerated rate of fibrosis progression with the development of cirrhosis and worse outcome has been documented during long-term follow-up of HCV-infected HCT recipients [99,100]. Owing to this risk, antiviral therapy is recommended. The classical therapy is based on interferon-α2b-containing regimens. For these regimens, the recommendation has been that HCT patients should be in complete remission, ≥2 years post-HCT, without evidence of GvHD, and off immunosuppression for ≥6 months[43]. However in a prospective cohort study, there was no indication that interferon-α2b-based therapy worsened chronic GvHD[99]. Today the situation is rapidly changing since several new antivirals are or will be approved in the near future. Therefore, expert advice should be sought prior to initiating HCV antiviral therapy.

Controversies and Expert Insight

1. *Should CMV serologic status of the donor be considered during donor selection?*

    That a CMV-seronegative donor should be chosen to a CMV-seronegative patient has been established for decades. The optimal donor for a CMV-seropositive patient has been controversial. However, a recent large registry study showed decreased survival and reduced NRM when a CMV-seropositive unrelated donor was used for a patient after the MAC regimen suggesting that donor serostatus should be one factor to consider in selecting the best donor.

2. *Does CMV replication have an impact on the risk for relapse?*

Several studies have now showed statistical evidence that patients with proven CMV replication have a reduced risk for relapse. The mechanism for this positive effect on relapse is still unknown. It is possible that the ongoing phase 3 trials with new antiviral drugs and CMV vaccine will elucidate the underlying mechanism.

3. *RSV therapy: systemic or inhaled ribavirin?*

There is no randomized, controlled trial large enough to show that any therapy is effective against RSV in HCT recipients. Retrospective, cohort studies have,

however, suggested efficacy. Treatment traditions have been different with some centers treating with inhaled ribavirin and other centers using either oral or intravenous ribavirin. It is unlikely that a controlled trial will be performed so today both forms of therapy can be attempted while waiting for new and possibly more effective antivirals.

4. *BK virus viremia: should preemptive therapy be given?*

There is a clear association between BK virus and HC although whether this is a direct virus effect or whether the immune response has a role is still not resolved. BK viremia can be detected in most patients developing severe HC but it is unclear if preemptive therapy would reduce the risk for or severity of the cystitis. Currently no optimal antiviral drug is licensed but brincidofovir might be studied in the future in this context.

References

1. Schmidt-Hieber M, Labopin M, Beelen D, Volin L, Ehninger G, Finke J, et al. CMV serostatus has still an important prognostic impact in de novo acute leukemia patients after allogeneic stem cell transplantation: a report from the acute leukemia working party of EBMT. *Blood.* 2013;122(19):3359–64.

2. Mariotti J, Maura F, Spina F, Roncari L, Dodero A, Farina L, et al. Impact of cytomegalovirus replication and cytomegalovirus serostatus on the outcome of patients with B cell lymphoma after allogeneic stem cell transplantation. *Biol Blood Marrow Transplant.* 2014;20(6):885–90.

3. Nichols WG, Corey L, Gooley T, Davis C, Boeckh M. High risk of death due to bacterial and fungal infection among cytomegalovirus (CMV)-seronegative recipients of stem cell transplants from seropositive donors: evidence for indirect effects of primary CMV infection. *J Infect Dis.* 2002;185(3):273–82.

4. Pergam SA, Xie H, Sandhu R, Pollack M, Smith J, Stevens-Ayers T, et al. Efficiency and risk factors for CMV transmission in seronegative hematopoietic stem cell recipients. *Biol Blood Marrow Transplant.* 2012;18(9):1391–400.

5. Ljungman P, Brand R, Hoek J, de la Camara R, Cordonnier C, Einsele H, et al. Donor CMV status influences the outcome of allogeneic stem cell transplantation; a study by the European Group for Blood and Marrow

Transplantation. *Clin Infect Dis.* 2014;59(4):473–81.

6. Ljungman P, Einsele H, Frassoni F, Niederwieser D, Cordonnier C. Donor CMV serological status influences the outcome of CMVseropositive recipients after unrelated donor stem cell transplantation: An EBMT Megafile analysis. *Blood.* 2003;102:4255–60.

7. Boeckh M, Nichols WG. The impact of cytomegalovirus serostatus of donor and recipient before hematopoietic stem cell transplantation in the era of antiviral prophylaxis and preemptive therapy. *Blood.* 2004;103(6):2003–8.

8. Preiksaitis JK, Hayden RT, Tong Y, Pang XL, Fryer JF, Heath AB, et al. Are we there yet? Impact of the first international standard for cytomegalovirus DNA on the harmonization of results reported on plasma samples. *Clin Infect Dis.* 2016;63(5):583–9.

9. Boeckh M, Ljungman P. How we treat cytomegalovirus in hematopoietic cell transplant recipients. *Blood.* 2009;113(23):5711–9.

10. Lilleri D, Gerna G, Furione M, Bernardo ME, Giorgiani G, Telli S, et al. Use of a DNAemia cut-off for monitoring human cytomegalovirus infection reduces the number of pre-emptively treated children and young adults receiving haematopoietic stem cell transplantation as compared to qualitative pp65-antigenemia. *Blood.* 2007;110(7):2757–60.

11. Milano F, Pergam SA, Xie H, Leisenring WM, Gutman JA, Riffkin I, et al.

Intensive strategy to prevent CMV disease in seropositive umbilical cord blood transplant recipients. *Blood.* 2011;118(20):5689–96.

12. Reusser P, Einsele H, Lee J, Volin L, Rovira M, Engelhard D, et al. Randomized multicenter trial of foscarnet *versus* ganciclovir for preemptive therapy of cytomegalovirus infection after allogeneic stem cell transplantation. *Blood.* 2002;99(4):1159–64.

13. Goodrich JM, Mori M, Gleaves CA, Du Mond C, Cays M, Ebeling DF, et al. Early treatment with ganciclovir to prevent cytomegalovirus disease after allogeneic bone marrow transplantation. *N Engl J Med.* 1991;325(23):1601–7.

14. Volin L, Barkholt L, Nihtinen A, Aschan J, Uotinen H, Hägglund H, et al. An open-label randomised study of oral valganciclovir *versus* intravenous ganciclovir for pre-emptive therapy of cytomegalovirus infection after allogeneic stem cell transplantation. *Bone Marrow Transplantation.* 2008;42(Suppl.1):S47.

15. Ljungman P, Perez-Bercoff L, Jonsson J, Avetisyan G, Sparrelid E, Aschan J, et al. Risk factors for the development of cytomegalovirus disease after allogeneic stem cell transplantation. *Haematologica.* 2006;91(1):78–83.

16. Milano F, Campbell AP, Guthrie KA, Kuypers J, Englund JA, Corey L, et al. Human rhinovirus and coronavirus detection among allogeneic hematopoietic stem cell transplantation

recipients. *Blood.* 2010;115(10):2088–94.

17. Winston D, Young J, Pullarkat V, Papanicolaou G, Vij R, E V, *et al.* Maribavir prophylaxis for prevention of cytomegalovirus infection in allogeneic stem cell transplant recipients: a multicenter randomized, double-blind, placebo-controlled, dose-ranging study. *Blood.* 2008;111:5403–10.

18. Marty FM, Ljungman P, Papanicolaou GA, Winston DJ, Chemaly RF, Strasfeld L, *et al.* Maribavir prophylaxis for prevention of cytomegalovirus disease in recipients of allogeneic stem-cell transplants: a phase 3, double-blind, placebo-controlled, randomised trial. *Lancet Infect Dis.* 2011;11(4):284–92.

19. Chemaly RF, Ullmann AJ, Stoelben S, Richard MP, Bornhauser M, Groth C, *et al.* Letermovir for cytomegalovirus prophylaxis in hematopoietic-cell transplantation. *N Engl J Med.* 2014;370(19):1781–9.

20. Marty FM, Winston DJ, Rowley SD, Vance E, Papanicolaou GA, Mullane KM, *et al.* CMX001 to prevent cytomegalovirus disease in hematopoietic-cell transplantation. *N Engl J Med.* 2013;369(13):1227–36.

21. Kharfan-Dabaja M, Boeckh M, Wilck M, Langston A, Chu A, Wloch M, *et al.* Phase 2 Trial of TransVax™, a Therapeutic DNA Vaccine for Control of Cytomegalovirus in Hematopoietic Cell Transplant Recipients 50th ICAAC; Boston, 2010: p. G1-1661a.

22. Chou S. Cytomegalovirus UL97 mutations in the era of ganciclovir and maribavir. *Rev Med Virol.* 2008;18(4):233–46.

23. Chou SW. Cytomegalovirus drug resistance and clinical implications. *Transplant Infect Dis.* 2001;3 (Suppl 2):20–4.

24. Avery RK, Marty FM, Strasfeld L, Lee I, Arrieta A, Chou S, *et al.* Oral maribavir for treatment of refractory or resistant cytomegalovirus infections in transplant recipients. *Transplant Infectious Dis.* 2010;12(6):489–96.

25. Avery RK, Mossad SB, Poggio E, Lard M, Budev M, Bolwell B, *et al.* Utility of leflunomide in the treatment of complex cytomegalovirus syndromes. *Transplantation.* 2010;90(4):419–26.

26. Avery RK, Bolwell BJ, Yen-Lieberman B, Lurain N, Waldman WJ, Longworth DL, *et al.* Use of leflunomide in an allogeneic bone marrow transplant recipient with refractory cytomegalovirus infection. *Bone Marrow Transplant.* 2004;34(12):1071–5.

27. Kaptein SJ, Efferth T, Leis M, Rechter S, Auerochs S, Kalmer M, *et al.* The anti-malaria drug artesunate inhibits replication of cytomegalovirus in vitro and in vivo. *Antiviral Res.* 2006;69(2):60–9.

28. Lönnqvist B, Ringdén O, Ljungman P, Wahren B, Gahrton G. Reduced risk of recurrent leukaemia in bone marrow transplant recipients after cytomegalovirus infection. *Br J Haematol.* 1986;63(4):671–9.

29. Elmaagacli AH, Steckel NK, Koldehoff M, Hegerfeldt Y, Trenschel R, Ditschkowski M, *et al.* Early human cytomegalovirus replication after transplantation is associated with a decreased relapse risk: evidence for a putative virus-*versus*-leukemia effect in acute myeloid leukemia patients. *Blood.* 2011;118(5):1402–12.

30. Styczynski J, Reusser P, Einsele H, de la Camara R, Cordonnier C, Ward KN, *et al.* Management of HSV, VZV and EBV infections in patients with hematological malignancies and after SCT: guidelines from the Second European Conference on Infections in Leukemia. *Bone Marrow Transplant.* 2009;43(10):757–70.

31. Styczynski J, Gil L, Tridello G, Ljungman P, Donnelly JP, van der Velden W, *et al.* Response to rituximab-based therapy and risk factor analysis in Epstein Barr Virus-related lymphoproliferative disorder after hematopoietic stem cell transplant in children and adults: a study from the Infectious Diseases Working Party of the European Group for Blood and Marrow Transplantation. *Clin Infect Dis.* 2013;57(6):794–802.

32. Leong HN, Tuke PW, Tedder RS, Khanom AB, Eglin RP, Atkinson CE, *et al.* The prevalence of chromosomally integrated human herpesvirus 6 genomes in the blood of UK blood donors. *J Med Virol.* 2007;79(1):45–51.

33. Hall CB, Caserta MT, Schnabel K, Shelley LM, Marino AS, Carnahan JA, *et al.* Chromosomal integration of human herpesvirus 6 is the major mode of congenital human herpesvirus 6 infection. *Pediatrics.* 2008;122(3):513-20.

34. Schmidt-Hieber M, Schwender J, Heinz WJ, Zabelina T, Kuhl JS, Mousset S, *et al.* Viral encephalitis after allogeneic stem cell transplantation: a rare complication with distinct characteristics of different causative agents. *Haematologica.* 2011;96(1):142–9.

35. Seeley WW, Marty FM, Holmes TM, Upchurch K, Soiffer RJ, Antin JH, *et al.* Post-transplant acute limbic encephalitis: clinical features and relationship to HHV6. *Neurology.* 2007;69(2):156–65.

36. Zerr DM, Gooley TA, Yeung L, Huang ML, Carpenter P, Wade JC, *et al.* Human herpesvirus 6 reactivation and encephalitis in allogeneic bone marrow transplant recipients. *Clin Infect Dis.* 2001;33(6):763–71.

37. Zerr DM, Fann JR, Breiger D, Boeckh M, Adler AL, Xie H, *et al.* HHV-6 reactivation and its effect on delirium and cognitive functioning in hematopoietic cell transplantation recipients. *Blood.* 2011;117(19):5243–9.

38. Scheurer ME, Pritchett JC, Amirian ES, Zemke NR, Lusso P, Ljungman P. HHV-6 encephalitis in umbilical cord blood transplantation: a systematic review and meta-analysis. *Bone Marrow Transplant.* 2013;48(4):574–80.

39. Zerr DM. Human herpesvirus 6 and central nervous system disease in hematopoietic cell transplantation. *J Clin Virol.* 2006;37 (Suppl. 1): S52–6.

40. Muta T, Fukuda T, Harada M. Human herpesvirus-6 encephalitis in hematopoietic SCT recipients in Japan: a retrospective multicenter study. *Bone Marrow Transplant.* 2009;43(7):583–5

41. Zerr DM, Corey L, Kim HW, Huang ML, Nguy L, Boeckh M. Clinical outcomes of human herpesvirus 6 reactivation after hematopoietic stem cell transplantation. *Clin Infect Dis.* 2005;40(7):932–40.

42. Zerr DM, Gupta D, Huang ML, Carter R, Corey L. Effect of antivirals on human herpesvirus 6 replication in hematopoietic stem cell transplant recipients. *Clin Infect Dis.* 2002;34(3):309–17.

43. Tomblyn M, Chiller T, Einsele H, Gress R, Sepkowitz K, Storek J, *et al.* Guidelines for preventing infectious complications among hematopoietic cell transplant recipients: a global

perspective. Preface. *Bone Marrow Transplant.* 2009;44(8):453–5.

44. Erard V, Guthrie KA, Varley C, Heugel J, Wald A, Flowers ME, et al. One-year acyclovir prophylaxis for preventing varicella-zoster virus (VZV) disease following hematopoietic cell transplantation: no evidence of rebound VZV disease after drug discontinuation. *Blood.* 2007;110(8):3071–7.

45. Feuchtinger T, Lucke J, Hamprecht K, Richard C, Handgretinger R, Schumm M, et al. Detection of adenovirus-specific T cells in children with adenovirus infection after allogeneic stem cell transplantation. *Br J Haematol.* 2005;128(4):503–9.

46. Guerin-El Khourouj V, Dalle JH, Pedron B, Yakouben K, Bensoussan D, Cordeiro DJ, et al. Quantitative and qualitative CD4 T cell immune responses related to adenovirus DNAemia in hematopoietic stem cell transplantation. *Biol Blood Marrow Transplant.* 2011;17(4):476–85.

47. Zandvliet ML, van Liempt E, Jedema I, Kruithof S, Kester MG, Guchelaar HJ, et al. Simultaneous isolation of CD8(+) and CD4(+) T cells specific for multiple viruses for broad antiviral immune reconstitution after allogeneic stem cell transplantation. *J Immunother.* 2011;34(3):307–19.

48. Lion T, Kosulin K, Landlinger C, Rauch M, Preuner S, Jugovic D, et al. Monitoring of adenovirus load in stool by real-time PCR permits early detection of impending invasive infection in patients after allogeneic stem cell transplantation. *Leukemia.* 2010;24(4):706–14.

49. Ohrmalm L, Lindblom A, Omar H, Norbeck O, Gustafson I, Lewensohn-Fuchs I, et al. Evaluation of a surveillance strategy for early detection of adenovirus by PCR of peripheral blood in hematopoietic SCT recipients: incidence and outcome. *Bone Marrow Transplant.* 2011;46(2):267–72.

50. Matthes-Martin S, Feuchtinger T, Shaw PJ, Engelhard D, Hirsch HH, Cordonnier C, et al. European guidelines for diagnosis and treatment of adenovirus infection in leukemia and stem cell transplantation: summary of ECIL-4 (2011). *Transplant Infect Dis.* 2012;14(6):555–63.

51. Lion T, Baumgartinger R, Watzinger F, Matthes-Martin S, Suda M, Preuner S, et al. Molecular monitoring of adenovirus in peripheral blood after allogeneic bone marrow transplantation permits early diagnosis of disseminated disease. *Blood.* 2003;102(3):1114–20.

52. Florescu DF, Pergam SA, Neely MN, Qiu F, Johnston C, Way S, et al. Safety and efficacy of CMX001 as salvage therapy for severe adenovirus infections in immunocompromised patients. *Biol Blood Marrow Transplant.* 2012;18(5):731–8.

53. Grimley M, Prasad V, Kurtzberg J, Chemaly R, Brundage T, Wilson C, et al. Twice-Weekly Brincidofovir (CMX001) shows promising antiviral activity in immunocompromised transplant recipients with asymptomatic adenovirus viremia. *Biol Blood Marrow Transplant.* 2104;20(2 Suppl).

54. Campbell AP, Guthrie KA, Englund JA, Farney RM, Minerich EL, Kuypers J, et al. Clinical outcomes associated with respiratory virus detection before allogeneic hematopoietic stem cell transplant. *Clin Infect Dis.* 2015;61(2):192–202.

55. Lehners N, Schnitzler P, Geis S, Puthenparambil J, Benz MA, Alber B, et al. Risk factors and containment of respiratory syncytial virus outbreak in a hematology and transplant unit. *Bone Marrow Transplant.* 2013;48(12):1548–53.

56. Kim YJ, Guthrie KA, Waghmare A, Walsh EE, Falsey AR, Kuypers J, et al. Respiratory syncytial virus in hematopoietic cell transplant recipients: factors determining progression to lower respiratory tract disease. *J Infect Dis.* 2014;209(8):1195–204.

57. Boeckh M, Englund J, Li Y, Miller C, Cross A, Fernandez H, et al. Randomized controlled multicenter trial of aerosolized ribavirin for respiratory syncytial virus upper respiratory tract infection in hematopoietic cell transplant recipients. *Clin Infect Dis.* 2007;44(2):245–9.

58. Shah DP, Ghantoji SS, Shah JN, El Taoum KK, Jiang Y, Popat U, et al. Impact of aerosolized ribavirin on mortality in 280 allogeneic haematopoietic stem cell transplant recipients with respiratory syncytial virus infections. *J Antimicrob Chemother.* 2013;68(8):1872–80.

59. Shah JN, Chemaly RF. Management of RSV infections in adult recipients of hematopoietic stem cell transplantation. *Blood.* 2011;117(10):2755–63.

60. Seo S, Campbell AP, Xie H, Chien JW, Leisenring WM, Englund JA, et al. Outcome of respiratory syncytial virus lower respiratory tract disease in hematopoietic cell transplant recipients receiving aerosolized ribavirin: significance of stem cell source and oxygen requirement. *Biol Blood Marrow Transplant.* 2013;19(4):589–96.

61. Tramontana AR, George B, Hurt AC, Doyle JS, Langan K, Reid AB, et al. Oseltamivir resistance in adult oncology and hematology patients infected with pandemic (H1N1) 2009 virus, Australia. *Emerg Infect Dis.* 2010;16(7):1068–75.

62. Mohty B, Thomas Y, Vukicevic M, Nagy M, Levrat E, Bernimoulin M, et al. Clinical features and outcome of 2009-influenza A (H1N1) after allogeneic hematopoietic SCT. *Bone Marrow Transplant.* 2012;47(2):236–42.

63. Lagler H, Wenisch JM, Tobudic S, Gualdoni GA, Rodler S, Rasoul-Rockenschaub S, et al. Pandemic influenza A H1N1 vaccine in recipients of solid organ transplants: immunogenicity and tolerability outcomes after vero cell derived, non-adjuvanted, whole-virion vaccination. *Vaccine.* 2011;29(40):6888–93.

64. Ljungman P, Ward KN, Crooks BN, Parker A, Martino R, Shaw PJ, et al. Respiratory virus infections after stem cell transplantation: a prospective study from the Infectious Diseases Working Party of the European Group for Blood and Marrow Transplantation. *Bone Marrow Transplant.* 2001;28(5):479–84.

65. Ljungman P, de la Camara R, Perez-Bercoff L, Abecasis M, Nieto Campuzano JB, Cannata-Ortiz MJ, et al. Outcome of pandemic H1N1 infections in hematopoietic stem cell transplant recipients. *Haematologica.* 2011;96(8):1231–5.

66. Casper C, Englund J, Boeckh M. How I treat influenza in patients with hematologic malignancies. *Blood.* 2010;115(7):1331–42.

67. Ljungman P, Avetisyan G. Influenza vaccination in hematopoietic SCT recipients. *Bone Marrow Transplant.* 2008;42(10):637–41.

68. Rubin LG, Levin MJ, Ljungman P, Davies EG, Avery R, Tomblyn M, et al. 2013 IDSA clinical practice guideline

for vaccination of the immunocompromised host. *Clin Infect Dis.* 2014;58(3):309–18.

69. Machado CM, Cardoso MR, da Rocha IF, Boas LS, Dulley FL, Pannuti CS. The benefit of influenza vaccination after bone marrow transplantation. *Bone Marrow Transplant.* 2005;36(10):897–900.

70. Engelhard D, Mohty B, de la Camara R, Cordonnier C, Ljungman P. European guidelines for prevention and management of influenza in hematopoietic stem cell transplantation and leukemia patients: Summary of ECIL-4 (2011). *Transplant Infecti Dis.* 2013;15(3):219–32.

71. Chemaly RF, Hanmod SS, Rathod DB, Ghantoji SS, Jiang Y, Doshi A, *et al.* The characteristics and outcomes of parainfluenza virus infections in 200 patients with leukemia or recipients of hematopoietic stem cell transplantation. *Blood.* 2012;119(12):2738–45; quiz 969.

72. Srinivasan A, Wang C, Yang J, Inaba H, Shenep JL, Leung WH, *et al.* Parainfluenza virus infections in children with hematologic malignancies. *Pediatr Infect Dis J.* 2011;30(10):855–9.

73. Ustun C, Slaby J, Shanley RM, Vydra J, Smith AR, Wagner JE, *et al.* Human parainfluenza virus infection after hematopoietic stem cell transplantation: risk factors, management, mortality, and changes over time. *Biol Blood Marrow Transplant.* 2012;8(10):1580–8.

74. Srinivasan A, Wang C, Yang J, Shenep JL, Leung WH, Hayden RT. Symptomatic parainfluenza virus infections in children undergoing hematopoietic stem cell transplantation. *Biol Blood Marrow Transplant.* 2011;17(10):1520–7.

75. Seo S, Xie H, Campbell AP, Kuypers JM, Leisenring WM, Englund JA, *et al.* Parainfluenza virus lower respiratory tract disease after hematopoietic cell transplant: viral detection in the lung predicts outcome. *Clin Infect Dis.* 2014;58(10):1357–68.

76. Raza K, Ismailjee SB, Crespo M, Studer SM, Sanghavi S, Paterson DL, *et al.* Successful outcome of human metapneumovirus (hMPV) pneumonia in a lung transplant recipient treated with intravenous ribavirin. *J Heart Lung Transplant.* 2007;26(8):862–4.

77. Englund JA, Boeckh M, Kuypers J, Nichols WG, Hackman RC, Morrow RA, *et al.* Brief communication: fatal human metapneumovirus infection in stem-cell transplant recipients. *Ann Intern Med.* 2006;144(5):344–9.

78. Renaud C, Xie H, Seo S, Kuypers J, Cent A, Corey L, *et al.* Mortality rates of human metapneumovirus and respiratory syncytial virus lower respiratory tract infections in hematopoietic cell transplantation recipients. *Biol Blood Marrow Transplant.* 2013;19(8):1220–6.

79. Seo S, Martin E, Xie H, Kuypers J, Campbell A, Choi S-M, *et al.* Human rhinovirus RNA detection in the lower respiratory tract of hematopoietic cell transplant recipients: association with mortality. *Biol Blood Marrow Transplant.* 2013;19(2 Suppl.):S167–S8.

80. Lee YJ, Zheng J, Kolitsopoulos Y, Chung D, Amigues I, Son T, *et al.* Relationship of BK polyoma virus (BKV) in the urine with hemorrhagic cystitis and renal function in recipients of T cell-depleted peripheral blood and cord blood stem cell transplantations. *Biol Blood Marrow Transplant.* 2014;20(8):1204-10.

81. Leung AY, Suen CK, Lie AK, Liang RH, Yuen KY, Kwong YL. Quantification of polyoma BK viruria in hemorrhagic cystitis complicating bone marrow transplantation. *Blood.* 2001;98(6):1971–8.

82. Gilis L, Morisset S, Billaud G, Ducastelle-Lepretre S, Labussiere-Wallet H, Nicolini FE, *et al.* High burden of BK virus-associated hemorrhagic cystitis in patients undergoing allogeneic hematopoietic stem cell transplantation. *Bone Marrow Transplant.* 2014;49(5):664–70.

83. Erard V, Kim HW, Corey L, Limaye A, Huang ML, Myerson D, *et al.* BK DNA viral load in plasma: evidence for an association with hemorrhagic cystitis in allogeneic hematopoietic cell transplant recipients. *Blood.* 2005;106(3):1130–2.

84. Laskin BL, Denburg M, Furth S, Diorio D, Goebel J, Davies SM, *et al.* BK viremia precedes hemorrhagic cystitis in children undergoing allogeneic hematopoietic stem cell transplantation. *Biol Blood Marrow Transplant.* 2013;19(8):1175–82.

85. Cesaro S, Facchin C, Tridello G, Messina C, Calore E, Biasolo MA, *et al.* A prospective study of BK-virus-associated haemorrhagic cystitis in paediatric patients undergoing allogeneic haematopoietic stem cell transplantation. *Bone Marrow Transplant.* 2008;41(4):363–70.

86. Cesaro S, Hirsch HH, Faraci M, Owoc-Lempach J, Beltrame A, Tendas A, *et al.* Cidofovir for BK virus-associated hemorrhagic cystitis: a retrospective study. *Clin Infect Dis.* 2009;49(2):233–40.

87. Kwon HJ, Kang JH, Lee JW, Chung NG, Kim HK, Cho B. Treatment of BK virus-associated hemorrhagic cystitis in pediatric hematopoietic stem cell transplant recipients with cidofovir: a single-center experience. *Transplant Infect Dis.* 2013;15(6):569–74.

88. Ganguly N, Clough LA, Dubois LK, McGuirk JP, Abhyankar S, Aljitawi OS, *et al.* Low-dose cidofovir in the treatment of symptomatic BK virus infection in patients undergoing allogeneic hematopoietic stem cell transplantation: a retrospective analysis of an algorithmic approach. *Transplant Infect Dis.* 2010;12(5):406–11.

89. Chen XC, Liu T, Li JJ, He C, Meng WT, Huang R. Efficacy and safety of leflunomide for the treatment of BK virus-associated hemorrhagic cystitis in allogeneic hematopoietic stem cell transplantation recipients. *Acta Haematol.* 2013;130(1):52–6.

90. Versluis J, Pas SD, Agteresch HJ, de Man RA, Maaskant J, Schipper ME, *et al.* Hepatitis E virus: an underestimated opportunistic pathogen in recipients of allogeneic hematopoietic stem cell transplantation. *Blood.* 2013;122(6):1079–86.

91. Hammond SP, Borchelt AM, Ukomadu C, Ho VT, Baden LR, Marty FM. Hepatitis B virus reactivation following allogeneic hematopoietic stem cell transplantation. *Biol Blood Marrow Transplant.* 2009;15(9):1049–59.

92. Onozawa M, Hashino S, Izumiyama K, Kahata K, Chuma M, Mori A, *et al.* Progressive disappearance of anti-hepatitis B surface antigen antibody and reverse seroconversion after allogeneic hematopoietic stem cell transplantation in patients with previous hepatitis B virus infection. *Transplantation.* 2005;79(5):616–9.

93. Arai S, Lee LA, Vogelsang GB. A systematic approach to hepatic complications in hematopoietic stem cell transplantation. *J Hematother Stem Cell Res.* 2002;11(2):215–29.

94. Lalazar G, Rund D, Shouval D. Screening, prevention and treatment of viral hepatitis B reactivation in patients with haematological malignancies. *Br J Haematol.* 2007;136(5):699–712

95. Mallet V, van Bömmel F, Doerig C, Pischke S, Hermine O, Locasciulli A, *et al.* Management of viral hepatitis in patients with haematological malignancy and in patients undergoing haemopoietic stem cell transplantation: recommendations of the 5th European Conference on Infections in Leukaemia (ECIL-5). *Lancet Infect Dis.* 2016;16(5):606–17.

96. Mahale P, Kontoyiannis DP, Chemaly RF, Jiang Y, Hwang JP, Davila M, *et al.* Acute exacerbation and reactivation of chronic hepatitis C virus infection in cancer patients. *J Hepatol.* 2012;57(6):1177–85.

97. Tomblyn M, Chen M, Kukreja M, Aljurf MD, Al Mohareb F, Bolwell BJ, *et al.* No increased mortality from donor or recipient hepatitis B- and/or hepatitis C-positive serostatus after related-donor allogeneic hematopoietic cell transplantation. *Transplant Infect Dis.* 2012;14(5):468–78.

98. Mahale P, Okhuysen PC, Torres HA. Does chemotherapy cause viral relapse in cancer patients with hepatitis C infection successfully treated with antivirals? *Clin Gastroenterol Hepatol.* 2014;12(6):1051–4 e1.

99. Ljungman P, Locasciulli A, de Soria VG, Bekassy AN, Brinch L, Espigado I, *et al.* Long-term follow-up of HCV-infected hematopoietic SCT patients and effects of antiviral therapy. *Bone Marrow Transplant.* 2012;47(9):1217 21.

100. Peffault de Latour R, Levy V, Asselah T, Marcellin P, Scieux C, Ades L, *et al.* Long-term outcome of hepatitis C infection after bone marrow transplantation. *Blood.* 2004;103(5):1618–24.

Chapter

18

Prevention and Treatment of Fungal Infections in Hematopoietic Cell Transplants

Lakshmikanth Katragadda and John R. Wingard

Introduction

Invasive fungal infections (IFI) are a major cause of morbidity and mortality (10–20%) in patients with hematologic malignancies undergoing hematopoietic cell transplant (HCT). Recent data show a trend towards increase in overall number of transplants, unrelated transplants, mismatched related transplants, and older age of recipients[1]. Several host, disease, transplant variables and complications are being identified as possible risk factors for IFI (Table 18.1). Efforts continue to study trends in the incidence of specific IFIs during various post-transplant periods[2]. Definitions of IFI were revised for uniformity across various centers and reproducibility in clinical trials and have added newer diagnostics[3].

Several single-center studies report an increase in incidence of mucormycosis. However, aspergillosis continues to be the most common IFI in comparison to candidiasis, which was more prevalent prior to the era of fluconazole prophylaxis[2]. There is continued emphasis on primary and secondary prophylaxis of IFI with the incorporation of newer antifungal agents. In most of the available literature and in our current chapter the focus is on allogeneic (allo) HCT.

IFI in HCT patients can be broadly divided into molds and yeast (Figure 18.1). Molds include Aspergillus, mucormycosis, Fusarium and others. Our discussion will emphasize strategies of prevention and treatment of Candida and Aspergillus, the most common yeast and mold infections respectively.

Antifungal Agents

Polyenes

Drugs from this class work by damaging the cell membrane of the fungus by binding to ergosterol and forming pores or by causing oxidative damage. Various formulations of amphotericin B are listed below. They are typically used as an intravenous (IV) formulation and have the widest spectrum of antifungal activity of all the antifungal drugs. As a group they are associated with considerable nephrotoxicity which is dose and duration dependent and have infusion reactions with the initial doses, which usually abate with future dosing.

Table 18.1 High risk for mold infection

Prior invasive fungal infection <6 months

Neutropenia for >3 weeks

Prior allogeneic hematopoietic cell transplant <6 months

Prednisone >1 mg/kg per day or similar for ≥3 weeks

Acute leukemia not in complete remission

More than one attempt at remission for AML

Cord blood transplant

T-cell depletion

Acute GvHD grade ≥3

Combination of other risk factors:

 Unrelated donor

 Mismatched related donor

 Acute GvHD grade 1–2

 Chronic GvHD

 Chronic prednisone >20 mg/day

 Prednisone >2 mg/kg for more than 1 week

 CMV infection

 Iron overload

 Recurrent neutropenia

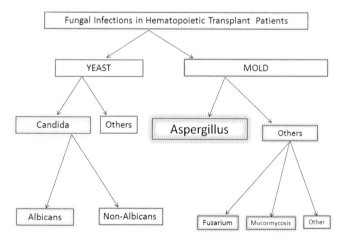

Figure 18.1. Common post-transplant fungal infections.

Table 18.2 Common cytochrome P-450 drug–drug interactions of triazoles

	Fluconazole[a]	Itraconazole[a]	Voriconazole[a]	Posaconazole[a]
Drug levels ↑ by azole	Cyclosporine, tacrolimus (50)	Cyclosporine (50), tacrolimus (66)	Cyclosporine (50), tacrolimus (66)	Cyclosporine (75), tacrolimus (66)
	Sirolimus	Sirolimus (×)	Sirolimus (×)	Sirolimus (×)
	Vincristine	Vincristine (×)	Vincristine (×)	Vincristine (×)
		Cyclophosphamide	Cyclophosphamide	Cyclophosphamide
↑ Level of azole		Grapefruit	Proton pump inhibitors, cimetidine	

List is not all inclusive and focuses on only common medications used in BMT.
[a] Approximate recommended dose reduction (%) when used in combination.
(×) Generally avoided.

Table 18.3 Triazoles for antifungal therapy

	Fluconazole	Itraconazole	Voriconazole	Posaconazole
Available forms	Oral, IV	Capsule, liquid, IV[a]	Tablet, liquid, IV[a]	Liquid, tablets, IV[a]
Fasting state[b]	NA	Yes – liquid	Yes	No
Acidic beverage[b]	NA	Yes – capsule	Decrease	Yes – liquid
Fatty food[b]	NA	Yes – capsule	Decrease	Yes – liquid
Proton pump[b] inhibitors	NA	Decrease – capsule	Increase	Decrease – liquid
Metabolism	Hepatic-minor	Hepatic	Hepatic	Hepatic
Dose adjustment	Renal	Hepatic	Hepatic	Hepatic
Level (µg/mL)[c]	NA	>0.5	2–6[d]	0.5–1.2[d]

[a] Caution with IV forms in renal failure as the cyclodextrin carrier could accumulate.
[b] Enhances absorption.
[c] Done after 7 days of treatment.
[d] Controversial.

Amphotericin B deoxycholate (Amb): This is the conventional older version with over 50 years of experience used at doses ranging between 0.3 and 1.5 mg/kg per day but it has fallen out of favor due to nephrotoxicity and infusional adverse events.

Lipid formulations of amphotericin (LF-Amb): The mid-1990s have seen the emergence of lipid formulations namely: liposomal amphotericin B (L-Amb/Ambisome), amphotericin B lipid complex (ABLC/Abelcet), and amphotericin B cholesteryl sulfate/amphotericin colloidal dispersion (ABCD/Amphotec). An allergic reaction to one of the lipid formulations does not preclude the use of others.

In comparison to Amb, all LF-Amb are substantially less nephrotoxic and associated with fewer infusion-related toxicities (except that ABCD had higher infusion reactions in a study), permitting use of higher doses. However, even with higher doses (3–5 mg/kg per day) clearly superior outcomes have been difficult to demonstrate[4].

Triazoles

Since the arrival of fluconazole in 1990, three other newer extended-spectrum azoles itraconazole, voriconazole, and posaconazole were Food and Drug Administration (FDA) approved. Azoles preferentially inhibit fungal cell membrane formation by interfering with fungal cytochrome P450 activity and decreasing ergosterol synthesis[5]. Due to their cytochrome P450-mediated mechanism they have several drug–drug interactions (Table 18.2). There is variability of bioavailability of the oral extended-spectrum azoles and checking levels is advisable after a week of treatment.

Fluconazole: It has good yeast activity but no mold activity. Some *Candida* species are less sensitive (*C. glabrata*) and some are resistant (*C. krusei*). Oral bioavailability is about 90% compared to IV fluconazole. It achieves excellent urine concentrations[6].

Itraconazole: It has both *Candida* and mold coverage including *Aspergillus*. IV itraconazole has been associated with negative inotropic effects and is not available in the United States. Proton pump inhibitors and H2 blockers inhibit absorption of capsule formulation. The oral solution with hydroxypropyl-b-cyclodextrin has more uniform bioavailability, and is better absorbed in a fasting state. Owing to poor absorption of the capsule formulation and GI intolerance with the oral solution, itraconazole has fallen out of favor (Table 18.3).

Voriconazole: Since approval in 2002 it has become the preferred first-line therapy for invasive aspergillosis. It has activity against scedosporiosis and fusariosis but not mucormycosis. The IV formulation is complexed to sulfobutyl-ether cyclodextrin. Visual disturbances and hallucinations may occasionally occur early after initiation of therapy and periostitis may occur after prolonged use.

Posaconazole: It has been available since 2007, has broader activity than voricaonzole, and is additionally active against mucormycosis. The oral solution has been best studied; the bioavailability is dependent on eating and can be variable. A delayed release tablet in November 2013 and an IV formulation in March 2014 were added to the oral solution, approved for prevention of *Candida* and *Aspergillus* infections. The delayed release tablets offer better bioavailability and tolerance over the oral solution and less reliance on eating for absorption. The dose schedule of the new formulations differs from the oral solution and they are given in a loading dose of 300 mg twice a day for 1 day and then 300 mg daily. Owing to high (up to 60%) incidence of thrombophlebitis when the IV formulation is given through a peripheral IV line it is recommended that it is administered through a central line[7].

Echinocandins

The echinocandins, caspofungin, micafungin, and anidulafungin, have fungicidal activity against *Candida* as compared to azoles that have a fungistatic activity. They also have some activity against *Aspergillus*. They act by inhibiting synthesis of 1,3-beta-glucan, a polysaccharide present in the cell wall of many pathogenic fungi responsible for cell wall strength, shape, and thereby cell division. They do not have activity on fungi which do not rely on glucan polymers. They are available in IV form only and their half-life allows once a day dosing. They are well tolerated with minimal drug–drug interactions. They are metabolized in the liver except for anidulafungin. Only caspofungin needs dose adjustment for hepatic impairment. The echinocandins have a broad spectrum of activity against most *Candida* species and represent excellent options for invasive *Candida* treatment. They also have anti-*Aspergillus* activity and are commonly used for salvage therapy for invasive aspergillosis. One study suggests there may be benefit in combination with voriconazole as first-line therapy for invasive aspergillosis.

Prophylaxis

Historically, IFIs were associated with a very high mortality and antifungal prophylaxis had become a standard during the post-transplant period. Here we will discuss available antifungal drugs and their appropriateness for use and the level of evidence from various published studies. The duration of consideration for prophylaxis is a minimum of 100 days or until the end of usage of immunosuppression. The decision to use *Candida* prophylaxis or mold-active prophylaxis is based on the extent of risk for IFI and is an evolving field[8].

Fluconazole

It is effective at a dose of 200–400 mg daily for prophylaxis and treatment of *Candida*. Its usage has the potential to lead to the emergence of resistant non-*albicans* species[9], but generally resistance in the HCT population has been infrequent. When fluconazole prophylaxis was extended to 75 days post-transplant in a double-blind randomized clinical trial (RCT), in addition to the decrease in incidence of IFI and empiric use of Amb there was a survival benefit compared to placebo[10]. Unless mold coverage is needed fluconazole is the preferred drug for primary prophylaxis of IFI[8] (Table 18.1).

Itraconazole

It is given as a 200-mg oral solution every 12 hours. A multicenter open-label RCT showed that in comparison to fluconazole, primary prophylaxis until day 100 with itraconazole showed significantly decreased proven IFI by either yeasts or molds but had significantly increased GI side effects. There was no overall survival advantage but there were fewer deaths from IFI[11]. In another open-label RCT aimed to assess mold protection, itraconazole when compared to fluconazole till day 180 was poorly tolerated due to GI toxicity and hepatotoxicity and had a higher rate of discontinuation. Although there were fewer IFI while on treatment, overall IFIs were similar. It provided superior mold protection but candidiasis was similar[12]. There was no survival benefit. Itraconazole showed limited efficacy for secondary prophylaxis in a multinational uncontrolled nonintervention study[13].

Itraconazole oral solution (not capsules) was as effective as or better than fluconazole for prophylaxis for IFI but intolerance has limited its success as a prophylactic agent.

Voriconazole

It is given at a dose of 4 mg/kg or 200 mg every 12 hours. A RCT double-blind study comparing voriconazole to fluconazole for primary prophylaxis in mostly standard-risk disease patients under intense monitoring and structured empiric antifungal therapy showed that despite trends towards fewer overall IFIs, *Aspergillus* infections, empiric treatment, fungus-free survival (FFS), OS, and AE were similar. Post hoc analyses showed significantly fewer IFI and improved FFS in acute myeloid leukemia (AML) patients who received HCT[14]. Another trial indicated better tolerance than itraconazole but similar rates of IFI and OS[15].

A prospective single-arm study showed efficacy in high-risk cord blood transplant recipients and for secondary prophylaxis [16,17]. A retrospective study suggests that it is more effective than fluconazole or itraconazole in patients receiving steroids[18].

Voriconazole is at least as effective as fluconazole for primary prophylaxis. It is preferred over fluconazole for primary mold prophylaxis but RCTs in high-risk settings are lacking.

Posaconazole

The oral solution is given as 200 mg of posaconazole in an oral suspension three times daily. Most of the studies were done on the oral solution. They are no RCTs for the immediate post-transplant period. For primary prophylaxis in HCT patients with severe graft-*versus*-host disease (GvHD), posaconazole was compared to fluconazole in a double-blind RCT. There was no significant difference in overall incidence of IFI and OS but there was significantly less IA and deaths related to IFI[19]. Important to note, some patients had positive galactomannan tests at baseline, and the benefit was seen only in patients with positive galactomannan tests before study entry.

A single-center small observation study showed prophylaxis until day 100 with posaconazole led to a lower incidence of proven or probable IFI, a high probability of FFS, and improved OS when compared to itraconazole. Three patients in the posaconazole group had primary engraftment failure from non-drug-related causes[20]. Other "real life setting" retrospective studies showed posaconazole to be safe and effective in the first 100 days post-transplant[21–23]. The delayed release tablets and IV form may overcome the GI limitations.

Caspofungin

Caspofungin is usually given at a dose of 50 mg IV daily. There are very few uncontrolled primary IFI prophylaxis studies in HCT patients with caspofungin. Single-center retrospective studies showed its efficacy as primary prophylaxis for IFI (mostly *Candida*) even in high-risk settings – on steroids, T-cell depletion, and with GvHD[24]. A phase 2 study evaluating caspofungin for secondary IFI prophylaxis was found to be safe with efficacy[13,25].

Caspofungin has efficacy in both primary and secondary prophylaxis of IFI based on level 2 studies.

Micafungin

Micafungin is administered at a dose of 50 mg IV daily. A double-blind RCT comparing micafungin to fluconazole during the pre-engraftment period reported it to be superior during the neutropenic phase and there was a trend to fewer episodes of aspergillosis[26]. An open-label RCT showed that it was non inferior to itraconazole solution[27]. A retrospective single-center study showed no difference in efficacy between micafungin 50 mg, 100 mg, and 150 mg[28].

Based on the above RCT and other nonrandomized trials micafungin appears to be superior to fluconazole mostly by reducing *Candida* IFIs.

Echinocandins are an attractive group for primary IFI prophylaxis until engraftment due to very few side effects, drug–drug interactions, and better mold coverage than fluconazole with the limitation that they are only available in oral form.

Amphotericin B

Recent studies evaluated weekly doses of lipid formulations of amphotericin B for primary prophylaxis taking advantage of its longer half-life. A pilot study with ABCD at 4 mg/kg twice weekly starting at day 30 for patients on prednisone $\geq$ 30 mg/day was effective and well tolerated[29]. Higher doses of L-Amb at 10 mg/kg weekly could not be tolerated in the PROPHYSOME study[30]. L-Amb every other day in autologous transplant patients was well tolerated and effective[31].

An RCT comparing inhaled L-Amb given twice a week to a placebo found that it was effective in prophylaxis of invasive pulmonary aspergillosis with cough and difficulty with inhalation being the causes for discontinuation[32]. Important to note, fluconazole was given concomitantly to prevent *Candida* IFI.

Amphotericin B given IV in a low dose twice a week and as inhalation therapy may occasionally serve as an alternative when other drugs could not be given due to toxicity, cost, or insurance issues.

Treatment Considerations

Host factors, aggressive diagnostic assessment, early initiation of therapy, timely surgical intervention when appropriate, center-specific epidemiology, the types of antifungal drugs on formulary in the center, proper dosing of the drug, tolerability of the drug right dosing, and adequate drug levels all play a role in influencing treatment outcomes. Host factors include duration and degree of neutropenia, prior IFI, status of the primary disease, if not in CR the chances of getting into one, if on steroids and or immunosuppression the expected duration of treatment, and coexisting infections like CMV.

Empiric Antifungal Therapy

Empiric antifungal therapy refers to use in patients with unexplained persistent neutropenic fever despite taking broad-spectrum antibiotics for $\geq$ 3–7 days for suspected IFI. Conventional amphotericin B was the gold standard until the advent of newer drugs. We discuss here studies on empiric antifungal therapy.

Double-blind RCTs showed that LF-Amb was as efficacious as Amb[33], and less toxic. L-Amb and ABCL were equally effective[34], but L-Amb was less toxic. Other open-label RCTs showed voriconazole and caspofungin were equally efficacious to L-Amb[35,36]. There are no RCTs using micafungin as empiric therapy but a retrospective, observational, sequential cohort study found micafungin and caspofungin to be equally effective[37]. Another recent single-arm prospective study confirmed its efficacy[38].

Treatment of Invasive Candidiasis

Most of the typical antifungals need loading doses for treatment. Fluconazole 800 mg then 400 mg (6 mg/kg) daily, micafungin IV 100 mg daily, caspofungin IV 70 mg then 50 mg daily, anidulafungin 200 mg then 100 mg daily, LF-Amb IV 3–5 mg/kg daily, voriconazole 6 mg/kg twice a day for 1 day followed by 4 mg/kg twice daily, itraconazole 200 mg three times a day for 3 days then 200 mg (3 mg/kg) once or twice a day. Posaconazole oral solution is given 200 mg three times a day or 400 mg twice a day and amphotericin deoxycholate 0.5–1 mg/kg.

Echinocandins and lipid formulation amphotericin B are the preferred regimens in critically ill patients. If not critically ill and not on recent azoles, fluconazole can be used.

Esophageal candidiasis is treated with higher doses of micafungin (150 mg) and anidulafungin (200 mg) based on studies in HIV patients. Candidemia is generally treated for 2 weeks beyond clearance on blood cultures. Chronic disseminated candidiasis is treated for weeks or months until clearance of lesions[39].

Species-specific considerations: For *C. glabrata* an echinocandin is preferred as there is dose-dependent response or resistance to azoles[6]. Transition from echinocandin to an azole should only be done after reviewing susceptibility. For *C. krusei* an echinocandin or fluconazole or lipid formulation amphotericin B is preferred. Although rare, Candida parapsilosis can be resistant to echinocandin.

Comparative evidence of efficacy: It is important to note that most Candida treatment studies were performed in non-neutropenic patients. Neutropenic patients and HCT patients accounted for only a small percentage in these studies.

Fluconazole 200–600 mg daily compared to a matched cohort who received Amb showed similar day 2, day 5, and overall response and was better tolerated[40]. A double-blind RCT found caspofungin to be as effective as Amb[41]. A prospective international study showed micafungin to be effective alone or in combination[42]. A double-blind RCT showed micafungin to be as effective as L-Amb and caspofungin. A higher dose of micafungin was no better than 100 mg [43,44].

Based on the results from an RCT in non-neutropenic patients and a small number of neutropenic cases in another trial, voriconazole is thought to be effective for treatment of candidiasis including in salvage setting[35,45,46]. Posaconazole was studied in HIV patients with esophageal candidiasis.

Treatment of Invasive Aspergillosis

Voriconazole is currently the preferred drug for invasive aspergillosis (IA) based on an RCT comparing voriconazole to Amb. Alternative agents that can be used for intolerance to voriconazole or for salvage treatment are: LF-Amb (ABLC 5 mg/kg per day, ABCD 3–4 mg/kg per day, L-Amb 3–5 mg/kg per day), posaconazole, itraconazole, caspofungin, and micafungin. Itraconazole is not recommended for voriconazole refractory IA.

Posaconazole is approved in Europe for treatment of IA. Caspofungin is not so effective for disseminated aspergillosis.

A mold-active triazole is preferred for *A. terreus*, due to resistance to amphotericin B. Treatment should be continued for 6 weeks beyond resolution of the immunosuppressive state and should be resumed during high-risk states. A change in drug class may be beneficial in refractory IA.

Adjunctive surgical resection may be needed with systemic therapy in certain situations: lesions close to the heart or great vessels, pericardial infection, endocarditis, sinusitis, osteomyelitis, and cerebral lesions, but this has not been systematically studied.

Comparative evidence of efficacy: Voriconazole was found to be superior and better tolerated than Amb and improved OS bases on an RCT[47]. It is effective in all forms of IA. LF-Amb was effective[48]. Several multicenter studies carried out during the mid-1990s showed that itraconazole was effective for treatment of IA, but the lack of an IV formulation in the United States and variable absorption of the oral solution makes this an unsatisfactory option. Two retrospective salvage studies which included some voriconazole refractory patients showed effectiveness of posaconazole[49,50].

Controversies

Posaconazole Drug Levels

Major interindividual and intraindividual variations in the posaconazole levels are well known. Although initial studies suggested that one should target a trough level of >0.5 μg/mL based on an MIC 90 for most *Aspergillus* species, a *post hoc* analysis of the two RCTs of posaconazole by the FDA suggested a level of 0.7 μg/mL would be preferable as the failure rate was higher if levels were <0.7[51]. A salvage study of posaconazole in IA showed that a level >1.2 correlated with a good response[49]. Others suggest an optimal level of between 0.5 and 1.5 μg/mL[52]. Studies have suggested that levels of >0.25, 0.35 on days 2–3 are predictive of a future "therapeutic level" of 0.5 μg/mL[53]. A recent IV posaconazole study targeted levels between 0.5 and 2.5 μg/mL[7].

It is believed that the posaconazole oral solution has saturable absorption and so splitting the 800 mg/day dose and administering up to four times/day doubles the bioavailability[52]. Levels were a little higher in patients getting a treatment dose *versus* prophylactic doses[54]. Increasing the dose from 200 to 400 mg three times a day increased the level in some patients but not in "poor absorbers"[55]. So it is generally felt that doses >800 mg/day may not always improve levels. Despite frequent lower levels, breakthrough IFIs were uncommon. It is unclear whether the 20 times higher concentrations in the alveolar cells compared to plasma concentrations could explain some of this.

The case for checking levels in prophylaxis is not very clear unless there are GI issues (inability to eat or diarrhea) that would raise a concern for poor bioavailability[8]. Much of the concern about bioavailability with the oral solution is substantially less with the slow-release tablet formulation. Until future studies incorporating IV posaconazole during periods of GI concerns are done to assess outcomes based on levels, we may have to settle with a level of between 0.5 and 1.2 μg/mL.

Voraconazole Drug Levels

Several studies reported wide inter- and intrapatient variations despite not having any organ dysfunction. This is thought to be from several factors including association with food, drug–drug interactions, polymorphisms of CYP2C19, and extensive saturable hepatic metabolism resulting in a nonlinear pharmacokinetic profile. Levels could not be predicted despite weight-based dosing.

Based on the outcomes report from initial prospective studies in IA and FDA briefing report a trough level >0.5 μg/mL was suggested[56]. Others suggested levels >1.0 μg/mL, based on a MIC 90 for most fungal infections and >50% protein binding of voriconazole[57]. Recent studies report better outcome with levels >2–2.5 μg/mL[58,59]. An upper limit of 5.5–6 μg/mL is where abnormal LFT or neurologic symptoms were reported. A recent study suggested that a trough/MIC level of between 2 and 5 was associated with maximal probability of response[60].

Close to a quarter of patients have levels <2 μg/mL and another quarter have levels >6 μg/mL. A single initial or terminal therapeutic value does not guarantee a future therapeutic value, so serial monitoring of therapeutic levels is generally practiced. But other studies have reported that failure and response have not always correlated with levels and dose adjustments based on levels did not affect outcome.

Until prospective RCTs are done checking levels at designated times and with any dose changes and assessing outcomes, we may have to settle with a target level of between 2 and 6 μg/mL.

Combination Antifungal Therapy

Invasive Aspergillosis

In-vitro and animal models and retrospective studies showed some synergistic activity of echinocandins and azoles against IA. An open-label noncomparative multicenter trial showed that combination of caspofungin with a polyene or an azole is safe and effective in treating IA[61]. Similar results were reported with micafungin[62]. But *in-vitro* and *in-vivo* studies in rabbit actually showed antagonism with combination of posaconazole and amphotericin for treatment of IA[63]. Results of a recent double-blind RCT (the first in combination therapy) in HCT and hematologic malignancy patients with proven and probable IA comparing voriconazole plus placebo *versus* voriconazole plus anidulafungin were reported. Combination therapy was given for 2–4 weeks and then can be switched to voriconazole monotherapy to complete 6 weeks of therapy. There was a trend towards improved OS at 6 weeks with combination therapy. A *post hoc* analysis of only patients with a positive galactomannan (n=218) showed a statistically significant improvement in OS[64].

Invasive Mucormycosis

As *Rhizopus*, one of the common causes of mucormycosis, expresses 1, 3-glucan synthase, echinocandins may have a role in their treatment. Combination of an echinocandin and amphotericin was found to be beneficial in mouse models. In a retrospective study that involved a very small number of transplant patients, a combination of caspofungin and amphotericin was found to be better than monotherapy with amphotericin[65]. One of the possible reasons for echinocandin activity in other members of Mucorales was thought to be enhancement of neutrophil activity. One could question this utility in a neutropenic patient. Preclinical data did not show benefit of combination of posaconazole and amphotericin for mucormycosis when the appropriate dose of amphotericin was used.

Data on efficacy of combination therapy are limited and are mostly from non-RCTs. Of these few studies most of the data are preclinical or for salvage treatment of mucormycosis. Recommendations in mucormycosis are mostly expert opinion. For mucormycosis combination antifungal therapy is being used before transitioning to posaconazole monotherapy due to concerns of unpredictable pharmacokinetics of oral posaconazole and the need to get adequate initial therapy. Now that IV posaconazole is available this could certainly change. At this time there is limited data to suggest the benefit of combination therapy and more studies are needed. There may be a limited role for an echinocandin with another class of antifungal for salvage therapy.

Single Nucleotide Polymorphisms to Define Risk and Guide Preventive Strategies

Recipients of donors with homozygous haplotype (h2/h2) for the three SNPs (+281A/G, +734A/C, +1449A/G) in the PTX3 gene were associated with increased risk of invasive aspergillosis. Similarly TLR5-Stop SNP in recipients was reported as a risk factor for IA after HCT[66]. Incidence of IA was not increased after HCT if either recipient or donor exhibited one of the two TLR4 gene variants (1063A/G and 1363C/T). In addition, recipients with these TLR gene variants and IA showed a delayed T-cell and NK-cell immune reconstitution. An association was reported between donor TLR4 haplotype S4 and the risk of IA among recipients of HCT from an unrelated donor[67].

Although there is growing interest in SNPs, which show promise, as with other diseases they will not be part of routine assessment until further confirmational studies have been carried out and there is easy availability of testing.

References

1. Pasquini MC, Wang Z, Horowitz MM, Gale RP. Report from the Center for International Blood and Marrow Transplant Research (CIBMTR): current uses and outcomes of hematopoietic cell transplants for blood and bone marrow disorders. *Clinical Transplants.* 2010:87–105.

2. Girmenia C, Raiola AM, Piciocchi A, Algarotti A, Stanzani M, Cudillo L, *et al.* Incidence and outcome of invasive fungal diseases after allogeneic stem cell transplantation: a prospective study of the Gruppo Italiano Trapianto Midollo Osseo (GITMO). *Biology of Blood and Marrow Transplantation: Journal of the American Society for Blood and Marrow Transplantation.* 2014;20(6):872–80.

3. De Pauw B, Walsh TJ, Donnelly JP, Stevens DA, Edwards JE, Calandra T, *et al.* Revised definitions of invasive fungal disease from the European Organization for Research and Treatment of Cancer/Invasive Fungal Infections Cooperative Group and the National Institute of Allergy and Infectious Diseases Mycoses Study Group (EORTC/MSG) Consensus Group. *Clinical Infectious Diseases: An Official Publication of the Infectious Diseases Society of America.* 2008;46(12):1813–21.

4. Wingard JR. Lipid formulations of amphotericins: are you a lumper or a splitter? *Clinical Infectious Diseases: An Official Publication of the Infectious Diseases Society of America.* 2002;35(7):891–5.

5. Dodds Ashley ES, Lewis R, Lewis JS, Martin C, Andes D. Pharmacology of systemic antifungal agents. *Clinical Infectious Diseases: An Official Publication of the Infectious Diseases Society of America.* 2006;43:S28–39.

6. Walsh TJ, Anaissie EJ, Denning DW, Herbrecht R, Kontoyiannis DP, Marr KA, *et al.* Treatment of aspergillosis: clinical practice guidelines of the Infectious Diseases Society of America. *Clinical Infectious Diseases: An Official Publication of the Infectious Diseases Society of America.* 2008;46(3):327–60.

7. Maertens J, Cornely OA, Ullmann AJ, Heinz WJ, Krishna G, Patino H, *et al.* Phase 1B study of the pharmacokinetics and safety of posaconazole intravenous solution in patients at risk for invasive fungal disease. *Antimicrobial Agents and Chemotherapy.* 2014;58(7):3610–7.

8. Girmenia C, Barosi G, Piciocchi A, Arcese W, Aversa F, Bacigalupo A, *et al.* Primary prophylaxis of invasive fungal diseases in allogeneic stem cell transplantation: revised recommendations from a consensus process by Gruppo Italiano Trapianto Midollo Osseo (GITMO). *Biology of Blood and Marrow Transplantation: Journal of the American Society for Blood and Marrow Transplantation.* 2014;20(8):1080–8.

9. Wingard JR, Merz WG, Rinaldi MG, Johnson TR, Karp JE, Saral R. Increase in Candida krusei infection among patients with bone marrow transplantation and neutropenia treated prophylactically with fluconazole. *The New England Journal of Medicine.* 1991;325(18):1274–7.

10. Marr KA, Seidel K, Slavin MA, Bowden RA, Schoch HG, Flowers ME, *et al.* Prolonged fluconazole prophylaxis is associated with persistent protection against candidiasis-related death in allogeneic marrow transplant recipients: long-term follow-up of a randomized, placebo-controlled trial. *Blood.* 2000;96(6):2055–61.

11. Winston DJ, Maziarz RT, Chandrasekar PH, Lazarus HM, Goldman M, Blumer JL, *et al.* Intravenous and oral itraconazole *versus* intravenous and oral fluconazole for long-term antifungal prophylaxis in allogeneic hematopoietic stem-cell transplant recipients. A multicenter, randomized trial. *Annals of Internal Medicine.* 2003;138(9):705–13.

12. Marr KA, Crippa F, Leisenring W, Hoyle M, Boeckh M, Balajee SA, *et al.* Itraconazole *versus* fluconazole for prevention of fungal infections in patients receiving allogeneic stem cell transplants. *Blood.* 2004;103(4):1527–33.

13. Vehreschild JJ, Sieniawski M, Reuter S, Arenz D, Reichert D, Maertens J, *et al.* Efficacy of caspofungin and itraconazole as secondary antifungal prophylaxis: analysis of data from a multinational case registry. *International Journal of Antimicrobial Agents.* 2009;34(5):446–50.

14. Wingard JR, Carter SL, Walsh TJ, Kurtzberg J, Small TN, Baden LR, *et al.* Randomized, double-blind trial of fluconazole *versus* voriconazole for prevention of invasive fungal infection after allogeneic hematopoietic cell transplantation. *Blood.* 2010;116(24):5111–8.

15. Marks DI, Pagliuca A, Kibbler CC, Glasmacher A, Heussel CP, Kantecki M, *et al.* Voriconazole *versus* itraconazole for antifungal prophylaxis following allogeneic haematopoietic stem-cell transplantation. *British Journal of Haematology.* 2011;155(3):318–27.

16. Takagi S, Araoka H, Uchida N, Uchida Y, Kaji D, Ota H, *et al.* A prospective feasibility study of primary prophylaxis against invasive fungal disease with voriconazole following umbilical cord blood transplantation with fludarabine-based conditioning. *International Journal of Hematology.* 2014;99(5):652–8.

17. Cordonnier C, Rovira M, Maertens J, Olavarria E, Faucher C, Bilger K, *et al.* Voriconazole for secondary prophylaxis of invasive fungal infections in allogeneic stem cell transplant recipients: results of the VOSIFI study. *Haematologica.* 2010;95(10):1762–8.

18. Gergis U, Markey K, Greene J, Kharfan-Dabaja M, Field T, Wetzstein G, *et al.* Voriconazole provides effective prophylaxis for invasive fungal infection in patients receiving glucocorticoid therapy for GvHD. *Bone Marrow Transplantation.* 2010;45(4):662–7.

19. Ullmann AJ, Lipton JH, Vesole DH, Chandrasekar P, Langston A, Tarantolo SR, *et al.* Posaconazole or fluconazole for prophylaxis in severe graft-*versus*-host disease. *The New England Journal of Medicine.* 2007;356(4):335–47.

20. Sanchez-Ortega I, Patino B, Arnan M, Peralta T, Parody R, Gudiol C, *et al.* Clinical efficacy and safety of primary antifungal prophylaxis with posaconazole vs itraconazole in allogeneic blood and marrow transplantation. *Bone Marrow Transplantation.* 2011;46(5):733–9.

21. Winston DJ, Bartoni K, Territo MC, Schiller GJ. Efficacy, safety, and breakthrough infections associated with standard long-term posaconazole antifungal prophylaxis in allogeneic stem cell transplantation recipients. *Biology of Blood and Marrow Transplantation: Journal of the American Society for Blood and Marrow Transplantation.* 2011;17(4):507–15.

22. Chaftari AM, Hachem RY, Ramos E, Kassis C, Campo M, Jiang Y, et al. Comparison of posaconazole versus weekly amphotericin B lipid complex for the prevention of invasive fungal infections in hematopoietic stem-cell transplantation. Transplantation. 2012;94(3):302–8.

23. Hahn J, Stifel F, Reichle A, Holler E, Andreesen R. Clinical experience with posaconazole prophylaxis: a retrospective analysis in a haematological unit. Mycoses. 2011;54 (Suppl 1):12–6.

24. Chou LS, Lewis RE, Ippoliti C, Champlin RE, Kontoyiannis DP. Caspofungin as primary antifungal prophylaxis in stem cell transplant recipients. Pharmacotherapy. 2007;27(12):1644–50.

25. de Fabritiis P, Spagnoli A, Di Bartolomeo P, Locasciulli A, Cudillo L, Milone G, et al. Efficacy of caspofungin as secondary prophylaxis in patients undergoing allogeneic stem cell transplantation with prior pulmonary and/or systemic fungal infection. Bone Marrow Transplantation. 2007;40(3):245–9.

26. van Burik JA, Ratanatharathorn V, Stepan DE, Miller CB, Lipton JH, Vesole DH, et al. Micafungin versus fluconazole for prophylaxis against invasive fungal infections during neutropenia in patients undergoing hematopoietic stem cell transplantation. Clinical Infectious Diseases: An Official Publication of the Infectious Diseases Society of America. 2004;39(10):1407–16.

27. Huang X, Chen H, Han M, Zou P, Wu D, Lai Y, et al. Multicenter, randomized, open-label study comparing the efficacy and safety of micafungin versus itraconazole for prophylaxis of invasive fungal infections in patients undergoing hematopoietic stem cell transplant. Biology of Blood and Marrow Transplantation: Journal of the American Society for Blood and Marrow Transplantation. 2012;18(10):1509–16.

28. Ziakas PD, Kourbeti IS, Mylonakis E. Systemic antifungal prophylaxis after hematopoietic stem cell transplantation: a meta-analysis. Clinical Therapeutics. 2014;36(2):292–306 e1.

29. Jansen J, Akard LP, Wack MF, Thompson JM, Dugan MJ, Leslie JK, et al. Delayed ABLC prophylaxis after allogeneic stem-cell transplantation. Mycoses. 2006;49(5):397–404.

30. Cordonnier C, Mohty M, Faucher C, Pautas C, Robin M, Vey N, et al. Safety of a weekly high dose of liposomal amphotericin B for prophylaxis of invasive fungal infection in immunocompromised patients: PROPHYSOME Study. International Journal of Antimicrobial Agents. 2008;31(2):135–41.

31. Penack O, Schwartz S, Martus P, Reinwald M, Schmidt-Hieber M, Thiel E, et al. Low-dose liposomal amphotericin B in the prevention of invasive fungal infections in patients with prolonged neutropenia: results from a randomized, single-center trial. Annals of Oncology: Official Journal of the European Society for Medical Oncology/ESMO. 2006;17(8):1306–12.

32. Rijnders BJ, Cornelissen JJ, Slobbe L, Becker MJ, Doorduijn JK, Hop WC, et al. Aerosolized liposomal amphotericin B for the prevention of invasive pulmonary aspergillosis during prolonged neutropenia: a randomized, placebo-controlled trial. Clinical Infectious Diseases: An Official Publication of the Infectious Diseases Society of America. 2008;46(9):1401–8.

33. Walsh TJ, Finberg RW, Arndt C, Hiemenz J, Schwartz C, Bodensteiner D, et al. Liposomal amphotericin B for empirical therapy in patients with persistent fever and neutropenia. National Institute of Allergy and Infectious Diseases Mycoses Study Group. The New England Journal of Medicine. 1999;340(10):764–71.

34. Wingard JR, White MH, Anaissie E, Raffalli J, Goodman J, Arrieta A, et al. A randomized, double-blind comparative trial evaluating the safety of liposomal amphotericin B versus amphotericin B lipid complex in the empirical treatment of febrile neutropenia. L Amph/ABLC Collaborative Study Group. Clinical Infectious Diseases: An Official Publication of the Infectious Diseases Society of America. 2000;31(5):1155–63.

35. Walsh TJ, Pappas P, Winston DJ, Lazarus HM, Petersen F, Raffalli J, et al. Voriconazole compared with liposomal amphotericin B for empirical antifungal therapy in patients with neutropenia and persistent fever. The New England Journal of Medicine. 2002;346(4):225–34.

36. Walsh TJ, Teppler H, Donowitz GR, Maertens JA, Baden LR, Dmoszynska A, et al. Caspofungin versus liposomal amphotericin B for empirical antifungal therapy in patients with persistent fever and neutropenia. The New England Journal of Medicine. 2004;351(14):1391–402.

37. Kubiak DW, Bryar JM, McDonnell AM, Delgado-Flores JO, Mui E, Baden LR, et al. Evaluation of caspofungin or micafungin as empiric antifungal therapy in adult patients with persistent febrile neutropenia: a retrospective, observational, sequential cohort analysis. Clinical Therapeutics. 2010;32(4):637–48.

38. Yamaguchi M, Kurokawa T, Ishiyama K, Aoki G, Ueda M, Matano S, et al. Efficacy and safety of micafungin as an empirical therapy for invasive fungal infections in patients with hematologic disorders: a multicenter, prospective study. Annals of Hematology. 2011;90(10):1209–17.

39. Chen SC, Slavin MA, Sorrell TC. Echinocandin antifungal drugs in fungal infections: a comparison. Drugs. 2011;71(1):11–41.

40. Anaissie EJ, Vartivarian SE, Abi-Said D, Uzun O, Pinczowski H, Kontoyiannis DP, et al. Fluconazole versus amphotericin B in the treatment of hematogenous candidiasis: a matched cohort study. The American Journal of Medicine. 1996;101(2):170–6.

41. Mora-Duarte J, Betts R, Rotstein C, Colombo AL, Thompson-Moya L, Smietana J, et al. Comparison of caspofungin and amphotericin B for invasive candidiasis. The New England Journal of Medicine. 2002;347(25):2020–9.

42. Ullmann AJ, Akova M, Herbrecht R, Viscoli C, Arendrup MC, Arikan-Akdagli S, et al. ESCMID* guideline for the diagnosis and management of Candida diseases 2012: adults with haematological malignancies and after haematopoietic stem cell transplantation (HCT). Clinical Microbiology and Infection: The Official Publication of the European Society of Clinical Microbiology and Infectious Diseases. 2012;18 (Suppl 7):53–67.

43. Pappas PG, Rotstein CM, Betts RF, Nucci M, Talwar D, De Waele JJ, et al. Micafungin versus caspofungin for treatment of candidemia and other forms of invasive candidiasis. Clinical

Infectious Diseases: an Official Publication of the Infectious Diseases Society of America. 2007;45(7):883–93.

44. Kuse ER, Chetchotisakd P, da Cunha CA, Ruhnke M, Barrios C, Raghunadharao D, et al. Micafungin *versus* liposomal amphotericin B for candidaemia and invasive candidosis: a phase III randomised double-blind trial. *Lancet.* 2007;369(9572):1519–27.

45. Ostrosky-Zeichner L, Oude Lashof AM, Kullberg BJ, Rex JH. Voriconazole salvage treatment of invasive candidiasis. *European Journal of Clinical Microbiology & Infectious Diseases: Official Publication of the European Society of Clinical Microbiology.* 2003;22(11):651–5.

46. Kullberg BJ, Sobel JD, Ruhnke M, Pappas PG, Viscoli C, Rex JH, et al. Voriconazole *versus* a regimen of amphotericin B followed by fluconazole for candidaemia in non-neutropenic patients: a randomised non-inferiority trial. *Lancet.* 2005;366(9495):1435–42.

47. Herbrecht R, Denning DW, Patterson TF, Bennett JE, Greene RE, Oestmann JW, et al. Voriconazole *versus* amphotericin B for primary therapy of invasive aspergillosis. *The New England Journal of Medicine.* 2002;347(6):408–15.

48. Bowden R, Chandrasekar P, White MH, Li X, Pietrelli L, Gurwith M, et al. A double-blind, randomized, controlled trial of amphotericin B colloidal dispersion *versus* amphotericin B for treatment of invasive aspergillosis in immunocompromised patients. *Clinical Infectious Diseases: An Official Publication of the Infectious Diseases Society of America.* 2002;35(4):359–66.

49. Walsh TJ, Raad I, Patterson TF, Chandrasekar P, Donowitz GR, Graybill R, et al. Treatment of invasive aspergillosis with posaconazole in patients who are refractory to or intolerant of conventional therapy: an externally controlled trial. *Clinical Infectious Diseases: An Official Publication of the Infectious Diseases Society of America.* 2007;44(1):2–12.

50. Heinz WJ, Grau A, Ulrich A, Helle-Beyersdorf A, Zirkel J, Schirmer D, et al. Impact of benzodiazepines on posaconazole serum concentrations: a population-based pharmacokinetic study on drug interaction. *Current Medical Research and Opinion.* 2012;28(4):551–7.

51. Jang SH, Colangelo PM, Gobburu JV. Exposure-response of posaconazole used for prophylaxis against invasive fungal infections: evaluating the need to adjust doses based on drug concentrations in plasma. *Clinical Pharmacology and Therapeutics.* 2010;88(1):115–9.

52. Andes D, Pascual A, Marchetti O. Antifungal therapeutic drug monitoring: established and emerging indications. *Antimicrobial Agents and Chemotherapy.* 2009;53(1):24–34.

53. Heinz WJ, Einsele H, Helle-Beyersdorf A, Zirkel J, Grau A, Schirmer D, et al. Posaconazole concentrations after allogeneic hematopoietic stem cell transplantation. *Transplant Infectious Disease: An Official Journal of the Transplantation Society.* 2013;15(5):449–56.

54. Lebeaux D, Lanternier F, Elie C, Suarez F, Buzyn A, Viard JP, et al. Therapeutic drug monitoring of posaconazole: a monocentric study with 54 adults. *Antimicrobial Agents and Chemotherapy.* 2009;53(12):5224–9.

55. Cornely OA, Helfgott D, Langston A, Heinz W, Vehreschild JJ, Vehreschild MJ, et al. Pharmacokinetics of different dosing strategies of oral posaconazole in patients with compromised gastrointestinal function and who are at high risk for invasive fungal infection. *Antimicrobial Agents and Chemotherapy.* 2012;56(5):2652–8.

56. Denning DW, Ribaud P, Milpied N, Caillot D, Herbrecht R, Thiel E, et al. Efficacy and safety of voriconazole in the treatment of acute invasive aspergillosis. *Clinical Infectious Diseases: An Official Publication of the Infectious Diseases Society of America.* 2002;34(5):563–71.

57. Pascual A, Calandra T, Bolay S, Buclin T, Bille J, Marchetti O. Voriconazole therapeutic drug monitoring in patients with invasive mycoses improves efficacy and safety outcomes. *Clinical Infectious Diseases: An Official Publication of the Infectious Diseases Society of America.* 2008;46(2):201–11.

58. Park WB, Kim NH, Kim KH, Lee SH, Nam WS, Yoon SH, et al. The effect of therapeutic drug monitoring on safety and efficacy of voriconazole in invasive

fungal infections: a randomized controlled trial. *Clinical Infectious Diseases: An Official Publication of the Infectious Diseases Society of America.* 2012;55(8):1080–7.

59. Ueda K, Nannya Y, Kumano K, Hangaishi A, Takahashi T, Imai Y, et al. Monitoring trough concentration of voriconazole is important to ensure successful antifungal therapy and to avoid hepatic damage in patients with hematological disorders. *International Journal of Hematology.* 2009;89(5):592–9.

60. Troke PF, Hockey HP, Hope WW. Observational study of the clinical efficacy of voriconazole and its relationship to plasma concentrations in patients. *Antimicrobial Agents and Chemotherapy.* 2011;55(10):4782–8.

61. Maertens J, Glasmacher A, Herbrecht R, Thiebaut A, Cordonnier C, Segal BH, et al. Multicenter, noncomparative study of caspofungin in combination with other antifungals as salvage therapy in adults with invasive aspergillosis. *Cancer.* 2006;107(12):2888–97.

62. Kontoyiannis DP, Ratanatharathorn V, Young JA, Raymond J, Laverdiere M, Denning DW, et al. Micafungin alone or in combination with other systemic antifungal therapies in hematopoietic stem cell transplant recipients with invasive aspergillosis. *Transplant Infectious Disease: An Official Journal of the Transplantation Society.* 2009;11(1):89–93.

63. Meletiadis J, Petraitis V, Petraitiene R, Lin P, Stergiopoulou T, Kelaher AM, et al. Triazole-polyene antagonism in experimental invasive pulmonary aspergillosis: in-vitro and in vivo correlation. *The Journal of Infectious Diseases.* 2006;194(7):1008–18.

64. Marr KA, Schlamm H, Rottinghaus ST, Jagannatha S, Bow EJ, Wingard JR, et al. A randomised, double-blind study of combination antifungal therapy with voriconazole and anidulafungin versus voriconazole monotherapy for primary treatment of invasive aspergillosis. European Congress of Clinical Microbiology and Infectious Diseases (ECCMID), March–April, 2012.

65. Reed C, Bryant R, Ibrahim AS, Edwards J, Jr., Filler SG, Goldberg R, et al. Combination polyene-caspofungin

treatment of rhino-orbital-cerebral mucormycosis. *Clinical Infectious Diseases: An Official Publication of the Infectious Diseases Society of America.* 2008;47(3):364–71.

66. Cunha C, Aversa F, Lacerda JF, Busca A, Kurzai O, Grube M, *et al.*

Genetic PTX3 deficiency and aspergillosis in stem-cell transplantation. *The New England Journal of Medicine.* 2014;370(5):421–32.

67. Bochud PY, Chien JW, Marr KA, Leisenring WM, Upton A,

Janer M, *et al.* Toll-like receptor 4 polymorphisms and aspergillosis in stem-cell transplantation. *The New England Journal of Medicine.* 2008;359(17):1766–77.

Chapter 19

Chronic Graft-*versus*-Host Disease: Consensus, Challenges, and Controversies

Iskra Pusic and Steven Z. Pavletic

Introduction

Chronic graft-*versus*-host disease (GvHD) is the most common late complication and the leading cause of treatment-related mortality (TRM) and morbidity after allogeneic hematopoietic cell transplant (HCT). It occurs in 30–70% of people surviving >1 year after allogeneic HCT and has a 5-year mortality rate of 30–50%. Chronic GvHD is characterized by immunosuppression and immune dysregulation resulting in decreased organ function, increased risk of infection, and reduced quality of life (QoL) in patients otherwise cured of their cancer. A continued rise in the number of allogeneic HCT performed and improved early post-transplant survival have resulted in an increased number of people at risk for developing chronic GvHD[1].

One of the major obstacles to clinical research in chronic GvHD has been the lack of standardized criteria for the diagnosis, staging, and measurements of response to therapy. In 2005 the National Institutes of Health (NIH) Consensus Conference consolidated expert opinions and standardized recommendations for diagnosis and staging, histopathology, biomarkers, response criteria, ancillary therapy and supportive care, and design of clinical trials. The Chronic GvHD Consortium was subsequently established to conduct multicenter studies on chronic GvHD and many retrospective and prospective longitudinal studies have been published over the last 9 years further validating the NIH Consensus Conference criteria[2–19]. In 2014, now with 9 years of experience, the experts met again to update and improve on the original recommendations and clarify controversies. The 2014 NIH criteria provide greater specificity and more accurate measures of the disease burden[20–25].

Pathophysiology

Although major progress has been achieved in understanding the pathophysiology of acute GvHD, the pathophysiology of chronic GvHD is less well defined. Major factors limiting our understanding of chronic GvHD pathophysiology have been the lack of clinically relevant animal models, heterogeneity of chronic GvHD, and its insidious onset. The exact role of, and interactions among, different T- and B-cell subsets and influence of cytokines has not been fully elucidated. Chronic GvHD is considered to be a disease of immune dysregulation where donor-derived immune cells react against host cell populations and tissues. It is likely that unique donor–recipient immune factors play a role in the development of chronic GvHD. Alloreactivity mediated by donor T-cells is considered a key component for initiation of the processes. Immune dysregulation ensues through the disruption of both central and peripheral mechanisms of tolerance. Degeneration of the thymus, due to age, prior acute GvHD, or transplant conditioning, results in decrease in negative selection of alloreactive CD4+ T-cells. In addition, peripheral tissue damage from previous acute GvHD or inflammation may lead to release of normally sequestrated, cryptic auto-antigens to the periphery. T-cell dysregulation then leads to cytokine response with increased production of interleukin (IL)-4, -5, and -11, and release of fibrogenic cytokines such as IL-2, transforming growth factor-β1 and TNF-α, resulting in immunodeficiency, target organ injury, and fibrosis. CD4+CD25+ regulatory T-cells (Tregs) are generated in the thymus and are thought to play a key role in the maintenance of immunologic self-tolerance. In preclinical studies, these Tregs have been shown to prevent GvHD by suppressing alloreactive donor T-cells, while preserving graft-*versus*-leukemia (GvL) effect[26]. In human studies, patients noted to have a higher relative frequency of Tregs after HCT had lower rate and severity of GvHD, lower rate of nonrelapse mortality, and equivalent relapse mortality[27]. Finally, there is increasing evidence of the role of B-cell dysregulation, with production of autoreactive antibodies. It has been suggested that B-cell activation may result from high levels of B-cell activating factor (BAFF) in the lymphoid microenvironment [28]. These observations may explain occasional responses of chronic GvHD to the therapy with rituximab. Better understanding of the biologic events, which initiate and promote the development of chronic GvHD, and of its most severe clinical presentations, are a major question for researchers.

Risk Factors

The ability to predict who will develop chronic GvHD, and how severe it will become, could potentially be of great clinical importance. A number of factors have been reported to be associated with a higher risk of developing chronic GvHD (Table 19.1)[16,29–37]. It is important to note that many of

Table 19.1 Risk factors for the development of chronic GvHD

Most important risk factor	Prior acute GvHD
Frequently reported risk factors	Greater HLA disparity Increased recipient age Use of female donors for male recipients Use of mobilized peripheral blood HPSC Use of donor lymphocyte infusion
Less frequently reported risk factors	Higher infused CD34$^+$ cell dose in peripheral blood transplantation Lower infused CD34$^+$ cell dose in bone marrow transplantation Faster achievement of complete hematopoietic chimerism Corticosteroids in GvHD prophylaxis Transplantation for chronic myeloid leukemia and aplastic anemia Cytomegalovirus seropositivity

GvHD, graft-*versus*-host disease; HLA, human leukocyte antigen; HPSC, hematopoietic progenitor and stem cells.

the older studies used the traditional definition of chronic GvHD, as any GvHD developing after day 100. Thus, persistent, recurrent, or late acute GvHD, according to the NIH criteria, would have been classified as chronic GvHD. Flowers *et al.* performed large comparative multivariate analysis of risk factors for acute and chronic GvHD according to the 2005 NIH consensus criteria[16]. The profiles of risk factors for acute and chronic GvHD were similar, but with some notable differences. Main risks for the development of chronic GvHD were female donor for male recipients, use of mobilized peripheral blood hematopoietic progenitor and stem cells (HPSC), and older recipient age. Risk factors associated with chronic GvHD were not changed after adjustment for prior acute GvHD, suggesting that chronic GvHD is not simply an evolution of acute GvHD.

The most influential and established risk factor for chronic GvHD is prior history of acute GvHD. The degree of human leukocyte antigen (HLA) mismatch between the donor and recipient significantly influences the risk for the development of acute and chronic GvHD. Incidence of GvHD is lowest after HLA-matched sibling HCT and higher after use of mismatched related donors or unrelated donors[31,37]. According to recent Center of International Blood and Marrow Transplantation Research (CIBMTR) analysis 1-year probability of chronic GvHD was approximately 30% after HLA-identical sibling HCT, 25–46% after one-antigen HLA-mismatched sibling HCT, and approximately 44–51% after HLA-matched unrelated HCT[30]. In addition, minor HLA antigen mismatches may also play a role in the development of chronic GvHD, particularly H-Y antigen.

Another important factor affecting the incidence of chronic GvHD is the HPSC source. A large meta-analysis evaluating results after HLA-matched sibling HCT demonstrated the increased incidence of chronic GvHD in patients who received

peripheral blood HPSC instead of bone marrow[33]. Two recent randomized trials, one in a related and one in an unrelated donor setting, also demonstrated the increased risk of chronic GvHD after transplantation of mobilized peripheral blood HPSC when comparing to bone marrow, however without significantly different survival or relapse incidence[34,35]. For patients who lack a suitable HLA-matched donor, umbilical cord HCT and more recently haploidentical HCT have become a favored approach (see Chapters 59 and 60).

The impact of conditioning on chronic GvHD incidence has been difficult to assess due to several factors: absence of prospective trials due to fundamental differences in the groups receiving reduced intensity conditioning (RIC) *versus* myeloablative, use of a variety of RIC regimens, lack of uniform GvHD prophylaxis, and inconsistent criteria for the diagnosis and staging of chronic GvHD. Acute GvHD after RIC regimen occurs often in a delayed fashion, leading to an overlap syndrome of acute and chronic GvHD that might have been classified as "chronic" in previous trials. In addition, early achievement of complete donor chimerism is frequently delayed after RIC that may affect the incidence and severity of chronic GvHD[38]. Other factors that appear to have an impact on development of chronic GvHD are the use of antithymocyte globulin (ATG) and alemtuzumab during conditioning. A large prospective clinical trial comparing addition of ATG to preparatory chemotherapy regimen to prevent development of severe GvHD is ongoing. The impact of ex-vivo T-cell depletion on the incidence of chronic GvHD is less clear (see Chapter 29)[39].

Diagnosis and Clinical Manifestations

Symptoms of chronic GvHD occur gradually, starting on average between 3 months and 2 years after HCT. Chronic GvHD targets the skin, eyes, mouth, gut, liver, lungs, joints, and genitourinary system. It may be restricted to a single site, but frequently several organ systems are involved. Early diagnosis is important because the goal of treatment is control of symptoms and the prevention of irreversible organ damage.

The diagnosis of chronic GvHD is sometimes challenging due to frequent coexistence of acute GvHD, polymorphic presentation, and lack of adequate biomarkers. According to the NIH criteria, the diagnosis of chronic GvHD requires at least one *diagnostic* sign (manifestation that establishes the diagnosis of chronic GvHD without the need for further testing) *or* at least one *distinctive* sign (manifestation highly suggestive of chronic GvHD but insufficient alone to establish the diagnosis) confirmed by biopsy, laboratory test, or by radiology in the same or another organ (Table 19.2)[20]. In addition, it is important to make a distinction from acute GvHD (maculopapular erythematous rash, elevated liver function tests, diarrhea-nausea-vomiting) and exclude other possible diagnoses (such as infections, drug toxicities, new cancers). Other features can be recognized as part of chronic GvHD only if the diagnosis is confirmed. Common features are found in both acute and chronic GvHD and cannot be used to distinguish between the two disorders.

Table 19.2 Signs and symptoms of chronic GvHD

Organ or Site	Diagnostic (sufficient to establish the diagnosis of chronic GvHD)	Distinctive (seen in chronic GvHD, but insufficient alone to establish a diagnosis)	Other features (can be recognized as part of chronic GvHD if diagnosis is confirmed)	Common features (seen with both acute and chronic GvHD)
Skin	• Poikiloderma • Lichen planus-like features • Sclerotic features • Morphea-like features • Lichen sclerosus-like features	• Depigmentation • Papulosquamous lesions	• Sweat impairment • Ichthyosis • Keratosis pilaris • Hypopigmentation • Hyperpigmentation	• Erythema • Maculopapular rash • Pruritus
Nails		• Dystrophy • Longitudinal ridging, splitting, or brittle features • Onycholysis • Pterygium unguis • Nail loss (usually symmetric)		
Scalp and body hair		• New onset of scarring or nonscarring scalp alopecia (after recovery from chemoradiotherapy) • Loss of body hair • Scaling	• Thinning scalp hair, typically patchy, coarse, or dull (not explained by other causes) • Premature gray hair	
• Mouth	• Lichen planus-like changes	• Xerostomia • Mucocele • Mucosal atrophy • Pseudomembranes • Ulcers		• Gingivitis • Mucositis • Erythema • Pain
• Eyes		• New onset dry, gritty, or painful eyes • Cicatricial conjunctivitis • Keratoconjunctivitis sicca • Confluent areas of punctate keratopathy	• Photophobia • Periorbital hyperpigmentation • Blepharitis (erythema of the eyelids with edema)	
Genitalia *Females* *Males*	• Lichen planus-like features • Lichen sclerosus-like features • Vaginal scarring or stenosis • Phimosis or urethral/meatus scarring or stenosis	• Erosions • Fissures • Ulcers		
GI tract	• Esophageal web • Strictures or stenosis in the upper to mid-third of the esophagus		• Exocrine pancreatic insufficiency	• Anorexia • Nausea, vomiting • Diarrhea • Weight loss • Failure to thrive
Liver				• Total bilirubin, ALP >2 x ULN ALT> 2 x ULN

Table 19.2 (cont.)

Organ or Site	Diagnostic (sufficient to establish the diagnosis of chronic GvHD)	Distinctive (seen in chronic GvHD, but insufficient alone to establish a diagnosis)	Other features (can be recognized as part of chronic GvHD if diagnosis is confirmed)	Common features (seen with both acute and chronic GvHD)
Lung	• Bronchiolitis obliterans diagnosed lung biopsy • Bronchiolitis obliterans syndrome[a]	• Air trapping and bronchiectasis on chest CT	• Cryptogenic organizing pneumonia[b] • Restrictive lung disease[b]	
Muscles, fascia, joints	• Fasciitis • Joint stiffness or contractures secondary to fasciitis or sclerosis	• Myositis or polymyositis	• Edema • Muscle cramps • Arthralgia or arthritis	
Hematopoietic and immune			• Thrombocytopenia • Eosinophilia • Lymphopenia • Hypo- or hyper-gammaglobulinemia • AIHA and ITP • Raynaud's phenomenon	
Other			• Pericardial or pleural effusions • Ascites • Peripheral neuropathy • Nephrotic syndrome • Myasthenia gravis • Cardiac conduction abnormality or cardiomyopathy	

[a] Bronchiolitis obliterans syndrome (BOS) can be diagnostic for lung chronic GvHD only if distinctive sign or symptom present in another organ.
[b] Pulmonary entities under investigation or unclassified.
ALP, alkaline phosphatase; ALT, alanine aminotransferase; PFTs, pulmonary function tests; AIHA, autoimmune hemolytic anemia; ITP, idiopathic thrombocytopenic purpura; ULN, upper limit of normal.
Modified from Jagasia MH *et al.* National Institutes of Health Consensus Development Project on Criteria for Clinical Trials in Chronic Graft-*versus*-Host Disease: I. Diagnosis and Staging Working Group. Biol Blood Marrow Transplant 2015;21:389–401.

Chronic GvHD diagnosis is primarily clinical and histologic confirmation is not mandatory if the patient has at least one diagnostic sign. Further testing is recommended to confirm chronic GvHD in situations where distinctive but non-diagnostic signs are present or alternative diagnoses are considered. A detailed color-atlas and classification of the skin and oral chronic GvHD is available at www.asbmt.org/, Practice Resources on NIH Chronic GvHD Consensus Project.

Classification

Acute *versus* Chronic

Historically, any manifestations of GvHD present after day +100 following HCT were arbitrarily defined as chronic GvHD. However, that definition is not biologically or clinically accurate since signs typical of acute GvHD can develop well after day 100, especially in patients who received RIC regimen or donor lymphocyte infusion (DLI). The NIH Consensus Conference recognizes two major categories of GvHD, each one with two subcategories (Table 19.3). Chronic GvHD is separated from acute GvHD not by time frame from HCT, but by the presence of diagnostic and distinctive clinical manifestations. In the absence of histologic or clinical signs characteristic of chronic GvHD, persistence, recurrence or new onset of maculopapular erythematous rash, gastrointestinal symptoms, or cholestatic hepatitis should be classified as acute GvHD, regardless of the time after transplantation. The 2014 NIH consensus criteria have defined the *overlap* category as the presence of acute GvHD manifestations in a patient diagnosed with chronic GvHD. The *overlap* syndrome is often transient and depends on a degree of immunosuppression: in patients who present with the *overlap* syndrome acute GvHD features can resolve with treatment while chronic GvHD may persist; likewise acute GvHD may flare in patients with chronic features when immunosuppression is tapered.

Type of Onset

"Progressive" chronic GvHD (20–30%) evolves directly from acute GvHD and carries the most unfavorable prognosis, and

Table 19.3 Classification of GvHD

Category	Onset of symptoms after HCT or DLI	Presence of acute GvHD features	Presence of chronic GvHD features
Acute GvHD			
Classic acute GvHD	≤100 days	Yes	No
Persistent, recurrent, or late-onset acute GvHD	>100 days	Yes	No
Chronic GvHD			
Classic chronic GvHD	No time limit	No	Yes
Overlap syndrome	No time limit	Yes	Yes

GvHD, graft-*versus*-host disease; DLI, donor lymphocyte infusion; HCT, hematopoietic cell transplantation.
Modified from Filipovich A *et al*. National Institutes of Health Consensus Development Project on Criteria for Clinical Trials in Chronic Graft-*versus*-Host Disease: I. Diagnosis and staging Working Group. Biol Blood Marrow Transplant 2005; 11:945–956.

"quiescent" chronic GvHD (30–40%) develops after a period of resolution of symptoms and has an intermediate prognosis. *De novo* chronic GvHD (30–40%) develops without previous history of acute GvHD and carries the best prognosis.

Scoring System

Historically, the most commonly used staging system for chronic GvHD has been "limited/extensive" classification, as proposed by a Seattle group in 1980. This classification was formulated on the basis of the results of a retrospective analysis of patients who were transplanted in the late 1970s before cyclosporine was in use. The aim of this classification was to identify patients who require systemic immunosuppression. "Limited" chronic GvHD was described as localized skin involvement and/or liver dysfunction and "extensive" as generalized skin involvement, liver histology showing aggressive hepatitis, or involvement of any other target organ. However, it provided little information on type and severity of organ involvement, and is becoming largely obsolete. Several other prognostic scales have since been developed for predicting nonrelapse mortality (NRM); however, none provided sufficient information about the extent of the disease or functional impairment.

The NIH criteria for scoring of chronic GvHD provide meaningful information on disease severity and functional impairment of key organ systems in patients with chronic GvHD and are the current standard[20,40]. This scoring system can be applied *only after* the diagnosis of chronic GvHD has been established. Eight organs are assessed: skin, eyes, mouth, GI tract, liver, lungs, joints and fascia, and genital tract (Figure 19.1). Each organ is scored according to a 4-point scale (0–3) with 0 representing no involvement and 3 reflecting severe impairment. The NIH global severity for chronic GvHD (mild, moderate, severe) is then derived by combining organ-specific scores (Table 19.4).

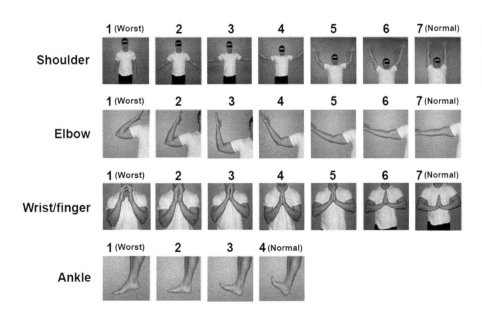

Figure 19.1. Organ scoring of chronic GvHD. Modified from Jagasia MH *et al*. National Institutes of Health Consensus Development Project on Criteria for Clinical Trials in Chronic Graft-*versus*-Host Disease: I. Diagnosis and Staging Working Group. Biol Blood Marrow Transplant 2015; 21:389–401.

Table 19.4. NIH global severity of chronic GvHD[a]

Mild chronic GvHD	Involves one or two organ systems with maximum score of 1 (except lung)
Moderate chronic GvHD	Involves at least one organ system with score of 2, or three or more organs with score of 1, or lung with score of 1
Severe chronic GvHD	Involves at least one organ system with score of 3, or lung with score of 2 or 3

[a] If the entire abnormality in an organ system is unequivocally explained by a non-GvHD documented cause, that organ is not included for calculation of the global severity. If the abnormality in an organ system is attributed to multifactorial causes (GvHD plus other causes) the scored organ will be used for calculation of the global severity regardless of the contributing causes.
Modified from Jagasia MH *et al*. National Institutes of Health Consensus Development Project on Criteria for Clinical Trials in Chronic Graft-*versus*-Host Disease: I. Diagnosis and Staging Working Group. Biol Blood Marrow Transplant 2015; 21:389–401.

Scoring criteria are intended for baseline and cross-sectional use during the course of chronic GvHD. Several studies have demonstrated that 2004 NIH organ-specific scoring and global severity are reliable measures of chronic GvHD disease burden[4–6,13]. However, the score assignment did not take into account other possible causes of organ damage that could serve as potential confounders and result in overestimation in the organ scoring. In a recent prospective study, Aki *et al*. evaluated the impact of confounders in organ scoring and showed that approximately 40% of patients had abnormalities not attributed to chronic GvHD in at least one organ[17]. After those changes were taken into account there was a modest downgrade of global severity of chronic GvHD. The 2014 revised NIH criteria changed the scoring such that sites or organs with abnormality entirely explained by non-GvHD causes are not included in computing the overall global severity. However, the data are still collected in the scoring form by checking the box "Abnormality present but explained entirely by non-GvHD documented cause" (Figure 19.1).

Prognostic Factors

Chronic GvHD usually lasts about 2–3 years, but 10–15% of patients may have active disease beyond 5 years after diagnosis. Features most consistently associated with TRM in patients with chronic GvHD are progressive onset, thrombocytopenia ($< 100000/\mu L$), higher percentage of skin involvement at the time of diagnosis, involvement of multiple organs, hyperbilirubinemia, and decreased clinical performance score[3,4,16,18,39,41]. Several prospective studies using the 2005 NIH criteria have shown that skin, lung, and gastrointestinal score each predict higher risk of TRM among patients with chronic GvHD [5,8,9,19]. The persistent, recurrent or late acute GvHD has been shown to be highly associated with poor survival[14,15]. The overlap GvHD subcategory has been associated with worse survival compared to classic chronic GvHD in several[2,11,14], but not all, studies[7,12,42].

Prevention

The most attractive approach for controlling chronic GvHD would be the prevention of the most severe and irreversible clinical manifestations while maintaining GvL effect. The major barrier in developing effective preventive measures for chronic GvHD is our still limited understanding of chronic GvHD pathophysiology. Advances in pharmacologic prevention and treatment of acute GvHD, the major risk factor for chronic GvHD, have not resulted in a corresponding decrease in incidence of chronic GvHD. Although some recipient, donor, and transplant characteristics are modifiable to minimize the risk of chronic GvHD, the majority of these approaches have very limited impact. Selective modulation of alloreactive response and inflammation, rather than general immunosuppression, appears to be the most promising mechanism for reducing GvHD while preserving GvL. Some of these measures include the use of bone marrow grafts, post-transplant high-dose cyclophosphamide (Chapter 12 and 29), selective T-cell depletion (TCD) (Chapter 30), and possibly incorporating ATG in the conditioning.

Treatment

Approaches to the treatment of chronic GvHD are complex and the field is rapidly advancing. Successful management and supportive care of patients with chronic GvHD require close follow-up to identify complications before they limit organ function or threaten mortality. Chronic GvHD and its treatment further results in increased risk of infection, impaired organ function, and reduced QoL. The goal of therapy is to stop destructive immunologic process, improve symptoms, and eventually establish immunologic tolerance with ultimate withdrawal of immunosuppressive therapy. Approximately 85% of patients who survive beyond 5 years after diagnosis are able to stop systemic therapy[43]. However, patients with chronic GvHD remain at increased risk of late complications of HCT even after permanent withdrawal of immunosuppression. Symptomatic mild chronic GvHD can often be treated with local therapies alone, allowing for a delay in the start of systemic immunosuppression, or for systemic agent dose reduction. Systemic therapy is generally indicated for patients with moderate and severe chronic GvHD.

Primary Therapy

For more than three decades the most widely used first-line systemic therapy of chronic GvHD has been prednisone alone or in conjunction with calcineurin inhibitors (cyclosporine [CSA] or tacrolimus [TAC]). The addition of CSA or TAC allows for more effective prednisone taper. Prednisone is usually started at 1mg/kg per day as a single oral dose. CSA or TAC is given twice a day and the dose is adjusted to maintain therapeutic level. If chronic GvHD is improving after 1 or 2 weeks of therapy, prednisone is tapered by 25% per week, over the following 4 weeks, to a target dose of

1 mg/kg every other day; the calcineurin inhibitor continues on a daily dosing schedule. Alternate-day administration of prednisone can mitigate some of the steroid toxicities and facilitate adrenal recovery. Patients are evaluated for response every 3 months after alternate-day dosing has been achieved. If the disease has resolved, patients are slowly weaned off the medications, with dose reductions approximately every 2 weeks, starting with prednisone. Patients with incomplete repose are kept on the same dose of steroids for an additional 3 months and then re-evaluated. Once optimal response is achieved, therapy is continued for another 3 months and then steroids are slowly tapered. If there is an exacerbation during the taper, the dose of prednisone may be increased by two levels with a shift to daily administration. Those patients who have not responded after 3 months of therapy or who progress are candidates for second-line therapeutic regimens.

Secondary Therapy

Second-line therapy is indicated for patients who fail to respond or progress through steroid-based therapy[44,45]. About 50% of patients with chronic GvHD will fail to achieve complete or partial response to steroid therapy by 1 year after diagnosis. Steroid-refractory disease is defined as: failure to improve despite up to 12 weeks of sustained therapy; progression after initiation of steroids; inability to taper steroids without exacerbation of GvHD. Most commonly used secondary therapies are outlined below and include: CSA, TAC, mycophenolate mofetil (MMF), sirolimus, rituximab, and extracorporeal photopheresis (ECP)[46–49]. A number of small phase 2 studies of secondary therapies have been published, most of them with incomplete and brief responses (Table 19.5). However, there is no standard of care second-line therapy for chronic GvHD and when possible, those patients should be treated on clinical trials.

CSA and TAC: CSA and TAC are classes of drugs called calcineurin inhibitors. CSA capsules are available as 25 and 100 mg and TAC as 0.5, 1, 5, and 10 mg. Usual dosing is twice a day (BID), adjusted according to the therapeutic level (target trough: CSA 150–250 ng/mL, TAC 5–10 ng/mL). CSA and TAC are used in combination with other drugs because, as single agents, they produce low responses. There are several possible drug interactions with CSA and TAC, most important being those with azoles, therefore requiring dose reductions. Toxicities include nephrotoxicity, neurotoxicity, hypertension, changes in glucose metabolism, gingival hyperplasia, and thrombotic microangiopathy (see Chapter 21).

MMF: MMF inhibits the *de novo* pathway of purine synthesis. It is available as 250 and 500 mg tablets; usually started as 500 mg BID, and may be increased up to 1500 mg BID. MMF is in part renally excreted and needs to be adjusted for renal function. Toxicities include gastrointestinal symptoms or rarely gastrointestinal bleeding, leukopenia, and risk of infections (see Chapter 70).

Sirolimus: Sirolimus is an mTOR inhibitor. It is available as 1 and 2 mg tablets, and dosing is daily or BID, adjusted according to the level (target trough: 5–15 ng/mL). It should be avoided with voriconazole because of significant drug reactions; if used together then the dose of sirolimus will require reduction. Toxicities include hyperlipidemia, peripheral edema, thrombocytopenia, leukopenia, delayed wound healing, noninfectious pneumonitis, stomatitis, hepatotoxicity, and thrombotic microangiopathy especially in combination with calcineurin inhibitors (see Chapter 70).

ECP: The mechanism by which ECP works is not clearly understood. It is thought to affect the balance of T-helper type 1 and 2 lymphocytes and dendritic cells. It is generally very well tolerated, but requires the patient to return to the apheresis center for treatment weekly to every other week. The best results have been reported in patients with mouth, skin, or liver involvement. Complications are mostly related to the central venous catheter and iron deficiency anemia associated with prolonged ECP.

Rituximab: There is increasing evidence of the role of B-cells and production of autoantibodies in the pathogenesis of chronic GvHD. Rituximab has been shown to be effective and safe in patients with steroid-refractory chronic GvHD. The best responses are noted in patients with cutaneous, mucosal, and musculoskeletal involvement. It is given at a standard dose of 375 mg/m² once a week for at least 4 consecutive weeks. The dose can be repeated at 3-month intervals (see Chapters 28 and 65).

High-dose pulse steroids: Use of high-dose pulse steroid is an option in situations when rapid response in chronic GvHD is required. The most frequently used regimen is methylprednisolone at 10 mg/kg per day for 4 consecutive days.

Ancillary Therapy and Supportive Care

Ancillary therapy and supportive care are the central components in the long-term multidisciplinary management of patients with chronic GvHD, employed as an adjunct to systemic GvHD treatment (Table 19.6)[21]. The term "ancillary therapy and supportive care" refers to any nonsystemic therapy intervention directed at control of organ-specific and systemic symptoms, prevention of infections, optimizing nutrition, functional performance, and psychosocial support. Occasionally symptomatic mild chronic GvHD can be treated with local therapies alone, allowing for a delay in the start of systemic immunosuppression. Information on specific dispensary guidelines is available at www.asbmt.org, Practice Resources on NIH Chronic GvHD Consortium.

Antimicrobial Prophylaxis

Chronic GvHD and systemic immunosuppressive therapy both impair immune defenses, resulting in the higher risk for opportunistic infections. Therefore, patients with active chronic GvHD who are on immunosuppressive therapy should receive infection prophylaxis. Patients with chronic

Table 19.5. Second-line therapies for chronic GvHD

Agent	Mechanism of action	Common and serious side effects	Comments
Ibrutinib	Reversible small molecule inhibitor of Bruton's tyrosine kinase	Fatigue, rash, arthralgia, diarrhea	Granted Breakthrough Designation for chronic GvHD by FDA, phase III trial is in progress
Pentostatin	Nucleoside analog	Nausea, vomiting, infections, renal failure	Activity in treatment of both acute and chronic GvHD
Low-dose methotrexate	Antimetabolite, anti-inflammatory	Myelosuppression, liver toxicity	Cannot be used in renal failure
Imatinib	Multi-kinase inhibitor targeting PDGFR and TGF-β	Myelosuppression, hepatitis	Best responses in skin and pulmonary GvHD
Psoralen and ultraviolet A	8-methoxypsolaren and untraviolet A irradiation	Nausea, photosensitivity, skin cancers	No systemic effect, best for skin lichen planus lesions
Hydroxychloroquine	Antimalarial agent	Gastrointestinal, renal failure, polyneuropathy	Best results in mucocutaneous and liver GvHD
Montelukast	Leukotriene antagonist	Headache, nausea	Lung GvHD
Acitretin	Retinoid	Skin dryness, alopecia, night blindness, pancreatitis, hyperlipidemia	Skin GvHD
Pulse cyclophosphamide	Alkylating agent	Myelosuppression, hemorrhagic cystitis	Effective for skin, liver, oral GvHD; toxicity profile acceptable
Clofazimine	Antimycobacterial	GI symptoms, hyperpigmentation	Best responses in mucocutaneous GvHD
Total lymphoid irradiation	Low-dose 100 cGy ionizing irradiation	Leukopenia, infections	Best responses in fasciitis and oral GvHD; rarely used today
Bortezomib	Proteasome inhibitor	Diarrhea, neuropathy	Small studies, responses in GI and skin GvHD
Daclizumab	Humanized anti-IL-2 receptor monoclonal antibody	GI symptoms, headache, insomnia, fatigue, infections	Limited reports, responses in skin GvHD
Infliximab	Chimeric anti-TNF-a monoclonal antibody	Hypersensitivity, infections	Limited reports
Etanercept	Recombinant human soluble TNF receptor fusion protein	Infections	Small studies, use in overlap syndrome with GI and skin GvHD
Low-dose IL2	Cytokine; induces Treg expansion	Constitutional symptoms, thrombotic microangiopathy	Best responses in skin and joint GvHD
Thalidomide	Anti-inflammatory, immunomodulatory	Neuropathy, somnolence, constipation, neutropenia, teratogenic, DVT	Disappointing as primary therapy; toxicity is a limitation
Alefacept	Dimeric anti-CD2 LFA-3 fusion protein	Infection risk	Limited reports, last resort
Alemtuzumab	Unconjugated IgG1 monoclonal antibody	Infection risk	Limited reports, last resort

GvHD, graft-*versus*-host disease; GI, gastrointestinal; DVT, deep venous thrombosis; PDGFR, platelet-derived growth factor receptor; Treg, regulatory T-cell

GvHD are considered at high risk for infections, even after the complete withdrawal of immunosuppression, and infections are the most common cause of mortality in those patients. Details on prevention and treatment of infections, as well as revaccination strategies are laid out in subsequent chapters (see Chapters 16–18, 22, and 70).

Measuring Therapeutic Response in Clinical Trials

Improvement in overall survival and survival with discontinuation of systemic immunosuppression are ultimate goals of treatment for chronic GvHD; however, these goals are

Table 19.6. Ancillary therapy and supportive care interventions in chronic GvHD

Organ system	Organ-specific intervention
Skin and appendages	• Photoprotection, sunscreens, avoidance of sun exposure; surveillance for malignancy • **For intact skin**: topical emollients (ointments and creams are better than lotions), corticosteroids (triamcinolone cream 0.1% tid to body; hydrocortisone cream 1.0% bid to face, axial, and groin), antipruritic agents, PUVA, calcineurin inhibitors • **For erosions/ulcerations:** topical antimicrobials, protective films or other dressings, debridement, hyperbaric oxygen, wound care specialist consultation
Mouth and oral cavity	• Maintain good oral/dental hygiene. Routine dental cleaning and endocarditis prophylaxis. Surveillance for infection and malignancy. Nutritional counseling. • Topical high and ultra-high potency corticosteroids (fluocinonide gel 0.05%, triamcinolone 0.1%), analgesics (mouthwash: 1 part dexamethasone + 2 parts viscous lidocaine, follow by tap water rinse), topical tacrolimus ointment 0.1%. Therapy for xerostomia (fluoride, saliva substitutes, cevimeline, pilocarpine)
Eyes	• Photoprotection, regular ophthalmology exams by eye specialist • Artificial tears and ointments, topical corticosteroids or cyclosporine, punctal occlusion, humidified environment, occlusive eye wear, moisture chamber glasses, tarsorraphy, gas-permeable scleral contact lens, autologous serum, topical antimicrobials, doxycycline
Musculoskeletal	• Surveillance for decreased range of motion, yearly bone densitometry, calcium levels and 25-OH vitamin D • Physical therapy, calcium, vitamin D, bisphosphonates
Gastrointestinal tract and liver	• Surveillance for infection (viral, fungal) • Eliminate other etiologies. Dietary modification, enzyme supplementation for malabsorption, gastroesophageal reflux management, esophageal dilatation, pancreatic enzyme replacement for pancreatic insufficiency, topical corticosteroids, bile salts resins
Lungs	• Surveillance for infection • Eliminate other etiologies. Inhaled glucocorticoids, bronchodilators, supplementary oxygen. Pulmonary rehabilitation. Consider lung transplantation for appropriate candidates
Hematopoietic	• Eliminate other etiologies, surveillance for infection • Hematopoietic growth factors, immunoglobulin
Neurologic	• Calcineurin drug level monitoring. Seizure prophylaxis including blood pressure control, electrolyte replacement, anticonvulsants • Occupational and physical therapy, treatment of neuropathic syndromes with tricyclic antidepressants, selective serotonin reuptake inhibitors, or anticonvulsants
Vulva and vagina	• Surveillance for estrogen deficiency, infection, and malignancy • Water-based lubricants, topical estrogens, topical corticosteroids or calcineurin inhibitors, dilators, surgery for extensive synechiae or obliteration
Immunologic and infectious disease	• Immunizations and prophylaxis against PCP, VZV, and encapsulated bacteria. Consider immunoglobulin replacement. Surveillance for infection • Organism-specific antimicrobials and empiric broad-spectrum antibiotics for fever

Modified from Carpenter PA *et al.* NIH Consensus Development Project on Criteria for Clinical Trials in Chronic Graft-*versus*-Host Disease: V. The 2014 Ancillary Therapy and Supportive Care Working Group Report. Biol Blood Marrow Transplant. 2015;21(7):1167–87.

not suitable for early phase drug development studies (see Chapter 69). Short-term measures of the therapeutic efficacy, such as partial or complete organ response, might serve as better potential outcome assessments. The 2005 NIH Consensus Conference provided, for the first time, standardized measures for assessing response to therapy of chronic GvHD. Provisional definitions of complete response, partial response, and progression were proposed for each organ and for overall outcome. Based on the publications over the last 9 years, the 2014 NIH Consensus Conference has updated its new and simplified recommendations[24,25]. Standardization of response measures should enhance uniformity of data collection and chronic GvHD assessments in clinical trials. It is imperative that response criteria measures are always established at the beginning of the trial, before the recruitment of patients. Response assessment involves a comparison of chronic GvHD activity at two time points. Measurements should be made at regular intervals and whenever a new systemic immunosuppression therapy is added, and efforts to document the durability of response are encouraged.

Table 19.7. Follow-up of patients with chronic GvHD

Category	Specific assessment	Minimum frequency
Interval history	Symptoms assessment (including psychosocial) and medication review	Every 3 mo
Physical exam	Weight	Every 3 mo
	Height	Every 12 mo
	Performance score	Every 3–6 mo
	Nutritional assessment	Every 3–6 mo
	General	Every 3–6 mo
	Skin	Every 3–6 mo
	Oral	Every 3–6 mo
	Range of motion	Every 3–6 mo
Laboratory	General blood work: CBC and differential Comprehensive metabolic panel Magnesium serum level L liver function tests	Every visit; more frequently during change of therapy
	Therapeutic drug levels	Weekly after starting or changing therapy, then twice monthly until stable, then monthly
	IgG level	Every 1–3 mo until normal levels independent of replacement therapy
	Lipid profile	Every 6–12 mo during treatment with corticosteroids or sirolimus
	Iron indices	Every 6–12 mo if requiring transfusions or if iron overload has been documented previously
	Thyroid function tests	Every 12 mo
Specific tests	Pulmonary function tests	Every 3–6 mo
	Bone Health: DEXA densitometry Serum calcium 25-OH Vitamin D	Every 12 mo
Subspecialty evaluations	Ophthalmology: Schirmer test Glaucoma test	Every 3–-2 mo
	Dental/oral medicine	Every 6–12 mo
	Dermatology	As clinically indicated
	Gynecology	As clinically indicated
	Physical Therapy	As clinically indicated
	Neuropsychologic	As clinically indicated

Modified from Carpenter PA *et al.* NIH Consensus Development Project on Criteria for Clinical Trials in Chronic Graft-*versus*-Host Disease: V. The 2014 Ancillary Therapy and Supportive Care Working Group Report. Biol Blood Marrow Transplant. 2015;21(7):1167–8.

Monitoring of Patients with Chronic GvHD and Long-Term Follow-Up

Close serial monitoring of all organs and sites potentially affected by chronic GvHD is recommended to facilitate early detection, prevent progression, and assess therapy response (Table 19.7). In addition, patients after HCT, and especially those with chronic GvHD, are at risk for developing other malignant and nonmalignant disorders. The scope and frequency of monitoring should be individualized as clinically indicated.

- Patients without chronic GvHD should be monitored at least every 3 months for the first year, every 6 months during the second year, and then annually for 5 years after HCT.
- Patients with active chronic GvHD should be monitored every 1 to 3 months or sooner if clinically indicated.

- Patients who responded well to therapy for chronic GvHD with subsequent discontinuation of systemic immunosuppression should be monitored every 1 to 3 months for 6 months, every 3 to 6 months for 1 year, every 6 to 12 months for 1 year, then annually.

Biomarkers

Biomarkers in chronic GvHD are critically needed to facilitate development and evaluation of new therapies. Unfortunately, there are no reliable laboratory indicators of the onset or severity of chronic GvHD. Potential areas for applications of biomarkers in chronic GvHD include: predicting risk for development of chronic GvHD, diagnosis and assessment of chronic GvHD, predicting response to therapy, and as a surrogate endpoint in clinical trials. Approaches to identification of biomarkers include hypothesis driven testing and discovery-based methods analyzing large numbers of samples in prospective clinical trials. Several candidate biomarkers have been proposed for further investigation including soluble BAFF, Tregs, antidouble strand DNA, soluble IL2-receptor alpha, soluble CD13, and soluble CXCL9. However, their ability to diagnose chronic GvHD or predict response to therapy is not well defined. The 2015 NIH Biomarker Working Group Report provides a framework for biomarker investigation including identification, verification, qualification, and application[23].

Quality of Life

Chronic GvHD is frequently associated with significant impairment of QoL and reduction of functionality, resulting both from the disease itself and immunosuppressive therapy [8,10,50]. QoL measures reflect patient experience of the disease, rather than the disease severity. These questionnaires are typically administered as self-reported assessments that provide a measure of overall satisfaction with life and sense of well-being. A very practical 30-item chronic GvHD symptom-specific QoL questionnaire has been developed and validated for use in practice and clinical trials of chronic GvHD[50]. The questionnaire asks patients to indicate the degree of bother that they experienced during the past 4 weeks due to the chronic GvHD. Published evidence supports its validity and sensitivity for the assessment of chronic GvHD severity. Further details on QoL after HCT are discussed in Chapter 71.

Graft-*versus*-Leukemia Effect

Chronic GvHD is associated with an important GvL therapeutic effect. Patients who developed chronic GvHD, regardless of its severity, have lower rates of malignancy relapse than those without chronic GvHD. Although NRM increases significantly with severe chronic GvHD, mild chronic GvHD does not increase mortality while preserving GvL effect[31]. Therefore, overly aggressive immunosuppressive therapy of mild chronic GvHD may potentially attenuate GvL effect and increase the risk of relapse, while putting the patient at additional risk for opportunistic infections. Strategies to augment GvL effect are discussed in Chapter 65.

Controversies and Future Directions

Research into the pathogenesis and therapy of acute GvHD has attracted funding from government and industry sources, while studies of the chronic GvHD biology have been noticeably lacking. Currently there is no FDA-approved treatment for chronic GvHD, and the incidence of this complication among the transplant population is rising. The 2005 NIH consensus criteria provided guidelines and a platform to study chronic GvHD for the very first time. Many papers have been published validating and exploring these criteria. The research field in chronic GvHD is now better organized and research momentum has intensified. Thus, it is an ideal time to pursue basic and translation studies which can enhance our understanding of the mechanisms of this complex disorder with the hope of improving treatment options for affected patients. Development of more effective treatments for chronic GvHD is an urgent unmet clinical need. In addition, it is essential to develop response criteria qualified for regulatory approval of new agents. Identification and characterization of measurable primary endpoints for clinical trials, without the need for years of follow-up, is essential. The 2014 NIH Consensus Conference provides further evidence-based refinement, clarifications, and standardization of criteria for diagnosis and staging, histopathology, biomarkers, measurement of response to therapy, ancillary and supportive care, and design of clinical trials, and hopefully will help the field move forward. However, these recommendations will still need to be tested in further prospective chronic GvHD therapeutic trials. Methods are needed to differentiate active chronic GvHD from irreversible damage. In addition, patients with chronic GvHD often have multifactorial etiologies to explain their abnormalities. Currently, on these occasions the abnormality is scored as if the entire deficit is due to GvHD, although it might not entirely be so. This limitation of the scoring system is unavoidable until better quantitative tests are available to assess chronic GvHD. Another source of controversy has been the new subclassification of chronic GvHD and the inclusion of "overlap" syndrome, for features of acute GvHD in a patient diagnosed with chronic GvHD. This subcategory has been associated with worse survival compared to "classic" chronic GvHD is some studies. However, the overlap syndrome is often transient, highly dependable on the degree of immunosuppression, and a potential cause of confusion among investigators. The 2014 NIH criteria recommend documentation of all clinical features in patients with chronic GvHD that are relevant for prognosis or treatment guidance. Ultimately, the development and validation of laboratory biomarkers reflecting chronic GvHD activity will be needed to enhance clinical assessment.

References

1. Arai S, Arora M, Wang T, Spellman SR, He W, Courie DR, et al. Increasing incidence of chronic graft-*versus*-host disease in allogeneic transplantation: A report from the Center for International Blood and Marrow Transplant Research. *Biol Blood Marrow Transplant*. 2015;21(2):266–74. PubMed PMID: WOS:000348632700009. English.

2. Perez-Simon JA, Encinas C, Silva F, Arcos MJ, Diez-Campelo M, Sanchez-Guijo FM, et al. Prognostic factors of chronic graft-*versus*-host disease following allogeneic peripheral blood stem cell transplantation: the national institutes health scale plus the type of onset can predict survival rates and the duration of immunosuppressive therapy. *Biol Blood Marrow Transplant*. 2008;14(10):1163–71. PubMed PMID: 18804047.

3. Kuzmina Z, Eder S, Bohm A, Pernicka E, Vormittag L, Kalhs P, et al. Significantly worse survival of patients with NIH-defined chronic graft-*versus*-host disease and thrombocytopenia or progressive onset type: results of a prospective study. *Leukemia*. 2012;26(4):746–56. PubMed PMID: 21926960.

4. Arai S, Jagasia M, Storer B, Chai X, Pidala J, Cutler C, et al. Global and organ-specific chronic graft-*versus*-host disease severity according to the 2005 NIH Consensus Criteria. *Blood*. 2011;118(15):4242–9. PubMed PMID: 21791424. Pubmed Central PMCID: 3204740.

5. Jacobsohn DA, Kurland BF, Pidala J, Inamoto Y, Chai X, Palmer JM, et al. Correlation between NIH composite skin score, patient-reported skin score, and outcome: results from the Chronic GVHD Consortium. *Blood*. 2012;120(13):2545–52; quiz 774. PubMed PMID: 22773386. Pubmed Central PMCID: 3460679.

6. Inamoto Y, Chai X, Kurland BF, Cutler C, Flowers ME, Palmer JM, et al. Validation of measurement scales in ocular graft-*versus*-host disease. *Ophthalmology*. 2012;119(3):487–93. PubMed PMID: 22153706. Pubmed Central PMCID: 3294118.

7. Arora M, Pidala J, Cutler CS, Chai X, Kurland B, Jacobsohn DA, et al. Impact of prior acute GvHD on chronic GvHD outcomes: a chronic graft *versus* host

disease consortium study. *Leukemia*. 2013;27(5):1196–201. PubMed PMID: 23047477.

8. Pidala J, Kurland B, Chai X, Majhail N, Weisdorf DJ, Pavletic S, et al. Patient-reported quality of life is associated with severity of chronic graft-*versus*-host disease as measured by NIH criteria: report on baseline data from the Chronic GvHD Consortium. *Blood*. 2011;117(17):4651–7. PubMed PMID: 21355084. Pubmed Central PMCID: 3099579.

9. Pidala J, Chai X, Kurland BF, Inamoto Y, Flowers ME, Palmer J, et al. Analysis of gastrointestinal and hepatic chronic grant-*versus*-host disease manifestations on major outcomes: a chronic grant-*versus*-host disease consortium study. *Biol Blood Marrow Transplant*. 2013;19(5):784–91. PubMed PMID: 23395601. Pubmed Central PMCID: 3896215.

10. Pidala J, Kurland BF, Chai X, Vogelsang G, Weisdorf DJ, Pavletic S, et al. Sensitivity of changes in chronic graft-*versus*-host disease activity to changes in patient-reported quality of life: results from the Chronic Graft-*versus*-Host Disease Consortium. *Haematologica*. 2011;96(10):1528–35. PubMed PMID: 21685473. Pubmed Central PMCID: 3186315.

11. Pidala J, Vogelsang G, Martin P, Chai X, Storer B, Pavletic S, et al. Overlap subtype of chronic graft-*versus*-host disease is associated with an adverse prognosis, functional impairment, and inferior patient-reported outcomes: a Chronic Graft-*versus*-Host Disease Consortium study. *Haematologica*. 2012;97(3):451–8. PubMed PMID: 22058206. Pubmed Central PMCID: 3291602.

12. Vigorito AC, Campregher PV, Storer BE, Carpenter PA, Moravec CK, Kiem HP, et al. Evaluation of NIH consensus criteria for classification of late acute and chronic GVHD. *Blood*. 2009;114(3):702–8. PubMed PMID: 19470693. Pubmed Central PMCID: 2713471.

13. Baird K, Steinberg SM, Grkovic L, Pulanic D, Cowen EW, Mitchell SA, et al. National Institutes of Health chronic graft-*versus*-host disease staging in severely affected patients: organ and global scoring correlate with established indicators of disease severity and prognosis. *Biol Blood Marrow Transplant*. 2013;19(4):632–9. PubMed

PMID: 23340040. Pubmed Central PMCID: 3619213.

14. Jagasia M, Giglia J, Chinratanalab W, Dixon S, Chen H, Frangoul H, et al. Incidence and outcome of chronic graft-*versus*-host disease using National Institutes of Health consensus criteria. *Biol Blood Marrow Transplant*. 2007;13(10):1207–15. PubMed PMID: 17889358.

15. Arora M, Nagaraj S, Witte J, DeFor TE, MacMillan M, Burns LJ, et al. New classification of chronic GvHD: added clarity from the consensus diagnoses. *Bone Marrow Transplant*. 2009;43(2):149–53. PubMed PMID: 18794869.

16. Flowers ME, Inamoto Y, Carpenter PA, Lee SJ, Kiem HP, Petersdorf EW, et al. Comparative analysis of risk factors for acute graft-*versus*-host disease and for chronic graft-*versus*-host disease according to National Institutes of Health consensus criteria. *Blood*. 2011;117(11):3214–9. PubMed PMID: 21263156. Pubmed Central PMCID: 3062319.

17. Aki SZ, Inamoto Y, Barry; S, Carpenter P, Lee S, Martin P, et al. Confounding Factors Affecting the National Institutes of Health (NIH) Chronic GVHD Organ-Specific Score and Global Severity. *Biol Blood Marrow Transplant*. 2014;20:265.

18. Arora M, Klein JP, Weisdorf DJ, Hassebroek A, Flowers ME, Cutler CS, et al. Chronic GVHD risk score: a Center for International Blood and Marrow Transplant Research analysis. *Blood*. 2011;117(24):6714-20. PubMed PMID: 21493797. Pubmed Central PMCID: 3123030.

19. Palmer J, Williams K, Inamoto Y, Chai X, Martin PJ, Tomas LS, et al. Pulmonary symptoms measured by the national institutes of health lung score predict overall survival, nonrelapse mortality, and patient-reported outcomes in chronic graft-*versus*-host disease. *Biol Blood Marrow Transplant*. 2014;20(3):337–44. PubMed PMID: 24315845. Pubmed Central PMCID: 3973401.

20. Jagasia MH, Greinix HT, Arora M, Williams KM, Wolff D, Cowen EW, et al. National Institutes of Health Consensus Development Project on Criteria for Clinical Trials in Chronic Graft-*versus*-Host Disease: I. The 2014 Diagnosis and Staging Working Group Report. *Biol Blood Marrow Transplant*. 2015;21(3):389–401 e1.

PubMed PMID: 25529383. Pubmed Central PMCID: 4329079.

21. Carpenter PA, Kitko CL, Elad S, Flowers ME, Gea-Banacloche JC, Halter JP, *et al.* National Institutes of Health Consensus Development Project on Criteria for Clinical Trials in Chronic Graft-*versus*-Host Disease: V. The 2014 Ancillary Therapy and Supportive Care Working Group Report. *Biol Blood Marrow Transplant.* 2015 Mar 31. PubMed PMID: 25838185.

22. Shulman HM, Cardona DM, Greenson JK, Hingorani S, Horn T, Huber E, *et al.* NIH Consensus development project on criteria for clinical trials in chronic graft-*versus*-host disease: II. The 2014 Pathology Working Group Report. *Biol Blood Marrow Transplant.* 2015;21(4):589–603. PubMed PMID: 25639770. Pubmed Central PMCID: 4359636.

23. Paczesny S, Hakim FT, Pidala J, Cooke KR, Lathrop J, Griffith LM, *et al.* National Institutes of Health Consensus Development Project on Criteria for Clinical Trials in Chronic Graft-*versus*-Host Disease: III. The 2014 Biomarker Working Group Report. *Biol Blood Marrow Transplant.* 2015;21(5):780–92. PubMed PMID: 25644957. Pubmed Central PMCID: 4408233.

24. Lee SJ, Wolff D, Kitko C, Koreth J, Inamoto Y, Jagasia M, *et al.* Measuring Therapeutic Response in Chronic Graft-*versus*-Host Disease. National Institutes of Health Consensus Development Project on Criteria for Clinical Trials in Chronic Graft-*versus*-Host Disease: IV. The 2014 Response Criteria Working Group Report. *Biol Blood Marrow Transplant.* 2015;21(6):984–99. PubMed PMID: 25796139.

25. Martin PJ, Lee SJ, Przepiorka D, Horowitz MM, Koreth J, Vogelsang GB, *et al.* National Institutes of Health Consensus Development Project on Criteria for Clinical Trials in Chronic Graft-*versus*-Host Disease: VI. The 2014 Clinical Trial Design Working Group Report. *Biol Blood Marrow Transplant.* 2015 May 15. PubMed PMID: 25985921.

26. Choi J, Ziga ED, Ritchey J, Collins L, Prior JL, Cooper ML, *et al.* IFNgammaR signaling mediates alloreactive T-cell trafficking and GVHD. *Blood.* 2012;120(19):4093-103. PubMed PMID: 22972985. Pubmed Central PMCID: 3496960.

27. Magenau JM, Qin X, Tawara I, Rogers CE, Kitko C, Schlough M, *et al.* Frequency of CD4(+)CD25(hi)FOXP3(+) regulatory T cells has diagnostic and prognostic value as a biomarker for acute graft-*versus*-host-disease. *Biol Blood Marrow Transplant.* 2010;16(7):907-14. PubMed PMID: 20302964. Pubmed Central PMCID: 2916071.

28. Allen JL, Fore MS, Wooten J, Roehrs PA, Bhuiya NS, Hoffert T, *et al.* B cells from patients with chronic GVHD are activated and primed for survival via BAFF-mediated pathways. *Blood.* 2012;120(12):2529–36. PubMed PMID: 22896003. Pubmed Central PMCID: 3448264.

29. Subramaniam DS, Fowler DH, Pavletic SZ. Chronic graft-*versus*-host disease in the era of reduced-intensity conditioning. *Leukemia.* 2007 Mar 22. PubMed PMID: 17377592. eng.

30. Valcarcel D, Sierra J, Wang T, Kan F, Gupta V, Hale GA, *et al.* One-antigen mismatched related *versus* HLA-matched unrelated donor hematopoietic stem cell transplantation in adults with acute leukemia: Center for International Blood and Marrow Transplant Research results in the era of molecular HLA typing. *Biol Blood Marrow Transplant.* 2011;17(5):640–8. PubMed PMID: 20674756. Pubmed Central PMCID: 3355271.

31. Lee SJ, Klein JP, Barrett AJ, Ringden O, Antin JH, Cahn JY, *et al.* Severity of chronic graft-*versus*-host disease: association with treatment-related mortality and relapse. *Blood.* 2002;100(2):406-14. PubMed PMID: 12091329. eng.

32. Moore J, Nivison-Smith I, Goh K, Ma D, Bradstock K, Szer J, *et al.* Equivalent survival for sibling and unrelated donor allogeneic stem cell transplantation for acute myelogenous leukemia. *Biol Blood Marrow Transplant.* 2007;13(5):601–7. PubMed PMID: 17448920.

33. al Jurf M, Aranha F, Annassetti C, Apperley JF, Baynes R, Bensinger WI, *et al.* Allogeneic peripheral blood stem-cell compared with bone marrow transplantation in the management of hematologic malignancies: An individual patient data meta-analysis of nine randomized trials. *J Clin Oncol.* 2005;23(22):5074–87.

34. Anasetti C, Logan BR, Lee SJ, Waller EK, Weisdorf DJ, Wingard JR, *et al.* Peripheral-blood stem cells *versus* bone marrow from unrelated donors. *N Engl J Med.* 2012;367(16):1487–96. PubMed PMID: 23075175. Pubmed Central PMCID: 3816375.

35. Morton J, Hutchins C, Durrant S. Granulocyte-colony-stimulating factor (G-CSF)-primed allogeneic bone marrow: significantly less graft-*versus*-host disease and comparable engraftment to G-CSF-mobilized peripheral blood stem cells. *Blood.* 2001;98(12):3186–91. PubMed PMID: 11719353. eng.

36. Majhail NS, Chitphakdithai P, Logan B, King R, Devine S, Rossmann SN, *et al.* Significant improvement in survival after unrelated donor hematopoietic cell transplantation in the recent era. *Biol Blood Marrow Transplant.* 2015;21(1):142–50. PubMed PMID: 25445638. Pubmed Central PMCID: 4272902.

37. Weisdorf DJ, Nelson G, Lee SJ, Haagenson M, Spellman S, Antin JH, *et al.* Sibling *versus* unrelated donor allogeneic hematopoietic cell transplantation for chronic myelogenous leukemia: refined HLA matching reveals more graft-*versus*-host disease but not less relapse. *Biol Blood Marrow Transplant.* 2009;15(11):1475–8. PubMed PMID: 19822308. Pubmed Central PMCID: 2929002.

38. Balon J, Halaburda K, Bieniaszewska M, Reichert M, Bieniaszewski L, Piekarska A, *et al.* Early complete donor hematopoietic chimerism in peripheral blood indicates the risk of extensive graft-*versus*-host disease. *Bone Marrow Transplant.* 2005;35(11):1083–8. PubMed PMID: 15821766. eng.

39. Pavletic SZ, Carter SL, Kernan NA, Henslee-Downey J, Mendizabal AM, Papadopoulos E, *et al.* Influence of T-cell depletion on chronic graft-*versus*-host disease: results of a multicenter randomized trial in unrelated marrow donor transplantation. *Blood.* 2005;106(9):3308-13. PubMed PMID: 16046530. eng.

40. Filipovich AH, Weisdorf D, Pavletic S, Socie G, Wingard JR, Lee SJ, *et al.* National Institutes of Health consensus development project on criteria for clinical trials in chronic graft-*versus*-host disease: I. Diagnosis and staging working group report. *Biol Blood Marrow Transplant.* 2005;11(12):945-56. PubMed PMID: 16338616.

41. Jacobsohn DA, Arora M, Klein JP, Hassebroek A, Flowers ME, Cutler CS,

et al. Risk factors associated with increased nonrelapse mortality and with poor overall survival in children with chronic graft-*versus*-host disease. *Blood.* 2011;118(16):4472–9. PubMed PMID: 21878671. Pubmed Central PMCID: 3204914.

42. Cho BS, Min CK, Eom KS, Kim YJ, Kim HJ, Lee S, *et al.* Feasibility of NIH consensus criteria for chronic graft-*versus*-host disease. *Leukemia.* 2009;23 (1):78–84. PubMed PMID: 18830253.

43. Stewart BL, Storer B, Storek J, Deeg HJ, Storb R, Hansen JA, *et al.* Duration of immunosuppressive treatment for chronic graft-*versus*-host disease. *Blood.* 2004 1;104(12):3501–6. PubMed PMID: 15292060.

44. Wolff D, Schleuning M, von Harsdorf S, Bacher U, Gerbitz A, Stadler M, *et al.* Consensus Conference on Clinical Practice in Chronic GVHD: Second-Line Treatment of Chronic Graft-*versus*-Host Disease. *Biol Blood Marrow Transplant.* 2011;17(1):1–17. PubMed PMID: 20685255.

45. Inamoto Y, Flowers ME. Treatment of chronic graft-*versus*-host disease in 2011. *Curr Opin Hematol.* 2011;18 (6):414-20. PubMed PMID: 21912257. Pubmed Central PMCID: 3276600.

46. Cutler C, Miklos D, Kim HT, Treister N, Woo SB, Bienfang D, *et al.* Rituximab for steroid-refractory chronic graft-*versus*-host disease. *Blood.* 2006;108(2):756-62. PubMed PMID: 16551963.

47. Lopez F, Parker P, Nademanee A, Rodriguez R, Al-Kadhimi Z, Bhatia R, *et al.* Efficacy of mycophenolate mofetil in the treatment of chronic graft-*versus*-host disease. *Biol Blood Marrow Transplant.* 2005;11(4):307-13. PubMed PMID: 15812396.

48. Couriel D, Hosing C, Saliba R, Shpall EJ, Andelini P, Popat U, *et al.* Extracorporeal photopheresis for acute and chronic graft-*versus*-host disease: does it work? *Biol Blood Marrow Transplant.* 2006 (1 Suppl 2):37–40. PubMed PMID: 16399600. eng.

49. Couriel DR, Saliba R, Escalon MP, Hsu Y, Ghosh S, Ippoliti C, *et al.* Sirolimus in combination with tacrolimus and corticosteroids for the treatment of resistant chronic graft-*versus*-host disease. *Br J Haematol.* 2005;130(3):409-17. PubMed PMID: 16042691.

50. Lee SJ, Kim HT, Ho VT, Cutler C, Alyea EP, Soiffer RJ, *et al.* Quality of life associated with acute and chronic graft-*versus*-host disease. *Bone Marrow Transplant.* 2006;38(4):305-10. PubMed PMID: 16819438.

Chapter 20

Epstein–Barr Virus-Driven Lymphoproliferation: Surveillance and Therapy

Lode J. Swinnen

Introduction

Epstein–Barr virus (EBV)-driven lymphoproliferations are a complication of immunosuppression following solid organ transplantation, allogeneic hematopoietic cell transplant (allo-HCT), and congenital immunodeficiency states. A range of histopathologies is embodied in the current WHO classification of post-transplantation lymphoproliferative disorder (PTLD), extending from hyperplasia to monomorphic histologies resembling diffuse large B-cell lymphoma and multiple myeloma. Lymphoproliferations following allo-HCT are typically of B-cell origin. Following allo-HCT, the vast majority of lymphoproliferations occur in the first post-transplant year, whereas in solid organ recipients, the cumulative incidence continues to increase over time. This difference has been ascribed to the fact that immunosuppressives are not continued indefinitely in allograft recipients. In the organ transplant setting, it has been recognized that PTLD occurring at very late time points may be quite different from what is seen earlier after transplantation, manifesting as primarily monomorphic histologies, with T-cell or EBV-negative tumors[1]. A recent study of a large cohort of patients reported to the Center for International Blood and Marrow Transplant Research (CIBMTR) of almost 27 000 allotransplant recipients, among whom 127 cases of PTLD were identified, provides some quantitative data on incidence, risk factors, and the occurrence of late PTLD following HCT[2]. The peak in incidence was at 2 to 3 months after transplantation and incidence declined rapidly after that. No cases of polymorphic lymphoproliferation were seen later than 18 months. However, new cases of PTLD were seen beyond 10 years following transplantation, with chronic GvHD identified as a risk factor for such late presentation. EBV-driven lymphoproliferation in latently infected B-cells is believed to result from a reduction in EBV-specific T-cell mediated immunity.

Risk Factors and Patterns of EBV-Driven Lymphoproliferation

The overall incidence of PTLD after allo-HCT is low at approximately 1%[3]. A number of risk factors for lymphoproliferative disease following allo-HCT have been identified from small series and large-scale registry data[2]. T-cell

Table 20.1 Risk factors for EBV-driven lymphoproliferation after allogeneic HCT

Selective T-cell depletion of allograft

Antithymocyte globulin (ATG)

HLA-mismatched allograft

Graft-versus-host disease (GvHD)

Age >50 years

EBV naïve donor

depletion of the graft, the use of antithymocyte globulin (ATG), unrelated or HLA-mismatched allografts, the occurrence of graft-versus-host disease (GvHD), and patient age greater than 50 years were all found to be associated with an increased risk of PTLD (Table 20.1). Selective T-cell depletion of the allograft carried an 8–15 times higher risk, and was the single greatest risk factor. The incidence of PTLD was 0.2% in patients without identified risk factors, 1.1%, 3.6%, and 8.1% in patients with 1, 2, and more than three risk factors, respectively. What is of particular value in the recent large study by Landgren et al. is the quantitative assessment of risk, and an exploration of why mismatched or unrelated transplantation might confer risk. Increased risk among mismatched or unrelated donor allografts was only found in the setting of T-cell depletion or ATG use. Furthermore, T-cell-depletion strategies that deplete both B-cells and T-cells carried less risk. Highly potent and selective T-cell depletion by means of monoclonal anti-T-cell antibodies has been used in the past, but has been abandoned in part because of the very high risk of lymphoproliferation[3,4]. Further emphasizing the importance of the specific regimens used is the report of a single-center experience of 526 HLA haplotype matched or unrelated donor transplants using post-transplant cyclophosphamide; no cases of PTLD were seen during the first post-transplant year. Preservation of pre-existing antiviral T-cell immunity was suggested as a possible contributory mechanism[5]. A recent retrospective study in organ transplant recipients suggests that specific immunosuppressive agents may affect not only the incidence of PTLD, but also its clinical manifestation[6]. The use of mycophenolate mofetil was associated with a higher likelihood of central nervous system involvement, and the concurrent use

Table 20.2 Therapeutic modalities for EBV-driven lymphoproliferation after allogeneic HCT

Immunosuppressive reduction

Rituximab

Donor-derived EBV-specific CTL[a]

Third-party HLA-matched EBV-specific CTL*

Cytotoxic chemotherapy

[a] See Chapter 64.

of calcineurin inhibitors appeared to protect against such involvement. Following solid organ transplantation, an initial EBV infection occurring in the setting of impaired immunity has long been recognized as the single strongest risk factor for PTLD[7]. Pretransplantation EBV seronegativity, of the donor in the case of allo-HCT, is a concern mainly encountered in the pediatric group as the vast majority of adults are EBV seropositive. Interestingly, a roughly fourfold higher incidence of PTLD has recently been reported following unrelated cord blood transplantation (CBT) for adult recipients. The allograft in this case is not expected to have been exposed to EBV, while more than 90% of the adult recipients were EBV seropositive. All the lymphoproliferations tested were EBV-associated and of donor origin[8]. Both myeloablative and reduced intensity conditioning (RIC) was used, with a number of different conditioning regimens. The risk was highest after RIC regimen at 12.6% 3-year cumulative incidence; the use of ATG with CBT had previously been identified as a particular risk factor[9].

Treatment of EBV-Driven Lymphoproliferation: Immunosuppression Withdrawal and Rituximab

The management of EBV-driven lymphoproliferation following allo-HCT has been studied less extensively than is the case for PTLD following solid organ transplantation. However, several recent studies in large numbers of patients specifically addressing the problem in the setting of allo-HCT have provided useful data on outcome for specific treatment modalities. PTLD following solid organ transplantation can be managed with immunosuppressive reduction, rituximab monotherapy, or cytotoxic chemotherapy, usually applied in a progressive fashion[10,11] (Table 20.2). Cytotoxic chemotherapy has been problematic due to immunodeficiency and marrow reserve; no specific regimens can be recommended beyond what is generally used in the immunocompetent population.

A large retrospective study by the European Group for Blood and Marrow Transplantation (EBMT) assessed treatment results for 144 PTLD cases among 4466 transplant recipients[12]. All patients received rituximab, typically weekly, for a median of three doses. In 355 cases, immunosuppressive reduction, defined as >20% reduction in daily immunosuppressive dosage, was also applied. Disease resolution was seen in 84% of patients treated with both immunosuppressive reduction and rituximab, and in 61% of cases treated with rituximab alone. Chemotherapy was used for disease not responsive to rituximab in 31 patients, of whom 52% were deemed to have survived PTLD, although only 35% survived overall. Overall mortality for PTLD in this series was 30.6%, considerably better than the 88% mortality reported in a large series that predated the use of rituximab[3]. Of note, patients in whom immunosuppressive reduction was applied had a 2.8-fold lower PTLD mortality than those in whom it was not.

T-Cell Therapy: How Effective and Will It Cause GvHD?

A number of adoptive T-cell immunotherapy strategies have been effective in the treatment of EBV-associated lymphoproliferative disorder following allo-HCT. Restoration of EBV-directed immunocompetence has been achieved by infusion of unmanipulated donor peripheral blood mononuclear cells in pediatric recipients of T-cell-depleted allografts who developed PTLD. A dose of 105 to 106 CD3+ cells/kg was administered. Response rates of 40–90% are reported. Although one tenth or less of the dose usually used for donor lymphocyte infusion (DLI) was administered, the development of subsequent acute or chronic GvHD remains a significant problem[12–16]. The administration of EBV-specific cytotoxic T-cells (CTL) rather than unselected donor T-cells is therefore an attractive approach (see Chapter 64). Polyclonal donor T-cells stimulated with irradiated EBV-transformed lymphoblastoid cells and expanded *in-vitro* have been used successfully for the treatment of PTLD[17–19]. A comparison of unmanipulated donor lymphocytes and EBV-specific CTL showed an acute GvHD rate of 17% compared to none, with comparable response rates of around 70% [16]. Lymphoproliferations resistant to rituximab have responded to T-cell therapy. Treatment failure has been associated with poor *in-vivo* expansion of the infused cells, and with the emergence of nonshared HLA alleles. Recently reported approaches using methods other than antigenic stimulation by EBV-transformed lymphoblastoid cells promise to shorten production time from the current 2 weeks or more[20–22].

Third-Party EBV-Specific T-Cells: Production Time, GvHD, and Efficacy?

The time required to generate EBV-specific CTL is a significant drawback, as PTLD is often rapidly progressive following allogeneic HCT. In addition, many pediatric donors, the occasional adult donor, and all cord blood donors are EBV naïve, with no pre-existing EBV-specific CTLs to collect and expand. For all these reasons, a bank of immediately available third-party HLA-matched EBV-specific CTLs would be desirable.

Such a bank of 100 CTLs was created from Scottish blood donors, allowing at least partial HLA-matching to the majority of the UK population. A pilot trial and subsequent phase 2 study were performed for the treatment of PTLD refractory to other treatments, almost entirely in solid organ transplant recipients. Among 33 patients, the response rate was 52% at 6 months. Long-term follow-up of the pilot trial participants showed durability of complete responses, with 89% of CR patients remaining in remission at 4–9 years[23–25]. Cell banks using relatively few donors but representing HLA types seen at high frequency in the relevant population have been established[26–28]. Calcineurin-resistant EBV-specific CTL with activity was created in a murine model of PTLD despite continuation of immunosuppressive therapy[29]. Response to third-party EBV-CTL therapy has been correlated with the extent of HLA matching, the dose of cells given, and the extent to which cells proliferated following infusion. HLA matching is likely to be more problematic in populations with more heterogeneous demographics. Toxicity of EBV-specific CTLs, whether third party or expanded from the marrow donor, has been very limited. GvHD has not clearly been a problem, although one case of systemic inflammatory response syndrome has been reported[30].

Controversies

Trigger for Preemptive Intervention, Best Preemptive Protocol and Prophylactic NOT Preemptive Therapy: Do We Know the Best Strategy?

Even in the case of a bank with pre-existing product, timing remains important: among 37 enquiries, 13 patients died before cells could be issued[26]. The ability to screen for the development of EBV-driven lymphoproliferation, and intervene preemptively, would therefore be desirable. Some evidence that early intervention is effective exists, in the form of a study of allo-HCT recipients deemed to be at high-risk (Table 20.1). Outcome was compared to historical controls [31]. EBV viral load (EBV–DNAemia by PCR) monitoring, resulting in preemptive therapy (viral load >1000 copies/mL with negative CT scan for lymphadenopathy) or treatment (viral load >1000 copies/mL with positive biopsy) at an earlier stage of disease, was believed to have resulted in a reduced mortality from EBV-related lymphoproliferation of 6% *versus*

the 29% (OR 0.2; 95% CI 0.05–0.9, $P=0.03$) seen in historical controls. In the same study, if the EBV load <1000 copies/mL without clinical signs or symptoms of PTLD then need for close monitoring was indicated, with a second EBV test by PCR being performed within 2–3 days. A study of 64 patients using EBV viral load monitoring following allo-HCT to trigger a stepwise preemptive strategy consisting of immunosuppressive reduction and antiviral therapy followed, if necessary, by rituximab administration, has been reported[32]. EBV DNA was considered positive when the copies were more than or equal to 500 copies/mL and patients experiencing blood EBV DNA-positive twice consecutively were considered for preemptive therapy. Response was defined as control of the EBV DNA viremia. Thirty-seven percent of patients responded to immunosuppressive reduction plus antiviral therapy; 14/15 treated with rituximab responded. However, the investigators advocated against antiviral therapy but early employment of rituximab in high-risk populations for PTLD (Table 20.1). A retrospective study (n=55) of post-transplantation rituximab 200 mg (fixed dose) on day+5 of ATG-based allo-HCT ("prophylactic *Not* preemptive") showed a significant reduction in the frequency of EBV viremia (56 *versus* 85%, $P=0.0004$), and also a reduced incidence of acute GvHD (20 *versus* 38%, $P=0.02$) in the group that received rituximab compared to the group who did not (n=68)[33]. The investigators concluded that the optimal dose and timing remains to be determined in a prospective trial.

Conclusion

EBV viral load monitoring is widely used following allo-HCT or solid organ transplantation. Neither methodologies for EBV viral load monitoring nor the precise parameters to apply are well defined. The efficacy of preemptive intervention is based on small series with varying methodologies. At this point in time, some form of EBV viral load monitoring appears to be warranted, particularly in high-risk subgroups (Table 20.1), if only to heighten clinical awareness of the possibility of PTLD in this group of patients. Although immunosuppressive reduction may be problematic, the preemptive use of rituximab has shown some efficacy and has so far not been associated with negative consequences in terms of engraftment or GvHD[34].

References

1. Leblond V, Davi F, Charlotte F, Dorent R, Bitker MO, Sutton L et al. Post-transplant lymphoproliferative disorders not associated with Epstein–Barr virus: a distinct entity? *J Clin Oncol* 1998; 16(6):2052-2059.

2. Landgren O, Gilbert ES, Rizzo JD, Socie G, Banks PM, Sobocinski KA et al. Risk factors for lymphoproliferative

disorders after allogeneic hematopoietic cell transplantation. *Blood* 2009; 113(20):4992-5001.

3. Curtis RE, Travis LB, Rowlings PA, Socie G, Kingma DW, Banks PM et al. Risk of lymphoproliferative disorders after bone marrow transplantation: a multi-institutional study. *Blood* 1999; 94(7):2208-2216.

4. Swinnen LJ, Costanzo-Nordin MR, Fisher SG, O'Sullivan EJ, Johnson MR,

Heroux AL et al. Increased incidence of lymphoproliferative disorder after immunosuppression with the monoclonal antibody OKT3 in cardiac-transplant recipients. *New Engl J Med* 1990; 323:1723-1728.

5. Kanakry JA, Kasamon YL, Bolanos-Meade J, Borrello IM, Brodsky RA, Fuchs EJ et al. Absence of post-transplantation lymphoproliferative disorder after allogeneic blood or

marrow transplantation using post-transplantation cyclophosphamide as graft-*versus*-host disease prophylaxis. *Biol Blood Marrow Transplant* 2013; 19(10):1514-1517.

6. Crane G, Powell H, Kostadinov R, Ambinder RF, Swinnen LJ, Borrowitz M et al. A Rise in CNS lymphoproliferative disease incidence reveals a protective role of calcineurin inhibitors. *Proc ASH* 2014;3020.

7. Ho M, Jaffe R, Miller G, Breinig MK, Dummer JS, Makowka L et al. The frequency of Epstein–Barr virus infection and associated lymphoproliferative syndrome after transplantation and its manifestations in children. *Transplantation* 1988; 45:719-727.

8. Sanz J, Arango M, Senent L, Jarque I, Montesinos P, Sempere A et al. EBV-associated post-transplant lymphoproliferative disorder after umbilical cord blood transplantation in adults with hematological diseases. *Bone Marrow Transplant* 2014; 49(3):397-402.

9. Blaes AH, Cao Q, Wagner JE, Young JA, Weisdorf DJ, Brunstein CG. Monitoring and preemptive rituximab therapy for Epstein–Barr virus reactivation after antithymocyte globulin containing nonmyeloablative conditioning for umbilical cord blood transplantation. *Biol Blood Marrow Transplant* 2010; 16(2):287-291.

10. Swinnen LJ, LeBlanc M, Grogan TM, Gordon LI, Stiff PJ, Miller AM et al. Prospective study of sequential reduction in immunosuppression, interferon alpha-2B, and chemotherapy for posttransplantation lymphoproliferative disorder. *Transplantation* 2008; 86(2):215-222.

11. Trappe R, Oertel S, Leblond V, Mollee P, Sender M, Reinke P et al. Sequential treatment with rituximab followed by CHOP chemotherapy in adult B-cell post-transplant lymphoproliferative disorder (PTLD): the prospective international multicentre phase 2 PTLD-1 trial. *Lancet Oncol* 2012; 13(2):196-206.

12. Styczynski J, Gil L, Tridello G, Ljungman P, Donnelly JP, van d, V et al. Response to rituximab-based therapy and risk factor analysis in Epstein Barr Virus-related lymphoproliferative disorder after hematopoietic stem cell transplant in children and adults: a study from the Infectious Diseases Working Party of the European Group for Blood and Marrow Transplantation. *Clin Infect Dis* 2013; 57(6):794-802.

13. Papadopoulos EB, Ladanyi M, Emanuel D, Mackinnon S, Boulad F, Carabasi MH et al. Infusions of donor leukocytes to treat Epstein–Barr virus-associated lymphoproliferative disorders after allogeneic bone marrow transplantation. *N Engl J Med* 1994; 330(17):1185-1191.

14. O'Reilly RJ, Small TN, Papadopoulos E, Lucas K, Lacerda J, Koulova L. Biology and adoptive cell therapy of Epstein–Barr virus-associated lymphoproliferative disorders in recipients of marrow allografts. [Review] [186 refs]. *Immunol Rev* 1997; 157:195-216.

15. Bollard CM, Rooney CM, Heslop HE. T-cell therapy in the treatment of post-transplant lymphoproliferative disease. *Nat Rev Clin Oncol* 2012; 9(9):510-519.

16. Doubrovina E, Oflaz-Sozmen B, Prockop SE, Kernan NA, Abramson S, Teruya-Feldstein J et al. Adoptive immunotherapy with unselected or EBV-specific T cells for biopsy-proven EBV+ lymphomas after allogeneic hematopoietic cell transplantation. *Blood* 2012; 119(11):2644-2656.

17. Bollard CM, Savoldo B, Rooney CM, Heslop HE. Adoptive T-cell therapy for EBV-associated post-transplant lymphoproliferative disease. *Acta Haematol* 2003; 110(2-3):139-148.

18. Rooney CM, Smith CA, Ng CY, Loftin SK, Sixbey JW, Gan Y et al. Infusion of cytotoxic T cells for the prevention and treatment of Epstein–Barr virus-induced lymphoma in allogeneic transplant recipients. *Blood* 1998; 92(5):1549-1555.

19. Gottschalk S, Ng CY, Perez M, Smith CA, Sample C, Brenner MK et al. An Epstein–Barr virus deletion mutant associated with fatal lymphoproliferative disease unresponsive to therapy with virus-specific CTLs. *Blood* 2001; 97(4):835-843.

20. Icheva V, Kayser S, Wolff D, Tuve S, Kyzirakos C, Bethge W et al. Adoptive transfer of Epstein-Barr virus (EBV) nuclear antigen 1-specific t cells as treatment for EBV reactivation and lymphoproliferative disorders after allogeneic stem-cell transplantation. *J Clin Oncol* 2013; 31(1):39-48.

21. Gerdemann U, Katari UL, Papadopoulou A, Keirnan JM, Craddock JA, Liu H et al. Safety and clinical efficacy of rapidly-generated trivirus-directed T cells as treatment for adenovirus, EBV, and CMV infections after allogeneic hematopoietic stem cell transplant. *Mol Ther* 2013; 21(11):2113-2121.

22. Papadopoulou A, Gerdemann U, Katari UL, Tzannou I, Liu H, Martinez C et al. Activity of broad-spectrum T cells as treatment for AdV, EBV, CMV, BKV, and HHV6 infections after HCT. *Sci Transl Med* 2014; 6(242):242ra83.

23. Haque T, Wilkie GM, Taylor C, Amlot PL, Murad P, Iley A et al. Treatment of Epstein–Barr-virus-positive post-transplantation lymphoproliferative disease with partly HLA-matched allogeneic cytotoxic T cells. *Lancet* 2002; 360(9331):436-442.

24. Haque T, Wilkie GM, Jones MM, Higgins CD, Urquhart G, Wingate P et al. Allogeneic cytotoxic T-cell therapy for EBV-positive posttransplantation lymphoproliferative disease: results of a phase 2 multicenter clinical trial. *Blood* 2007; 110(4):1123-1131.

25. Haque T, McAulay KA, Kelly D, Crawford DH. Allogeneic T-cell therapy for Epstein–Barr virus-positive posttransplant lymphoproliferative disease: long-term follow-up. *Transplantation* 2010; 90(1):93-94.

26. Vickers MA, Wilkie GM, Robinson N, Rivera N, Haque T, Crawford DH et al. Establishment and operation of a Good Manufacturing Practice-compliant allogeneic Epstein–Barr virus (EBV)-specific cytotoxic cell bank for the treatment of EBV-associated lymphoproliferative disease. *Br J Haematol* 2014; 167(3):402-410.

27. Leen AM, Bollard CM, Mendizabal AM, Shpall EJ, Szabolcs P, Antin JH et al. Multicenter study of banked third-party virus-specific T cells to treat severe viral infections after hematopoietic stem cell transplantation. *Blood* 2013; 121(26):5113-5123.

28. Gallot G, Vollant S, Saiagh S, Clemenceau B, Vivien R, Cerato E et al. T-cell therapy using a bank of EBV-specific cytotoxic T cells: lessons from a phase I/II feasibility and safety study. *J Immunother* 2014; 37(3):170-179.

29. Ricciardelli I, Blundell MP, Brewin J, Thrasher A, Pule M, Amrolia PJ. Towards gene therapy for EBV-associated posttransplant lymphoma with genetically modified EBV-specific cytotoxic T cells. *Blood* 2014; 124(16):2514-2522.

30. Papadopoulou A, Krance RA, Allen CE, Lee D, Rooney CM, Brenner MK *et al.* Systemic inflammatory response syndrome after administration of unmodified T lymphocytes. *Mol Ther* 2014; 22(6):1134-1138.

31. van d, V, Mori T, Stevens WB, de Haan AF, Stelma FF, Blijlevens NM *et al.* Reduced PTLD-related mortality in patients experiencing EBV infection following allo-SCT after the introduction of a protocol incorporating preemptive rituximab. *Bone Marrow Transplant* 2013; 48(11):1465-1471.

32. Liu Q, Xuan L, Liu H, Huang F, Zhou H, Fan Z *et al.* Molecular monitoring and stepwise preemptive therapy for Epstein–Barr virus viremia after allogeneic stem cell transplantation. *Am J Hematol* 2013; 88(7):550-555.

33. Dominietto A, Tedone E, Soracco M, Bruno B, Raiola AM, Van Lint MT *et al.* In vivo B-cell depletion with rituximab for alternative donor hemopoietic SCT. *Bone Marrow Transplant* 2012; 47(1):101-106.

34. Laport G, Wu J, Logan BR, Bachanova V, Hosing CM, Fenske TS *et al.* Reduced intensity conditioning (RIC) with rituximab yields excellent outcomes after allogeneic hematopoietic cell transplantation (alloHCT) for relapsed follicular lymphoma (FL): a phase ii multicenter trial from the Blood and Marrow Transplant Network (BMT CTN 0701). *Proc ASH* 2014;682.

Chapter

21 Organ-Specific Complications after Hematopoietic Cell Transplants: Practical Considerations and Controversies

Enric Carreras

Introduction

Hematopoietic cell transplantation (HCT) is the therapy of choice for a number of malignant and nonmalignant conditions. Unfortunately, the success of this procedure is limited by several early and late side effects of multifactorial origin, mainly regimen-related toxicity, infections, and graft-*versus*-host disease (GvHD). Early complications are the most relevant because of their immediate impact on survival but, at present, the initial morbi-mortality has decreased notably because of improvements in the patient and donor selection, conditioning regimens, and prevention and management of GvHD. When patients survive for a longer time after HCT, they are at risk of developing late complications related to pre-, peri-, and post-transplant exposures. These complications can cause substantial morbidity, impair quality of life, and contribute to late mortality. Several large studies have shown that, compared with the general population, the mortality rate is 4 to 10 times higher for at least 30 years after HCT and that life expectancy is an estimated 30% lower[1,2].

This chapter analyzes the most controversial and not so well-defined aspects of main organ-specific complications not attributable to infection, GvHD, or malignancy, which are analyzed in other chapters in this book (Table 21.1).

Lungs

Diffuse lung injury remains a significant problem following HCT. It can be observed in the immediate post-HCT period or months and years later in 25–50% of HCT recipients and accounts for about 50% of mortality[3]. We focus on the most relevant complications, idiopathic pneumonia syndrome (IPS) and diffuse alveolar hemorrhage (DAH). The data and controversies are discussed.

Has There Been Improvement in Establishing the Diagnosis of IPS?

IPS is defined as a widespread alveolar injury following HCT in which active lower respiratory tract infection, cardiac dysfunction, acute renal failure, and iatrogenic fluid overload have been excluded[4]. Consequently, to establish the diagnosis, all requirements listed in Table 21.2 must be present [4]. Thanks to improvements in diagnostic methods, the incidence and the median time of onset of IPS declined from 20–25% in earlier series of allo-HCT to <10% (8% after

MAC regimen and 2% after RIC) and from days +40–50 to days +18–21[3,4,5].

What Is the Role of Bronchoscopy to Exclude Other Diagnoses and Is Timing of the Procedure Important?

Pulmonary complications are common and constitute an independent risk factor for mortality, stressing the importance of an appropriate clinical management. A recent prospective interventional study using systematic methodology (including noninvasive tests, imaging and fiberoptic bronchoscopy (FOB)) showed that this approach offered an etiologic diagnosis in 83% of cases (59% thanks to non invasive methods)[6]. The use of FOB is more controversial but its diagnostic yield is of 67%, increasing to 78% for pulmonary infections. Especially relevant is that 28% of infectious episodes could only be diagnosed by means of FOB. Additionally, FOB could prove the presence of unsuspected microorganisms in 24% of patients with positive noninvasive tests. In patients with pulmonary infections, early FOB, performed when the patient does not respond after 48–72 hours of empirical treatment, offers a superior yield (78%) to those that were performed later (23%) (P=0.02)[6].

Can We Differentiate Several Subtypes of IPS?

Yes. The American Thoracic Society proposed a classification of lung complications after HCT according to their primary tissue injury and etiology distinguishing three different subtypes of IPS[4] (Table 21.2). Additionally, from a clinical point of view, some IPS are relatively easy to differentiate from the classical IPS occurring from days +18 to +21. This would be true for the diagnosis of DAH. DAH is characterized by a progressive bloodier return of successive aliquots of bronchoalveolar lavage fluid, indicating blood in the alveoli. BOS and COP are obstructive and restrictive pulmonary complications, respectively, that could be observed late after HCT (COP, around day + 100; BOS, after day +120), and clearly related to upper respiratory tract infections and chronic GvHD, respectively[4,7,8].

Has There Been Any Progress with IPS Treatment?

Unfortunately not. The treatment of IPS is based on supportive care measures (including noninvasive and invasive mechanical ventilation and continuous venovenous hemofiltration),

Table 21.1 Early and late tissue and organ toxicity after HCT *not* directly related to infections, GvHD, or malignancy

Organ	Early complication (<day +120)	Late complications
Eyes	- Sicca syndrome[a]	- Cataracts - Keratoconjunctivitis sicca[a] - Microvascular retinopathy (also please refer to Table 21.6)
Gut	- Oral mucositis, diarrhea - Pancreatitis - Sicca syndrome[a]	- Caries
Lungs	- Idiopathic pneumonia syndrome	- Cryptogenic organizing pneumonia - Bronchiolitis obliterans syndrome
Cardiovascular – endothelial	- Leak capillary syndrome - Diffuse alveolar hemorrhage - Engraftment syndrome - Thrombotic microangiopathy	- Cardiotoxicity - Late vascular complications - Metabolic syndrome
Liver	- Sinusoidal obstruction syndrome	- Iron overload
Genitourinary system	- Hemorrhagic cystitis - Acute kidney disease	- Chronic kidney disease
Bones		- Osteopenia/osteoporosis - Avascular necrosis
Endocrine organs		- Hypothyroidism - Hypogonadism - Growth retardation - Adrenal dysfunction - Infertility
Muscle	- Myopathy	- Myopathy - Muscle cramps
Nervous system	- Calcineurin inhibitors toxicity	- Leukoencephalopathy - Peripheral neuropathy - Guillain–Barré syndrome - Neurocognitive deficits

[a] Occasionally observed after autologous HCT.

Table 21.2 Definition of idiopathic pneumonia syndrome

I: Evidence of widespread alveolar injury:

a. Multilobar infiltrates on routine chest radiographs or CT
b. Symptoms and signs of pneumonia (cough, dyspnea, tachypnea, rales)
c. Evidence of abnormal pulmonary physiology
    1. Increased alveolar to arterial oxygen difference
    2. New or increased restrictive PFTs abnormality

II: Absence of active lower respiratory tract infection based upon:

a. BAL negative for significant bacterial pathogens including acid-fast bacilli, Nocardia, and *Legionella* species
b. BAL negative for pathogenic nonbacterial microorganisms:
    1. Routine culture for viruses and fungi
    2. Shell vial culture for CMV and respiratory RSV
    3. Cytology for CMV inclusions, fungi, and *Pneumocystis jirovecii*
    4. Direct fluorescence staining with antibodies against CMV, RSV, HSV, VZV, influenza virus, parainfluenza virus, adenovirus, and other organisms
c. Other organisms/tests to also consider:
    1. Polymerase chain reaction for human metapneumovirus, rhinovirus, coronavirus, and HHV6
    2. Polymerase chain reaction for *Chlamydia*, *Mycoplasma*, and *Aspergillus* species
    3. Serum galactomannan ELISA for *Aspergillus* species[a]
d. Transbronchial biopsy if condition of the patient permits

Table 21.2 (*cont.*)

III: Absence of:

Cardiac dysfunction, acute renal failure, or iatrogenic fluid overload as etiology for pulmonary dysfunction

Classification of IPS according to the primary tissue injury and etiology

Pulmonary parenchyma	- Acute interstitial pneumonitis - Acute respiratory distress syndrome - Delayed pulmonary toxicity syndrome
Vascular endothelium	- Peri-engraftment respiratory distress syndrome - Capillary leak syndrome - Diffuse alveolar hemorrhage
Airway epithelium	- Crytogenetic organizing pneumonia (COP) - Bronchiolitis obliterans syndrome (BOS)

a Nowadays, some authors include galactomannan in BAL.
PCR = polymerase chain reaction; BAL = bronchoalveolar lavage; CMV = cytomegalovirus; HSV = herpes simplex virus; RSV = respiratory syncytial virus; VZV = varicella-zoster virus.
Adapted from references [3] and [4].

broad-spectrum antimicrobial agents, and corticosteroids. Low (≤ 2 mg/kg) or high (> 4 mg/kg) doses of methylprednisolone seem to have limited efficacy (except in COP, some cases of BOS and DAH)[4]. Unfortunately, 60–80% of patients with an early form of IPS will die (95% if requiring mechanical ventilation) after a median time of 2 weeks from progressive impairment of respiratory function. Despite the initial expectations, a recent trial has shown that etanercept does not improve the results obtained with steroids alone[9], although this result should be evaluated carefully because the study was interrupted before the planned recruitment was complete, precluding any definitive conclusion about effectiveness.

Is Treatment of DAH Satisfactory with Steroids?

Although the overall response to steroids remains disappointing[10], no other therapeutic measures have proved to be more effective in DAH[11]. The usual treatment is methylprednisolone 250–500 mg every 6 hours for 5 days and tapering off for 2–4 weeks plus aminocaproic acid. Despite the fact that fewer than 15% of patients die as a direct consequence of DAH, the frequent evolution to multiorgan failure (MOF) increases the mortality to >60%. The addition of rh-Factor VIIa does not confer advantages to the corticosteroids alone[12].

Vascular Endothelial

A number of early complications may be triggered by injury to the vascular endothelium. Usually observed in the first 30–60 days after HCT, these complications have imprecise diagnostic criteria and overlapping clinical features. The best-defined syndromes resulting from such endothelial damage are sinusoidal obstruction syndrome (SOS) (see Liver); capillary leak syndrome; engraftment syndrome (ES); DAH (see Lung); and HCT-associated thrombotic microangiopathy[13,14]. Endothelial injury probably plays a role as well in the development of acute GvHD[15]. The impact of early endothelial damage on late cardiovascular complications after HCT is unknown.

Engraftment Syndrome (ES)
When to Suspect ES and What Is the Best Diagnostic Criterion?

We must suspect an ES when a patient undergoing an autologous HCT presents, during neutrophil recovery, a high and well-tolerated fever that does not respond to empirical antibiotic therapy. The presence of skin rash, hypoxemia, or diarrhea is also frequently observed[16]. When applied correctly (timing around engraftment), the Maiolino criteria (Table 21.3) are better than those published by Speizer for establishing an early diagnosis[16,17,18]. The abrupt and significant increase in C-reactive protein (CRP) level, higher than that observed in infection, can help establish the diagnosis[16].

Does ES Predominate in Certain Groups of Patients Undergoing HCT?

Yes. Most cases of ES have been described after the introduction of growth factors and peripheral blood-HCT. However, nowadays, ES is observed mainly in patients with low-intensity (or any) chemotherapy before auto-HCT, as occurs in breast cancer, AL amyloidosis, myeloma, POEMS syndrome, or autoimmune diseases [16,19].

How About ES in Recipients of Allogeneic HCT: Does It Portend Poor Prognosis?

Yes. ES (occasionally denominated peri-engraftment syndrome) is recognized with increased frequency (10–13%) after allo-HCT and in up to 50% of double-unit cord blood transplants (dUCBT)[20,21]. In these cases, the differential diagnosis with aGvHD, which is frequently associated, could be very difficult due to the similarity of clinical manifestations (fever, maculopapular skin rash, diarrhea). When observed after allo-HCT, ES generally implies a poor prognosis[22]. A recent study among 927 patients demonstrated that persons who developed ES (13%) experienced significantly higher cumulative incidence of grade 2 to 4 aGvHD at day 100 (75% *versus*

Table 21.3 Diagnostic criteria for endothelial complications after HCT

Recommended diagnostic criteria of endothelial syndromes after HCT

Engraftment syndrome

Maiolino criteria	Noninfectious fever[a] 24h before or at any time after engraftment[b] + any of the following: - Cutaneous rash (maculopapular exanthema > 25% body surface) - Pulmonary infiltrates (by X-ray or CT without other causes)[c] - Diarrhea (> episodes/day with negative cultures)

Thrombotic microangiopathy associated with HCT

Probable TMA criteria	1. Increased percentage (≥4%) of schistocytes in peripheral blood 2. Concurrent increased serum lactate dehydrogenase(LDH) 3. Thrombocytopenia <50 x 10⁹/L or a ≥50% decrease in platelet count 4. Negative direct and indirect Coombs test 5. Decrease in serum haptoglobin concentration 6. Absence of coagulopathy

Sinusoidal obstruction syndrome

Baltimore criteria (adults)	Before day +21, jaundice + 2 or 3 of the following: - Jaundice - Weight gain >5% - Hepatomegaly - Ascites
Modified criteria (children)	Before day +30, 2 or 3 of the following: - Jaundice - Weight gain >5% - Hepatomegaly - Ascites
Severe SOS	Baltimore clinical criteria + one of the following criteria of MOF: - Lung: SO₂ <90% in room air and/or ventilator dependence - Kidney: doubling of baseline creatinine and/or dialysis dependence - CNS: confusion, encephalopathy, or coma

[a] New fever (>38°C) without clinical or microbiologic documentation or response to antimicrobial treatment.
[b] The original sentence "24h before or after" is confusing and has generated incorrect interpretations in some papers.
[c] Without signs of infection, cardiac failure, or pulmonary embolism.

34%, $P<0.001$) and higher nonrelapse mortality at 2 years (38% *versus* 19%, $P<0.001$) compared with non-ES patients, resulting in lower overall survival at 2 years (38% *versus* 54%, $P<0.001$). There was no significant difference in relapse at 2 years (26% *versus* 31%, $P=0.772$)[22].

How Should ES Be Managed?

G-CSF should be stopped immediately, performing any complementary studies necessary to discard an infection (cultures, image studies), and starting the empirical antibiotic therapy used at the center[5]. If after a maximum of 48 hours fever does not respond and cultures are negative, start methylprednisolone 1mg/kg every 12 hours for 3 days with progressive tapering off over 1 week. In the auto-HCT setting, when introduced early, steroids produce a complete resolution in 1–5 days in >80% of patients[16].

HCT-Associated Thrombotic Microangiopathy (TMA)

What Are the Best Clinical Criteria for TMA Diagnosis?

From a practical point of view, probably the best policy would be to use the recently described criteria of "probable TMA" (Table 21.3) that allows the clinician to suspect this diagnosis earlier, and adopt immediate therapeutic measures[23]. Other published criteria are more specific but may hinder an early diagnosis[24,25].

Why Do We Observe a Higher Incidence of TMA and SOS when Using Sirolimus?

In-vitro studies show that sirolimus *per se* does not damage endothelia but, when associated with calcineurin inhibitors (CNI), it boosts their well-known endothelial toxicity[26]. This observation must be validated with protocols using sirolimus without CNI (see Chapter 70).

How Can We Prevent or Treat TMA?

The only reasonable measure to prevent TMA is close observation (2–3 times per week) of CNI, LDH, proteinuria, and creatinine levels. If any of these markers increases, haptoglobin level, peripheral blood smear, and direct and indirect antiglobulin tests and levels of C5b-9 fraction of complement should be evaluated[5]. Experts insist on the relevance and high frequency of elevated blood pressure, diarrhea secondary to intestinal TMA and proteinuria, and the possible absence of renal and neurologic symptoms[27]. The most effective therapeutic measure is to stop the CNI immediately (not to reduce the dosage), changing GvHD prophylaxis. If we are in front of a CNI-associated TMA the prognosis after stopping CNI is excellent. Unfortunately, when TMA is not associated with CNI toxicity (TMA mimicking hemolytic uremic syndrome or fulminating multifactorial TMA) the prognosis is very bad and most cases have a fatal evolution to MOF[28]. Plasma exchange usually offers a poor response[5]. Some authors have reported successful results with defibrotide (DF), rituximab, daclizumab, basiliximab, and eculizumab therapies[28].

Late Cardiovascular Events (CV)

Which Data that Support Late Cardiovascular Events Are Related to HCT?

Late CV events after HCT fall into a group of complications in which an unequivocal relationship with the transplant procedure is more difficult to demonstrate. CV accidents have a relatively low incidence, are observed among the general population, and would be expected to occur decades after HCT. For these reasons, CV events after HCT are probably underreported[29,30,31]. A possible explanation is the higher incidence of CV risk factors among HCT recipients. The metabolic syndrome (obesity, hypertriglyceridemia, low HDL cholesterol levels, high blood pressure, and high fasting glucose)[32] was found in 23–49% of HCT survivors *versus* 4–8% in leukemia controls; these values represent a > twofold increase in prevalence compared with population controls [32,33]. In a study from a single center, the cumulative incidence rates of these risk factors 10 years after HCT were: hypertension, 38%; diabetes, 18%; dyslipidemia, 47%; and multiple risk factors, 31%[34]. Acute GvHD and TBI can also play a role in late CV events. GvHD is associated with an increased risk of developing arterial hypertension, diabetes, and dyslipidemia (relative risk (RR), 9.1, 5.8, and 3.2, respectively). TBI is associated with diabetes and dyslipidemia (RR, 1.5 and 1.4, respectively)[34]. The effect of these risk factors is additive (5%, 7%, and 11% for patients with 0, 1, and ≥2 factors, respectively). Proof of the impact of GvHD and its prevention is the 7-fold increase in CV risk after allo-HCT compared with auto-HCT[29]. The role that CNI can have in these late CV events is unknown.

How Best to Prevent Late CV Event?

Prevention is based on avoiding or treating risk factors as in the general population. Surprisingly, many patients with these risk factors are not treated, probably because of the false belief that these conditions will improve spontaneously with time, especially after withdrawal of immunosuppressive treatment[31,35]. Table 21.4 summarizes the measures internationally recommended to prevent late complications after HCT.

Liver

The most relevant complications not related to infection, GvHD, or malignancy affecting the liver after HCT are sinusoidal obstruction syndrome (SOS) and iron overload.

Sinusoidal Obstruction Syndrome (SOS)
What Is the Best Clinical Criteria for SOS Diagnosis?

As in 42% of adult patients with two of the Seattle criteria, SOS could not be confirmed by hemodynamic studies compared with only 9% using the Baltimore criteria[36–38]. For this reason, and because almost 100% of adults with a classical SOS present with jaundice, most groups treating adults prefer the Baltimore criteria (Table 21.3). However, pediatricians prefer the modified Seattle criteria (similar to the Baltimore criteria but without hiperbilirubinemia as a prerequisite) (Table 21.3), because jaundice does not occur in children in up to 40% in some series[39]. Remember that neither criterion considers the case of late SOS appearing after day +21–30 and up to day +40 to +50. These cases are not infrequent in patients

receiving alkylating agents (e.g., busulfan (Bu) plus melphalan or thiotepa) as conditioning and could represent a diagnostic problem, especially when SOS develops after discharge (one-third of cases) or when only weight gain and edema are present[40,41].

When Must SOS Be Considered Severe?

Fortunately, in most patients (75–80%), SOS progressively resolves over a 2- to 3-week period. Nevertheless, severe SOS is a potentially life-threatening complication associated with a high mortality rate (>80%)[42–44]. The clinical criteria can establish the diagnosis of SOS but cannot predict whether it will be severe. Classically, SOS severity was described using the Seattle criteria, which classified SOS cases retrospectively as mild, moderate, or severe[42]. However, this classification is not useful for the clinician because it lacks prognostic value. Based on retrospective analyses, the presence of MOF affecting the kidneys, lungs, or central nervous system (see definition in Table 21.3) has emerged as the best clinical marker of severe SOS[43]. A working group of the EBMT is preparing a more realistic diagnostic criterion and severity grading of a suspected SOS in adults and children.

What Are the Most Relevant Risk Factors for SOS?

The incidence of SOS is clearly related to the intensity of the conditioning regimen, previous liver damage, the alloreactivity presence of several additional risk factors (mainly a previous liver damage and the degree of alloreactivity) and the clinical criteria used for SOS diagnosis (Table 21.5)[42–45]. The current incidence of SOS is around 10–15% after allogeneic HCT using myeloablative conditioning regimens (MAC regimen) and <5% after reduced intensity conditioning (RIC) or autologous HCT[42–44]. The incidence of SOS after MAC–HCT or RIC–HCT is clearly influenced by alloreactivity. Thus, the incidence of SOS is higher in allogeneic (*versus* autologous), unrelated (*versus* sibling), mismatched (*versus* matched), or unmanipulated (*versus* T-cell-depleted) HCT[46,47].

How Best to Prevent the Development of Severe SOS?

Most patient-related risk factors (such as patients undergoing a second HCT, or with a previous liver disease or radiation, or treated with gemtuzumab ozogamicin) are impossible to reverse; all of these patients have a high risk of developing SOS and should be included in prophylactic programs. The most easily reversible risk factors are iron overload, which should be reduced as much as possible with iron chelators before HCT[48], and the avoidance of hepatotoxic drugs (a classical example being progestogens)[49].

Transplant-related risk factors can, occasionally, be modified. Thus, the use of RIC–HCT has clearly reduced the incidence of SOS[44] and, currently, this modality of HCT provides results similar to those of MAC–HCT for many diseases. It is also possible to reduce the toxicity of MAC regimen, as occurs with the combination of intravenous Bu

Table 21.4 Summary of recommendations for screening and prevention of organ-specific late complications[a]

Recommended screening	6 mo	1 y	An	Comments
Ocular:				- Immediate exam if visual symptoms
- Clinical symptoms evaluation	1	1	1	- Special attention to *sicca* syndrome
- Visual acuity & fundus exam	+	1	+	
Oral:				- Preventive oral health education
- Clinical assessment	1	1	1	- Avoid smoking, sugar beverages, or oral piercing
- Dental assessment	+	1	1	- If oral cGvHD high-risk squamous cell cancer; evaluation every 6m
Respiratory:				- Active or passive*
- Clinical pulmonary assessment	1	1	1	- If chronic GvHD, spirometry test in each control (recommended by many
- Smoking tobacco avoidance*	1	1	1	authors)
- Pulmonary function testing	+	+	+	
- Chest radiography	+	+	+	
Cardiac and vascular				- Active treatment of risk factors
- CV risk factors assessment	+	1	1	- Counseling on heart healthy life style
Liver:				- Additional testing if high ferritin levels (MRI/FerriScan®)
- Liver function testing	1	1	+	
- Serum ferritin testing		1	+	
Kidney:				- Treat hypertension
- Blood pressure screening	1	1	1	- Avoid nephrotoxins
- Urine protein screening	1	1	1	
- BUN/creatinine testing	1	1	1	
Muscle and connective tissue:				- If risk of cGvHD, test joint mobility and touch skin to detect sclerotic changes
- Evaluation muscle weakness	2	2	2	- Treat cramps symptomatically
- Physical activity counseling	1	1	1	
Skeletal:				- Prevent bone loss and fractures with exercise, vitamin D, and calcium
- Bone density testing[b]		1	+	
Nervous system:				- Special attention of cognitive development in pediatric patients
- Neurologic clinical evaluation	+	1	1	
- Evaluate cognitive development		1	1	
Endocrine:				- Annual gynecologic evaluation in women
- Thyroid function testing	1	1	1	- Hormonal replacement if necessary
- Growth velocity in children		1	1	
- Gonadal function assessment[c]		1	1	
- Gonadal function assessment[d]		1	+	
Mucocutaneous:				- Avoid sunlight without adequate protection
- Skin self-exam & sun counseling	1	1	1	
- Gynecologic exam in women		+	+	

[a] Similar recommendations but focused in children have been elaborated by the Children's Oncology Group http://www.survivorshipguidelines.org.
[b] Adult women, all allo-HCT, and patients at high-risk for bone loss.
[c] Prepubertal men and women.
[d] Postpubertal women and men.
An = annually; 1 = recommended for all transplant recipients; 2 = recommended for patients with ongoing chronic GvHD or immunosuppression; + = reassessment recommended for abnormal testing in a previous time period or for new signs/symptoms.
Adapted with permission from reference [35].

and fludarabine instead of the classical oral Bu and cyclophosphamide (Cy)[50]. Another possibility, based on the physiopathology of SOS, is to change the order of the drugs (Cy/Bu instead of Bu/Cy)[51]. The alloreactive phenomena can be prevented by the use of donors with the maximum degree of

HLA compatibility, or the use of T-cell depleted grafts[46,47]. Finally, by avoiding CNI we also can reduce the risk of developing SOS[52].

The third approach is to use pharmacologic measures to prevent SOS. The most relevant agents tested are low

Table 21.5 Main risk factors for SOS after HCT

Risk factor	Lower risk < higher risk
Transplant-related factors	
Type of HCT	Syngeneic/autologous < allogeneic
Grade of compatibility	Match < minor mismatch < major mismatch
Origin of stem cells	T-cell depleted < non-T-cell depleted
Conditioning regimen:	
- Total dose	Cy < Fluda-BulV < Cy-fTBI + < 12 Gy < Cy-fTBI + > 12Gy < BVC RIC < MAC regimen
- Busulfan	IV < PO dose targeted < PO nonadjusted
- Order of administration	Other combinations < busulfan first than Cy
GvHD prophylaxis	Without CNI < with CNI < CNI + sirolimus
HCT number	First < second
Patient-related factors	
Diagnosis	Nonmalignancy < malignancy < some malignancies[a]
Status of the disease	Remission < relapse
AST level before HCT	Normal < high
Previous liver radiation	No < yes
Liver status	Normal < fibrosis, cirrhosis, tumor
Previous drugs	Gemtuzumab or inotuzumab ozogamicin

[a] Hemophagocytic lymphohistiocytosis, adrenoleukodystrophy, osteopetrosis. Cy = cyclophosphamide; fTBI = fractionated total body irradiation; Gy = greys; BVC (BCNU, etoposide, cyclophosphamide); GvHD = graft-*versus*-host disease; CNI = calcineurin inhibitors.

molecular weight heparin, antithrombin III, prostaglandin E1, pentoxifylline, ursodeoxycholic acid (UDCA), and defibrotide (DF). All of them are suboptimal except UDCA and DF[53]. Despite the inconclusive results of prevention with UDCA, it is evident that all the studies show that patients receiving this prophylaxis have less liver toxicity, less GvHD, and better survival rates[54]. With respect to DF, as it is the best drug available for SOS treatment, it will probably be the best one for its prophylaxis. Several nonrandomized and randomized studies have shown its effectiveness[35]. For that reason, DF should also be considered for SOS prophylaxis. In fact, recent guidelines of the British Society for Blood and Marrow Transplantation recommend its use in children (IA) and adults (IIB) with a high risk of SOS (pre-existing hepatic disease, second

MAC–HCT, allogeneic HCT for leukemia beyond second relapse, conditioning with Bu-containing regimens, prior treatment with gemtuzumab ozogamicin, or diagnosis of primary hemophagocytic lymphohistiocytosis, adrenoleukodystrophy, or osteopetrosis)[53].

How Best to Manage Persons Who Develop SOS?

SOS treatment should be based on the following steps[55]:

First, purposefully look for clinical data suggesting SOS. A careful daily weight measurement and checking of the fluid balance should be performed during the conditioning regimen, and maintained, as a minimum, up to day 14–21 after HCT. Ultrasound could be very useful to detect hepatomegaly and ascites.

Second, establish the diagnosis using the Baltimore criteria (adults) or the modified Seattle criteria (children). As characteristic symptoms and signs of this complication could be produced by other causes, a precise differential diagnosis must be established. In patients receiving alkylating agents, remember that these sets of criteria do not consider the possibility of late SOS appearing after day +21–30. In doubtful cases, the measurement of the hepatic venous gradient pressure (HVGP) through the jugular vein could be very useful[56]. Additionally, we must carefully check if there are any data of multiorgan failure that define severe SOS (Table 21.3).

Third, treat severe cases of SOS, as well as the apparently nonsevere cases that do not improve after 2–3 days, with an adequate fluid and sodium balance, avoidance of hepato- or nephrotoxic drugs, and a prudent use of diuretics, with defibrotide (6.25 mg/kg IV every 6 hours, 14–21 days)[53].

Iron Overload

Is Phlebotomy Indicated for Iron Overload after HCT?

Because iron overload decreases spontaneously in the years after HCT, mild iron overload (<700–800 ng/mL) does not require therapy. Those patients with higher ferritin levels (>1000 ng/mL) not attributable to other causes of increasing acute-phase reactant levels are candidates for phlebotomy (350–400 mL every 3–4 weeks until achieving a ferritin level <700 ng/mL) and/or chelation therapy. MRI, FerriScan®, or liver biopsy can help with the differential diagnosis but they are not a prerequisite. Phlebotomy has the advantages of better compliance, fewer side effects, and lower cost. If a low hemoglobin level prevents the use of phlebotomy, iron chelation therapy or administration of rh-EPO can be useful [7]. Adequate iron depletion significantly decreases transaminase levels and may improve liver fibrosis and cardiac function[7,8,42].

Kidneys and Urinary Tract

Acute and chronic kidney disease, a consequence of kidney damage during the pre-, peri-, and post-HCT periods, and hemorrhagic cystitis (HC) can be a major cause of morbidity and mortality after HCT[57].

Hemorrhagic Cystitis (HC)

In recent years, we have witnessed an increase in the incidence of this complication, probably as a consequence of new HCT modalities. Thus late HC has been reported in a recent series in 7% of patients with RIC, in 17% of those with MAC regimen, but in up to 58% of patients receiving an haploidentical HCT with post-HCT Cy for GvHD prophylaxis[58,59].

Must Mesna Be Used Systematically, and How Should It Be Administered?

Although most centers use mesna as a prophylaxis when using Cy-based regimens, several randomized studies have shown that this drug does not offer additional benefits if hydration and diuresis are adequate[60]. The recommended daily dose for hydration is 3 L/m^2. If used, the daily dose of mesna should be 1.0–1.5 times the daily dose of Cy administered IV as a continuous infusion, bolus injections after each Cy dose, or a mixture of both. Mesna should be maintained for 24 hours after the last dose of Cy because of the persistence of acrolein in the bladder[5,60].

Any Relevant Improvements in the Treatment of HC?

Unfortunately not. The most relevant advances have been the observation that systemic or intravesical instillation of cidofovir, ciprofloxacin (reduces BK virus replication), or ribavirin could be useful for cases of HC attributable to BK virus or adenovirus[5,57,58]. With persistent and nonresponsive HC, the selective embolization of bladder arteries has proved to be one of the most effective measures in the hands of an expert angioradiologist[61].

Chronic Kidney Disease (CKD)

Is It Best to Screen for CKD in Recipients of HCT?

Yes. As international recommendations indicate (Table 21.4), urine protein, BUN, and creatinine must be checked 6 and 12 months after HCT and yearly thereafter[35]. Blood pressure should be screened more frequently. Additionally all nephrotoxic drugs should be avoided and arterial hypertension intensively treated. Some authors consider the presence of albuminuria on day +100 as an early marker of CKD[57,62,63].

Bones

Osteoporosis

Is Osteoporosis after HCT a Relevant Complication?

Yes. About 33–50% of patients develop osteopenia and 18–25% develop osteoporosis 12–18 months after HCT. Additionally, nontraumatic fractures can occur in up to 10% of patients[7,8,35]. Bone loss results from impaired bone mineralization through disturbances of calcium and vitamin D homeostasis, osteoclast and osteoblast function, and deficiencies in growth hormone or gonadal hormone secretion[64].

Can We Prevent Bone Loss in Recipients of HCT?

Yes. All patients must be evaluated 1 year after HCT by means of dual-photon densitometry (see Chapter 71). This control acquires special relevance in older people, women, patients with low body weight, physically inactive patients, and those receiving extended CNI or corticosteroid therapy[7,35,62]. Treatment is based on active exercise that combines aerobic weight-bearing and resistive exercises, calcium and vitamin D supplementation, estrogen replacement in women, and reduction of the dosage of steroids and other immunosuppressants to the maximum extent possible. Bisphosphonates should be considered, while keeping in mind the risk of osteonecrosis of the jaw and fractures of the femur[35].

Endocrine Organs

Patients undergoing HCT are at risk of developing multiple endocrine abnormalities. The most relevant are hypothyroidism, gonadal failure, and growth retardation.

When Are Replacement Therapies Indicated and When Best to Stop Them?

Thyroidal hormones should be tested at 6, 12 months, and thereafter yearly. The median time to diagnosis of overt hypothyroidism is around 4 years after HCT, but some patients are diagnosed up to 28 years later, and 7–15% of patients can present a subclinical compensated hypothyroidism during the first year after HCT. The incidence of overt hypothyroidism (thyroid function tests (TFTs) show elevated thyroid-stimulating hormone (TSH) and low FT4 and FT3 levels) is 30–60% among patients receiving single-dose TBI, 15–25% after fractionated TBI, and 11% after conditioning with Bu/Cy. Patients with overt hypothyroidism should receive hormonal substitution with periodic dose adjustments[8,35,64,65].

In symptomatic men with low testosterone levels or with loss of bone mass, replacement therapy may be necessary. A transdermal patch is the most effective method, but prolonged use can cause hepatic peliosis and hepatic adenoma. Polycythemia, prostatic hypertrophy, and cancer have also been described. Other side effects are male pattern baldness, tachycardia, nausea, and LFT abnormalities. Treatment should be stopped for 2 months at regular intervals to check for gonadal recovery[35,64].

In women, the risk of developing ovarian failure after HCT is higher (95–100%) than in men. Despite its possible side effects, hormonal replacement (estrogen combined with progestin) is recommended in patients with menopausal symptoms, bone loss, and growth and development delay, until the age of 50. Hormonal therapy increases the risk of breast cancer, coronary heart disease, stroke, and venous thromboembolism but decreases the risk of bone fractures and colon cancer. Treatment should be stopped for 2 months at regular intervals to check for gonadal recovery[35].

The benefits of growth hormone supplementation are unclear, probably because of the multifactorial origin of growth retardation and the inconsistent results published [35]. Despite these concerns, treatment with recombinant GH must be considered in children younger than 10 years at HCT with demonstrated GH deficiency[66].

Infertility

The crude birth rate was 1.7 per 1000 among patients surviving >4 months after HCT (normal US population 10 per 1000 in 2013) in the largest evaluated series. However, most patients who conceive after HCT should have uncomplicated pregnancies and give birth to normal babies[7,8,62,67].

Any Advances in Preventing Infertility?

The use of less-intensive conditioning regimens and access to new methods of fertility preservation can improve this panorama. The most common and well-established method in adult women and pubertal females is embryo cryopreservation using in-vitro fecundation (IVF). The time necessary for oocyte retrieval, the availability of a partner, and the overall cost limit this approach. Despite being used for many groups, the use of contraceptives or gonadotropin-releasing hormone agonists could not be considered an option to preserve fertility after HCT. The development of vitrification allows us to cryopreserve oocytes without irreversible damage during freezing and thawing. This technique does not require embryo cryopreservation but does need time to obtain the oocytes and has the added costs of IVF. The time necessary to obtain oocytes and their further cryopreservation could be avoided by means of ovarian tissue banking. The reimplantation of this tissue after HCT allows ovarian activity to be restored in 3–6 months. Unfortunately, this procedure could not be recommended for patients with leukemia or other malignancies that could involve the ovaries[68].

Muscle
What Is the Etiology of Muscle Cramps after HCT?

Cramps are normally associated with myopathy, neuropathy, or metabolic abnormalities but may also occur as an isolated complication. If occurring daily (>50% of patients) and long lasting (1–10 minutes), cramps can interfere significantly with the patient's normal activities. Classically, cramps were considered secondary to cGvHD but, in our experience and in the large series of Seattle, they are also frequent among patients after receiving auto-HCT[8]. Cramps occurs once (or more) per day, typically at rest or at night, and affect the hamstring, hand, forearm, thoracic, and even jaw muscles. The etiology remains unclear. Cramps are treated with little success with stretching exercises, adequate hydration, magnesium supplementation, muscle relaxant-anticonvulsants (clonazepam, gabapentin, pregabalin, or carbamazepine), and quinine sulfate. The latter is one of the most effective treatments (response rate of about 40%), but is considered off-label by the FDA because of its serious adverse effects[8,69].

Ocular Problems

Ocular problems and their potential solutions after HCT are reviewed in Table 21.1 and Table 21.6.

Table 21.6 Ocular problems and their potential solution

1. Anterior segment complications

1.1. Keratoconjunctivitis due to sicca syndrome

Incidence: Up to 10% in patients w/o cGvHD; 40–50% in patients with cGvHD
Symptoms: Burning, irritation, pain, foreign body sensation, blurred vision, photophobia
Risk factors: cGvHD, females, TBI, older age
Diagnosis: Symptoms + positive Schirmer's test (<10 mm in 5 min)
Treatment: Artificial tears, occlusion of tear duct puncta, temporal tarsorraphia, scleral lens can be useful (never use contact lens!), topical steroids or CNI, autologous serum

1.2. Cataracts (mainly posterior subcapsular)

Incidence: CT alone – 5–20% at 5 yr
TBI single-dose: 80–90%
TBI fractionated: 25–40% at 10 yr
Risk factors: TBI (single > fractionated), MAC regimen, older age, use of steroids for GvHD >3 months, allo-SCT
Symptoms: Decrease in vision (bright/low light) and contrast, altered color perception
Diagnosis: By slit lamp examination
Treatment: Surgical

2. Posterior segment complications

2.1. Ischemic microvascular retinopathy

Incidence: <10% (usually within first 6 months after HCT)
Symptoms: Decreased visual acuity and scotoma (usually bilateral and symmetrical)
Risk factors: Almost exclusively seen after allo-HCT with TBI and CSA, hypertension, diabetes
Diagnosis: Fundus examination – cotton wool spots, optic disc edema, microaneurysms, superficial and intraretinal hemorrhages
Treatment: Reduction/stop of immunosuppression (reversible in most cases)

Recommendations:

- Ocular clinical symptoms evaluation: 6 mon, 1 yr, annually for Auto + Allo
- Ocular fundus exam: at 1 yr for allo-HCT, annually (if previous abnormalities)
- If cGvHD → ophthalmologist evaluation before first yr
- If visual symptoms → ocular examination immediately

References

1. Martin PJ, Counts GW Jr, Appelbaum FR, *et al*. Life expectancy in patients surviving more than 5 years after hematopoietic cell transplantation. *J Clin Oncol*. 2010; 28: 1011–6.

2. Bhatia S, Francisco L, Carter A, *et al*. Late mortality after allogeneic hematopoietic cell transplantation and functional status of long-term survivors: report from the Bone Marrow Transplant Survivor Study. *Blood*. 2007; 110: 3784–92.

3. Cooke KR, Yanik GA. Lung injury following hematopoietic cell transplantation. In: Appelbaum FR, Forman SJ, Negrin SJ, Blume KG, eds. *Thomas' Hematopoietic Cell Transplantation* , 4th edn. Malden, MA, Blackwell Publishing, 2009, pp 1456–71.

4. Panoskaltsis-Mortari A, Griese M, Madtes DK, *et al*. An official American Thoracic Society research statement: noninfectious lung injury after hematopoietic stem cell transplantation: idiopathic pneumonia syndrome. *Am J Respir Crit Care Med*. 2011; 183: 1262–79.

5. Carreras E. Early complications after HSCT. In: Apperley J, Carreras E, Gluckman E, Mazzi T, eds. *EBMT Handbook of Hematopoietic Stem Cell Transplantation*. Genoa, Italy, Forum Service Editore, 2012, pp 177–94.

6. Lucena CM, Torres A, Rovira M, *et al*. Pulmonary complications in hematopoietic SCT: a prospective study. *Bone Marrow Transplant*. 2014 Jul 21. doi:10.1038/bmt.2014.151. [Epub ahead of print] PubMed PMID: 25046219.

7. Socié G, Salooja N, Cohen A, *et al* Nonmalignant late effects after allogeneic stem cell transplantation. *Blood*. 2003; 101: 3373–85.

8. Flowers MED, Deeg HJ. Delayed non-malignant complications after hematopoietic cell transplantation. In: Appelbaum FR, Forman SJ, Negrin SJ, Blume KG, eds. *Thomas' Hematopoietic Cell Transplantation* , 4th edn. Malden, MA, Blackwell Publishing, 2009, pp 1620–36.

9. Yanik GA, Horowitz MM, Weisdorf DJ, *et al*. Randomized, double-blind, placebo-controlled trial of soluble tumor necrosis factor receptor: Enbrel (etanercept) for the treatment of idiopathic pneumonia syndrome after allogeneic stem cell transplantation:

10. blood and marrow transplant clinical trials network protocol. *Biol Blood Marrow Transplant*. 2014; 20: 858–64.

10. Afessa B, Tefferi A, Litzow MR, Krowka MJ, Wylam ME, Peters SG. Diffuse alveolar hemorrhage in hematopoietic stem cell transplant recipients. *Am J Respir Crit Care Med*. 2002; 166: 641–5.

11. Majhail NS, Parks K, Defor TE, Weisdorf DJ. Diffuse alveolar hemorrhage and infection-associated alveolar hemorrhage following hematopoietic stem cell transplantation: related and high-risk clinical syndromes. *Biol Blood Marrow Transplant*. 2006; 12:1038–46.

12. Elinoff JM, Bagci U, Moriyama B, *et al*. Recombinant human factor VIIa for alveolar hemorrhage following allogeneic stem cell transplantation. *Biol Blood Marrow Transplant*. 2014; 20: 969–78.

13. Carreras E, Diaz-Ricart M. The role of the endothelium in the short-term complications of hematopoietic SCT. *Bone Marrow Transplant*. 201; 46: 1495–502.

14. Paczesny S, Diaz-Ricart M, Carreras E, Cooke KR. Translational research efforts in biomarkers and biology of early transplant-related complications. *Biol Blood Marrow Transplant*. 2011; 17 (Suppl): S101–8.

15. Penack O, Socié G, van den Brink MR. The importance of neovascularization and its inhibition for allogeneic hematopoietic stem cell transplantation. *Blood*. 2011; 117: 4181–9.

16. Carreras E, Fernández-Avilés F, Silva L, *et al*. Engraftment syndrome alters auto-SCT: analysis of diagnostic criteria and risk factors in a large series from a single center. *Bone Marrow Transplant*. 2010; 45: 1417–22.

17. Maiolino A, Biasoli I, Lima J, *et al*. Engraftment syndrome following autologous hematopoietic stem cell transplantation: definition of diagnostic criteria. *Bone Marrow Transplant*. 2003; 31: 393–7.

18. Speizer TR. Engraftment syndrome following hematopoietic stem cell transplantation. *Bone Marrow Transplant*. 2001; 27: 893–8.

19. Cornell RF, Hari P, Zhang MJ, *et al*. Divergent effects of novel immunomodulatory agents and cyclophosphamide on the risk of

engraftment syndrome after autologous peripheral blood stem cell transplantation for multiple myeloma. *Biol Blood Marrow Transplant*. 2013; 19: 1368–73.

20. Gorak E, Geller N, Srinivasan R, *et al*. Engraftment syndrome after nonmyeloablative allogeneic hematopoietic stem cell transplantation: incidence and effects on survival. *Biol Blood Marrow Transplant*. 2005; 11: 542–50.

21. Hong KT, Kang HJ, Kim NH, *et al*. Peri-engraftment syndrome in allogeneic hematopoietic SCT. *Bone Marrow Transplant*. 2013; 48: 523–8.

22. Chang L, Frame D, Braun T, *et al*. Engraftment syndrome after allogeneic hematopoietic cell transplantation predicts poor outcomes. *Biol Blood Marrow Transplant*. 2014; 20: 1407–17.

23. Cho BS, Yahng SA, Lee SE, *et al*. Validation of recently proposed consensus criteria for thrombotic microangiopathy after allogeneic hematopoietic stem-cell transplantation. *Transplantation*. 2010; 90: 918–26.

24. Ruutu T, Barosi G, Benjamin RJ, *et al*. Diagnostic criteria for hematopoietic stem cell transplant-associated microangiopathy: results of a consensus process by an International Working Group. *Haematologica*. 2007; 92: 95–100.

25. Ho VT, Cutler C, Carter S, *et al*. Blood and Marrow Transplant Clinical Trials Network Toxicity Committee consensus summary: thrombotic microangiopathy after hematopoietic stem cell transplantation. *Biol Blood Marrow Transplant*. 2005; 11: 571–5.

26. Carmona A, Díaz-Ricart M, Palomo M, *et al*. Distinct deleterious effects of cyclosporine and tacrolimus and combined tacrolimus-sirolimus on endothelial cells: protective effect of defibrotide. *Biol Blood Marrow Transplant*. 2013; 19: 1439–45.

27. Laskin BL, Goebel J, Davies SM, Jodele S. Small vessels, big trouble in the kidneys and beyond: hematopoietic stem cell transplant associated-thrombotic microangiopathy. *Blood*. 2011; 118: 1452–62.

28. Daly AS, Xenocostas A, Lipton JH. Transplantation-associated thrombotic microangiopathy: twenty-two years

later. *Bone Marrow Transplant.* 2002; 30: 709–15.

29. Tichelli A, Bucher C, Rovó A, et al., Premature cardiovascular disease after allogeneic hematopoietic stem-cell transplantation. *Blood.* 2007; 110: 3463–71.

30. Tichelli A, Passweg J, Wójcik D, et al. Late cardiovascular events after allogeneic hematopoietic stem cell transplantation: a retrospective multicenter study of the Late Effects Working Party of the EBMT. *Haematologica.* 2008; 93: 1203–10.

31. Chow EJ, Wong K, Lee SJ, et al. Late cardiovascular complications after hematopoietic cell transplantation. *Biol Blood Marrow Transplant.* 2014; 20: 794–800.

32. Baker KS, Chow E, Steinberger J. Metabolic syndrome and cardiovascular risk in survivors after hematopoietic cell transplantation. *Bone Marrow Transplant.* 2012; 47: 619–25.

33. Baker KS, Ness KK, Steinberger J, et al. Diabetes, hypertension, and cardiovascular events in survivors of hematopoietic cell transplantation: a report from the bone marrow transplantation survivor study. *Blood.* 2007; 109: 1765–72.

34. Armenian SH, Sun CL, Vase T, et al., Cardiovascular risk factors in hematopoietic cell transplantation survivors: role in development of subsequent cardiovascular disease. *Blood.* 2012; 120: 4505–12.

35. Majhail NS, Rizzo JD, Lee SJ, et al. Recommended screening and preventive practices for long-term survivors after hematopoietic cell transplantation. *Biol Blood Marrow Transplant.* 2012; 18: 348–71.

36. McDonald GB, Sharma P, Matthews DE, Shulman HM, Thomas ED. Venocclusive disease of the liver after bone marrow transplantation: diagnosis, incidence, and predisposing factors. *Hepatology* 1984; 4: 116–22.

37. Jones RJ, Lee KS, Beschorner WE, et al. Venoocclusive disease of the liver following bone marrow transplantation. *Transplantation* 1987; 44: 778–83.

38. Carreras E, Grañena A, Navasa M, et al. On the reliability of clinical criteria for the diagnosis of hepatic veno-occlusive disease. *Ann Hematol.* 1993; 66: 77–80.

39. Corbacioglu S, Cesaro S, Faraci M, et al. Defibrotide for prophylaxis of hepatic veno-occlusive disease in paediatric haemopoietic stem-cell transplantation: an open-label, phase 3, randomised controlled trial. *Lancet.* 2012; 379: 1301–9.

40. Lee JL, Gooley T, Bensinger W, Schiffman K, McDonald GB. Veno-occlusive disease of the liver after busulfan, melphalan, and thiotepa conditioning therapy: incidence, risk factors, and outcome. *Biol Blood Marrow Transplant.* 1999; 5: 306–15.

41. Carreras E, Fernández-Avilés F, Silva L, et al. Engraftment syndrome alter auto-SCT: analysis of diagnostic criteria and risk factors in a large series from a single center. *Bone Marrow Transplant.* 2010; 45: 1417–22.

42. Strasser SI, McDonald GB. Gastrointestinal and hepatic complications. In: Appelbaum FR, Forman SJ, Negrin SJ, Blume KG, eds. *Thomas' Hematopoietic Cell Transplantation* , 4th edn. Malden, MA, Blackwell Publishing, 2009, pp 1434–55.

43. Coppell JA, Richardson PG, Soiffer R, et al. Hepatic veno-occlusive disease following stem cell transplantation: incidence, clinical course, and outcome. *Biol Blood Marrow Transplant.* 2010; 16: 157–68.

44. Carreras E, Díaz-Beyá M, Rosiñol L, et al. The incidence of veno-occlusive disease following allogeneic hematopoietic stem cell transplantation has diminished and the outcome improved over the last decade. *Biol Blood Marrow Transplant.* 2011; 17: 1713–20.

45. Carreras E, Bertz H, Arcese W, et al. Incidence and outcome of hepatic veno-occlusive disease after blood or marrow transplantation: a prospective cohort study of the EBMT. *Blood.* 1998; 92: 3599–604.

46. Soiffer RJ, Dear K, Rabinowe SN, et al. Hepatic dysfunction following T-cell-depleted allogeneic bone marrow transplantation. *Transplantation.* 1991; 52: 1014–9.

47. Moscardó F, Urbano-Ispizua A, Sanz GF, et al. Positive selection for CD34+ reduces the incidence and severity of veno-occlusive disease of the liver after HLA-identical sibling allogeneic peripheral blood stem cell transplantation. *Exp Hematol.* 2003; 31: 545–50.

48. Vallejo C, Batlle M, Vazquez L, et al. Phase IV open-label study of the efficacy and safety of deferasirox after allogeneic stem cell transplantation. *Haematologica.* 2014; Jul 4. [Epub ahead of print] PubMed PMID: 24997153.

49. Hägglund H, Remberger M, Klaesson S, Lönnqvist B, Ljungman P, Ringden O. Norethisterone treatment, a major risk factor for veno-occlusive disease in the liver after allogeneic bone marrow transplantation. *Blood.* 1998; 92: 4568 72.

50. Daly A, Savoie ML, Geddes M, et al. Fludarabine, busulfan, antithymocyte globulin, and total body irradiation for pretransplantation conditioning in acute lymphoblastic leukemia: excellent outcomes in all but older patients with comorbidities. *Biol Blood Marrow Transplant.* 2012; 18: 1921–6.

51. Cantoni N, Gerull S, Heim D, et al. Order of application and liver toxicity in patients given BU and CY containing conditioning regimens for allogeneic hematopoietic SCT. *Bone Marrow Transplant.* 2011; 46: 344–9.

52. Deeg HJ, Shulman HM, Schmidt E, Yee GC, Thomas ED, Storb R. Marrow graft rejection and veno-occlusive disease of the liver in patients with aplastic anemia conditioned with cyclophosphamide and cyclosporine. *Transplantation.* 1986; 42: 497–501.

53. Dignan FL, Wynn RF, Hadzic N, et al. BCSH/BSBMT guideline: diagnosis and management of veno-occlusive disease (sinusoidal obstruction syndrome) following haematopoietic stem cell transplantation. *Br J Haematol.* 2013; 163: 444–57.

54. Ruutu T, Juvonen E, Remberger M, et al. Improved survival with ursodeoxycholic acid prophylaxis in allogeneic stem cell transplantation: long-term follow-up of a randomized study. *Biol Blood Marrow Transplant.* 2014; 20: 135–8.

55. Carreras E. How I treat sinusoidal obstruction syndrome after hematopoietic cell transplantation. *Br J Haematol.* 2015; 168: 481–91.

56. Carreras E, Grañena A, Navasa M, et al. Transjugular liver biopsy in BMT. *Bone Marrow Transplant.* 1993; 11: 21–6.

57. Hingorani S. Kidney and bladder complications of hematopoietic cell transplantation. In: Appelbaum FR, Forman SJ, Negrin SJ, Blume KG, eds. *Thomas' Hematopoietic Cell*

Transplantation; 4th edn. Malden, MA, Blackwell Publishing, 2009, pp 1473–86.

58. Silva L de P, Patah PA, Saliba RM, *et al.* Hemorrhagic cystitis after allogeneic hematopoietic stem cell transplants is the complex result of BK virus infection, preparative regimen intensity and donor type. *Haematologica.* 2010; 95: 1183–90.

59. Raiola AM, Dominietto A, Ghiso A, *et al.* Unmanipulated haploidentical bone marrow transplantation and posttransplantation cyclophosphamide for hematologic malignancies after myeloablative conditioning. *Biol Blood Marrow Transplant.* 2013; 19: 117–22.

60. Shepherd JD, Pringle LE, Barnett MJ, Klingemann HG, Reece DE, Phillips GL. Mesna *versus* hyperhydration for the prevention of cyclophosphamide-induced hemorrhagic cystitis in bone marrow transplantation. *J Clin Oncol.* 1991; 9: 2016–20.

61. Giné E, Rovira M, Real I, *et al.* Successful treatment of severe hemorrhagic cystitis after hemopoietic cell transplantation by selective embolization of the vesical arteries. *Bone Marrow Transplant.* 2003; 31: 923–5.

62. Tichelli A, Socié G. Late effects in patients treated with HSCT. In: Apperley J, Carreras E, Gluckman E, Mazzi T eds. *EBMT Handbook of Hematopoietic Stem Cell Transplantation.* Genoa, Italy, Forum Service Editore, 2012, pp 249–67.

63. Choi M, Sun CL, Kurian S, *et al.* Incidence and predictors of delayed chronic kidney disease in long-term survivors of hematopoietic cell transplantation. *Cancer.* 2008; 113: 1580–7.

64. Kandeel FR. Endocrine complications following hematopoietic cell transplantation. In: Appelbaum FR, Forman SJ, Negrin SJ, Blume KG, eds. *Thomas' Hematopoietic Cell Transplantation;* 4th edn. Malden, MA, Blackwell Publishing, 2009, pp 1487–522.

65. Sanders JE, Hoffmeister PA, Woolfrey AE, *et al.* Thyroid function following hematopoietic cell transplantation in children: 30 years' experience. *Blood.* 2009; 113: 306–8.

66. Sanders JE. Growth and development after hematopoietic cell transplantation. In: Appelbaum FR, Forman SJ, Negrin SJ, Blume KG, eds, *Thomas' Hematopoietic Cell Transplantation;* 4th edn. Malden, MA, Blackwell Publishing, 2009, pp 1608–16.

67. Loren AW, Chow E, Jacobsohn DA, *et al.* Pregnancy after hematopoietic cell transplantation: a report from the late effects working committee of the Center for International Blood and Marrow Transplant Research (CIBMTR). *Biol Blood Marrow Transplant.* 2011; 17: 157–66.

68. Joshi S, Savani BN, Chow EJ, *et al.* Clinical guide to fertility preservation in hematopoietic cell transplant recipients. *Bone Marrow Transplant.* 2014; 49: 477–84.

69. Kraus PD, Wolff D, Grauer O, *et al.* Muscle cramps and neuropathies in patients with allogeneic hematopoietic stem cell transplantation and graft-versus-host disease. *PLoS One.* 2012; 7: e44922.

Immune Paralysis and Reconstitution after Hematopoietic Cell Transplants

Stephane Eeckhoudt, Aurore Saudemont, and Alejandro Madrigal

Introduction

Allogeneic hematopoietic cell transplant (allo-HCT) is now a standard treatment for a variety of malignant and nonmalignant hematologic diseases. Bone marrow (BM), mobilized peripheral blood (PB) following administration of cytokines such as granulocyte-colony stimulating factor (G-CSF), and umbilical cord blood (UCB) are currently used as a source of hematopoietic stem and progenitor cells (HSPC) for transplantation. Whatever the HSPC source, the main complications of allo-HCT are infections, relapse, graft-*versus*-host disease (GvHD), and to a lesser extent autoimmune diseases and secondary malignancies. Some of these complications are due to the fact that after allo-HCT patients experienced a partial or complete deficiency of the immune system, which can persist for a long period of time, up to 1−2 years post-allo-HCT.

Numerous factors impact on the rapidity and intensity of immune reconstitution; they are summarized in Table 22.1. They can be separated into pre-, peri-, and post-transplantation factors. Pretransplant factors include the underlying disease, prior chemotherapy and/or radiation, nutritional status, patient and donor age, and previous exposure to pathogens. Peritransplant factors correspond to the conditioning regimen (type and dose of chemotherapy, total body irradiation, administration of antilymphocyte globulin), graft manipulation, HSPC source, donor−recipient matching

Table 22.1 Factors impacting kinetics of immune reconstitution after HCT

Pretransplant factors	Peritransplant factors	Post-transplant factors
Underlying disease	Conditioning regimen	GvHD prophylaxis
Prior chemotherapy	Graft manipulation	DLI
Radiation treatment	Graft source	Antibiotics treatment
Nutritional status Patient age Donor age Infectious medical history	HLA matching ABO matching Peritransplant infections	GvHD treatment

for human leukocyte antigen (HLA), and non-HLA (ABO and CMV) and peritransplant infection. Post-transplant factors include the type of prophylaxis used for GvHD (see Chapters 12, 13, and 19), donor lymphocyte infusion (DLI) (see Chapter 25), antibiotic treatment and prophylaxis (see Section 5), development of GvHD, and the type of immunosuppressive regimen used. Therefore, immune reconstitution is a very complex and multifactorial phenomenon (Figure 22.1) that must be further studied to improve outcome of patients after allo-HCT. In the next sections, we will review the quantitative and qualitative recovery of the innate and adaptive immune system and discuss some of the factors that influence immune reconstitution after HCT.

Recovery Tempo and Assessment of Immune Reconstitution

Definition of Immune Reconstitution: What Is It?

There is currently no clear definition to establish that a transplanted patient has recovered an effective immune system. Some authors define immune reconstitution as a general concept leading to the recovery of antigen-specific T-cell function, production of cytokines, and antibody production by B-cells. However, this definition is quite limited as a potent ("recovered") immune reconstitution also requires reconstitution of all components of the innate immune system to reduce risks of infection and relapse. The reconstitution of different immune cell subsets after HCT occurs at different time points and tempo. Overall, cells of the adaptive immune system recover more slowly than innate immune cells after HCT, and functional deficiencies can be detected years after normal cell counts have been reached. Forcina *et al.* suggested that it is key to distinguish between quantitative and qualitative aspects of immune reconstitution; quantitative repopulation of immune cells may be assessed by flow cytometry methods (FCM) and quality of immune recovery by a set of functional assays relevant to the cell type of interest[1].

Absolute Lymphocyte Count

Absolute lymphocyte count (ALC) is the first biomarker used to evaluate immune reconstitution. ALC can be measured by FCM from whole blood and is used to predict clinical outcome

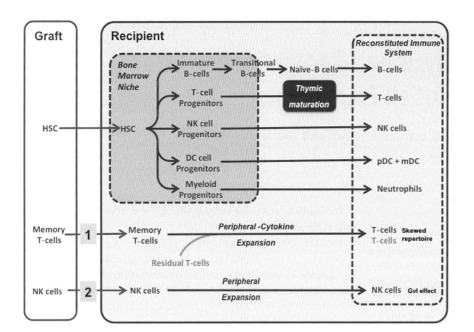

Figure 22.1. Reconstitution of immunity after HCT. B-cell, NK cell, and dendritic cell (DC) reconstitution occurs via recipient's bone marrow maturation of donor's hematopoietic cells mainly. Reconstitution of T-cell subsets requires thymus maturation of T-cell progenitors emerging from the recipient's bone marrow. Peripheral cytokine expansion of mature T-cells contained in the graft and/or residual mature T-cells from the recipient also occurs (pathway 1) but leads to the generation of T-cells with a skewed T-cell receptor (TCR) repertoire. Pathway 1 is minor in case of T-cell-depleted HCT or CBT. UCB graft contains a high proportion of functional NK cells, which induce a GvL effect (pathway 2).

of patients after HCT. However, different groups have proposed and used different ALC thresholds to determine levels of immune recovery, and no clear consensus has been achieved yet. For example, in the case of T-cell-depleted allo-HCT from an HLA-matched sibling, an ALC above 450 cells/μL 30 days post-transplant correlated with a lower transplant-related mortality (TRM), longer disease-free survival and overall survival (OS)[2]. Similar results have been obtained using an arbitrary threshold of 1000 cells/μL after T-cell-replete allo-HCT from unrelated matched donor or following infusion of purified CD34+ cells from haplotype matched donors[3]. More recently, Michelis *et al.* reported that an ALC above 500 cells/μL at day 28 post-transplant correlated with a reduced risk of relapse in patients transplanted with mobilized PB for acute myeloid leukemia[4]. Finally, Burke *et al.* have proposed to use an arbitrary threshold of 200 cells/μL following UCB transplantation (CBT)[5]. It should be noted that Komanduri *et al.* showed that, despite a prolonged lymphopenia after CBT, some patients exhibited functional CMV-specific T-cells by day 100[6].

Practice Points

These studies highlight the fact that numeration of lymphocyte populations is not sufficient to predict immune recovery and that functional assays should also be performed to assess immune reconstitution in transplanted patients.

Reconstitution of the Innate Immune System: *Do We Really Know What Constitutes Recovery?*
Myeloid-Derived Cells

Erythrocytes, granulocytes, platelets, and other cells of the myeloid lineage such as monocytes and macrophages are the first cells to recover and to differentiate from the graft. Notably, neutrophil recovery occurs between 14 and 30 days post-transplant depending on the type of graft used. However, despite a rapid numerical recovery, the functions of the newly produced cells can be abnormal especially if HCT complications develop. For example, it has been shown that neutrophil functions (e.g., chemotaxis, phagocytosis, and bacterial killing) can be impaired for several months post-HCT in patients with GvHD.

Dendritic cells (DCs) are known as professional antigen-presenting cells (APCs) that play a central role in the initiation of immune responses. In particular, DCs are key in the initiation of GvHD and of the graft-*versus*-leukemia (GvL) effect after allo-HCT. DCs are divided into two main subsets: plasmacytoid DCs (pDCs) that are lin−MHCII+CD11c−CD123+BDCA2+ and myeloid DCs (mDCs) lin−MHCII+CD11c+CD123−BDCA1+. These cells develop progressively from restricted BM progenitors although the precise contribution of common myeloid or common lymphoid marrow progenitors in the generation of DC lineages is still a matter of debate[7]. Even if DCs differentiate relatively quickly from the graft, subtype deficiencies have been demonstrated. In particular, pDCs are rare in the periphery of transplanted patients even 1 year post-transplant whereas mDCs generally recover in the first 6 months post-HCT.

Natural Killer Cells

Natural killer (NK) cells are CD56+CD3− innate immune cells that can eliminate tumor cells or virus-infected cells without prior stimulation. The role of donor NK cells in the outcome of haplotype matched HCT was demonstrated by Ruggeri *et al.*, whereby donor-*versus*-recipient NK cell alloreactivity not only resulted in GvL, but also in depletion of recipient

DCs and T-cells facilitating engraftment and protecting against GvHD, allowing for reduction of the conditioning regimen pre-HCT[8,9]. In addition, these studies also highlighted the importance of killer cell Ig-like receptor (KIR) ligand in haplotype matched HCT.

After HCT, NK cells recover more slowly than myeloid-derived cells but are actually the first lymphocytes to recover; their absolute count usually takes 1 to 2 months to normalize according to the type of graft used. While in the blood of healthy donors NK cells exhibit mostly a CD56^{dim} phenotype with only a minority of NK cells being CD56^{bright}, NK cell recovery after HCT is mainly based on the expansion of the CD56^{bright} NK cell subset, constituting most of the NK cells in the periphery of transplanted subjects for several months. Importantly, Chang and Huang proposed to use NK cell recovery as a biomarker of outcome after haplotype matched HCT as they showed that patients with high levels of CD56^{bright} NK cells at day 14 post-transplantation had a higher survival rate[10]. In addition, Della Chiesa et al. have recently reviewed the impact of CMV infection on NK cell development and function after HCT[11]. They found that CMV infection/reactivation accelerated NK cell maturation in transplanted patients by inducing the differentiation of a subset of NK cells characterized by a KIR+NKG2A- and NKG2C+ mature phenotype (see Chapters 17, 23, and 63). These results highlight that complications such as infection will also impact and shape immune reconstitution in patients post-HCT.

Reconstitution of Adaptive Immunity: Cells, Thymus, and TCR Repertoire

B-cells

B-cells are CD19$^+$ lymphocytes that differentiate into antibody producing cells upon activation. B-cells are important effector cells after HCT as they not only protect the patients against infection from encapsulated bacteria such as Haemophilus influenza and Streptococcus pneumoniae but also from viral infection such as varicella-zoster virus (VZV)[12]. After allo-HCT, it can take up to a year for B-cell count to normalize whatever the type of graft used. However, functions of B-cells can be compromised for up to 2 years. It has been shown that patients present a high level of transitional B-cells but low numbers of memory B-cells in peripheral blood for an extended time after transplantation, suggesting a defect in memory cell formation after allo-HCT. The different protective antibody subclasses emerge in a distinct order in adults mimicking normal neonatal development, with IgM levels recovering first within a few months post-allo-HCT, followed by IgG and finally IgA.

T-cells

The two major T-lymphocyte subsets are helper T-lymphocytes (T$_H$) and cytotoxic T-lymphocytes (CTLs), which express the antigen receptor $\alpha\beta$. Most T$_H$ cells express CD4 antigen and most CTLs express CD8 antigen. T-cells express TCR (T-cell receptor), a molecule restricted to the recognition of peptides bound to major histocompatibility complex (MHC) molecules presented by APCs.

Reconstitution of T-cell subsets after HCT occurs via two different pathways. The first one is thymus-independent and relies on homeostatic expansion of mature T-cells from the graft. The second one is thymus-dependent and requires de novo generation of recent T-cell emigrants from donor lymphoid progenitors[13]. During the first 6 months after transplantation, T-cell counts are mainly derived from cytokine-mediated expansion of naïve and memory T-cells from the donor. This early peripheral expansion produces a restricted T-cell population with a limited TCR repertoire against infectious agents (Figure 22.1)[14].

CD4+ and CD8+ T-cell counts after HCT are commonly used to study immune reconstitution. A CD4+ T-cell count above 200/μL at day +90 post-transplantation was associated with a lower NRM, less opportunistic infections, and longer OS[15]. Other studies have confirmed the role of the rapid CD4+ T-cell reconstitution in protecting the patient from transplant-related mortality and morbidity. More recently, Fedele et al. have suggested that a threshold of 115 CD4+ T-cells/μL at day +20 post-transplant correlated with a better outcome after allo-HCT[16]. Overall, most studies have focused on the predictive value of the CD4+ T-cell count recovery on the outcome of HCT not CD8+ T-cells recovery.

The diversity of the TCR repertoire after allo-HCT has been mainly studied using the CDR3 spectratyping method. Alterations in the TCR repertoire have been demonstrated even in patients receiving large doses of T-cells. Skewing of the TCR repertoire was mostly confined to early memory T-cells. Moreover, CD4+ and CD8+ T-cell subsets showed differences in their CDR3 distribution after HCT, essentially due to the rapid reconstitution of naïve CD4+ T-cells. Overall, the homeostatic expansion of CD8+ T-cells occurs faster than for CD4+T-cells resulting in a reverse CD4/CD8 ratio during the first months after transplantation. Recent advances in molecular biology such as next-generation sequencing (NGS) will allow further study of T-cell maturation during immune reconstitution[17].

The long-term reconstitution of a naïve T-cell repertoire able to respond to a broad range of pathogens and tumor antigens implies an effective thymic function to recover a complete T-cell ontogeny. Age, transplant conditioning regimen, and GvHD are the three main impediments to normal thymus function after HCT[18]. A method believed to measure thymic output more reliably in the context of HCT is the quantification of TCR excision circles (TRECs). TRECs are stable, episomal, nonreplicative DNA circles generated during TCR α chain rearrangement during the excision of the locus D. Righoffer et al. have shown that it took more than 2 years after HCT to restore the pretransplant thymic proliferation capacity mainly in T-cell depleted (70% of the cohort) HCT [19]. They assessed the thymus-dependent pathway by combining measurements and assessment of single joint TREC (sjTREC) and β TREC (βTREC) ratio in an improved quantitative light-cycler hybridization PCR assay. In another study by Toubert et al. pretransplant TRECs above the threshold of 172/150 000 CD3+ T-cells is an independent factor associated with a lower infection rate, including CMV reactivation and a longer OS after allo-HCT[20].

Type of Transplant and Immune Reconstitution: It Does Matter

Autologous Hematopoietic Cell Transplantation

In the past decade, the number of autologous HCT (auto-HCT) performed has increased (see Chapter 2). Auto-HCT is mainly used to treat hematologic diseases but it is also used for autoimmune diseases (See Chapter 56). Immune reconstitution after auto-HCT can be considered as a gold standard regarding the rapidity and the quality of immune reconstitution, as the patient's own cells are used. NK cells recover first after auto-HCT, with values for NK cell counts being normal as soon as 1 month after transplant[21]. B-cells recover later, with normal values observed 6 months after transplant. Regarding T-cell subsets, CD8+ T-cells appear first and normal cell counts are observed within a month while CD4+ T-cell counts are still below normal values 24 months post-HCT. Muraro et al. confirm these results showing that neither naïve nor memory CD4+ T-cells recover to baseline values by 24 months post-HCT[22]. In contrast, naïve and memory CD8+ T-cells recovered to normal values by 6 months.

Haplotype Matched Hematopoietic Cell Transplantation

Currently, different types of graft can be used for haplotype matched HCT such as BM or mobilized PB that can be T-cell depleted or repleted, which will impact differently on immune reconstitution. Regardless of the type of graft used, neutrophils reconstitute quickly at a median time of 11 days when T-cells are depleted from the graft or after 21 days when BM is used. Recovery of NK cells is based on the expansion of the CD16⁻CD56^bright NK cells whether T-cells are depleted from the graft or not. The absolute number of NK cells usually recovers after 30 days but may be impacted by the development of GvHD. NK cell cytotoxicity is lower after haplotype matched HCT and is associated with modification of expression of activating and inhibitory receptors.

The first 90 days after haplotype matched HCT are characterized by a low thymic function, which renders patients particularly susceptible to viral and fungal infections. T-cell recovery after haplotype matched transplant is impacted by the pretreatment applied to the graft. TCD (by CD34-positive- or or CD3/CD19-negative selection) seems to induce a slower T-cell recovery than unmanipulated grafts. The recovery of CD4+ memory T-cells is slower than for CD8+ memory T-cells and relies more on de novo thymic production of naïve

T-cells from donor T-cell progenitors. Better outcomes after T cell-replete haplotype matched transplants have been reported compared to T-cell-depleted haplotype matched transplants[23].

Umbilical Cord Blood Transplantation

CBT is associated with a delayed engraftment, poor immune reconstitution, and consequently a higher infection rate compared to other graft sources. This is due to qualitative and quantitative differences in the composition of UCB grafts. Neutrophil and platelet engraftment are linked to the total nucleated cell dose, which is clearly lower in obtained UCB as compared to BM or mobilized PB. Therefore, the time to neutrophil engraftment is prolonged to 30 days compared to 14 or 21 days when mobilized PB or BM is used, respectively. NK cells recover very rapidly after CBT through expansion of CD16⁻CD56^bright cells with total NK cell counts returning to normal values within 30 days.

UCB is characterized by a high proportion of antigen-inexperienced naïve T-cells and the presence of very few memory T-cells[24]. Early T-cell reconstitution can therefore only occur via the more stringent priming, activation, and proliferation of the limited naïve T-cell repertoire from the graft. However, CBT is characterized by a slower thymopoiesis compared to other HSC sources. Escalon has suggested that this delay is induced by the limited dose of lymphoid precursors in UCB grafts[25].

Impact of the Transplant Conditioning Regimen on Immune Reconstitution

Standard "myeloablative" conditioning (MAC regimen) for allo-HCT has been associated with a high rate of TRM. To address this issue, less toxic conditioning regimens including nonmyeloablative conditioning (NMA) and reduced intensity conditioning (RIC) have been developed. The concept is to deliver adequate immunosuppression to allow successful engraftment of donor hematopoietic cells and to eradicate the underlying malignancy while minimizing transplant-related toxicities.

After MAC regimen, allo-HCT recipients experience a period of profound pancytopenia lasting days to weeks depending on the HSPC source, the longest being after CBT. The degree of myelotoxicity is milder after NMA or RIC regimen (see Chapter 3), but the depth and extent of lympho-depletion seems to be similar. This could be due to the fact that lymphocyte recovery is a long process requiring engraftment and maturation of hematopoietic precursors in the BM or the thymus for B-cells and T-cells, respectively.

In addition, treatments used for GvHD prophylaxis (Chapter 12) also impact on immune reconstitution. Gärtner et al. have recently demonstrated that using 10 or 20mg of alemtuzumab instead of 40mg in the conditioning regimen supports early regeneration of NK cells after allo-HCT, which may have a positive effect on OS[26]. However, this approach didn't impact on the kinetic of recovery of other lymphocyte subpopulations such as CD4+ and CD8+ T-cells.

Controversies and Future Directions

The restoration of a functional immune system is one of the main factors influencing clinical outcome of transplanted patients. Impaired immune reconstitution results in increased susceptibility to lethal infection and reduces the patient's ability to generate an anticancer immune response. Many groups have studied immune reconstitution following HCT, but there is a clear lack of consensus concerning biomarkers and thresholds that must be used to evaluate the immunologic status of patients whichever graft and conditioning regimen is used. There is a clear need to determine specific guidelines regarding time points to be analyzed and thresholds to consider for each cell type in order to establish that the immune system of a given patient has been restored.

The flow cytometry method is a powerful tool to evaluate the reconstitution of immune cell subsets. It is extensively used to study immune recovery of specific cell subsets. However, the complexity of the technology together with the diversity of equipment, reagents, and many other preanalytical factors such as specimen age, compensation settings, and analytical factors such as gating strategies can also increase the variability observed when comparing results between different studies. Multicenter flow cytometry studies are needed to define immune cell subsets to focus on during immune reconstitution

and to clarify the analytical and preanalytical variables that could affect the quality of flow cytometry results. Such a study has been recently published about the standardization of whole blood immune phenotype monitoring for clinical trials aiming to promote renal allografts[27] and it will be essential to perform such a study to standardize the way we analyze immune reconstitution post-HCT.

Kinetics of immune reconstitution differs according to the graft and conditioning regimen used. However, substantial progress has been made to accelerate and improve immune reconstitution following HCT with the development of approaches such as DLI (see Chapter 25), cytokine administration, preemptive transfer of NK cells, genetically modified donor T-cell infusion, and adoptive transfer of pathogen-specific T-cells. These methods are discussed in detail in Section 17 of this book. Multicenter trials are needed to investigate when and which one of these strategies must be applied to transplanted patients. In addition, pilot studies are also required to assess which one of these strategies is the most effective to improve immune reconstitution regarding the different HSPC sources and conditioning regimens and to determine the impact on the recovery of each immune cell subset. It is clear that a predictive subset-guided strategy to accelerate immune reconstitution might improve outcome of transplanted patients. Therefore, we think that more in-depth clinical and preclinical studies are warranted to allow a better immune reconstitution of patients after HCT.

References

1. M. Bosch, and J. Storek. Immune reconstitution after hematopoietic cell transplantation. *Curr Opin Hematol* 2012; 19:324–35.

2. B. N. Savani, S. Adams, M. Uribe, *et al.* Rapid natural killer cell recovery determines outcome after T-cell-depleted HLA-identical stem cell transplantation in patients with myeloid leukemias but not with acute lymphoblastic leukemia. *Leukemia* 2007; 21:2145–52.

3. K. Le Blanc, M. Schaffer, H. Hägglund, *et al.* Lymphocyte recovery is a major determinant of outcome after matched unrelated myeloablative transplantation for myelogenous malignancies. *Biol Blood Marrow Transplant* 2009; 15:1108–15.

4. F. V. Michelis, D. Loach, J. Uhm, *et al.* Early lymphocyte recovery at 28 d post-transplant is predictive of reduced risk of relapse in patients with acute myeloid leukemia transplanted with peripheral blood stem cell grafts. *Eur J Haematol* 2014; 93(4):273–80. .

5. M. J. Burke, S. K. Janardan, C. Brunstein, *et al.* Early lymphocyte recovery and outcomes after umbilical cord blood transplantation (UCBT) for hematologic malignancies. *Biol Blood Marrow Transplant* 2011; 17:831–40.

6. K. V. Komanduri, M. de Lima, J. McMannis, *et al.* Delayed immune reconstitution after cord blood transplantation is characterized by impaired thymopoiesis and late memory T-cell skewing. *Blood* 2007; 110:4543–51.

7. A. T. Satpathy, J. C. Albring, and K. M. Murphy. Re(de)fining the dendritic cell lineage. *Nat Immunol* 2012; 13:1145–54.

8. L. Ruggeri, E. Urbani, K. Perruccio, *et al.* Effectiveness of donor natural killer cell alloreactivity in mismatched hematopoietic transplants. *Science* 2002; 295:2097–100.

9. L. Ruggeri, E. Burchielli, M. Capanni M, *et al.* NK cell alloreactivity and allogeneic hematopoietic stem cell transplantation. *Blood Cells Mol Dis* 2008; 40:84–90.

10. Y. J. Chang, and X. J. Huang. Effects of the NK cell recovery on outcomes of unmanipulated haploidentical blood and marrow transplantation for patients with hematologic malignancies. *Biol Blood Marrow Transplant* 2008; 14:323–34.

11. M. Della Chiesa, L. Muccio, A. Bertaina, *et al.* Impact of HCMV infection on NK cell development and function after HCT. *Front Immunol* 2013; 4:458.

12. C. Gudiol, M. Arnan, I. Sánchez-Ortega, *et al.* Etiology, clinical features and outcomes of pre-engraftment and post-engraftment bloodstream infection in hematopoietic SCT recipients. *Bone Marrow Transplant* 2014; 49:824–30.

13. C. Mackall, R. Gress, K. Peggs, *et al*; Center for International Blood and Marrow Transplant Research (CIBMTR); National Marrow Donor Program (NMDP); European Blood and Marrow Transplant Group (EBMT); American Society of Blood and Marrow Transplantation (ASBMT); Canadian Blood and Marrow Transplant Group (CBMTG); Infectious Disease Society of America

(IDSA); Society for Healthcare Epidemiology of America (SHEA); Association of Medical Microbiology and Infectious Diseases Canada (AMMI); Centers for Disease Control and Prevention (CDC). Background to hematopoietic cell transplantation, including post transplant immune recovery. *Bone Marrow Transplant* 2009; 44:457–62.

14. C. Fozza. T-cell receptor repertoire usage in hematologic malignancies. *Crit Rev Oncol Hematol* 2013; 86:201–11.

15. D. H. Kim, D. I. Won, N. Y. Lee, *et al*. Rapid helper T-cell recovery above 200 x 10 6/l at 3 months correlates to successful transplant outcomes after allogeneic stem cell transplantation. *Bone Marrow Transplant* 2006; 37:1119–28.

16. R. Fedele, C. Garreffa, G. Messina, *et al*. The impact of early CD4+ lymphocyte recovery on the outcome of patients who undergo allogeneic bone marrow or peripheral blood stem cell transplantation. *Blood Transfus* 2012; 10:174–80.

17. A. Six A, W. Chaara, S. Magadan, *et al*. The past, present, and future of immune repertoire biology — the rise of next-generation repertoire analysis. *Front Immunol* 2013; 4:413.

18. W. Krenger, and G. A. Holländer. Thymic T-cell development in allogeneic stem cell transplantation. *Blood* 2011; 117:6758–76.

19. S. Ringhoffer, H. Döhner, D. Bunjes, *et al*. T-cell reconstitution after allogeneic stem cell transplantation: assessment by measurement of the sjTREC/βTREC ratio and thymic naive T cells. *Haematologica* 2013; 98:1600–8.

20. A. Toubert, C. Douay, and E. Clave. Thymus and immune reconstitution after allogeneic hematopoietic stem cell transplantation in humans: never say never again. *Tissue Antigens* 2012; 79:83–9.

21. J. Rueff, D. Heim, J. Passweg, *et al*. Lymphocyte subset recovery and outcome after autologous hematopoietic stem cell transplantation for plasma cell myeloma. *Biol Blood Marrow Transplant* 2014; 20:869–9.

22. P. Muraro, S. Malhotra, M. Howell, *et al*. T cell repertoire following autologous stem cell transplantation for multiple sclerosis. *J Clin Invest* 2014; 124:1168–72.

23. S. O. Ciurea, R. M. Saliba, U. D. Bayraktar, *et al*. Improved early outcomes using a T cell replete graft compared with T cell depleted haploidentical hematopoietic stem cell transplantation. *Biol Blood Marrow Transplant* 2012; 18:1835–44.

24. P. Chevallier, M. Illiaquer, J. Esbelin, *et al*. Characterization of various blood and graft sources: a prospective series. *Transfusion* 2013; 53:2020–6.

25. M. P. Escalón. Cord blood transplantation: evolving strategies to improve engraftment and immune reconstitution. *Curr Opin Oncol* 2010; 22:122–9.

26. F. Gärtner, J. Finke, and H. Bertz. Lowering the alemtuzumab dose in reduced intensity conditioning allogeneic hematopoietic cell transplantation is associated with a favorable early intense natural killer cell recovery. *Cytotherapy* 2013; 15:1237–44.

27. M. Streitz, M. Kapinsky, M. Reed, *et al*. Standardization of whole blood immune phenotype monitoring for clinical trials: panels and methods from the ONE study. *Transplant Res* 2013; 2:17.

Chapter

23

Preventing Relapse Post-Transplant: When and How to Best Intervene?

Basem M. William, Christopher S. Hourigan, and Marcos de Lima

Introduction

Relapse is a devastating event in patients with hematologic malignancies treated with hematopoietic cell transplantation (HCT). Patients frequently have limited options if they relapse after HCT. In the allogeneic transplant setting, because of the development of reduced intensity conditioning (RIC) regimens, advances in supportive care, and better patient selection strategies, transplant-related mortality (TRM) has diminished significantly over the past few decades[1]. As TRM rates have decreased, disease relapse is the leading cause of mortality after HCT[2,3]. Autologous HCT (auto-HCT) is the current standard of care for medically fit patients with plasma cell myeloma who sustained at least a partial response after induction therapy; however, it is not curative and a significant proportion of patients relapse at some point after HCT (see Section 13). Auto-HCT is the current standard of care for relapsed lymphomas and as a consolidation therapy for certain lymphomas that are at a high risk of relapse after induction therapy (see Chapter 41). The introduction of rituximab improved survival in diffuse large B-cell lymphoma (DLBCL), the commonest subtype of non-Hodgkin lymphoma (NHL). However, most patients with DLBCL who relapse after rituximab and anthracycline-based induction therapy have poor outcomes with progression-free survival of 23% even after auto-HCT (see Chapter 43)[4].

Refinement of methods of detection of minimal residual disease (MRD) is critical in early detection of relapse and in assessing efficacy of maintenance therapies (see Chapter 24). Historically, enthusiasm for maintenance therapies was decreased by toxicity and lack of efficacy[2]. However, we now have less toxic new agents, and there is renewed interest in maintenance after HCT. In this chapter, we will discuss MRD measurements as applicable to the post-transplant setting followed by a discussion of the role of maintenance therapies after auto-HCT and allogeneic (allo)-HCT.

Minimal or "Measurable" Residual Disease (MRD)

Clinically evident recurrence of malignancy after HCT is described as relapse, a concept predicated on the concept of remission. Remission is defined as the absence of detectable disease, which is of course dependent on the sensitivity of the modality used for disease detection. Minimal (or more accurately measurable[5]) residual disease (MRD) therefore refers to that disease that is present below the threshold set for a remission in traditional clinical response criteria. Such traditional response criteria thresholds are based not on any underlying biologic reality but rather on the technical sensitivity of tests used for disease detection. This artificial dichotomy between clinical remission and relapse, based only on low sensitivity measurements, has the consequence that patients with the same disease achieving a "complete remission" may have dramatically different risks of subsequent relapse. Such highly heterogeneous clinical outcomes are not unexpected given the wide range in residual disease burden in patients in a standard "complete remission" (see Chapter 24).

Fortunately there are many methods available for measuring residual disease with greater sensitivity than traditional standard morphologic examination (Figure 23.1). These include techniques with low/intermediate sensitivity ($\sim 10^{-2}$ detection limit) such as fluorescent *in-situ* hybridization (FISH) for cytogenetic abnormalities and (in the post-allo-HCT setting) donor cell chimerism and also higher sensitivity methods ($\sim 10^{-3}$ to 10^{-4}, in some cases up to 10^{-5}) such as flow cytometry and quantitative polymerase chain reaction (RQ-PCR)-based methods to quantify overexpressed genes (e.g., WT1 in acute leukemia). Additionally, extremely high-sensitivity methods ($\sim 10^{-5}$ to 10^{-6} detection limit and beyond) are now increasingly available including PCR for mutated (e.g., NPM1) and translocated sequence (e.g., t(9;22) BCR-ABL in chronic myeloid leukemia [CML] and some ALL), or t(15:17) PML/RARA in acute promyelocytic leukemia (APL) or deep sequencing using next-generation technology for clonally rearranged sequence (e.g., immunoglobulin heavy chain in lymphoid malignancies)[6].

These techniques to MRD burden with high sensitivity are available for almost all the malignant diseases where HCT is indicated (see Table 23.1) such as multiple myeloma[7], acute lymphoblastic leukemia (ALL)[8], chronic lymphocytic leukemia (CLL)[9], lymphomas[10,11], CML[12], APL[13] (where MRD monitoring is already considered standard of care), non-APL AML[14], and MDS[15] where MRD monitoring is the

Table 23.1 Use of MRD in malignancies treated with transplantation

Disease	MRD methods available[a]	Notes
AML	PCR-mut PCR-GE MFC Cytogenetics NGS	Standard of care in APL Multiple clinical trials ongoing using MRD Lack of universal target in non-APL AML makes MRD assessment challenging
MDS	PCR-GE MFC FISH	Use of donor chimerism for MDS MRD well-established but generally underdeveloped area of research
ALL	PCR-mut (Ph+) NGS MFC	25-year history of being able to detect MRD in ALL. Deeply integrated into clinical trials for a decade
CLL	NGS PCR MFC	Well established, with multiple modalities available
CML	PCR-mut (Ph+)	Standard of care
MM	PCR-mut NGS MFC Imaging	As therapy in MM has become more effective, MRD measurements have become integrated in standard response criteria definitions

[a] Donor chimerism analysis post-allo-HCT is an MRD-testing option in all listed disease indications.
Abbreviations: AML, acute myeloid leukemia; MDS, myelodysplastic syndrome; ALL, acute lymphoblastic leukemia; CLL, chronic lymphoid leukemia; CML, chronic myeloid leukemia; MM, multiple myeloma; MFC, multiparametric flow cytometry; PCR-GE, PCR for gene overexpressed in disease compared to healthy tissue; PCR-mut, PCR for sequence, somatic mutation, or splice variant specific to tumor; Ph+, Philadelphia positive,i.e., Bcr:Abl translocation; NGS, next-generation sequencing; FISH, fluorescent in-situ hybridization.
Adapted from Hourigan et al. (2014)[2].

subject of much active research[16]. Concerns regarding competing platforms and modalities, standardization, and inter-center variability have limited the widespread adoption of high-sensitivity MRD measurements into the clinical standard of care. The greatest successes in implementation have come in those malignancy subtypes with a single invariant, pathognomonic genetic feature (e.g., CML, APL) or diseases of sufficient rarity that they are typically treated only at tertiary centers with a critical mass of pathologist expertise, experience, and capacity to correctly interpret more complex flow cytometry data (e.g., pediatric ALL). Increasingly, however, sophisticated high-sensitivity MRD data are becoming available on a commercial basis without the need for expensive patient-specific personalization, local laboratory set-up, or highly trained pathologist expertise to interpret the results (e.g., next-generation sequencing for clonally rearranged immune receptor sequence in lymphoid malignancies[6,17], a development which may change the landscape of how MRD can be used in routine clinical care).

MRD measurements integrate many different factors into a single estimate of residual disease burden and the results from such testing must be used judiciously. In particular technical, patient, and disease-specific factors should be considered when considering personalization of treatment based on MRD-testing (Figure 23.2). Firstly, different MRD assays have different sensitivities and therefore have different capacity to pick up a rare, but potentially clinical relevant, malignancy. Negative MRD-testing enriches for patients who may be cured and hence at no risk of relapse but does not in itself equate to cure; it is possible to be MRD-negative using even the most high-sensitivity tools currently available and still later experience clinical relapse[17]. The site, volume, and timing of sampling can also have a profound impact on MRD-testing results. MRD-testing offers a landmark "snapshot" of the

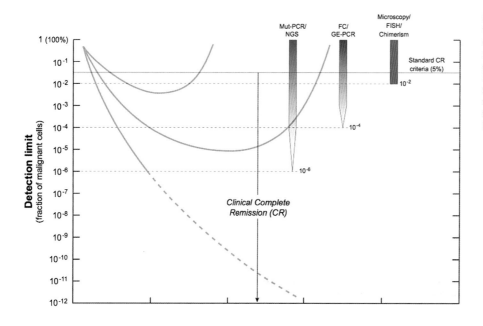

Figure 23.1. Higher sensitivity MRD techniques give a more complete description of residual disease burden. Abbreviations: FC, multi parameter flow cytometry; GE-PCR, PCR for gene overexpressed in disease compared to healthy tissue (e.g., WT1); mut-PCR, PCR for sequence, somatic mutation or splice variant specific to tumor; NGS, next-generation sequencing; FISH, fluorescent in-situ hybridization. Figure adapted from Hourigan and Karp (2013)[14].

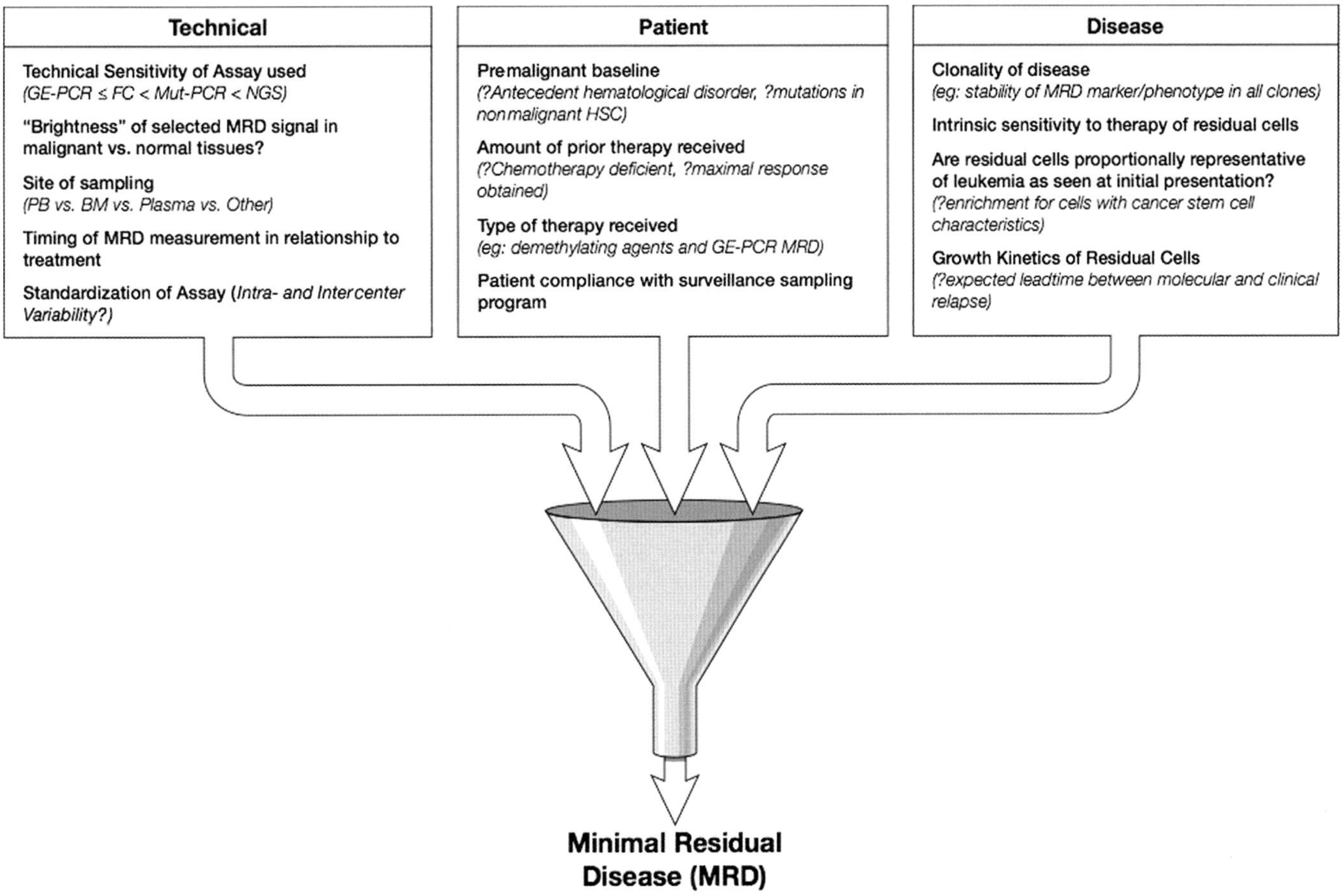

Technical	Patient	Disease
Technical Sensitivity of Assay used (GE-PCR ≤ FC < Mut-PCR < NGS)	Premalignant baseline (?Antecedent hematological disorder, ?mutations in non malignant HSC)	Clonality of disease (eg: stability of MRD marker/phenotype in all clones)
"Brightness" of selected MRD signal in malignant vs. normal tissues?	Amount of prior therapy received (?Chemotherapy deficient, ?maximal response obtained)	Intrinsic sensitivity to therapy of residual cells
Site of sampling (PB vs. BM vs. Plasma vs. Other)	Type of therapy received (eg: demethylating agents and GE-PCR MRD)	Are residual cells proportionally representative of leukemia as seen at initial presentation? (?enrichment for cells with cancer stem cell characteristics)
Timing of MRD measurement in relationship to treatment	Patient compliance with surveillance sampling program	Growth Kinetics of Residual Cells (?expected leadtime between molecular and clinical relapse)
Standardization of Assay (Intra- and Intercenter Variability?)		

Minimal Residual Disease (MRD)

Figure 23.2. Factors influencing MRD assessment.

disease currently present; this value is not static and is subject over time to either increase (e.g., due to malignant clonal outgrowth) or decline (e.g., secondary to therapeutic intervention or the impact of antimalignant immune responses). Changes in detectable MRD due to therapy or immune response may represent true declines in total malignant disease burden or changes in the phenotype of the population of residual malignant cells (e.g., decreased clonality and/or selective pressure leading to outgrowth of escape mutants) and requires careful selection of the MRD marker(s) to be followed (potentially multiple markers) given that the clone responsible for clinical relapse may well differ from the predominant clone at presentation. Finally, the presence of MRD at post-treatment time points has often been shown to be more prognostic than the pretreatment descriptors of disease biology that are typically used to risk-stratify patients into different categories of relapse risk. Nevertheless, the characteristics, including chemosensitivity and growth kinetics, of residual cells at the MRD level mean that comparison between absolute levels of MRD between patients within broad disease diagnosis groups may be less informative than the study of changes in MRD over time in a single patient.

Measurement of MRD levels can have utility in the context of hematopoietic cell transplantation in several different ways.

Firstly, they can help triage patients to HCT as consolidative therapy; there is increasing evidence that measurement of residual disease burden after chemotherapy may have greater utility than pretreatment cytogenetic and molecular correlates of disease biology in predicting future relapse risk (e.g., a patient with favorable-risk AML based on translocation 8,21 cytogenetics, but a suboptimal response to chemotherapy, is at high risk of relapse). Secondly, MRD measurements can help quantify, in the context of clinical trials, the efficacy interventions such as different transplantation and/or maintenance therapy approaches. Finally, it may be possible to personalize transplantation (conditioning and/or immunosuppression regimens) and maintenance (cytotoxic, targeted, immune, or cellular "therapy given to patients in a CR after completion of standard therapy to prevent future relapse"[2]) approaches based on residual disease levels observed immediately before or following transplantation to minimize risk of clinical relapse.

Preventing Relapse after Autologous Hematopoietic Cell Transplants

Auto-HCT is a form of therapy for high-risk hematologic malignancies including high-risk or relapsed/refractory lymphomas, leukemias, and myeloma. Myeloablative doses of chemotherapy are given to destroy the tumor with an infusion of hematopoietic cells to rescue the patient from the marrow-toxic effects of the high-dose regimen. There is no immunologic graft-*versus*-tumor effect accompanying auto-HCT, unlike allo-HCT. Thus auto-HCT relies on the dose-intensive effects of the treatment regimen, resulting in a higher relapse risk when compared with allo-HCT. However, allo-HCT is often complicated by graft-*versus*-host disease (GvHD), resulting in higher TRM rates. Thus, strategies have been developed to increase antitumor effects after auto-HCT to decrease relapse. An early study demonstrated that relapse may occur due to infusion of cancer cells in the graft[18]. Other studies have demonstrated that the major source of relapse after auto-HCT is endogenous tumor remaining in the patient and therefore *positive selection* for CD34+ hematopoietic cells[19], or purging of tumor cells by immunomagnetic bead selection[20], does not result in improved survival (see Chapter 41). Over the past 3 decades, different strategies have been tested in efforts to improve auto-HCT outcomes, including purging of the graft and post-auto-HCT treatments to decrease relapse incidence.

The use of post-auto-HCT treatments is attractive, since the "burden of malignant cells" in the recipient is frequently low after auto-HCT. There has been limited success using monoclonal antibodies as maintenance therapy for B-cell NHL. Neither B4-blocked ricin (anti-CD19 conjugated with ricin) nor rituximab improved event-free survival or OS in this setting (Table 23.2)[4,21,22]. Rituximab improved PFS in follicular lymphoma patients but had no effect on OS. Induction of an antitumor immune response by immunostimulatory agents has been tested. A phase I/II trial is currently ongoing and is aiming to examine the role of lenalidomide maintenance in prevention of relapse after auto-HCT for refractory or other high-risk lymphomas (NCT01035463). Tyrosine kinase inhibitors (TKIs) have been used as part of induction, consolidation, and maintenance therapy for Ph+ ALL. Generally, TKIs (imatinib and dasatinib) have been well tolerated after auto-HCT. The GALGB 10001 study showed that auto-HCT followed by TKI resulted in similar outcomes to allo-HCT in subjects with Ph+ ALL and without sibling donor[23]. Post-transplant maintenance or consolidation therapies for myeloma are described in detail in Chapter 47.

Other strategies for maintaining response include the use of antibody–drug conjugates, such as brentuximab vedotin (anti-CD30 and auristatin), inotuzumab ozogamicin (anti-CD22 and calicheamicin), and gemtuzumab ozogamicin[24–26]. The latter is not available for clinical use in the United States, but a pediatric AML study showed that it could be used to decrease the burden of MRD[26]. A phase 2 clinical trial is currently ongoing examining the role of brentuximab vedotin maintenance in the prevention of relapse after auto-HCT for Hodgkin's lymphoma (NCT01874054). Chimeric antigen receptor T-cells (CAR T-cells) and "immune checkpoint blockade therapy" with anti-PD-1 antibodies represent other novel

strategies for preventing relapse after auto-HCT and are discussed in Chapters 38 and 62. Prevention of relapse in mantle cell lymphoma following auto-HCT is discussed in Chapter 42.

Preventing Relapse after Allogeneic Hematopoietic Cell Transplants

The hypothesis that the graft-*versus*-leukemia (GvL) effect can be completely dissociated from GvHD has driven a significant part of hematopoietic cell transplantation research over the last 20 years, with limited success. Most post-HCT interventions have aimed at preventing GvHD while attempting to preserve antitumor activity.

Azacitidine, a DNA methyl transferase inhibitor, is arguably the drug that has been most extensively studied in the post-allo-HCT setting (and is the only one currently in a phase 3 clinical trial). In 2003, we hypothesized that low doses of this agent could decrease the risk of relapse after allo-HCT in MDS and AML, based on a series of experiments in the 1980s and early 1990s showing that *in-vitro* after exposure to hypomethylating agents increases the expression of tumor antigens and HLA molecules in leukemia cells. In addition, growing evidence at the time suggested a malignant cell differentiating effect of decitabine. Clinical and laboratory studies showed that longer exposure to lower doses were sufficient for demethylation and activation of tumor suppressor gene promoters and were more effective than higher doses that induced classic cytotoxic effects. We have shown, in a phase 1 trial, that azacitidine at the dose of $32 mg/m^2$ daily for 5 days was well tolerated and also suggested that the risk of chronic GvHD incidence was decreased among patients receiving longer schedules of the drug (administered in 30-day cycles)[27]. Subsequently, investigators showed in murine models that decitabine or azacitidine could induce tolerance, possibly by increasing the numbers of T-regulatory cells (Tregs)[28,29]. Craddock *et al.* then showed that AML patients receiving low-dose azacitidine had an increase in CD8 + T-cell response to a variety of tumor antigens and also augmented reconstitution of Tregs after T cell-depleted transplantation[30]. Longer follow-up of the British multicenter study showed that no patient developed severe acute GvHD or chronic extensive GvHD. A subsequent analysis of longitudinal recovery of Tregs in 12 patients treated with varying numbers of azacitidine cycles, after T cell-replete HCT, failed to show expansion of Tregs (Komanduri, personal communication). It is possible that the T-cell depletion used in the British trial would account for the difference between the two studies. Interestingly, azacitidine induced a CD8 + T-cell response to at least one tumor-specific peptide in 16 of 31 patients who received more than three treatment cycles, and this T-cell response was linked to improved 1-year OS (Craddock, personal communication). Moving forward, these studies suggest that a control group would be necessary to determine the actual influence of azacitidine on Tregs and GvL/

Table 23.2 Phase 3 studies comparing maintenance therapy or consolidation *versus* observation after autologous hematopoietic cell transplantation

Study	Disease	Intervention	Benefit on EFS/PFS	Benefit in OS
Furman *et al.*[21]	B-cell NHL	B4 blocked ricin	No difference	Favors observation
Gisselbrecht *et al.*[4]	DLBCL	Rituximab	No difference	No difference
Pettengell *et al.*[22]	FL	Rituximab	Favors rituximab	No difference
Thompson *et al.*[36]	NHL low, intermediate, high	IL-2	No difference	No difference
Bolaños-Meade *et al.*[37]	Poor-risk NHL	CSA IFN-γ, IL-2 to generate autologous GvHD	No difference	No difference
Simonsson *et al.*[38]	AML	Linomide	No difference	No difference
Attal *et al.*[39]	MM	Thalidomide	Favors thalidomide	Favors thalidomide
Barlogie *et al.*[40]	MM	Thalidomide	Favors thalidomide	Trend to thalidomide
Lokhorst *et al.*[41]	MM	Thalidomide	Favors thalidomide	No difference
Morgan *et al.*[42]	MM	Thalidomide	Favors thalidomide	No difference
Spencer *et al.*[43]	MM	Thalidomide and prednisone	Favors thalidomide	No difference
Krishnan *et al.*[44]	MM	Thalidomide and dexamethasone	Trend towards thalidomide	No difference
Maiolino *et al.*[45]	MM	Thalidomide and dexamethasone	Favors thalidomide	No difference
Stewart *et al.*[46]	MM	Thalidomide and prednisone	Favors thalidomide	No difference
McCarthy *et al.*[47]	MM	Lenalidomide	Favors lenalidomide	Favors lenalidomide
Attal *et al.*[48]	MM	Lenalidomide	Favors lenalidomide	No difference
Boccadoro *et al.*[49]	MM	Lenalidomide	Favors lenalidomide	Favors lenalidomide
Sonneveld *et al.*[50]	MM	Bortezomib *versus* thalidomide	Favors bortezomib in del 17p and in patients with renal failure	Favors bortezomib in del 17p and in patients with renal failure
Cavo *et al.*[51]	MM	Bortezomib and thalidomide *versus* thalidomide	Favors bortezomib and thalidomide	No difference
Mellqvist *et al.*[52]	MM	Bortezomib	Favors bortezomib	No difference
Palumbo *et al.*[53]	MM	Lenalidomide	Favors lenalidomide	No difference

Abbreviations: NHL, non-Hodgkin lymphoma; FL, follicular lymphoma; DLBCL, diffuse large B-cell lymphoma; AML, acute myeloid leukemia; MM, multiple myeloma; EFS, event-free survival; PFS, progression-free survival; OS, overall survival; CSA, cyclosporine A; IL-2, interleukin-2; IFN-γ, interferon-gamma; GvHD, graft-*versus*-host disease.
Adapted from Hourigan *et al.* (2014)[2].

GvH balance. Indeed, a phase 3 study comparing 1 year of low-dose azacitidine maintenance therapy *versus* standard of care (no maintenance) is ongoing at MD Anderson Cancer Center (Table 23.3). This study aims at improving EFS of patients receiving allo-HCT for high-risk AML and MDS.

FLT-3 inhibitors are also under active investigation as maintenance therapy after HCT (Table 23.3). The rationale is similar to the use of these drugs to treat AML, i.e., patients bearing the ITD mutation have a higher likelihood of relapse, and maintenance therapy with FLT-3 inhibitors could reduce recurrence rates after HCT. As with other drugs, tolerance and medication interactions after HCT are potential problems to be addressed in future studies. Bug *et al.* in Germany are investigating the deacetylase inhibitor panobinostat after allo-

Table 23.3 Highlighted maintenance studies after hematopoietic cell transplantation

Trial title	Clinicaltrials.gov Responsible part/sponsor
Randomized controlled study of post-transplant azacitidine for prevention of acute myelogenous leukemia and myelodysplastic syndrome relapse (VZ-AML-PI-0129)	NCT00887068 MD Anderson Cancer Center
Safety study of oral azacitidine (cc-486) as maintenance therapy after allogeneic hematopoietic cell transplantation in subjects with acute myeloid leukemia or myelodysplastic syndromes	NCT01835587 Celgene Corporation. University Hospitals Case Medical Center Anderson Cancer Center; Queen Elizabeth Hospital, Birmingham, UK; Fred Hutchinson Cancer Research Center; Memorial Sloan Kettering Cancer Center
Decitabine maintenance for acute myelogenous leukemia (AML) and myelodysplastic syndrome (MDS) post-transplant (AML MDS)	NCT00986804 Washington University School of Medicine
Dose-finding study of post-BMT decitabine maintenance treatment in higher risk MDS and MDS/AML (PODAC)	NCT01277484 Seoul St. Mary's Hospital
VIDAZA-DLI Preemptive azacitidine and donor lymphocyte infusions following allogeneic hematopoietic cell transplantation for high-risk acute myeloid leukemia and myelodysplastic syndrome	NCT01541280 Nantes University Hospital
Phase 1/2 study with oral panobinostat maintenance therapy following allogeneic hematopoietic cell transplant in patients with high-risk myelodysplastic syndrome (MDS) or acute myeloid leukemia (AML) (PANOBEST)	NCT01451268 Johann Wolfgang Goethe University Hospitals
Protocol in acute myeloid leukemia with FLT3-ITD (midostaurin)	NCT01477606 University of Ulm
Standard of care +/− midostaurin to prevent relapse post-stem cell transplant in patients with FLT3-ITDemutated AML (ARMOR)	NCT01883362 Novartis Pharmaceuticals/multicenter
Sorafenib maintenance therapy for patients with AML after allogeneic hematopoietic cell transplant	NCT01398501 Massachusetts General Hospital
A study of AC220 given after transplant in subjects with acute myeloid leukemia (AML) Dose-finding of lenalidomide as maintenance in multiple myeloma Safety and efficacy of lenalidomide as maintenance therapy in patients with newly diagnosed multiple myeloma following a tandem autologous-allogeneic transplant	NCT01468467 Sponsor: Ambit Biosciences Corporation NCT00778752 Universitätsklinikum Hamburg-Eppendorf NCT01264315 Fondazione Neoplasie Sangue Onlus
Azacitidine after allo blood and marrow transplantation (BMT) for chronic myelogenous leukemia (CML)	NCT00813124 MD Anderson Cancer Center
Allotransplant followed by lenalidomide and sirolimus maintenance in high-risk multiple myeloma (MM)	NCT01303965 Indiana University School of Medicine
Lenalidomide after donor stem cell transplant and bortezomib in treating patients with high-risk multiple myeloma	NCT01954784 Case Comprehensive Cancer Center
Ofatumumab induction and maintenance in elderly patients with poor-risk CLL in the context of allogeneic transplantation Study of dasatinib to treat Philadelphia-positive acute lymphoblastic leukemia (DASA-TRAS)	NCT01809847 Technische Universität Dresden/Multicenter NCT01310010 Grupo Espanol de trasplantes hematopoyeticos y terapia celular
Brentuximab vedotin after donor stem cell transplantation in treating patients with hematologic malignancies	NCT01620229 Fred Hutchinson Cancer Research Center
PF-04449913 For Patients With Acute Leukemia at High-Risk of Relapse After Donor Stem Cell Transplant	NCT01841333 University of Colorado, Denver
Lenalidomide as Maintenance Therapy After Combination Chemotherapy With or Without Rituximab and Stem Cell Transplant in Treating Patients With Persistent or Recurrent Non-Hodgkin Lymphoma That is Resistant to Chemotherapy	NCT01035463 University of Nebraska Medical Center University Hospitals Case Medical Center University of Kansas Medical Center

Adapted from Hourigan et al. (2014)[2].

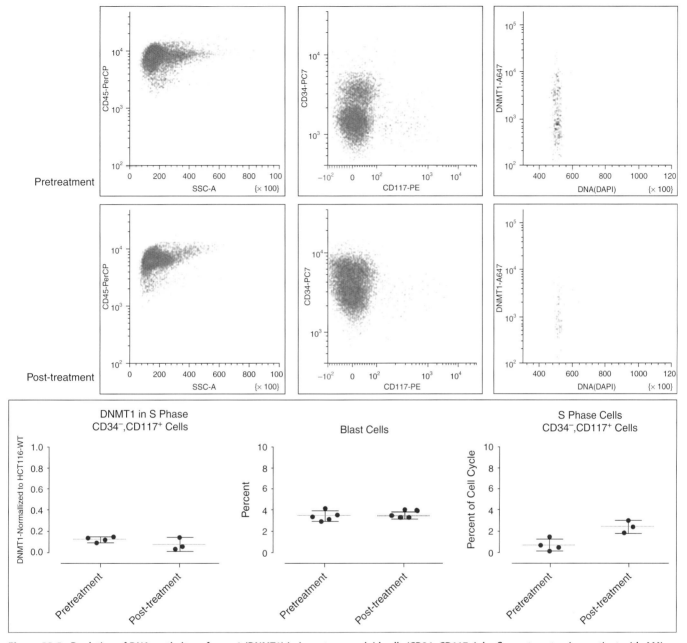

Figure 23.3. Depletion of DNA methyltransferase-1 (DNMT1) in immature myeloid cells (CD34+CD117+), by flow cytometry, in a patient with AML, in remission, treated with oral azacitidine maintenance after allo-HCT (on protocol NCT01835587). Pretreatment peripheral blood sample was collected at T+85 after myeloablative allo-HCT and before starting oral azacitidine (300mg PO daily for 1 week). Post-treatment sample was collected on day 8. DNMT1 level is determined in CD34+CD117+ and S-phase cells by flow cytometry.

HCT for AML or MDS. This drug has immunomodulatory effects and is moderately active against myeloid leukemias.

The dose-limiting toxicity was colitis and nausea at the 30mg three times weekly maximum tolerated dose[32].

The hypothesis that newer pharmacologic interventions could have an additive effect with cellular treatments post-HCT is fascinating and opens a wide array of questions. Conceivably, antigen-specific or nonspecific cellular maintenance strategies could be magnified by concomitant administration of drugs that might enhance the effects of cellular therapy or modulate GvHD *versus* GvL effects.

Several groups are currently investigating this possibility (Table 23.3).

Controversies

Controversy #1: Does MRD Affect the Decision to Proceed to Allo-HCT or Change the Outcomes of Allo-HCT in Acute Leukemias?

Depends on the disease; there are recent data that adult patients with Ph-ALL treated with a pediatric regimen and achieving MRD negativity after induction may not need consolidation with allo-HCT[33]. For AML, MRD positivity (even at minute amounts) was associated with worse outcomes after myeloablative allo-HCT for AML[34]. Currently, MRD positivity is not part of the decision-making in proceeding to allo-HCT in AML as some patients who have even refractory AML can benefit from allo-HCT especially with the addition of post-transplant maintenance azacitidine[27].

Controversy#2: Does Azacitidine Improve Treg Reconstitution after Allo-HCT?

Goodyear *et al.* have shown that azacitidine does enhance the reconstitution of Treg cells after T-cell depleted allo-HCT and such expansion was proportionate to the number of azacitidine cycles given[30]. However, no control group was employed in this study and improved reconstitution of Treg cells was not demonstrated in T-cell replete allo-HCT(Komanduri, personal communication). A randomized controlled trial of post-allo-HCT azacitidine versus placebo would be the only setting where such a question can be conclusively answered.

Controversy#3: Is There a Benefit in "Sandwiching" Azacitidine and Donor Lymphocyte Infusions (DLI) to Treat Relapse After Allo-HCT?

Yes, although the data remain limited. The largest series was of 115 patients treated with azacitidine and DLI for relapse of AML and myeloproliferative disease. The overall response rate was 36% with 29% complete remission. Interestingly, incidence and severity of acute GvHD (overall: 25%, grade I: 10%, grade II: 6%, grade III: 7%, grade IV: 2%) and chronic GvHD (overall 23%, limited 19%, extensive 4%) were low and mild as compared to what had been historically observed after DLI[35].

The relative contribution of azacitidine and DLI, individually, to the observed benefit remains unclear however.

Controversy#4: Should Maintenance Azacitidine Be Routinely Recommended for Patients with High-Risk MDS/AML after RIC Allo-HCT?

Probably – although prospective randomized controlled trials are needed before maintenance azacitidine can be recommended as the standard of care. Relapse rates after allo-HCT for MDS/AML are as high at 30% and are likely higher in patients who receive RIC, as compared to myeloablation, and when patients have refractory disease pre-allo-HCT[1]. The initial phase I study of azacitidine maintenance after allo-HCT for MDS/AML showed a 1-year event-free and overall survival of 58% and 77% despite the fact that many of the patients on this trial had refractory disease with only 33% being in remission at the time of allo-HCT[27]. FLT3 inhibitor and other targeted therapies may have a role here as well.

Conclusions and Future Directions

Post-transplantation treatments are under active investigation. We should keep in mind that the burden of the proof falls on the investigators and that significant costs are associated with maintenance therapy. Therefore, well-conducted prospective, controlled clinical trials will be necessary to demonstrate the benefits and risks of these new approaches.

Acknowledgments

This work was supported by the Intramural Research Program of the National Heart, Lung, Blood Institute of the National Institutes of Health (C.S.H.) and the American Cancer Society IRG-91-022-18 (B.M.W.).

References

1. William BM, de Lima M. Advances in conditioning regimens for older adults undergoing allogeneic stem cell transplantation to treat hematologic malignancies. *Drugs & Aging.* 2013;30(6):373–81.

2. Hourigan CS, McCarthy P, de Lima M. Back to the future! The evolving role of maintenance therapy after hematopoietic stem cell transplantation. *Biology of Blood and Marrow Transplantation: Journal of the American Society for Blood and Marrow Transplantation.* 2014;20(2):154–63.

3. de Lima M, Porter DL, Battiwalla M, Bishop MR, Giralt SA, Hardy NM, *et al.* Proceedings from the National Cancer Institute's Second International Workshop on the Biology, Prevention, and Treatment of Relapse After Hematopoietic Stem Cell Transplantation: part III. Prevention and treatment of relapse after allogeneic transplantation. *Biology of Blood and Marrow Transplantation: Journal of the American Society for Blood and Marrow Transplantation.* 2014;20(1):4–13.

4. Gisselbrecht C, Schmitz N, Mounier N, Singh Gill D, Linch DC, Trneny M, *et al.* Rituximab maintenance therapy after autologous stem-cell transplantation in patients with relapsed CD20(+) diffuse large B-cell lymphoma: final analysis of the collaborative trial in relapsed aggressive lymphoma. *Journal of Clinical Oncology: Official Journal of the American Society of Clinical Oncology.* 2012;30(36):4462–9.

5. Goldman JM, Gale RP. What does MRD in leukemia really mean? *Leukemia: Official Journal of the Leukemia Society of America, Leukemia Research Fund, UK.* 2014;28(5):1131.

6. Hourigan CS. Next Generation MRD. *Biology of Blood and Marrow Transplantation: Journal of the American Society for Blood and Marrow Transplantation.* 2014;20(9):1259–60.

7. Puig N, Sarasquete ME, Balanzategui A, Martinez J, Paiva B, Garcia H, *et al.* Critical evaluation of ASO RQ-PCR for minimal residual disease evaluation in multiple myeloma. A comparative analysis with flow cytometry. *Leukemia.* 2014;28(2):391–7.

8. Bruggemann M, Raff T, Kneba M. Has MRD monitoring superseded other

prognostic factors in adult ALL? *Blood.* 2012;120(23):4470–81.

9. Richardson SE, Khan I, Rawstron A, Sudak J, Edwards N, Verfuerth S, et al. Risk-stratified adoptive cellular therapy following allogeneic hematopoietic stem cell transplantation for advanced chronic lymphocytic leukaemia. *British Journal of Haematology.* 2013;160(5):640–8.

10. Pott C, Bruggemann M, Ritgen M, van der Velden VH, van Dongen JJ, Kneba M. MRD detection in B-cell non-Hodgkin lymphomas using Ig gene rearrangements and chromosomal translocations as targets for real-time quantitative PCR. *Methods in Molecular Biology (Clifton, NJ).* 2013;971:175–200.

11. Gimenez E, Chauvet M, Rabin L, Puteaud I, Duley S, Hamaidia S, et al. Cloned IGH VDJ targets as tools for personalized minimal residual disease monitoring in mature lymphoid malignancies; a feasibility study in mantle cell lymphoma by the Groupe Ouest Est d'Etude des Leucemies et Autres Maladies du Sang. *British Journal of Haematology.* 2012;158(2):186–97.

12. Radich JP. Monitoring response to tyrosine kinase inhibitor therapy, mutational analysis, and new treatment options in chronic myelogenous leukemia. *Journal of the National Comprehensive Cancer Network.* 2013;11(5 Suppl):663–6.

13. O'Donnell MR, Tallman MS, Abboud CN, Altman JK, Appelbaum FR, Arber DA, et al. Acute myeloid leukemia, version 2.2013. *Journal of the National Comprehensive Cancer Network.* 2013;11(9):1047–55.

14. Hourigan CS, Karp JE. Minimal residual disease in acute myeloid leukaemia. *Nature Reviews Clinical Oncology.* 2013;10(8):460–71.

15. Qin YZ, Zhu HH, Liu YR, Wang YZ, Shi HX, Lai YY, et al. PRAME and WT1 transcripts constitute a good molecular marker combination for monitoring minimal residual disease in myelodysplastic syndromes. *Leukemia & Lymphoma.* 2013;54(7):1442–9.

16. Grimwade D, Freeman SD. Defining minimal residual disease in acute myeloid leukemia: which platforms are ready for "Prime Time"? *Blood.* 2014;124(23):3345–55.

17. Logan AC, Vashi N, Faham M, Carlton V, Kong K, Buno I, et al. Immunoglobulin and T cell receptor gene high-throughput sequencing quantifies minimal residual disease in acute lymphoblastic leukemia and predicts post-transplantation relapse and survival. *Biology of Blood and Marrow Transplantation: Journal of the American Society for Blood and Marrow Transplantation.* 2014;20(9):1307–13.

18. Brenner MK, Rill DR, Moen RC, Krance RA, Mirro J, Jr., Anderson WF, et al. Gene-marking to trace origin of relapse after autologous bone-marrow transplantation. *Lancet.* 1993;341(8837):85–6.

19. Stewart AK, Vescio R, Schiller G, Ballester O, Noga S, Rugo H, et al. Purging of autologous peripheral-blood stem cells using CD34 selection does not improve overall or progression-free survival after high-dose chemotherapy for multiple myeloma: results of a multicenter randomized controlled trial. *Journal of Clinical Oncology: Official Journal of the American Society of Clinical Oncology.* 2001;19(17):3771–9.

20. Schouten HC, Qian W, Kvaloy S, Porcellini A, Hagberg H, Johnsen HE, et al. High-dose therapy improves progression-free survival and survival in relapsed follicular non-Hodgkin's lymphoma: results from the randomized European CUP trial. *Journal of Clinical Oncology: Official Journal of the American Society of Clinical Oncology.* 2003;21(21):3918–27.

21. Furman RR, Grossbard ML, Johnson JL, Pecora AL, Cassileth PA, Jung SH, et al. A phase III study of anti-B4-blocked ricin as adjuvant therapy post-autologous bone marrow transplant: CALGB 9254. *Leukemia & Lymphoma.* 2011;52(4):587–96.

22. Pettengell R, Schmitz N, Gisselbrecht C, Smith G, Patton WN, Metzner B, et al. Rituximab purging and/or maintenance in patients undergoing autologous transplantation for relapsed follicular lymphoma: a prospective randomized trial from the lymphoma working party of the European group for blood and marrow transplantation. *Journal of Clinical Oncology: Official Journal of the American Society of Clinical Oncology.* 2013;31(13):1624–30.

23. Wetzler M, Watson D, Stock W, Koval G, Mulkey FA, Hoke EE, et al. Autologous transplantation for Philadelphia chromosome-positive acute lymphoblastic leukemia achieves outcomes similar to allogeneic transplantation: results of CALGB Study 10001 (Alliance). *Haematologica.* 2014;99(1):111–5.

24. Younes A, Bartlett NL, Leonard JP, Kennedy DA, Lynch CM, Sievers EL, et al. Brentuximab vedotin (SGN-35) for relapsed CD30-positive lymphomas. *The New England Journal of Medicine.* 2010;363(19):1812–21.

25. Rytting M, Triche L, Thomas D, O'Brien S, Kantarjian H. Initial experience with CMC-544 (inotuzumab ozogamicin) in pediatric patients with relapsed B-cell acute lymphoblastic leukemia. *Pediatric Blood and Cancer.* 2014;61(2):369–72.

26. O'Hear C, Inaba H, Pounds S, Shi L, Dahl G, Bowman WP, et al. Gemtuzumab ozogamicin can reduce minimal residual disease in patients with childhood acute myeloid leukemia. *Cancer.* 2013;119(22):4036–43.

27. de Lima M, Giralt S, Thall PF, de Padua Silva L, Jones RB, Komanduri K, et al. Maintenance therapy with low-dose azacitidine after allogeneic hematopoietic stem cell transplantation for recurrent acute myelogenous leukemia or myelodysplastic syndrome: a dose and schedule finding study. *Cancer.* 2010;116(23):5420–31.

28. Choi J, Ritchey J, Prior JL, Holt M, Shannon WD, Deych E, et al. In vivo administration of hypomethylating agents mitigate graft-*versus*-host disease without sacrificing graft-*versus*-leukemia. *Blood.* 2010;116(1):129–39.

29. Sanchez-Abarca LI, Gutierrez-Cosio S, Santamaria C, Caballero-Velazquez T, Blanco B, Herrero-Sanchez C, et al. Immunomodulatory effect of 5-azacytidine (5-azaC): potential role in the transplantation setting. *Blood.* 2010;115(1):107–21.

30. Goodyear OC, Dennis M, Jilani NY, Loke J, Siddique S, Ryan G, et al. Azacitidine augments expansion of regulatory T cells after allogeneic stem cell transplantation in patients with acute myeloid leukemia (AML). *Blood.* 2012;119(14):3361–9.

31. Garcia-Manero G, Gore SD, Cogle C, Ward R, Shi T, Macbeth KJ, et al. Phase I study of oral azacitidine in myelodysplastic syndromes, chronic myelomonocytic leukemia, and acute myeloid leukemia. *Journal of Clinical Oncology: Official Journal of the American Society of Clinical Oncology.* 2011;29(18):2521–7.

32. Burchert A, Nicolaus K, Huenecke S, Duenzinger U, Wolf A, Bader P, et al. Post-transplant maintenance with the deacetylase inhibitor panobinostat in patients with high-risk AML or MDS: results of the phase I part of the panobest trial. *Blood.* 2013;122(21):3315.

33. Dhedin N, Huynh A, Maury S, Tabrizi R, Beldjord K, Asnafi V, et al. Role of allogeneic stem cell transplantation in adult patients with Ph-negative acute lymphoblastic leukemia. *Blood.* 2015;125(16):2486–96; quiz 586.

34. Walter RB, Buckley SA, Pagel JM, Wood BL, Storer BE, Sandmaier BM, et al. Significance of minimal residual disease before myeloablative allogeneic hematopoietic cell transplantation for AML in first and second complete remission. *Blood.* 2013;122(10):1813–21.

35. Schroeder T, Czibere A, Platzbecker U, Bug G, Uharek L, Luft T, et al. Azacitidine and donor lymphocyte infusions as first salvage therapy for relapse of AML or MDS after allogeneic stem cell transplantation. *Leukemia.* 2013;27(6):1229–35.

36. Thompson JA, Fisher RI, Leblanc M, Forman SJ, Press OW, Unger JM, et al. Total body irradiation, etoposide, cyclophosphamide, and autologous peripheral blood stem-cell transplantation followed by randomization to therapy with interleukin-2 *versus* observation for patients with non-Hodgkin lymphoma: results of a phase 3 randomized trial by the Southwest Oncology Group (SWOG 9438). *Blood.* 2008;111(8):4048–54.

37. Bolanos-Meade J, Garrett-Mayer E, Luznik L, Anders V, Webb J, Fuchs EJ, et al. Induction of autologous graft-*versus*-host disease: results of a randomized prospective clinical trial in patients with poor risk lymphoma. *Journal of Clinical Oncology: Official Journal of the American Society of Clinical Oncology.* 2007;13(10):1185–91.

38. Simonsson B, Totterman T, Hokland P, Lauria F, Carella AM, Fernandez MN, et al. Roquinimex (Linomide) vs placebo in AML after autologous bone marrow transplantation. *Bone Marrow Transplant.* 2000;25(11):1121–7.

39. Attal M, Harousseau JL, Leyvraz S, Doyen C, Hulin C, Benboubker L, et al. Maintenance therapy with thalidomide improves survival in patients with multiple myeloma. *Blood.* 2006;108(10):3289–94.

40. Barlogie B, Pineda-Roman M, van Rhee F, Haessler J, Anaissie E, Hollmig K, et al. Thalidomide arm of Total Therapy 2 improves complete remission duration and survival in myeloma patients with metaphase cytogenetic abnormalities. *Blood.* 2008;112(8):3115–21.

41. Lokhorst HM, van der Holt B, Zweegman S, Vellenga E, Croockewit S, van Oers MH, et al. A randomized phase 3 study on the effect of thalidomide combined with adriamycin, dexamethasone, and high-dose melphalan, followed by thalidomide maintenance in patients with multiple myeloma. *Blood.* 2010;115(6):1113–20.

42. Morgan GJ, Davies FE, Gregory WM, Bell SE, Szubert AJ, Cook G, et al. Long-term follow-up of MRC Myeloma IX trial: Survival outcomes with bisphosphonate and thalidomide treatment. *Clin Cancer Res.* 2013;19(21):6030–8.

43. Spencer A, Prince HM, Roberts AW, Prosser IW, Bradstock KF, Coyle L, et al. Consolidation therapy with low-dose thalidomide and prednisolone prolongs the survival of multiple myeloma patients undergoing a single autologous stem-cell transplantation procedure. *Journal of Clinical Oncology: Official Journal of the American Society of Clinical Oncology.* 2009;27(11):1788–93.

44. Krishnan A, Pasquini MC, Logan B, Stadtmauer EA, Vesole DH, Alyea E, 3rd, et al. Autologous haemopoietic stem-cell transplantation followed by allogeneic or autologous haemopoietic stem-cell transplantation in patients with multiple myeloma (BMT CTN 0102): a phase 3 biological assignment trial. *The Lancet Oncology.* 2011;12(13):1195–203.

45. Maiolino A, Hungria VT, Garnica M, Oliveira-Duarte G, Oliveira LC, Mercante DR, et al. Thalidomide plus dexamethasone as a maintenance therapy after autologous hematopoietic stem cell transplantation improves progression-free survival in multiple myeloma. *Am J Hematol.* 2012;87(10):948–52.

46. Stewart AK, Trudel S, Bahlis NJ, White D, Sabry W, Belch A, et al. A randomized phase 3 trial of thalidomide and prednisone as maintenance therapy after ASCT in patients with MM with a quality-of-life assessment: the National Cancer Institute of Canada Clinicals Trials Group Myeloma 10 Trial. *Blood.* 2013;121(9):1517–23.

47. McCarthy PL, Owzar K, Hofmeister CC, Hurd DD, Hassoun H, Richardson PG, et al. Lenalidomide after stem-cell transplantation for multiple myeloma. *The New England Journal of Medicine.* 2012;366(19):1770–81.

48. Attal M, Lauwers-Cances V, Marit G, Caillot D, Moreau P, Facon T, et al. Lenalidomide maintenance after stem-cell transplantation for multiple myeloma. *The New England Journal of Medicine.* 2012;366(19):1782–91.

49. Boccadoro M, Cavallo, F., Gay, F. Melphalan/prednisone/lenalidomide (MPR) *versus* high-dose melphalan and autologous transplantation MEL200) plus lenalidomide maintenance or no maintenance in newly diagnosed multiple myeloma (MM) patients. *Journal of Clinical Oncology.* 2013;(Suppl): Abstract 8509.

50. Sonneveld P, Schmidt-Wolf IG, van der Holt B, El Jarari L, Bertsch U, Salwender H, et al. Bortezomib induction and maintenance treatment in patients with newly diagnosed multiple myeloma: results of the randomized phase III HOVON-65/GMMG-HD4 trial. *Journal of Clinical Oncology: Official Journal of the American Society of Clinical Oncology.* 2012;30(24):2946–55.

51. Cavo M, Pantani L, Petrucci MT, Patriarca F, Zamagni E, Donnarumma D, et al. Bortezomib-thalidomide-dexamethasone is superior to

thalidomide-dexamethasone as consolidation therapy after autologous hematopoietic stem cell transplantation in patients with newly diagnosed multiple myeloma. *Blood.* 2012;120(1):9–19.

52. Mellqvist UH, Gimsing P, Hjertner O, Lenhoff S, Laane E, Remes K, *et al.* Bortezomib consolidation after autologous stem cell transplantation in multiple myeloma: a Nordic Myeloma Study Group randomized phase 3 trial. *Blood.* 2013;121(23):4647–54.

53. Palumbo A, Cavallo F, Gay F, Di Raimondo F, Ben Yehuda D, Petrucci MT, *et al.* Autologous transplantation and maintenance therapy in multiple myeloma. *The New England Journal of Medicine.* 2014;371(10):895–905.

Chapter

24

Minimal Residual Disease in Acute Leukemias: Are We on the Right Path?

Elisabeth Paietta and Mark Litzow

The Definition of Response

The principle of assessing response in leukemia relies on the detection of aberrancies in morphology, immunophenotype, or the genetic make-up of leukemic cells in individual patients at the time of presentation and allows one to distinguish them from normal hematopoietic cells when they are present at low numbers after treatment. Evaluation of bone marrow morphology by the human eye remains an integral part of response definition. In adult treatment trials of the US National Cancer Trial Network (NCTN), the accepted definition of a complete response (CR) in acute leukemia is still based on normal bone marrow morphology with $\leq 5\%$ blasts, absence of circulating blasts, peripheral count recovery, and absence of extramedullary disease[1]. Half a century ago, Freireich et al.[2] demonstrated that patients with acute myeloid leukemia (AML) who achieved a durable morphologic CR survived longer than those who did not. Clinical experience over the years has taught us, however, that there are clear limitations to this approach. After all, 30–50% of morphologically defined remitters relapse sooner or later, usually with catastrophic consequences. Conventional CR criteria suffer from limited sensitivity, disagreements among pathologists, and sheer difficulties in the distinction of normal regenerating blasts from residual leukemic blasts when counting blast cells by light microscopy. A reduction of the leukemic burden to below the level of morphologic detection ($< 10^9$ cells) by induction chemotherapy leaves patients with, as we know now, largely varied amounts of disease. In fact, the wide range of levels of disease remaining in patients in morphologic CR offers an opportunity for post-therapeutic risk classification.

In the early days of antibody development to hematopoietic antigens, Bradstock et al.[3] provided evidence that bone marrows from T-lineage acute lymphoblastic leukemia (ALL) patients in morphologic CR have measurable disease. This observation was revolutionary. Until today, the accepted hypothesis remains that the predominant root of relapse is the persistence of such subclinical minimal residual disease, or MRD, that remains after treatment at levels too low to be detected under the microscope. The level of MRD reflects the quality of the remission and, therefore, serves as a post-therapy prognosticator closely associated with outcome.

The discovery of MRD has changed the definition of CR and of treatment response in general. MRD has also been implicated in the CR subcategory, CR with incomplete blood count recovery (CRi), and its subset, CR with incomplete platelet recovery (to less than 100000/μL) (CRp)[1]. Patients with CRp have poorer long-term survival than true responders [4]. MRD levels in the marrows of CRi patients are significantly higher than in CR or CRp patients, paralleled by higher risk of relapse[5]. Chen et al.[5] suggested that rather than delaying therapy to await count recovery, the diagnosis of CRp or Cri should prompt immediate further therapy to eradicate MRD, which they blamed for the impaired hematopoiesis. Freeman et al.[6] confirmed the high incidence of MRD positivity in CRp patients and reported that absent platelet count recovery lost its prognostic value in multivariate analysis after adjustment for MRD status.

While it is widely accepted that the morphologic definition of CR is not sufficiently reliable in predicting outcome, it is disappointing that with currently available routine methods of MRD detection, approximately 25% of patients in MRD-negative (MRD^{NEG}) morphologic CR will relapse while about the same proportion in MRD-positive (MRD^{POS}) morphologic CR will not. Despite considerably higher sensitivity, efforts, and costs, we still fail to consistently recognize MRD^{NEG} CR patients who require additional, enhanced, or, more likely, alternative treatment as well as those who should be spared such measures although they present with MRD after treatment. There are multiple potential reasons for cases in which outcome is unexpected given the MRD status (Table 24.1). Technical difficulties or errors in the definition of MRD status may account for a significant proportion of patients whose long-term outcome is unpredictable given their post-therapy MRD data. As a result, what is primarily needed is the optimization of MRD assays to make MRD results "trustworthy enough" for physicians to base treatment decisions on, even if these results disagree with morphology. Furthermore, there exist alternate proposed mechanisms to explain MRD-independent prognostication[7–9].

Biologic reasons for favorable outcome in apparently MRD^{POS} patients could be therapy-induced leukemic cell differentiation, leading to apoptotic cell death, or immune surveillance preventing small numbers of leukemic cells from

Table 24.1 Potential reasons for leukemia outcome unexplained by MRD results

MRD^{NEG} patients experience poorer outcome than expected

Patient falsely characterized as MRD^{NEG} due to problems with MRD assay itself or lacking operator skills

With a given therapy, the threshold used for defining MRD-negativity is not clinically relevant and must be re-established

Changes in MRD target (e.g., oligoclonality or clonal evolution of molecular targets, change in antigen profiles with therapy, outgrowth of immunophenotypic subpopulation) lead to inability to detect MRD

MRD negativity is based on the absence of leukemic bulk cells; leukemic stem cells or preleukemic stem cells, however, have remained and lead to relapse

Frequency of MRD-testing in patients in apparently MRD^{NEG} remission does not match the kinetics of the relapse leukemic clone

Existence of MRD-independent prognosticators (e.g., BCR/ABL1-like phenotype, gene polymorphisms)

MRD^{POS} patients do better than expected

Patient falsely characterized as MRD^{POS} due to problems with MRD assay itself or lacking operator skills (e.g., misinterpretation of hematogones as lymphoblasts)

The threshold used for defining MRD positivity does not apply to a new therapy and must be set lower given the higher efficacy of that therapy

Time point of MRD positivity was clinically not impactful (e.g., subsequent therapy was able to abrogate negative MRD effect)

Therapy-induced differentiation of blast cells leading to apoptotic cell death yields temporary MRD positivity which resolves without further clinical intervention (e.g., persistent PML/RARα transcripts with retinoid acid therapy in APL)

MRD positivity was based on the persistence of a molecular signature found in the original leukemic cell; after therapy, this signature remains in a clone which lacks other genetic mutations required for relapse

Successful immune surveillance of low levels of MRD cells prevents relapse

growing to the critical mass necessary for relapse. The hypothesis that leukemic cells can undergo prolonged dormancy is supported by children who relapse >10 years after ALL diagnosis with IgH or TCR gene rearrangements identical to those present at diagnosis[10]. Reasons for relapse in apparently MRD^{NEG} patients include instability of the diagnostic mutated clone, which is missed at relapse, or reappearance of a leukemic clone with particularly rapid relapse kinetics, which is missed by too infrequent MRD sampling[11].

Among MRD-independent prognostication, Kang *et al.* [7] suggested that a combination of their prognostic gene-classifier with end-induction MRD level, determined by multiparametric flow cytometry (MFC), had enhanced clinical utility, as they retained independent prognostic significance in the presence of other pretreatment characteristics associated with poor outcome in pediatric ALL (e.g., age >10 years, presenting white blood cell count >50 000/μL, high-risk cytogenetic aberrations, IKZF1 alterations, etc.). Yang *et al.*[8] identified germline variations which distinguished children at risk of relapse despite an excellent early response to therapy. Of the 134 single nucleotide polymorphisms associated with relapse, 14 were associated with unfavorable pharmacokinetics of commonly used antileukemic drugs. Such polymorphisms could explain surprising clinical data, such as significantly better outcome in relapsed ALL children induced with mitoxantrone *versus* idarubicin without apparent difference in postinduction MRD levels[12]. On the other hand, Butturini *et al.*[13] warned about applying a definition of MRD status which was

established in a given clinical situation in a random fashion to other settings. In other words, MRD thresholds that are prognostically significant in children with *de novo* ALL treated with standard therapy may not be applicable to children in relapse treated with experimental regimens. In both B- and T-ALL, high-risk genetics, including IKZF1 gene deletions, and poor early MRD response independently predict relapse[9]. Regrettably, in that study, B-ALL patients were not evaluated for the unfavorable BCR/ABL1-like phenotype, which frequently presents with IKZF1 mutations[14]. Both BCR/ABL-like gene signature and IKZF1 gene mutations have independent prognostic value[15]. Though BCR/ABL1-like phenotype and MRD contribute independently to risk of relapse with contemporary therapies (C. Willman, personal communication), data may look different once BCR/ABL1-like patients are treated optimally, according to their kinase-activating aberrations[16]. In Philadelphia-chromosome^{POS} (BCR/ABL^{POS}) ALL, on the other hand, the addition of tyrosine kinase inhibitors (TKI) to chemotherapy has altered the MRD kinetics and made MRD the most powerful predictor for long-term outcome[17–19].

The Importance of Sample Quality in MRD Detection

In the comparison of morphology and MRD results, a critical overlooked factor is that the pathologist has the advantage of counting blasts in a bone marrow smear from a first pull aspirate which has the highest likelihood of containing spicules, given the common practice to send the first aspirate to the local pathology laboratory and to continue aspirating from the same puncture site for additional studies. This practice further increases the underrepresentation of leukemic cells in the aspirate, which might already be caused by marrow fibrosis, cell adherence, or other factors. In an elegant, though little noticed study, Helgestad et al.[20] demonstrated that the technique of marrow aspiration dramatically influenced MRD levels in AML. Even a second pull from the same aspiration site reduced leukemic cells by almost 50% due to hemodilution. These data on sample quality are of crucial importance for multi-institutional trials with central MRD evaluation. At least in AML and B-lineage ALL, MRD levels are drastically lower in blood than bone marrow[21,22]. Several NCTN protocols involving central MRD determinations, therefore, now require that aspirates from a separate puncture site be submitted to the reference laboratory by redirecting the needle after the first pull. The problem of hemodilution of aspirates for accurate MRD measurements is rarely directly addressed in publications[23]. Even with the best assay and perfect standardization, it is the quality of the aspirate that determines the accuracy of MRD results. Loken et al.[24] proposed the normalization of aspirates for hemodilution flow cytometrically based on the proportion of dim-staining CD16-positive maturing myeloid cells to a level observed in bone marrow biopsies, based on an average mature neutrophil composition, a proposal that has not found widespread application. Buccisano et al.[25] suggested that MRD levels of >0.015% in the blood were associated with a high likelihood of subsequent relapse. Unfortunately, in a large fraction of B-ALL[22] and AML patients (E. Paietta, unpublished data), MRD is undetectable by MFC in the blood, while substantial levels of disease remain measurable in the marrow.

Morphology Differs from MRD Results

We have established above that sample quality is one main reason why in some patients who failed to achieve a morphologic CR MFC cannot detect measurable MRD[6,26,27]. On the other hand, in discordant cases, erroneous interpretation of blast cells by morphology must be considered. In ALL, hematologists have difficulties distinguishing between residual leukemic lymphoblasts and nonmalignant B-lymphoid precursor cells (hematogones), which are particularly frequent at the end of intensive induction therapy[28] and can present at various stages of maturation[29–31]. In Children's Oncology Group (COG) AML trials, NCT00070174[26] and NCT00372593[32], approximately one-third of patients had morphologic disease after induction therapy but were MRD[NEG] by MFC. These patients did as well as patients in morphologic CR on both trials[26,32].

These data prompt the question whether MFC-MRD[NEG] morphologic response failures represent a distinct biologic subgroup. A possible explanation for this phenomenon lies in slower regression of the leukemic clone, possibly due to

therapy-induced differentiation of leukemic cells and a resultant discordance between morphology and antigen expression [27,32]. Induction of differentiation would agree with the favorable outcome of these patients since maturing blasts are doomed to undergo apoptosis. In acute promyelocytic leukemia treated with all-*trans* retinoic acid, early MRD assessment by polymerase chain reaction (PCR) amplification for PML/RARα is not informative because the transcript persists in leukemic promyelocytes undergoing maturation[33]. Similar complications in MRD measurements can be expected from other differentiation-inducing therapies, such as inhibitors targeting IDH2 mutant AML[34].

Whatever the answer, the result of counting immature cells under the microscope must no longer be the determining factor in the decision as to whether to measure MRD. At a minimum, MRD should be measured in all patients post induction chemotherapy, not only in the cohort in morphologic CR.

MRD Detection Methods

Any definition of CR must be reproducible, reliable, and technically feasible within the time and cost restraints of therapeutic decision-making and today's medical climate, respectively, whether it relies on morphology, MFC, quantitative PCR, or next-generation sequencing (NGS). Given our understanding of the limited clinical value of a morphologically defined CR and ample, though mostly retrospective, data suggesting that MRD has a decisive role in treatment stratification, one cannot help but ask why the implementation of MRD into clinical practice remains a major challenge. The common answer lies in methodologic aspects of MRD assays commonly used in clinical laboratories. Comparative analyses have found that MFC and PCR are equally effective in identifying patients at high risk of relapse[27,28,35]. The biggest concern on the part of treating physicians and regulatory agencies remains the lack of assay standardization. It seems illogical when one thinks of the enormous efforts (and costs) that are being spent on the near impossible task of standardizing MRD measurements vis-a-vis the completely unregulated, evaluator-dependent, though accepted method of counting 'blast cells' under the microscope. However, we certainly agree that efforts regarding assay standardization, such as those undertaken by several European groups, are commendable and the guidelines of the EuroMRD Group for DNA-based MRD diagnostics are a big step towards broad clinical application at least in ALL [36]. The EuroFlow project on standardized flow cytometric immunophenotyping of leukemias and lymphomas across laboratories and countries, designed in 2004, has recently culminated in the publication of the EuroFlow Educational Book[37].

The main limitation for MFC is the need for data interpretation which, in the hands of the untrained, is as subjective as the morphologic assessment of bone marrow smears. Knowledge of the expression of antigens during normal differentiation along all hematopoietic cell lineages is an absolute prerequisite. With proper training and experience, MFC and PCR provide comparable results provided that the level of MRD is $\geq 0.01\%$; thus, the choice of MRD methodology depends on facilities and expertise available, clinical need for fast results (MFC is the fastest), and budget (MFC is the cheapest). The fact that the majority of ALL cases have somatic antigen receptor gene rearrangements suitable for MRD monitoring by PCR represents an important difference between ALL and AML, given that most AML cases lack comparative immunogenotypes[38]. Suitable fusion genes as the result of chromosomal rearrangements are more frequent in ALL (especially BCR/ABL), while gene mutations are increasingly being used for MRD detection in AML (e.g., FLT3, NPM1, DNMT3A gene mutations). The vast majority of ALL and AML patients have leukemic blasts with immunophenotypic characteristics distinct enough to allow for their reliable recognition when present at very low level among an overwhelming number of normal cells. This high degree of applicability of MFC is a critical factor in the selection of MRD assessment technique. Allele-specific oligonucleotide (ASO) real-time quantitative PCR analysis of rearranged immunoglobulin (Ig) and T-cell receptor (TCR) genes requires the development of patient-specific probes, which is laborious, expensive, and time-consuming. Furthermore, ASO-PCR is limited to Ig/TCR gene rearrangements with junctional regions that yield sufficient sensitivity[36]. In comparison, deep sequencing or NGS of the antigen receptor repertoire in ALL uses consensus primers to universally amplify and sequence all rearranged Ig/TCR genes, thus does not require the design of patient-specific probes, and exceeds the lower limit of detection provided by standard ASO-PCR or MFC by 1 to 2 orders of magnitude[39]. A good concordance across the three methodologic platforms has been seen both in ALL[40] and multiple myeloma[41]. It is important to remember that the sensitivity of all three assays is dependent upon the quality of the specimen as well as the number of cells or the amount and purity of DNA analyzed[13,41]. Each MRD methodology faces its own challenges and we will address some, particularly those affecting MFC.

While PCR for Ig/TCR gene rearrangements and recurrent gene mutations are regulated by proficiency testing (PT) programs, there are currently no PT programs available in the United States for MFC-MRD. We take advantage of the PT for MFC-based MRD in B-ALL offered by the UK National External Quality Assessment Service (NEQAS) Leukemia Immunophenotyping and Diagnostic Interpretation Program[42]. The NIH-led effort of standardizing and optimizing MFC-MRD assays in the US MRD Working Group, which includes reference laboratories from all NCTN groups with leukemia trials, takes advantage of the COG experience[43,44] and is a laudable approach to export a successful assay into the medical community.

Important for MFC-MRD is that flow cytometrists are aware of antecedent antibody therapy potentially resulting in the loss of the antigens targeted by the antibody. In patients treated with gemtuzumab, CD33 expression persisted at relapse in most cases[45]. In contrast, after rituximab therapy, more than one-third of cases lost CD20 expression[46]. With the bispecific CD3/CD19 targeting antibody, blinatumomab, loss of CD19 expression occurred with treatment and at the time of relapse[47].

After managing all technical issues of MFC-MRD, one has to decide whether to monitor MRD based on leukemia-associated immunophenotypes (LAIP)[25,28,48–50], established in the diagnostic specimen, or by using the different-from-normal approach, which does not require knowledge of the presenting immunophenotype[6,43,44]. The latter tactic may benefit from the discovery of novel markers with substantially abnormal gene expression levels in leukemic cells when compared to normal maturation stages[51]. Which strategy to use is personal preference and a combination of the two might be the way to go. One major advantage of the different-from-normal route is its independence from immunophenotypic changes due to therapy. Immunophenotypic switches occur more commonly in AML[21,25], either as a result of maturational changes[52] or clonal selection[53].

Clonal evolution also plagues ASO-PCR commonly used to amplify Ig/TCR gene rearrangements in ALL[27,40,54]. At presentation, genetic diversity often exists at multiple Ig/TCR genes. NGS, but not ASO-PCR, allows for the tracking of the evolution of all gene rearrangements during therapy[39,40,55]. With respect to common gene mutations, PCR- and sequencing-based MRD monitoring confirmed heterogeneity and clonal instability between diagnosis and relapse with selective outgrowth of mutated clones (oligoclonality), in particular, for FLT3-ITD[56], while NPM1, DNMT3A, and IDH2 mutations were found to be more stable[56–60]. These findings have cautionary clinical implications, especially for FLT3-ITD AML when treated with FLT3 kinase inhibitors.

The threshold for defining MRD positivity is crucial. In the literature, the value used to dichotomize into MRD^{POS} and MRD^{NEG} patients is consistently 10 times lower in ALL (0.01%) than AML (0.1%). There are data in pediatric B-ALL suggesting that ultralow MRD levels ($<0.001\%$) reachable with NGS are clinically relevant[61]. In AML, on the other hand, patients with slow blast cell clearance whose MRD levels are $> 0.1\%$ but $<1\%$ postinduction do as well long term as patients with MRD levels $<0.1\%$[27,62–64]. The level of MRD that influences AML outcome may be lowered by enhanced induction chemotherapy[25]. On the other hand, high-dose *versus* low-dose cytarabine during induction did not affect postinduction MRD levels in pediatric AML[63], and neither did doubling of the daunorubicin dose in adults[65], although the latter resulted in prolonged OS[66]. These data imply that with any novel, improved therapy, the MRD level with clinical efficacy needs to be re-established retrospectively, a requirement that complicates the introduction of MRD-guided interventions. A biologic feature of, at least, some subtypes of AML may be persistent MRD in patients in long-term CR[60,67].

Salipante et al.[60] found NPM1-mutation positive MRD by NGS in six out of six randomly selected AML patients after therapy though they were MFC-MRD-negative. Such low-level, temporarily dormant, "disease" most probably reflects therapy-resistant preleukemic stem cells carrying preleukemic mutations in landscaping genes (e.g., NPM1, RUNX1/RUNXT1, CBFβ/MYH11, DNMT3A, IDH1/IDH2), which during remission contribute to normal hematopoiesis but could potentially provide a reservoir for leukemic progression[68–70]. With increased usage of deep-sequencing techniques for MRD detection, we will learn about the clinical significance of such extremely low-level latent disease. However, sequencing technologies also require workflow standardization and clear bioinformatics guidelines for optimal performance and true utility in the clinic[71].

MRD Targets

It is surprising that commonly used MFC-MRD assays, which solely measure residual cells from the original leukemic bulk, provide clinically relevant information. MFC also provides a means to monitor leukemic stem cells (LSCs) which, in contrast to the elusive preleukemic stem cells introduced above, can be detected based on a CD34^{POS}CD38^{NEG} surrogate phenotype[72]. The frequency of these cells at diagnosis of ALL[73] and AML[74–76] predicts for high MRD levels. Different from AML, the immunophenotype of LSCs in ALL remains imprecisely characterized[77]. That LSCs in MLL-rearranged leukemias have distinct surface antigen expression patterns of CD34, CD38, CD19, and CD33, dependent on gene fusion partners[78], suggests that the CD34^{POS}CD38^{NEG} cell pool may not uniquely contain LSCs.

Both in ALL and AML [69,70,79–82], genetically diverse subclones exist at presentation. The relapse clone is either derived from a minor subclone with genetic alterations distinct from those of the predominant clone at diagnosis or it shares lesions with the predominant clone at diagnosis, indicating a common "ancestral" or preleukemic origin[83]. Current methodologies to isolate and characterize preleukemic stem cells are out of the reach of routine clinical laboratories. However, the novel understanding of which mutations arise early in leukemia development (e.g., DNMT3A, IDH1/2 or TET2[70,84]) allows a prediction as to which mutations will persist in the preleukemic stem cells after therapy. These cells and the founder mutations they harbor represent the real MRD that must be targeted. With the development of drugs that effectively target those mutations[85,86] these preleukemic cells might be eliminated before they acquire additional mutations that lead to relapse. Along the same path are efforts to identify and subsequently target antigens selectively expressed by LSCs, such as IL1RAP[87,88]. Collectively, these data propose clinical success when the MRD marker is not only a tool to assess the quality of response but also the target for therapy and thus a predictor for response to available MRD-targeting therapy.

An excellent example for this concept is BCR/ABL^{POS} ALL. Remission induction therapy which includes TKIs results in much lower MRD levels at the end of induction than regimens which lack TKIs[19], and BCR/ABL^{POS} ALL patients have a better outcome if they become MRD-negative with TKIs and chemotherapy than patients who remain MRD-positive[18]. TKIs given during[17] or after induction [89] abrogated the negative prognostic impact of end-induction MRD, and imatinib administration prior to allogeneic hematopoietic cell transplant (allo-HCT) converted MRD^{POS} patients to MRD^{NEG}[90]. In the pre-TKI era, BCR/ABL positivity before HCT predicted relapse[91]. Recent data have shown that patients who turned MRD^{NEG} with TKIs prior to HCT could safely receive reduced intensity conditioning (RIC) and even experienced overall survival superior to that of patients who received myeloablative conditioning regimen (MAC regimen)[92]. On the other hand, MRD^{POS} patients pre-HCT had a higher risk of relapse with RIC than MAC regimens. It has been suggested that BCR/ABL^{POS} children who achieve MRD^{NEG} status with TKIs at the end of remission induction may no longer require allogeneic HCT[19,90]. Wetzler et al.[93] demonstrated that purging in-vivo with imatinib prior to stem cell collection and TKI maintenance following an autologous HCT yielded results comparable to those of allogeneic HCT. Although cohorts were small, this study suggested that MRD levels equal to or lower than a major molecular response (≤0.001) on day +120, after autologous HCT and imatinib maintenance, resulted in prolonged survival. This vital importance of accurately assessing MRD status in BCR/ABL^{POS} ALL emphasizes the need for a standardized, reliable MRD assay. In fact, Ravandi et al.[18] reported that >50% of MRD specimens in their patient cohort were BCR/ABL^{POS} by PCR but negative by MFC. These findings are in agreement with those of others who found that MRD levels by MFC and/or PCR amplification of antigen receptor genes are largely equivalent but different from BCR/ABL transcript quantification[19]. Multilineage involvement with the presence of BCR/ABL in non-ALL cells[94] could account in part for this finding. More recently, suppression of BCR/ABL protein translation in LSCs which carry BCR/ABL transcripts has been reported in imatinib-refractory chronic myeloid leukemia (CML) resulting from the modulation of LSC metabolism by the environment in the stem cell niche[95]. The detection of MRD which is represented by residual LSCs is essential for long-term outcome in BCR/ABL^{POS} disease. Whether second-generation TKIs, such as dasatinib, nilotinib, or ponatinib, a multitargeted kinase inhibitor with activity against mutated BCR/ABL[96], are effective against LSC-based MRD will need to be established. A potential marker of BCR/ABL^{POS} LSC, dipeptidylpeptidase IV (CD26), has been proposed as a follow-up parameter at least in TKI-treated CML and lymphoid blast crisis of CML[97].

MRD detection in BCR/ABL^{POS} ALL and monitoring of disease at optimal, still to be determined, frequency is also imperative given the availability of TKIs for preemptive therapy when re-emerging disease is detected[96]. In fact, prophylactic imatinib reduced the incidence of molecular recurrence in BCR/ABL^POS ALL post-allogeneic HCT and reduced the probability of relapse significantly compared with imatinib given in response to re-emerging MRD [98].

Pretherapeutic Risk Factors and MRD

The level of MRD depends on a patient's pretherapeutic risk factors which include those represented by the characteristics of the leukemic cells (e.g., somatic gene mutations, gene polymorphisms) as well as a patient's inherent features (e.g., age, comorbidities). Most recently, obesity during induction of pediatric B-ALL patients has been associated with risk of end-induction MRD, irrespective of other predictors of response[99]. Obesity in mice substantially impaired the antileukemic effect of L-asparaginase in that adipocytes were found to protect leukemia cells both from the asparaginase effect and asparagine/glutamine starvation by producing and secreting glutamine[100]. Furthermore, several adipocyte-derived chemokines serve as attractants to normal and leukemia lymphocytes thus providing an environment that protects leukemia cells from chemotherapy[101], which may explain the observation that a child's body mass index also contributed significant additional risk for relapse independent of end-induction MRD[99].

Within each conventional risk category, MRD status adds independent prognostic information. Particularly in standard intermediate-risk patients, MRD allows for stratification into prognostic subgroups[23,25,63,65,102–104]. Conflicting data exist with respect to the value of MRD in favorable standard-risk patients. TEL/AML1 ALL patients will do much more poorly if they remain MRD^POS after therapy than favorable-risk patients without detectable post-therapy disease[104]. In core-binding factor (CBF) AML, Inaba et al.[27] reported several cases of RUNX1/RUNX1T1 and CBFβ/MYH11 AML, which at the end of induction were MRD^POS for their respective leukemia transcripts but MRD^NEG by MFC. Moreover, PCR results did not identify patients with worse outcome, suggesting persistence of fusion transcripts in preleukemic cells or in differentiating leukemic cells without leukemogenic potential[28]. The critical time point for identifying patients at risk of relapse by PCR in CBF-AML warrants further studies [105–109]. The French AML Intergroup[107] found that PCR-MRD levels after the first of three courses of high-dose cytarabine consolidation were associated with a lower risk of relapse and longer relapse-free survival. In multivariate analysis, including KIT and FLT3 gene mutations, this MRD response remained the unique predictor of relapse, possibly an indication that increased cytarabine susceptibility may be the determining factor in response in CBF-AML. These observations disagreed with those of the UK Medical Research Council AML-15 protocol, which demonstrated a predictive value of quantitative PCR-MRD in CBF-AML already after induction

as well as after first consolidation chemotherapy, possibly because of the use of gemtuzumab[108]. Buccisano et al. [109] corroborated the significance of positive MFC-based MRD in CBF leukemias at the end of postremission therapy. On the other hand, not yet published data from NCTN intergroup trial, NCT00049517[66], suggest that CBF-AML patients with MFC-MRD levels of <0.1% postinduction therapy have significantly better survival probability than patients with MRD >0.1% or those with MRD levels of ≥1% (Ganzel et al., in preparation). In pediatric CBF-AML, MFC-MRD levels of >0.1% after first induction were rare (approximately 15% of patients) but without effect on disease-free survival (S. Meshinchi, personal communication).

Even in poor-risk patients, the integration of pretherapeutic prognostic features, e.g., expression of CD25 in FLT3-ITD AML[110] or presence of Ikaros gene alterations in ALL [111] with MRD status, may optimize our ability to predict relapse. The expression level of CD25, a hallmark of BCR/ABL^POS ALL[112], by lymphoblasts at diagnosis was directly correlated with the level of end-induction MRD, at least in the pre-TKI era, and outcome. In BCR/ABL^POS CML, CD25 expression by CD34^POS CD38^NEG LSCs has been identified as a marker of LSCs with multilineage differentiation potential and a potential MRD target in combination with TKIs[113].

While there is little question that accurate risk allocation of leukemia patients depends on knowing their postremission MRD status, increased knowledge of pretherapeutic indicators of MRD may identify patients who could benefit from intensified induction therapy.

Controversies

While MRD detection strives for simple targets, such as a single mutation or one immunophenotypic clone, the genetic landscape of leukemias is increasingly found to be heterogeneous, thus complicating MRD-monitoring efforts. The pressure to incorporate MRD monitoring into every leukemia trial, while allegedly stalled by methodologic issues, is hampered by these forces pulling in opposite directions. Further heterogeneity in response predictors among as well as within genetic subgroups, the influence of nongenomic covariates of response, as well as the differential effects of new agents on MRD in leukemic subpopulations defined by classic risk standards have revealed a previously unanticipated complexity of MRD. For MRD detection to gauge treatment response in routine patient care, MRD assays have to be technically feasible in hospital laboratories, sufficiently standardized to be amenable to proficiency testing and regulatory surveillance and thus reimbursable by third-party payers, cost-effective, and fast. The degree of complexity in the molecular pathogenesis of the acute leukemias, however, presents laboratories with countless MRD targets, which can further change from diagnosis to remission to relapse due to clonal changes.

Whether or not isolated extramedullary relapse can be predicted by MRD in the BM has remained a contested though important issue, particularly in ALL[114,115]. We did not discuss the issue of preemptive therapy in response to MRD reappearance during hematologic CR, in part, because of the paucity of suitable treatment options for this situation.

In fact, the biggest obstacle to incorporating MRD into leukemic trials is the paucity of MRD-targeting treatment options and the mostly disappointing results obtained with standard treatment strategies. Particularly at the stage of hematologic remission, the quest for preemptive therapy in response to re-emerging MRD presents a difficult situation to treating oncologists. How to prevent relapse without hurting patients who are without obvious symptoms of disease? There is a true paucity of MRD-targeted preemptive therapies. Arsenic trioxide has proven to be a well-tolerated and successful intervention in acute promyelocytic leukemia patients who were predicted to experience relapse on the basis of molecular MRD monitoring[116]. Epigenetic modification, e.g., with azacitidine[117,118], antibody-based immunotherapy, e.g., with calicheamicin-conjugated anti-CD33 antibody, gemtuzumab ozogamicin[119,120], anti-CD22 antibodies[121], or the bispecific T-cell engaging (BiTE) CD19/CD3 antibody blinatumomab[122], all have converted MRD^{POS} to MRD^{NEG} status in acute leukemias. The ECOG-ACRIN NCTN group currently investigates the efficacy of blinatumomab in adult B-lineage ALL in MRD^{NEG} versus MRD^{POS} morphologic remission (NCT02003222).

A review of clinicaltrials.gov reveals >100 acute leukemia trials which address or at least utilize MRD as a marker for therapeutic success. The following are examples of studies which search for novel MRD-targeting alternatives. Greatly exciting is the further development of immunotherapy in some form, such as the anti-CD22 recombinant immunotoxin moxetumomab pasudotox (NCT02338050), or the adoptive transfer of genetically modified CD19-specific T-cells (NCT01044069) to eliminate B-lymphoblasts. Along the same lines is adoptive immunotherapy with expanded natural killer cells in B-lineage ALL (NCT02185781) and AML or T-ALL (NCT02123839) and trials of immune reactivity of autologous dendritic cells to leukemic myeloblasts in the MRD setting (NCT00965224). The COG is recruiting patients to a large randomized phase 3 trial which will explore the efficacy of the proteosome inhibitor bortezomib (NCT01371981). Taking advantage of other drug mechanisms, the clinical benefit of high-dose pegylated asparaginase plus other drugs (NCT02067143, NCT00549848) is studied in ALL, and the effect of the hypomethylating agent, azacitidine, on MRD in AML continues to be explored in the preemptive setting (NCT01462578).

If we consider the multistep development of leukemias, the extensive clonal heterogeneity at diagnosis and recent whole genome sequencing studies exploring how and why people with leukemia relapse, it would be extraordinarily unlikely to expect that the genotype and/or phenotype of MRD would be static or resemble cells at diagnosis. Accordingly, it seems unlikely that MRD-testing will be a foolproof method of predicting relapse. Furthermore, many or most leukemia relapses occur from a LSC or preleukemic stem cell whose genotype and phenotype are still barely known to us and therefore not the target of current MRD-testing.

References

1. Cheson BD, Bennett JM, Kopecky KJ, et al. Revised recommendations of the International Working Group for Diagnosis, Standardization of Response Criteria, Treatment Outcomes, and Reporting Standards for Therapeutic Trials in Acute Myeloid Leukemia. J Clin Oncol 2003;21:4642–9.

2. Freireich EJ, Gehan EA, Sulman D, et al. The effect of chemotherapy on acute leukemia in the human. J Chronic Dis 1961;14:593–608.

3. Bradstock KF, Janossy G, Tidman N, et al. Immunological monitoring of residual disease in treated thymic acute lymphoblastic leukemia. Leuk Res 1981;5:301–9.

4. Walter RB, Kantarjian HM, Huang X, et al. Effect of complete remission and responses less than complete remission on survival in acute myeloid leukemia: a combined Eastern Cooperative Oncology Group, Southwest Oncology Group, and M. D. Anderson Cancer Center Study. J Clin Oncol 2010;28:1766–71.

5. Chen X, Xie H, Bohm C, et al. The relation of clinical response and minimal residual disease and their prognostic impact on outcome in acute myeloid leukemia. J Clin Oncol 2015;33:1258-64.

6. Freeman SD, Virgo P, Couzens S, et al. Prognostic relevance of treatment response measured by flow cytometric residual disease detection in older patient with acute myeloid leukemia. J Clin Oncol 2013;31:4123–31.

7. Kang H, Chen I-M, Wilson CS, et al. Gene expression classifiers for relapse-free survival and minimal residual disease improve risk-classification and outcome prediction in pediatric B-precursor acute lymphoblastic leukemia. Blood 2010;115:1394–405.

8. Yang JJ, Cheng C, Devidas M, et al. Genome-wide association study identifies Germline polymorphisms associated with relapse of childhood acute lymphoblastic leukemia. Blood 2012;120:4197–204.

9. Beldjord K, Chevret S, Asnafi V, et al. Oncogenetics and minimal residual disease are independent outcome predictors in adult patients with acute lymphoblastic leukemia. Blood 2014;123:3739–49.

10. Vora A, Frost L, Goodeve A, et al. Late relapsing childhood lymphoblastic leukemia. Blood 1998;92:2334–7.

11. Ommen HB, Schnittger S, Jovanovic JV, et al. Strikingly different molecular relapse Grimwadekinetics in NPM1c, PML-RARA, RUNX1-RUNX1T1, and CBFB-MYH11 acute myeloid leukemias. Blood 2010;115:198–205.

12. Parker C, Waters R, Leighton C, et al. Effect of mitoxantrone on outcome of children with first relapse of acute lymphoblastic leukemia (ALL R3): an

open-label randomized trial. *The Lancet* 2010;376:2009–17.

13. Butturini A, Klein J, Gale RP. Modeling minimal residual disease (MRD)-testing. *Leuk Res* 2003;27:293–300.

14. Mulligan CG, Su X, Zhang J, *et al*. Deletion of IKZF1 and prognosis in acute lymphoblastic leukemia. *N Engl J Med* 2009;360:470–80.

15. van der Veer A, Waanders E, Pieters R, *et al*. Independent prognostic value of BCR-ABL1-like signature and IKZF1 deletion, but not high CRLF2 expression, in children with B-cell precursor ALL. *Blood* 2013;122:2622–9.

16. Roberts KG, Li Y, Payne-Turner D, *et al*. Targetable kinase-activating lesions in Ph-like acute lymphoblastic leukemia. *N Engl J Med* 2014;371:1005–15.

17. Lee S, Kim D-W, Cho B-S, *et al*. Impact of minimal residual disease kinetics during imatinib-based treatment on transplantation outcome in Philadelphia chromosome-positive acute lymphoblastic leukemia. *Leukemia* 2012;26:2367–74.

18. Ravandi F, Jorgensen JL, Thomas DA, *et al*. Detection of MRD may predict the outcome of patients with Philadelphia chromosome-positive ALL treated with tyrosine kinase inhibitors plus chemotherapy. *Blood* 2013;122:1214–21.

19. Jeha S, Coustan-Smith E, Pei D, *et al*. Impact of tyrosine kinase inhibitors on minimal residual disease and outcome in childhood Philadelphia chromosome-positive acute lymphoblastic leukemia. *Cancer* 2014;120:1514–9.

20. Helgestad J, Rosthøj S, Johansen P, *et al*. Bone marrow aspiration technique may have an impact on therapy stratification in children with acute lymphoblastic leukemia. *Pediatr Blood Cancer* 2011;57:224–6.

21. Paietta E. Minimal residual disease in AML: coming of age. *Hematol Am Soc Hematol Educ Program* 2012;2012:35–42.

22. Paietta E. Minimal residual disease in acute leukaemia: a guide to precision medicine ready for prime time? *In Treatment Strategies Haematology*, Vol 4, issue 2, 2014, pp 45-48.

23. Grimwade D, Freeman SD. Defining minimal residual disease in acute myeloid leukemia: which platforms are ready for "prime time"? *Blood* 2014;124:3345–55.

24. Loken MR, Chu S-C, Fritschle W, *et al*. Normalization of bone marrow aspirates for hemodilution in flow cytometric analyses. *Cytometry Part B (Clin Cytometry)* 2009;76B:27–36.

25. Buccisano F, Maurillo L, Del Principe MI, *et al*. Prognostic and therapeutic implications of minimal residual disease detection in acute myeloid leukemia. *Blood* 2012;119:332–41.

26. Loken MR, Alonzo TA, Pardo L, *et al*. Residual disease detected by multidimensional flow cytometry signifies high relapse risk in patients with de novo acute myeloid leukemia: a report from Children's Oncology Group. *Blood* 2012;120:1581–8.

27. Inaba H, Coustan-Smith E, Cao X, *et al*. Comparative analysis of different approaches to measure treatment response in acute myeloid leukemia. *J Clin Oncol* 2012;30:3625–32.

28. Campana D, Coustan-Smith E. Measurements of treatment response in childhood acute leukemia. *Korean J Hematol* 2012;47:245–54.

29. McKenna RW, Washington LT, Aquino DB, *et al*. Immunophenotypic analysis of hematogones (B-lymphocyte precursor) in 662 consecutive bone marrow specimens by 4-color flow cytometry. *Blood* 2001;98:2498–507.

30. Sevilla DW, Colovai AI, Emmons FN, *et al*. Hematogones: a review and update. *Leuk Lymphoma* 2010;51:10–19.

31. Sedek L, Bulsa J, Sonsala A, *et al*. The immunophenotypes of blast cells in B-cell precursor acute lymphoblastic leukemia: how different are they from their normal counterparts? *Cytometry B Clin Cytom* 2014;86:329–39.

32. Loken MR, Alonzo TA, Pardo L, *et al*. Multidimensional flow cytometry significantly improves upon the morphologic assessment of post-induction marrow remission status-comparison of morphology and multidimensional flow cytometry: a report from the Children's Oncology Group AML Protocol AAML0531. *Blood* 2012;120(8):1581–8.

33. Grimwade D, Tallman M. Should minimal residual disease monitoring be the standard of care for all patients with acute promyelocytic leukemia? *Leuk Research* 2011;35:3–7.

34. Wang F, Travis J, DeLaBarre B, *et al*. Targeted inhibition of mutant IDH2 in leukemia cells induces cellular differentiation. *Science* 2013;340:622–6.

35. Gaipa G, Cazzaniga G, Valsecchi MG, *et al*. Time point-dependent concordance of flow cytometry and real-time quantitative polymerase chain reaction for minimal residual disease detection in childhood acute lymphoblastic leukemia. *Haematologica* 2012;97:1582–93.

36. Van der Velden VHJ, Cazzaniga G, Schrauder A, *et al*. Analysis of minimal residual disease by Ig/TCR gene rearrangements: guidelines for interpretation of real-time quantitative PCR data. *Leukemia* 2007;21:604–11.

37. van Dongen JJM. *EuroFlow Educational Book* 2012; Rotterdam: Macmillan.

38. Boeckx N, Willemse MJ, Szczepanski T, *et al*. Fusion gene transcripts and Ig/TCR gene rearrangements are complementary but infrequent targets for PCR-based detection of minimal residual disease in acute myeloid leukemia. *Leukemia* 2002;16:368–75.

39. Warren EH, Matsen IV FA, Chou J. High-throughput sequencing of B- and T-lymphocyte antigen receptors in hematology. *Blood* 2013;122:19–22.

40. Faham M, Zheng J, Moorhead M, *et al*. Deep-sequencing approach for minimal residual disease detection in acute lymphoblastic leukemia. *Blood* 2012;120:5173–80.

41. Martinez-Lopez J, Lahuerta JJ, Pepin F, *et al*. Prognostic value of deep sequencing method for minimal residual disease detection in multiple myeloma. *Blood* 2014;123:3073–9.

42. UK NEQAS. www.ukneqas.org.uk

43. Wood B. Flow cytometric assessment of MRD. Presented at the FDA Public Workshop on Minimal Residual Disease, FDA White Oak Campus, Silver Spring, MD, April 18, 2012.

44. Wood BL. Flow cytometric monitoring of residual disease in acute leukemia. In M. Czader (ed) *Hematological Malignancies: Methods in Molecular Biology*, vol 999. 2013; New York: Springer, pp. 123–36.

45. Chevallier P, Robillard N, Ayari S, *et al*. Persistence of CD33 expression at relapse in CD33(+) acute myeloid leukaemia patients after receiving Gemtuzumab in the course of the disease. *Br J Haematol* 2008;143:744–6.

46. Chu PG, Chen YY, Molina A, *et al.* Recurrent B-cell neoplasms after Rituximab therapy: an immunophenotypic and genotypic study. *Leuk Lymphoma* 2002;43:2335–41.

47. Topp MS, Kufer P, Gökbuget N, *et al.* Targeted therapy with the T-cell-engaging antibody blinatumomab of chemotherapy-refractory minimal residual disease in B-lineage acute lymphoblastic leukemia patients results in high response rate and prolonged leukemia-free survival. *J Clin Oncol* 2011;29:2493–8.

48. Campana D. Should minimal residual disease monitoring in acute lymphoblastic leukemia be standard of care? *Curr Hematol Malig Rep* 2012;7:170–7.

49. van Dongen JJM, Lhermitte L, Böttcher S, *et al.* EuroFlow antibody panels for standardized *n*-dimensional flow cytometric immunophenotyping of normal, reactive and malignant leukocytes. *Leukemia* 2012;26:1908–75.

50. Zeijlemaker W, Gratama JW, Schuurhuis GJ. Tumor heterogeneity makes AML a "moving target" for detection of residual disease. *Cytometry B Clin Cytom* 2014;86:3–14.

51. Coustan-Smith E, Song G, Clark C, *et al.* New markers for minimal residual disease detection in acute lymphoblastic leukemia. *Blood* 2011;117:6267–76.

52. Langebrake C, Brinkmann I, Teigler-Schlegel A, *et al.* Immunophenotypic differences between diagnosis and relapse in childhood AML: implications for MRD monitoring. *Cytometry B Clin Cytom* 2005;63B:1–9.

53. Macedo A, San Miguel JF, Vidriales MB, *et al.* Phenotypic changes in acute myeloid leukemia: implications in the detection of minimal residual disease. *J Clin Pathol* 1996;49:15–18.

54. Brüggemann M, Raff T, Kneba M. Has MRD monitoring superseded other prognostic factors in adult ALL? *Blood* 2012;120:4470–81.

55. Wu D, Emerson RO, Sherwood A, *et al.* Detection of minimal residual disease in B lymphoblastic leukemia by high-throughput sequencing of IGH. *Clin Cancer Res* 2014;20:4540–8.

56. Thol F, Kölking B, Damm F, *et al.* Next-generation sequencing for minimal residual disease monitoring in acute myeloid leukemia patients with FLT3-ITD or NPM1 mutations. *Genes Chromosom Cancer* 2012;51:689–95.

57. Bachas C, Schuurhuis GJ, Assaraf YG, *et al.* The role of minor subpopulations within the leukemic blast compartment of AML patients at initial diagnosis in the development of relapse. *Leukemia* 2012;26:1313–20.

58. Hou H-A, Kuo Y-Y, Liu C-Y, *et al.* DNMT3A mutations in acute myeloid leukemia: stability during disease evolution and clinical implications. *Blood* 2012;119:559–68.

59. Im AP, Sehgal AR, Carroll MP, *et al.* DNMT3A and IDH mutations in acute myeloid leukemia and other myeloid malignancies: associations with prognosis and potential treatment strategies. *Leukemia* 2014;28:1774–83.

60. Salipante SJ, Fromm JR, Shendure J, *et al.* Detection of minimal residual disease in NPM1-mutated acute myeloid leukemia by next-generation sequencing. *Mod Pathol* 2014;27:1438–46.

61. Stow P, Key L, Chen X, *et al.* Clinical significance of low levels of minimal residual disease at the end of remission induction therapy in childhood acute lymphoblastic leukemia. *Blood* 2010;115:4657–63.

62. Maurillo L, Buccisano F, Del Principe MI, *et al.* Toward optimization of postremission therapy for residual disease-positive patients with acute myeloid leukemia. *J Clin Oncol* 2008;26:4944–51.

63. Rubnitz JE, Inaba H, Dahl G, *et al.* Minimal residual disease-directed therapy for childhood acute myeloid leukemia: results of the AML02 multicentre trial. *The Lancet* 2010;11:543–52.

64. Terwijn M, van Putten WLJ, Kelder A, *et al.* High prognostic impact of flow cytometric minimal residual disease detection in acute myeloid leukemia: Data from the HOVON/SAKK AML 42A study. *J Clin Oncol* 2013;31:3889–97.

65. Ganzel C, Sun Z, Gönen M, *et al.* Minimal residual disease assessment by flow cytometry in AML is an independent prognostic factor even after adjusting for cytogenetic/molecular abnormalities. *Blood* 2014;124:1016.

66. Fernandez HF, Sun Z, Yao X, *et al.* Anthracycline dose intensification in acute myeloid leukemia: Results of ECOG Study E1900. *N Engl J Med* 2009;361:1249–59.

67. Perea G, Lasa A, Aventin A, *et al.* Prognostic value of minimal residual disease (MRD) in acute myeloid leukemia (AML) with favorable cytogenetics [t(8;21) and inv(16)]. *Leukemia* 2006;20:87–94.

68. Miyamoto T, Weissman IL, Akashi K. AML1/ETO-expressing nonleukemic stem cells in acute myelogenous leukemia with 8;21 chromosomal translocation. *Proc Natl Acad Sci USA* 2000;97:7521–6.

69. Corces-Zimmerman MR, Hong W-J, Weissman IL, *et al.* Preleukemic mutations in human acute myeloid leukemia affect epigenetic regulators and persist in remission. *Proc Natl Acad Sci USA* 2014;111:2548–53.

70. Shlush LI, Zandi S, Mitchell A, *et al.* Identification of pre-leukaemic haematopoietic stem cells in acute leukaemia. *Nature* 2014;506:328–33.

71. Bodini M, Ronchini C, Giacò L, *et al.* The hidden genomic landscape of acute myeloid leukemia: subclonal structure revealed by undetected mutations. *Blood* 2015;125:600–5.

72. Will B, Steidl U. Multi-parameter fluorescence-activated cell sorting and analysis of stem and progenitor cells in myeloid malignancies. *Best Pract Res Clin Haematol* 2010;23:391–401.

73. Ebinger M, Witte K-E, Ahlers J, *et al.* High frequency of immature cells at diagnosis predicts high minimal residual disease level in childhood acute lymphoblastic leukemia. *Leuk Res* 2010;34:1139–42.

74. Terwijn M, Kelder A, Snel AN, *et al.* Minimal residual disease detection defined as the malignant fraction of the total primitive stem cell compartment offers additional prognostic information in acute myeloid leukemia. *Int J Lab Hem* 2012;34:432–41.

75. Gerber JM, Smith BD, Ngwang B, *et al.* A clinically relevant population of leukemic CD34+CD38- cells in acute myeloid leukemia. *Blood* 2012;119:3571–7.

76. Roug AS, Larsen HØ, Nederby L, *et al.* hMICL and CD123 in combination with a CD45/CD34/CD117 backbone – a universal marker combination for the detection of minimal residual

disease in acute myeloid leukemia. *Br J Haematol* 2014;164:212–22.

77. DiGiuseppe JA. CD34+/CD38- cells and minimal residual disease in childhood lymphoblastic leukemia. *Leuk Res* 2010;34:1125–6.

78. Aoki Y, Watanabe T, Saito Y, *et al.* Identification of CD34$^+$ and CD34$^-$ leukemia-initiating cells in MLL-rearranged human acute lymphoblastic leukemia. *Blood* 2014;125:967–80.

79. Mullighan CG, Phillips LA, Su X, *et al.* Genomic analysis of the clonal origins of relapsed acute lymphoblastic leukemia. *Science* 2008;322:1377–80.

80. Notta F, Mullighan CG, Wang JC, *et al.* Evolution of human *BCR-ABL1* lymphoblastic leukaemia-initiating cells. *Nature* 2011;469:362–7.

81. Clappier E, Gerby B, Sigaux F, *et al.* Clonal selection in xenografted human T cell acute lymphoblastic leukemia recapitulates gain of malignancy at relapse. *J Exp Med* 2011;208:653–61.

82. Klco JM, Spencer DH, Miller CA, *et al.* Functional heterogeneity of genetically defined subclones in acute myeloid leukemia. *Cancer Cell* 2014;25:379–92.

83. Inaba H, Greaves M, Mullighan CG. Acute lymphoblastic leukemia. *Lancet* 2013;381:1943–55.

84. Chan SM, Majeti R. Role of DNMT3A, TET2, and IDH1/2 mutations in pre-leukemic stem cells in acute myeloid leukemia. *Int J Hematol* 2013;98:648–57.

85. Peloquin GL, Chen YB, Fathi AT. The evolving landscape in the therapy of acute myeloid leukemia. *Protein Cell* 2013;4:735–46.

86. Li KK, Luo LF, Shen Y, *et al.* DNA methyltransferases in hematologic malignancies. *Semin Hematol* 2013;50:48–60.

87. Barreyro L, Will B, Bartholdy B, *et al.* Overexpression of IL-1 receptor accessory protein in stem and progenitor cells and outcome correlation in AML and MDS. *Blood* 2012;120:1290–8.

88. Askmyr M, Ågerstam H, Hansen N, *et al.* Selective killing of candidate AML stem cells by antibody targeting of IL1RAP. *Blood* 2013;121:3709–13.

89. Schultz KR, Bowman WP, Aledo A, *et al.* Improved early event-free survival with imatinib in Philadelphia chromosome-positive acute lymphoblastic leukemia: a Children's Oncology Group study. *J Clin Oncol* 2009;27:5175–81.

90. Manabe A, Kawasaki H, Shimada H, *et al.* Imatinib use immediately before stem cell transplantation in children with Philadelphia chromosome-positive acute lymphoblastic leukemia: Results from Japanese Pediatric Leukemia/Lymphoma Study Group (JPLSG) Study Ph+ALL04. *Cancer Med* 2015; Jan 31. doi: 10.1002/cam4.383. [Epub ahead of print]

91. Lee HJ, Thompson JE, Wang ES, Wetzler M. Philadelphia chromosome-positive acute lymphoblastic leukemia. *Cancer* 2011;117:1583–94.

92. Bachanova V, Marks DI, Zhang M-J, *et al.* Ph+ ALL patients in first complete remission have similar survival after reduced intensity and myeloablative allogeneic transplantation: Impact of tyrosine kinase inhibitor and minimal residual disease. *Leukemia* 2014;28:658–65.

93. Wetzler M, Watson D, Stock W, *et al.* Autologous transplantation for Philadelphia chromosome-positive acute lymphoblastic leukemia achieves outcomes similar to allogeneic transplantation: results of CALGB Study 10001 (Alliance). *Haematologica* 2014;99:111–5.

94. Schenk TM, Keyhani A, Böttcher S, *et al.* Multilineage involvement of Philadelphia chromosome positive acute lymphoblastic leukemia. *Leukemia* 1998;12:666–74.

95. Rovida E, Peppicelli S, Bono S, *et al.* The metabolically-modulated stem cell niche: a dynamic scenario regulating cancer cell phenotype and resistance to therapy. *Cell Cycle* 2014;13:3169–75.

96. Ribera J-M. Optimal approach to treatment of patients with Philadelphia chromosome-positive acute lymphoblastic leukemia: how to best use all the available tools. *Leuk Lymphoma* 2013;54:21–7.

97. Herrmann H, Sadovnik I, Cerny-Reiterer S, *et al.* Dipeptidylpeptidase IV (CD26) defines leukemic stem cells in chronic myeloid leukemia. *Blood* 2014;123:3951–62.

98. Pfeifer H, Wassmann B, Bethge W, *et al.* Randomized comparison of prophylactic and minimal residual disease-triggered imatinib after allogeneic stem cell transplantation for BCR-ABL1-positive acute lymphoblastic leukemia. *Leukemia* 2013;27:1254–62.

99. Orgel E, Tucci J, Alhushki W, *et al.* Obesity is associated with residual leukemia following induction therapy for childhood B-precursor acute lymphoblastic leukemia. *Blood* 2014;124:3932–8.

100. Ehsanipour EA, Sheng X, Behan JW, *et al.* Adipocytes cause leukemia cell resistance to L-asparaginase via release of glutamine. *Cancer Res* 2013;73:2998–3006.

101. Pramanik R, Sheng X, Ichihara B, *et al.* Adipose tissue attracts and protects acute lymphoblastic leukemia cells from chemotherapy. *Leuk Res* 2013;37:503–9.

102. Borowitz MJ, Devidas M, Hunger SP, *et al.* Clinical significance of minimal residual disease in childhood acute lymphoblastic leukemia and its relationship to other prognostic factors: a Children's Oncology Group study. *Blood* 2008;111:5477–85.

103. Möricke A, Reiter A, Zimmermann M, *et al.* Risk-adjusted therapy of acute lymphoblastic leukemia can decrease treatment burden and improve survival: treatment results of 2169 unselected pediatric and adolescent patients enrolled in the trial ALL-BFM 95. *Blood* 2008;111:4477–89.

104. Conter V, Bartram CR, Valsecchi MG, *et al.* Molecular response to treatment redefines all prognostic factors in children and adolescents with B-cell precursor acute lymphoblastic leukemia: results in 3184 patients of the AIEOP-BFM ALL 2000 study. *Blood* 2010;115:3206-14.

105. Corbacioglu A, Scholl C, Schlenk RF, *et al.* Prognostic impact of miminal residual disease in CBFB-MYH11-positive acute myeloid leukemia. *J Clin Oncol* 2010;28:3724–9.

106. Zhu H-H, Zhang X-H, Qin Y-Z, *et al.* MRD-directed risk stratification treatment may improve outcomes of t (8;21) AML in the first complete remission: results from the AML05 multicenter trial. *Blood* 2013;121:4056–62.

107. Jourdan E, Boissel N, Chevret S, *et al.* Prospective evaluation of gene mutations and minimal residual disease in patients with core binding factor acute myeloid leukemia. *Blood* 2013;121:2213–23.

108. Liu Yin JA, O'Brien MA, Hills RK, *et al.* Minimal residual disease monitoring by RT-qPCR in core-binding factor AML allows risk-stratification and predicts relapse: results of the UK MRC AML-15 trial. *Blood* 2012;120:2826–35.

109. Buccisano F, Maurillo L, Spagnoli A, *et al.* Cytogenetic and molecular diagnostic characterization combined to post-consolidation minimal residual disease assessment by flow-cytometry improves risk stratification in adult acute myeloid leukemia. *Blood* 2010;116:2295–303.

110. Gönen M, Sun Z, Figueroa ME, *et al.* CD25 expression status improves prognostic risk classification in AML independent of established biomarkers: ECOG phase III trial, E1900. *Blood* 2012;120:2297–306.

111. Waanders E, van der Velden VHJ, van der Schoot CE, *et al.* Integrated use of minimal residual disease classification and IKZF1 alteration status accurately predicts 79% of relapses in pediatric acute lymphoblastic leukemia. *Leukemia* 2011;25:254–8.

112. Geng H, Brennan S, Milne TA, *et al.* Integrative epigenomic analysis of adult B-acute lymphoblastic leukemia identifies biomarkers and therapeutic targets. *Cancer Discovery* 2012;2:1004–23.

113. Kobayashi CI, Takubo K, Kobayashi H, *et al.* The IL-2/CD25 axis maintains distinct subsets of chronic myeloid leukemia-initiating cells. *Blood* 2014;123:2540–9.

114. Hagedorn N, Acquaviva C, Fronkova E, *et al.* Submicroscopic bone marrow involvement in isolated extramedullary relapses in childhood acute lymphoblastic leukemia: a more precise definition of "isolated" and its possible clinical implications, a collaborative study of the Resistant Disease Committee of the International BFM study group. *Blood* 2007;110:4022–9.

115. Patel B, Rai L, Buck G, *et al.* Minimal residual disease is a significant predictor of treatment failure in non T-lineage adult acute lymphoblastic leukaemia: final results of the international trial UKALL XII/ECOG2993. *Br J Haematol* 2009;148:80–9.

116. Grimwade D, Jovanovic JV, Hills RK, *et al.* Prospective minimal residual disease monitoring to predict relapse of acute promyelocytic leukemia and to direct pre-emptive arsenic trioxide therapy. *J Clin Oncol* 2009;27:3650–8.

117. Sockel K, Wermke M, Radke J, *et al.* Minimal residual disease-directed preemptive treatment with azacitidine in patients with NPM1-mutant acute myeloid leukemia and molecular relapse. *Haematologica* 2011;96:1568–70.

118. Platzbecker U, Wermke M, Radke J, *et al.* Azacitidine for treatment of imminent relapse in MDS or AML patients after allogeneic HSCT: results of the RELAZA trial. *Leukemia* 2012;26:381–9.

119. Rubnitz J, Inaba H, Dahl G, *et al.* Minimal residual disease-directed therapy for childhood acute myeloid leukaemia: results of the AML02 multicentre trial. *Lancet Oncol* 2010;11:543–52.

120. O'Hear C, Inaba H, Punds S, *et al.* Gemtuzumab ozogamicin can reduce minimal residual disease in patients with childhood acute myeloid leukemia. *Cancer* 2013;119:4036–43.

121. Annesley CE, Brown P. Novel agents for the treatment of childhood acute leukemia. *Ther Adv Hematol* 2015;6:61–79.

122. Topp M, Gökbuget N, Zugmaier G, *et al.* Long-term follow-up of hematologic relapse-free survival in a phase 2 study of blinatumomab in patients with MRD in B-lineage ALL. *Blood* 2012;120:5185–7.

Chapter

25

Donor Lymphocyte Infusion: Rationale, Benefits, and Limitations

Donal P. McLornan, Victoria T. Potter, and Francesco Dazzi

Introduction

Donor lymphocyte infusions (DLIs) are extremely effective for cytogenetic relapses or chronic phase relapses of chronic myelogenous leukemia (CML), but are less effective in acute leukemias or other hematologic malignancies. The DLIs are associated with a significant risk of morbidity and mortality due to graft-*versus*-host disease (GvHD) and occasionally pancytopenia. Current research focuses on optimal cell doses, prophylactic or preemptive infusions, selective depletion of CD8+ lymphocytes, and addition of agents to augment DLI effect as methods of diminishing associated toxicities and maximizing benefits. In this chapter we will review the use of donor lymphocyte infusions (DLI), summarize their efficacy and applicability in specific disease groups, and discuss current indications and future developments.

What Have We Learned from DLI Given in CML?

It is widely accepted that one of the major therapeutic components of allogeneic hematopoietic cell transplant (allo-HCT) is the graft-*versus*-leukemia (GvL) effect induced by donor lymphocytes administered with the hematopoietic cell preparation. Initially reflected by the high incidence of leukemia relapse in patients receiving T-cell-depleted (TCD) transplants, direct evidence supporting the GvL effect was provided by the successful use of DLI in restoring disease remission (see Chapters 29 and 30)[1,2]. CML has provided the best platform to evaluate DLI and identify factors influencing clinical efficacy and toxicity. CML is highly sensitive to immune recognition, the disease pace in the chronic phase is slow, and the disease can be accurately quantitated using different, yet complimentary, approaches (molecular, cytogenetic, and hematologic).

In CML, DLI may induce durable remissions even longer than those achievable following the primary transplant procedure[3], thus leading to a redefinition of leukemia-free survival (LFS) to take account of successful treatment of relapse (current leukemia-free survival)[4].

The major factor influencing responses to DLI in CML is disease stage. Patients treated in molecular relapse fare better than those treated when relapse is diagnosed at a cytogenetic or hematologic level, indicating that either early disease is qualitatively more sensitive to DLI and/or that bulky disease is more difficult to eradicate[3,5,6]. In this regard, an often neglected issue is the DLI dosage to be used. It is conceivable that at a fixed DLI dose the ratio between the number of donor CD3+ lymphocytes infused and the number of leukemic cells at molecular, cytogenetic, and hematologic relapse varies extensively (see Chapter 65).

Effective Cell Dose of DLI: What Factors Influence It?

There are two major factors influencing the effective DLI dose required to produce molecular remission (termed the *effective cell dose* (ECD)). Primarily, we need to consider the donor type; patients receiving an HLA-matched unrelated donor require a lower ECD as compared to patients infused with HLA-matched sibling derived-DLI[7]. This is consistent with the fact that differences in minor histocompatibility antigens are likely to be more extensive in unrelated than sibling donor–recipient pairings, thus making the frequency of 'alloreactive' T-cells – and of potential antileukemia effectors – higher. In accord with this notion, the other major factor affecting ECD is disease stage at time of DLI. Patients with more advanced disease necessitate a higher ECD than those in early (molecular/cytogenetic) relapses. Therefore, it is not surprising that overall the number of responding patients increase with higher doses. These data strongly indicate that dose escalation enhances the chance of responding.

Escalating Dose Regimen: Rationale?

Initial studies of DLI often involved a single, relatively large, and random dose of lymphocytes called a *bulk dose regimen* (BDR)[6]. In recent years a shift in practice has occurred towards usage of an *escalating dose regimen* (EDR); an attempt to maximize antileukemic efficacy with less GvHD. Pioneered at the Sloan Kettering Transplant Centre[5], EDR was later tested on a large cohort of patients at the Hammersmith Hospital, London and showed that, without affecting the probability of achieving remission, the incidence of GvHD was much lower using EDR[8]. Moreover, when subset analyses of both BDR and EDR patients receiving equivalent total lymphoid cell doses were evaluated, the incidence and severity of both acute and chronic GvHD were significantly lower for recipients treated by EDR than for recipients treated by BDR. These findings suggest that the incidence of GvHD associated with the EDR is low, not because the final cell dose is smaller, but because lymphocytes are administered over a prolonged period of time. This concept was further confirmed in a subsequent study evaluating the factors affecting the incidence and severity of GvHD following EDR DLI[9]. Here, it was actually observed that the DLI dose received was not associated with increased GvHD. In contrast, the time between the original allo-HCT and DLI was found to be one of the major factors predictive of severe GvHD. Although apparently counterintuitive, these results are consistent with the notion that the cytokine storm generated in the post-transplant period plays a key role in the development of GvHD[10,11].

General Obstacles and Controversies in DLI for Non-CML Hematologic Malignancies

Despite the very important lessons learned from the CML platform, several questions remain unanswered, particularly because most of the advantages of DLI usage in CML are not as evident in other conditions (Table 25.1). For example, the impact of timing DLI on GvHD has been confirmed in other conditions whereby low cell doses administered early after transplantation may cause GvHD while larger doses administered more than 1 year post-allo-HCT may be delivered safely (Figure 25.1)[9]. Unfortunately, the use of DLI to treat or prevent relapse cannot be delayed in aggressive malignancies like high-risk AML in which relapses occur early after the transplant. Bar *et al.* have recently published the results of a large retrospective review of 255 patients with a variety of hematologic malignancies receiving DLI for relapsed disease in an attempt to correlate dose of DLI with outcome[12]. In terms of GvHD rates, higher DLI doses ($>10 \times 10^7$ CD3+ lymphocytes/kg) and time to administration of less than 1 year were associated with increased GvHD risks confirming the results of earlier studies. In this study, higher doses of DLI did not result in additional clinical benefit, thus suggesting that disease intrinsic factors impede the application of CML-type DLI strategies to diseases like acute leukemias.

Another important aspect that must be considered is whether other hematologic malignancies are as sensitive as CML to the GvL effect and/or whether the time required for donor T-cells to expand *in-vivo* after the infusion is sufficient to compete with leukemic cell proliferation. This question ties in with the role of procedures potentially associated with DLI acquisition or administration, such as the use of granulocyte colony-stimulating factor (G-CSF)-mobilized DLI or of cytoreduction to create hematopoietic "space" for DLI expansion.

Practice Points

Despite the many difficulties in delivering a safe and efficacious treatment, DLI is being considered as playing a prominent role as salvage treatment because of the large proportion of patients undergoing reduced intensity conditioning regimens and/or TCD transplants; the likelihood of relapses in these conditions

is high. However, there is no convincing evidence that DLI is a life-saving procedure for patients who relapse. Therefore, at least in high-risk conditions, DLI has been proposed as a prophylactic approach to prevent the development of otherwise untreatable stages. In contrast to therapeutic DLI (tDLI) – in which DLI is used after relapse has already occurred – *or* preemptive DLI (pDLI) – most commonly given for low or falling CD3+ cell chimerism or molecular/cytogenetic relapses, prophylactic DLI is administered in the absence of a specific indicator. For example, the use of prophylactic DLI has been described as part of a sequential conditioning approach for patients with high-risk disease or those that are not in remission[13]. In this context, pDLI can be used as part of the platform provided by TCD protocols in an attempt to engineer relapse prevention while minimizing GvHD toxicity. However, it is essential to note that significant variation exists across institutions and countries as to the use of TCD or not, the type of TCD employed, and the dose of TCD agents. Finally, the timing of cessation of immunosuppression prior to DLI is also of extreme importance, with general consensus being that at least 4 weeks of immunosuppression in the absence of GvHD is required before DLI administration. It is evident that in order for progress to occur in this area standardization of protocols and prospective studies are urgently required.

Specific Diseases and Role of DLI
DLI for Myeloid Malignancies
Acute Myeloid Leukemia and Myelodysplasia

The response rates achieved in relapsed acute myeloid leukemia (AML) or myelodysplastic syndromes (MDS) are certainly inferior to CML (Table 25.2). Retrospective work from the Acute Leukaemia working party of the European Blood and Marrow Transplant (EBMT) group compared outcomes in 399 patients with AML who were in first relapse after predominantly myeloablative transplants[14]. A total of 171 patients received DLI as part of relapse management, 75% of whom received chemotherapy in addition. More than two-thirds of the DLI group had active leukemia at the time of infusion. Following adjustment for risk stratification, DLI treatment was associated with significantly improved survival on multivariate analysis (2-year survival of 21% for DLI cohort *versus* 9% for patients not receiving DLI). Achievement of response to preadministration chemotherapy and lower tumor burden at time of DLI administration was a major predictor of response. This study confirmed an established role for DLI in the management of relapsed AML post-allo-HCT (see Chapters 23, 26, and 34).

A definitive role for DLI for relapsed MDS post-transplant has also been established in multiple studies but conclusions have been limited by small cohort size and inconsistent DLI regimens and dosing (see Chapter 35)[15,16]. A recent retrospective study from our institution analyzed the outcome of pDLI and tDLI in 113 patients who had undergone a TCD-RIC

Table 25.1 Summary of pivotal trials describing the outcomes of DLI according to disease type

Disease type	Number of patients	Donor lymphocyte approach	Responses	GvHD rates	Survival outcomes	References
AML in 1st Relapse post-allo-HCT	171 received DLI 228 did not receive DLI	75% received DLI in combination with chemotherapy. A total of 61% received 1 infusion; 39% between 2 and 11 infusions	In DLI cohort: 34% achieved a CR	Overall incidence: aGvHD: 43% cGvHD: 46%	2-year OS: DLI: 21% +/− 3% No DLI: 9% +/− 2%	[14]
MDS and AML post-TCD-RIC allo-HCT	pDLI: 62 patients tDLI: 51 patients	Planned escalating dose regimen pDLI: median time to 1st DLI 180 days tDLI: median time to 1st DLI 277 days	Not reported	pDLI: 5-year incidence of GvHD of 31% tDLI: 5-year incidence of GvHD 45%	pDLI: 5-year OS of 80%; EFS of 65% tDLI: 5-year OS of 40%; relapse/ progression rate of 69%	[17]
AML and MDS	n=30 (28 AML; 2 MDS) 22/30 patients received DLI	1st DLI given after second cycle of 5'-azacitidine. Median of 3 courses; range 1–8 cycles	CR rate of 23% was achieved PR rate of 7%; SD rate of 17%	11 patients (37%) developed aGvHD	2-year OS rate of 17%	[19]
Myelofibrosis	17 patients: pDLI: n=9; tDLI: n=8	pDLI for MRD persistence tDLI for clinical relapse (salvage)	CMR of 100% in pDLI cohort CMR of 44% in salvage arm	No GvHD pDLI arm aGvHD II–IV: 18%	Not reported	[21]
Low-grade Lymphoid Disorders	28 patients Progressive disease +/− MC: n =17 MC: n=11	Escalating dose regimen planned at 3-monthly intervals	13 patients demonstrated response. Cumulative response rate of 76%	Cumulative incidence of aGvHD was 14.7%; extensive cGvHD was 31.4%	17 patients treated for disease progression. The projected 5-year OS was 87.8%; PFS 76.2%	[24]
Hodgkin's Lymphoma post-TCD –RIC allo-HCT	46 patients: n=24 relapsed (10 received concomitant cytoreduction) n= 22 for MC	Escalating dose regimen 3-monthly intervals. Median time to 1st DLI was 287 days	79% of those receiving DLI for relapse responded	MC: 13/19 who converted to full MC had no GvHD	4-year OS from relapse was 59%	[26]
CLL post-TCD-RIC allo-HCT	n=31: pDLI 15; tDLI 16	Escalating dose regimen at 3-monthly intervals	9/16 receiving DLI for persistent or relapsed disease attained MRD-negative CR	4-year cumulative incidence of GvHD was 30%	4-year current PFS was 65% and OS was 75%	[29]
Multiple Myeloma post-RIC-allo-HCT (50% received TCD)	63 patients Relapsed disease (n=48) Persistent disease (n=15)	12/63 received cytoreductive therapy pre-DLI	Total response rates (CR+PR) to DLI were 38%	Significant rates of both aGvHD (38%) and cGvHD (43%)	In responders, PFS after DLI was 27.8 months	[33]

Abbreviations: AML: acute myeloid leukemia, MDS: myelodysplasia, DLI: donor lymphocyte infusions, CR: complete response, PR: partial response, aGvHD: acute graft-*versus*-host disease, cGvHD: chronic GvHD, OS: overall survival, EFS: event-free survival, PFS: progression-free survival, pDLI: preemptive DLI, tDLI: therapeutic DLI, TCD: T-cell deplete, RIC: reduced intensity conditioning, MRD: minimal residual disease, CMR: complete metabolic response, MC: mixed chimerism, CLL: chronic lymphocytic leukemia.

Table 25.2 Novel approaches to DLI in the post-allogeneic HCT setting

1. DLI in combination with hypomethylating agents

2. DLI in combination with immunomodulatory drugs, e.g., lenalidomide

3. DLI in combination with novel targeted agents, e.g., brentuximab vedotin

4. CD8+ lymphocyte-depleted DLI

5. Natural killer cell-enhanced DLI

6. Co-infusion of dendritic cells and DLI

7. Thymidine kinase suicide gene transduced DLI

8. Regulatory T-cell-depleted DLI

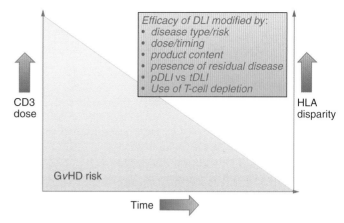

Figure 25.1 DLI toxicity (GvHD risk) and efficacy are influenced by CD3+ cell dose, timing of DLI dose, and degree of HLA mismatch. Another important factor remains disease type with most established efficacy for CML. Presence of residual disease, and other prognostic factors such as karyotype are also important to consider when assessing the utility of DLI for a particular patient.

allo-HCT for either MDS or AML[17]. T-cell-depletion strategies included alemtuzumab (100 mg; n=99) in the HLA-matched unrelated setting or ATG (6 mg/kg; n=14) in the HLA-matched sibling setting. In this study, recipients of tDLI (n=51), most usually involving a combined approach with chemotherapy, had an OS 5-year of 40%, an encouraging result given the high-risk features of this population. Those receiving pDLI (n=62) had an estimated 5-year overall survival (OS) of 80% and an event-free survival of 65%, suggesting durable remissions can be achieved following this approach. GvHD rates were not considered excessive (31% at 5 years) despite more than half receiving pDLI within 6 months of allo-HCT. Our data are in contrast to the much higher GvHD rates (47% of pDLI recipients developed GvHD) in the 15 acute leukemia patients (including some acute lymphoblastic leukemia (ALL) patients) receiving pDLI following alemtuzumab conditioning as reported by Liga *et al.*, perhaps reflective of the lower alemtuzumab dose in that particular study[18].

DLI for relapsed AML or MDS is being increasingly combined with hypomethylating agents such as 5′-azacitidine (see Chapters 23 and 65). Not only do hypomethylating agents combat the underlying disease but they also seem to exhibit immunomodulatory activity that stimulates cytotoxic T-lymphocytes. Schroeder *et al.* recently reported a prospective multicentre study (AZARELA trial) investigating DLI in combination with 5′-azacitidine in 30 patients who had relapsed post-allo-HCT (AML; n=28 and MDS; n=2)[19]. The median time to relapse was 175 days (range 19–1688). A median of three courses of 5′-azacitidine (100 mg/m² for 5 days; range 1–8 cycles) was administered, with 22 patients (73%) also receiving DLI. Despite many patients displaying high-risk disease characteristics, a CR rate of 23% was achieved. This suggests that successful salvage with this approach is achievable. However, the exact sequencing and dosing of the combination requires further clarification. Some centers, including ours, are using this combined approach post-allo-HCT in a preemptive manner for patients with high-risk disease and cumulative data are anticipated with much interest.

DLI for Myelofibrosis and Other Myeloproliferative Neoplasms

Initial proof in support of graft-*versus*-myelofibrosis emerged from small studies correlating grade II–IV GvHD with reduced treatment failure, and successful salvage of relapsed disease with DLI (reviewed in [20])(see Chapter 37). Subsequently, Kröger *et al.* reported their experience on 17 patients receiving either salvage DLI (n=9 for clinical relapse) or pDLI (n=8 for MRD persistence) and confirmed higher rates of molecular responses with pDLI (100%) over tDLI (44%) (Table 25.2) [21]. No grade II–IV aGvHD was noted in the eight patients treated with pDLI. With the advent of specific robust platforms for monitoring post-allo-HCT MRD (*JAK2*, *MPL*, *CALR*, etc.), pDLI is likely to be employed more frequently. Few data exist for DLI in other 'Ph chromosome' negative myeloproliferative neoplasms, although limited evidence supporting a beneficial DLI effect on relapsed juvenile myelomonocytic leukemia (JMML) has been suggested in a small cohort of pediatric patients [22].

DLI for Lymphoid Malignancies

Data concerning the applicability of DLI in the setting of allo-HCT for non-Hodgkin Lymphoma (NHL), Hodgkin lymphoma (HL), and chronic lymphocytic leukemia (CLL) are often limited by cohort size and heterogeneity in both disease stage and type. However, several clear messages are emerging. El-Jurdi *et al.* performed a comprehensive systematic review of the published literature[23]. Although limited by a lack of disease-specific characterization, complete response rates appeared higher when DLI was used for relapsed NHL, HL, or CLL in comparison to both acute lymphoblastic leukemia (ALL) and multiple myeloma (see Chapters 38 and 41–44).

DLI for Non-Hodgkin's Lymphoma and Hodgkin's Lymphoma

Bloor *et al.* demonstrated the feasibility and safety of using DLI in the management of 28 patients with predominantly relapsed indolent lymphoma (17 with relapsed disease and 11 with mixed chimerism (MC) (Table 25.2)[24]. An escalating dose strategy was implemented until obtainment of disease stabilization or full donor chimerism. The cumulative response rate to treat progressive disease and persistent MC were 76.5% and 91.6%, respectively. These data were also corroborated by a subsequent study in patients with follicular lymphoma undergoing T-cell-depleted RIC regimen whereby DLI demonstrated significant efficacy and durable responses in 9 of 13 patients with current progression-free survival at 4 years of 76% for the whole cohort[25] (see Chapter 41). Similarly, in a study involving 46 patients with Hodgkin's lymphoma, both pDLI for MC and tDLI for relapsed disease demonstrated reductions in the rate of relapse and achievement of durable antitumor clinical responses. Nearly 89% of patients responded with a 4-year overall survival of 59%[26]. However, treatment of relapsed HL remains challenging and very recently encouraging results have been reported with the combined use of DLI with adjuvant therapies[27,28] (see Chapter 38). Brentuximab vedotin, and anti-CD30 antibody coupled to the antitubulin agent monomethylauristatin E, induces the release of cytokines such as interleukin-6, chemokine ligand 17, and tumor necrosis factor α. Administered with DLI, this approach induced marked clinical and metabolic responses in a small number of patients. In an attempt to debulk the underlying disease before DLI, another study treated 18 patients with bendamustine before EDR DLI and obtained a significant overall response rate of 55%, with 70% of responding patients alive at 1 year.

DLI for Chronic Lymphocytic Leukemia, ALL and ATLL

As regards CLL, Richardson *et al.* investigated the use of both pDLI and tDLI in 50 patients, 42 of whom had high-risk disease, who had undergone alemtuzumab-containing RIC regimens[29]. A total of 19 patients received pDLI for either MC (n=15) or MRD (n=4) whereas 16 patients received tDLI for either persistent or progressive disease. Progression-free survival was improved by the use of pDLI for MC and 68% of patients with stable, persistent, or progressive disease responded to tDLI. The 4-year cumulative incidence of severe acute or extensive chronic GvHD was around 30% of all those receiving DLI (see Chapter 39). The combination of DLI with novel agents and further immunotherapeutic approaches may improve the prevention and management of relapse in CLL (Table 25.2).

Despite initial enthusiasm in relapsed ALL, the evidence in favor of DLI efficacy in this context is less robust and more contradictory than for myeloid disorders[30]. Initial studies failed to suggest durable responses despite substantial proof in support of a GvL effect in ALL[31, 32]. It is now well established that the presence of GvHD post-all-HCT for both T- and B-lineage ALL is associated with decreased risk of relapse. Nevertheless, clinical efficacy of DLI at relapse remains limited (see Chapters 31–33). In addition, our own experience suggests limited efficacy of DLI for relapsed adult T-cell leukemia/lymphoma (ATLL), probably as a consequence of disease aggressiveness. Larger prospective studies are warranted to better understand the role of pDLI for these high-risk disorders.

DLI for Plasma Cell Dyscrasias

The last, and possibly most uncertain area of DLI-based therapy, is multiple myeloma (see Chapter 18). Despite the well-documented graft-*versus*-myeloma effect, historical data indicate that the beneficial effect produced by DLI is almost invariably associated with severe GvHD and responses are not durable. A seminal study reported on the treatment of 63 patients who had received nonmyeloablative conditioning and had either relapsed (n=48) or persistent disease (n=15) (Table 25.2)[33]. Just over 50% of these recipients had received T-cell depletion with either alemtuzumab or ATG. Only 12 patients received debulking combination chemotherapy prior to DLI. Varying T-cell dosages were employed, with the vast majority commencing with doses $<1 \times 10^7$ T-cells/kg. Total response rates (CR+PR) to DLI were 38%. Significant rates of both aGvHD (38%) and cGvHD (43%) were noted with this approach and durable remissions were restricted to the minority who achieved a CR. This is compounded by the fact that only a small proportion received debulking therapy (see Chapter 48).

However, independently of DLI administration, a very recent EBMT retrospective analysis demonstrated that plasma cell disorders, in general, appear largely refractory to any beneficial allo-immune effects occurring with either aGvHD or limited cGvHD and reductions in the relapse rate after transplantation appears to be only modest[34]. Whether this also applies to DLI is as yet unknown. In a recent study performed in 10 high-risk patients who received low-dose DLI, a correlation was observed between the frequency of Wilms' tumor 1 (WT1)-specific cytotoxic T-lymphocytes and responders to DLI[35]. All patients responded in the absence of GvHD. These data suggest the potential for developing WT-1-specific T-cell adoptive therapies for high-risk plasma cell disorders (see Chapter 62).

Strategies to Augment DLI: Does It Work?

A number of approaches are being investigated to improve the efficacy and reduce toxicity of DLI regimens (Table 25.2). They can be divided into those aimed at selecting T-cell subsets prior to infusion and those involving the administration of additional therapies in combination.

Cytokine Addition

Interferon-alpha or IL-2 have both been used in the post-allo-HCT setting to augment the potential immune response mediated by DLI, but the data, thus far, have been unconvincing[36].

Furthermore, the use of cytokines is limited by their short-range pharmacokinetics and toxicity. Furthermore, more recent work has suggested a synergistic effect of lenalidomide in combination with DLI for high-risk myeloma[37].

NK Cells

Natural killer (NK) cell-enhanced DLI (see Chapter 63) has been tested in a heterogeneous group of 30 patients following TCD nonmyeloablative allografts with 3–6/6 HLA-matched related donors[38]. Standardized NK cell enrichment was achieved in the lymphocyte preparations using the *CliniMACs system* with resultant high levels of purity and low levels of CD8+ and γδ T-cells (see Chapters 29, 30, and 59). At 8 weeks post-allograft, and in the absence of GvHD, NK-enriched DLIs were administered between 2 and 3 times at 8-week intervals. Infusions were associated with low rates of aGvHD. Long-term responders demonstrated improved T-cell recovery and possibly improved survival.

Dendritic Cells with Cytokines

More recently, dendritic cells have been tested as a DLI adjuvant in a phase I trial. *Ex-vivo* generated DCs were administered intravenously in 16 patients with hematologic cancers followed by DLI a day later. While the observed toxicity was very limited, 4 out of 14 evaluable patients achieved durable remissions (see Chapter 65)[39].

CD4+ Cells and Beyond

An alternative approach to DLI manipulation is based upon selectively eliminating the T-cells responsible for GvHD. One of the first strategies was CD8+ T-cell depletion. Although used since the mid 2000s, updates have only recently been presented. In one series, a total of 53 of 134 patients received at least one dose of CD8+ T-cell-depleted (CD8^{DEPL}) DLI, administered prophylactically with planned dose escalation and a starting dose of 1×10^6 CD4+ T-cells/kg, following a TCD-RIC allo-HCT[40]. A significant survival advantage was evident at the 3-year mark favoring the DLI cohort (overall survivalof 63.8% *versus* 30.1% in the non-DLI cohort, P= 0.002), which was more apparent in the MDS/AML cohort. This approach also favored achievement of full donor chimerism.

The depletion of antihost reactivity represents an interesting approach to reduce the potential of generating GvHD, particularly in the haploidentical setting (see Chapter 59). Various approaches have been developed, all based on the selective elimination of alloreactive donor T-cells *ex-vivo* using immunotoxins and/or magnetic beads targeting antigens like CD25, CD71, or CD137[41,42]. Large-scale clinical trials are awaited to validate this technology.

Of note, the control of T-cells responsible for GvHD can also be achieved *in-vivo*. Ciceri *et al.* were the first to report on the use of donor lymphocytes transduced with the herpes simplex thymidine kinase (TK) gene (TK-DLI) in 23 patients who had relapsed following HLA-matched sibling allo-HCT

[43]. Of the 17 patients evaluable, approximately one-third achieved a CR, a PR, or had progressive disease, respectively. The extent of *in-vivo* expansion of TK-DLI correlated with clinical response, although the numbers involved were small. The use of ganciclovir, used to kill donor lymphocytes, produced attenuation of GvHD when needed. Long-term follow-up data have recently been reported and included results on a further 34 patients receiving TK-DLI to expedite immune reconstitution following HLA-haplotype mismatch transplant. Collectively, over 50% achieved clinical benefit by either improvements in chimerism, immune reconstitution, or a GvL response. GvHD overall occurred in 22% of recipients and in all cases it was successfully controlled by SGT[44]. An alternative approach using caspase 9 (iCas9) encoding gene offers the possibility of inducing apoptosis in T-cells in cases of GvHD and has also demonstrated promise[45].

Future Directions

The notion that GvL is crucially involved in the efficacy of allo-HCT has provoked a fundamental rethinking of transplant modalities and paved the way to RIC protocols whereby the role of conditioning is confined to the establishment of host-*versus*-graft tolerance to allow the use of DLI to prevent and control disease relapse. Unfortunately, efficacy and toxicity of DLI for current indications are not as good as originally experienced in CML. Firstly, there is very limited evidence that DLI, at least administered therapeutically or preemptively, is a life-saving approach in acute leukemias and lymphomas. Secondly, therapeutic efficacy is very often associated with severe GvHD.

These aspects are probably sufficient to discourage further pursuit of DLI in its current use. However, there are a number of possible avenues that can improve its therapeutic potential. We think major benefits could derive from (Table 25.2):

1. **Prophylactic use of DLI.** The rationale to test this approach is to improve the outcome in conditions in which relapse rate is very high.
2. **Progressing towards fractionated DLI.** Although unfractionated DLI offers the benefit of a large repertoire of GvL effectors because it recognizes minor histocompatibility antigen polymorphisms, toxicity seems unacceptable and the use of selective population, either by depletion of alloreactive T-cells or choosing antigen-specific subsets, could reduce the severity of GvHD.
3. **Combining DLI with immunostimulating drugs.** Early data discussed in this chapter seem to support an increased antitumor activity.
4. **Developing better strategies to control GvHD.** An alternative approach is to maximize the GvL activity and act on the GvHD only when remission is achieved. The use of suicide gene approaches or cellular therapies like mesenchymal stromal cells (see Chapter 68) may contribute to a successful outcome.

Finally, one may wonder whether there is still a need for DLI once chimeric-antigen-receptor-transduced cells come to fruition. Although the results seem very exciting there are still major limitations related to the cost of personalized medicine. However, the initiative to engineer third-party cells devoid of HLA molecules will pave new pathways that will probably make allo-HCT much less used.

References

1. Goldman JM, Gale RP, Horowitz MM, Biggs JC, Champlin RE, Gluckman E, et al. Bone marrow transplantation for chronic myelogenous leukemia in chronic phase. Increased risk for relapse associated with T-cell depletion. *Ann Intern Med.* 1988;108(6):806–14. PubMed PMID: 3285744.

2. Kolb HJ, Mittermuller J, Clemm C, Holler E, Ledderose G, Brehm G, et al. Donor leukocyte transfusions for treatment of recurrent chronic myelogenous leukemia in marrow transplant patients. *Blood.* 1990;76(12):2462–5. PubMed PMID: 2265242.

3. Dazzi F, Szydlo RM, Cross NC, Craddock C, Kaeda J, Kanfer E, et al. Durability of responses following donor lymphocyte infusions for patients who relapse after allogeneic stem cell transplantation for chronic myeloid leukemia. *Blood.* 2000;96(8):2712–6. PubMed PMID: 11023502.

4. Craddock C, Szydlo RM, Klein JP, Dazzi F, Olavarria E, van Rhee F, et al. Estimating leukemia-free survival after allografting for chronic myeloid leukemia: a new method that takes into account patients who relapse and are restored to complete remission. *Blood.* 2000;96(1):86–90. PubMed PMID: 10891435.

5. Mackinnon S, Papadopoulos EB, Carabasi MH, Reich L, Collins NH, Boulad F, et al. Adoptive immunotherapy evaluating escalating doses of donor leukocytes for relapse of chronic myeloid leukemia after bone marrow transplantation: separation of graft-*versus*-leukemia responses from graft-versus-host disease. *Blood.* 1995;86(4):1261–8. PubMed PMID: 7632930.

6. van Rhee F, Savage D, Blackwell J, Orchard K, Dazzi F, Lin F, et al. Adoptive immunotherapy for relapse of chronic myeloid leukemia after allogeneic bone marrow transplant: equal efficacy of lymphocytes from sibling and matched unrelated donors. *Bone Marrow Transplant.* 1998;21(10):1055–61. PubMed PMID: 9632281.

7. Simula MP, Marktel S, Fozza C, Kaeda J, Szydlo RM, Nadal E, et al. Response to donor lymphocyte infusions for chronic myeloid leukemia is dose-dependent: the importance of escalating the cell dose to maximize therapeutic efficacy. *Leukemia.* 2007;21(5):943–8. PubMed PMID: 17361226. Epub 2007/03/16. eng.

8. Dazzi F, Szydlo RM, Craddock C, Cross NC, Kaeda J, Chase A, et al. Comparison of single-dose and escalating-dose regimens of donor lymphocyte infusion for relapse after allografting for chronic myeloid leukemia. *Blood.* 2000;95(1):67–71. PubMed PMID: 10607686.

9. Fozza C, Szydlo RM, Abdel-Rehim MM, Nadal E, Goldman JM, Apperley JF, et al. Factors for graft-*versus*-host disease after donor lymphocyte infusions with an escalating dose regimen: lack of association with cell dose. *Bri J Haematol.* 2007;136(6):833–6. PubMed PMID: 17341269. Epub 2007/03/08. eng.

10. Ferrara JL, Levine JE, Reddy P, Holler E. Graft-*versus*-host disease. *Lancet.* 2009;373(9674):1550–61. PubMed PMID: 19282026. Pubmed Central PMCID: 2735047. Epub 2009/03/14. eng.

11. Vianello F, Cannella L, Coe D, Chai JG, Golshayan D, Marelli-Berg FM, et al. Enhanced and aberrant T cell trafficking following total body irradiation: a gateway to graft-*versus*-host disease? *Br J Haematol.* 2013;162(6):808–18. PubMed PMID: 23855835.

12. Bar M, Sandmaier BM, Inamoto Y, Bruno B, Hari P, Chauncey T, et al. Donor lymphocyte infusion for relapsed hematological malignancies after allogeneic hematopoietic cell transplantation prognostic relevance of the initial CD3+ T cell dose. *Biol Blood Marrow Transplant.* 2013 19(6):949–57.

13. Schmid C, Schleuning M, Hentrich M, Markl GE, Gerbitz A, Tischer J, et al. High antileukemic efficacy of an intermediate intensity conditioning regimen for allogeneic stem cell transplantation in patients with high-risk acute myeloid leukemia in first complete remission. *Bone Marrow Transplant.* 2008;41(8):721–7.

14. Schmid C, Labopin M, Nagler A, Bornhauser M, Finke J, Fassas A et al. Donor lymphocyte infusion in the treatment of first hematological relapse after allogeneic stem-cell transplantation in adults with acute myeloid leukemia: a retrospective risk factors analysis and comparison with other strategies by the EBMT Acute Leukemia Working Party. *J Clin Oncol.* 2007;25:4938–45.

15. Campregher PV, Gooley T, Scott BL, Moravec C, Sandmaier B, Martin PJ, et al. Results of donor lymphocyte infusions for relapsed myelodysplastic syndrome after hematopoietic cell transplantation. *Bone Marrow Transplant.* 2007;40(10):965–71.

16. Elliott MA, Tefferi A, Hogan WJ, Letendre L, Gastineau DA, Ansell SM, et al. Allogeneic stem cell transplantation and donor lymphocyte infusions for chronic myelomonocytic leukemia. *Bone Marrow Transplant.* 2006; 37(11):1003–8.

17. Krishnamurthy P, Potter VT, Barber LD, Kulasekararaj AG, Lim ZY, Pearce RM, de Lavallade H, et al. Outcome of donor lymphocyte infusion after T cell-depleted allogeneic hematopoietic stem cell transplantation for acute myelogenous leukemia and myelodysplastic syndromes. *Biol Blood Marrow Transplant.* 2013;19(4):562–8.

18. Liga M, Triantafyllou E, Tiniakou M, Lambropoulou P, Karakantza M, Zoumbos NC, et al. High alloreactivity of low-dose prophylactic donor lymphocyte infusion in patients with acute leukemia undergoing allogeneic hematopoietic cell transplantation with an alemtuzumab-containing conditioning regimen. *Biol Blood Marrow Transplant.* 2013;19(1):75–81.

19. Schroeder T, Fröbel J, Cadeddu RP, Czibere A, Dienst A, Platzbecker U, et al. Salvage therapy with azacitidine increases regulatory T cells in

peripheral blood of patients with AML or MDS and early relapse after allogeneic blood stem cell transplantation. *Leukemia.* 2013;27(9):1910–3.

20. McLornan DP, Mead AJ, Jackson G, Harrison CN. Allogeneic stem cell transplantation for myelofibrosis in 2012. *Br J Haematol.* 2012;157(4):413–25.

21. Kröger N, Alchalby H, Klyuchnikov E, Badbaran A, Hildebrandt Y, Ayuk F, *et al.* JAK2-V617F-triggered preemptive and salvage adoptive immunotherapy with donor-lymphocyte infusion in patients with myelofibrosis after allogeneic stem cell transplantation. *Blood.* 2009;113(8):1866–8.

22. Yoshimi A, Bader P, Matthes-Martin S, Stary J, Sedlacek P, Duffner U *et al.* Donor leukocyte infusion after hematopoietic stem cell transplantation in patients with juvenile myelomonocytic leukemia. *Leukemia* 2005;19:971–7.

23. El-Jurdi N, Reljic T, Kumar A, Pidala J, Bazarbachi A, Djulbegovic B, *et al.* Efficacy of adoptive immunotherapy with donor lymphocyte infusion in relapsed lymphoid malignancies. *Immunotherapy.* 2013;5(5):457–66.

24. Bloor AJ, Thomson K, Chowdhry N, Verfuerth S, Ings SJ, Chakraverty R, *et al.* High response rate to donor lymphocyte infusion after allogeneic stem cell transplantation for indolent non-Hodgkin lymphoma. *Biol Blood Marrow Transplant.* 2008;14(1):50–8.

25. Thomson KJ, Morris EC, Milligan D, Parker AN, Hunter AE, Cook G, *et al.* T-cell-depleted reduced-intensity transplantation followed by donor leukocyte infusions to promote graft-*versus*-lymphoma activity results in excellent long-term survival in patients with multiply relapsed follicular lymphoma. *J Clin Oncol.* 2010;28(23):3695–700.

26. Peggs KS, Kayani I, Edwards N, Kottaridis P, Goldstone AH, Linch DC *et al.* Donor lymphocyte infusions modulate relapse risk in mixed chimeras and induce durable salvage in relapsed patients after T-cell-depleted allogeneic transplantation for Hodgkin's lymphoma. *J Clin Oncol.* 2011;29(8):971–8.

27. Theurich S, Malcher J, Wennhold K, Shimabukuro-Vornhagen A, Chemnitz J, Holtick U, *et al.* Brentuximab vedotin

combined with donor lymphocyte infusions for early relapse of Hodgkin lymphoma after allogeneic stem-cell transplantation induces tumor-specific immunity and sustained clinical remission. *J Clin Oncol.* 2013;31(5):e59-63.

28. Sala E, Crocchiolo R, Gandolfi S, Bruno-Ventre M, Bramanti S, Peccatori J, *et al.* Bendamustine combined with donor lymphocytes infusion in Hodgkin's lymphoma relapsing after allogeneic hematopoietic stem cell transplantation. *Biol Blood Marrow Transplant.* 2014;20(9):1444–7.

29. Richardson SE, Khan I, Rawstron A, Sudak J, Edwards N, Verfuerth S, *et al.* Risk-stratified adoptive cellular therapy following allogeneic hematopoietic stem cell transplantation for advanced chronic lymphocytic leukaemia. *Br J Haematol.* 2013;160(5):640–8.

30. Slavin S, Naparstek E, Nagler A, Ackerstein A, Samuel S, Kapelushnik J *et al.* Allogeneic cell therapy with donor peripheral blood cells and recombinant human interleukin-2 to treat leukemia relapse after allogeneic bone marrow transplantation. *Blood* 1996; 87:2195–204.

31. Collins RH Jr., Goldstein S, Giralt S, Levine J, Porter D, Drobyski W *et al.* Donor leukocyte infusions in acute lymphocytic leukemia. *Bone Marrow Transplant.* 2000;26:511–16.

32. Medd PG, Peniket AJ, Littlewood TJ, Pearce R, Perry J, Kirkland KE et al; British Society of Blood and Marrow Transplantation. Evidence for a GVL effect following reduced-intensity allo-SCT in ALL: a British Society of Blood and Marrow Transplantation study. *Bone Marrow Transplant.* 2013;48(7):982–7.

33. van de Donk NW, Kröger N, Hegenbart U, Corradini P, San Miguel JF, Goldschmidt H, *et al.* Prognostic factors for donor lymphocyte infusions following non-myeloablative allogeneic stem cell transplantation in multiple myeloma. *Bone Marrow Transplant.* 2006;37(12):1135–41.

34. Stern M, de Wreede LC, Brand R, van Biezen A, Dreger P, Mohty M, *et al.* Sensitivity of hematological malignancies to graft-versus-host effects: an EBMT megafile analysis. *Leukemia.* 2014; Apr 30. [Epub ahead of print]

35. Tyler EM, Jungbluth AA, O'Reilly RJ, Koehne G. WT1-specific T-cell responses in high-risk multiple myeloma patients undergoing allogeneic T cell-depleted hematopoietic stem cell transplantation and donor lymphocyte infusions. *Blood.* 2013;121(2):308–17.

36. Cooper, N., Rao, K., Goulden, N., Amrolia, P. and Veys, P. Alpha interferon augments the graft-*versus*-leukaemia effect of second stem cell transplants and donor lymphocyte infusions in high-risk paediatric leukaemias. *Br J Haematol.* 2012;156:550–2.

37. El-Cheikh J, Crocchiolo R, Furst S, Ladaique P, Castagna L, Faucher C, *et al.* Lenalidomide plus donor-lymphocytes infusion after allogeneic stem-cell transplantation with reduced-intensity conditioning in patients with high-risk multiple myeloma. *Exp Hematol.* 2012;40(7):521–7.

38. Rizzieri DA, Storms R, Chen DF, Long G, Yang Y, Nikcevich DA *et al.* Natural killer cell-enriched donor lymphocyte infusions from A 3–6/6 HLA-matched family member following nonmyeloablative allogeneic stem cell transplantation. *Biol Blood Marrow Transplant.* 2010;16(8):1107–14.

39. Ho VT, Kim HT, Kao G, Cutler C, Levine J, Rosenblatt J, *et al.* Sequential infusion of donor-derived dendritic cells with donor lymphocyte infusion for relapsed hematologic cancers after allogeneic hematopoietic stem cell transplantation. *Am J Hematol.* 2014; Aug 13. [Epub ahead of print]

40. Wagner E, Wehler D, Kolbe K, Theobald M, Herr W and Meyer R. Impact of Prophylactic CD8-Depleted Donor-Lymphocyte Infusions After Allogeneic Hematopoietic Stem Cell Transplantation and Alemtuzumab Mediated T-Cell Depletion. Abstract 4109. American Society of Hematology Annual Meeting 2013.

41. Samarasinghe S, Mancao C, Pule M, Nawroly N, Karlsson H, Brewin J, *et al.* Functional characterization of alloreactive T cells identifies CD25 and CD71 as optimal targets for a clinically applicable allodepletion strategy. *Blood.* 2010;115(2):396–407.

42. Solomon SR, Mielke S, Savani BN, Montero A, Wisch L, Childs R, *et al.* Selective depletion of alloreactive donor lymphocytes: a novel method to reduce

the severity of graft-*versus*-host disease in older patients undergoing matched sibling donor stem cell transplantation. *Blood*. 2005;106(3):1123–9. Epub 2005 Apr 7.

43. Ciceri F, Bonini C, Marktel S, Zappone E, Servida P, Bernadi M *et al*. Anti-tumor effect of HSV-TK engineered donor lymphocytes after allogeneic stem cell transplantation. *Blood*. 2007;109:4698–707.

44. Ciceri F, Lupo-Stanghellini M, Oliveira G, Greco R *et al*. Long-term safety and survival outcomes after TK-expressing donor lymphocyte infusion (TK-DLI) in allogeneic hematopoietic stem cell transplantation (HSCT).*J Clin Oncol*. 2013;31(Suppl): abstr 7007.

45. Di Stasi A, Tey SK, Dotti G, Fujita Y, Kennedy-Nasser A, Martinez C, Vago L, Bondanzo A *et al*. Inducible apoptosis as a safety switch for adoptive cell therapy. *N Engl J Med*. 2011;365(18):1673–83.

26

Post-Transplant Relapse and Graft Failure: Does a Second Allogeneic Hematopoietic Cell Transplant Work?

Sebastian Mayer and Koen van Besien

Introduction

In the last two decades, the outcome of allogeneic hematopoietic cell transplant (allo-HCT) for hematologic malignancies has improved, mainly due to decreases in nonrelapse mortality (NRM) with disease recurrence remaining the most common cause for failure[1,2]. Graft failure is historically a less common problem but with the increasing use of alternative hematopoietic cell sources and expanding indication of allo-HCT for nonmalignant diseases it is more widely encountered[3–6]. In such circumstances, an attempt at second allo-HCT is increasingly undertaken, but represents unique challenges and is the focus of this chapter.

Second Allo-HCT for Relapsed Disease: How and When or Yes or No?

Acute leukemia and other hematologic malignancies relapsing after allo-HCT have a poor prognosis with median survival of 2 to 6 months without further therapy[7–10]. The nontransplant approaches are usually applied upon relapse but the CR rates and sustainable remissions are extremely rare.

Nontransplant Approaches Remain Suboptimal for Relapsed Disease after Allo-HCT

A number of nontransplant approaches have been employed in the treatment of leukemic relapse post transplant and will be briefly described:

A. *Cessation of immunosuppression*

   Withdrawal of immunosuppression in the hope of igniting a graft-*versus*-malignancy effect: This is restricted to early relapses when the patient is still on immunosuppression and only a few anecdotal reports of a successful remission induction are available. There is, however, also a risk of GvHD occurrence or flare up [11,12,13].

B. *Myeloid growth factors*

   Following the premise of donor cell stimulation by granulocyte colony-stimulating factor (G-CSF), growth factor administration led to remissions in three of seven patients with relapsed leukemia after allo-HCT (six acute myeloid leukemia (AML) and myelodysplastic syndrome

(MDS), one chronic myeloid leukemia (CML)) but no long-term follow-up is available[14]. Another case report described an infant with congenital AML who relapsed 6 months after cord blood transplant, was treated with GM-CSF (granulocyte-macrophage colony-stimulating factor) and obtained a 24 months sustained CR[15].

C. *Remission induction with various pharmacologic agents*

   i. Hypomethylating agents:

      Several smaller studies have evaluated azacytidine for recurrent AML/MDS after allo-HCT. Overall remission rates were 16–23% and 2-year survival rates between 15% and 23%. Of note, most of the patients had also received donor lymphocyte infusion (DLI), and thus the effect cannot be ascribed to the azacytidine alone (see Chapters 23 and 25). Nonetheless, the survival data are not very encouraging and long-term outcome data are not available[16,17,18].

   ii. Conventional chemotherapy:

      Reinduction of a complete remission (CR) is feasible with various chemotherapeutic regimens and CR rates vary between 20% and 80%[19] but the long-term outcome is very poor[8,20].

   iii. Targeted therapies:

      For patients harboring *FLT3-ITD* mutation, sorafenib as single agent and in combination with chemotherapy has been studied in the setting of relapse post-allo-HCT resulting in CR rates between 0 and 30%, many of the remissions being sustained. However, there are significant discrepancies between studies, possibly due to patient selection[21,22].

D. **Donor lymphocyte infusion: limitations?**

   DLI has emerged as a highly effective intervention for smoldering and chronic phase CML after allo-HCT with CR rates between 60% and 86%[23,24,25] (see Chapter 36), but the results in acute leukemias have been sobering with CR rates ranging between 13% and 23% and 2-year survivals ranging from 0 to 23% (see Chapter 25)[26–29]. The largest study of DLI for AML to date showed a 2-year survival of 21% for patients after DLI *versus* 9% for those who did not receive DLI[26], an outcome that is far worse than in CML. A study concerned with the long-term outcome of patients who achieve a CR with DLI showed a 38% event-free survival (EFS) at 2 years for patients with AML, MDS (see Chapters 34 and 35), or acute lymphoblastic leukemia (ALL) (see Chapters 32 and 33). Relapse, infections, and GvHD-related complications were frequent[30]. Given suboptimal outcomes with DLI and frequent unavailability of donor lymphocytes in the case of HLA-matched unrelated donors and cord blood transplant, second allo-HCT is often considered.

Important Consideration before Second Allo-HCT for Relapsed Disease

The first question relates to what criteria to use for patient selection and how they differ from those for the initial transplant eligibility. Studies of comorbidity, and performance status-related risk, of pretransplant CRP or ferritin are lacking in this setting but it seems prudent to utilize these parameters as well for a second transplantation, in particular since the patient's overall health may have declined considerably after the initial HCT.

Other patient- and disease-related prognostic information can be extracted from several large retrospective studies reported over the last 10 years and are summarized in Table 26.1[31–39,104–106].

Although the clinical circumstances vary among the cited studies, OS is comparable at 18–33%, with follow-up periods between 1 and 5 years. Despite a shift from "myeloablative" to reduced intensity conditioning in the last 10 years, TRM rates have remained unchanged at around 30%, and relapse of the underlying malignancy remains the most common cause of failure across all studies[31,32,39,105,106].

The following prognostic factors have been identified and can be helpful in deciding whether to offer a second allo-HCT for recurrent or relapsed leukemia:

1. *Duration of CR1:* The factor most consistently predictive of outcome was the duration of the time from first allo-HCT to relapse, with a very poor outcome for those relapsing early (within 6 or 12 months depending on the study), highlighting the aggressiveness of the malignancy as a major determinant of the patients' outcome[31–34,38,39,105,106]. Not surprisingly, CR at the time of second allo-HCT was associated with improved survival in several series[31,32,40,104–106].

2. *Age:* Younger age was associated with better survival in three reports but the difference in cut-offs was quite large (<20, <60, and <65 years)[31,34,39]. Given the increasingly recognized importance of comorbidities and performance status for transplant-related mortality (TRM) in first transplant, age may no longer be as prominent an independent factor as in the past[41,42]. While most studies on second HCT do not provide prognostic information of these health-related parameters, 2 large studies demonstrated that a poor performance status was predictive of a bad outcome in second allo-HCT[39,106].

Practice Points

With the above findings in mind it is reasonable to consider a relapse-free interval of more than 6 months a condition for consideration for second allo-HCT. Failure to attain a CR prior to a second allo-HCT predicts for poor outcomes in most studies. Lastly, extrapolating from widely published and accepted standards for first allo-HCT, the absence of major comorbidities and a good performance status should be mandatory for patients undergoing a second allo-HCT [39,41,42,106].

Controversies for Second Allo-HCT for Relapsed Disease

Controversy#1: What Is the Best Conditioning Regimen for Second Allo-HCT?

While older studies have shown a decreased relapse rate with "myeloablative" conditioning regimen (MAC regimen)[39,43], in recent years reduced intensity condition regimens (RIC) or even non myeloablative (NMA) approaches (see Chapters 3 and 27) were applied in the majority of patients without finding a difference in OS between conditioning intensities[32,37].

Two studies have even shown superior OS for NMA second allo-HCT, but in one of them the data is confounded by the inclusion of patients with prior autologous hematopoietic cell transplant into the study group[44,106]. RIC regimen was found to lead to better OS in another report; however, many of the second transplants in this series were done for graft failure and 15% of patients had noncancerous hematologic disorders such as aplastic anemia[45]. The role of total body irradiation (TBI) in second allo-HCT has not been systematically studied, and while an older report showed that toxicities can be decreased by alternating non-TBI-based with TBI-containing regimens[46], most recent studies have not shown a benefit of one over the other modality[32,38,39]. Only one report showed superiority for TBI-containing regimens, which must be interpreted with caution as the study group included patients with prior history of autologous transplants and the authors did not distinguish between MAC regimen and NMA TBI dosing[44]. Therefore, the optimal preparative regimen for second allo-HCT is still not known but RIC regimen will be more universally applicable.

Controversy#2: The Best Donor for the Second Allo-HCT?

While procurement of graft from an HLA-matched sibling is usually straightforward, repeat collections from unrelated donors are subject to strict regulation and may be impossible within a reasonable time frame[47]. In case of previously performed cord blood transplant an alternative graft source is sought (see Chapters 60, 61, and 66). In the case of HLA-matched sibling donor, some centers collect an excess amount of hematopoietic cells and cryopreserve them for later use (DLI and second allo-HCT). However, the hope to harness a more pronounced graft-*versus*-malignancy effect leads some

Table 26.1 Studies evaluating second allogeneic hematopoietic cell transplant for relapsed disease

Reference	Year	Number of patients	Median age (range)	Disease	Regimen	Donor	Same donor	GvHD prophylaxis	aGvHD Grade 2–4	cGvHD	TRM	Relapse	Outcome	Predictors of improved survival
Tachibana et al.[104]	2016	60	35 (18–60)	AML/ALL	MA (15) RIC (45)	MRD (20) MMRD (7) MUD (27) CBU (6)	Missing	CNI based (95%) None (5%)	32%	41%	40% at 2 years	30% at 2 years	OS 30% at 2 years	MRD CR at SCT 2 RIC
Orti et al.[105]	2016	116	38 (4–69)	AML/MDS/MPN	MA (42) NMA (67)	MRD (96) UD (13) MMRD (5) Syngeneic (2)	83%	CSA based (57%) Other (43%)	39%	15% ltd 17% ext	32% at 5 years	38% at 5 years	OS 32% at 5 years	MRD CR at SCT 2 Interval after SCT 1 >430 days
Vrhovac et al. [106]	2016	234	52 (20–74)	AML/ALL	RIC (234)	MRD (99) MUD (106) Haplo (27)	43%	CNI based (64%) Other/missing (36%)	32%	12% ltd 13% ext	22% at 2 years	64% at 2 years	OS 20% at 2 years	CR at SCT 2 CR after SCT 1 >225 days KPS >80 NMA
Fan et al. [39]	2014	65	47 (11–73)	AML/MDS (49)	RIC (61)	MRD (33) MUD (21) Haplo-CBU (11)		TCD (71%)	23%[a]	8%	31%	40%	OS 33.8% at 1 year	CR at SCT 2 CR after SCT 1 >12 months Age < 60
Christopeit et al.[32]	2013	179	39 (16–68)	AML/MDS	MA (50) RIC (59) NMA (64) Missing (6)	MRD (46) MUD (133)	46%	CSA based (72%) Other (28%)	46.1 %	30.2%	35% at 4 years	54% at 4 years	OS 25% at 2 years	MRD CR at SCT 2 CR after SCT 1 >6 months
Leung et al. [33]	2013	108	37 (16–57)	AML/ALL	RIC (108)	MRD (97) MUD (11)	100%	Incomplete	55% [a]		17%	67%	OS 26% at 2 years	CR/Cri after HCT 2 GvHD CR after HCT 1 >11 months
Christopoulos et al.[34]	2013	58	53 (23–69)	AML/MDS	RIC (58)	MRD (2) MUD (41) MMUD (15)	3%	CSA based (100%)	41%	12% ltd 37% ext	31% at 3 years	56% at 3 years	OS 18% at 3 years	Age <65 CR after HCT 1 >12 months cGvHD

Poon et al.[35]	2012	31	26 (7-49)	ALL	MA (11) RIC (20)	MRD (19) MUD (8) MMUD (2) CBU (2)	52%	Incomplete	26%	10% ltd 16% ext	41% at 1 year	36% at 1 year	OS 11% at 3 years	Longer CR after SCT 1 (HR=0.93/month)
Spyridonidis et al.[36]	2012	93	32 (18-66)	ALL	Missing	Missing	Missing	Missing	Missing	Missing	Missing	Missing	Median OS 12.6 months OS at 41 months 6%	Not done
Hartwig et al. [37]	2009	25	45 (4-46)	AML/MDS (20) MPN (5)	RIC (23) MA (2)	MRD (3) MMRD (1) MUD (10) MMUD (11)	40%	CI based (100%)	44%	21% ltd 16% ext	32% at 18 months	44% at 18 months	OS 32% at 18 months	No multivariate analysis
Shaw et al.[38]	2008	71	43 (8-69)	AML/MDS (57) LPD (9) MM(2) MPN(3)	RIC (71)	MRD (49) MUD (18) MMRD (4)	80%	CSA based (89%)	26%	27% ltd 15% ext	27% (2 years)	56% (2 years)	OS 28% at 2 years	CR after HCT 1 >11 months cGvHD
Eapen et al. [39]	2004	279	25	AML (125) ALL (72) CML (82)	MA (234) RIC (45)	MRD (279)	85%	CSA based (93%)	29%	41% at 5 years	30% at 5 years	42% at 5 years	OS 28% at 5 years	CR after HCT 1 >6 months Age ≤20

[a] No grading given in reference.
Abbreviations: MA: myeloablative, RIC: reduced intensity conditioning, NMA: nonmyeloablative, AML: acute myeloid leukemia, MDS: myelodysplastic syndrome, ALL: acute lymphoblastic leukemia, MM: multiple myeloma, MPN: myeloproliferative disease, CML: chronic myeloid leukemia, LPD: lymphoproliferative neoplasm, CBU: cord blood unit, CSA: cyclosporin A, CI: calcineurin inhibitor, aGvHD: acute graft-versus-host disease, cGvHD: chronic graft-versus-host disease, MUD: matched unrelated donor, MMUD: mismatched unrelated donor, MRD: matched related donor, MMRD: mismatched related donor, MUD: matched related donor, SCT: stem cell transplant, CR: complete remission, CRi: complete remission with incomplete platelet recovery, ltd: limited, ext: extensive. disease, TRM: transplant-related mortality, OS: overall survival,

physicians to routinely opt for an alternative ("different") donor. In the case of a sibling transplant, changing to another sibling does not influence the outcome[39]. A more recent study has specifically addressed the question of donor change for relapsed acute leukemia after first allo-HCT[32]. The outcome was significantly better for patients who initially were transplanted from a related donor compared to an unrelated donor (2 years OS 37% *versus* 16%). Donor change did not alter the prognosis, regardless of whether the first allo-HCT was performed with a related or unrelated donor, but second allo-SCT from a matched related donor was superior, findings that were both confirmed this year[105]. In all practicality, the choice of donor is based on availability, giving preference to a matched related donor.

Controversy#3: What Should Be the GvHD Prophylaxis with Second Allo-HCT?

After initial failure of the desired graft-*versus*-leukemia effect it may be tempting to curtail the graft-*versus*-host prophylaxis to attain stronger antileukemic activity. Moreover, it has been hypothesized that given persistence of a mixed chimerism (if true) the risk of GvHD may be lower after a second transplant, at least in the case of the same donor. In one series, it was shown that one could safely omit GvHD prophylaxis if there had been no GvHD with the first transplant[48], a strategy leading to a very high incidence of severe and sometimes fatal GvHD in another report[49]. Consistent with an earlier report [48] showing decreased relapse with chronic GvHD, three more recent studies even show a survival benefit associated with the development of this complication[3,34,38]; however, the follow-up periods are only between 2 and 3 years and just recently chronic GvHD was shown to have a detrimental effect on OS that becomes apparent only after prolonged follow up [50] and persists for many years after transplant[51]. Therefore, the beneficial role of chronic GvHD should not be over-estimated and attempts to dilute GvHD prophylaxis are probably misguided. In fact, all the recent series have almost uniformly employed a calcineurin inhibitor (CNI)-based anti-GvHD strategy[31–39].

Controversy#4: Graft Source from Bone Marrow or Peripheral Blood?

There are no recent studies addressing the issue of graft source in second transplant but a few older studies did not show a conclusive difference in survival utilizing either BM or PB[39], and others have conflicting results either in favor of BM[52] or PB[53]. It is possible that the higher lymphocyte dose in graft obtained from PB may confer a stronger GvL effect compared with BM but at the cost of higher rates of GvHD [54]. PB graft is the most commonly used source in current practice and given the relative logistic ease and decreased burden on the donor there is little reason to advocate for BM over PB[55]. One approach currently pursued by our own group is to utilize cord blood donors, often associated with

lower recurrence rates, for second transplant. Our data are, however, very preliminary.

Practice Points

In summary, second allo-HCT for relapsed leukemia is increasingly recognized as a potentially curative modality and has become available to a larger patient population, especially due to the feasibility of treating older patients as seen by the increase of the median age of patients in the last 20 years from 25 to 45[31–39,104–106]. Paradoxically, it may be offered to more patients due to the improvement in the pharmaceutical repertoire for acute leukemia leading to higher remission rates after failed initial allo-HCT. The lessons that can be learned are that in patients who relapse early, and in particular those whose health has suffered from the initial transplant, either a palliative approach or an investigational treatment would be more appropriate given the extremely high relapse rates after second allo-HCT but also increased TRM[32,39]. Furthermore, given the already high TRM rates it seems advisable to preferentially use RIC regimens with few rare exceptions. Lastly, the speculation that donor change or decreased GvHD prophylaxis may confer a stronger GvL effect should give way to choosing the most readily available donor and using well-established CNI-based GvHD prophylaxis, respectively.

Second Allo-HCT for Graft Failure
Incidence of Graft Failure: Where Do We Stand?

Sustained engraftment is routinely achieved after allogeneic transplantation from an HLA-identical related donor for patients with hematologic malignancies. In the rare cases of graft failure, a technical problem during collection or processing, or an occult hematologic problem in the donor (cases of familial MDS/AML syndromes are increasingly described) should be suspected[56]. Therefore, the majority of graft failures occur in transplants from unrelated or mismatched donors or in transplantation for nonmalignant disorders such as aplastic anemia or hemoglobinopathies (see Chapters 9, 52, 54, and 55)[6,57,58].

Primary graft failure (PGF) is usually defined as the inability to achieve an absolute neutrophil count of at least 500/µL by day 28 post-HCT or day 42 after cord blood transplant[59]. Between the years 1990 and 2005, the rates for PGF in transplants from matched unrelated adult donors reported to the NMDP have continuously dropped from 8.2% to 3.6%, likely due to refinement of HLA typing in donor selection and in conditioning (see Chapters 7, 8, and 9)[60]. The rates of graft failure/rejection are higher in recipients of mismatched grafts (10%), T-cell depleted transplants, and matched unrelated bone marrow grafts (9%) compared to PB allografts (3%) [3,61–63]. The increasingly widespread use of alternative sources of allo-graft such as cord blood and HLA-haplotype mismatched donors has also been burdened by relatively higher rates of graft failure ranging from 12% to 20%[4,64–67].

Primary Graft Failure: Why Does This Happen?

In PGF, no recovery of hematopoiesis occurs. In such cases, no-donor engraftment can be detected in any hematopoietic lineage including myeloid, erythroid, and lymphoid lineages. The underlying biology of this phenomenon is not yet fully understood and likely there is more than one mechanism. Poor graft potency due to prolonged transport usually at room temperature seems to be a factor in unrelated donor BM grafts (see Chapter 11). No such correlation was found for unrelated PB grafts, which usually are transported at 4°C and tend to require fewer manipulations upon arrival at the transplant center[68]. In a smaller report by Lioznov et al., cryopreservation of PB grafts but not BM had deleterious effects on graft activity as measured by aldehyde dehydrogenase levels and was associated with significantly higher graft failure rates (see Chapter 11)[69]. Both studies implicate an intrinsic defect in the graft and technical issues in its preparation rather than host-related factors. Studies of unit predominance in double cord blood transplant have also provided some insight into potential mechanisms of graft failure: in the "myeloablative" setting only the CD3+ cell dose of the CBU was predictive of dominance; in "nonablative" transplants HLA match was equally important, suggesting an immunologic mechanism of graft rejection, in keeping with studies of BM transplant showing graft failure rates to be directly proportional to the degree of HLA mismatch[63,70].

Building on the hypothesis of immunologic graft rejection, early studies in dogs suggest a cellular mechanism[71,72], but more recent work in murine models as well as observational studies in clinical cohorts have highlighted a humoral mechanism of graft rejection, in particular the effect of donor-specific anti-HLA antibodies (see Chapter 9)[65,66,73–77]. However, given contradicting reports in the literature, this area is still a matter of controversy [78,79].

Secondary Graft Failure

Secondary graft rejection occurs after an initial period of engraftment. While immunologically mediated graft rejection can play a role in secondary graft failure, some cases are characterized by persistent donor chimerism but ineffective donor hematopoiesis. The pathophysiology of such poor graft function is very poorly understood.

Prognosis for Allograft Failure

The prognosis for PGF is dismal with a 1-year survival rate of about 1% without further intervention in the largest reported series[60] and various therapeutic approaches have been studied in this situation.

Outcomes of Second Allo-HCT for Graft Failure

The published data must be interpreted with caution due to significant heterogeneity with respect to diagnoses as well as transplant modalities not only within the study groups but also between the various studies. Furthermore, in one study a small fraction of patients did not undergo a second transplant at all or had an autologous cell infusion[80]. Finally, most series are relatively small with only four publications including more than 50 patients[60,80–82]. Table 26.2 summarizes the latest published studies of second transplants for graft failure[60,80–86]. With one exception[85] they are all retrospective, mostly registry-based reports.

Despite the difficulty in comparing the various published studies on primary and secondary graft failure there are some common findings across most series. Firstly, transplant-related mortality is higher than with first allo-HCT and patients usually succumb to infections despite relatively high rates of neutrophil engraftment (66–100% for PB graft and 40–45% for CB grafts)[60,80–82,84–86,107]. Secondly, younger adults and those with nonmalignant disease do significantly better[45,87].

Survival Outcomes

The OS data reported by Schriber et al. for the NMDP (unrelated donor for both transplants) was 11% at 1 year, while a study by Ferrà et al. showed a 1-year survival of 50%. However, the study population in the latter report was more heterogeneous, with patients having undergone second allo-HCTs from related, unrelated, and cord blood sources[60,80]. Two Japanese studies evaluated the outcome of CBT after graft failure and both showed a comparable 1-year survival of about 30% [81,82,107]. Some smaller reports show higher OS rates of 80–90% at 3 years but they either had a comparably higher proportion of nonmalignant diseases[83] or did not have enough patients to draw firm conclusions[84].

Treatment-Related Mortality

TRM rates are generally high, ranging between 30% and 86%, with the predominant cause of death being infection[60,80–82]. In part, the high TRM may be due to carry-over toxicities from the first transplant resulting in poor performance status, reduced organ function reserve, as well as sustained immunosuppression.

Predictors of Outcome

Several clinical variables have been examined in order to define the best candidates and best approach to second allo-HCT for graft failure.

Graft Source

Studies have addressed the impact of changing to an alternative donor for second allo-HCT in the adult donor setting but have failed to show any improvement in engraftment or survival[60,80,83]. A series of 220 patients with graft failure after CBT showed superior outcomes for second allo-HCT from PB grafts over a second CBT (1-year OS 58% versus 28%)[81]. In this study only a relatively small number (n=24) of patients received a second graft from PB. Another study showed that

Table 26.2 Studies evaluating second allogeneic hematopoietic cell transplant after primary or secondary allograft failure

Reference	Year	No	Age median (range)	Disease	First donor	Second donor	Graft source 2	Same donor	Conditioning intensity	Time between first and second allo-HCT median (range)	TRM	Engraftment	Outcome	Predictors of improved survival (multivariate analyses)
Lund et al. [107]	2015	95	10 (0.9–69)	Malignant: 36 Nonmalignant: 67	Not specified	MRD: 9 Haplo: 7 URD: 70	CBU: 44 PBHC: 18 BM: 33	28	Not available	60 days (19–1751)	46% (one year)	45% (neutropenic GF) 88% (non-neutropenic GF)	OS 1 year: 44% 27% for neutropenic GF 76% for non-neutropenic GF	Non-neutropenic graft failure
Ferrà et al. [80] (GETH)	2014	89	35 (1–68)	AML/MDS: 48 ALL: 14 Lymphoma: 11 MPN: 6 Nonmalignant: 10	RD: 41 UD: 20 CBU: 28	(n=75)	PBHC: 61 CBU: 8 BM: 6	38	Not available	69 days (24–652)	52% (5 years)	79% (of 62)	OS 5 years: 31%	Age <18 (trend)
Fuji et al. [81]	2012	220	42.5 (0–75)	AML/MDS: 123 ALL: 40 CML: 8 Lymphoma: 31 Other: 18	CBU: 220	MMRD: 24 MMRD: 13 MRD: 1 MUD: 2	CBU: 180 PBHC: 24 BM: 16	0	MA: 5 RIC: 122 NMA: 77	11 days (0–89)[a]	29% (1 year)	CBU: 39% PB graft: 71% BM: 75%	OS 1 year CBT: 28% PBHC: 58% BM: 38%	PB versus CBT
Waki et al. [82]	2011	80	51 (17–68)	AML/MDS: 63 ALL: 13 Other: 14	RD: 5 UD: 16 CBU: 59		CBU: 80	0	RIC: 80	47 days 15 days [a]	56% (1 year)	56%	OS 1 year 33%	Standard-risk disease No carry over organ toxicity >2
Schriber et al.[60] (NMDP)	2010	122	29 (2–62)	AML/MDS: 99 SAA: 20 Other: 3	MUD	MUD	BM: 51% PBHC: 49%	98	MA: 36 RIC: 44 None: 14 Missing: 28	48 (18–126)	86% (1 year) malignant disease only	66% (of 79 pts)	OS 1 year 11%	
Remberger et al.[83]	2011	20	16 (1.5–65)	Nonmalignant: 10 AML/MDS/CML: 10	MRD: 3 MUD: 14 MMUD: 3	MRD: 3 MUD: 13 MMUD: 4	BM: 11 PBHC: 7 CBU: 2	11	RIC: 19 MA: 1	43 days (9–270) [a]	30% (1 year)	90%	OS 3 years 60%	Nonmalignant disorder

Study	Year	N	Age (range)	Disease	Donor	Graft		Conditioning	Time to engraftment[a]			Outcome	
Byrne et al. [84]	2008	11	(20–68)	AML/MDS/ CML/MPD: 6 NHL: 2 RCC: 2 Thalassemia: 1	MRD: 2 MMRD: 9	All PB grafts	4	NMA: 11	70 days (51–774)	18%	81%	OS 45% (29 months)	
Jabbour et al.[85]	2007	9	42 (26–75)	CML: 5 AML/MDS: 4	MRD: 2 MMRD: 4 MUD: 2	PB grafts: 8 CBU: 1	8	NMA: 9	54 days (31–140)	67%	67%	Median survival 7 months	
Chewning et al.[86]	2007	16	22 (4–59)	AL/MDS: 13 CML: 2 FA: 1	MRD: 3 MMRD: 8 MUD: 5 MMUD: 6	BM: 3 PB grafts: 13	MRD: 2 MMRD: 9 MUD: 2 MMUD: 1 6	NMA:	45 days (31–85)	56%	100%	OS 3 years 35%	Age <20 years

[a] Denotes time between graft failure and second transplantation.
Abbreviations: AML: acute myeloid leukemia, MDS: myelodysplastic syndrome, ALL: acute lymphoblastic leukemia, CML: chronic myeloid leukemia, SAA: severe aplastic anemia, MPN: Myeloproliferative neoplasm, NHL: non-Hodgkin lymphoma, RCC: renal cell carcinoma, FA: Fanconi anemia, CBU: cord blood unit, MUD: matched unrelated donor, MMUD: mismatched unrelated donor, MRD: matched related donor, MMRD: mismatched unrelated donor, BM: bone marrow, PBHC: peripheral blood hematopoietic cells, MA: myeloablative, RIC: reduced intensity conditioning, NMA: nonmyeloablative, OS: overall survival, SCT: stem cell transplantation, GETH: Grupo Espanol de Trasplante Hematopoyetico, NMDP: National Marrow Donor Program.

engraftment from a CBT can be achieved also after initially failed engraftment from an adult hematopoietic cell source with a 1-year OS of 33%[82].

Cell Dose

Increasing the cell dose for a second allo-HCT may seem logical in an attempt to increase the chances of engraftment but the NMDP data show no improvement in survival with this approach[60]. Not surprisingly, the number of transplanted cells in second CBT was indeed relevant, a finding well established for initial transplantations, and the infusion of total nucleated cells (TNCs) $\geq 2.5 \times 10^7$/kg led to neutrophil engraftment in 80% compared to 50% with lower TNC doses[82].

Controversies for Second Allo-HCT for Graft Failure

Controversy#1: What Is the Role of Hematopoietic Growth Factors?

Granulocyte colony-stimulating factor has been administered to patients with graft failure, with short-term (75 days) improvement in neutrophil counts in 9 out of 15 patients [88,89]. Responses were only seen in the granulocytic lineage and in patients with more than 10% bone marrow cellularity. Long-term data are less encouraging with only 1 in 6 patients alive at 22 months for PGF and 3 out of 13 surviving 5 years after secondary graft failure in a report from MD Anderson Cancer Center[59]. Romiplostim has been successfully used for delayed platelet recovery as well as in secondary failure of platelet recovery with a complete response in all patients; however, both case series were quite small with less than 10 patients[90,91]. In this particular setting, this drug should not be used outside of a clinical trial.

Controversy#2: DLI for Allograft Failure – Yes or No?

There are few anecdotal reports of DLI reversing incipient graft failure – defined by progressive pancytopenia and decreasing donor chimerism – in the TCD allo-HCT setting[92]. The only systematic attempt at utilizing DLI for this scenario was performed in seven patients with thalassemia with only two low-risk patients showing a response[93].

Controversy#3: How About Autologous Hematopoietic Cell Infusion, if Available?

When available, previously collected (so-called "back-up," i.e., lymphomas and multiple myeloma) autologous hematopoietic cells can be infused[94,95]. This represents a reasonably safe salvage modality usually resulting in hematopoietic recovery within 10–14 days after infusion. Unfortunately, back-up autologous graft is available in only a minority of cases and even then, there is a considerable risk of recurrence of the underlying hematologic disorder given the risk of a graft contaminated with tumor cells (and the lack of a graft-*versus*-malignancy effect) resulting in very poor long-term

outcomes[96]. Thus, this can be seen mostly as a measure of temporary "count" stabilization.

Controversy#4: What About Additional Donor Cell Infusion "Boost"?

For patients with poor hematopoiesis but persistent donor chimerism the infusion of additional CD34+ cells from the original donor has been studied with varying success but a high rate of severe acute GvHD[87,97]. The CD34+ selected cells approach (via any method) in this context seems to be a promising technique of reducing the risk of GvHD[98].

Controversy#5: Watch and Wait/Observation for Allograft Failure?

Some studies of second allo-HCT have shown a better outcome if there was a prolonged interval between the first and second allo-HCT[83,99]. This raises the question whether an initial "watch and wait" position can be taken. The rationale in this case would be to give the patient some time to recover from the toxicities of the initial transplant.

Controversy#6: What Should Be GvHD Prophylaxis with Second Allo-HCT for Allograft Failure?

Most series are either too small to analyze the impact of different approaches to GvHD prophylaxis[83–85] or, as in the NMDP data, the methods were too similar to find differences with 83% of all patients having received a calcineurin inhibitor-based regimen[60]. Only the study by Ferrà *et al.* shows improved survival for patients receiving cyclosporine. As 63% received cyclosporine and 23% had no GvHD prophylaxis, this could also be simply due to higher rates of fatal GvHD in the no prophylaxis group. Unfortunately, the details on the remaining 14% of patients are not available[80]. Interestingly, in the only prospective trial of second allo-HCT for graft failure, there was an excessive death rate due to GvHD (5/9) in the setting of a nonmyeloablative approach and posttransplant cyclosporine only[85]. Given the already high rates of TRM in this patient population, these findings argue for stringent GvHD prophylaxis.

Controversy#7: Is There an "Ideal" Conditioning Regimen for Allograft Failure?

There are no comparative studies between different conditioning regimens but the use of a fludarabine-based nonmyeloablative- or reduced intensity conditioning could achieve engraftment in the majority of patients[82,84,86]. Ferrà *et al.* suggest a higher TRM for fludarabine in combination with antithymocyte globulin (ATG), a finding not confirmed in any other study. As less than a third of the study population received fludarabine and ATG, this finding needs to be interpreted with caution[80]. A Japanese report on CBT for graft failure in 80 patients showed superior engraftment for the combination of fludarabine and an alkylating agent over all other conditioning regimens[82]. No study was powered or designed to show an impact of conditioning intensity and given the already high TRM it appears reasonable to avoid the toxicities of MAC regimens.

Controversy#8: Is the Time from Graft Failure to Second Allo-HCT Relevant?

An older study by Guardiola *et al.* found an improved survival in patients with an inter-transplant period of more than 80 days. This finding cannot be universally applied as 54 of the 82 patients had secondary graft failure and thus had time to both recover from the initial transplant toxicities and had some time of neutrophil protection. Thus, the criterion of a prolonged inter-transplant period may just select patients who were generally healthier[99]. Other larger studies could not find an association between times from first to second transplant[60,80] and given the poor outcome for patients without a second transplant [59,60], one should expeditiously set a plan for donor procurement in motion while the patient is recovering from transplant-related toxicities. Early identification of patients at risk can be aided by a white blood count (WBC) on day 16 of less than 200/μL, which has been shown to be highly predictive of PGF in transplantation from adult graft sources[100].

Practice Points

Graft failure remains one of the most daunting complications of allo-HCT and given the mostly poor outcomes of second allo-HCT, every effort should be undertaken to minimize the risk of this complication occurring (see Chapters 23, 24, and 65). This will encompass optimization of logistics to minimize avoidable delays as well as cryopreservation-related damage to graft (see Chapter 11)[68,69,101]. Furthermore, screening for donor-specific anti-HLA antibodies and, if positive, their incorporation in the selection of CBUs or mismatched donors is important (see Chapter 9)[102]. Emerging techniques will be helpful in better defining CBU viability and potency, and these along with strict quality control of the cryopreservation process as well as a uniform accreditation process for cord blood banks should lead to standardized criteria of cord selection and hopefully reduce the rate of graft failure in UCB transplantation (see Chapters 7, 8, 60, and 66)[103]. Lastly, given the extremely high rates of TRM with second allo-HCT for graft failure it is advisable to rigorously implement the patient selection criteria already established for initial allo-HCT.

References

1. Gooley TA, Chien JW, Pergam SA, *et al.* Reduced mortality after allogeneic hematopoietic-cell transplantation. *N Engl J Med.* 2010;363(22):2091–101.

2. Horan JT, Logan BR, Agovi-Johnson MA, *et al.* Reducing the risk for transplantation-related mortality after allogeneic hematopoietic cell transplantation: how much progress has been made? *J Clin Oncol.* 2011;29(7):805–13.

3. Anasetti C, Logan BR, Lee SJ, *et al.* Blood and Marrow Transplant Clinical Trials Network. Peripheral-blood stem cells *versus* bone marrow from unrelated donors. *N Engl J Med.* 2012;367(16):1487–96.

4. Rocha V, Labopin M, Sanz G, *et al.* Acute Leukemia Working Party of European Blood and Marrow Transplant Group; Eurocord-Netcord Registry. Transplants of umbilical-cord blood or bone marrow from unrelated donors in adults with acute leukemia. *N Engl J Med.* 2004;351(22):2276–85.

5. Locatelli F, Kabbara N, Ruggeri A, *et al.* Outcome of patients with hemoglobinopathies given either cord blood or bone marrow transplantation from an HLA-identical sibling. *Blood.* 2013;122(6):1072–8.

6. Bernaudin F, Socie G, Kuentz M, *et al.* SFGM-T: .Long-term results of related myeloablative stem-cell transplantation to cure sickle cell disease. *Blood.* 2007;110(7):2749–56.

7. Porter DL, Alyea EP, Antin JH, *et al.* NCI First International Workshop on the Biology, Prevention, and Treatment of Relapse after Allogeneic Hematopoietic Stem Cell Transplantation: Report from the Committee on Treatment of Relapse after Allogeneic Hematopoietic Stem Cell Transplantation. *Biol Blood Marrow Transplant.* 2010;16(11):1467–503.

8. Schmid C, Labopin M, Nagler A, *et al.* Acute Leukaemia Working Party of the European Group for Blood and Marrow Transplantation (EBMT). Treatment, risk factors, and outcome of adults with relapsed AML after reduced intensity conditioning for allogeneic stem cell transplantation. *Blood.* 2012;119(6):1599–606.

9. Pollyea DA, Artz AS, Stock W, *et al.* Outcomes of patients with AML and MDS who relapse or progress after reduced intensity allogeneic hematopoietic cell transplantation. *Bone Marrow Transplant.* 2007;40(11):1027–32.

10. Kenkre VP, Horowitz S, Artz AS, *et al.* T-cell-depleted allogeneic transplant without donor leukocyte infusions results in excellent long-term survival in patients with multiply relapsed Lymphoma. Predictors for survival after transplant relapse. *Leuk Lymphoma.* 2011;52(2):214–22.

11. Elmaagacli AH, Beelen DW, Schaefer UW. A retrospective single centre study of the outcome of five different therapy approaches in 48 patients with relapse of chronic myelogenous leukemia after allogeneic bone marrow transplantation. *Bone Marrow Transplant.* 1997;20(12):1045–55.

12. Mehta J, Powles R, Kulkarni S, *et al.* Induction of graft-*versus*-host disease as immunotherapy of leukemia relapsing after allogeneic transplantation: single-center experience of 32 adult patients. *Bone Marrow Transplant.* 1997;20(2):129–35.

13. Higano CS, Brixey M, Bryant EM, *et al.* Durable complete remission of acute nonlymphocytic leukemia associated with discontinuation of immunosuppression following relapse after allogeneic bone marrow transplantation. A case report of a probable graft-versus-leukemia effect. *Transplantation.* 1990;50(1):175–7.

14. Giralt S, Escudier S, Kantarjian H, *et al.* Preliminary results of treatment with filgrastim for relapse of leukemia and myelodysplasia after allogeneic bone marrow transplantation. *N Engl J Med.* 1993;329(11):757–61.

15. Worth LL, Mullen CA, Choroszy M, *et al.* Treatment of leukemia relapse

with recombinant granulocyte-macrophage colony stimulating factor (rhGM-CSF) following unrelated umbilical cord blood transplant: Induction of graft-vs.-leukemia. *Pediatr Transplant*. 2002;6(5):439–42.

16. Jabbour E, Giralt S, Kantarjian H, *et al.* Low-dose azacitidine after allogeneic stem cell transplantation for acute leukemia. *Cancer*. 2009;115(9):1899–905.

17. Bolaños-Meade J, Smith BD, Gore SD, *et al.* 5-azacytidine as salvage treatment in relapsed myeloid tumors after allogeneic bone marrow transplantation. *Biol Blood Marrow Transplant*. 2011;17(5):754–8.

18. Czibere A, Bruns I, Kröger N, *et al.* 5-Azacytidine for the treatment of patients with acute myeloid leukemia or myelodysplastic syndrome who relapse after allo-SCT: a retrospective analysis. *Bone Marrow Transplant*. 2010;45(5):872–6.

19. Fathi AT, Chen YB. Treatment of relapse of acute myeloid leukemia after allogeneic hematopoietic stem cell transplantation. *Curr Hematol Malig Rep*. 2014;9(2):186–92.

20. Giralt SA, Champlin RE. Leukemia relapse after allogeneic bone marrow transplantation: a review. *Blood*. 1994;84(11):3603–12.

21. Sharma M, Ravandi F, Bayraktar UD, *et al.* Treatment of FLT3-ITD-positive acute myeloid leukemia relapsing after allogeneic stem cell transplantation with sorafenib. *Biol Blood Marrow Transplant*. 2011;17(12):1874–7.

22. Metzelder SK, Schroeder T, Finck A, *et al.* High activity of sorafenib in FLT3-ITD-positive acute myeloid leukemia synergizes with allo-immune effects to induce sustained responses. *Leukemia*. 2012;26(11):2353–9.

23. Kolb HJ, Mittermüller J, Clemm C, *et al.* Donor leukocyte transfusions for treatment of recurrent chronic myelogenous leukemia in marrow transplant patients. *Blood*. 1990;76(12):2462–5.

24. Kolb HJ, Schattenberg A, Goldman JM, *et al.* European Group for Blood and Marrow Transplantation Working Party Chronic Leukemia: Graft-*versus*-leukemia effect of donor lymphocyte transfusions in marrow grafted patients. *Blood*. 1995;86(5):2041–50.

25. Porter DL, Collins RH Jr, Hardy C, *et al.* Treatment of relapsed leukemia after unrelated donor marrow transplantation with unrelated donor leukocyte infusions. *Blood*. 2000;95(4):1214–21.

26. Schmid C, Labopin M, Nagler A, *et al.* EBMT Acute Leukemia Working Party. Donor lymphocyte infusion in the treatment of first hematological relapse after allogeneic stem-cell transplantation in adults with acute myeloid leukemia: a retrospective risk factors analysis and comparison with other strategies by the EBMT Acute Leukemia Working Party. *J Clin Oncol*. 2007;25(31):4938–45.

27. Schroeder T, Czibere A, Platzbecker U, *et al.* Azacitidine and donor lymphocyte infusions as first salvage therapy for relapse of AML or MDS after allogeneic stem cell transplantation. *Leukemia*. 2013;27(6):1229–35.

28. Hasskarl J, Zerweck A, Wäsch R, *et al.* Induction of graft *versus* malignancy effect after unrelated allogeneic PBSCT using donor lymphocyte infusions derived from frozen aliquots of the original graft. *Bone Marrow Transplant*. 2012;47(2):277–82.

29. Warlick ED, DeFor T, Blazar BR, *et al.* Successful remission rates and survival after lymphodepleting chemotherapy and donor lymphocyte infusion for relapsed hematologic malignancies postallogeneic hematopoietic cell transplantation. *Biol Blood Marrow Transplant*. 2012;18(3):480–6.

30. Porter DL, Collins RH Jr, Shpilberg O, *et al.* Long-term follow-up of patients who achieved complete remission after donor leukocyte infusions. *Biol Blood Marrow Transplant*. 1999;5(4):253–61.

31. Fan Y, Liu H, Artz A *et al.* The outcomes of second allogeneic stem cell transplantation for disease relapse after T cell depleted allogeneic stem cell transplantation: A single center experience, University of Chicago. *Blood*. 2014;124:2509.

32. Christopeit M, Kuss O, Finke J, *et al.* Second allograft for hematologic relapse of acute leukemia after first allogeneic stem-cell transplantation from related and unrelated donors: the role of donor change. *J Clin Oncol*. 2013;31(26):3259–71.

33. Leung AY, Tse E, Hwang YY, *et al.* Primary treatment of leukemia relapses

after allogeneic hematopoietic stem cell transplantation with reduced-intensity conditioning second transplantation from the original donor. *Am J Hematol*. 2013;88(6):485–91.

34. Christopoulos P, Schmoor C, Waterhouse M, *et al.* Reduced-intensity conditioning with fludarabine and thiotepa for second allogeneic transplantation of relapsed patients with AML. *Bone Marrow Transplant*. 2013;48(7):901–7.

35. Poon LM, Bassett R Jr, Rondon G, *et al.* Outcomes of second allogeneic hematopoietic stem cell transplantation for patients with acute lymphoblastic leukemia. *Bone Marrow Transplant*. 2013;48(5):666–70.

36. Spyridonidis A, Labopin M, Schmid C, *et al.* Immunotherapy Subcommittee of Acute Leukemia Working Party. Outcomes and prognostic factors of adults with acute lymphoblastic leukemia who relapse after allogeneic hematopoietic cell transplantation. An analysis on behalf of the Acute Leukemia Working Party of EBMT. *Leukemia*. 2012;26(6):1211–7.

37. Hartwig M, Ocheni S, Asenova S, *et al.* Second allogeneic stem cell transplantation in myeloid malignancies. *Acta Haematol*. 2009;122(4):185–92.

38. Shaw BE, Mufti GJ, Mackinnon S, *et al.* Outcome of second allogeneic transplants using reduced-intensity conditioning following relapse of haematological malignancy after an initial allogeneic transplant. *Bone Marrow Transplant*. 2008;42(12):783–9.

39. Eapen M, Giralt SA, Horowitz MM, *et al.* Second transplant for acute and chronic leukemia relapsing after first HLA-identical sibling transplant. *Bone Marrow Transplant*. 2004;34(8):721–7.

40. Chueh HW, Lee SH, Sung KW, *et al.* Second allogeneic stem cell transplantation in hematologic malignancies: a single-center experience. *J Pediatr Hematol Oncol*. 2013;35(6):424–9.

41. Sorror ML. Comorbidities and hematopoietic cell transplantation outcomes. *Hematology Am Soc Hematol Educ Program*. 2010;2010:237–47.

42. Artz AS, Pollyea DA, Kocherginsky M, *et al.* Performance status and comorbidity predict transplant-related mortality after allogeneic hematopoietic

cell transplantation. *Biol Blood Marrow Transplant*. 2006;12(9):954–64.

43. Kishi K, Takahashi S, Gondo H, *et al.* Second allogeneic bone marrow transplantation for post-transplant leukemia relapse: results of a survey of 66 cases in 24 Japanese institutes. *Bone Marrow Transplant*. 1997;19(5):461–6.

44. Hill BT, Bolwell BJ, Rybicki L, *et al.* Nonmyeloablative second transplants are associated with lower nonrelapse mortality and superior survival than myeloablative second transplants. *Biol Blood Marrow Transplant*. 2010;16(12):1738–46.

45. Kedmi M, Resnick IB, Dray L, *et al.* A retrospective review of the outcome after second or subsequent allogeneic transplantation. *Biol Blood Marrow Transplant*. 2009;15(4):483–9.

46. Wagner JE, Vogelsang GB, Zehnbauer BA, *et al.* Relapse of leukemia after bone marrow transplantation: effect of second myeloablative therapy. *Bone Marrow Transplant*. 1992;9(3):205–9.

47. Hurley CK, Raffoux C; World Marrow Donor Association. World Marrow Donor Association: international standards for unrelated hematopoietic stem cell donor registries. *Bone Marrow Transplant*. 2004;34(2):103–10.

48. Barrett AJ, Locatelli F, Treleaven JG, *et al.* Second transplants for leukaemic relapse after bone marrow transplantation: high early mortality but favourable effect of chronic GVHD on continued remission. A report by the EBMT Leukaemia Working Party. *Br J Haematol*. 1991;79(4):567–74.

49. Al-Qurashi F, Ayas M, Al Sharif F, *et al.* Second allogeneic bone marrow transplantation after myeloablative conditioning analysis of 43 cases from single institution. *Hematology*. 2004;9(2):123–9.

50. Storb R, Gyurkocza B, Storer BE, *et al.* Graft-*versus*-host disease and graft-*versus*-tumor effects after allogeneic hematopoietic cell transplantation. *J Clin Oncol*. 2013;31(12):1530–8

51. Bhatia S, Francisco L, Carter A, *et al.* Late mortality after allogeneic hematopoietic cell transplantation and functional status of long-term survivors: report from the Bone Marrow Transplant Survivor Study. *Blood*. 2007;110(10):3784–92.

52. Bosi A, Laszlo D, Labopin M, *et al.* Acute Leukemia Working Party of the European Blood and Marrow Transplant Group. Second allogeneic bone marrow transplantation in acute leukemia: results of a survey by the European Cooperative Group for Blood and Marrow Transplantation. *J Clin Oncol*. 2001;19(16):3675–84.

53. Russell JA, Bowen T, Brown C, *et al.* Second allogeneic transplants for leukemia using blood instead of bone marrow as a source of hemopoietic cells. *Bone Marrow Transplant*. 1996;18(3):501–5.

54. Körbling M, Huh YO, Durett A, *et al.* Allogeneic blood stem cell transplantation: peripheralization and yield of donor-derived primitive hematopoietic progenitor cells (CD34+ Thy-1dim) and lymphoid subsets, and possible predictors of engraftment and graft-*versus*-host disease. *Blood*. 1995;86(7):2842–8.

55. Stroncek DF, Lopez AM, Maharaj D, *et al.* Acute toxicities of unrelated bone marrow *versus* peripheral blood stem cell donation: results of a prospective trial from the National Marrow Donor Program. *Blood*. 2013;121(1):197–206.

56. Churpek JE, Nickels E, Marquez R, *et al.* Identifying familial myelodysplastic/acute leukemia predisposition syndromes through hematopoietic stem cell transplantation donors with thrombocytopenia. *Blood*. 2012;120(26):5247–9.

57. Srinivasan R, Takahashi Y, McCoy JP, *et al.* Overcoming graft rejection in heavily transfused and allo-immunised patients with bone marrow failure syndromes using fludarabine-based haematopoietic cell transplantation. *Br J Haematol*. 2006;133(3):305–14.

58. Champlin RE, Horowitz MM, van Bekkum DW, *et al.* Graft failure following bone marrow transplantation for severe aplastic anemia: risk factors and treatment results. *Blood*. 1989;73(2):606–13.

59. Rondón G, Saliba RM, Khouri I, *et al.* Long-term follow-up of patients who experienced graft failure post allogeneic progenitor cell transplantation. Results of a single institution analysis. *Biol Blood Marrow Transplant*. 2008;14(8):859–66.

60. Schriber J, Agovi MA, Ho V, *et al.* Second unrelated donor hematopoietic cell transplantation for primary graft failure. *Biol Blood Marrow Transplant*. 2010;16(8):1099–106.

61. Fleischhauer K, Locatelli F, Zecca M, *et al.* Graft rejection after unrelated donor hematopoietic stem cell transplantation for thalassemia is associated with nonpermissive HLA-DPB1 disparity in host-*versus*-graft direction. *Blood*. 2006;107(7):2984–92.

62. Young JW, Papadopoulos EB, Cunningham I, *et al.* T-cell-depleted allogeneic bone marrow transplantation in adults with acute nonlymphocytic leukemia in first remission. *Blood*. 1992;79(12):3380–7.

63. Anasetti C, Amos D, Beatty PG, *et al.* Effect of HLA compatibility on engraftment of bone marrow transplants in patients with leukemia or lymphoma. *N Engl J Med*. 1989;320(4):197–204.

64. Ruggeri A, Labopin M, Sormani MP, *et al.* Engraftment kinetics and graft failure after single umbilical cord blood transplantation using myeloablative conditioning regimen. *Haematologica*. 2014;99:1509–15.

65. Ciurea SO, de Lima M, Cano P, *et al.* High risk of graft failure in patients with anti-HLA antibodies undergoing haploidentical stem-cell transplantation. *Transplantation*. 2009;88(8):1019–24.

66. Cutler C, Kim HT, Sun L, *et al.* Donor-specific anti-HLA antibodies predict outcome in double umbilical cord blood transplantation. *Blood*. 2011;118(25):6691–7.

67. Laughlin MJ, Eapen M, Rubinstein P, *et al.* Outcomes after transplantation of cord blood or bone marrow from unrelated donors in adults with leukemia. *N Engl J Med*. 2004;351(22):2265–75.

68. Lazarus HM, Kan F, Tarima S, *et al.* Rapid transport and infusion of hematopoietic cells is associated with improved outcome after myeloablative therapy and unrelated donor transplant. *Biol Blood Marrow Transplant*. 2009;15(5):589–96.

69. Lioznov M, Dellbrügger C, Sputtek A, *et al.* Transportation and cryopreservation may impair haematopoietic stem cell function and engraftment of allogeneic PBSCs, but not BM. *Bone Marrow Transplant*. 2008;42(2):121–8.

70. Ramirez P, Wagner JE, DeFor TE, *et al.* Factors predicting single-unit predominance after double umbilical cord blood transplantation. *Bone Marrow Transplant.* 2012;47(6):799–803.

71. Storb R, Epstein RB, Rudolph RH, Thomas ED. The effect of prior transfusion on marrow grafts between histocompatible canine siblings. *J Immunol.* 1970;105(3):627–33.

72. Storb R, Rudolph RH, Graham TC, Thomas ED. The influence of transfusions from unrelated donors upon marrow grafts between histocompatible canine siblings. *J Immunol.* 1971;107(2):409–13.

73. Xu H, Chilton PM, Tanner MK, *et al.* Humoral immunity is the dominant barrier for allogeneic bone marrow engraftment in sensitized recipients. *Blood.* 2006;108(10):3611–9.

74. Taylor PA, Ehrhardt MJ, Roforth MM, *et al.* Preformed antibody, not primed T cells, is the initial and major barrier to bone marrow engraftment in allosensitized recipients. *Blood.* 2007;109(3):1307–15.

75. Takanashi M, Atsuta Y, Fujiwara K, *et al.* The impact of anti-HLA antibodies on unrelated cord blood transplantations. *Blood.* 2010;116(15):2839–46.

76. Spellman S, Bray R, Rosen-Bronson S, *et al.* The detection of donor-directed, HLA-specific alloantibodies in recipients of unrelated hematopoietic cell transplantation is predictive of graft failure. *Blood.* 2010;115(13):2704–8.

77. Ruggeri A, Rocha V, Masson E, *et al.* Impact of donor-specific anti-HLA antibodies on graft failure and survival after reduced intensity conditioning-unrelated cord blood transplantation: a Eurocord, Société Francophone d'Histocompatibilité et d'Immunogénétique (SFHI) and Société Française de Greffe de Moelle et de Thérapie Cellulaire (SFGM-TC) analysis. *Haematologica.* 2013;98(7):1154–60.

78. Storb R. B-cells *versus* T cells as primary barrier to hematopoietic engraftment in allosensitized recipients. *Blood.* 2009;113(5):1205.

79. Brunstein CG, Noreen H, DeFor TE, *et al.* Anti-HLA antibodies in double umbilical cord blood transplantation. *Biol Blood Marrow Transplant.* 2011;17(11):1704–8.

80. Ferrà C, Sanz J, Díaz-Pérez MA, *et al.* Outcome of graft failure after allogeneic stem cell transplantation: Study of 89 patients. *Leuk Lymphoma.* 2014;10:1–24.

81. Fuji S, Nakamura F, Hatanaka K, *et al.* Peripheral blood as a preferable source of stem cells for salvage transplantation in patients with graft failure after cord blood transplantation: a retrospective analysis of the registry data of the Japanese Society for Hematopoietic Cell Transplantation. *Biol Blood Marrow Transplant.* 2012;18(9):1407–14.

82. Waki F, Masuoka K, Fukuda T, *et al.* Feasibility of reduced-intensity cord blood transplantation as salvage therapy for graft failure: results of a nationwide survey of adult patients. *Biol Blood Marrow Transplant.* 2011;17(6):841–51.

83. Remberger M, Mattsson J, Olsson R, Ringdén O. Second allogeneic hematopoietic stem cell transplantation: a treatment for graft failure. *Clin Transplant.* 2011;25(1):E68–76.

84. Byrne BJ, Horwitz M, Long GD, *et al.* Outcomes of a second non-myeloablative allogeneic stem cell transplantation following graft rejection. *Bone Marrow Transplant.* 2008;41(1):39–43.

85. Jabbour E, Rondon G, Anderlini P, *et al.* Treatment of donor graft failure with nonmyeloablative conditioning of fludarabine, antithymocyte globulin and a second allogeneic hematopoietic transplantation. *Bone Marrow Transplant.* 2007;40(5):431–5.

86. Chewning JH, Castro-Malaspina H, Jakubowski A, *et al.* Fludarabine-based conditioning secures engraftment of second hematopoietic stem cell allografts (HSCT) in the treatment of initial graft failure. *Biol Blood Marrow Transplant.* 2007;13(11):1313–23.

87. Remberger M, Ringdén O, Ljungman P, Hägglund H, *et al.* Booster marrow or blood cells for graft failure after allogeneic bone marrow transplantation. *Bone Marrow Transplant.* 1998;22(1):73–8.

88. Appelbaum FR, Nemunaitis J, Singer JW, *et al.* Use of recombinant human granulocyte macrophage colony-stimulating factor to speed engraftment and treat graft failure following marrow transplantation in man. *Haematol Blood Transfus.* 1990;33:736–40.

89. Nemunaitis J, Singer JW, Buckner CD, *et al.* Use of recombinant human granulocyte-macrophage colony-stimulating factor in graft failure after bone marrow transplantation. *Blood.* 1990;76(1):245–53.

90. Poon LM, Di Stasi A, Popat U, *et al.* Romiplostim for delayed platelet recovery and secondary thrombocytopenia following allogeneic stem cell transplantation. *Am J Blood Res.* 2013;3(3):260–4.

91. Calmettes C, Vigouroux S, Tabrizi R, Milpied N. Romiplostim (AMG531, Nplate) for secondary failure of platelet recovery after allo-SCT. *Bone Marrow Transplant.* 2011;46(12):1587–9.

92. Díez-Martín JL, Gómez-Pineda A, Serrano D, *et al.* Successful treatment of incipient graft rejection with donor leukocyte infusions, further proof of a graft *versus* host lymphohaemopoietic effect. *Bone Marrow Transplant.* 2004;33(10):1037–41.

93. Frugnoli I, Cappelli B, Chiesa R, *et al.* Escalating doses of donor lymphocytes for incipient graft rejection following SCT for thalassemia. *Bone Marrow Transplant.* 2010;45(6):1047–51.

94. Mehta J, Powles R, Singhal S, *et al.* Outcome of autologous rescue after failed engraftment of allogeneic marrow. *Bone Marrow Transplant.* 1996;17(2):213–7.

95. Pottinger B, Walker M, Campbell M, *et al.* The storage and re-infusion of autologous blood and BM as back-up following failed primary hematopoietic stem-cell transplantation: a survey of European practice. *Cytotherapy.* 2002;4(2):127–35.

96. Stelljes M, van Biezen A, Slavin S, *et al.* The harvest and use of autologous back-up grafts for graft failure or severe GvHD after allogeneic hematopoietic stem cell transplantation: a survey of the European Group for Blood and Marrow Transplantation. *Bone Marrow Transplant.* 2008;42(11):739–42.

97. Min CK, Kim DW, Lee JW, *et al.* Additional stem cell therapy for graft failure after allogeneic bone marrow transplantation. *Acta Haematol.* 2000;104(4):185–92.

98. Larocca A, Piaggio G, Podestà M, *et al.* Boost of CD34+-selected peripheral

blood cells without further conditioning in patients with poor graft function following allogeneic stem cell transplantation. *Haematologica*. 2006;91(7):935–40.

99. Guardiola P, Kuentz M, Garban F, *et al*. Second early allogeneic stem cell transplantations for graft failure in acute leukaemia, chronic myeloid leukaemia and aplastic anaemia. French Society of Bone Marrow Transplantation. *Br J Haematol* 2000;111(1):292–302.

100. Mehta J, Powles R, Singhal S, *et al*. Early identification of patients at risk of death due to infections, hemorrhage, or graft failure after allogeneic bone marrow transplantation on the basis of the leukocyte counts. *Bone Marrow Transplant*. 1997;19(4):349–55.

101. van Besien K, Shore T, Cushing M. Peripheral-blood *versus* bone marrow stem cells. *N Engl J Med*. 2013;368(3):287–8.

102. Gergis U, Mayer S, Gordon B, *et al*. A strategy to reduce donor-specific HLA Abs before allogeneic transplantation. *Bone Marrow Transplant*. 2014;49(5):722–4.

103. van Besien K. Advances in umbilical cord blood transplant: an overview of the 12th International Cord Blood Symposium, San Francisco, 5–7 June 2014. *Leuk Lymphoma*. 2014;18:1–5.

104. Tachibana T, Matsumoto K, Tanaka M *et al*. Outcome and prognostic factors among patients who underwent a second transplantation for disease relapse post the first allogeneic cell transplantation. Leuk Lymphoma.; in press.

105. Orti G, Sanz J, Bermudez A, *et al*. Outcome of second allogeneic hematopoietic cell transplantation after relapse of myeloid malignancies following allogeneic hematopoietic cell transplantation: a retrospective cohort on behalf of the Grupo Español de Trasplante Hematopoyetico. *Biol Blood Marrow Transplant*. 2016;22(3):584–8.

106. Vrhovac R, Labopin M, Ciceri F, *et al*. Acute Leukemia Working Party of the European Society for Blood and Marrow Transplantation (EBMT). Second reduced intensity conditioning allogeneic transplant as a rescue strategy for acute leukaemia patients who relapse after an initial RIC allogeneic transplantation: analysis of risk factors and treatment outcomes. *Bone Marrow Transplant*. 2016;51(2):186–93.

107. Lund TC, Liegel J, Bejanyan N, *et al*. Second allogeneic hematopoietic cell transplantation for graft failure: poor outcomes for neutropenic graft failure. *Am J Hematol*. 2015;90(10): 892–6.

245

27 Conditioning Regimens: Do They Really Matter?

Charles Craddock

Introduction

Conditioning regimens, a compendious term referring to combinations of chemo- and radiotherapy delivered immediately prior to CD34+ hematopoietic cell infusion, play a central role in determining the outcome of autologous and allogeneic hematopoietic cell transplant (HCT)[1]. In autologous transplants, the curative capacity of which are predicated on the dose intensification permitted by CD34+ hematopoietic cell rescue, the conditioning regimen is the primary determinant of both antitumor activity and regimen-related toxicity. Thus identification of the preferred conditioning regimen is dependent on balancing the survival benefits delivered by increased tumor kill with the extramedullary toxicity consequent upon dose escalation. Considerations concerning the design of the optimal conditioning regimen in allogeneic transplant recipients are, however, more nuanced given the conditioning regimen's twin role in delivering both a direct antitumor effect and immunosuppression required for durable engraftment of donor stem cells and the genesis of a graft-*versus*-tumor (GvT) effect[2]. Recently, the increased awareness of the importance of the GvT effect in determining the curative potential of an allogeneic transplant, has led to the development of reduced intensity conditioning (RIC) regimens which aim to utilize an immunologically mediated antitumor activity as the dominant curative mechanism. In the last 20 years, RIC regimens have

moved from an experimental animal model to become a key component of the transplant physician's armamentarium, particularly in older patients in whom myeloablative conditioning (MAC) regimens are associated with excessive toxicity.

Important Questions: Answers?

Important questions still remain in the design of conditioning regimens in both autografts and allografts. Disease relapse remains the commonest cause of treatment failure after autologous transplants and the development of novel conditioning regimens represents the most promising approach to improve long-term survival. These include either the delivery of established components of the conditioning regimen, such as busulfan (Bu) or total body irradiation (TBI), in different formulations or alternatively the utilization of novel chemotherapeutic agents so that the antitumor activity of the conditioning regimen is increased without a concomitant rise in transplant toxicity. The future utilization of the genomic characteristics of the underlying tumor to inform the choice of the conditioning regimen may represent an additional route towards reducing relapse risk.

The challenges faced in the development of novel conditioning regimens in allogeneic transplants are more complex (Tables 27.1 to 27.3). Firstly, transplant toxicity after an

Table 27.1 Plasma cell myeloma: allogeneic transplant-conditioning regimens — controversies and future directions

Disease	Common myeloablative (MAC) regimens	Common non-MAC (NMA/RIC) regimens	Indication/ rationale for non-MAC	Controversies	Future directions
Plasma cell myeloma	MAC regimens are not widely used although these may be considered in exceptional circumstances in very young patients, particularly those with skeletal disease	• Flu/low-dose TBI • Flu/Bu/ATG • Flu/Cy	Non-MAC regimens are utilized in the great majority of patients	The importance of performing an auto-HCT transplant as a prelude to a RIC allograft has not been determined. The impact of *in-vivo* TCD on transplant outcome? ATG or alemtuzumab is the preferred agent?	Novel GvHD prophylaxis regimens, potentially utilizing agents such as bortezomib? Post-transplant strategies?

ATG, antithymocyte globulin; Bu, busulfan; Cy, cyclophosphamide; Flu, fludarabine.

Table 27.2 Acute leukemias: allogeneic transplant conditioning regimens — controversies and future directions

Disease	Common MAC regimens	Common non-MAC (NMA/RIC) regimens	Indication/rationale for non-MAC	Controversies	Future directions
Acute lymphoblastic leukemia	• Cy/TBI • VP-16/TBI • Bu/Cy	• Flu/Bu/ATG • Flu/Mel/alemtuzumab • Flu/low-doseTBI (Seattle NMA protocol)	Indicated in older adults (>45 years) or those with significant comorbidities. Use unclear (<45 years) and the results of ongoing prospective studies are awaited	What is the optimal MAC regimen? What is the optimal CNS prophylaxis in patients transplanted using a RIC regimen? Does a RIC allograft confer a survival advantage compared with chemotherapy in older patients with ALL? Should patients with significant levels of MRD pretransplant receive additional cytoreduction prior to transplant?	Prospective studies examining the outcomes of older adults with high-risk ALL transplanted using RIC regimen compared with chemotherapy alone are required. Studies examining the potential role of RIC allografts in younger patients according to disease risk stratification and patient fitness will inform the decision concerning whether selected younger patients may benefit from RIC allograft. Whether additional cytoreductive therapy decreases the risk of relapse post-transplant in MRD +ve patients?
Acute myeloid leukemia	• Cy/TBI • iv Bu/Cy • Flu/iv Bu4	• Flu/Bu/ATG • Flu/Bu • Flu/Mel/alemtuzumab • Flu/low-dose TBI (Seattle protocol) • FLAMSA/Bu	There remains lack of clarity concerning the impact of patient age and comorbidities on outcome after specific non-MAC regimens. In which patients should a non-MAC regimen be preferred? The possibility that non-MAC regimens might result in, relative at least, fertility preservation in younger female patients requires further evaluation	The optimal non-MAC regimen in AML requires determination in prospective studies. Importance of TCD? Optimal strategy for TCD?	Prospective studies evaluating the impact of additional chemotherapy pretransplant, different conditioning regimens The role of "intensified" RIC regimens, such as FLAMSA, requires examination in prospective trials

allograft is multifactorial and determined by a complex interplay between the conditioning regimen, graft source, the degree of donor:patient alloreactivity and the intensity of post-transplant immunosuppression. It is increasingly recognized that a critical determinant of transplant-related mortality (TRM) in allogeneic transplants is patient fitness. This is currently, somewhat crudely, assessed by comorbidity scoring and much work remains to be done not only to define more precise assessment tools but also to determine the specific impact of

factors such as age and the HCT-CI index on transplant outcome in the setting of defined conditioning regimens[3] (see Chapter 4). At the same time the extent to which the underlying malignancy is susceptible to a G*v*T (see Chapter 65) effect coupled with the extent to which this is compromised by strategies utilized for graft-*versus*-host disease (GvHD) prophylaxis (see Chapter 12), such as T-cell depletion (TCD) (see Chapters 29 and 30), remain important and largely undefined determinants of relapse and long-term disease-free-survival.

Table 27.3 Lymphomas: allogeneic transplant conditioning regimens – controversies and future directions

Disease	Common myeloablative (MAC) regimens	Common non-MAC (NMA/ RIC) regimens	Indication/ rationale for non-MAC	Controversies	Future directions
Hodgkin lymphoma	Not widely used	• Flu/Bu/ATG • Flu/Mel/ Campath • Flu/low-dose TBI • Flu/Cy	MA regimens are not indicated in the great majority of clinical settings	Outcome after allo-HCT compared with an autograft requires prospective evaluation	The impact of adjunctive brentuximab on outcome after allograft requires evaluation
B-cell non-Hodgkin lymphomas	• Cy/TBI • Intravenous Bu/Cy	• Flu/low-dose TBI • Flu/Mel • Flu/Mel/ alemtuzumab	Preferred especially in older patients and recipients of a previous autograft	The survival benefit of allo-HCT in high-risk B-NHL requires evaluation in a prospective study. It remains unclear which, if any, patients may benefit from transplantation using a MAC regimen	Incorporation of radioimmunotherapy into RIC or MAC regimens Optimize a GvL effect immediately post-allograft Consequently studies which address whether or not TCD should be utilized are required in addition to trials designed to develop novel forms of GvHD prophylaxis, potentially utilizing agents with additional antitumor activity, such as bortezomib

Controversies and Possible Solutions

Controversy #1: Conditioning Regimens in Autologous Transplants – Opportunities?

Autologous HCT (auto-HCT) remains a centrally important treatment modality in patients with plasma cell myeloma and lymphomas. Autografts also have the capacity to deliver long-term disease-free survival (DFS) in patients with acute myeloid leukemia (AML) second CR – particularly in the setting of acute promyelocytic leukemia and AML associated with favorable cytogenetics such as t(8;21) and inv[4].

The major consideration in the design of conditioning regimens in autologous transplants is to achieve maximal dose intensification without excessive toxicity, which typically manifest as either gastrointestinal (mucositis and diarrhea) or pulmonary complications. The advent of agents with the capacity to reduce the severity of mucositis, such as palifermin, represents a potentially important strategy allowing further dose escalation of the conditioning regimen[5]. Agents with the potential to reduce relapse risk include the monoclonal antibodies, yttrium-90 ibritumomab tiuxetan and iodine-131 tositumomab, which have been utilized in combination with standard conditioning regimens such as BEAM (BCNU (carmustine), etoposide, cytosine arabinoside, and melphalan) in patients autografted for lymphoma (see Chapters 28, 38, and 40–44), although their utilization is complicated by practical considerations and cost[6]. In plasma cell disorders the adjunctive use of bortezomib is feasible but awaits examination in prospective clinical trials (see Chapters 46 and 49). The

potential of co-infused tumor cells to contribute to disease relapse as supported by retroviral tagging studies has also led to the development of numerous approaches aimed at purging the graft of contaminating malignant cells[7]. While CD34+ selection strategies reduce tumor load in CD34+ hematopoietic cell harvests from patients with both non-Hodgkin lymphomas and plasma cell disorders there is no convincing randomized evidence that this maneuver improves outcome. *In-vivo* purging using rituximab represents an alternative approach to reduce the risk of disease relapse after auto-HCT for follicular lymphoma (see Chapter 41) and in phase 2 studies has been reported to increase the incidence of molecular remission[8].

Controversy #2: Choices of Conditioning Regimens for Autologous Transplants in Lymphomas: Prospective Data?

There are limited prospective randomized data on which to base the choice of autologous conditioning regimens in patients with relapsed lymphoma or, given the evidence of a potent GvT effect in lymphoid malignancies, which patients should instead be allografted. Currently BEAM (BCNU (carmustine), etoposide, cytosine arabinoside, and melphalan 140 mg/m^2) is a widely used preparative regimen in patients with relapsed follicular, diffuse large B-cell lymphoma (DLBCL) and Hodgkin lymphoma. Alternative regimens include BEAC (carmustine, etoposide, cytosine arabinoside, and cyclophosphamide)[9] and CBV (cyclophosphamide, carmustine, and etoposide) and TBI-based regimens[10]. A recent Center for International Blood and Marrow Transplant Research (CIBMTR) analysis reported an increased risk of interstitial pneumonia syndrome with both TBI and CBV regimens[11]. Furthermore, a number of studies have reported an increased risk of secondary malignancies, particularly AML and myelodysplastic syndromes, in patients transplanted using TBI-based conditioning regimens, such as TBI/etoposide[12]. This has led to the restriction in the use of TBI-based regimens. Specifically their use is contraindicated in patients with Hodgkin lymphoma, particularly those who have received previous mantle radiotherapy, where it is associated with excessive pulmonary toxicity. The complex interplay between disease histology, disease stage, and conditioning regimen, coupled with the impact of recent advances in nontransplant therapy, such as the introduction of rituximab into standard care, in determining disease relapse post-transplant make it impossible to use retrospective studies to inform the choice of optimal conditioning regimen in lymphoma and the delivery of carefully designed prospective randomized studies remains a priority.

Controversy #3:Conditioning Regimen for Autologous Transplant in Myeloma: Can We Improve on Current Standard of Melphalan 200 mg/m²?

High-dose melphalan (200 mg/m^2) remains the standard conditioning regimen in myeloma autografts[13]. This regimen is generally well tolerated with an observed 100-day TRM of 3% or less. The commonest serious adverse event is gastrointestinal toxicity, particularly abdominal pain and diarrhea. Cardiotoxicity and encephalopathy are rarely observed although there are some data that suggest there may be an increased risk of cardiac complications at melphalan doses of 220 mg/m^2 or higher. Because of concern about increased TRM in patients on hemodialysis, many centers choose to reduce the melphalan dose to 140 mg/m^2 in this patient population (see Chapters 46 and 70). A very small number of patients autografted for plasma cell myeloma achieve long-term disease-free-survival, but given the fact that relapse is almost universally observed there is a compelling case for the development of more effective conditioning regimens. A randomized comparison between melphalan 200 mg/m^2 and a TBI (8Gy)/melphalan (140 mg/m^2) regimen demonstrated that no benefit was associated with the use of TBI[14]. A number of phase II studies have demonstrated improved outcomes using combinations of melphalan and Bu[15], and this combination as well as the incorporation of bortezomib into a melphalan-based regimen is currently undergoing prospective evaluation. Tellingly, however, more than four decades after its first use in conditioning regimens we cannot confidently state what the optimal dose of melphalan should be in patients with myeloma undergoing autologous transplants or how this agent might best be combined with other alkylators and a comprehensive program of prospective randomized trials are required to answer this fundamental question. Please refer to Table 27.1 for highlights of controversies and future directions related to conditioning regimens for allograft in plasma cell myeloma.

Controversy #4:Conditioning Regimens in Solid Tumors and Nonmalignant Diseases: A Work in Progress

Autologous transplant has the capacity to deliver long-term survival in patients with relapsed germ cell tumors and neuroblastoma (see Chapters 50 and 51). Varying combinations of melphalan, Bu, thiotepa, and TBI are used but there are limited data concerning the optimal combination of agents. In the setting of neuroblastoma, there is also emerging evidence that adjunctive post-transplant retinoids improve outcome. There is increasing interest in the role of autografting as a disease-modifying therapy in autoimmune diseases such as scleroderma and rheumatoid arthritis and recent evidence also supports a potential benefit for autologous transplant in advanced multiple sclerosis (see Chapters 56 and 57). The mechanism of activity of autologous transplant in this group of nonmalignant diseases remains unknown but it is postulated that the conditioning regimen plays a critical role in delivering augmented immunosuppression[16] (see Chapters 52–55).

Controversy #5:Progress in Defining Conditioning Regimen Intensity for Allogeneic Transplants: Not Just Semantics

In the setting of allogeneic HCT, the conditioning regimen has conventionally been viewed to serve two central purposes: immunosuppression designed to abrogate a host-*versus*-graft reaction, ensuring sustained engraftment of donor cells, and "myeloablation" in order to achieve tumor eradication. While a number of refinements have been made over the past three decades to the design and delivery of MAC regimens they remain associated with significant toxicity, which limits their use in patients older than 50–55 years. Perversely this has prevented the delivery of a potentially curative GvL effect to older patients whose outcome with conventional chemotherapy is particularly poor. Consequently, the demonstration in the late 1990s that durable donor hematopoietic engraftment can be reliably achieved using a highly immunosuppressive but nonmyeloablative preparative regimen represented a major advance[4]. The more recent confirmation that RIC allografts demonstrate the capacity to deliver a potent GvT effect, as evidenced by the observation that the relapse risk after such a procedure is both reduced in the presence of chronic GvHD and proportional to the degree of post-transplant immunosuppression, confirms their importance as a major development in allogeneic transplant[17,18].

Until recently the nomenclature used to describe this important new class of conditioning regimens was confusing. However a consensus has now been reached which classifies a "reduced intensity" conditioning regimen as one which "utilizes lower doses of chemotherapy or radiotherapy (an arbitrary 30% reduction has been identified), than those employed in conventional myeloablative conditioning regimens and may or may not result in cytopenias requiring CD34+ hematopoietic cell support." A separate group of "nonmyeloablative" conditioning regimens which result in modest and transient cytopenias and do not require CD34+ hematopoietic cell support has

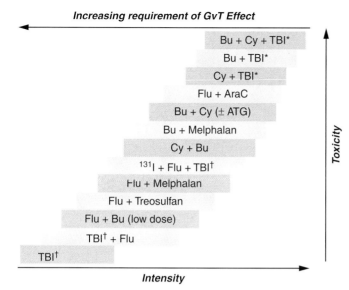

Figure 27.1 Comparison of conditioning regimens according to dose intensity and toxicity. AraC, cytosine arabinoside; ATG, antithymocyte globulin; 131I, anti-CD45 antibody conjugated to 131I; Bu, busulfan; Cy, cyclophosphamide; Flu, fludarabine.*High-dose TBI (800–1320 cGy); †low-dose TBI (200–400 cGy)[20].

also been agreed (Figure 27.1) (see Chapter 3)[19,20]. It is important, however, to remember that there is no necessary correlation between the myelosuppressive properties of an individual regimen and its toxicity. Thus the most important factors determining outcome after an allograft are patient comorbidities, patient:donor HLA disparity, graft source, and GvHD prophylaxis regimen, none of which necessarily correlate with the myelosuppressive properties of the conditioning regimen[21]. Taken together these considerations support the emerging consensus that in future individual conditioning regimens should be classified according to their predicted toxicity, irrespective of their myelosuppressive properties or to put it another way: "reduced toxicity" rather than "reduced intensity".

Controversy #6: Identifying an Optimal Myeloablative Conditioning Regimen in Acute Leukemia for Allograft: Are We There Yet?

Combinations of Cy with either TBI or oral Bu have been the most widely used myeloablative conditioning regimens in patients allografted for leukemia. More recently the advent of intravenous (iv) preparations of Bu have led to its substitution for oral Bu in the Bu/Cy regimen, as well as the design of novel combinations of iv Bu with other agents, notably the potently immunosuppressive fludarabine (Flu)[22,23]. To date, prospective randomized studies of myeloablative conditioning regimens in patients with acute leukemia have compared Cy/TBI with Bu/Cy utilizing oral preparations of Bu. These trials demonstrated broad equivalence of oral Bu/Cy and TBI in patients allografted with early phase disease (AML or ALL in CR1 or CML first chronic phase) but showed improved survival in patients with advanced phase disease who were transplanted using Cy/TBI[24]. However recent registry studies are

consistent with improved outcomes in patients transplanted with iv BU/Cy compared to Cy/TBI in patients transplanted for AML[22,23]. There is no evidence that addition of Bu to a Cy/TBI regimen improves survival because of excessive early transplant toxicity. Of note preliminary results obtained combining myeloablative doses of iv Bu with Flu have demonstrated a low TRM and encouraging disease-free-survival in patients with high-risk AML[25]. Of interest, Flu augments the ability of alkylating agents such as Bu to induce DNA cross-links raising the possibility that, in addition to its important role in securing donor engraftment, it may also reduce disease relapse. A recent small randomized trial comparing iv Bu/Cy with iv Bu/Flu failed to demonstrate benefit of this novel combination but the results of a number of larger ongoing prospective studies of these two myeloablative conditioning regimens in patients with acute leukemia are keenly awaited (Table 27.2)[26].

Characterizing the Properties of Different RIC Regimens

The confirmation that myeloablation was not required in order to achieve durable donor stem cell engraftment has led to the development of a range of novel reduced toxicity conditioning regimens, which are summarized below:

Low-Dose (2Gy) TBI-Containing Regimens

The original Seattle nonmyeloablative conditioning regimen utilized low-dose (2 Gy) TBI coupled with post-transplant cyclosporine and mycophenolate mofetil and was associated with a significant risk of failure, particularly in patients who had received only modest doses of chemotherapy prior to transplant. The addition of Flu has resulted in a regimen which reliably delivers durable hematopoietic engraftment in recipients of sibling and adult unrelated grafts with modest early transplant toxicity, and has the capacity to result in long-term DFS in both acute and chronic leukemias and lymphoid malignancies (Tables 27.2 and 27.3)[27]. There is, however, a significant risk of extensive chronic GvHD with this T-cell-replete regimen which represents a cause of mortality and long-term morbidity, especially in older patients transplanted using an alternative graft source.

Fludarabine and Alkylating Agent Combinations

While the low-dose TBI/Flu regimen represents the archetypal nonmyeloablative conditioning regimen, combinations of Flu and the alkylating agents Bu or melphalan now form the backbone of many reduced intensity conditioning regimens [28,29]. The original Flu/Bu regimen has now been adapted to include iv Bu with encouraging long-term survival reported in patients with high-risk AML and ALL and lymphomas. More recently combinations of Flu with treosulfan, a novel alkylating agent initially developed for the treatment of breast cancer, have generated encouraging survival rates, particularly in patients with myelodysplastic syndromes and myelofibrosis

(A)

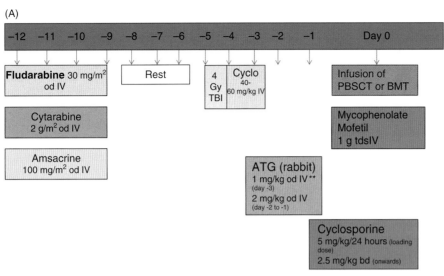

(B)

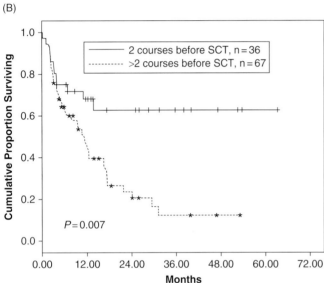

Figure 27.2 (A) Graphical representation of the components and timing of the FLAMSA conditioning regimen[37]. (B) Outcome after allogeneic transplantation using a FLAMSA sequential conditioning regimen in patients with primary refractory AML according to the number of courses of induction chemotherapy[38].

(see Chapters 37 and 35)[30]. Clofarabine, another immuno-suppressive purine analog, has been used in place of Flu in patients allografted for high-risk myeloid malignancies in the hope that its additional antitumor activity will reduce the risk of disease relapse[31].The combination of Flu and Cy is also effective in facilitating long-term hematopoietic engraftment with modest toxicity and has been reported to be associated with encouraging long-term survival in patients with AML and, intriguingly, in solid tumors including renal cell carcinoma[32,33]. The use of a T-cell-replete graft in all of these Flu-based RIC regimens is associated with a substantial risk of acute and chronic extensive GvHD. This has led to the increasing use of *in-vivo* T-cell depletion (TCD), utilizing alemtuzumab or antithymocyte globulin (ATG), in the above regimens a maneuver which substantially reduces the risk of both acute and chronic GvHD but may increase the risk of relapse in certain settings[34,35].

In lymphoid diseases the combination of BEAM-type regimen and alemtuzumab, with additional Flu in patients transplanted using an unrelated donor, represents a promising conditioning regimen with the capacity to deliver durable hematopoietic engraftment with modest rates of GvHD in patients with relapsed Hodgkin disease and follicular and diffuse large B-cell lymphoma[36].

Sequential Regimens: The FLAMSA Regimen

The development of the sequential FLAMSA RIC regimen, which aims to maximize pretransplant cytoreduction while delivering a potent GvT effect through the delivery of early donor lymphocyte infusions (DLI), represents an important conceptual development in the design of RIC regimens for the management of patients with high-risk myeloid malignancies (see Chapter 25)[37]. In its original iteration, the FLAMSA regimen utilized a 5-day course of amsacrine and cytosine arabinoside chemotherapy followed, after a 4-day rest, by a low-dose TBI (4Gy)-based conditioning regimen. Patients with no evidence of GvHD who had discontinued immunosuppression received DLI at 120 days post-transplant (Figure 27.2A).

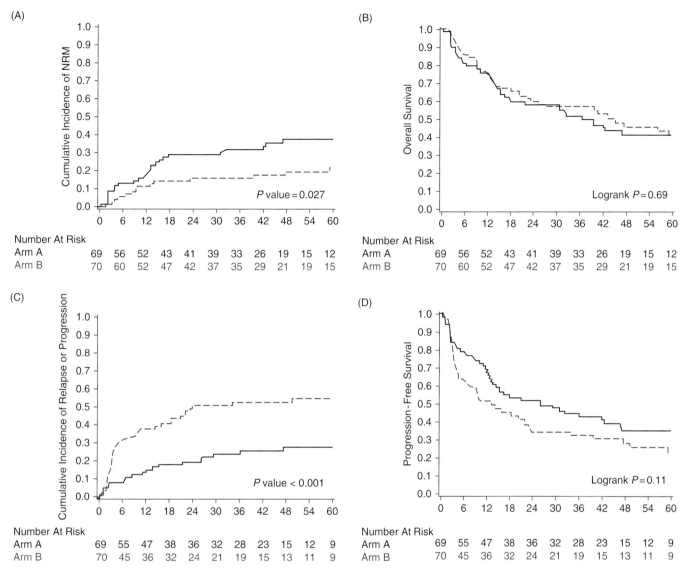

Figure 27.3 Outcomes after a randomized study of two reduced intensity conditioning strategies for human leukocyte antigen-matched, related allogeneic peripheral blood stem cell transplantation[42]. Solid lines indicate fludarabine with busulfan and rabbit antithymocyte globulin; dashed lines, fludarabine with total body irradiation.

Phase 2 studies demonstrated encouraging relapse-free survival rates in patients with high-risk AML or primary refractory disease (Figure 27.2B). In an effort to further reduce relapse rates and improve tolerability, iv Bu, at an age-adjusted dose, has been substituted for low-dose TBI and the results of an ongoing UK prospective randomized trial are awaited.

Total Lymphoid Irradiation-Based Regimens

In murine models the Stanford group has demonstrated that total lymphoid irradiation (TLI) coupled with *in-vivo* lymphocyte depletion facilitated hematopoietic engraftment and was associated with an expansion of regulatory natural killer T-cells and a low incidence of GvHD. This model has been successfully translated into the clinical setting and a TLI/ATG conditioning regimen has been shown to be associated with modest toxicity and low rates of acute and chronic GvHD

in recipients of both sibling and unrelated donor grafts[39]. In patients with lymphoid malignancies, particularly those in remission, disease control is promising and recent data suggest that this well-tolerated regimen may also have a role in the management of myeloid malignancies[40].

Controversies Continued

Controversy #7: What Is the Optimal RIC Regimen in the Management of Older Adults with AML?

The evidence of a potent GvT effect in patients allografted for AML using a MAC regimen supported the exploration of the activity of a wide range of RIC regimens in older patients with high-risk AML. It was only recently that a recent UK study confirmed, using a donor-*versus*-no-donor analysis, that RIC regimen transplants possess the capacity to improve overall

1) Minimize pretransplant disease burden
2) Optimize cytotoxic properties of the conditioning regimen
3) Target leukemia-specific antigens post-transplant:
   -adjunctive biological therapies with direct antitumor effect
   -optimizing a GvL effect

Figure 27.4 Pharmacologic strategies to reduce the risk of disease relapse after an allogeneic hematopoietic cell transplant for AML.

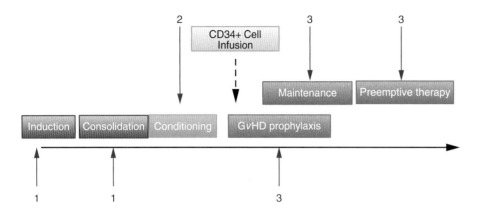

survival in patients with AML although the benefit was limited to patients with intermediate risk cytogenetics in CR at the time of transplant[41]. However, it remains the case that despite more than 15 years of experience with a variety of RIC regimens no consensus exists concerning the optimal conditioning regimen in this patient population. Phase II studies of RIC regimens in AML have identified disease relapse and GvHD as the major causes of treatment failure. One of the only randomized comparisons of RIC regimens in AML has highlighted contrasting activities of the Seattle low-dose TBI/Flu regimen and a Flu/Bu/ATG regimen with regard to toxicity and relapse[42](Figure 27.3). While the TBI/Flu regimen was associated with a reduced 100-day TRM this failed to translate into a survival benefit because of an increased risk of disease relapse. Strategies to reduce the risk of disease relapse in AML patients transplanted using a RIC regimen include increasing the intensity of the conditioning regimen (without concomitantly increasing transplant toxicity), optimizing a GvT effect, and the use of adjunctive post-transplant pharmacologic therapies (Figure 27.4). An alternative approach with the potential to increase the antileukemic properties of the conditioning regimen includes the addition of targeted radiotherapy utilizing radiolabeled antibodies such as anti-CD45, and this approach is the subject of ongoing studies (see Chapter 28)[43]. The post-transplant administration of agents with direct antitumor activity, such as the FLT3 inhibitor sorafenib, represents a promising approach alternative approach[44]. Alternatively the administration of azacitidine, which up-regulates expression of tumor antigens on leukemic blasts, may allow the GvT effect to be augmented without a concomitant increase in the risk of GvHD (see Chapters 23, 24, 26, and 65)[45].

The knotty problem remains of defining the optimal form of GvHD prophylaxis in patients undergoing a RIC allograft for AML. Although the risk of significant GvHD-related morbidity and mortality utilizing a T-replete regimen remains substantial there are conflicting registry data concerning whether in-vivo TCD using ATG or alemtuzumab can increase the risk of disease relapse[35,46]. As a consequence the role of TCD in RIC allografts remains controversial (see Chapters 29 and 30). When deployed it is important to adjust the degree of post-transplant immunosuppression accordingly given the observation that elevated post-transplant cyclosporine levels are associated with an increased relapse risk after an alemtuzumab-based RIC regimen in patients with AML[18]. Furthermore, given the increased incidence of mixed T-cell chimerism after alemtuzumab-based regimens the adjunctive use of DLI should be considered as a potentially important strategy to reduce relapse[47]. In murine models T-regulatory cells have been shown to play an important role in ameliorating both the incidence and severity of GvHD (see Chapters 12 and 13). A number of groups are therefore pursuing strategies including either early infusion of T-regulatory cells post-transplant or the administration of pharmacologic agents such as azacitidine both of which have the potential to accelerate the reconstitution of T-regulatory cells post-transplant[45,48]. It is not possible to recommend an optimal conditioning regimen in the commonest indication of RIC regimen at present. A similar paucity of prospective randomized data blights rational decision-making in other indications for RIC allografts. As a consequence, now that well-tolerated RIC regimens have been established in a range of common hematologic malignancies, the transplant community have a shared obligation to accelerate the delivery of a portfolio of prospective randomized trials, which is essential if patients are to maximally benefit from the recent potentially transformative developments in clinical practice.

References

1. Appelbaum FR. Hematopoietic-cell transplantation at 50. *N Engl J Med*. 2007;357(15):1472–5. Epub 2007/10/12. doi: 357/15/1472 [pii]10.1056/NEJMp078166. PubMed PMID: 17928594.

2. Lazarus HM, Phillips GL, Herzig RH, Hurd DD, Wolff SN, Herzig GP. High-dose melphalan and the development of hematopoietic stem-cell transplantation: 25 years later. *J Clin Oncol*. 2008;26(14):2240–3. doi: 10.1200/JCO.2007.14.7827. PubMed PMID: 18467711.

3. Sorror ML, Maris MB, Storb R, Baron F, Sandmaier BM, Maloney DG, et al. Hematopoietic cell transplantation (HCT)-specific comorbidity index: a new tool for risk assessment before allogeneic HCT. *Blood*. 2005;106(8):2912–9. PubMed PMID: 15994282.

4. McSweeney PA, Niederwieser D, Shizuru JA, Sandmaier BM, Molina AJ, Maloney DG, et al. Hematopoietic cell transplantation in older patients with hematologic malignancies: replacing high-dose cytotoxic therapy with graft-*versus*-tumor effects. *Blood*. 2001;97(11):3390–400. PubMed PMID: 11369628.

5. Abidi MH, Agarwal R, Tageja N, Ayash L, Deol A, Al-Kadhimi Z, et al. A phase I dose-escalation trial of high-dose melphalan with palifermin for cytoprotection followed by autologous stem cell transplantation for patients with multiple myeloma with normal renal function. *Biol Blood Marrow Transplant*. 2013;19(1):56–61. doi: 10.1016/j.bbmt.2012.08.003. PubMed PMID: 22892551; PubMed Central PMCID: PMC3786738.

6. Vose JM, Bierman PJ, Loberiza FR, Enke C, Hankins J, Bociek RG, et al. Phase II trial of 131-Iodine tositumomab with high-dose chemotherapy and autologous stem cell transplantation for relapsed diffuse large B cell lymphoma. *Biol Blood Marrow Transplant*. 2013;19(1):123–8. doi: 10.1016/j.bbmt.2012.08.013. PubMed PMID: 22940055.

7. Brenner MK, Rill DR, Holladay MS, Heslop HE, Moen RC, Buschle M, et al. Gene marking to determine whether autologous marrow infusion restores long-term haemopoiesis in cancer patients. *Lancet*. 1993;342(8880):1134–7. PubMed PMID: 7901474.

8. Arcaini L, Montanari F, Alessandrino EP, Tucci A, Brusamolino E, Gargantini L, et al. Immunochemotherapy with in vivo purging and autotransplant induces long clinical and molecular remission in advanced relapsed and refractory follicular lymphoma. *Ann Oncol*. 2008;19(7):1331–5. doi: 10.1093/annonc/mdn044. PubMed PMID: 18344536.

9. Philip T, Guglielmi C, Hagenbeek A, Somers R, Van der Lelie H, Bron D, et al. Autologous bone marrow transplantation as compared with salvage chemotherapy in relapses of chemotherapy-sensitive non-Hodgkin's lymphoma. *New Engl J Med*. 1995;333(23):1540–5. doi: 10.1056/NEJM199512073332305. PubMed PMID: 7477169.

10. Weaver CH, Appelbaum FR, Petersen FB, Clift R, Singer J, Press O, et al. High-dose cyclophosphamide, carmustine, and etoposide followed by autologous bone marrow transplantation in patients with lymphoid malignancies who have received dose-limiting radiation therapy. *J Clin Oncol*. 1993;11(7):1329–35. PubMed PMID: 8315430.

11. Chen YB, Lane AA, Logan B, Zhu X, Akpek G, Aljurf M, et al. Impact of conditioning regimen on outcomes for patients with lymphoma undergoing high-dose therapy with autologous hematopoietic cell transplantation. *Biol Blood Marrow Transplant*. 2015. doi: 10.1016/j.bbmt.2015.02.005. PubMed PMID: 25687795.

12. Kalaycio M, Rybicki L, Pohlman B, Sobecks R, Andresen S, Kuczkowski E, et al. Risk factors before autologous stem-cell transplantation for lymphoma predict for secondary myelodysplasia and acute myelogenous leukemia. *J Clin Oncol*. 2006;24(22):3604–10. doi: 10.1200/JCO.2006.06.0673. PubMed PMID: 16877727.

13. Shaw PJ, Nath CE, Lazarus HM. Not too little, not too much-just right! (Better ways to give high dose melphalan). *Bone Marrow Transplant*. 2014. doi: 10.1038/bmt.2014.186. PubMed PMID: 25133893.

14. Moreau P, Facon T, Attal M, Hulin C, Michallet M, Maloisel F, et al. Comparison of 200 mg/m(2) melphalan and 8 Gy total body irradiation plus 140 mg/m(2) melphalan as conditioning regimens for peripheral blood stem cell transplantation in patients with newly diagnosed multiple myeloma: final analysis of the Intergroupe Francophone du Myelome 9502 randomized trial. *Blood*. 2002;99(3):731–5. PubMed PMID: 11806971.

15. Moreau P, Attal M, Harousseau JL. New developments in conditioning regimens before auto-HCT in multiple myeloma. *Bone Marrow Transplant*. 2011;46(7):911–5. doi: 10.1038/bmt.2011.20. PubMed PMID: 21358678.

16. Atkins HL, Muraro PA, van Laar JM, Pavletic SZ. Autologous hematopoietic stem cell transplantation for autoimmune disease – is it now ready for prime time? *Biol Blood Marrow Transplant*. 2012;18(1 Suppl):S177–83. doi: 10.1016/j.bbmt.2011.11.020. PubMed PMID: 22226104.

17. Baron F, Labopin M, Niederwieser D, Vigouroux S, Cornelissen JJ, Malm C, et al. Impact of graft-*versus*-host disease after reduced-intensity conditioning allogeneic stem cell transplantation for acute myeloid leukemia: a report from the Acute Leukemia Working Party of the European group for blood and marrow transplantation. *Leukemia*. 2012;26(12):2462–8. doi: 10.1038/leu.2012.135. PubMed PMID: 22699419.

18. Craddock C, Nagra S, Peniket A, Brookes C, Buckley L, Nikolousis E, et al. Factors predicting long-term survival after T-cell depleted reduced intensity allogeneic stem cell transplantation for acute myeloid leukemia. *Haematologica*. 2010;95(6):989–95. Epub 2009/12/03. doi: 10.3324/haematol.2009.013920. PubMed PMID: 19951968; PubMed Central PMCID: PMC2878799.

19. Bacigalupo A, Ballen K, Rizzo D, Giralt S, Lazarus H, Ho V, et al. Defining the intensity of conditioning regimens: working definitions. *Biol Blood Marrow Transplant*. 2009;15(12):1628–33. doi: 10.1016/j.bbmt.2009.07.004. PubMed PMID: 19896087; PubMed Central PMCID: PMC2861656.

20. Deeg HJ, Sandmaier BM. Who is fit for allogeneic transplantation? *Blood*. 2010;116(23):4762–70. doi: 10.1182/blood-2010-07-259358. PubMed PMID: 20702782; PubMed Central PMCID: PMC3253743.

21. Sorror ML, Giralt S, Sandmaier BM, De Lima M, Shahjahan M, Maloney DG, *et al.* Hematopoietic cell transplantation specific comorbidity index as an outcome predictor for patients with acute myeloid leukemia in first remission: combined FHCRC and MDACC experiences. *Blood.* 2007;110(13):4606–13. PubMed PMID: 17873123.

22. Copelan EA, Hamilton BK, Avalos B, Ahn KW, Bolwell BJ, Zhu X, *et al.* Better leukemia-free and overall survival in AML in first remission following cyclophosphamide in combination with busulfan compared with TBI. *Blood.* 2013;122(24):3863–70. doi: 10.1182/blood-2013-07-514448. PubMed PMID: 24065243; PubMed Central PMCID: PMC3854108.

23. Nagler A, Rocha V, Labopin M, Unal A, Ben Othman T, Campos A, *et al.* Allogeneic hematopoietic stem-cell transplantation for acute myeloid leukemia in remission: comparison of intravenous busulfan plus cyclophosphamide (Cy) *versus* total-body irradiation plus Cy as conditioning regimen – a report from the acute leukemia working party of the European group for blood and marrow transplantation. *J Clin Oncol.* 2013;31(28):3549–56. doi: 10.1200/JCO.2013.48.8114. PubMed PMID: 23980086.

24. Socie G, Clift RA, Blaise D, Devergie A, Ringden O, Martin PJ, *et al.* Busulfan plus cyclophosphamide compared with total-body irradiation plus cyclophosphamide before marrow transplantation for myeloid leukemia: long-term follow-up of 4 randomized studies. *Blood.* 2001;98(13):3569–74. PubMed PMID: 11739158.

25. Andersson BS, de Lima M, Thall PF, Wang X, Couriel D, Korbling M, *et al.* Once daily i.v. busulfan and fludarabine (i.v. Bu-Flu) compares favorably with i.v. busulfan and cyclophosphamide (i.v. BuCy2) as pretransplant conditioning therapy in AML/MDS. *Biol Blood Marrow Transplant.* 2008;14(6):672–84. doi: 10.1016/j.bbmt.2008.03.009. PubMed PMID: 18489993.

26. Lee JH, Joo YD, Kim H, Ryoo HM, Kim MK, Lee GW, *et al.* Randomized trial of myeloablative conditioning regimens: busulfan plus cyclophosphamide *versus* busulfan plus fludarabine. *J Clin Oncol.* 2013;31(6):701–9. doi: 10.1200/JCO.2011.40.2362. PubMed PMID: 23129746.

27. Ram R, Storb R, Sandmaier BM, Maloney DG, Woolfrey A, Flowers ME, *et al.* Non-myeloablative conditioning with allogeneic hematopoietic cell transplantation for the treatment of high-risk acute lymphoblastic leukemia. *Haematologica.* 2011;96(8):1113–20. Epub 2011/04/22. doi: 10.3324/haematol.2011.040261. PubMed PMID: 21508120; PubMed Central PMCID: PMC3148904.

28. Slavin S, Nagler A, Naparstek E, Kapelushnik Y, Aker M, Cividalli G, *et al.* Nonmyeloablative stem cell transplantation and cell therapy as an alternative to conventional bone marrow transplantation with lethal cytoreduction for the treatment of malignant and nonmalignant hematologic diseases. *Blood.* 1998;91(3):756–63. PubMed PMID: 9446633.

29. Giralt S, Estey E, Albitar M, van Besien K, Rondon G, Anderlini P, *et al.* Engraftment of allogeneic hematopoietic progenitor cells with purine analog-containing chemotherapy: harnessing graft-*versus*-leukemia without myeloablative therapy. *Blood.* 1997;89(12):4531–6. PubMed PMID: 9192777.

30. Nemecek ER, Guthrie KA, Sorror ML, Wood BL, Doney KC, Hilger RA, *et al.* Conditioning with treosulfan and fludarabine followed by allogeneic hematopoietic cell transplantation for high-risk hematologic malignancies. *Biol Blood Marrow Transplant.* 2011;17(3):341–50. doi: 10.1016/j.bbmt.2010.05.007. PubMed PMID: 20685259; PubMed Central PMCID: PMC2974965.

31. Chevallier P, Labopin M, Buchholz S, Ganser A, Ciceri F, Lioure B, *et al.* Clofarabine-containing conditioning regimen for allo-HCT in AML/ALL patients: a survey from the Acute Leukemia Working Party of EBMT. *Eur J Haematol.* 2012;89(3):214–9. doi: 10.1111/j.1600-0609.2012.01822.x. PubMed PMID: 22702414.

32. Childs R, Chernoff A, Contentin N, Bahceci E, Schrump D, Leitman S, *et al.* Regression of metastatic renal-cell carcinoma after nonmyeloablative allogeneic peripheral-blood stem-cell transplantation. *New Engl J Med.* 2000;343(11):750–8. doi: 10.1056/NEJM200009143431101. PubMed PMID: 10984562.

33. Childs R, Clave E, Contentin N, Jayasekera D, Hensel N, Leitman S, *et al.* Engraftment kinetics after nonmyeloablative allogeneic peripheral blood stem cell transplantation: full donor T-cell chimerism precedes alloimmune responses. *Blood.* 1999;94(9):3234–41. PubMed PMID: 10556212.

34. Kottaridis PD, Milligan DW, Chopra R, Chakraverty RK, Chakrabarti S, Robinson S, *et al.* In vivo CAMPATH-1H prevents GvHD following nonmyeloablative stem-cell transplantation. *Cytotherapy.* 2001;3(3):197–201. PubMed PMID: 12171726.

35. Soiffer RJ, Lerademacher J, Ho V, Kan F, Artz A, Champlin RE, *et al.* Impact of immune modulation with anti-T-cell antibodies on the outcome of reduced-intensity allogeneic hematopoietic stem cell transplantation for hematologic malignancies. *Blood.* 2011;117(25):6963–70. doi: 10.1182/blood-2011-01-332007. PubMed PMID: 21464372; PubMed Central PMCID: PMC3128486.

36. Lush RJ, Haynes AP, Byrne J, Cull GM, Carter GI, Pagliuca A, *et al.* Allogeneic stem-cell transplantation for lymphoproliferative disorders using BEAM-CAMPATH (+/- fludarabine) conditioning combined with post-transplant donor-lymphocyte infusion. *Cytotherapy.* 2001;3(3):203–10. Epub 2002/08/13. doi: 10.1080/146532401753174034. PubMed PMID: 12171727.

37. Schmid C, Schleuning M, Ledderose G, Tischer J, Kolb HJ. Sequential regimen of chemotherapy, reduced-intensity conditioning for allogeneic stem-cell transplantation, and prophylactic donor lymphocyte transfusion in high-risk acute myeloid leukemia and myelodysplastic syndrome. *J Clin Oncol.* 2005;23(24):5675–87. PubMed PMID: 16110027.

38. Schmid C, Schleuning M, Schwerdtfeger R, Hertenstein B, Mischak-Weissinger E, Bunjes D, *et al.* Long-term survival in refractory acute myeloid leukemia after sequential treatment with chemotherapy and reduced-intensity conditioning for allogeneic stem cell transplantation.

Blood. 2006;108(3):1092–9. PubMed PMID: 16551971.

39. Kohrt HE, Turnbull BB, Heydari K, Shizuru JA, Laport GG, Miklos DB, *et al.* TLI and ATG conditioning with low risk of graft-*versus*-host disease retains antitumor reactions after allogeneic hematopoietic cell transplantation from related and unrelated donors. *Blood.* 2009;114(5):1099–109. doi: 10.1182/blood-2009-03-211441. PubMed PMID: 19423725; PubMed Central PMCID: PMC2721787.

40. Benjamin J, Chhabra S, Kohrt HE, Lavori P, Laport GG, Arai S, *et al.* Total lymphoid irradiation-antithymocyte globulin conditioning and allogeneic transplantation for patients with myelodysplastic syndromes and myeloproliferative neoplasms. *Biol Blood Marrow Transplant.* 2014;20(6):837–43. doi: 10.1016/j.bbmt.2014.02.023. PubMed PMID: 24607552.

41. Russell NH, Kjeldsen L, Craddock C, Pagliuca A, Yin JA, Clark RE, *et al.* A comparative assessment of the curative potential of reduced intensity allografts in acute myeloid leukaemia. *Leukemia.* 2014. doi: 10.1038/leu.2014.319. PubMed PMID: 25376374.

42. Blaise D, Tabrizi R, Boher JM, Le Corroller-Soriano AG, Bay JO, Fegueux N, *et al.* Randomized study of 2 reduced-intensity conditioning strategies for human leukocyte antigen-matched, related allogeneic peripheral blood stem cell transplantation: prospective clinical and socioeconomic evaluation. *Cancer.* 2013;119(3):602–11. doi: 10.1002/cncr.27786. PubMed PMID: 22893313.

43. Pagel JM, Gooley TA, Rajendran J, Fisher DR, Wilson WA, Sandmaier BM, *et al.* Allogeneic hematopoietic cell transplantation after conditioning with 131I-anti-CD45 antibody plus fludarabine and low-dose total body irradiation for elderly patients with advanced acute myeloid leukemia or high-risk myelodysplastic syndrome. *Blood.* 2009;114(27):5444–53. doi: 10.1182/blood-2009-03-213298. PubMed PMID: 19786617; PubMed Central PMCID: PMC2798861.

44. Chen YB, Li S, Lane AA, Connolly C, Del Rio C, Valles B, *et al.* Phase I trial of maintenance sorafenib after allogeneic hematopoietic stem cell transplantation for fms-like tyrosine kinase 3 internal tandem duplication acute myeloid leukemia. *Biol Blood Marrow Transplant.* 2014;20(12):2042–8. doi: 10.1016/j.bbmt.2014.09.007. PubMed PMID: 25239228; PubMed Central PMCID: PMC4253683.

45. Goodyear OC, Dennis M, Jilani NY, Loke J, Siddique S, Ryan G, *et al.* Azacitidine augments expansion of regulatory T cells after allogeneic stem cell transplantation in patients with acute myeloid leukemia (AML). *Blood.* 2012;119(14):3361–9. Epub 2012/01/12. doi: 10.1182/blood-2011-09-377044. PubMed PMID: 22234690.

46. Baron F, Labopin M, Blaise D, Lopez-Corral L, Vigouroux S, Craddock C, *et al.* Impact of in-vivo T-cell depletion on outcome of AML patients in first CR given peripheral blood stem cells and reduced-intensity conditioning allo-HCT from a HLA-identical sibling donor: a report from the Acute Leukemia Working Party of the European Group for Blood and Marrow Transplantation. *Bone Marrow Transplant.* 2014;49(3):389–96. doi: 10.1038/bmt.2013.204. PubMed PMID: 24419525.

47. Peggs KS, Sureda A, Qian W, Caballero D, Hunter A, Urbano-Ispizua A, *et al.* Reduced-intensity conditioning for allogeneic haematopoietic stem cell transplantation in relapsed and refractory Hodgkin lymphoma: impact of alemtuzumab and donor lymphocyte infusions on long-term outcomes. *Br J Haematol.* 2007;139(1):70–80. doi: 10.1111/j.1365–2141.2007.06759.x. PubMed PMID: 17854309.

48. Negrin RS. Role of regulatory T cell populations in controlling graft vs host disease. *Best Pract Res Clin Haematol.* 2011;24(3):453–7. doi: 10.1016/j.beha.2011.05.006. PubMed PMID: 21925098; PubMed Central PMCID: PMC3176418.

28 Controversies in Radioimmunotherapy for Hematopoietic Cell Transplantation

Sarah A. Buckley and John M. Pagel

Background

The concept that hematopoietic stem cell rescue could facilitate dose escalation to curative levels was supported by the work of Thomas and colleagues, who, in the early 1970s, first defined a role for hematopoietic cell transplantation (HCT) in the treatment of acute leukemia. Clinical trials conducted in Seattle demonstrated the antileukemic effect of total body irradiation (TBI) in combination with high-dose chemotherapy for bone marrow transplantation (BMT)[1]. Importantly, higher doses of TBI correlated with a reduced risk of disease recurrence after transplant. In two randomized trials, patients with either acute myeloid leukemia (AML)[2] or chronic myeloid leukemia (CML)[3] were given cyclophosphamide (CY) and either 12 Gy or 15.75 Gy of TBI conditioning prior to allogeneic sibling matched HCT. The rate of post-transplant relapse dropped from 35% to 13% in the AML population, and from 30% to 7% in the CML group for those patients receiving the higher dose of TBI. These studies clearly demonstrated the potential for higher doses of radiation to generate more durable responses; however, those in the higher dose group experienced a significant increase in severe or fatal toxicities. Owing to the increased frequency of toxicity (most often radiation-induced pneumonitis, mucositis, or hepatic damage), the higher doses of TBI did not improve overall survival. Nonetheless, Thomas' studies demonstrated a steep dose–response curve of the leukemia to radiation and supported the need for improved methods of selectively delivering radiation to malignant cells. To this end, monoclonal antibodies (MAb) conjugated to therapeutic radionuclides have been used in the management of hematologic malignancies for over two decades. Despite this experience, radioimmunotherapy (RIT) is not currently widely applied as treatment for these diseases. In this chapter we review the current state of RIT in HCT and outline ongoing controversies in the field.

Clinical RIT and Current Controversies

A variety of radioimmunoconjugates have been employed for the treatment of hematologic malignancies, yet the optimal approach remains controversial. Most investigators have utilized CD20 or CD22 as a target for RIT of non-Hodgkin lymphoma (NHL) and either CD33, CD66, or CD45 for myeloid neoplasms[4]. In particular, studies of RIT for lymphoma have escalated the doses of radioimmunoconjugates targeting CD20 to myeloablative levels and relied on autologous HCT to reconstitute hematopoiesis. With this approach, most relapsed lymphoma patients achieved objective remissions, with the vast majority of these being complete remissions[5], many of which have lasted for over a decade. Furthermore, outcomes using anti-CD20 radiolabeled Ab-based regimens combined with high-dose chemotherapy and autologous HCT have suggested superior progression-free and overall survival compared to identical doses of chemotherapy with TBI, albeit in a non-randomized setting[6]. Despite these encouraging results, the widespread use of the RIT-based autologous approach has proven to be controversial as relapse remains a challenge, particularly for high-risk patients. Therefore, some investigators have used high-dose RIT as part of an allogeneic HCT conditioning regimen to gain the benefit of a graft-*versus*-malignancy effect while mitigating the potential for a contaminated stem cell product. In particular, investigators have demonstrated the feasibility of using targeted delivery of high and standard dose radiotherapy combined with standard high-dose preparative regimens for treatment of patients with AML, ALL, MDS, and NHL respectively.

Despite the enormous potential for targeted therapy, problems were identified soon after the early clinical RIT trials were completed. Initially it was thought that any tumor could be targeted efficiently with a MAb and that specific antigen targeting with radiolabeled antibodies (RAb) could produce a biodistribution profile favoring radiation delivery to malignant cells. In reality, however, the long circulatory half-life of RAb and the fact that a portion of the radioimmunoconjugate remains unbound in the circulation cause prolonged high background activity levels and lead to nonspecific irradiation of normal tissues. The relative radiation exposure of target and nontarget tissues, or biodistribution, is thus a key factor impacting both on- and off-target response to RIT. Biodistribution of RAb, which can be estimated *via* imaging and has been delineated through both preclinical animal studies and patient trials, is impacted by the target antigen, features and dosing of the antibody, the chosen radionuclide, and the labeling procedure. Thus, efforts to expand RIT to more widespread use in HCT currently focus on the therapeutic target as well as the optimal drug delivery and radioisotopes.

Controversy #1: How Should We Select the Optimal Target Antigen for RIT?

Appropriate target antigen selection is crucial to achieve a favorable RAb biodistribution. Ideally, the target antigen will be homogeneously displayed on all malignant cells, including malignant stem cells, is not shed into the circulation, and will not be expressed on any normal cells. Unfortunately, the rarity of tumor-specific cell surface antigens and the antigenic heterogeneity of some hematopoietic malignancies are obstacles to choosing this ideal target. Targeting lineage-specific antigens (e.g., CD20, CD45) can be successful in the setting of marrow rescue by HCT. In fact, targeting these more widely distributed antigens can provide a beneficial crossfire effect on antigen-negative tumor cell variants and rare diseased cells within the marrow that may not be directly accessible to antibody[7].

Antigen density is directly correlated with distribution of MAb at tumor sites[1]. When the number of antigenic sites is less than 10000/cell, target saturation occurs at a relatively low MAb dose. As each MAb molecule can be labeled with only a limited amount of radionuclide before immunoreactivity is impaired, target saturation is a potentially significant limitation. Low antigen density may pose less of a problem for alpha-emitting radionuclides, which require only a single DNA "hit" to kill a cell, than for the more commonly used beta-emitting radionuclides, which require multiple hits to induce irreparable DNA strand breaks. Another factor in antigen selection is the degree to which the receptor is internalized following binding: while some antigens remain on the cell surface, others are rapidly endocytosed and transported to lysosomes for proteolytic degradation, after which the receptor density may remain low for several days[8,9]. One of the best studied radionuclides, ^{131}I, is not optimal for targeting internalizing receptors because rapid lysosomal metabolism of the conjugate leads to release of free radioiodine from cells[10,11], thereby reducing the ratio of radiation effect on malignant to normal cells. When internalized antibodies are labeled with ^{111}In or ^{90}Y, however, small molecular weight cationic metabolites remain trapped within the lysosomes, and they retain their therapeutic impact[12]. Surface antigens that are not internalized following antigen—immunoconjugate complex formation exhibit minimal variation in cellular retention of ^{131}I, ^{111}In, and ^{90}Y[12,13]. Currently the ideal target antigen for RIT remains an open question but likely depends upon disease state, disease burden, and radionuclide used. In the next section, we will outline both of the commonly used targets.

Target Antigens Used for RIT

CD20 is one of the most frequently targeted receptors for B-cell neoplasms and possesses many of the favorable attributes noted above, including a high-expression density on more than 90% of B-cell tumors, stability on the cell surface after antibody binding, and minimal shedding into the circulation. One potential limitation of anti-CD20 RIT includes inferior response rates in patients with B-cell depletion and higher serum levels of the unconjugated anti-CD20 MAb rituximab [14], as CD20 blocking may obstruct the RAb target[15]. Furthermore, CD20 is not universal on NHL and thus this strategy could only be applied to select patients.

An alternative approach is targeting the pan-hematopoietic antigen CD45[15]. CD45 (leukocyte common antigen) is a cell surface glycoprotein with tyrosine phosphatase activity[16] that is restricted to the hematopoietic compartment and is expressed on almost all hematopoietic cell lineages. In addition, CD45 is expressed by most hematologic malignancies, including 85–90% of acute lymphoid and myeloid leukemias [17–19], at a relatively high copy number (200000 binding sites per cell) and is not appreciably internalized or shed after ligand binding[12,20].

Like CD45, CD66 antigens are neither internalized nor shed[21]. They are expressed on members of the carcinoembryonic-antigen-related cell adhesion molecule (CEACAM) family of proteins that play a role in various intercellular-adhesion and intracellular signaling-mediated effects involved in cellular growth and differentiation[22]. Some isoforms of CD66 are expressed on hematopoietic cells but can also be found on epithelial or endothelial cells. CD66 antigens are found in myeloid cells from the late myeloblast or early promyelocyte stage and reach their highest levels in myelocytes and metamyelocytes but are not found on early myeloid progenitors or multipotent progenitors[23–25]. Only a minority of AML cells express CD66, but many B-cell acute lymphoblastic leukemias and some cases of lymphoid blast crisis CML express these antigens[24,26]. While studies with a CD66c-specific MAb suggested restriction primarily to CD10-positive early B-cell acute lymphoblastic leukemia (ALL)[27], many anti-CD66 MAb recognize several CD66 antigens (e.g., BW 250/183, the most widely used MAb for CD66-targeted RIT, recognizes multiple CD66 isoforms[28]), and thus the differential expression patterns between the individual CD66 antigens may be of limited significance for radioimmunotherapeutic approaches[22,28].

The myeloid differentiation antigen CD33 (SIGLEC-3) is an attractive target as it is displayed on a subset of leukemic blasts in most AML patients and possibly on leukemic stem cells in some patients[29,30]. Both CD33 and CD45 are expressed by normal as well as malignant cells, and so MAb targeting these antigens can deliver radiation to marrow, spleen, and lymph nodes in patients with measureable disease as well as in patients in remission. Malignant cells that do not express these antigens may be killed if they are surrounded predominantly by nonmalignant hematopoietic cells because of the bystander effect. This bystander effect is particularly important for RIT of myeloid leukemia using CD66, as these antigens are commonly not expressed by the malignant clone.

Besides, CD33, CD45, and CD66, a number of other antigens have been used in clinical and preclinical studies of RIT for hematologic malignancies. These will be discussed with new approaches below.

Controversy #2: How Should We Design the Optimal Antibody for RIT?

Appropriate biodistribution of a RAb depends not only on the target antigen selected, but also on MAb immunoreactivity, stability, and dosing. Low antibody immunoreactivity may lead to insufficient levels in target tissues and a relatively nonspecific pattern of distribution. In the HCT setting where accumulation in the marrow is reversible, cross-reactivity in organs like lung and liver are frequently dose limiting; in the non-HCT setting, on the other hand, myelosuppression frequently limits dose escalation. MAb stability is another important factor as susceptibility to damage or agglutination during the labeling process often leads to antibody accumulation in the liver. In early studies, MAb with high avidity were presumed to be optimal for RIT[31]; subsequent findings, however, suggest that very high avidity may promote preferential uptake at the most peripheral perivascular target sites leading to heterogeneous MAb deposition. This so-called binding site barrier[32] was subsequently demonstrated in a nonhuman primate study employing two different CD45 MAb in which the MAb with higher avidity preferentially localized to the most easily accessible antigen-positive cells, was more rapidly cleared from the circulation (t½ 0.6 versus 2.7 hours), and consequently resulted in lower uptake in the lymph nodes[33]. One proposed strategy to improve tissue penetration and overall distribution of RAb has been to use smaller antibody moieties, which can be produced by enzyme digestion of intact MAb or through cloning and expression of the Fv portions of the immunoglobulin light and heavy chains in *E. coli*[34,35]. Their small size, however, results in rapid clearance compared to intact IgG antibody[36–40], leading to lower intratumoral concentrations and undesirable renal accumulation[41].

Another potential obstacle in the development of effective RAb is development of a humoral immune response with formation of a neutralizing human antimouse antibody (HAMA). HAMA can cause rapid circulatory clearance and increased hepatic uptake of the resultant immune complexes, resulting in an altered RAb biodistribution. Fortunately, patients with hematologic malignancies undergoing HCT are at relatively low risk for development of HAMA because they lack a robust immune system to respond to new antigens, their use of immunosuppressive agents hampers antibody production, and they complete RIT conditioning over a short time and thus do not have the prolonged exposure required to elicit neutralizing antibodies. While development of humanized or chimeric molecules for use in RIT may limit the HAMA response, there is actually some evidence that development of HAMA after RIT in the non-HCT setting may be associated with improved survival[42], and so it is currently unclear whether the same association holds true in the HCT setting

and whether elimination of HAMA production should be a goal in creation of the RAb.

Opinions vary on the optimal antibody design for use in RIT, and further studies will be needed to optimize antigen binding, antibody stability, and effective tumor penetration in the case of lymphomas. Furthermore, the role of HAMA in response to RAb remains controversial. In the next section, we will lay out some of the complexities involving how these RAb are dosed for effective biodistribution.

Controversy #3: What Is the Most Effective Radionuclide?

Most RIT experience is with ^{131}I and ^{90}Y, both β-particle-emitting isotopes linked with a murine CD20-directed MAb (^{131}I-tositumomab and ^{90}Y-ibritumomab) initially approved for treatment of relapsed or refractory B-cell NHL, although the former was withdrawn from the market in 2013 due to declining sales. While there are theoretical advantages to both isotopes, it should be noted that no randomized controlled trial comparing them has been performed. ^{131}I, which has a half-life of 8 days, emits both β particles and γ rays allowing it to be used for both imaging (due to high energy γ emission) and therapy. It is also relatively low cost, has a long history of treating hematologic and solid tumor malignancies, and has well-understood chemistry for protein labeling. On the other hand, ^{131}I-labeled proteins are rapidly degraded upon endocytosis, resulting in release of free ^{131}I and ^{131}I-tyrosine into the bloodstream, thus adding to the radiation exposure time [11,43]. Furthermore, γ rays emitted by ^{131}I may pose a potential safety risk to healthcare workers and family, and patients must be hospitalized for radiation isolation to receive large doses, such as those required for HCT. ^{90}Y, on the other hand, is a radiometal with a short half-life (2.7 days) that emits β particles that are four times as energetic as those from ^{131}I, but virtually no γ rays; hence it cannot be easily imaged with a gamma camera, and dosimetry is reliant on the administration of a surrogate γ−emitting radionuclide, such as ^{111}In. One particular advantage is that, as β particles do not leave the patient's body, there is less potential for caregivers to be exposed to radiation. Conversely, ^{90}Y is less abundant and more expensive than ^{131}I and has been shown to accumulate nonspecifically in liver and bone[44]. Other β and γ emitters under investigation include the radiometals ^{177}Lu, ^{67}Cu, ^{186}Re, and ^{188}Re. As a group, the radiometals, including ^{90}Y, offer several advantages over ^{131}I, including better retention by target cells after antibody endocytosis. Details of each radionuclide are listed in Table 28.1.

In contrast to the relatively long range of β-emitting radio-isotopes, the shorter emission range (path length <0.1 mm) and higher linear energy transfer (LET) of the much larger α-emitting radioisotopes (approximately 100 keV//μm versus 0.2 keV/μm) may allow for more potential to produce double-stranded DNA breaks and thus more potent and selective tumor cell killing[45]. Furthermore, unlike β-emitters, damage

Table 28.1 Radionuclides in clinical use or under consideration for use in RIT

Radionuclide	Emission	Range (mm)	Energy (MeV)	Details
Beta-emitters				
Iodine-131	β, γ	0.8 (mean) 2.3 (max)	0.66 β	Half-life 8.1 days Inexpensive Well-studied Releases free radionuclide into bloodstream after endocytosis
Yttrium-90	β	2.7 (mean) 11.3 (max)	2.3 β	Half-life 2.7 days Stable when internalized No gamma Accumulates in liver and bone More uniform uptake in larger tumors than ^{117}Lu
Lutetium-177	β, γ	0.22 (mean) 1.8 (max)	0.50 β	Half-life 6.7 days Reduced potential for radiation to caregivers Stable when internalized May provide better irradiation to small tumors
Rhenium-188	β, γ	2.4 (mean) 10.4 (max)	4.4 β	Half-life 17 hours (short), which may limit utility
Rhenium-186	β, γ	0.98 (mean) 4.8 (max)	1.8 β	Half-life 89 hours
Copper-67	β, γ	0.24 (mean) 2.1 (max)	0.57 β	Half-life 2.6 days Stable when internalized Can image with PET Expense, limited access
Alpha-emitters				
Bismuth-213	α	0.05–0.08 (mean)	5.84 α	Half-life 46 minutes
Astatine-211	α	0.05–0.08 (mean)	5.87 α	Half-life 7.2 hours Difficult to produce
Actinium-225	α	0.05–0.08 (mean)	5.75–8.7 α	Half-life 10 days Daughters a potential problem if released into circulation
Auger electron emitters				
Indium-111	Electron, γ	Nanometers	<100 keV	

caused by α-emitters is independent of tumor hypoxia[46]. The absence of a significant bystander effect may not be optimal for larger tumors, but it is favorable for targeting small tumors or tumor deposits and individual tumor cells (such as leukemia with low burden of disease)[47–49]. For this reason, α-emitters have considerable promise for RIT. On the other hand, they have significantly shorter half-lives and their radiolabeling chemistry is more challenging; notwithstanding, a number of trials have been conducted successfully with ^{221}At ($t_{1/2}$ = 7.2 hours), ^{225}Ac ($t_{1/2}$ = 10 days), and ^{213}Bi ($t_{1/2}$ = 45.6 minutes)[46,50]. Individual properties of these radionuclides are outlined in Table 28.1.

A third type of radionuclide, the Auger-emitter, represents a new approach with the potential to reduce nonspecific toxicity. Auger emission, which results when electrons fall from higher to lower energy shells causing release of energy in the form of an ejected electron, is low energy with particle ranges less than a cell diameter. Though not yet tested clinically, in-vitro studies of an anti-CD33 MAb modified with a peptide harboring a nuclear localizing sequence and labeled with the Auger-emitter ^{111}In demonstrated improved routing of the radioimmunoconjugate to the nucleus and enhanced killing of leukemia cells compared to MAb constructs lacking the nuclear localization sequence[51,52].

In summary, the choice of radionuclide for RIT depends upon multiple factors, including radioisotope availability, tumor type and bulk of disease, as well as healthcare resources available for facilitation of RAb administration. Radionuclide properties that can affect RAb efficacy include type of particulate radiation produced (α-particles, β-particles, and Auger electrons), emission energy, half-life, ability to be conjugated, ease of use, and capacity for imaging. The merits of various radionuclides are still debated, with controversy over use of ^{131}I *versus* ^{90}Y or use of β-particle *versus* α-particle emitting radioisotopes being fueled by lack of randomized trials comparing these modalities. That said, rather than striving to find one ideal radionuclide, we should consider whether the breadth of radionuclides presented here could offer the possibility of personalizing therapy to the needs of an individual patient.

Radiolabeling Strategies

Great care must be taken during the radiolabeling process, which is very sensitive to external factors including fluctuations in temperature and pH, to ensure production of a successful RAb with its desired reactivity. Moreover, radiolabeling procedures must be efficient, reproducible, and affordable in order to achieve mainstream use. While ^{131}I fulfils requirements for commercial development and can be covalently conjugated to antibodies on a tyrosine residue by either the chloramine-T or Iodogen™ methods, these approaches do not protect against rapid metabolism and release of free radioiodine when the RAb is endocytosed. Alternative processes to prevent intracellular degradation have therefore been developed, including using a tyramine cellobiose adduct as a bridge between the MAb and the halogen radionuclide, which promotes cellular retention of the radioligand[53]. Metallic radionuclides (^{90}Y, ^{111}In, ^{67}Cu, and ^{177}Lu) cannot be readily linked to antibodies and require chelation chemistry for attachment, generally with isothiocyanotobenzyl DTPA or 1,4,7,10-tetra-azacyclododecane-N,N^1,N^{11},N^{111}-tetracetic acid (DOTA).

RAb Dosing

The importance of appropriate RAb dosing in achieving optimal biodistributions has been studied in preclinical models and in human subjects. Dosing RAb too low may result in poor distribution to lymph nodes and bulky tumors, while excessive dosing may increase toxicity from off-target effects[9,54]. It is important to note that the precise MAb dose that will deliver the optimal radiation exposure to tumor sites and limit exposure to normal organs in a given clinical scenario may also depend on the burden of antigen-expressing cells (tumor load) and presence of persistent prior antibody (e.g., rituximab) that may compete for target antigens and Fc receptors[15]. In addition to dose of RAb administered, dosing schedule can be modulated to achieve a desired effect. For example, to allow for re-expression of an internalizing antigenic site on the cell surface (CD33), a model in which 2–4 divided doses are delivered at 48–72-hour intervals has been studied in patients with AML and yields appropriate biodistribution with antileukemic effects[55]. Fractionation has also been evaluated for B-NHL with a noninternalizing target (CD20) to allow a delivery of a higher total absorbed dose[56]. Another strategy to improve biodistribution is to deliver a pretreatment dose of an unlabeled antibody to clear circulating cells expressing the target antigen. Animal studies have suggested that this strategy could lead to improved marrow localization and decreased uptake by the liver[57]. Patient trials have yielded inconsistent results, with one group reporting no benefit of this approach in

an anti-CD45 MAb (BC8; murine IgG1) model in terms of hepatic uptake and clearance[58] and another demonstrating preferential marrow targeting in an anti-CD45 MAb (YAML568; rat IgG2a) model[59].

In order to ensure appropriate and safe levels of radiation to normal and target tissues during RIT, individualized biodistribution data must be obtained. Dosimetry involves injection of a trace-labeled dose of antibody followed by single photon emission computed tomography or planar imaging to generate depth dose curves. Based on the measured biodistribution of the RAb, tables have been developed that allow estimation of the mean absorbed dose over a specific organ volume for any radionuclide administered[60]; accuracy of these methods can be further enhanced by radiographically quantified individualized organ volumes[61]. This approach, which has been validated in animal models[54], confirms tumor uptake and estimates absorbed dose to various organs to ensure that delivered doses remain within a safe range. Some limitations of this technique include decreased accuracy for small, deep-seated tumors and for whole organs or large tumor volumes in which signal averaging occurs such that information on distribution heterogeneity is lost. More recently, positron emission tomography has been used in conjunction with photon emitting radionuclides to improve the localization of radionuclide uptake[62]. It must also be noted that, given the high energy of α-particles delivered over a short range, this system for calculating dosimetry may not yield meaningful information. Alternative methods involving microdosimetry have been developed[63].

Radiation Effects

Because leukemias and lymphomas are exquisitely radiosensitive, external-beam TBI is an effective component of many transplant conditioning regimens. Standard TBI, however, delivers the same radiation to normal organs as it does to tumor, thus limiting the safe dose to 12–15.75 Gy, typically delivered as fractionated doses of 1–2 Gy at 7–25 cGy/minute [64]. Though the peak rate of radiation delivery with RIT is substantially lower than with TBI, there is continuous exposure of tumor cells to radiation rather than intermittent exposure as with fractionated TBI, and the radiation delivered is exponentially decreasing at a rate dependent on the chosen particle's half-life. The low rate and exponential drop-off of radiation delivery with RIT could allow radiation delivery at higher doses to the tumor and lower doses to normal organs than TBI. For example, the maximum tolerated dose of ^{131}I-tositumomab is 25 Gy, substantially higher than that given with TBI. Another theoretic benefit to continuous radiation as delivered with RAb *versus* fractionated dosing with TBI is that with steady dosing, there are no intervals during which cellular DNA repair can occur[2]. Consistent with this theory, human solid tumor xenograft experiments have demonstrated RAb to have equivalent or even enhanced antitumor activity compared to external-beam radiation[65,66].

Another explanation for this finding involves the "inverse dose-rate effect," whereby lower doses of radiation are observed to be more cytotoxic than higher doses. It is theorized that this seemingly paradoxical finding is related to the ability of cells to progress through G2 phase in the presence of low-dose radiation only to be held up by mitotic delay. This progression redistributes cells to a particularly radiosensitive phase of the cell cycle, the G2/M interface, and thus even lower dose radiation can have quite toxic effects[67]. Likewise, there is preclinical evidence to suggest that low-dose-rate radiation may best synergize with chemotherapeutics that interfere with single-strand DNA repair such as the nucleoside analogs[68].

Controversy #4: Can We Overcome the Obstacles to Promote More Widespread Use of RIT as Part of HCT Conditioning for Hematologic Malignancies?

Despite improvements in supportive care, relapse remains the main cause of transplant failure for hematologic malignancies, and efforts to improve upon pretransplant conditioning have been a cogent way of improving transplant outcomes. In this vein, the rationale for creating a method of targeting radiation directly to the site of highly radiosensitive tumors (and thus away from normal tissue) has been highly appealing for use during HCT. Now, with several decades of clinical data in support of as well as FDA approval of RIT in some contexts, we may be entering an era in which its use becomes significantly more widespread. Challenges remain, however, in bringing RIT into mainstream HCT therapy and the techniques we use have substantial room for improvement. Nevertheless, the clinical progress described in this section for autologous and allogeneic HCT provides strong evidence for further study of RIT in this setting.

Early data demonstrating that the addition of RIT to conditioning regimens for autologous HCT may improve outcomes over standard conditioning come from nonrandomized trials in relapsed lymphoma showing that myeloablative doses of anti-CD20-mediated RIT plus high-dose etoposide and cyclophosphamide followed by stem cell rescue outperformed TBI plus identical doses of chemotherapy in terms of 2-year PFS (68% versus 36%) and OS (83% versus 53%)[6]. In fact, in multiple studies on high-risk relapsed/refractory non-Hodgkin lymphoma, responses with anti-CD20 RIT followed by stem cell rescue have been encouraging. Objective remissions have been seen in 85% to 90% of such patients, with 75% to 80% experiencing durable CR, often lasting 5 to almost 20 years[5,6,69,70]. Even in older, heavily pretreated patients, 3-year PFS over 50% has been noted[71]. More recently, randomized controlled trials have compared conditioning regimens with and without RIT. In particular, two studies compared BEAM or R-BEAM to BEAM plus ^{90}Y-ibritumomab tiuxetan (Zevalin®; Z-BEAM) and one compared R-BEAM to BEAM plus ^{131}I-tositumomab (Bexxar®; B-BEAM) as conditioning prior to autologous HCT for aggressive lymphomas. Together, these studies showed that RIT-based regimens were associated with similar or perhaps slightly improved PFS and OS, though any improvement seen was at most of borderline statistical significance. Strongest results were obtained with Z-BEAM, which yielded 2-year PFS 59% versus 37% ($P=0.2$) and OS 91% versus 62% ($P=0.05$). It should be noted that Z-BEAM and B-BEAM were no more toxic than standard BEAM conditioning, with no difference in treatment-related mortality, infection, or engraftment[72–74].

In the same vein, targeted radiotherapy can be used to bolster conditioning in allogeneic HCT. This strategy was employed using standard dose anti-CD20 RIT with fludarabine plus 200 cGy TBI conditioning for high-risk lymphoma, proving to be safe overall and effective in a subset of heavily pretreated patients[75]. In fact, it may be possible that TBI could be replaced entirely with a RAb; this strategy was employed by investigators in Seattle and at the University of Tubingen (Tubingen, Germany), who demonstrated in a canine model ^{213}Bi-anti-CD45 MAb could be used in a TBI-free allogeneic reduced intensity HCT[76]. RIT has also been used as HCT conditioning for myeloid malignancies in early phase trials targeting CD33[56,77], CD45[59,78–80], and CD66[28,81–83]. While results from this work have been mixed, overall the addition of radioimmunoconjugates to conditioning has resulted in tolerable toxicities and antileukemic activity. The lack of well-controlled trials, however, limits our understanding of whether RIT improves outcomes of HCT for myeloid malignancies. To this end, a multicenter randomized phase 3 trial has been designed for older patients with refractory AML. The design is simple: 75 patients will be treated with ^{131}I-anti-CD45 MAb (BC8) and HCT while the other 75 control patients will be treated with conventional care. The primary endpoint is durable CR rates. For ethical considerations, the FDA requested a crossover aspect to the trial where if a complete response cannot be achieved for the standard of care arm, the patient will be allowed to cross over to the ^{131}I-BC8 and HCT study arm (Figure 28.1).

Though results from these studies appear generally promising and the randomized phase 3 refractory older AML trial will merit anti-CD45 RIT over continued cytotoxic chemotherapy, it remains clear that further investigation is needed in conducting randomized trials to assess the benefit of RIT over standard conditioning, to determine the optimal antigenic target and radionuclide, and to develop novel strategies for improving the efficacy of this technology. This last point is of paramount importance: given the technical difficulties and hurdles involved in bringing RIT to the mainstream, it is likely that we will have to see substantial improvements in efficacy before RIT becomes a component of standard therapy. In the next section, we will focus on new channels of research that may offer drastic improvements in our ability to deliver RIT safely and effectively.

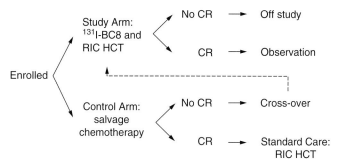

Figure 28.1. Proposed trial evaluating RIT *versus* standard therapy for relapsed AML. Design of a proposed randomized controlled trial for older patients with refractory AML comparing upfront RIT-based nonmyeloablative HCT to standard salvage chemotherapy. This trial allows crossover for patients who did not achieve CR after standard therapy. RIT will involve ^{131}I-BC8, a radiolabeled CD45 MAb. Abbreviations: RIC, reduced intensity conditioning; HCT, hematopoietic cell transplantation; CR, complete remission; AML, acute myeloid leukemia; RIT, radioimmunotherapy; MAb, monoclonal antibody.

Future Directions

Preclinical studies in experimental rodents and primates were instrumental in demonstrating the feasibility and potential efficacy of RIT[84]. Undoubtedly, preclinical studies remain critical for the development of radioimmunotherapeutic approaches. This research will focus its efforts in several different directions, including the identification of alternative target antigens and radionuclides that demonstrate enhanced efficacy for RIT, offer improved specificity for tumor targeting, and enhance tumor penetration in the case of bulky or inaccessible disease.

The number of antigens targeted with RIT may expand significantly over the next years with the aim of optimizing the therapeutic index of RIT by improving biodistribution ratios in favor of target cells. A number of pharmaceutical and academic research centers are focusing on the identification of new antigenic targets that are highly expressed on malignant cells and minimally expressed on normal tissues. Many new antigenic targets are under active investigation, including HLA-DR, CD22, CD25, CD30, and CD52. For example, even though CD25 has so far not gained major importance for RIT of leukemias[85], it remains an attractive target due to its relatively selected expression on a high proportion of malignant cells in certain forms of lymphoid neoplasms, including adult T-cell leukemia, as well as on AML[86]. Given this expression pattern, alpha-particle therapy may be particularly appealing in an attempt to spare normal hematopoietic tissue. To this end, a [211]At-labeled murine anti-CD25 IgG2a MAb (7G7/B6) has been developed and tested with promising results in immunodeficient mice bearing CD25-positive leukemia and lymphoma cells[87]. Using a similar model, the same group also achieved promising results using a [211]At-labeled murine anti-CD30 IgG1 MAb (HeFi-1) in prolonging survival of immunodeficient mice bearing tumors that express CD30, an antigen that is found on some lymphocyte subsets but is also expressed on some lymphoid neoplasms[88]. Together, these findings may set the foundation for progression to clinical studies using [211]At-labeled RAb for the treatment of patients with either CD25- or CD30-expressing leukemias. CD52 is normally expressed on B- and T-lymphocytes, monocytes, macrophages, eosinophils, natural killer cells, dendritic cells, as well as on cells of the male reproductive tract[89]. However, CD52 is also expressed by a variety of lymphoid as well as some myeloid neoplasms and has thus been exploited as a target for MAb-based therapies, in particular for CLL. Alemtuzumab (Campath-1H), a humanized rat IgG1 MAb directed against CD52, has shown activity alone and in combination with other therapeutics for untreated and previously treated patients with CLL[89–91]. More recently, this MAb has been explored for RIT using [188]Re. Preclinical studies found [188]Re-alemtuzumab to have good *in-vitro* stability and showed high uptake in blood with bi-exponential clearance and some increased uptake observed in kidneys and heart[92]. Among the targets explored for treatment of CLL is also CD23. A unconjugated anti-CD23 MAb, lumiliximab (IDEC-152), has shown promising activity in clinical studies[91,93,94], and it is conceivable that this, or other MAb under development, may be used to deliver radiation to tumor sites. CD22 has also been studied as an antigenic target for RIT in patients with aggressive lymphoma outside of the transplant setting in conjunction with an unconjugated CD20 antibody yielding objective responses in over half the patients[95].

Parallel efforts are ongoing to identify novel radionuclides and radionuclide–antibody conjugates and define their antitumor properties. For example, a [213]Bi-labeled anti-CD45 MAb (YAML568) is under preclinical development that shows interesting properties regarding induction of apoptosis and breakage of chemoresistance and radioresistance by overcoming DNA repair mechanisms in leukemia cells[96]. The high LET of [213]Bi RIT may also provide synergistic cytotoxic activity when combined with antileukemic chemotherapeutics, for example for the treatment of CLL[97]. The increased availability of beta-emitting radionuclides with favorable physical characteristics, such as ^{177}Lu and [67]Cu, may provide an avenue for future investigations. Alpha-emitters, including those with longer half-lives such as [225]Ac, also show great promise[98]. Radioimmunoconjugates currently being considered for use in the clinical setting include ^{90}Y-B4, ^{90}Y-BU12, and ^{90}Y-HD37 (mouse IgG1 anti-CD19 MAb), ^{90}Y-RFB4 (mouse IgG1 anti-CD22 MAb), [211]At-hTac (humanized anti-CD25 MAb), [213]Bi-rituximab (humanized anti-CD20 MAb), ^{177}Lu-labeled anti-CD20, anti-CD22, and anti-HLA-DR MAb[99–105].

A number of novel approaches are also being explored to improve the ratio of target to nontarget exposure. As noted previously, dose escalation in high-dose RIT for HCT is limited by nonspecific irradiation of normal tissues due to both the slow distribution of the RAb to target cells and the presence of unbound labeled MAb persisting in the circulation. One approach, pretargeted RIT (PRIT), is a process in which patients are initially treated with tumor-reactive MAb that are not bound to therapeutic radionuclides, allowing localization

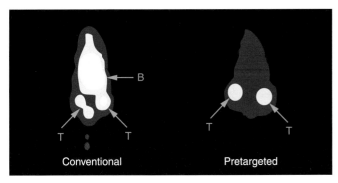

Figure 28.2. *In-vivo* demonstration of pretargeted RIT. Efficacy of pretargeting as demonstrated by planar gamma camera images of Burkitt lymphoma xenograft tumors in athymic mice. Animals were injected with either directly labeled ^{111}In-anti-CD20 Ab (on left) or pretargeted with anti-CD20-SA conjugate followed 24 hours later by clearing agent and then by ^{111}In-DOTA-biotin (on right). Arrows indicate radioactivity in tumors (T), and blood pool (B) 24 hours after injection of ^{111}In-reagents. Bladder activity is also seen in the conventional mouse.

to tumor sites without subjecting the rest of the body to nonspecific irradiation. After maximal accumulation of MAb in the tumor, a low molecular weight radioactive moiety with high affinity for the tumor-reactive MAb is administered. Because of its small size, this second reagent penetrates tumors rapidly where it binds to the pretargeted MAb. The unbound molecules of the radioactive reagent are small enough to be rapidly cleared from the blood and excreted in the urine within minutes. To further improve the targeted delivery of the radioimmunoconjugate, preclinical studies show that a clearing agent can be injected shortly before the radiolabeled small molecule to remove unbound MAb from the bloodstream [106,107]. The high-affinity binding that occurs between the pretargeted MAb and subsequently administered radiolabeled small molecule can be achieved through a number of proposed mechanisms. One of the most promising mechanisms exploits the exceptionally high affinity of avidin for biotin. Other proposed approaches include bispecific MAb that recognize both tumor antigen and radiolabeled hapten and MAb conjugated to an oligonucleotide that can bind to a radiolabeled complementary oligomer. In animal models, PRIT has generated therapeutic tumor-to-normal organ ratios of greater than 10:1 (Figure 28.2) and cures have been achieved in 100% of animals with lymphoma and solid tumor xenografts[106,108]. Early patient trials have exhibited similarly encouraging findings in both solid tumors and lymphoma[109–111]. A trial combining PRIT with allogeneic HCT for patients with relapsed/refractory AML is ongoing in Seattle (NCT00988715).

Similar to PRIT, extracorporeal adsorption therapy (ECAT) offers another promising means for optimizing biodistribution. In this process, RAb are injected and allowed 24–48 hours to circulate and distribute to antigen-bearing cells. Patients then undergo a hemodialysis-like procedure during which their blood volume is circulated across an avidin–agarose column, removing biotin-conjugated RAb that

remain in the circulation and minimizing nonspecific radiation to normal organs. In a small safety and efficacy trial conducted in Sweden, seven patients with relapsed or refractory B-cell NHL received biotin-conjugated ^{90}Y-rituximab, followed 24–48 hours later by ECAT filtration. The procedure was demonstrated to be safe and effectively cleared ~96% of the unbound ^{90}Y-rituximab–biotin from the blood[112].

Nanomaterials have enormous potential in a wide range of applications associated with HCT, including for the delivery of radiation. Owing to their nanostructured surfaces offering a large surface area and greater reactivity, nanovectors are potentially ideal for targeted RIT[113,114]. Nanoparticle materials can be synthetically modified for RIT using well-established techniques after radionuclide loading. Multiple studies over the past decade have been performed to determine the efficacy of nanoparticle carriers for drug delivery (i.e., radiopharmaceutical and chemical). While initial studies determined that blood circulation time and hepatic clearance were primarily dependent on nanoparticle size[113,115,116], a number of more recent studies have shown that there are many factors that determine circulation time and clearance, for example, surface coating and surface charge[114,117–120], presence of high immunologic protein concentration on the particle surface[121–123], as well as particle size [114,116,117,124,125]. In fact, the term "stealth particle" has been coined to describe the characteristics necessary in a successful carrier nanoparticle: it should be targeted for delivery of its payload, have a sufficient contact time with the target, and not be removed by the reticuloendothelial system (RES) so that toxic levels of drug, radiation, or particles are not accumulated in the liver and spleen[113]. To target blood-borne cancer cells, mediated by an antibody or peptide located on the surface, a radiolabeled nanoparticle must have an appropriately long circulation time and have its accumulation in the RES (liver and spleen) and uptake on the bone surfaces slowed sufficiently to maximize therapeutic efficacy and minimize dose to healthy tissues.

Other new avenues to explore for delivery of targeted radiation to sites of disease include the development of small synthetic multidentate ligands that mimic properties of MAb by binding to cell surface antigens with high affinity and specificity, and, due to smaller size, may provide better tumor penetration[126,127]. An alternative approach to increase accessibility of tumors to radioimmunoconjugates lies in the manipulation of tumor blood flow, and early studies with interleukin-2 suggest that increasing vascular permeability to achieve this goal might be a valid strategy worth exploring[128].

Conclusions

An increasing number of proof-of-principle clinical studies demonstrate that RIT in HCT is safe, feasible, and has acceptable toxicities, even in older adults. Research over the last few decades established important principles of directing RAb to malignancies and provided encouraging results. Nevertheless, RIT is a complex, multidisciplinary effort that still faces many challenges; significant obstacles remain that must be overcome to achieve optimal targeting and elimination of target cells by radioimmunoconjugates. In particular, the optimal therapeutic radionuclide-antibody-antigen combination for RIT remains controversial, and controlled trials will ultimately be required to address this question and to determine whether addition of radioimmunoconjugates truly improves patient outcomes over standard treatment. Undoubtedly, future studies will explore alternative antigenic targets and novel radionuclides to improve imaging, dosimetry, and therapy. Furthermore, innovative strategies such as PRIT and ECAT may optimize the administration of radionuclide therapy and allow more widespread use of alpha-emitters with short half-lives. RIT-based approaches may become an important means to improve transplant outcomes, and innovations such as those enumerated above will no doubt further enhance the feasibility, safety, and efficacy of RIT, with and without HCT.

References

1. Thomas, E.D., Storb, R., Clift, R.A., *et al.*, Bone-marrow transplantation (second of two parts). *N Engl J Med*, 1975. 292(17): p. 895–902.

2. Clift, R.A., Buckner, C., Appelbaum, F.R., *et al.*, Allogeneic marrow transplantation in patients with acute myeloid leukemia in first remission: a randomized trial of two irradiation regimens. *Blood*, 1990. 76(9): p. 1867–71.

3. Clift, R.A., Buckner, C., Appelbaum, F.R., *et al.*, Allogeneic marrow transplantation in patients with chronic myeloid leukemia in the chronic phase: a randomized trial of two irradiation regimens. *Blood*, 1991. 77(8): p. 1660–5.

4. Gyurkocza, B. and Sandmaier, BM. Conditioning regimens for hematopoietic cell transplantation: one size does not fit all. *Blood*, 2014. 124(3): p. 344–53.

5. Liu, S.Y., Eary, J.F., Petersdorf, S.H., *et al.*, Follow-up of relapsed B-cell lymphoma patients treated with iodine-131- labeled anti-CD20 antibody and autologous stem-cell rescue. *J Clin Oncol*, 1998. 16(10): p. 3270–8.

6. Press, O.W., Eary, J.F., Gooley, T., *et al.*, A phase I/II trial of iodine-131-tositumomab (anti-CD20), etoposide, cyclophosphamide, and autologous stem cell transplantation for relapsed B-cell lymphomas. *Blood*, 2000. 96(9): p. 2934–42.

7. Nourigat, C., Badger C.C., and Bernstein, I.D. Treatment of lymphoma with radiolabeled antibody: elimination of tumor cells lacking target antigen. *J Natl Cancer Inst*, 1990. 82(1): p. 47–50.

8. Press, O.W., Hansen, J.A., Farr, A., *et al.*, Endocytosis and degradation of murine anti-human CD3 monoclonal antibodies by normal and malignant T-lymphocytes. *Cancer Res*, 1988. 48(8): p. 2249–57.

9. Press, O.W., Eary, J.F., Badger, C.C., *et al.*, Treatment of refractory non-Hodgkin's lymphoma with radiolabeled MB-1 (anti-CD37) antibody. *J Clin Oncol*, 1989. 7(8): p. 1027–38.

10. Geissler, F., Anderson, S.K., and Press, O. Intracellular catabolism of radiolabeled anti-CD3 antibodies by leukemic T cells. *Blood*, 1991. 78(7): p. 1864–74.

11. Geissler, F., Anderson, S.K., Venkatesan, P., *et al.*, Intracellular catabolism of radiolabeled anti-mu antibodies by malignant B cells. *Cancer Res*, 1992. 52(10): p. 2907–15

12. van der Jagt, R.H., Badger, C.C., Appelbaum, F.R., *et al.*, Localization of radiolabeled antimyeloid antibodies in a human acute leukemia xenograft tumor model. *Cancer Res*, 1992. 52(1): p. 89–94.

13. Press, O.W., Grogan, T.M., and Fisher, R.I. Evaluation and management of mantle cell lymphoma. *Adv Leuk Lymphoma*, 1996. 6: p. 3–11.

14. Winter, J.N., Inwards, D.J., Spies, S., *et al.*, Yttrium-90 ibritumomab tiuxetan doses calculated to deliver up to 15 Gy to critical organs may be safely combined with high-dose BEAM and autologous transplantation in relapsed or refractory B-cell non-Hodgkin's lymphoma. *J Clin Oncol*, 2009. 27(10): p. 1653–9.

15. Gopal, A.K., Press, O.W., Wilbur, S.M., *et al.*, Rituximab blocks binding of radiolabeled anti-CD20 antibodies (Ab) but not radiolabeled anti-CD45 Ab. *Blood*, 2008. 112(3): p. 830–5.

16. Omary, M.B., Trowbridge, I.S., and BattiforaH.A. Human homologue of murine T200 glycoprotein. *J Exp Med*, 1980. 152(4): p. 842–52.

17. Andres, T.L. and Kadin, M.E. Immunologic markers in the differential diagnosis of small round cell tumors from lymphocytic lymphoma and leukemia. *Am J Clin Pathol*, 1983. 79(5): p. 546–52.

18. Nakano, A., Harada, T., Morikawa, S., *et al.*, Expression of leukocyte common antigen (CD45) on various human leukemia/lymphoma cell lines. *Acta Pathol Jpn*, 1990. 40(2): p. 107–15.

19. Taetle, R., Ostergaard, H., Smedsrud, M., *et al.*, Regulation of CD45 expression in human leukemia cells. *Leukemia*, 1991. 5(4): p. 309–14.

20. Press, O.W., Howell-Clark, J., Anderson, S., *et al.*, Retention of B-cell-specific monoclonal antibodies by human lymphoma cells. *Blood*, 1994. 83(5): p. 1390–7.

21. Becker, W., Goldenberg, D.M., and Wolf, F. The use of monoclonal antibodies and antibody fragments in the imaging of infectious lesions. *Semin Nucl Med*, 1994. 24(2): p. 142–53.

22. Gray-Owen, S.D. and Blumberg, R.S. CEACAM1: contact-dependent control of immunity. *Nat Rev Immunol*, 2006. 6(6): p. 433–46.

23. Wahren, B., Gahrton, G., and Hammarstrom, S. Nonspecific cross-reacting antigen in normal and leukemic myeloid cells and serum of leukemic patients. *Cancer Res*, 1980. 40(6): p. 2039–44.

24. Noworolska, A., Harlozinska, A., Richter, R., *et al.*, Non-specific cross-reacting antigen (NCA) in individual maturation stages of myelocytic cell series. *Br J Cancer*, 1985. 51(3): p. 371–7.

25. Watt, S.M., Sala-Newby, G., Hoang, T., *et al.*, CD66 identifies a neutrophil-specific epitope within the hematopoietic system that is expressed by members of the carcinoembryonic antigen family of adhesion molecules. *Blood*, 1991. 78(1): p. 63–74.

26. Carrasco, M., Munoz, L., Bellido, M., et al., CD66 expression in acute leukaemia. *Ann Hematol*, 2000. 79(6): p. 299–303.

27. Boccuni, P., Di Noto, R., Lo Pardo, C., et al., CD66c antigen expression is myeloid restricted in normal bone marrow but is a common feature of CD10+ early-B-cell malignancies. *Tissue Antigens*, 1998. 52(1): p. 1–8.

28. Bunjes, D., 118Re-labeled anti-CD66 monoclonal antibody in stem cell transplantation for patients wth high-risk acute myeloid leukemia. *Leuk Lymphoma*. 2002. 43(11): p. 2125–31.

29. Pollard, J.A., Alonzo, T.A., Loken, M., et al., Correlation of CD33 expression level with disease characteristics and response to gemtuzumab ozogamicin containing chemotherapy in childhood AML. *Blood*. 2012. 119(16): p. 3705-11.

30. Walter, R.B., Appelbaum, F.R., Estey, E.H., et al., Acute myeloid leukemia stem cells and CD33-targeted immunotherapy. *Blood*. 2012. 119(26): p. 6198–208.

31. Schlom, J., Eggensperger, D., Colcher, D., et al., Therapeutic advantage of high-affinity anticarcinoma radioimmunoconjugates. *Cancer Res*, 1992. 52(5): p. 1067–72.

32. Fujimori, K., Covell, D.G., Fletcher, J.E., et al., A modeling analysis of monoclonal antibody percolation through tumors: a binding-site barrier. *J Nucl Med*, 1990. 31(7): p. 1191–8.

33. Matthews, D.C., Appelbaum, F.R., Eary, J.F., et al., Radiolabeled anti-CD45 monoclonal antibodies target lymphohematopoietic tissue in the macaque. *Blood*, 1991. 78(7): p. 1864–74.

34. Colcher, D., Bird, R., Rosselli, M., et al., In vivo tumor targeting of a recombinant single-chain antigen-binding protein. *J Natl Cancer Inst*, 1990. 82(14): p. 1191–7.

35. Larson, S.M., Improved tumor targeting with radiolabeled, recombinant, single-chain, antigen-binding protein. *J Natl Cancer Inst*, 1990. 82(14): p. 1173–4.

36. Yokota, T., Milenic, D.E., Whitlow, M., et al., Rapid tumor penetration of a single-chain Fv and comparison with other immunoglobulin forms. *Cancer Res*, 1992. 52(12): p. 3402–8.

37. Matthews, D.C., Badger, C.C., Fisher, D.R., et al., Selective radiation of hematolymphoid tissue delivered by anti-CD45 antibody. *Cancer Res*, 1992. 52(5): p. 1228–34.

38. King, D.J., Turner, A., Farnsworth, A.P., et al., Improved tumor targeting with chemically cross-linked recombinant antibody fragments. *Cancer Res*, 1994. 54(23): p. 6176–85.

39. Nieroda, C.A., Milenic, D.E., Carrasquillo, J.A., et al., Improved tumor radioimmunodetection using a single-chain Fv and gamma- interferon: potential clinical applications for radioimmunoguided surgery and gamma scanning. *Cancer Res*, 1995. 55(13): p. 2858–65.

40. Milenic, D.E., Yokota, T., Filpula, D.R., et al., Construction, binding properties, metabolism, and tumor targeting of a single-chain Fv derived from the pancarcinoma monoclonal antibody CC49. *Cancer Res*, 1991. 51(23 Pt 1): p. 6363–71.

41. Larson, S.M., El-Shirbiny, A.M., Divgi, C.R., et al., Single chain antigen binding protein (sFv CC49): first human studies in colorectal carcinoma metastatic to liver. *Cancer*,1997. 80(12 Suppl): p. 2458–68.

42. Lamborn, K.R., DeNardo, G.L., DeNardo, S.J., et al., Treatment-related parameters predicting efficacy of Lym-1 radioimmunotherapy in patients with B-lymphocytic malignancies. *Clin Cancer Res*. 1997. 3(8):1253–60.

43. Press, O.W., Shan, D., Howell-Clark, J., et al., Comparative metabolism and retention of iodine-125, yttrium-90, and indium-111 radioimmunoconjugates by cancer cells. *Cancer Res*, 1996. 56(9): p. 2123–9.

44. Wilder, R.B., DeNardo, G.L., and DeNardo, S.J. Radioimmunotherapy: recent results and future directions. *J Clin Oncol*, 1996. 14(4): p. 1383–400.

45. Humm, J.L. and Chin, L.M. A model of cell inactivation by alpha-particle internal emitters. *Radiat Res*, 1993. 134(2): p. 143–50.

46. Zalutsky, M.R. and Pozzi, O.R. Radioimmunotherapy with alpha-particle emitting radionuclides. *Q J Nucl Med Mol Imaging*, 2004. 48(4): p. 289–96.

47. Zhang, M., Yao, Z., Garmestani, K., et al., Pretargeting radioimmunotherapy of a murine model of adult T-cell leukemia with the alpha-emitting radionuclide, bismuth 213. *Blood*, 2002. 100(1): p. 208–16.

48. McDevitt, M.R., Ma, D., Lai, L.T., et al., Tumor therapy with targeted atomic nanogenerators. *Science*, 2001. 294(5546): p. 1537–40.

49. Macklis, R.M., Kaplan, W.D., Ferrara, J.L., et al., Biodistribution studies of anti-Thy 1.2 IgM immunoconjugates: implications for radioimmunotherapy. *Int J Radiat Oncol Biol Phys*, 1988. 15(2): p. 383–9.

50. Couturier, O., Supiot, S., Degraef-Mougin, M., et al., Cancer radioimmunotherapy with alpha-emitting nuclides. *Eur J Nucl Med Mol Imaging*, 2005. 32(5): p. 601–14.

51. Chen, P., Wang, J., Hope, K., et al., Nuclear localizing sequences promote nuclear translocation and enhance the radiotoxicity of the anti-CD33 monoclonal antibody HuM195 labeled with 111In in human myeloid leukemia cells. *J Nucl Med*, 2006. 47(5): p. 827–36.

52. Kersemans, V., Cornelissen, B., Minden, M.D., et al., Drug-resistant AML cells and primary AML specimens are killed by 111In-anti-CD33 monoclonal antibodies modified with nuclear localizing peptide sequences. *J Nucl Med*, 2008. 49(9): p. 1546–54.

53. Ali, S.A., Warren, S.D., Richter, K.Y., et al., Improving the tumor retention of radioiodinated antibody: aryl carbohydrate adducts. *Cancer Res*, 1990. 50(4): p. 1243–50.

54. Nemecek, E.R., Hamlin, D.K., Fisher, D.R., et al., Biodistribution of yttrium-90-labeled anti-CD45 antibody in a nonhuman primate model. *Clin Cancer Res*, 2005. 11(2 Pt 1): p. 787–94.

55. Burke, J.M., Caron, P.C., Papadopoulos, E.B., et al., Cytoreduction with iodine-131-anti-CD33 antibodies before bone marrow transplantation for advanced myeloid leukemias. *Bone Marrow Transplant*, 2003. 32(6): p. 549–56.

56. Illidge, T.M., Bayne, M., Brown, N.S., et al., Phase 1/2 study of fractionated (131)I-rituximab in low-grade B-cell lymphoma: the effect of prior rituximab dosing and tumor burden on subsequent radioimmunotherapy. *Blood*, 2009. 113(7): p. 1412–21.

57. Bianco, J.A., Sandmaier, B., Brown, P.A., et al., Specific marrow localization of an 131I-labeled anti-myeloid antibody in normal dogs: effects of a "cold" antibody pretreatment dose on marrow localization. *Exp Hematol*, 1989. 17(9): p. 929–34.

267

58. Matthews, D.C., Appelbaum, F.R., Eary, J.F., *et al.*, Development of a marrow transplant regimen for acute leukemia using targeted hematopoietic irradiation delivered by 131I-labeled anti-CD45 antibody, combined with cyclophosphamide and total body irradiation. *Blood*, 1995. 85(4): p. 1122–31.

59. Glatting, G., Muller, M., Koop, B., *et al.*, Anti-CD45 monoclonal antibody YAML568: A promising radioimmunoconjugate for targeted therapy of acute leukemia. *J Nucl Med*, 2006. 47(8): p. 1335–41.

60. Fisher, D.R., Internal dosimetry for systemic radiation therapy. *Semin Radiat Oncol*, 2000. 10(2): p. 123–32.

61. Rajendran, J.G., Fisher, D.R., Gopal, A.K., *et al.*, High-dose I-131 tositumomab (anti-CD20) radioimmunotherapy for Non-Hodgkin's Lymphoma: Adjusting radiation absorbed dose to actual organ volumes. *J. Nucl Med*, 2004. 45(6):1059–64.

62. Carrasquillo, J.A., Pandit-Taskar, N., O'Donoghue, J.A., *et al.*, (124)I-huA33 antibody PET of colorectal cancer. *J Nucl Med*, 2011. 52(8): p. 1173–80.

63. Mulford, D.A., Scheinberg, D.A., and Jurcic, J.G. The promise of targeted {alpha}-particle therapy. *J Nucl Med*, 2005. 46(Suppl 1): p. 199S–204S.

64. Clift, R.A., Buckner, C.D., Appelbaum, F.R., *et al.*, Long-term follow-up of a randomized trial of two irradiation regimens for patients receiving allogeneic marrow transplants during first remission of acute myeloid leukemia. *Blood*, 1998. 92(4): 1455–6.

65. Knox, S.J., Levy, R., Miller, R.A., *et al.*, Determinants of the antitumor effect of radiolabeled monoclonal antibodies. *Cancer Res*, 1990. 50(16): p. 4935–40.

66. Wessels, B.W., Vessella, R.L., Palme, D.F., *et al.*, Radiobiological comparison of external beam irradiation and radioimmunotherapy in renal cell carcinoma xenografts. *Int J Radiat Oncol Biol Phys*, 1989. 17(6): p. 1257–63.

67. Fowler, J.F., Radiobiological aspects of low-dose rates in radioimmunotherapy. *Int J Radiat Oncol Biol Phys*, 1990. 18(5): p. 1261–9.

68. Johnson, T.A. and Press, O.W. Synergistic cytotoxicity of iodine-131-anti-CD20 monoclonal antibodies and chemotherapy for treatment of B-cell lymphomas. *Int J Cancer*, 2000. 85(1): p. 104–12.

69. Press, O.W., Eary, J.F., Appelbaum, F.R., *et al.*, Radiolabeled-antibody therapy of B-cell lymphoma with autologous bone marrow support [see comments]. *N Engl J Med*, 1993. 329(17): p. 1219–24.

70. Press, O.W., Eary, J.F., Appelbaum, F.R., *et al.*, Phase II trial of 131I-B1 (anti-CD20) antibody therapy with autologous stem cell transplantation for relapsed B cell lymphomas. *Lancet*, 1995. 346(8971): p. 336–40.

71. Gopal, A.K., Rajendran, J.G., Gooley, T.A., *et al.*, High-dose [131] tositumomab (anti-CD20) radioimmunotherapy and autologous hematopoietic stem-cell transplantation for adults > or = 60 years old with relapsed or refractory B-cell lymphoma. *J Clin Oncol*, 2007. 25(11): p. 1396–402.

72. Berger, M.D., Branger, G., Klaeser, B., *et al.*, Zevalin and BEAM (Z-BEAM) versus rituximab and BEAM (R-BEAM) conditioning chemotherapy prior to autologous stem cell transplantation in patients with mantle cell lymphoma. *Hematol Oncol*, 2015. doi: 10.1002/hon.2197.

73. Shimoni, A., Avivi, I., Rowe, J.M., *et al.*, A randomized study comparing yttrium-90 ibritumomab tiuxetan (Zevalin) and high-dose BEAM chemotherapy *versus* BEAM alone as the conditioning regimen before autologous stem cell transplantation in patients with aggressive lymphoma. *Cancer*, 2012. 118(19): p. 4706–14.

74. Vose, J.M., Carter, S., Burns, L.J., *et al.*, Phase III randomized study of rituximab/carmustine, etoposide, cytarabine, and melphalan (BEAM) compared with iodine-131 tositumomab/BEAM with autologous hemtopoietic cell transplantation for relapsed diffuse large B-cell lymphoma: results from the BMT CTN 0401 trial. *J Clin Oncol*, 2013. 31(13): p. 1662–8.

75. Gopal, A.K., Guthrie, K.A., Rajendran, J., *et al.*, 90Y-Ibritumomab tiuxetan, fludarabine, and TBI-based nonmyeloablative allogeneic transplantation conditioning for patients with persistent high-risk B-cell lymphoma. *Blood*, 2011. 118(4): p. 1132–9.

76. Bethge, W.A., Wilbur, D.S., and Sandmaier, B.M. Radioimmunotherapy as non-myeloablative conditioning for allogeneic marrow transplantation. *Leuk Lymphoma*, 2006. 47(7): p. 1205–14.

77. Appelbaum, F.R., Matthews, D.C., Eary, J.F., *et al.*, The use of radiolabeled anti-CD33 antibody to augment marrow irradiation prior to marrow transplanatation for acute myelogenous leukemia. *Transplantation*, 1992. 54(5): p. 829–33.

78. Pagel, J.M., Appelbaum, F.R., Eary, J.F., *et al.*, 131I-anti-CD45 antibody plus busulfan and cyclophosphamide before allogeneic hemtopoietic cell transplantation for treatment of acute myeloid leukemia in first remission. *Blood*, 2006. 107(5): p. 2184–91.

79. Pagel, J.M., Gooley, T.A., Rajendran, J., *et al.* Allogeneic hemtopoietic cell transplantation after conditioning with 131I-anti-CD45 antibody plus fludarabine and low-dose total body irradiation for elderly patients with advanced acute myeloid leukemia or high-risk myelodysplastic syndrome. *Blood*, 2009. 114(27): p. 5444–53.

80. Mawad, R., Gooley, T.A., Rajendran, J., *et al.*, Radiolabeled-anti-CD45 antibody with reduced-intensity conditioning and allogeneic transplantation for younger patients with advanced acute myeloid leukemia or myelodysplastic syndrome. *Biol Blood Marrow Transplant*, 2014. 20(9): p. 1363–8.

81. Klein, S.A., Hermann, S., Dietrich, J.W., *et al.*, Transplantation-related toxicity and acute intestinal graft-*versus*-host disease after conditioning regimens intensified with Rhenium 188-labeled anti-CD66 monoclonal antibodies. *Blood*, 2002. 99(6): p. 2270-1.

82. Ringhoffer, M., Blumstein, N., Neumaier, B., *et al.*, 118Re or 90Y-labelled anti-CD66 antibody as part of a dose-reduced conditioning regimen for patients with acute leukemia or myelodysplastic syndrome over the age of 55: results of a phase I-II study. *Br J Haematol*, 2005. 130(4): p. 604–13.

83. Koenecke, C., Hofmann, M., Bolte, O., *et al.*, Radioimmunotherapy with [(188) Re]-labelled anti-CD66 antibody in the conditioning for allogeneic stem cell transplantation for high-risk acute myeloid leukemia. *Int J Hematol*, 2008. 87(4): p. 414–21.

84. Grossbard, M.L., Press, O.W., Applebaum, F.R., *et al.*, Monoclonal

antibody-based therapies of leukemia and lymphoma. *Blood*, 1992. 80(4): p. 863–78.

85. Waldmann, T.A., White, J.D., Carrasquillo, J.A., *et al.*, Radioimmunotherapy of interleukin-2R alpha-expressing adult T-cell leukemia with Yttrium-90-labeled anti-Tac. *Blood*, 1995. 86(11): p. 4063–75.

86. Waldmann, T.A., Daclizumab (anti-Tac, Zenapax) in the treatment of leukemia/lymphoma. *Oncogene*, 2007. 26(25): p. 3699–703.

87. Zhang, M., Yao, Z., Zhang, Z., *et al.*, The anti-CD25 monoclonal antibody 7G7/B6, armed with the alpha-emitter 211At, provides effective radioimmunotherapy for a murine model of leukemia. *Cancer Res*, 2006. 66(16): p. 8227–32.

88. Zhang, M., Yao, Z., Patel, H., *et al.*, Effective therapy of murine models of human leukemia and lymphoma with radiolabeled anti-CD30 antibody, HeFi-1. *Proc Natl Acad Sci U S A*, 2007. 104(20): p. 8444–8.

89. Alinari, L., Lapalombella, R., Andritsos, L., *et al.*, Alemtuzumab (Campath-1H) in the treatment of chronic lymphocytic leukemia. *Oncogene*, 2007. 26(25): p. 3644–53.

90. Tam, C.S. and Keating, M.J. Chemoimmunotherapy of chronic lymphocytic leukemia. *Best Pract Res Clin Haematol*, 2007. 20(3): p. 479–98.

91. Robak, T., Recent progress in the management of chronic lymphocytic leukemia. *Cancer Treat Rev*, 2007. 33(8): p. 710–28.

92. De Decker, M., Bacher, K., Thierens, H., *et al.*, In vitro and in vivo evaluation of direct rhenium-188-labeled anti-CD52 monoclonal antibody alemtuzumab for radioimmunotherapy of B-cell chronic lymphocytic leukemia. *Nucl Med Biol*, 2008. 35(5): p. 599–604.

93. Mavromatis, B. and Cheson, B.D., Monoclonal antibody therapy of chronic lymphocytic leukemia. *J Clin Oncol*, 2003. 21(9): p. 1874–81.

94. Cheson, B.D., Monoclonal antibody therapy of chronic lymphocytic leukemia. *Cancer Immunol Immunother*, 2006. 55(2): p. 188–96.

95. Witzig, T.E., Tomblyn, M.B., Misleh, J.G., *et al.*, Anti-CD22 90Y-epratuzumab tetraxetan combined with anti-CD20 veltuzumab: a phase I study in patients with relapsed/refractory,

aggressive non-Hodgkin lymphoma. *Haematologica*, 2014. 99(11): p. 1738–45.

96. Friesen, C., Glatting, G., Koop, B., *et al.*, Breaking chemoresistance and radioresistance with [213Bi]anti-CD45 antibodies in leukemia cells. *Cancer Res*, 2007. 67(5): p. 1950–8.

97. Vandenbulcke, K., Thierens, H., De Vos, F., *et al.*, In vitro screening for synergism of high-linear energy transfer 213Bi radiotherapy with other therapeutic agents for the treatment of B-cell chronic lymphocytic leukemia. *Cancer Biother Radiopharm*, 2006. 21(4): p. 364–72.

98. Scheinberg, D.A. and McDevitt, M.R. Actinium-225 in targeted alpha-particle therapeutic applications. *Curr Radiopharm*, 2011. 4(4): p. 306–20.

99. Ma, D., McDevitt, M.R., Barendswaard, E., *et al.*, Radioimmunotherapy for model B cell malignancies using 90Y-labeled anti-CD19 and anti-CD20 monoclonal antibodies. *Leukemia*, 2002. 16(1): p. 60–6.

100. Vallera, D.A., Elson, M., Brechbiel, M.W., *et al.*, Radiotherapy of CD19 expressing Daudi tumors in nude mice with Yttrium-90-labeled anti-CD19 antibody. *Cancer Biother Radiopharm*, 2004. 19(1): p. 11–23.

101. Vallera, D.A., Brechbiel, M.W., Burns, L.J., *et al.*, Radioimmunotherapy of CD22-expressing Daudi tumors in nude mice with a 90Y-labeled anti-CD22 monoclonal antibody. *Clin Cancer Res*, 2005. 11(21): p. 7920–8.

102. Wesley, J.N., McGee, E.C., Garmestani, K., *et al.*, Systemic radioimmunotherapy using a monoclonal antibody, anti-Tac directed toward the alpha subunit of the IL-2 receptor armed with the alpha-emitting radionuclides (212)Bi or (211)At. *Nucl Med Biol*, 2004. 31(3): p. 357–64.

103. Vandenbulcke, K., DeVos, F., Offner, F., *et al.*, In vitro evaluation of 213Bi-rituximab *versus* external gamma irradiation for the treatment of B-CLL patients: relative biological efficacy with respect to apoptosis induction and chromosomal damage. *Eur J Nucl Med Mol Imaging*, 2003. 30(10): p. 1357–64.

104. Michel, R.B., Andrews, P.M., Rosario, A.V., *et al.*, 177Lu-antibody conjugates for single-cell kill of B-lymphoma cells in vitro and for therapy of micrometastases in vivo. *Nucl Med Biol*, 2005. 32(3): p. 269–78.

105. Postema, E.J., Frielink, C., Oyen, W.J., *et al.*, Biodistribution of 131I-, 186Re-, 177Lu-, and 88Y-labeled hLL2 (Epratuzumab) in nude mice with CD22-positive lymphoma. *Cancer Biother Radiopharm*, 2003. 18(4): p. 525–33.

106. Press, O.W., Corcoran, M., Subbiah, K., *et al.*, A comparative evaluation of conventional and pretargeted radioimmunotherapy of CD20-expressing lymphoma xenografts. *Blood*, 2001. 98(8): p. 2535–43.

107. Pagel, J.M., Lin, Y., Hedin, N., *et al.*, Comparison of a tetravalent single-chain antibody-strepavidin fusion protein and an antibody-streptavidin chemical conjugate for pretargeted anti-CD20 radioimmunotherapy of B-cell lymphomas. *Blood*, 2006. 108(1): p. 328–36.

108. Axworthy, D.B., Reno, J.M., Hylarides, M.D., *et al.*, Cure of human carcinoma xenografts by a single dose of pretargeted yttrium-90 with negligible toxicity. *Proc Natl Acad Sci U S A*, 2000. 97(4): p. 1802–7.

109. Forero, A., Weiden, P.L., Vose, J.M., *et al.*, Phase 1 trial of a novel anti-CD20 fusion protein in pretargeted radioimmunotherapy for B-cell non-Hodgkin lymphoma. *Blood.*, 2004. 104(1): p. 227–36. Epub 2004 Mar 2.

110. Forero-Torres, A., Shen, S., Breitz, H., *et al.*, Pretargeted radioimmunotherapy (RIT) with a novel anti-TAG-72 fusion protein. *Cancer Biother Radiopharm*, 2005. 20(4): p. 379–90.

111. Knox, S.J., Goris, M.L., Tempero, M., *et al.*, Phase II trial of yttrium-90-DOTA-biotin pretargeted by NR-LU-10 antibody/streptavidin in patients with metastatic colon cancer. *Clin Cancer Res*, 2000. 6(2): p. 406–14.

112. Linden, O., Kurkus, J., Garkavij, M., *et al.*, A novel platform for radioimmunotherapy: extracorporeal depletion of biotinylated and 90Y-labeled rituximab in patients with refractory B-cell lymphoma. *Cancer Biother Radiopharm*, 2005. 20(4): p. 457–66.

113. Moghimi, S.M., Hunter, A.C., and Murray, J.C., Long-circulating and target-specific nanoparticles: theory to practice. *Pharmacol Rev*, 2001. 53(2): p. 283–318.

114. Zhang, H., Burnum, K.E., Luna, M.L., *et al.*, Quantitative proteomics analysis

of adsorbed plasma proteins classifies nanoparticles with different surface properties and size. *Proteomics*, 2011. 11(23): p. 4569–77.

115. Torchilin, V.P., Multifunctional nanocarriers. *Adv Drug Deliv Rev*, 2006. 58(14): p. 1532–55.

116. Alexis, F., Pridgen, E., Molnar, L.K., *et al.*, Factors affecting the clearance and biodistribution of polymeric nanoparticles. *Mol Pharm*, 2008. 5(4): p. 505–15.

117. Fang, C., Shi, B., Pei, Y.Y., *et al.*, In vivo tumor targeting of tumor necrosis factor-alpha-loaded stealth nanoparticles: effect of MePEG molecular weight and particle size. *Eur J Pharm Sci*, 2006. 27(1): p. 27–36.

118. Cole, A.J., David, A.E., Wang, J., *et al.*, Magnetic brain tumor targeting and biodistribution of long-circulating PEG-modified, cross-linked starch-coated iron oxide nanoparticles. *Biomaterials*, 2011. 32(26): p. 6291–301.

119. Goncalves, C., Torrado, E., Martins, T., *et al.*, Dextrin nanoparticles: studies on the interaction with murine macrophages and blood clearance.

Colloids Surf B Biointerfaces, 2010. 75(2): p. 483–9.

120. Karmali, P.P., Chao, Y., Park, J.H., *et al.*, Different effect of hydrogelation on antifouling and circulation properties of dextran-iron oxide nanoparticles. *Mol Pharm*, 2012. 9(3): p. 539–45.

121. Bartlett, D.W., Su, H., Hildebrandt, I.J., *et al.*, Impact of tumor-specific targeting on the biodistribution and efficacy of siRNA nanoparticles measured by multimodality in vivo imaging. *Proc Natl Acad Sci U S A*, 2007. 104(39): p. 15549–54.

122. Henriksen, G., Schoultz, B.W., Michaelsen, T.E., *et al.*, Sterically stabilized liposomes as a carrier for alpha-emitting radium and actinium radionuclides. *Nucl Med Biol*, 2004. 31(4): p. 441–9.

123. Jonasdottir, T.J., Fisher, D.R., Borrebaek, J., *et al.*, First in vivo evaluation of liposome-encapsulated 223Ra as a potential alpha-particle-emitting cancer therapeutic agent. *Anticancer Res*, 2006. 26(4B): p. 2841–8.

124. van Vlerken, L.E., Vyas, T.K., and Amiji, M.M. Poly(ethylene glycol)-

modified nanocarriers for tumor-targeted and intracellular delivery. *Pharm Res*, 2007. 24(8): p. 1405–14.

125. Kommareddy, S. and Amiji, M. Biodistribution and pharmacokinetic analysis of long-circulating thiolated gelatin nanoparticles following systemic administration in breast cancer-bearing mice. *J Pharm Sci*, 2007. 96(2): p. 397–407.

126. DeNardo, G.L., Hok, S., Van Natarajan, A., *et al.*, Characteristics of dimeric (bis) bidentate selective high affinity ligands as HLA-DR10 beta antibody mimics targeting non-Hodgkin's lymphoma. *Int J Oncol*, 2007. 31(4): p. 729–40.

127. Balhorn, R., Hok, S., Burke, P.A., *et al.*, Selective high-affinity ligand antibody mimics for cancer diagnosis and therapy: initial application to lymphoma/leukemia. *Clin Cancer Res*, 2007. 13(18 Pt 2): p. 5621s–5628s.

128. DeNardo, G.L., Kukis, D.L., DeNardo, S.J., *et al.*, Enhancement of 67Cu-2IT-BAT-LYM-1 therapy in mice with human Burkitt's lymphoma (Raji) using interleukin-2. *Cancer*, 1997. 80(12 Suppl): p. 2576–82.

29 T-Cell Depletion in Allogeneic Hematopoietic Cell Transplantation: Results, Barriers, and Future Directions

Robert J. Soiffer

Introduction

Acute and chronic graft-*versus*-host disease (GvHD) causes significant morbidity after allogeneic hematopoietic cell transplant (allo-HCT) and contributes to mortality either as a direct result of tissue damage or as a consequence of infectious complications prompted by immune suppressive therapy[1]. The central role of donor T-cells in the pathogenesis of GvHD has been recognized for over 40 years. Traditional pharmacologic approaches with calcineurin inhibitors (CNIs) target T-cell functional activity without necessarily reducing T-cell number. T-cell depletion (TCD), either by eliminating donor T-cells via *ex-vivo* graft manipulation or *in-vivo* T-cell destruction, offers the potential for prevention of GvHD often without the need for immune suppressive agents. The efficacy of TCD in experimental animal models in the 1970s spawned a plethora of clinical trials in the 1980s which demonstrated that TCD could substantially limit GvHD. However, in many of these early studies, the reduction in GvHD came at the price of unanticipated high rates of graft failure[2], EBV-associated lymphoproliferative disorders (EBV-LPD)[3], and disease recurrence with TCD[4,5]. Few prospective randomized studies evaluating TCD have been conducted and have not demonstrated a survival advantage[6]. TCD strategies have their strong proponents trumpeting the beneficial impact on chronic GvHD (cGvHD) and long-term quality of life as well as firm detractors who focus on several decades old reports of increased relapse rates. These supporters and opponents hold on to their beliefs often with intense passion.

The title of this chapter, "T-Cell Depletion in Allogeneic Hematopoietic Cell Transplants: Results, Barriers, and Future Directions," poses a question that cannot be answered in a blanket manner. Variables such as disease histology, disease stage, graft source, conditioning intensity, extent of TCD, and specificity of TCD all likely influence the impact of "TCD" on allo-HCT outcome (Table 29.1). This chapter will attempt to lend some perspective to the issue by presenting data that will allow the reader to draw his or her own conclusions on the matter.

Methodologies for TCD

A variety of TCD methodologies have been utilized since the introduction of this strategy, including *ex-vivo negative selection* approaches (e.g., monoclonal antibody ± complement, elutriation, lectin agglutination, or photodepletion), *ex-vivo positive selection* with CD34+ columns, or *in-vivo* administration of anti-T-cell antibody preparations such as antithymocyte globulin (ATG) and alemtuzumab (see Chapter 30). In some protocols, these strategies have been combined. Regulatory issues and other practical concerns have limited the number of approaches currently in use. There have been very few attempts to directly compare these different TCD methods to each other, though one study demonstrated no difference in outcomes of CD34+ selection *versus* alemtuzumab-based TCD in HLA haplotype mismatched transplantation[7] (see Chapters 59 and 61).

How important Is Extent and Specificity of TCD?

The TCD methods vary in the number of T-cells removed and the specific T-cells targeted. Limiting dilution assays suggest that at least a 2-log depletion of T-cells to 1×105 cells/kg is necessary to significantly reduce GvHD in an HLA-identical related bone marrow allo-HCT without resultant immune suppression[8,9]. The extent of TCD needed to prevent GvHD likely depends not only on T-cell burden, but also on donor source, type of graft, degree of major and minor HLA disparity, and polymorphisms in immune response genes present in donor and recipient pairs. G-CSF mobilized blood hematopoietic cell products contain approximately 10-fold more T-cells than bone marrow grafts. Consequently, methods removing only 2 logs of T-cells would likely be insufficient for GvHD prevention in peripheral blood (PB) grafts. CD34+ selection (positive selection) of peripheral blood progenitor cells (PBPCs) with a 3–4 log reduction in CD3+ count below 1×10^5 cells/kg is associated with low rates of GvHD in matched sibling transplantation[10]. The T-cell threshold to accomplish the desired benefit in persons receiving unrelated or HLA haplotype mismatched hematopoietic cell products may be considerably lower.

Other graft components may impact TCD allo-HCT outcomes as well. A report of persons receiving mobilized PB indicated that higher numbers of CD34+ cells were associated with lower nonrelapse mortality (NRM), improved overall survival (OS), and improved disease-free survival (DFS) after TCD, but not T-cell-replete, allo-HCT[11]. Natural killer (NK) cells (see Chapter 63), B-cells, and dendritic cells all play a role

Table 29.1 Studies and impact of T-cell depletion on transplant outcomes

TCD technique	*Ex vivo* negative selection TCD	*In vivo* TCD with ATG-Fresenius	*Ex vivo* positive selection TCD	*In vivo* TCD with ATG or alemtuzumab	*In vivo* TCD with ATG or alemtuzumab
Study design	Prospective randomized trial	Prospective randomized trial	Prospective contemporaneous trials	Retrospective registry analyses	Retrospective registry analyses
Patient population	Unrelated myeloablative BMT (Wagner *et al.*, 2005)[6]	Unrelated myeloablative BMT (Finke *et al.*, 2009)[52]	Related myeloablative PB-HCT (AML only) (Pasquini *et al.*, 2012)[30]	Related/Unrelated RIC HCT (Soiffer *et al.*, 2011)[64]	Related/Unrelated RIC HCT (AML only) (Baron *et al.*, 2012)[65]
Engraftment	No impact	No impact	No impact	Delayed ATG only	Not reported
Acute GvHD	Lower Gr 3-4	Lower Gr 2-4	Lower Gr 3-4	Lower Gr 2-4 Alemtuzumab only	Not reported
Extensive chronic GvHD	No impact	Lower	Lower	Lower ATG and alemtuzumab	Lower ATG and alemtuzumab
Non relapse mortality	No impact	No impact	No impact	TCD higher ATG only	No impact
Relapse	Higher CML No impact AML	No impact	No impact	TCD inferior ATG and alemtuzumab	TCD inferior ATG and alemtuzumab
Progression-free survival	No impact	No impact	No impact	TCD inferior ATG and alemtuzumab	TCD inferior Alemtuzumab only
Overall survival	No impact	No impact	No impact	TCD inferior ATG only	TCD inferior Alemtuzumab only

in immune surveillance, engraftment, and elimination of residual disease post-allo-HCT. TCD strategies can differ in their selectivity. One retrospective study formally analyzed the breadth of cellular specificity among TCD methods. The Center for International Blood and Marrow Transplant Research (CIBMTR) compared negative selection TCD techniques with "narrow" and "broad" spectra of reactivity in alternative donor bone marrow transplantation. Narrow specificity antibodies targeted mature T-cells only, such as anti-CD6, anti-CD5, or anti-CD8, whereas broad-specificity techniques included antibodies such as CAMPATH (anti-CD52), multiple antibody combinations, and physical separation techniques such as elutriation or lectin agglutination. Patients who received TCD marrow using narrow specificity antibodies had a superior 5-year leukemia-free survival (LFS) compared to those receiving broad-specificity depletion, due to a combination of increased relapse, graft failure, and transplant-related mortality (TRM) in the broad-specificity TCD cohort[12]. Selective CD8+ TCD had attracted particular interest as early recovery of CD8+ T-cells after allo-HCT is associated with subsequent development of GvHD[13]. A prospective randomized trial in HLA-matched related donor bone marrow graft suggested that CD8+ depletion with post-transplant cyclosporine alone could reduce the incidence and severity of GvHD without compromising GvL[14]. However, results of CD8+ depletion of mobilized PBPCs achieving a 2-log reduction have been disappointing, particularly in

the HLA-matched unrelated allo-HCT setting[15]. CD8+ TCD of donor lymphocyte infusions (see Chapter 25) has been used successfully after TCD allo-HCT as a prophylactic and therapeutic strategy for disease relapse and for falling donor T-cell chimerism[16,17]. In these uncontrolled studies, low relapse rates were noted in the absence of significant GvHD. Large-scale randomized trials to confirm impact of removal of CD8+ T-cells have not been conducted.

Ex-vivo TCD Strategies

Ex-vivo Negative Selection TCD: What Are the Data?

Early phase 2 trials of ex-vivo negative selection TCD with monoclonal antibodies plus complement or immunotoxins, which removed 2–3 logs of T-lymphocytes, decreased the incidence of GvHD to 10–20% after HLA-matched related donor bone marrow even in the absence of post-transplant immune suppression[18–20]. Addition of anti-CD52 antibody directly to the hematopoietic cell product as it is being infused (CAMPATH "in the bag") also resulted in a low incidence of GvHD [21]. Physical separation techniques with E-rosetting/soybean lectin agglutination, or counterflow centrifugal elutriation similarly yielded a substantial reduction in GvHD[9,21,22]. When unrelated donor transplants were initiated in the 1990s, the National Marrow Donor Program (NMDP) reported TCD was the most significant factor predicting freedom from severe (grade III–IV) acute GvHD (aGvHD)[23]. A subsequent analysis from the CIBMTR involving 1868 leukemia patients receiving *bone marrow* grafts from donors other than HLA-identical siblings revealed that the grade II–IV aGvHD incidence was 34% compared to 57% for the TCD and non-TCD cohort, respectively (P <0.0001)[12]. While TCD did appear to reduce aGvHD in unrelated marrow recipients, rates were not as low as those observed in the matched related donor setting. A large prospective trial in 410 unrelated BMT randomized recipients to receive either TCD bone marrow (by the monoclonal antibody $T_{10}B_9$ or counterflow centrifugal elutriation) with post-transplant cyclosporine alone *versus* T-cell-replete bone marrow with post-transplant cyclosporine and methotrexate[6]. Patients received cyclophosphamide and TBI for conditioning regimen; persons in the TCD arm received additional treatment to promote engraftment: ATG in the elutriation group and cytarabine in the $T_{10}B_9$ antibody group. Mean T-cell dose infused for the TCD was only 1 log lower than in the non-TCD arm. Primary graft failure (PGF) was similar in the two groups. Grades II–IV aGvHD was lower in the TCD arms (39% *versus* 63%, $P<0.0001$), as were rates of grades III–IV aGvHD (18% *versus* 37%, respectively, $P<0.0001$). Regimen-related toxicity was lower in the TCD arm. There was no difference in relapse rates in patients with acute leukemia whereas patients with CML were more much likely to relapse if they received TCD bone marrow. CMV infection rates were higher in the TCD group. The NRM, DFS, and OS at 3 years were similar. It is noteworthy that a reduction in acute GvHD did not positively impact TRM or OS (see Chapters 12 and 13). This trial did not demonstrate a reduction in cGvHD. The 1-log reduction in T-cells achieved by the methods described above appeared to be insufficient to protect against cGvHD.

Ex-vivo CD34+ Cell "Positive Selection" TCD: Does It Decrease TRM or Improve OS?

When mobilized PBPCs emerged as the most common graft source for allo-HCT in adults, there also occurred a shift in the techniques employed for *ex-vivo* TCD. Regulatory and commercial obstacles curtailed the use of negative selection strategies, replaced in large part by *ex-vivo* CD34+ selection technology. Initial studies of HLA-identical sibling PBPCs HCT using *ex-vivo* CD34+ selection reported a wide variation in aGvHD incidenc[24,25]. A study comparing three devices (CEPRATE, Isolex 300i, CliniMACS) found no apparent differences in the allograft composition or clinical outcomes, although ease of processing did differ[26]. Initial studies using CD34 selection columns showed that a 2-log reduction in T-cells from HLA-matched related donor progenitors was insufficient to control GvHD despite the use of post-transplant immune suppression[24]. When the T-cell content in the sibling PBPC graft was reduced by 3–4 logs, grades II–IV aGvHD were only 10%[25]. Single-institution studies demonstrated very low rates of acute and chronic GvHD with CD34+

selection when combined with sheep erythrocyte resetting to deplete residual donor T-cells[27].

One of the challenges of *ex-vivo* TCD has been reproducibility at different centers. In 2005, the Blood and Marrow Clinical Trials Network (BMT CTN) launched a multicenter trial at eight sites of CD34+ cell positive selection as the sole form of GvHD prophylaxis in 44 patients receiving HLA-matched related donor in persons with AML[28]. All patients engrafted. The incidence of grade II–IV and Grade III–IV aGvHD was 23% and 5%, respectively, while the incidence of extensive cGvHD was 7% at 24 months. All products infused met the prespecified goal of less than 1×10^5 CD3+ cells/kg recipient body weight and greater than 2×10^7 CD34+ cells/kg [29]. Differences in processing outcomes between centers were minimal. These clinical outcomes were compared to those of 84 AML patients receiving T-replete HLA-matched related donor grafts and pharmacologic immune suppression therapy (treated on contemporaneous trials sponsored by the CTN [30]). The 100-day rates of grades II–IV aGvHD were 23% and 39% with TCD and pharmacologic prophylaxis, respectively ($P=0.07$). The 2-year rates of overall cGvHD were lower with TCD compared to T-replete grafts (19% *versus* 50%, $P<0.001$). There were no differences in rates of graft rejection or leukemia relapse in the two cohorts. The TRM, DFS, and OS rates were also similar in the two groups. At 1 year, 54% and 12% of patients were still on immunosuppression in the T-replete and TCD allo-HCT cohorts, respectively. TCD led to a higher GvHD-free survival at 2 years (41% *versus* 19%, respectively; $P=0.006$). Subsequently, a joint retrospective study from Memorial Sloan Kettering Cancer Center and MD Anderson Cancer Center examined outcomes transplants for persons with AML, where TCD was utilized at one and conventional GvHD prophylaxis at the other. The incidences of grades II–IV aGvHD and cGvHD were significantly lower in the TCD graft group (5% *versus* 18% and 13% *versus* 53%). Three-year relapse-free and OS rates were comparable in recipients[31]. These two studies suggest that, at least in AML, TCD by *ex-vivo* CD34+ selection in the absence of post-transplant immune suppressive therapy improves cGvHD-free survival without significantly increasing relapse rates. Again, despite this advantage, OS was not improved.

HLA Haplotype Mismatched Transplant: Where Do We Stand with TCD?

Early studies of TCD in HLA-mismatched bone marrow transplants resulted in reasonable GvHD control with rates ranging from 13% to 40%[32,33]. Unfortunately, overall outcome was compromised by increases in graft failure, infection, and relapse. Improved engraftment with haplotype-matched HCT has been achieved through infusion of "mega" doses of mobilized PB cells depleted of T-cells after CD34+ selection[34,35]. Among 60 acute leukemia patients who underwent haplotype-matched transplant with an intensive high-dose conditioning regimen (myeloablative) coupled with extensive TCD and no post-transplant immune suppression, only four cases of GvHD were observed [34]. Results were particularly favorable in persons with AML. An European Bone Marrow Transplant Group (EBMT) survey of 173 adults undergoing haplotype-matched HCT after exhaustive TCD also showed favorable results[36]. Immunologic analysis of these HLA-haplotype-matched extensively TCD transplants led to an appreciation of the role of NK cells and killer immuno-globulin receptors (KIRs) in allo-recognition and GvHD [34,37,38] (see Chapters 7, 8, 63, and 65). The most frequently encountered limitation of this extensive TCD approach has been immune incompetence and increased risk of fatal infections. Attempts to address this stumbling block have focused on infu-sions of conventional donor T-cells either alone, after photode-pletion, or in conjunction with regulatory T-cells, with promising results reported in single-institution studies[39,40]. An alterna-tive graft engineering approach for HLA haplotype mismatch donors removing $\alpha\beta$ T-cell receptor and CD19+ cells expressed on T- and B cells, respectively, has been reported in children resulting in very low rates of GvHD, though graft failure was noted in 4/23 patients[41].

The more recent use of post-transplant cyclophosphamide to eliminate alloreactive T-cells following HLA haplotype mis-match HCT using bone marrow infusion has been associated with relatively low rates of GvHD and encouraging survival in the absence of major infectious risks[42,43]. The comparative ease of this approach coupled with its promising results has challenged other HLA haplotype mismatch TCD strategies. No major comparative analyses have yet been reported (see Chap-ters 59 and 61).

In-vivo Anti-T-Cell Antibody: Is This the Answer for Better Outcomes?

Myeloablative Conditioning

While *ex-vivo* methods of TCD may allow engineering of graft with a precise T-cell dose, *in-vivo* administration of anti-T-cell antibodies yields a level of T-cell reduction that is much less predictable, owing to the variable half-lives of these antibody preparations, the doses of antibodies used, the administration schedule, and the number of T-cells contained in the donor graft. There have recently been four products in general use. Three of these are polyclonal anti-T-cell antibody preparations that have been labeled antithymocyte globulins (ATG). These products are all different and must be evaluated individually. Atgam is produced from horses inoculated with human thy-mocytes. Thymoglobulin is also directed against human thy-mocytes but is raised in rabbits. ATG-Fresenius (now Neovii), also rabbit derived, is actually not an antithymocyte prepar-ation but is directed against a *Jurkat* T-cell leukemia line. The antigens targeted and cells eliminated by these ATGs will vary depending on antibody preparation used[44]. Alemtuzumab is a monoclonal antibody directed against CD52+ antigen, which is broadly expressed on T-cells as well as other cellular elem-ents including B-cells and dendritic cells.

A number of comparative retrospective studies of *in-vivo* TCD have been conducted. Russell *et al.* reported in a matched pair analysis that at a total thymoglobulin dose of 4.5 mg/kg, acute and chronic GvHD rates were significantly lower com-pared to immune suppressive therapy alone in HLA-matched related graft recipients following "myeloablative" doses of busulfan/fludarabine. Thymoglobulin was associated with a lower NRM and higher relapse rate. The OS was superior (66% *versus* 50%, $P=0.046$) not ATG recipients[45]. This report is the only study that has shown a survival advantage for *in-vivo* TCD. The CIBMTR conducted a matched pair analysis of thymoglobulin use in patients receiving busulfan plus cyclophosphamide. ATG was associated with lower aGvHD rates, but not cGvHD rates. The NRM was lower but relapse higher in the ATG cohort; in this series there was no difference in survival[46]. Mohty *et al.* reported a retrospective "myeloablative" analysis with or without thymoglobulin in an adult cohort. ATG recipients did not have a statistically sig-nificant reduction of aGvHD though there was a dramatic decrease in cGvHD[47]. There was no impact on relapse, NRM, LFS, or OS. In single-institution series utilizing alemtuzumab, lower GvHD rates but higher infection and relapse rates have been observed with no difference in OS [48]. The CIBMTR compared pediatric ALL patients undergo-ing "myeloablative" HCT receiving ATG preparations (n= 191), alemtuzumab (n=131), or without *in-vivo* TCD (n= 392). Doses and origin of ATG preparations were not speci-fied. Both ATG and alemtuzumab were associated with lower rates of acute and chronic GvHD. There was no effect on NRM or relapse rates. In-vivo TCD did not improve event-free or overall survival[49].

Up until recently only a limited number of prospective randomized controlled trials have been conducted. Bacigalupo *et al.* compared cyclosporine/methotrexate to cyclosporine plus ATG (15 mg/kg in one study, 7.5 mg/kg in the other) in patients receiving HLA-matched unrelated bone marrow HCT. Only the higher dose of ATG was associated with a significant reduction in grades III–IV aGvHD. However, this reduction in severe aGvHD did not improve outcomes because of a high rate of deaths from infections on the higher dose ATG[50]. However, there was a reduction in cGvHD for those receiving ATG with a reduction in long-term pulmonary complications and late deaths[51]. The largest reported prospective random-ized trial of *in-vivo* TCD compared patients randomized to conventional pharmacologic GvHD prophylaxis alone to those randomized to immune suppression plus ATG-Fresenius at a total dose of 60 mg/kg. Lower grades II–IV aGvHD (33% *versus* 51%, CI 25.1–43.5, $P=0.011$) and Grade II–IV rates (11.7% *versus* 24.5%, CI 0.25–1.01, $P=0.054$) were noted in the ATG-F group. Extensive cGvHD incidence was also lower (12.2% *versus* 42.6%, CI 0.10–0.39, $P<0.0001$). Relapse rates, NRM, DFS, and OS were not significantly different in the two groups [52]. Immune suppression free survival was markedly superior for the ATG-F group (16.9% *versus* 52.9%, CI 0.18–0.55, P< 0.000)[53]. It is interesting that some investigators have suggested that ATG-Fresenius, since it was raised against a tumor cell line, may have antitumor activity, including induction of antibody-dependent cell cytotoxicity (ADCC, complement-dependent cytotoxicity, and apoptosis, towards different hematologic malignancies[54]. As of 2014, two additional large prospective randomized trials have completed enrollment for an open-label trial assessing thymoglobulin in Canada and a blinded trial testing ATG-F in the United States and Australia. A preliminary report from the Canadian trial suggested an improvement in quality of life measures in patients receiving thymoglobulin[55]. If indeed survival differences are not marked, such quality of life assessments will be critical to assess value of ATG. Yu *et al.* previously demonstrated in a comparative series that ATG administration was associated not only with lower GvHD rates, but improved quality of life parameters[56].

Reduced Intensity Conditioning

The primary antitumor activity of reduced intensity conditioning (RIC) allogeneic HCT derives not from the cytotoxic effects of chemotherapy, but from the allo-immune effect of the donor cells. TCD in RIC regimen transplantation could conceptually defeat the entire purpose of the transplant if it substantially blunted the GvL effect. Nonetheless, both ATG and alemtuzumab have been used extensively to reduce GvHD in RIC allo-HCTs[57–59]. In a comparative analysis of two prospective, though not randomized, studies using either alemtuzumab/cyclosporine or cyclosporine/methotrexate as GvHD prophylaxis after RIC, there was a lower incidence of acute and cGvHD in patients receiving alemtuzumab, but more CMV reactivation and disease relapse/progression was observed[57]. However, long-term disease and overall-survival status were similar between the two cohorts when donor lymphocyte infusion (DLI) (see Chapter 25) was incorporated in the alemtuzumab arm. These data and others suggest that TCD can be used to induce a state of mixed chimerism with minimal GvHD, and provide a platform for additional adoptive immunotherapy interventions to bolster immune reactivity[17,60,61]. Lower levels of donor T-cell chimerism have been associated with higher relapse rates after RIC HCT[62] (see Chapter 27) and it may be necessary to build in strategies to increase donor T-cell recovery in this setting. When *ex-vivo* TCD has been studied in RIC HCT, both engraftment and disease relapse have been problems in the absence of additional donor lymphocyte infusion (see Chapter 25)[63].

Unfortunately, there has yet to be a large prospective randomized trial evaluating the consequence of *in-vivo* anti-T-cell antibody administration in RIC HCT. In a retrospective study, the CIBMTR examined 1676 adults undergoing RIC related and unrelated HCT for hematologic malignancies[64]. Outcomes after in-vivo TCD (n=584 ATG, n=213 alemtuzumab) were compared with T-cell-replete (n=879) transplantation. Engraftment was slightly inferior in recipients of ATG. GradesII to IV aGvHD were lower with alemtuzumab compared

with ATG or T-cell-replete regimens (19% *versus* 38% *versus* 40%, *P* < 0.0001). No CI for three-way comparison and chronic GvHD, lower with alemtuzumab and ATG regimens compared with T-replete approaches (24% *versus* 40% *versus* 52%, *P* < 0.0001). However, relapse was more frequent with alemtuzumab and ATG compared with T cell-replete regimens (49%, 51%, and 38%, respectively, *P* < 0.001). The DFS was lower with both alemtuzumab and ATG compared with T cell-replete regimens (30%, 25%, and 39%, respectively, *P* < 0.001). Probabilities of overall survival were 50%, 38%, and 46%, lower for ATG recipients (*P* = 0.008). The EBMT conducted a similar analysis in 1859 AML patients undergoing RIC HCT[65]. In-vivo T-cell depletion with ATG or alemtuzumab was successful at preventing extensive chronic GvHD (*P* < 0.001), but without improving OS for ATG and in this series worsening OS for alemtuzumab (HR=0.65; *P*=0.001). Another EBMT report suggested that a dose of ATG > 6 mg/kg in RIC HCT increased risk of relapse in this setting whereas lower doses did not[66]. A smaller retrospective study from Germany examining patients receiving pharmacologic prophylaxis with or without ATG-Fresenius demonstrated lower GvHD rates and higher EBV reactivation rates but no statistically significant impact on relapse, NRM, or survival[67]. These collective data suggest adopting a cautious approach to *in-vivo* T-cell depletion with RIC regimens and emphasize the need for randomized controlled trials in the RIC setting.

ATG Dose and Serum Levels: Does It Matter?

Doses of *in-vivo* T-cell antibodies influence both GvHD incidence and immune reconstitution (see Chapter 22). Retrospective French series in HLA-matched related donors examining doses of 2.5, 5.0, and 7.5–10 mg/kg ATG demonstrated that higher doses were associated with lower rates of acute and chronic GvHD, but that did not translate into an improvement in LFS or OS[68,69]. Fewer comparative studies have been performed with other ATG preparations, but one study of ATG-Fresenius suggested equivalent GvHD control can be achieved with lower doses than in standard use (30 mg/kg *versus* 60 mg/kg) with a suggestion of lower NRM with lower dose[70]. One prospective randomized study directly comparing 6 and 10 mg/kg of thymoglobulin in haplotype-matched transplant resulted in higher EBV reactivation (see Chapter 20) and lower GvHD rates with the higher ATG dose but no survival differences[71].

ATG levels may be influenced by a variety of factors including dose, schedule of administration, and antibody clearance. Remberger and Sundberg studied rabbit IgG levels early after HLA-matched unrelated donor HCT and found a correlation between high levels and protection from aGvHD[72]. Podgorny *et al.* reported that low levels of ATG at day 7 and 28 correlated with increased GvHD while high levels were associated with the development of PTLD. ATG levels though did not impact relapse or OS[73]. After cord blood transplantation (CBT), low serum levels of thymoglobulin on day +11 were associated with higher rates of grade II–IV aGvHD, higher NRM, but a lower incidence of relapse[74]. Hoegh-Petersen *et al.* examined day-7 serum levels of ATG antibodies specific for particular lymphoid subsets and found high levels of antibodies with specificities for conventional T- and B-cells were associated with lower aGvHD and higher viral infection rates, without relation to relapse. High level of globulins with specificities for both Treg and invariant NK T-cells (see Chapter 63) were linked to lower relapse rates[75]. Reports from solid organ transplant recipients suggest that the presence of antibodies to rabbit-derived globulin in the serum accelerates clearance and results in a lower serum level of ATG. Pediatric patients that developed IgG anti-ATG antibodies before day +22 had rapid clearance of ATG which was associated with faster T-cell recovery and a higher rate of aGvHD[76].

Beyond GvHD: Organ Damage, Engraftment Immune Compromise, and GvL Effect

Organ Damage

Most retrospective analyses and prospective randomized trials have established that both *ex-vivo* and *in-vivo* TCD reduce the incidence of GvHD. Additionally, TCD has been associated with lower rates of pulmonary and hepatic toxicity[77–79]. In the largest prospective randomized study of TCD, Wagner *et al.*, reported TCD marrow recipients experienced less regimen-related toxicity within the first 28 days of transplant, including stomatitis ($P<0.0001$), hepatic ($P=0.0003$), pulmonary ($P=0.012$), and CNS complications ($P=0.024$)[6]. However, despite the reduction in GvHD and organ dysfunction, TCD has not clearly led to a decrease in TRM or improvements in OS. This disappointing observation has often been attributed, not always justifiably, to increases in graft failure, infection, and disease relapse.

Engraftment

Registry analysis from the CIBMTR in the early 1990s identified a significantly increased risk for graft failure in TCD recipients compared to unmanipulated bone marrow transplantation (relative risk 9.29, $P<0.0001$)[23]. Host T-lymphocytes with donor-specific activity have been isolated from the blood of patients at the time of graft rejection [80,81]. TCD may remove cells that are important for promoting engraftment. However, it remains uncertain what roles specific donor cells play in establishing and maintaining a graft. Graft failure has been much less commonly observed with recent studies of TCD mobilized PB HCT. In one report, all patients transplanted with CD34+ selected TCD HLA-matched sibling mobilized PBPCs engrafted after conditioning with fractionated TBI, thiotepa, and fludarabine without ATG, despite only receiving a median of 0.99×10^3 cells/kg[82]. Other recent series from the past decade have likewise reported low graft failure rates[27,28]. Strategies to combat rejection after HCT have included increasing host immune suppression

and intensification of the conditioning regimen[21,32,83]. Other approaches have included narrowing the spectrum of TCD, infusion of increasing doses of CD34+ cells in the graft, and administration of DLI after HCT. There are no sizable randomized data available to support the use of any of these interventions.

Immune Compromise

Immune reconstitution (see Chapter 22) is delayed after *ex-vivo* T-cell depletion[84–87]. In general, total lymphocyte counts are lower in recipients of TCD grafts. Prolonged inversion of CD4+/CD8+ ratios are observed with delays in CD4+ T-cell recovery. The number of T-cells with memory phenotypes is decreased. Proliferative responses of PBPCs to mitogenic stimuli are impaired for a longer period[84]. T-lymphocytes from recipients of TCD-HCT have restricted variability in their T-cell receptor repertoires limiting the breadth of potential cellular responses[85]. Decreased numbers of thymic emigrants measured by TREC analysis post-TCD-HCT indicate impaired capacity to generate new T-cells [87,86]. Comparative studies on immune reconstitution after *in-vivo* TCD with ATG administration have demonstrated high ATG levels associated with slower T-cell, but more rapid B-cell and NK cell recovery[88]. Delayed immune reconstitution place TCD-HCT recipients at increased risk for opportunistic infections. CMV and EBV reactivation and adenovirus infections (see Chapter 17) occur more frequently after TCD transplants and in recipients of *in-vivo* anti-T-cell antibodies [57–59,89]. Higher incidences of severe CMV (28% *versus* 17%, $P=0.02$) and life-threatening *Aspergillus* (16% *versus* 7%, $P=0.01$) infections were observed in the patients receiving TCD compared to pharmacologic GvHD prophylaxis[6,90] though the overall rate of fatal infections did not differ between the TCD and T-replete arms in the randomized trial reported by Wagner *et al.* Recipients of CBT (see Chapters 60 and 61) appear to be at higher risk for EBV reactivation and PTLD if they are conditioned with a regimen that includes ATG[91,92]. Strategies to treat EBV reactivation have included rituximab [93,94] (see Chapter 20), DLI[95] (see Chapter 25), and EBV-specific cytotoxic T-cells[96] (see Chapter 64). The production of virus-specific T-lymphocytes with the capacity to recognize CMV, EBV, and adenovirus but without alloreactive potential is being studied in both the therapeutic and prophylactic settings[97,98] (see Chapter 64). Other strategies to accelerate recovery of T-cell immunity after TCD-HCT include attempts to improve thymic function through administration of interleukin-7 and LHRH antagonists and [99,100].

Graft-*versus*-Leukemia Effect

The major objection of detractors when discussing TCD is their fear of loss of GvL activity. In early studies of patients receiving HLA-matched sibling BMT for first chronic phase CML (see Chapter 36), the risk of relapse with TCD has been estimated to be 5- to 6-fold higher than conventional transplantation[4,5]. The incremental risk of relapse is less marked after TCD unrelated bone marrow transplant[101]. A study from the EBMT demonstrated that in patients with CML who received HLA-matched unrelated bone marrow transplant, TCD was not associated with a higher incidence of relapse in the multivariate analysis[102]. However, in the large US multicenter randomized trial in unrelated bone marrow recipients, the 3-year incidence of relapse was higher in the TCD patients transplanted for CML (20% *versus* 7%, *P* = 0.017)[6]. The risk of leukemia relapse may vary depending on the extent and specificity of TCD employed. The 5-year probability of leukemia relapse was 28% for recipients of narrow specificity TCD BMT, *versus* 51% for recipients of TCD by other techniques in a large CIBMTR cohort study (*P* < 0.001) [12]. The 5-year relapse rate for recipients of narrow specificity TCD was similar to that observed in patients who received unmanipulated bone marrow transplant. The increased incidence of CML relapse after TCD-HCT has been linked to the reduction in GvHD[103]. Direct evidence of the importance of donor T-cells in the GvL effect emanate from DLI studies (see Chapter 25) for patients with CML who have relapsed after allogeneic bone marrow transplant where complete remission rates of 70–80% are achieved[104,105]. In contrast to CML, TCD appears to have a less significant effect on the relapse rates of patients transplanted for acute leukemia[106,107]. In two separate randomized trials comparing TCD with methotrexate and cyclosporine as GvHD prophylaxis for patients undergoing HLA-matched related or unrelated bone marrow transplantation, a higher relapse rate was observed after TCD bone marrow transplant in patients with CML, not in patients with acute leukemia[6,108]. The comparative myeloablative studies of CD34+ TCD in AML patients reported by the BMT CTN and by Memorial Sloan Kettering and MD Anderson as well as the randomized ATG-Fresenius trial including AML, MDS, and ALL all showed no increase in relapse rate with either *ex-vivo* or *in-vivo* TCD[30,52,53]. These trials excluded patients with advanced disease and thus this observation should not be extrapolated to all patients. Nor should it be extended to patients receiving RIC conditioning as the retrospective analyses of CIBMTR and EBMT show a higher relapse rate for both ATG and/or alemtuzumab in this setting[64,65]. Efforts aimed at reducing leukemia relapse after TCD have primarily focused on immune-based strategies to enhance GvL activity without compromising GvHD prevention. Prophylactic DLI strategies may be useful after TCD-HCT using CD34+ selection, ATG, or alemtuzumab. While the incidence of GvHD after prophylactic DLI is similar to conventional transplantation, one report suggests that cGvHD

after T-cell add-back is associated with less mortality, but retains its protective effect on relapse[109]. Retrospective studies in patients with CML and multiple myeloma undergoing high-dose transplantation have suggested that TCD plus DLI is a reasonable alternative to conventional GvH prophylaxis, and may in some circumstances be associated with superior outcome[110–112]. A report on RIC HCT in Hodgkin's lymphoma suggests that with the addition of DLI, current DFS is superior for patients treated with cyclosporine/alemtuzumab compared to those receiving cyclosporine/methotrexate for GvHD prophylaxis[113].

TCD-HCT: Practice Implications and Future Directions

Although it is clear that TCD does reduce the incidence of acute and chronic GvHD (Table 29.1), there remains no broad consensus as to its place in transplantation. Prior prospective randomized *in-vivo* and *ex-vivo* TCD studies in "myeloablative" transplantation suggest that this reduction in GvHD does not reduce NRM, does not increase relapse for acute leukemia in remission, and does not improve OS. Both recent Canadian and US trials of the impact of ATG formulations on outcome have completed accrual and await final analysis. The interpretation of these trials may depend very much on what is considered the most critical endpoint. TCD may not pass the bar of improving OS given its failure to do so in several prior randomized and retrospective studies. However, if cGvHD-free long-term survival and quality of life are considered relevant and important endpoints, then these studies could firmly establish *in-vivo* TCD as part of the standard transplant regimen. As for *ex-vivo* TCD, BMT CTN 1301 will begin accrual in 2015. This trial will compare CD34+ selection without pharmacologic immune suppression to tacrolimus/methotrexate in AML, ALL, and MDS patients undergoing matched related or unrelated allogeneic HCT. This trial could definitively resolve the role of ex-vivo TCD in myeloablative HCT. The new wrinkle in this study is the inclusion of a third arm of patients receiving post *bone marrow* transplant cyclophosphamide without calcineurin inhibition, based on the encouraging results from Johns Hopkins and other institutions[43]. Even after assessing results in these important studies, we will still need to wait for definitive prospective trials of TCD to be conducted in RIC settings and in HLA-haplotype-matched donors. Investigators remain optimistic that graft engineering and targeted T-cell antibodies will one day fulfil the promise of separating GvH and GvL, leading to higher cure rates for our patients. The proof remains in the pudding.

References

1. Socie G, Stone JV, Wingard JR, *et al*: Long-term survival and late deaths after allogeneic bone marrow transplantation. Late Effects Working Committee of the International Bone Marrow Transplant Registry. *N Engl J Med* 341:14–21, 1999

2. Patterson J, Prentice HG, Brenner MK, *et al*: Graft rejection following HLA-matched T-lymphocyte depleted bone marrow transplantation. *Br J Haematol* 63:221–30, 1986

3. Zutter MM, Martin PJ, Sale GE, *et al*: Epstein–Barr virus lymphoproliferation

after bone marrow transplantation. *Blood* 72:520–9, 1988

4. Marmont AM, Horowitz MM, Gale RP, *et al*: T-cell depletion of HLA-identical transplants in leukemia. *Blood* 78:2120–30, 1991

5. Goldman JM, Gale RP, Horowitz MM, *et al*: Bone marrow transplantation for chronic myelogenous leukemia in chronic phase. Increased risk for relapse associated with T-cell depletion. *Ann Intern Med* 108:806–14, 1988

6. Wagner JE, Thompson JS, Carter SL, *et al*: Effect of graft-*versus*-host disease prophylaxis on 3-year disease-free survival in recipients of unrelated donor bone marrow (T-cell Depletion Trial): a multi-centre, randomised phase II-III trial. *Lancet* 366:733–41, 2005

7. Marek A, Stern M, Chalandon Y, *et al*: The impact of T-cell depletion techniques on the outcome after haploidentical hematopoietic SCT. *Bone Marrow Transplant* 49:55–61, 2014

8. Kernan NA, Collins NH, Juliano L, *et al*: Clonable T lymphocytes in T-cell depleted bone marrow transplants correlate with development of graft-*versus*-host disease. *Blood* 68:770–773, 1986

9. Wagner JE, Donnenberg AD, Noga SJ, *et al*: Lymphocyte depletion of donor bone marrow by counterflow centrifugal elutriation: results of a phase I clinical trial. *Blood* 72:1168–76, 1988

10. Urbano-Ispizua A, Rozman C, Pimentel P, *et al*: The number of donor CD3(+) cells is the most important factor for graft failure after allogeneic transplantation of CD34(+) selected cells from peripheral blood from HLA-identical siblings. *Blood* 97:383–7, 2001

11. Kanate AS, Craig M, Cumpston A, *et al*: Higher infused CD34+ cell dose and overall survival in patients undergoing in vivo T-cell depleted, but not t-cell repleted, allogeneic peripheral blood hematopoietic cell transplantation. *Hematol Oncol Stem Cell Ther* 4:149–56, 2011

12. Champlin RE, Passweg JR, Zhang MJ, *et al*: T-cell depletion of bone marrow transplants for leukemia from donors other than HLA-identical siblings: advantage of T-cell antibodies with narrow specificities. *Blood* 95:3996–4003, 2000

13. Soiffer RJ, Gonin R, Murray C, *et al*: Prediction of graft-*versus*-host disease by phenotypic analysis of early immune reconstitution after CD6-depleted allogeneic bone marrow transplantation. *Blood* 82:2216–23, 1993

14. Nimer SD, Giorgi J, Gajewski JL, *et al*: Selective depletion of CD8+ cells for prevention of graft-*versus*-host disease after bone marrow transplantation. A randomized controlled trial. *Transplantation* 57:82–7, 1994

15. Ho VT, Kim HT, Li S, *et al*: Partial CD8 + T-cell depletion of allogeneic peripheral blood stem cell transplantation is insufficient to prevent graft-*versus*-host disease. *Bone Marrow Transplant* 34:987–94, 2004

16. Alyea EP, Soiffer RJ, Canning C, *et al*: Toxicity and efficacy of defined doses of CD4(+) donor lymphocytes for treatment of relapse after allogeneic bone marrow transplant. *Blood* 91:3671–80, 1998

17. Meyer RG, Britten CM, Wehler D, *et al*: Prophylactic transfer of CD8-depleted donor lymphocytes after T-cell-depleted reduced-intensity transplantation. *Blood* 109:374–82, 2007

18. Antin JH, Bierer BE, Smith BR, *et al*: Selective depletion of bone marrow T lymphocytes with anti-CD5 monoclonal antibodies: effective prophylaxis for graft-*versus*-host disease in patients with hematologic malignancies. *Blood* 78:2139–49, 1991

19. Soiffer RJ, Murray C, Mauch P, *et al*: Prevention of graft-*versus*-host disease by selective depletion of CD6-positive T lymphocytes from donor bone marrow. *J Clin Oncol* 10:1191–200, 1992

20. Filipovich AH, Vallera D, McGlave P, *et al*: T cell depletion with anti-CD5 immunotoxin in histocompatible bone marrow transplantation. The correlation between residual CD5 negative T cells and subsequent graft-*versus*-host disease. *Transplantation* 50:410–5, 1990

21. Hale G, Jacobs P, Wood L, *et al*: CD52 antibodies for prevention of graft-*versus*-host disease and graft rejection following transplantation of allogeneic peripheral blood stem cells. *Bone Marrow Transplant* 26:69–76, 2000

22. Young JW, Papadopoulos EB, Cunningham I, *et al*: T-cell-depleted allogeneic bone marrow transplantation in adults with acute nonlymphocytic leukemia in first remission. *Blood* 79:3380–7, 1992

23. Kernan NA, Bartsch G, Ash RC, *et al*: Analysis of 462 transplantations from unrelated donors facilitated by the National Marrow Donor Program. *N Engl J Med* 328:593–602, 1993

24. Bensinger WI, Buckner CD, Shannon-Dorcy K, *et al*: Transplantation of allogeneic CD34+ peripheral blood stem cells in patients with advanced hematologic malignancy. *Blood* 88:4132–8, 1996

25. Urbano-Ispizua A, Solano C, Brunet S, *et al*: Allogeneic transplantation of selected CD34+ cells from peripheral blood: experience of 62 cases using immunoadsorption or immunomagnetic technique. Spanish Group of Allo-PBT. *Bone Marrow Transplant* 22:519–25, 1998

26. O'Donnell PV, Myers B, Edwards J, *et al*: CD34 selection using three immunoselection devices: comparison of T-cell depleted allografts. *Cytotherapy* 3:483–8, 2001

27. Jakubowski AA, Small TN, Kernan NA, *et al*: T cell-depleted unrelated donor stem cell transplantation provides favorable disease-free survival for adults with hematologic malignancies. *Biol Blood Marrow Transplant* 17:1335–42, 2011

28. Devine SM, Carter S, Soiffer RJ, *et al*: Low-risk of chronic graft-*versus*-host disease and relapse associated with T cell-depleted peripheral blood stem cell transplantation for acute myelogenous leukemia in first remission: results of the blood and marrow transplant clinical trials network protocol 0303. *Biol Blood Marrow Transplant* 17:1343–51, 2011

29. Keever-Taylor CA, Devine SM, Soiffer RJ, *et al*: Characteristics of CliniMACS (R) System CD34-enriched T cell-depleted grafts in a multicenter trial for acute myeloid leukemia-Blood and Marrow Transplant Clinical Trials Network (BMT CTN) protocol 0303. *Biol Blood Marrow Transplant* 18:690–7, 2012

30. Pasquini MC, Devine S, Mendizabal A, *et al*: Comparative outcomes of donor graft CD34+ selection and immune suppressive therapy as graft-*versus*-host disease prophylaxis for patients with acute myeloid leukemia in complete

remission undergoing HLA-matched sibling allogeneic hematopoietic cell transplantation. *J Clin Oncol* 30:3194–201, 2012

31. Bayraktar UD, de Lima M, Saliba RM, *et al*: Ex vivo T cell depleted versus unmodified allografts in patients with acute myeloid leukemia in first complete remission. *Biol Blood Marrow Transplant*,19:898–903, 2013

32. Soiffer RJ, Mauch P, Fairclough D, *et al*: CD6+ T cell depleted allogeneic bone marrow transplantation from genotypically HLA nonidentical related donors. *Biol Blood Marrow Transplant* 3:11–7, 1997

33. Mehta J, Singhal S, Gee AP, *et al*: Bone marrow transplantation from partially HLA-mismatched family donors for acute leukemia: single-center experience of 201 patients. *Bone Marrow Transplant* 33:389–96, 2004

34. Aversa F, Tabilio A, Velardi A, *et al*: Treatment of high-risk acute leukemia with T-cell-depleted stem cells from related donors with one fully mismatched HLA haplotype. *N Engl J Med* 339:1186–93, 1998

35. Marks DI, Khattry N, Cummins M, *et al*: Haploidentical stem cell transplantation for children with acute leukaemia. *Br J Haematol* 134:196–201, 2006

36. Ciceri F, Labopin M, Aversa F, *et al*: A survey of fully haploidentical hematopoietic stem cell transplantation in adults with high-risk acute leukemia: a risk factor analysis of outcomes for patients in remission at transplantation. *Blood* 112:3574–81, 2008

37. Ruggeri L, Capanni M, Casucci M, *et al*: Role of natural killer cell alloreactivity in HLA-mismatched hematopoietic stem cell transplantation. *Blood* 94:333–9, 1999

38. Hsu KC, Keever-Taylor CA, Wilton A, *et al*: Improved outcome in HLA-identical sibling hematopoietic stem-cell transplantation for acute myelogenous leukemia predicted by KIR and HLA genotypes. *Blood* 105:4878–84, 2005

39. Geyer MB, Ricci AM, Jacobson JS, *et al*: T cell depletion utilizing CD34(+) stem cell selection and CD3(+) addback from unrelated adult donors in paediatric allogeneic stem cell transplantation recipients. *Br J Haematol* 157:205–19, 2012

40. Di Ianni M, Falzetti F, Carotti A, *et al*: Tregs prevent GVHD and promote immune reconstitution in HLA-haploidentical transplantation. *Blood* 117:3921–8, 2011

41. Bertaina A, Merli P, Rutella S, *et al*: HLA-haploidentical stem cell transplantation after removal of alphabeta+ T and B cells in children with nonmalignant disorders. *Blood* 124:822–6, 2014

42. Bashey A, Solomon SR: T-cell replete haploidentical donor transplantation using post-transplant CY: an emerging standard-of-care option for patients who lack an HLA-identical sibling donor. *Bone Marrow Transplant* 49:999–1008, 2014

43. Luznik L, O'Donnell PV, Symons HJ, *et al*: HLA-haploidentical bone marrow transplantation for hematologic malignancies using nonmyeloablative conditioning and high-dose, posttransplantation cyclophosphamide. *Biol Blood Marrow Transplant* 14:641–50, 2008

44. Ayuk F, Maywald N, Hannemann S, *et al*: Comparison of the cytotoxicity of 4 preparations of anti-T-cell globulins in various hematological malignancies. *Anticancer Res* 29:1355–60, 2009

45. Russell JA, Turner AR, Larratt L, *et al*: Adult recipients of matched related donor blood cell transplants given myeloablative regimens including pretransplant antithymocyte globulin have lower mortality related to graft-versus-host disease: a matched pair analysis. *Biol Blood Marrow Transplant* 13:299–306, 2007

46. Bredeson CN, Zhang MJ, Agovi MA, *et al*: Outcomes following HSCT using fludarabine, busulfan, and thymoglobulin: a matched comparison to allogeneic transplants conditioned with busulfan and cyclophosphamide. *Biol Blood Marrow Transplant* 14:993–1003, 2008

47. Mohty M, Labopin M, Balere ML, *et al*: Antithymocyte globulins and chronic graft-vs-host disease after myeloablative allogeneic stem cell transplantation from HLA-matched unrelated donors: a report from the Societe Francaise de Greffe de Moelle et de Therapie Cellulaire. *Leukemia* 24:1867–74, 2010

48. Malladi RK, Peniket AJ, Littlewood TJ, *et al*: Alemtuzumab markedly reduces chronic GVHD without affecting overall survival in reduced-intensity conditioning sibling allo-SCT for adults with AML. *Bone Marrow Transplant* 43:709–15, 2009

49. Veys P, Wynn RF, Ahn KW, *et al*: Impact of immune modulation with in vivo T-cell depletion and myleoablative total body irradiation conditioning on outcomes after unrelated donor transplantation for childhood acute lymphoblastic leukemia. *Blood* 119:6155–61, 2012

50. Bacigalupo A, Lamparelli T, Bruzzi P, *et al*: Antithymocyte globulin for graft-versus-host disease prophylaxis in transplants from unrelated donors: 2 randomized studies from Gruppo Italiano Trapianti Midollo Osseo (GITMO). *Blood* 98:2942–7, 2001

51. Bacigalupo A, Lamparelli T, Barisione G, *et al*: Thymoglobulin prevents chronic graft-versus-host disease, chronic lung dysfunction, and late transplant-related mortality: long-term follow-up of a randomized trial in patients undergoing unrelated donor transplantation. *Biol Blood Marrow Transplant* 12:560–5, 2006

52. Finke J, Bethge WA, Schmoor C, *et al*: Standard graft-versus-host disease prophylaxis with or without anti-T-cell globulin in haematopoietic cell transplantation from matched unrelated donors: a randomised, open-label, multicentre phase 3 trial. *Lancet Oncol* 10:855–64, 2009

53. Socie G, Schmoor C, Bethge WA, *et al*: Chronic graft-versus-host disease: long-term results from a randomized trial on graft-versus-host disease prophylaxis with or without anti-T-cell globulin ATG-Fresenius. *Blood* 117:6375–82, 2011

54. Westphal S, Brinkmann H, Kalupa M, *et al*: Anti-tumor effects of anti-T-cell globulin. *Exp Hematol* 42:875–82, 2014

55. Walker I, Schultz KR, Toze CL, *et al*: Thymoglobulin decreases the need for immunosuppression at 12 months after myeloablative and nonmyeloablative unrelated donor transplantation: CBMTG 0801, a randomized, controlled trial. *Blood* 124:38, 2014

56. Yu ZP, Ding JH, Wu F, et al: Quality of life of patients after allogeneic hematopoietic stem cell transplantation with antihuman thymocyte globulin. *Biol Blood Marrow Transplant* 18:593–9, 2012

57. Perez-Simon JA, Kottaridis PD, Martino R, *et al*: Nonmyeloablative transplantation with or without alemtuzumab: comparison between 2 prospective studies in patients with lymphoproliferative disorders. *Blood* 100:3121–7, 2002

58. Chakrabarti S, Mackinnon S, Chopra R, *et al*: High incidence of cytomegalovirus infection after nonmyeloablative stem cell transplantation: potential role of Campath-1H in delaying immune reconstitution. *Blood* 99:4357–63, 2002

59. Mohty M, Jacot W, Faucher C, *et al*: Infectious complications following allogeneic HLA-identical sibling transplantation with antithymocyte globulin-based reduced intensity preparative regimen. *Leukemia* 17:2168–77, 2003

60. Peggs KS, Kayani I, Edwards N, *et al*: Donor lymphocyte infusions modulate relapse risk in mixed chimeras and induce durable salvage in relapsed patients after T-cell-depleted allogeneic transplantation for Hodgkin's lymphoma. *J Clin Oncol* 29:971–8, 2011

61. Thomson KJ, Morris EC, Milligan D, *et al*: T-cell-depleted reduced-intensity transplantation followed by donor leukocyte infusions to promote graft-*versus*-lymphoma activity results in excellent long-term survival in patients with multiply relapsed follicular lymphoma. *J Clin Oncol* 28:3695–700, 2010

62. Koreth J, Kim HT, Nikiforow S, *et al*: Donor chimerism early after reduced-intensity conditioning hematopoietic stem cell transplantation predicts relapse and survival. *Biol Blood Marrow Transplant* 20:1516–21, 2014

63. Baron F, Schaaf-Lafontaine N, Humblet-Baron S, *et al*: T-cell reconstitution after unmanipulated, CD8-depleted or CD34-selected nonmyeloablative peripheral blood stem-cell transplantation. *Transplantation* 76:1705–13, 2003

64. Soiffer RJ, Lerademacher J, Ho V, *et al*: Impact of immune modulation with anti-T-cell antibodies on the outcome of reduced-intensity allogeneic hematopoietic stem cell transplantation for hematologic malignancies. *Blood* 117:6963–70, 2011

65. Baron F, Labopin M, Niederwieser D, *et al*: Impact of graft-*versus*-host disease after reduced-intensity conditioning allogeneic stem cell transplantation for acute myeloid leukemia: a report from the Acute Leukemia Working Party of the European group for blood and marrow transplantation. *Leukemia* 26:2462–8, 2012

66. Baron F, Labopin M, Blaise D, *et al*: Impact of in vivo T-cell depletion on outcome of AML patients in first CR given peripheral blood stem cells and reduced-intensity conditioning allo-SCT from a HLA-identical sibling donor: a report from the Acute Leukemia Working Party of the European Group for Blood and Marrow Transplantation. *Bone Marrow Transplant* 49:389–96, 2014

67. Wolschke C, Zabelina T, Ayuk F, *et al*: Effective prevention of GvHD using in vivo T-cell depletion with anti-lymphocyte globulin in HLA-identical or -mismatched sibling peripheral blood stem cell transplantation. *Bone Marrow Transplant* 49:126–30, 2014

68. Devillier R, Crocchiolo R, Castagna L, *et al*: The increase from 2.5 to 5 mg/kg of rabbit anti-thymocyte-globulin dose in reduced intensity conditioning reduces acute and chronic GVHD for patients with myeloid malignancies undergoing allo-SCT. *Bone Marrow Transplant* 47:639–45, 2012

69. Mohty M, Bay JO, Faucher C, *et al*: Graft-*versus*-host disease following allogeneic transplantation from HLA-identical sibling with antithymocyte globulin-based reduced-intensity preparative regimen. *Blood* 102:470–6, 2003

70. Ayuk F, Diyachenko G, Zabelina T, *et al*: Comparison of two doses of antithymocyte globulin in patients undergoing matched unrelated donor allogeneic stem cell transplantation. *Biol Blood Marrow Transplant* 14:913–9, 2008

71. Wang Y, Fu HX, Liu DH, *et al*: Influence of two different doses of antithymocyte globulin in patients with standard-risk disease following haploidentical transplantation: a randomized trial. *Bone Marrow Transplant* 49:426–33, 2014

72. Remberger M, Sundberg B: Low serum levels of total rabbit-IgG is associated with acute graft-*versus*-host disease after unrelated donor hematopoietic stem cell transplantation: results from a prospective study. *Biol Blood Marrow Transplant* 15:996–9, 2009

73. Podgorny PJ, Ugarte-Torres A, Liu Y, *et al*: High rabbit-antihuman thymocyte globulin levels are associated with low likelihood of graft-vs-host disease and high likelihood of posttransplant lymphoproliferative disorder. *Biol Blood Marrow Transplant* 16:915–26, 2010

74. Remberger M, Persson M, Mattsson J, *et al*: Effects of different serum-levels of ATG after unrelated donor umbilical cord blood transplantation. *Transpl Immunol* 27:59–62, 2012

75. Hoegh-Petersen M, Amin MA, Liu Y, *et al*: Anti-thymocyte globulins capable of binding to T and B cells reduce graft-vs-host disease without increasing relapse. *Bone Marrow Transplant* 48:105–14, 2013

76. Jol-van der Zijde CM, Bredius RG, Jansen-Hoogendijk AM, *et al*: Antibodies to anti-thymocyte globulin in aplastic anemia patients have a negative impact on hematopoietic SCT. *Bone Marrow Transplant* 47:1256–8, 2012

77. Ho VT, Weller E, Lee SJ, *et al*: Prognostic factors for early severe pulmonary complications after hematopoietic stem cell transplantation. *Biol Blood Marrow Transplant* 7:223–9, 2001

78. Huisman C, van der Straaten HM, Canninga-van Dijk MR, *et al*: Pulmonary complications after T-cell-depleted allogeneic stem cell transplantation: low incidence and strong association with acute graft-*versus*-host disease. *Bone Marrow Transplant* 38:561–6, 2006

79. Moscardo F, Urbano-Ispizua A, Sanz GF, *et al*: Positive selection for CD34+ reduces the incidence and severity of veno-occlusive disease of the liver after HLA-identical sibling allogeneic peripheral blood stem cell transplantation. *Exp Hematol* 31:545–50, 2003

80. Voogt PJ, Fibbe WE, Marijt WA, *et al*: Rejection of bone-marrow graft by recipient-derived cytotoxic T lymphocytes against minor histocompatibility antigens. *Lancet* 335:131–4, 1990

81. Fleischhauer K, Kernan NA, O'Reilly RJ, *et al*: Bone marrow-allograft rejection by T lymphocytes recognizing a single amino acid difference in HLA-B44. *N Engl J Med* 323:1818–22, 1990

82. Jakubowski AA, Small TN, Young JW, et al: T cell depleted stem-cell transplantation for adults with hematologic malignancies: sustained engraftment of HLA-matched related donor grafts without the use of antithymocyte globulin. *Blood* 110:4552–9, 2007

83. Burnett AK, Hann IM, Robertson AG, et al: Prevention of graft-*versus*-host disease by ex vivo T cell depletion: reduction in graft failure with augmented total body irradiation. *Leukemia* 2:300–3, 1988

84. Roux E, Helg C, Dumont-Girard F, et al: Analysis of T-cell repopulation after allogeneic bone marrow transplantation: significant differences between recipients of T-cell depleted and unmanipulated grafts. *Blood* 87:3984–92, 1996

85. Wu CJ, Chillemi A, Alyea EP, et al: Reconstitution of T-cell receptor repertoire diversity following T-cell depleted allogeneic bone marrow transplantation is related to hematopoietic chimerism. *Blood* 95:352–9, 2000

86. Hochberg EP, Chillemi AC, Wu CJ, et al: Quantitation of T-cell neogenesis in vivo after allogeneic bone marrow transplantation in adults. *Blood* 98:1116–21, 2001

87. Small TN, Papadopoulos EB, Boulad F, et al: Comparison of immune reconstitution after unrelated and related T-cell-depleted bone marrow transplantation: effect of patient age and donor leukocyte infusions. *Blood* 93:467–80, 1999

88. Bosch M, Dhadda M, Hoegh-Petersen M, et al: Immune reconstitution after anti-thymocyte globulin-conditioned hematopoietic cell transplantation. *Cytotherapy* 14:1258–75, 2012

89. Avivi I, Chakrabarti S, Milligan DW, et al: Incidence and outcome of adenovirus disease in transplant recipients after reduced-intensity conditioning with alemtuzumab. *Biol Blood Marrow Transplant* 10:186–94, 2004

90. van Burik JA, Carter SL, Freifeld AG, et al: Higher risk of cytomegalovirus and aspergillus infections in recipients of T cell-depleted unrelated bone marrow: analysis of infectious complications in patients treated with T cell depletion *versus* immunosuppressive therapy to prevent graft-*versus*-host disease. *Biol Blood Marrow Transplant* 13:1487–98, 2007

91. Brunstein CG, Weisdorf DJ, DeFor T, et al: Marked increased risk of Epstein–Barr virus-related complications with the addition of antithymocyte globulin to a nonmyeloablative conditioning prior to unrelated umbilical cord blood transplantation. *Blood* 108:2874–80, 2006

92. Lindemans CA, Chiesa R, Amrolia PJ, et al: Impact of thymoglobulin prior to pediatric unrelated umbilical cord blood transplantation on immune reconstitution and clinical outcome. *Blood* 123:126–32, 2014

93. Kuehnle I, Huls MH, Liu Z, et al: CD20 monoclonal antibody (rituximab) for therapy of Epstein–Barr virus lymphoma after hemopoietic stem-cell transplantation. *Blood* 95:1502–5, 2000

94. Stevens SJ, Verschuuren EA, Pronk I, et al: Frequent monitoring of Epstein–Barr virus DNA load in unfractionated whole blood is essential for early detection of posttransplant lymphoproliferative disease in high-risk patients. *Blood* 97:1165–71, 2001

95. Papadopoulos EB, Ladanyi M, Emanuel D, et al: Infusions of donor leukocytes to treat Epstein–Barr virus-associated lymphoproliferative disorders after allogeneic bone marrow transplantation. *N Engl J Med* 330:1185–91, 1994

96. Doubrovina E, Oflaz-Sozmen B, Prockop SE, et al: Adoptive immunotherapy with unselected or EBV-specific T cells for biopsy-proven EBV+ lymphomas after allogeneic hematopoietic cell transplantation. *Blood* 119:2644–56, 2012

97. Gerdemann U, Keirnan JM, Katari UL, et al: Rapidly generated multivirus-specific cytotoxic T lymphocytes for the prophylaxis and treatment of viral infections. *Mol Ther* 20:1622–32, 2012

98. Leen AM, Myers GD, Sili U, et al: Monoculture-derived T lymphocytes specific for multiple viruses expand and produce clinically relevant effects in immunocompromised individuals. *Nat Med* 12:1160–6, 2006

99. Perales MA, Goldberg JD, Yuan J, et al: Recombinant human interleukin-7 (CYT107) promotes T-cell recovery after allogeneic stem cell transplantation. *Blood* 120:4882–91, 2012

100. Goldberg GL, Alpdogan O, Muriglan SJ, et al: Enhanced immune reconstitution by sex steroid ablation following allogeneic hemopoietic stem cell transplantation. *J Immunol* 178:7473–84, 2007

101. Hessner MJ, Endean DJ, Casper JT, et al: Use of unrelated marrow grafts compensates for reduced graft-*versus*-leukemia reactivity after T-cell-depleted allogeneic marrow transplantation for chronic myelogenous leukemia. *Blood* 86:3987–96, 1995

102. Devergie A, Apperley JF, Labopin M, et al: European results of matched unrelated donor bone marrow transplantation for chronic myeloid leukemia. Impact of HLA class II matching. Chronic Leukemia Working Party of the European Group for Blood and Marrow Transplantation. *Bone Marrow Transplant* 20:11–9, 1997

103. Sullivan KM, Weiden PL, Storb R, et al: Influence of acute and chronic graft-*versus*-host disease on relapse and survival after bone marrow transplantation from HLA-identical siblings as treatment of acute and chronic leukemia. *Blood* 73:1720–8, 1989

104. Kolb HJ, Mittermuller J, Clemm C, et al: Donor leukocyte transfusions for treatment of recurrent chronic myelogenous leukemia in marrow transplant patients. *Blood* 76:2462–5, 1990

105. Collins RH, Jr., Shpilberg O, Drobyski WR, et al: Donor leukocyte infusions in 140 patients with relapsed malignancy after allogeneic bone marrow transplantation. *J Clin Oncol* 15:433–44, 1997

106. Soiffer RJ, Fairclough D, Robertson M, et al: CD6-depleted allogeneic bone marrow transplantation for acute leukemia in first complete remission. *Blood* 89:3039–47, 1997

107. Papadopoulos EB, Carabasi MH, Castro-Malaspina H, et al: T-cell-depleted allogeneic bone marrow transplantation as postremission therapy for acute myelogenous leukemia: freedom from relapse in the absence of graft-*versus*-host disease. *Blood* 91:1083–90, 1998

108. Remberger M, Ringden O, Aschan J, et al: Long-term follow-up of a randomized trial comparing T-cell depletion with a combination of methotrexate and cyclosporine in adult

leukemic marrow transplant recipients. *Transplant Proc* 26:1829–30, 1994

109. Montero A, Savani BN, Shenoy A, *et al*: T-cell depleted peripheral blood stem cell allotransplantation with T-cell add-back for patients with hematological malignancies: effect of chronic GVHD on outcome. *Biol Blood Marrow Transplant* 12:1318–25, 2006

110. Soiffer RJ, Alyea EP, Hochberg E, *et al*: Randomized trial of CD8+ T-cell depletion in the prevention of graft-*versus*-host disease associated with

donor lymphocyte infusion. *Biol Blood Marrow Transplant* 8:625–32, 2002

111. Sehn LH, Alyea EP, Weller E, *et al*: Comparative outcomes of T-cell-depleted and non-T-cell-depleted allogeneic bone marrow transplantation for chronic myelogenous leukemia: impact of donor lymphocyte infusion. *J Clin Oncol* 17:561–8, 1999

112. Chalandon Y, Roosnek E, Mermillod B, *et al*: Can only partial T-cell depletion of the graft before hematopoietic stem cell transplantation mitigate graft-

versus-host disease while preserving a graft-*versus*-leukemia reaction? A prospective phase II study. *Biol Blood Marrow Transplant* 12:102–10, 2006

113. Peggs KS, Sureda A, Qian W, *et al*: Reduced-intensity conditioning for allogeneic haematopoietic stem cell transplantation in relapsed and refractory Hodgkin lymphoma: impact of alemtuzumab and donor lymphocyte infusions on long-term outcomes. *Br J Haematol* 139:70–80, 2007

Selection of Conditioning Regimen and Challenges with Different Types of T-Cell Depletion Methods

30
CD34+ Cell Selection: Current Concepts, Methods, and Controversies

Melody Smith and Miguel-Angel Perales

Introduction

Graft-*versus*-host disease (GvHD) is one of the primary factors contributing to transplant-related mortality (TRM) after allogeneic hematopoietic cell transplant (allo-HCT). The risk of grade II–IV acute GvHD ranges from 35–50% in recipients of HLA-matched related donor (MRD) and 40–70% in recipients of HLA-matched unrelated donor (MUD) grafts[1,2]. Given that donor-derived alloreactive T-cells have been shown to play a critical role in GvHD, T-cell depletion (TCD) has been investigated as an approach to attenuate GvHD[3–9]. T-cell depletion of the graft results in decreased GvHD as well as a decreased need for post-transplant immunosuppression. This chapter will elucidate the use of CD34 selection and *ex-vivo* T-cell depletion of the graft, as well as its impact on the recipients (Table 30.1).

Techniques to Deplete the Allograft of T-cells

Techniques used for TCD have varied over time and the specific approach used should be noted when analyzing data in this regard. There are several factors that may impact the effectiveness and degree of TCD, including the type of cells that are depleted, the source of hematopoietic cells, HLA-matching, and the use of post-transplant immunosuppression.

T-cell depletion of the graft can be performed by either positive or negative selection of CD34+ cells. Soybean lectin agglutination (SBA) followed by sheep red blood cell (sRBC)-rosette depletion (E-rosetting)[10], and counterflow elution [11,12] are physical methods that have been employed for "negative" selection of donor lymphocytes. Immunologic approaches to T-cell depletion have also been harnessed through the use of monoclonal antibodies, such as anti-CD6 monoclonal antibody-conjugated immunomagnetic beads[13]. The "negative" depletion techniques retain a larger number of effector lymphocytes, such as NK cells, in the allogeneic peripheral hematopoietic cell grafts compared to "positive" selection[14].

At present, however, CD34+ positive selection is the most common technique in clinical use to achieve TCD of the graft [5,6,15–18]. Although this was previously performed with the ISOLEX 300i magnetic cell selection system (Baxter, Deerfield, IL) followed by E-rosetting, the use of immunomagnetic beads with the CliniMACS CD34 Reagent System (Miltenyi Biotec, Bergisch Gladbach, Germany) is now the preferred approach [5,6,15]. Comparison of CD34 selection by ISOLEX 300i *versus* CliniMACS showed that the CliniMACS CD34 Reagent System yielded higher purity with fewer T-cells while the ISOLEX 300i contained fewer apoptotic cells[19]. The

Table 30.1 Pros and cons of negative and positive selection of CD34+ cells

Outcome	Pros	Cons
Engraftment		Potential increase in the risk of graft failure
Toxicity	Reduced mucositis (related to methotrexate) Reduced renal toxicity (related to calcineurin inhibitors)	
GvHD	Decrease in acute and chronic GvHD	
Immune recovery		Delay in immune recovery
Relapse	Survival and relapse comparable to conventional non-TCD grafts in subjects with ALL, AML, MDS, and NHL	Increase in risk of relapse in subjects with CML
Older patients, patients with comorbidities	Spare patients exposure to potentially toxic immunosuppressive drugs	
Quality of life	Expected better quality of life due to decreased morbidity associated with chronic GvHD	

CliniMACS CD34 Reagent System is able to achieve a 5-log depletion of the T-cells in the graft with a median viability of 98%[20]. With the use of different immunomagnetic beads, the CliniMACS system is also capable of depleting the graft of CD3+ T-cells[14,21], CD19+ B-cells[22], or T-cell receptor alpha/beta positive (TCRαβ⁺) T-cells[14,22].

Impact of TCD on Engraftment

One of the potential consequences of CD34+ positive selection of the allograft is a higher rate of graft failure (see Chapter 29). Initial studies of TCD grafts demonstrated a higher risk of graft failure compared to non-TCD ("unmanipulated" or "unmodified") allo-HCT[8,20,23], which reduced disease-free (DFS) and overall survival (OS). It has been postulated that, in unmodified transplants, donor T-cells in the graft marrow may help to sustain engraftment by eliminating host cells that could cause graft rejection[20]. In order to overcome this immunologic barrier in TCD allo-HCT, the addition of antithymocyte globulin (ATG) and thiotepa to the conditioning regimen has been shown to promote engraftment and result in rates of graft failure similar to those observed with unmodified marrow grafts in myeloablative and mainly in HLA-MSD (matched sibling donor) settings[7,9].

Impact of TCD on GvHD: What Is in the Log?

The main benefit of TCD is a significant decrease in both acute and chronic GvHD compared to conventional transplants [4,16,24–29]. However, the impact on GvHD is correlated with the degree of TCD of the graft. In recipients of peripheral blood (PB) HCT, a 4-log depletion of T-cells is required to reduce the risk of GvHD[30,31]. In contrast, only a 3-log depletion of T-cells results in decreased GvHD in recipients of bone marrow (BM) grafts. In contrast, lower degrees of TCD, in the order of 1–2 logs, do not result in a significant reduction in the incidence of GvHD and typically require post-transplant GvHD prophylaxis.

Correlation Between TCD and Disease Relapse: Does Disease Status and Intensity of Conditioning Regimen Matter?

One of the benefits of allo-HCT in patients with malignant diseases is the graft-versus-leukemia (GvL) effect (see Chapter 65). For example, post-transplant GvL plays a significant role in preventing disease relapse in chronic myelogenous leukemia (CML). In a retrospective analysis of the outcomes in patients with chronic phase CML, 46 patients who received a TCD transplant were compared with 40 patients who underwent a non-TCD transplant[32]. The 3-year probability of relapse for the TCD group was 2.5 times higher than the non-TCD group (62% *versus* 24%, P = 0.0003). However, complete remission was achieved after donor lymphocyte infusion (DLI) in 17 of 20 of the TCD recipients and 2 of 3 of the non-TCD recipients, resulting in similar OS (see Chapter 25).

Given the increased risk of relapse for patients with CML who receive TCD transplants, CD34 selected transplants are not routinely recommended for these patients (see Chapter 36).

In contrast, patients with AML or ALL appear to have similar rates of disease relapse and survival whether they receive TCD or unmodified allografts[5–7,16,28,33]. The Blood and Marrow Clinical Trials Network recently reported the results of a multicenter single-arm phase 2 study in 44 patients up to 65 years of age with AML in CR1 or CR2 who received TCD transplants using CD34 selection with the CliniMACS CD34 Reagent System (BMT CTN 0303)[16]. In patients with AML in CR1, the relapse rate was 17.4% at 36 months. A comparative analysis of patients with AML in CR who received MSD allo-HCT evaluated the 44 recipients of TCD grafts on BMT CTN 0303 *versus* 84 recipients of unmodified grafts who were given pharmacologic immune suppression therapy on BMT CTN 0201[29]. Although the rates of acute grade 2–4 and chronic GvHD were significantly decreased in the TCD *versus* the unmodified transplant groups, the study noted no difference in the rates of leukemia relapse, graft rejection, TRM, DFS, or OS. These results suggest that TCD may decrease TRM in patients with AML without increasing the rates of relapse in the myeloablative setting.

Furthermore, a retrospective evaluation compared clinical outcomes in patients with AML in CR1 who received TCD transplant (n = 115) at Memorial Sloan Kettering Cancer Center (MSKCC) with those who received unmodified allo-HCT (n=181) at MD Anderson Cancer Center (MDACC)[28]. There was no significant difference in the relapse rate between the TCD and unmodified transplant groups at 1 year (17% *versus* 21%, P = 0.4) and 3 years (18% *versus* 25%, P = 0.9). However, there was a significant reduction in the rate of grade 2–4 acute GvHD (5% *versus* 18%, p = 0.005) and chronic GvHD (13% *versus* 53%, P <0.001) in the TCD group compared to the unmodified graft group. Finally, a recent retrospective evaluation of 56 patients with ALL who underwent TCD allo-HCT noted a cumulative incidence of relapse of 0.23, with 2- and 5-year OS and DFS that were comparable to those reported in conventional transplants, but with lower rates of acute and chronic GvHD[33]. Thus, in our opinion CD34 selected transplants do not appear to place patients with ALL or AML at increased risk for relapse.

Impact of TCD on Immune Recovery

Immune recovery following allo-HCT is dependent upon the conditioning regimen, the allograft, and the thymic activity of the recipient[34,35] (see Chapter 22). In the initial post-transplant period, there is a decrease in thymic function as noted by a decrease in T-cell receptor rearrangement excision circles (TRECs)[36,37]. This finding is also associated with decreased diversity in the TCR repertoire and decreased CD4+ T-cells[36].

The use of TCD grafts results in delayed recovery of total and naïve CD4+ T-cells, as well as T-cell mitogen responses, and is associated with an increase in opportunistic infections, including Epstein–Barr virus-associated lymphoproliferative disorders (see Chapter 20), in the first 12 months post-transplant[38,39].

Comparison of TRECs in patients who received TCD *versus* conventional allografts noted lower TRECs in the TCD group[34]. However, the difference in TRECs normalized by 9 months post-transplant. Low TRECs are associated with increased susceptibility to opportunistic infections. In addition, quantitative assessment of the T-cell receptor (TCR) repertoire has also identified slower recovery in the diversity of the TCR repertoire in recipients of TCD *versus* unmodified grafts[40]. Comparison of the TCR repertoire at 6 months in recipients of cord blood transplants compared to CD34-selected PB allo-HCT noted that the TCR diversity in cord blood recipients was similar to healthy individuals whereas the diversity of CD4+ and CD8+ T-cells was 14- and 28-fold lower, respectively, in TCD recipients. Nevertheless, these differences also normalized by 12 months post-transplant[40].

As noted previously, while ATG can be used to promote engraftment in the TCD setting it also prolongs the time to T-cell reconstitution, and potentially increases the risk of opportunistic infections. A prospective study of 52 adult patients at MSKCC with various hematologic malignancies who received TCD PB allo-HCT from HLA-matched donors without the use of ATG aimed to address this issue[6]. The patients were administered a conditioning regimen of hyperfractionated total body irradiation (HFTBI), thiotepa, and fludarabine, where fludarabine was substituted for cyclophosphamide to increase immune suppression without ATG. Neither GvHD nor additional graft rejection prophylaxis were given. Consistent with prior studies, there was a low incidence of GvHD (grade 2 acute GvHD 8% and chronic GvHD 9%) and no graft failure. Although patients older than 50 years of age had slower recovery of CD4+ T-cells, the majority (66%) of patients regardless of age had a CD4+ count of ≥ 200 cells/μL by 1 year. There was also a low incidence of opportunistic infections.

Novel Strategies to Enhance Immune Recovery after TCD Allo-HCT

Following allo-HCT, patients are at a high risk for complications from viral and fungal infections. The delay in immune reconstitution associated with CD34+ selected transplants further increases the potential morbidity associated with infections. A number of strategies have been investigated to overcome this limitation.

T-cell add-backs have been investigated in recipients of CD34+ selected HCT in order to support engraftment and immune reconstitution without increasing GvHD[41]. In a study of 19 patients who received PB allo-HCT from MUD, T-cells were added back to achieve a total T-cell dose of $1.0–2.5 \times 10^5$ CD3+/kg without any significant deleterious effects.

Additional potential modalities to improve immune include keratinocyte growth factor (KGF), interleukin-7 (IL-7)[42], growth hormone, and alteration in sex steroids through the use of agents such as degarelix and leuprolide[43]. IL-7 plays a key role in the development and survival of T-cells and has been shown to improve immune recovery in murine models of allo-HCT. A phase 1 clinical trial at MSKCC administered escalating weekly doses of recombinant IL-7 (CYT107, Cytheris Inc) to 12 recipients of CD34-selected grafts from HLA-matched related or unrelated donors[42]. The study demonstrated that IL-7 increases functional T-cells and enhances TCR diversity without increasing GvHD. Finally, a randomized clinical trial in patients who have received TCD transplant and total body irradiation (TBI) is currently accruing patients to receive KGF plus leuprolide in order to assess whether these agents result in faster immune reconstitution (NCT01746849).

Clinical Benefits of CD34+ Cell Selection

The primary benefit of TCD allograft is decreased acute and chronic GvHD compared to conventional allografts[16,29] (see Chapter 29). The decrease in chronic GvHD associated with TCD from CD34+ cell "positive" selection also translates into a decrease in long-term morbidity[29]. Furthermore, patients do not require GvHD prophylaxis post-transplant and are therefore spared the potential toxicity of the prophylactic medications used in conventional transplants. The ability to eliminate the use of medications such as calcineurin inhibitors abrogates the need to exclude patients with underlying renal toxicity from transplant. Furthermore, the ability to avoid GvHD prophylaxis enables the use of ablative conditioning in older patients, given that the combined toxicity of ablative conditioning and GvHD prophylaxis is prohibitive in this population. As a result, older patients are often given nonmyeloablative or reduced intensity conditioning, which portend an increase in malignant relapse.

Practice Points
Optimal Patient Population for CD34+ Cell-Selected Allograft
Patients who receive HLA mismatched related or unrelated donor transplants are at a higher risk for post-transplant GvHD than patients who receive HLA-matched related donor transplants. Recipients of HLA mismatched grafts should therefore be given TCD transplants. Patients with nonmalignant conditions, such as sickle cell anemia (see Chapter 55) and severe combined immunodeficiency who do not benefit from GvL effects, should also be given CD34+ cell-selected HCT to decrease the morbidity of GvHD[44,45]. Although patients with CML who receive TCD transplants have an increased risk of disease relapse[32], there are several hematologic malignancies in which CD34+ selected grafts should be considered. Patients with MDS, AML, ALL, and high-grade NHL are optimal candidates for a CD34+ selected transplant given that these patients, in our opinion have similar rates of

survival and relapse as those who receive conventional transplants[5–7,16,28,33,46,47]. Hence, identifying the optimal patient for CD34+ selected allograft should assess the underlying disease as well as the HLA matching as key determinants in the decision process.

Negative Selection of CD34+ Cells: Where Is CliniMACS?

Although most of the current clinical data have been obtained through positive selection of CD34+ cells, negative selection may be achieved with CD3, CD3/CD19, and TCRαβ(+)/CD19 depletion strategies. In particular, recent studies with the CliniMACS system have investigated the depletion of TCRαβ+ and CD19+ cells[22] (see Chapter 59). The number of CD34+ cells recovered with this technique is comparable to that observed with CD34+ cell "positive" selection and CD3+/CD19+ depletion approaches. A study of HLA haplotype mismatch transplant in 29 patients who received CD3/CD19 depleted grafts noted rapid immune recovery and full donor chimerism within 2 to 4 weeks[48]. Furthermore, a prospective, multicenter phase 2 study of 61 patients who received CD3+/CD19+ depleted HLA haplotype mismatch grafts after reduced intensity conditioning also noted rapid engraftment with a median of 12 (range, 9–50) days to 0.5×10^9 granulocytes/L and 11 (range, 7–38) days for 20×10^9 platelets/L[49]. Finally, a randomized trial of matched sibling and matched unrelated donor transplant recipients who received CD3+/CD19+ depleted PB allo-HCT *versus* CD34+ "positive" selected grafts noted faster recovery of NK cells in the CD3+/CD19+ depleted group, which may aid in the antitumor response early after transplant[50].

Controversies and Future Directions

Although further randomized studies need to be performed in order to compare the outcomes of TCD to unmodified transplants, current data demonstrate the benefits of T-cell depletion in the appropriate patient population. Specifically, a multicenter, randomized phase 2/3 clinical trial in recipients of unrelated bone marrow donor transplants noted decreased grade III–IV acute G*v*HD (18% *versus* 37%) in TCD *versus* unmodified transplants, respectively[51]. Of note, patients who received TCD transplants also had decreased hospitalizations, whereas there was no difference in DFS and an increase in the rate of CMV infection[51].

T-cell depletion has been shown to decrease post-transplant morbidity and mortality. However, when considering this approach, several factors should be considered, including the technique for TCD, the manipulation of the graft, as well as the potential risks posed by ablative conditioning and delayed immune reconstitution. In addition, for those patients in whom post-transplant G*v*L is needed a TCD transplant should not be performed (see Chapters 25, 29, 36, and 65). Nonetheless, the potential of TCD to decrease TRM for recipients of allo-HCT, particularly as it relates to decreased GvHD, makes this approach promising in a selected patient population. BMT CTN is performing a phase 3 trial that will compare TCD with the CliniMACS CD34 Reagent System to the post-transplant cyclophosphamide approach, and a tacrolimus and methotrexate control arm in patients with acute leukemia and MDS undergoing a "myeloablative" conditioning transplant from an HLA-matched related or unrelated donor (BMT CTN 1301).

References

1. Nash RA, Antin JH, Karanes C, Fay JW, Avalos BR, Yeager AM, *et al*. Phase 3 study comparing methotrexate and tacrolimus with methotrexate and cyclosporine for prophylaxis of acute graft-*versus*-host disease after marrow transplantation from unrelated donors. *Blood*. 2000;96(6):2062–8. PubMed PMID: 10979948. Epub 2000/09/09. eng.

2. Inamoto Y, Flowers ME, Appelbaum FR, Carpenter PA, Deeg HJ, Furlong T, *et al*. A retrospective comparison of tacrolimus *versus* cyclosporine with methotrexate for immunosuppression after allogeneic hematopoietic cell transplantation with mobilized blood cells. *Biology of Blood and Marrow Transplantation: Journal of the American Society for Blood and Marrow Transplantation*. 2011;17(7):1088–92. PubMed PMID: 21421070. Pubmed Central PMCID: Pmc3114191. Epub 2011/03/23. eng.

3. Martin PJ, Rowley SD, Anasetti C, Chauncey TR, Gooley T, Petersdorf EW, *et al*. A phase I-II clinical trial to evaluate removal of CD4 cells and partial depletion of CD8 cells from donor marrow for HLA-mismatched unrelated recipients. *Blood*. 1999;94(7):2192–9. PubMed PMID: 10498588. Epub 1999/09/25. eng.

4. Alyea EP, Weller E, Fisher DC, Freedman AS, Gribben JG, Lee S, *et al*. Comparable outcome with T-cell-depleted unrelated-donor *versus* related-donor allogeneic bone marrow transplantation. *Biology of Blood and Marrow Transplantation: Journal of the American Society for Blood and Marrow Transplantation*. 2002;8(11):601–7. PubMed PMID: 12463479. Epub 2002/12/05. eng.

5. Jakubowski AA, Small TN, Kernan NA, Castro-Malaspina H, Collins N, Koehne G, *et al*. T cell-depleted unrelated donor stem cell transplantation provides favorable disease-free survival for adults with hematologic malignancies. *Biology of Blood and Marrow Transplantation: Journal of the American Society for Blood and Marrow Transplantation*. 2011;17(9):1335–42. PubMed PMID: 21232623. Pubmed Central PMCID: Pmc3094599. Epub 2011/01/15. eng.

6. Jakubowski AA, Small TN, Young JW, Kernan NA, Castro-Malaspina H, Hsu KC, *et al*. T cell depleted stem-cell transplantation for adults with hematologic malignancies: sustained engraftment of HLA-matched related donor grafts without the use of antithymocyte globulin. *Blood*. 2007;110(13):4552–9. PubMed PMID: 17717135. Pubmed Central PMCID: Pmc2234775. Epub 2007/08/25. eng.

7. Papadopoulos EB, Carabasi MH, Castro-Malaspina H, Childs BH, Mackinnon S, Boulad F, *et al*. T-cell-depleted allogeneic bone marrow transplantation as postremission therapy for acute myelogenous leukemia: freedom from relapse in the

absence of graft-*versus*-host disease. *Blood*. 1998;91(3):1083–90. PubMed PMID: 9446672. Epub 1998/02/03. eng.

8. Young JW, Papadopoulos EB, Cunningham I, Castro-Malaspina H, Flomenberg N, Carabasi MH, *et al.* T-cell-depleted allogeneic bone marrow transplantation in adults with acute nonlymphocytic leukemia in first remission. *Blood*. 1992;79(12):3380–7. PubMed PMID. 1596577. Epub 1992/06/15. eng.

9. Aversa F, Terenzi A, Carotti A, Felicini R, Jacucci R, Zei T, *et al.* Improved outcome with T-cell-depleted bone marrow transplantation for acute leukemia. *Journal of Clinical Oncology: Official Journal of the American Society of Clinical Oncology*. 1999;17(5):1545–50. PubMed PMID: 10334542. Epub 1999/05/20. eng.

10. Reisner Y, Kapoor N, Kirkpatrick D, Pollack MS, Dupont B, Good RA, *et al.* Transplantation for acute leukaemia with HLA-A and B nonidentical parental marrow cells fractionated with soybean agglutinin and sheep red blood cells. *Lancet*. 1981;2(8242):327–31. PubMed PMID: 6115110. Epub 1981/08/15. eng.

11. de Witte T, Hoogenhout J, de Pauw B, Holdrinet R, Janssen J, Wessels J, *et al.* Depletion of donor lymphocytes by counterflow centrifugation successfully prevents acute graft-*versus*-host disease in matched allogeneic marrow transplantation. *Blood*. 1986;67(5):1302–8. PubMed PMID: 3516253. Epub 1986/05/01. eng.

12. Wagner JE, Donnenberg AD, Noga SJ, Cremo CA, Gao IK, Yin HJ, *et al.* Lymphocyte depletion of donor bone marrow by counterflow centrifugal elutriation: results of a phase I clinical trial. *Blood*. 1988;72(4):1168–76. PubMed PMID: 3048436. Epub 1988/10/01. eng.

13. Sao H, Kitaori K, Kasai M, Shimokawa T, Kato C, Yamanishi H, *et al.* A new marrow T cell depletion method using anti-CD6 monoclonal antibody-conjugated magnetic beads and its clinical application for prevention of acute graft-vs.-host disease in allogeneic bone marrow transplantation: results of a phase I-II trial. *International journal of hematology*. 1999;69(1):27–35. PubMed PMID: 10641440. Epub 2000/01/21. eng.

14. Handgretinger R. Negative depletion of CD3(+) and TcRalphabeta(+) T cells. *Current Opinion in Hematology*. 2012;19(6):434–9. PubMed PMID: 22914586. Epub 2012/08/24. eng.

15. Aversa F, Terenzi A, Tabilio A, Falzetti F, Carotti A, Ballanti S, *et al.* Full haplotype-mismatched hematopoietic stem-cell transplantation: a phase II study in patients with acute leukemia at high risk of relapse. *Journal of Clinical Oncology: Official Journal of the American Society of Clinical Oncology*. 2005;23(15):3447–54. PubMed PMID: 15753458. Epub 2005/03/09. eng.

16. Devine SM, Carter S, Soiffer RJ, Pasquini MC, Hari PN, Stein A, *et al.* Low-risk of chronic graft-*versus*-host disease and relapse associated with T cell-depleted peripheral blood stem cell transplantation for acute myelogenous leukemia in first remission: results of the blood and marrow transplant clinical trials network protocol 0303. *Biology of Blood and Marrow Transplantation: Journal of the American Society for Blood and Marrow Transplantation*. 2011;17(9):1343–51. PubMed PMID: 21320619. Pubmed Central PMCID: Pmc3150599. Epub 2011/02/16. eng.

17. Finke J, Brugger W, Bertz H, Behringer D, Kunzmann R, Weber-Nordt RM, *et al.* Allogeneic transplantation of positively selected peripheral blood CD34+ progenitor cells from matched related donors. *Bone Marrow Transplantation*. 1996 Dec;18(6):1081–6. PubMed PMID: 8971376. Epub 1996/12/01. eng.

18. Urbano-Ispizua A, Brunet S, Solano C, Moraleda JM, Rovira M, Zuazu J, *et al.* Allogeneic transplantation of CD34+-selected cells from peripheral blood in patients with myeloid malignancies in early phase: a case control comparison with unmodified peripheral blood transplantation. *Bone Marrow Transplantation*. 2001;28(4):349–54. PubMed PMID: 11571506. Epub 2001/09/26. eng.

19. Watts MJ, Somervaille TC, Ings SJ, Ahmed F, Khwaja A, Yong K, *et al.* Variable product purity and functional capacity after CD34 selection: a direct comparison of the CliniMACS (v2.1) and Isolex 300i (v2.5) clinical scale devices. *British Journal of Haematology*. 2002;118(1):117–23. PubMed PMID: 12100134. Epub 2002/07/09. eng.

20. Martin PJ, Hansen JA, Buckner CD, Sanders JE, Deeg HJ, Stewart P, *et al.* Effects of in vitro depletion of T cells in HLA-identical allogeneic marrow grafts. *Blood*. 1985;66(3):664–72. PubMed PMID: 3896348. Epub 1985/09/01. eng.

21. Dykes JH, Toporski J, Juliusson G, Bekassy AN, Lenhoff S, Lindmark A, *et al.* Rapid and effective CD3 T-cell depletion with a magnetic cell sorting program to produce peripheral blood progenitor cell products for haploidentical transplantation in children and adults. *Transfusion*. 2007;47(11):2134–42. PubMed PMID: 17958543. Epub 2007/10/26. eng.

22. Schumm M, Lang P, Bethge W, Faul C, Feuchtinger T, Pfeiffer M, *et al.* Depletion of T-cell receptor alpha/beta and CD19 positive cells from apheresis products with the CliniMACS device. *Cytotherapy*. 2013;15(10):1253–8. PubMed PMID: 23993299. Epub 2013/09/03. eng.

23. Castro-Malaspina H, Harris RE, Gajewski J, Ramsay N, Collins R, Dharan B, *et al.* Unrelated donor marrow transplantation for myelodysplastic syndromes: outcome analysis in 510 transplants facilitated by the National Marrow Donor Program. *Blood*. 2002;99(6):1943–51. PubMed PMID: 11877264. Epub 2002/03/06. eng.

24. Laurent G, Maraninchi D, Gluckman E, Vernant JP, Derocq JM, Gaspard MH, *et al.* Donor bone marrow treatment with T101 Fab fragment-ricin A-chain immunotoxin prevents graft-*versus*-host disease. *Bone Marrow Transplantation*. 1989;4(4):367–71. PubMed PMID: 2789084. Epub 1989/07/01. eng.

25. Mitsuyasu RT, Champlin RE, Gale RP, Ho WG, Lenarsky C, Winston D, *et al.* Treatment of donor bone marrow with monoclonal anti-T-cell antibody and complement for the prevention of graft-*versus*-host disease. A prospective, randomized, double-blind trial. *Annals of Internal Medicine*. 1986;105(1):20–6. PubMed PMID: 3521427. Epub 1986/07/01. eng.

26. Prentice HG, Blacklock HA, Janossy G, Gilmore MJ, Price-Jones L, Tidman N, *et al.* Depletion of T lymphocytes in donor marrow prevents significant graft-*versus*-host disease in matched allogeneic leukaemic marrow transplant

recipients. *Lancet.* 1984;1(8375):472–6. PubMed PMID: 6142207. Epub 1984/03/03. eng.

27. Soiffer RJ, Fairclough D, Robertson M, Alyea E, Anderson K, Freedman A, *et al.* CD6-depleted allogeneic bone marrow transplantation for acute leukemia in first complete remission. *Blood.* 1997;89(8):3039–47. PubMed PMID: 9108425. Epub 1997/04/15. eng.

28. Bayraktar UD, de Lima M, Saliba RM, Maloy M, Castro-Malaspina HR, Chen J, *et al.* Ex vivo T cell-depleted *versus* unmodified allografts in patients with acute myeloid leukemia in first complete remission. *Biology of Blood and Marrow Transplantation: Journal of the American Society for Blood and Marrow Transplantation.* 2013;19(6):898–903. PubMed PMID: 23467126. Pubmed Central PMCID: Pmc4059063. Epub 2013/03/08. eng.

29. Pasquini MC, Devine S, Mendizabal A, Baden LR, Wingard JR, Lazarus HM, *et al.* Comparative outcomes of donor graft CD34+ selection and immune suppressive therapy as graft-*versus*-host disease prophylaxis for patients with acute myeloid leukemia in complete remission undergoing HLA-matched sibling allogeneic hematopoietic cell transplantation. *Journal of Clinical Oncology: Official Journal of the American Society of Clinical Oncology.* 2012;30(26):3194–201. PubMed PMID: 22869882. Pubmed Central PMCID: Pmc3434978. Epub 2012/08/08. eng.

30. Clarke E, Potter MN, Hale G, Waldmann H, Lankester A, Cornish JM, *et al.* Double T cell depletion of bone marrow using sequential positive and negative cell immunoaffinity or CD34+ cell selection followed by Campath-1M; effect on CD34+ cells and progenitor cell recoveries. *Bone Marrow Transplantation.* 1998;22(2):117–24. PubMed PMID: 9707017. Epub 1998/08/26. eng.

31. Butt NM, McGinnity N, Clark RE. CD34 positive selection as prophylaxis against graft *versus* host disease in allogeneic peripheral blood stem cell transplantation. *Leukemia & Lymphoma.* 2003;44(9):1509–13. PubMed PMID: 14565652. Epub 2003/10/21. eng.

32. Sehn LH, Alyea EP, Weller E, Canning C, Lee S, Ritz J, *et al.* Comparative outcomes of T-cell-depleted and non-T-cell-depleted allogeneic bone marrow transplantation for chronic myelogenous leukemia: impact of donor lymphocyte infusion. *Journal of Clinical Oncology: Official Journal of the American Society of Clinical Oncology.* 1999;17(2):561–8. PubMed PMID: 10080600. Epub 1999/03/18. eng.

33. Goldberg JD, Linker A, Kuk D, Ratan R, Jurcic J, Barker JN, *et al.* T cell-depleted stem cell transplantation for adults with high-risk acute lymphoblastic leukemia: long-term survival for patients in first complete remission with a decreased risk of graft-*versus*-host disease. *Biology of Blood and Marrow Transplantation: Journal of the American Society for Blood and Marrow Transplantation.* 2013;19(2):208–13. PubMed PMID: 22982534. Pubmed Central PMCID: Pmc3963704. Epub 2012/09/18. eng.

34. Lewin SR, Heller G, Zhang L, Rodrigues E, Skulsky E, van den Brink MR, *et al.* Direct evidence for new T-cell generation by patients after either T-cell-depleted or unmodified allogeneic hematopoietic stem cell transplantations. *Blood.* 2002;100(6):2235–42. PubMed PMID: 12200390. Epub 2002/08/30. eng.

35. McIver Z, Melenhorst JJ, Wu C, Grim A, Ito S, Cho I, *et al.* Donor lymphocyte count and thymic activity predict lymphocyte recovery and outcomes after matched-sibling hematopoietic stem cell transplant. *Haematologica.* 2013;98(3):346–52. PubMed PMID: 23065508. Pubmed Central PMCID: Pmc3659951. Epub 2012/10/16. eng.

36. Clave E, Busson M, Douay C, Peffault de Latour R, Berrou J, Rabian C, *et al.* Acute graft-*versus*-host disease transiently impairs thymic output in young patients after allogeneic hematopoietic stem cell transplantation. *Blood.* 2009;113(25):6477–84. PubMed PMID: 19258596. Epub 2009/03/05. eng.

37. Olkinuora H, von Willebrand E, Kantele JM, Vainio O, Talvensaari K, Saarinen-Pihkala U, *et al.* The impact of early viral infections and graft-*versus*-host disease on immune reconstitution following paediatric stem cell transplantation. *Scandinavian Journal of Immunology.* 2011;73(6):586–93. PubMed PMID: 21323694. Epub 2011/02/18. eng.

38. Small TN, Avigan D, Dupont B, Smith K, Black P, Heller G, *et al.* Immune reconstitution following T-cell depleted bone marrow transplantation: effect of age and posttransplant graft rejection prophylaxis. *Biology of Blood and Marrow Transplantation: Journal of the American Society for Blood and Marrow Transplantation.* 1997;3(2):65–75. PubMed PMID: 9267666. Epub 1997/06/01. eng.

39. Small TN, Papadopoulos EB, Boulad F, Black P, Castro-Malaspina H, Childs BH, *et al.* Comparison of immune reconstitution after unrelated and related T-cell-depleted bone marrow transplantation: effect of patient age and donor leukocyte infusions. *Blood.* 1999;93(2):467–80. PubMed PMID: 9885208. Epub 1999/01/13. eng.

40. van Heijst JW, Ceberio I, Lipuma LB, Samilo DW, Wasilewski GD, Gonzales AM, *et al.* Quantitative assessment of T cell repertoire recovery after hematopoietic stem cell transplantation. *Nature Medicine.* 2013;19(3):372–7. PubMed PMID: 23435170. Pubmed Central PMCID: Pmc3594333. Epub 2013/02/26. eng.

41. Geyer MB, Ricci AM, Jacobson JS, Majzner R, Duffy D, Van de Ven C, *et al.* T cell depletion utilizing CD34(+) stem cell selection and CD3(+) addback from unrelated adult donors in paediatric allogeneic stem cell transplantation recipients. *British Journal of Haematology.* 2012;157(2):205–19. PubMed PMID: 22313507. Epub 2012/02/09. eng.

42. Perales MA, Goldberg JD, Yuan J, Koehne G, Lechner L, Papadopoulos EB, *et al.* Recombinant human interleukin-7 (CYT107) promotes T-cell recovery after allogeneic stem cell transplantation. *Blood.* 2012;120(24):4882–91. PubMed PMID: 23012326. Pubmed Central PMCID: Pmc3520625. Epub 2012/09/27. eng.

43. Goldberg GL, Zakrzewski JL, Perales MA, van den Brink MR. Clinical strategies to enhance T cell reconstitution. *Seminars in Immunology.* 2007;19(5):289–96. PubMed PMID: 17964803. Pubmed Central PMCID: Pmc2696308. Epub 2007/10/30. eng.

44. Incefy GS, Flomenberg N, Heller G, Kernan NA, Brochstein J, Kirkpatrick D, *et al.* Evidence that appearance of thymulin in plasma follows lymphoid chimerism and precedes development of immunity in patients with lethal combined immunodeficiency

transplanted with T cell-depleted haploidentical marrow. *Transplantation*. 1990;50(1):55–61. PubMed PMID: 2368151. Epub 1990/07/01. eng.

45. Reisner Y, Kapoor N, Kirkpatrick D, Pollack MS, Cunningham-Rundles S, Dupont B, *et al.* Transplantation for severe combined immunodeficiency with HLA-A,B,D,DR incompatible parental marrow cells fractionated by soybean agglutinin and sheep red blood cells. *Blood*. 1983;61(2):341–8. PubMed PMID: 6217853. Epub 1983/02/01. eng.

46. Castro-Malaspina H, Jabubowski AA, Papadopoulos EB, Boulad F, Young JW, Kernan NA, *et al.* Transplantation in remission improves the disease-free survival of patients with advanced myelodysplastic syndromes treated with myeloablative T cell-depleted stem cell transplants from HLA-identical siblings. *Biology of Blood and Marrow Transplantation: Journal of the American Society for Blood and Marrow Transplantation*. 2008;14(4):458–68.

PubMed PMID: 18342789. Epub 2008/03/18. eng.

47. Perales MA, Jenq R, Goldberg JD, Wilton AS, Lee SS, Castro-Malaspina HR, *et al.* Second-line age-adjusted International Prognostic Index in patients with advanced non-Hodgkin lymphoma after T-cell depleted allogeneic hematopoietic SCT. *Bone Marrow Transplantation*. 2010;45(9):1408–16. PubMed PMID: 20062091. Pubmed Central PMCID: Pmc3076892. Epub 2010/01/12. eng.

48. Bethge WA, Faul C, Bornhauser M, Stuhler G, Beelen DW, Lang P, *et al.* Haploidentical allogeneic hematopoietic cell transplantation in adults using CD3/CD19 depletion and reduced intensity conditioning: an update. *Blood Cells, Molecules & Diseases*. 2008;40(1):13–9. PubMed PMID: 17869547. Epub 2007/09/18. eng.

49. Federmann B, Bornhauser M, Meisner C, Kordelas L, Beelen DW, Stuhler G, *et al.* Haploidentical allogeneic hematopoietic cell transplantation in

adults using CD3/CD19 depletion and reduced intensity conditioning: a phase II study. *Haematologica*. 2012;97(10):1523–31. PubMed PMID: 22491731. Pubmed Central PMCID: Pmc3487553. Epub 2012/04/12. eng.

50. Eissens DN, Schaap NP, Preijers FW, Dolstra H, van Cranenbroek B, Schattenberg AV, *et al.* CD3+/CD19+-depleted grafts in HLA-matched allogeneic peripheral blood stem cell transplantation lead to early NK cell cytolytic responses and reduced inhibitory activity of NKG2A. *Leukemia*. 2010;24(3):583–91. PubMed PMID: 20033055. Epub 2009/12/25. eng.

51. Wagner JE, Thompson JS, Carter SL, Kernan NA. Effect of graft-*versus*-host disease prophylaxis on 3-year disease-free survival in recipients of unrelated donor bone marrow (T-cell Depletion Trial): a multi-centre, randomised phase II-III trial. *Lancet*. 2005;366(9487):733–41. PubMed PMID: 16125590. Epub 2005/08/30. eng.

Chapter

31

Hematopoietic Cell Transplants for Children with Acute Lymphoblastic Leukemia

Sarah Dobrozsi, Julie-An Talano, and Bruce Camitta

Introduction

Treatment and prognosis for children with acute lymphoblastic leukemia (ALL) have improved dramatically in the last decades. Expected overall survival (OS) is >85% at 5 years from diagnosis[1]. Risk stratification uses clinical variables, immunophenotype, genetic or molecular lesions, and response to therapy to determine treatment intensity. The most intense treatment approach is reserved for patients with a very high risk of relapse, and has significantly improved outcomes in this challenging group of patients.

Currently, the use of hematopoietic cell transplant (HCT) for ALL in first remission (CR1) is reserved for a select group of very high-risk patients. The use of HCT for treatment of relapsed ALL is more common, but has declined as better outcomes with chemotherapy alone are achieved. This chapter will discuss the current evidence for use of HCT for children with ALL in first remission or after relapse. Gaps in our knowledge are highlighted and suggested approaches proposed.

HCT in First Remission (CR1)

Response to Treatment

Primary Induction Failure

Children with B-precursor ALL who experience induction failure, defined as greater than 5% blasts in the bone marrow (BM) at the end of induction, have a poor prognosis when treated with chemotherapy alone. In both retrospective and prospective analyses, the OS for children with primary induction failure improved to 60% when treated with HCT in CR1 compared to 30% with chemotherapy alone[2,3]. These data support the use of HCT for children with primary induction failure who achieve CR1 after additional chemotherapy.

Children with T-cell ALL with induction failure or prednisone poor response ($\geq$1000 blasts/µL in peripheral blood after 1 week of prednisone) have a poor prognosis when treated with chemotherapy alone. In two consecutive Berlin–Frankfurt–Munster (BFM) trials, 191 patients with high-risk T-cell ALL received HCT if a matched sibling donor (MSD) was available or chemotherapy alone. The 5-year disease-free survival (DFS) was 72 +/−11% for patients who had a MSD HCT *versus* 48 +/−6% for patients who received

chemotherapy (P=0.07)[4]. Based on these limited data, we recommend HCT for children with T-cell ALL who experience poor response to initial therapy. Further confirmatory evidence is needed.

Minimal Residual Disease

Evaluation for minimal residual disease (MRD) by flow cytometry or PCR detects the presence of small amounts of leukemia cells. Early response to therapy is an independent prognostic factor in childhood ALL; patients who fail to achieve MRD-negative status after induction therapy have increased risk of relapse[5–8]. MRD in early therapy is used as a clinical tool for treatment modification.

In the Children's Oncology Group (COG) high-risk trial AALL0232, 5-year event-free survival (EFS) for patients with positive MRD ($\geq$0.01%) at the end of induction was 63% *versus* 86% for MRD-negative patients. For MRD-positive patients, those who became negative by the end of consolidation had an improved 5-year EFS of 79% compared to 52% for those who remained positive (P=0.0012)[9]. Patients who are MRD-positive after induction should continue with chemotherapy and repeat MRD evaluation after consolidation. There are no data to suggest that HCT improves outcomes for patients who achieve MRD-negative status at this later time point. Patients who remain MRD-positive after consolidation have a high rate of relapse, and warrant consideration of HCT in CR1. However, the effectiveness of HCT in such patients remains to be shown.

Biology

Hypodiploid ALL

Hypodiploid ALL (fewer than 46 chromosomes in leukemia cells) has a poor prognosis when treated with conventional chemotherapy. Outcomes are worse in patients with $\leq$44 chromosomes. A review of 130 patients with $\leq$44 chromosomes treated by various cooperative groups and large single institutions demonstrated an 8-year EFS/OS of 38.5 +/−5.7% and 49.8 +/−6.0%. Nine of the 130 patients underwent HCT in CR1; five had an adverse event (relapse, second malignancy, or death) after transplantation. Overall survival and EFS did not differ significantly between those who underwent HCT and those who did not, though analysis was limited by small patient numbers[10]. The COG very high-risk ALL study (AALL0031) treated 40 children with hypodiploid ALL. Twenty-eight received chemotherapy alone and 12 underwent related donor HCT. The 4-year EFS was 50 +/−11% for chemotherapy alone and 65 +/−14% for HCT ($P=0.65$)[11]. Analysis was again limited by small patient numbers. A retrospective study of 78 children with hypodiploid ALL who underwent HCT demonstrated improved outcomes for patients transplanted in CR1, particularly for children with ≤ 43 chromosomes[12]. Mehta *et al.* reported on 78 children with hypodiploid ALL who underwent hematopoietic stem cell transplantation between 1990 and 2010[13]. Thirty-nine (50%) patients had ≤ 43 chromosomes, 12 (15%) had 44 chromosomes, and 27 (35%) had 45 chromosomes. Forty-three (55%) patients underwent transplantation in first remission (CR1) and 35 (45%) underwent transplantation in $\geq$ second remission (CR2). Twenty-nine patients (37%) received a graft from a related donor and 49 (63%) from an unrelated donor. All patients received a myeloablative conditioning regimen. The 5-year probabilities of leukemia-free survival, overall survival, relapse, and treatment-related mortality for the entire cohort were 51%, 56%, 27%, and 22%, respectively. Multivariate analysis confirmed that mortality risks were higher for patients who underwent transplantation in CR2 (hazard ratio, 2.16; $P=0.05$), with number of chromosomes ≤ 43 (hazard ratio, 2.15; $P=0.05$), and for those who underwent transplantation in the first decade of the study period (hazard ratio, 2.60; $P=0.01$). Similarly, treatment failure risks were higher with number of chromosomes ≤ 43 (hazard ratio, 2.28; $P=0.04$) and the earlier transplantation period (hazard ratio, 2.51; $P=0.01$). Further research is necessary to better define the role of HCT in these patients. However, given the high rate of postremission events and poor EFS in children with hypodiploid ALL treated with chemotherapy alone, we recommend consideration of HCT in first remission.

Philadelphia Chromosome-Positive (Ph+) ALL

The Philadelphia chromosome (Ph) results from the translocation t(9;22) and occurs in 3–5% of childhood ALL. Classically it was associated with a poor prognosis. Prior to the use of imatinib, children who underwent HCT in CR1 had a reduced risk of relapse or death in remission at 5 years compared to children who received aggressive chemotherapy alone (HR 0.32, 95% CI 0.20−0.52)[14]. Even with HCT the EFS/OS for Ph+ ALL of 43.5%/54% was significantly worse than for Ph-ALL[14]. The COG study AALL0031 treated all Ph+ patients with imatinib plus chemotherapy with marked improvement. Patients with HLA-matched related donors proceeded to HCT. The 5-year EFS for Ph+ patients treated with imatinib and chemotherapy was 71 +/−12% *versus* 64 +/−12% for those treated with an HCT ($P=0.77$). Patients who relapsed after treatment with chemotherapy plus imatinib achieved a second complete remission (CR2) at similar rates as patients treated without imatinib and proceeded to HCT in CR2[15,16]. Long-term follow-up for patients

transplanted in CR2 is not yet available. Given the improvement in treatment of Ph+ ALL, we recommend treatment with chemotherapy plus imatinib in children who attain a CR1. HCT should be reserved for salvage therapy of refractory or relapsed patients.

Mixed-Lineage-Leukemia (MLL) Gene Rearrangement

Rearrangements of the 11q23 chromosomal region, the site of the MLL gene, are seen in 8% of pediatric ALL. Patients with MLL gene rearrangements (MLL-R) demonstrate significant clinical heterogeneity, and age is the most important prognostic factor. Infants with any MLL-R experience significantly inferior EFS compared to older cohorts; EFS of children < 1 year at diagnosis is 19–40% *versus* 43–78% for children 1–9 years, and 39–60% for children ≥ 10 years[17]. Analysis of children with the t(4;11) translocation who underwent HCT compared to chemotherapy alone demonstrated worse DFS and OS for children who received HCT (DFS HR 1.61, 95% CI 1.10–2.35, $P=0.014$)[17]. Children > 1 year old with MLL-R should not undergo HCT in CR1 if MLL-R is the only risk factor. Further consideration should be given on a case by case basis for children with MLL-R and additional poor prognostic factors.

Infants with MLL-R represent a distinct subpopulation. Treatment recommendations are discussed below.

Infant ALL

Infants with ALL have a worse prognosis compared to older children, with cure rates of 40–50%. Outcomes are further stratified by patient age (younger patients fare worse), WBC count at diagnosis (higher WBC count worse), and the presence of MLL-R (rearranged worse). The prevalence of MLL-R is 70–80%, much higher than in older children.

The multinational Interfant-99 study evaluated intensive hybrid chemotherapy in infants with ALL. Infants without MLL-R had a 3-year EFS of 75%, infants ≥ 90 days old with MLL-R had a 3-year EFS of 47–53%, while infants < 90 days with MLL-R had a 3-year EFS of < 20%[18]. These data support treatment of non-MLL-R infant ALL with chemotherapy alone.

The use of HCT in infants with MLL-R ALL remains controversial. Studies demonstrate similar outcomes for infants with MLL-R ALL treated with HCT or chemotherapy in CR1 (EFS 40–50% for both groups)[18–20]. There is no question that infants with MLL-R ALL have dismal outcomes, particularly infants < 3 months. Current available data do not support a survival advantage for treatment with chemotherapy *versus* HCT. Ongoing investigation into novel treatment approaches for this group of patients is critical. Given the toxicities of both intensive chemotherapy and HCT in this patient age group (especially children < 3 months) without clear survival benefit of either approach, we recommend treatment with chemotherapy in CR1 for all infants with ALL regardless of MLL-R unless there are other considerations (such as MRD positivity).

iAMP21

Intrachromosomal amplification of chromosome 21 (iAMP21) is a gene amplification of *RUNX1* with a morphologically abnormal chromosome 21. iAMP21 is seen in 2% of childhood ALL and is a marker of inferior survival[21–23]. The 6-year EFS/OS for patients with iAMP21 is 26–38%/66−60%[21,24]. A retrospective analysis of patients stratified to SR or HR therapy without knowledge of iAMP21 status demonstrated that children who received HR therapy had similar outcomes regardless of iAMP21 status (4-year EFS 72.5% *versus* 80.8%, P =0.6670), while children with iAMP21 treated with SR therapy had worse outcomes than SR patients without iAMP21 (4-year EFS 72.7% *versus* 90.0 %, P <0.001)[23].

The presence of MRD in combination with iAMP21 is a robust predictor of risk of relapse. Patients with iAMP21 and negative MRD at days 33 and 78 had 100% RFS compared to patients with iAMP21 and positive MRD at either time point, whose RFS was 37 +/−16% (P=0.02)[24]. Given the rarity of iAMP21, trials comparing high-risk chemotherapy *versus* HCT in CR1 do not exist. The data demonstrate that patients with iAMP21 who remain MRD-positive after the first month of treatment have a high risk of relapse and inferior overall survival. We recommend consideration of HCT for patients with iAMP21 who are MRD-positive at the end of induction after additional chemotherapy to achieve an MRD-negative status. However, the effectiveness of HCT for these patients is not yet known.

IKAROS

Deletion or mutation of the gene encoding the transcription factor IKAROS is associated with elevated levels of MRD and high rates of relapse[25]. Patients with IKAROS mutation or deletion have a relapse-free survival rate (RFS) of 35% treated with high-risk therapy. The combination of the IKAROS mutation and elevated MRD after the initial phase of therapy resulted in significantly inferior 9-year RFS of 27% compared with patients who were MRD-positive but IKAROS negative, whose RFS was 96% (P <0.001)[26]. Similar to iAMP21, trials comparing treatment with high-risk chemotherapy *versus* HCT in CR1 do not exist. Owing to the increased risk of relapse for patients with IKAROS mutation/deletion with residual MRD after the initial phase of therapy, we recommend consideration of HCT after achievement of MRD-negative status with additional chemotherapy.

Early T-Cell Precursor (ETP) ALL

ETP ALL represents a distinct subpopulation of pediatric T-cell ALL (immunophenotype CD1a$^-$, CD8$^-$, CD5^{weak} with stem cell/myeloid markers). Historically, ETP ALL had a worse prognosis compared to other T-ALL when treated with conventional chemotherapy, with 10-year EFS/OS of 19%/22% *versus* 69%/84%[27]. Large studies of ETP patients treated with HCT are lacking, however many centers have elected to treat patients with HCT based upon superiority of HCT in other

high-risk T-ALL (induction failure or prednisone poor responders)[4]. Results of the European study UKALL 2003 (MRD used to risk-stratify patients) demonstrated a 4-year EFS/OS of 76.0%/84.1% for ETP ALL, a substantial improvement over historical controls[28]. Results from the AIEOP-Berlin-Frankfurt-Münster (AIEOP-BFM) protocols reveal similar results[29]. These recent data suggest that modern risk-directed chemotherapy is appropriate for children with ETP ALL. Ongoing investigation into optimal treatment for these patients is critical to better define best treatment approaches.

HCT in Second Remission (CR2)

Hematologic Relapse

The role of HCT for treatment of relapsed ALL has evolved over the last two decades. Current practice distinguishes between patients at high, intermediate, and low risk of treatment failure in relapse, refining the use of HCT in those groups.

Early Relapse

Early BM relapse is variably defined as relapse <36 months from initial diagnosis (COG) or within 6 months of completing therapy (European groups). Patients with B-precursor ALL and early relapse have an EFS of 14–20%[30]. EFS improves to 33 +/−5% (P <0.005) when treated with HCT after achievement of CR2 with reinduction therapy[30]. We recommend HCT for children with B-ALL and early BM relapse after achievement of CR2.

Late Relapse

Late BM relapse is defined as BM or combined relapse >36 months from diagnosis or >6 months after completion of treatment. The use of HCT in this group remains controversial. Uncontrolled series have favored either chemotherapy or HCT; however, the data are complicated by many factors including different chemotherapy protocols, transplantation regimens, histocompatibility of transplant donors, variable salvage after treatment failures, and inability to transplant some individuals due to poor performance status or relapse prior to transplantation.

MRD monitoring is useful to optimize the treatment approach in these patients. A prospective, blinded study of patients with late BM relapse treated molecular good responders (MRD < 10^{-3}) with HCT if a matched sibling donor (MSD) was available or continued with consolidation and maintenance chemotherapy. The EFS was not statistically different, at 80 +/−9% for the HCT group compared to 66 +/−6% for chemotherapy alone (P=0.45)[31]. Children with molecular poor response (MRD >10^{-3}) were eligible for HCT from MSD and matched unrelated donors (MUD): 83% of eligible patients underwent transplant with the remaining patients continuing chemotherapy. Outcomes improved significantly in the transplant cohort, with EFS of 64% compared to chemotherapy alone (EFS of 24%)[31]. There were no statistically significant differences in EFS/OS between molecular good responders who received chemotherapy alone and molecular poor responders who received HCT[31].

A separate analysis of a limited number of patients who received chemotherapy alone for treatment of first relapse demonstrated a 2-year second relapse rate of 81.5 +/−14.4% for MRD-positive patients at the end of induction compared to 25.0 +/−13.1% for MRD-negative patients ($P=0.004$)[32]. Based on these data, we recommend chemotherapy alone for children with late BM relapse with molecular good response after reinduction therapy and HCT for children with poor molecular response after reinduction therapy.

Extramedullary Relapse

Isolated CNS Relapse

Similar to BM relapse, CNS relapse that occurs early (<18 months from initial diagnosis) has a worse prognosis than later CNS relapse. Patients treated with intensive systemic chemotherapy plus radiation therapy with early relapse had significantly worse EFS (51.6% compared to 80.2% in late relapse, $P=0.027$), as did patients who were classified as high risk *versus* standard risk at initial presentation (4-year EFS 51.4% *versus* 80.2%, $P=0.0018$)[33]. These patients were compared to children who received MSD HCT in CR2 for treatment of isolated CNS relapse. The relapse rates were similar after chemotherapy or HCT for both groups, with an 8-year leukemia-free survival of 66% for chemotherapy plus irradiation and 58% for HCT[34]. Relapse rates were higher in older children aged 11–17 years (RR 2.81) and patients with early relapse (RR 3.89). Treatment-related mortality was higher after HCT (RR 4.28)[34]. For children with late isolated CNS relapse, we recommend treatment with chemotherapy plus radiation therapy. Current data do not support a clear survival benefit of HCT for children with early isolated CNS relapse. Treatment should be chosen based on physician and family preferences.

Isolated Testicular Relapse

Isolated testicular relapse is rare, occurring in ~2% of patients. Relapse is defined as early or late according to the same criteria as CNS relapse (<18 months or ≥ 18 months from initial diagnosis). The 6-year OS for early relapse is 52% and late relapse is 81% with chemotherapy plus orchiectomy or testicular irradiation[35–39], supporting treatment of late relapse patients without HCT. Transplant is often used as standard therapy for children with early isolated testicular relapse. However, there are very limited data to support this approach.

Relapsed T-ALL

Children with BM relapse of T-ALL have a significantly worse prognosis than patients with B-ALL; EFS after intensive reinduction chemotherapy is $<20%$ regardless of time to relapse [40–42]. We recommend treatment with HCT for all children with relapsed T-ALL, regardless of other clinical features of disease. However, more data are needed to confirm a benefit of HCT in these patients.

Decision Tree

In the absence of controlled clinical trials clearly delineating the outcomes for chemotherapy *versus* HCT in various settings of relapsed ALL, a decision tree analysis can be used. A diagram is made of all possible outcomes for each treatment, and each outcome is assigned two values: the frequency with which it occurs and the value of that outcome for a patient. By multiplying these and summing the numbers one arrives at the expected value (utility) of each initial choice. Investigators/patients can test how sensitive the analysis is to changes in frequencies of events or in values of outcomes to individual patients.

Decision tree analysis of chemotherapy *versus* stem cell transplantation for treatment of B-precursor ALL in CR2 is modeled in Figure 31.1. This model was created by the authors based on the best available data and predicts that the approaches produce equivalent long-term results. The equivalent long-term result in our model is supported by data comparing outcomes of COG chemotherapy with transplant results from the IBMTR[43]. EFS/OS were similar in patients treated initially with chemotherapy (59%/66%) or stem cell transplantation (60%/63%)[43].

It should be stressed that the decision model in Figure 31.1 does not account for patient preferences regarding risk taking nor does it account for physician preferences and center biases. That is with HCT the greatest period of risk is in the first 6 months of transplantation. In contrast, the risks of chemotherapy are spread out over a longer period of time. For some patients, immediate risk is less tolerable whereas for others, longer treatment with chemotherapy is less tolerable.

Controversies

What Is the Role of MRD in Preparation for HCT?

For children who warrant HCT for relapsed ALL, the presence or absence of MRD prior to HCT has important prognostic implications. In a study of 64 children with very high-risk ALL who underwent HCT in CR2, those with pretransplant MRD had a 5-year OS of 49% compared to 88% for those who were MRD-negative[44]. Sutton *et al.* analysed HCT outcomes in 81 children from the ANZCHOG ALL8 trial. Patients achieving bone marrow MRD negativity pre-HSCT had better outcomes (LFS 83%, OS 92%) than those with persistent MRD pre-HSCT (LFS 41%, OS 64%, $P<0·0001$) or post-HSCT (LFS 35%, OS 55%, $P<0·0001$)[45]. The prognostic significance of MRD on OS and EFS is proportional to the amount of MRD, patients with higher levels of pretransplant MRD being more likely to experience relapse[46,47]. We recommend consideration of MRD status, in combination with additional patient-specific factors, in determination of timing of HCT for children with relapsed ALL.

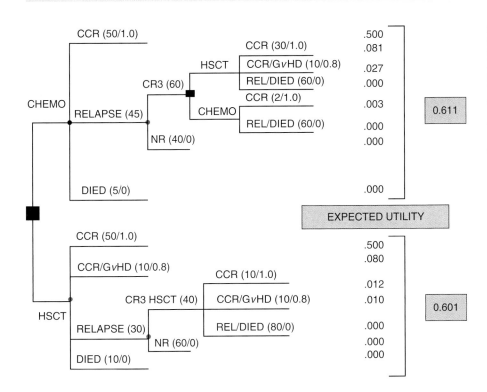

Figure 31.1 Decision tree analysis of chemotherapy *versus* stem cell transplantation for treatment of B-precursor acute lymphocytic leukemia in second remission after a late bone marrow relapse. Numbers in parentheses (/) indicate frequency of outcomes/value of that outcome to a patient. CCR = continued complete remission, chemo = chemotherapy, GvHD = graft-*versus*-host disease, NR = no response, REL = relapse, HSCT = stem cell transplant. For this analysis we have assigned patient values for CCR of 1, for relapse/death/no response of 0, and for alive in CCR with GvHD of 0.8.

How Aggressive Should We Be to Achieve MRD-Negative Status Prior to HCT?

Some patients with MRD who proceed to HCT achieve durable remission. MRD positivity should not be an absolute contraindication to HCT[44,48]. Debate continues regarding how aggressive to be to achieve MRD-negative status prior to HCT. A report of a small number of patients (n=8) used reduced dose clofarabine, cytarabine, and etoposide as "bridging therapy" for children with relapsed ALL with detectable MRD (>0.01%) prior to HCT. The regimen was well tolerated and effectively reduced pretransplant MRD[49]. It is too soon to tell how this or similar regimens should be used. Our current recommendation is consideration of MRD status, in combination with additional patient-specific factors, in determination of timing of HCT for children with relapsed ALL.

What Is the Optimal Donor Source?

The debate continues regarding the optimal donor source for patients with relapse. Early studies comparing MSD *versus* unrelated donor transplants demonstrated clear survival advantage with MSD (8-year OS 60.0% *versus* 13.5%, P= 0.0062)[50]. Improved supportive care practices and transplant center expertise with unrelated donor transplants has eliminated this disparity[51]. Considerations for donor source should include degree of match, timing and logistics of transplant, and expertise with various alternative donor transplant approaches at individual transplant centers[52].

References

1. Schrappe M, Nachman J, Hunger S, Schmeigelow K, Conter V, Masera G, *et al.* Educational symposium on long-term results of large prospective clinical trials for childhood acute lymphoblastic leukemia (1985–2000). *Leukemia.* 2010;24:253–4.

2. Schrappe M, Hunger S, Pui C-H, Saha V, Gaynon P, Baruchel A, *et al.* Outcomes after induction failure in childhood acute lymphoblastic leukemia. *New Engl J Med.* 2012;366:1371–81.

3. Balduzzi A, Valsecchi M, Uderzo C, De Lorenzo P, Klingbiel T, Peters C, *et al.* Chemotherapy *versus* allogeneic transplantation for very-high-risk childhood acute lymphoblastic leukemia in first complete remission: comparison by genetic randomisation in an international prospective study. *Lancet.* 2005;366:635–42.

4. Schrauder A, Reiter A, Gadner H, Niethammer D, Klingbiel T, Kremens B, *et al.* Superiority of allogeneic hematopoietic stem-cell transplantation compared with chemotherapy alone in high-risk childhood T-cell acute lymphoblastic leukemia: results from ALL-BFM 90 and 95. *J Clin Oncol.* 2006;36:5742–9.

5. van Dongen J, Seriu T, Panzer-Grumayer E, Biondi A, Pongers-Willemse M, Corral L, *et al.* Prognostic value of minimal residual disease in acute lymphoblastic leukemia. *Lancet.* 1998;352:1731–8.

6. Cave H, van de Werff T, Bosch J, Suciu S, Guidal C, Waterkeyn C, *et al.* Clinical significance of minimal residual disease in childhood acute lymphoblastic leukemia. European Organization for Research and Treatment of

Cancer – Childhood Leukemia Cooperative Group. *New Engl J Med.* 1998;339:591–8.

7. Jacquy C, Delepaut B, Van Daele S, Vaerman J, Zenebergh A, Brichard B, *et al.* A prospective study of minimal residual disease in childhood B-lineage acute lymphoblastic leukaemia: MRD level at the end of induction is a strong predictive factor of relapse. *Br J Haematol.* 1997;98:140–6.

8. Panzer-Grumayer E, Schneider M, Panzer S, Fasching K, Gadner H. Rapid molecular response during early induction chemotherapy predicts a good outcome in childhood acute lymphoblastic leukemia. *Blood.* 2000;95:790–4.

9. Borowitz MJ, Wood BL, Devidas M, Loh ML, Raetz EA, Salzer W, *et al.* Prognostic significance of minimal residual disease in high risk B-ALL: a report from Children's Oncology Group study AALL0232. *Blood.* 2015;126(8):964–71.

10. Nachman J, Heerema N, Sather H, Camitta B, Forestier E, Harrison C, *et al.* Outcome of treatment in children with hypodiploid acute lymphoblastic leukemia. *Blood.* 2007;110:1112–5.

11. Schultz K, Devidas M, Bowman W, Aledo A, Slayton W, Sather H, *et al.* Philadelphia chromosome-negative very high-risk acute lymphoblastic leukemia in cihldren and adolescents: results from Children's Oncology Group Study AALL0031. *Leukemia.* 2014;28:964–7.

12. Mehta P, Eapen M, Zhang M-J. Transplant outcomes for children with hypodiploid acute lymphoblastic leukemia: The CIBMTR experience. *Biol Blood Marrow Transplant.* 2014;20: S87–S.

13. Mehta PA, Zhang MJ, Eapen M, He W, Seber A, Gibson B, *et al.* Transplantation outcomes for children with hypodiploid acute lymphoblastic leukemia. *Biol Blood Marrow Transplant.* 2015;21(7):1273–7.

14. Arico M, Schrappe M, Hunger S, Carroll WL, Conter V, Galimberti S, *et al.* Clinical outcome in children with newly diagnosed Philadephia chromosome-positive acute lymphoblastic leukemia treated between 1995 and 2005. *J Clin Oncol.* 2010;28(31):4755–61.

15. Schultz K, Bowman W, Aledo A, Slayton W, Sather H, Devidas M, *et al.*

Improved early event-free survival with imatinib in Philadelphia chromosome-positive acute lymphoblastic leukemia: a Children's Oncology Group Study. *J Clin Oncol.* 2009;31:5175–81.

16. Schultz K, Carroll A, Heerema N, Bowman W, Aledo A, Slayton W, *et al.* Long-term follow up of imatinib in pediatric Philadelphia chromosome-positive acute lymphoblastic leukemia: Children's Oncology Group Study AALL0031. *Leukemia.* 2014:1–5.

17. Pui C-H, Gayson P, Boyett J, Chessells J, Baruchel A, Kamps W, *et al.* Outcome of treatment in childhood acute lymphoblastic leukaemia with rearrangements of the 11q23 chromosomal region. *Lancet.* 2002;359:1909–15.

18. Pieters R, Schrappe M, De Lorenzo P, Hann I, De Rossi G, Felice M, *et al.* A treatment protocol for infants younger than 1 year with acute lymphoblastic leukemia (Interfant-99): an observational study and a multicentre randomised trial. *Lancet* 2007;370:240–50.

19. Dreyer Z, Dinndorf P, Camitta B, Sather H, La M, Devidas M, *et al.* Analysis of the role of hematopoietic stem-cell transplantation in infants with acute lymphoblastic leukemia in first remission and MLL gene rearrangements: a report from the Children's Oncology Group. *J Clin Oncol.* 2011;29(2):214–22.

20. Koh K, Tomizawa D, Moriya Saito A, Watanabe T, Miyamura T, Hirayama M, *et al.* Early use of hematopoietic stem cell transplantation for infants with MLL gene-rearrangement-positive acute lymphoblastic leukemia. *Leukemia.* 2015;29(2):290–6.

21. Moorman A, Ensor H, Richards S, Chilton L, Schwab C, Kinsey S, *et al.* Prognostic effect of chromosomal abnormalities in childhood B-cell precursor acute lymphoblastic leukemia: results from the UK Medical Research Council ALL97/99 randomised trial. *Lancet Oncol.* 2010;11:429–38.

22. Moorman A, Richards S, Robinson H, Strefford J, Gibson B, Kinsey S, *et al.* Prognosis of children with acute lymphoblastic leukemia (ALL) and intrachromosomal amplification of chromosome 21 (iAMP21). *Blood.* 2007;109:2327–30.

23. Heerema N, Carroll A, Devidas M, Loh ML, Borowitz MJ, Gastier-Foster JM, *et al.* Intrachromosomal amplification of chromosome 21 is associated with inferior outcomes in children with acute lymphoblastic leukemia treated in contemporary standard-risk Children's Oncology Group Studies: A report from the Children's Oncology Group. *J Clin Oncol.* 2013;31:3397–402.

24. Attarbaschi A, Mann G, Panzer-Grumayer R, Rottgers S, Steiner M, Konig M, *et al.* Minimal residual disease values discriminate between low and high relapse risk in children with B-cell precursor acute lymphoblastic leukemia and an intracromosomal amplification if chromosome 21: The Austrian and German Acute Lymphoblastic Leukemia Berline-Frankfurt-Munster (ALL-BFM) Trials. *J Clin Oncol.* 2008;26:3046–50.

25. Mullighan C, Su Z, Zhang J, Radke I, Phillips L, Miller C, *et al.* Deletion of IKZF1 and prognosis in acute lymphoblastic leukemia. *NEJM.* 2009;360:470–80.

26. Waaders E, van der Velden V, van der Schoot C, van Leeuwen F, van Reijmersdal S, de Haas V, *et al.* Integrated use of minimal residual disease classification and IKZF1 alteration status accurately predicts 79% of relapses in pediatric acute lymphoblastic leukemia. *Leukemia.* 2011;25:254–8.

27. Coustan-Smith E, Mullighan C, Onciu M, Behm F, Raimondi S, Pei D, *et al.* Early T-cell precursor leukemia: a subtype of very high-risk acute lymphoblastic leukemia identified in two independent cohorts. *Lancet Oncol.* 2009;10(2):147–56.

28. Wade R, Goulden N, Mitchell C, Rowntree C, Hough RE, Vora AJ, editors. Characteristics and Outcome Of Children and Young Adults With Early T-Precursor (ETP) ALL Treated On UKALL 2003. ASH Annual Meeting, 15 November 2013, New Orleans, LA.

29. Conter V, Valsecchi MG, Buldini B, Parasole R, Locatelli F, Colombini A, *et al.* Early T-cell precursor acute lymphoblastic leukaemia in children treated in AIEOP centres with AIEOP-BFM protocols: a retrospective analysis. *Lancet Haematol.* 2016;3(2):e80–6.

30. Tallen G, Ratei R, Mann G, Kaspers G, Niggli F, Karachunsky A, *et al.*

Long-Term Outcome in Children with Relapsed Acute Lymphoblastic Leukemia After Time-Point and Site-of-Relapse Stratification and Intensified Short-Course Multidrug Chemotherapy: Results of Trial ALL-REZ BFM 90. *J Clin Oncol.* 2010;28:2339–47.

31. Eckert C, Henze G, Seeger K, Hagedorn N, Mann G, Panzer-Grumayer R, et al. Use of allogeneic hematopoietic stem-cell transplantation based on minimal residual disease response improves outcomes for children wiht relaped acute lymphoblastic leukemia in the Intermediate-Risk Group. *J Clin Oncol.* 2013;31(21):2736–42.

32. Coustan-Smith E, Gajjar A, Hijaya N, Razzouk B, Ribeiro R, Rivera G, et al. Clinical significance of minimal residual disease in childhood acute lymphoblastic leukemia after first relapse. *Leukemia.* 2004;18:499–504.

33. Barredo J, Devidas M, Lauer S, Billett A, Marymont M, Pullen J, et al. Isolated CNS relapse of acute lymphoblastic leukemia treated with intensive systemic chemotherapy and delayed CNS radiation: A pediatric oncology group study. *J Clin Oncol.* 2006;24:3142–9.

34. Eapen M, Zhang M-J, Devidas M, Raetz E, Barredo J, Ritchey A, et al. Outcomes after HLA-matched sibling transplantation or chemotherapy in children with acute lymphoblatic leukemia in a second remission after an isolated central nervous system relapse: a collaborative study of teh Children's Oncology Group and the Center for International Blood and Marrow Transplant Research. *Leukemia.* 2008;22:281–6.

35. Gaynon P, Qu R, Chappell R, Willoughby M, Tubergen D, Steinherz P, et al. Survival after relapse in childhood acute lymphoblastic leukemia: impact of site and time to first relapse – the Children's Cancer Group Experience. *Cancer.* 1998;82:1387–95.

36. van den Berg H, Langeveld N, Veenhof C, Behrendt H. Treatment of isolated testicular recurrence of acute lymphoblastic leukemia without radiotherapy. Report from the Dutch Late Effects Study Group. *Cancer.* 1997;79:2257–63.

37. Locatelli F, Schrappe M, Bernardo M, Rutella S. How I treat relapsed childhood acute lymphoblastic leukemia. *Blood.* 2012;120:2807–16.

38. Uderzo C, Grazia Zurlo M, Adamoli L, Zanesco L, Arico M, Calculli G, et al. Treatment of isolated testicular relapse in childhood acute lymphoblastic leukemia: an Italian multicenter study. Associazione Italiana Ematologia ed Oncologia Pediatrica. *J Clin Oncol.* 1990;8:672–7.

39. Thakar M, Talano J, Tower R, Kelly M, Burke M. Indications for transplantation in childhood acute leukemia and the impact of minimal residual disease on relapse: a review. *Clin Pract.* 2014;11(1):79–90.

40. Borgmann A, von Stackelberg A, Hartmann R, Ebell W, Klingbiel T, Peters C, et al. Unrelated donor stem cell transplantation compared with chemotherapy for children with acute lymphoblastic leukemia in a second remission: a matched-pair analysis. *Blood.* 2003;101(10):3835–9.

41. Einsiedel G, von Stackelberg A, Hartmann R, Fengler R, Schrappe M, Janka-Schaub G, et al. Long-term outcome in children with relapsed ALL by risk-stratified salvage therapy: results of Trial Acute Lymphoblastic Leukemia-Relapse Study of the Berlin-Frankfurt-Munster Group 87. *J Clin Oncol.* 2005;23(31):7942–50.

42. Reismuller B, Peters C, Dworzak M, Potschger U, Urban C, Meister B, et al. Third relapse of acute lymphoblastic leukemia (ALL): a population-based analysis of the Austrian ALL-BFM Study Group. *J Pediatr Hematol Oncol.* 2013;35:e200–4.

43. Eapen M, Raetz E, Zhang M, Muehlenbein C, Devidas M, Abshire T, et al. Outcomes after HLA-matched sibling transplantation or chemotherapy in children with B-precursor acute lymphoblastic leukemia in a second remission: a collaborative study of the Children's Oncology Group and the Center for International Blood and Marrow Transplant Research. *Blood.* 2006;107:4961–7.

44. Leung W, Pui C-H, Coustan-Smith E, Yang J, Pei D, Gan K, et al. Detectable minimal residual disease before hematopoietic cell transplantation is prognostic but does not preclude cure for children with very-high-risk leukemia. *Blood.* 2012;120:468–72.

45. Sutton R, Shaw PJ, Venn NC, Law T, Dissanayake A, Kilo T, et al. Persistent MRD before and after allogeneic BMT predicts relapse in children with acute lymphoblastic leukaemia. *Br J Haematol.* 2015;168(3):395–404.

46. Bader P, Kreyenberg H, Henze G, Eckert C, Reising M, Willasch A, et al. Prognostic value of minimal residual disease quantification before allogeneic stem-cell transplantation in relapsed childhood acute lymphoblastic leukemia: the ALL-REZ BFM Study Group. *J Clin Oncol.* 2009;27:377–84.

47. Paganin M, Zecca M, Fabbri G, Polato K, Biondi A, Rizzari C, et al. Minimal residual disease is an important predictive factor of outcome in children with relapsed 'high-risk' acute lymphoblastic leukemia. *Leukemia.* 2008;22:2193–200.

48. Wayne A, Radich J. Pretransplant MRD: the light is yellow, not red. *Blood.* 2012;120:244–6.

49. Gossai N, Vernaris M, Karras N, Gorman M, Patel N, Burke M. A clofarabine-based bridging regimen in patients with relapsed ALL and persistent minimal residual disease (MRD). *Bone Marrow Transplant.* 2014;49:440–2.

50. Bleakley M, Shaw P, Nielsen J. Allogeneic bone marrow transplantation for childhood relapsed acute lymphoblastic leukemia: comparison of outcome in patients with and without a matched family donor. *Bone Marrow Transplant.* 2002;30:1–7.

51. Saarinen-Pihkala U, Gustafsson G, Ringden O, Heilmann C, Glomstein A, Lonnerholm G, et al. No disadvantage in outcome of using matched unrelated donors as compared with matched sibling donors for bone marrow transplantation in children with acute lymphoblastic leukemia in second remission. *J Clin Oncol.* 2001;15:3406–14.

52. Peters C, Schrappe M, von Stackelberg A, Schrauder A, Bader P, Ebell W, et al. Stem-cell transplantation in children with acute lymphoblastic leukemia: A prospective international multicenter trial comparing sibling donors with matched unrelated donors: The ALL-SCT-BFM-2003 trial. *J Clin Oncol.* 2015;33(11):1265–74.

Chapter

32

Hematopoietic Cell Transplants for *BCR/ABL Negative* Acute Lymphocytic Leukemia

Michelle Limei Poon and Partow Kebriaei

Introduction

Acute lymphoblastic leukemia (ALL) is a neoplasm originating from B- or T-lymphocyte precursors which undergo malignant transformation. Despite advances in our understanding of the disease process, therapeutic progress for adult ALL has been relatively slow, with long-term leukemia-free survival being achieved only in about 30–40% of subjects[1]. Modern chemotherapeutic induction regimens achieve high remission rates of more than 80%[1,2] but disease relapse following first complete remission (CR1) remains a major issue. While allogeneic hematopoietic cell transplant (allo-HCT) remains the single most effective consolidative modality for prevention of relapse, the potent graft-*versus*-leukemia (G*v*L) effect of allo-HCT is balanced by significantly higher toxicity and complication rates. The prognostic stratification for determination of the "ideal" transplant candidate, graft source, and timing of allo-HCT for adult subjects is crucial. We review herein the growing and recently published data in the field of adult ALL in order to clarify the role of frontline allo-HCT in adult ALL.

Allogeneic HCT for Patients In First Complete Remission: Does One Size Fits All?

Since the description of allo-HCT for ALL in 1973, the G*v*L effect in this context has been demonstrated in several reports [3]. The indications of allo-HCT in ALL in CR1 remain controversial, and there are differing recommendations from guidelines of various major organizations[4,5]. What is clear is that despite high CR rates, relapse remains a major issue in adult ALL patients.

In patients who relapse, outcomes are dismal with long-term overall survival (OS) rates ranging between 3% and 24% in various series[6,7]. This is largely due to the inability to attain second complete remission (CR2) or to maintain fitness for allo-HCT following salvage therapy. Given the inherent heterogeneity of ALL, it is therefore crucial to identify prognostic indicators that would identify patients for whom frontline allo-HCT should be considered. These prognostic indicators are summarized in Table 32.1.

Table 32.1 Prognostic factors in adult ALL

Risk factors	Prognostic impact
Age[57]	Continuous variable, higher risk with increasing age; Age > 35 years old commonly used cut-off
WBC counts	Adverse prognostic marker: • B-Lineage ALL: $>30 \times 10^9$/L (high-risk) • T-Lineage ALL: $>100 \times 10^9$/L (high-risk)
Cytogenetics[58,59]	Good-risk prognostic marker: • Hyperdiploidy (51–65 chromosomes) • t(12;21)(p13;q22) Intermediate risk prognostic markers: • Trisomy chromosomes 21 or 8 • t(1;19)/E2A-PBX • Deletion (6q) High-risk prognostic marker: • t(9;22)(q34;q11.2) • t(v;11q23) (MLL rearrangement) • t(4;11)/MLL-AF4 • Monosomy of chromosome 7 • Low hypodiploidy or near tetraploidy • Complex cytogenetics (>5 chromosomal abnormalities)
Immunophenotyping [60]	Good prognostic marker: • Cortical T phenotype (CD1a positive) Poor prognostic marker: • Early T precursor ALL • CD20 expression
Time to response to induction therapy	Poor prognostic marker: • Failure to achieve complete remission within 4 weeks of induction treatment

Table 32.2 Summary of meta-analyses looking at the role of allo-HCT compared to autologous transplantation or chemotherapy in first complete remission in adult ALL

Meta-analyses	Time period included/ number of studies included	Conclusions
Yanada *et al.* 2006[8]	Before 2005/7 studies (n=1274 patients)	For high-risk patients: Improved OS in patients in the donor compared to no-donor groups Hazard ratio (HR): 1.42 and 95% CI (1.06–1.90) (P=0.019) Results inconclusive for SR patients, as the majority of studies included (n=6) did not provide data for this patient population
Orsi *et al.* 2007[61]	Between 2000 and 2007/4 studies (n= 772 patients)	For high-risk patients: Improved EFS in the donor arm, P=0.011 Cost-effectiveness profile acceptable Results inconclusive for SR patients, as studies included did not provide data for this patient population
Ram *et al.* 2010[11]	Before 2009/13 studies (n= 2648 patients)	Reduction in *all-cause mortality* (ACM) in the donor group compared to the no-donor group (RR, 0.88; 95% CI 0.8–0.97) This reduction in ACM and survival advantage was of greater statistical significance for patients with SR ALL (RR, 0.8; 95% CI 0.68–0.94) than for patients with HR ALL (RR, 0.88; 95% CI 0.76–1.01) Increased NRM (RR, 2.99; 95% CI 1.37–6.53) and a decrease in the relapse rate in the donor arm (RR, 0.52; 95% CI 0.33–0.83).
Pidala *et al.* 2011[12]	Between 1966 and 2010/14 studies (n=3157)	Improved overall survival In the donor-*versus*-no-donor group (HR 0.86; 95% CI 0.77 to 0.97; P=0.01). Improved EFS in the donor group (HR 0.82; 95% CI 0.72 to 0.94; P=0.004) Increased NRM (RR 2.8; 95% CI 1.66 to 4.73; P=0.001) in the donor group, and a decrease in relapse rates in the donor arm (RR 0.53; 95% CI 0.37 to 0.76; P=0.0004).
Gupta *et al.* 2013[13]	13 studies (n-2962)[a]	Improved overall survival in the donor group for patients <35 years of age (OR 0.79; 95% CI 0.70–0.90, P=0.0003) but not for those >35 years of age (OR 1.01; 95% CI 0.85–1.19, P=0.9)

[a] Individual patient data (IPD) from the relevant clinical studies were used which allowed assessment of the impact of important patient- and disease-related variables.

Limitations

There have been no trials in the allo-HCT field in which patients with an available donor have been randomized between allogeneic HCT and chemotherapy. Instead, most of the large prospective studies that have looked at this issue have used biologic randomization based on the availability of an HLA-matched sibling donor (MSD). Overall, data from these studies on the benefits of allo-HCT have been conflicting possibly due to the heterogeneity between the studies in terms of time period of trials, trial size, study population, definitions of risk categories, and/or treatment characteristics. Additionally, the results should be interpreted with caution since the definitions of prognostic groups are not uniform among studies.

Of note, while older trials and meta-analyses have suggested that only "high-risk" (HR) but not "standard-risk" (SR) patients benefit from allo-HCT in CR1[8], a number of recent large prospective studies have shown more pronounced benefits from allo-HCT in the SR group[9,10]. In one of the largest studies, Goldstone *et al.*[9] reported on the Medical Research Council (MRC) UKALLXII/ECOG 2993 study involving 1031 patients and showed using a donor *versus* no-donor analysis, an improved 5-year OS (53% *versus* 45%, P=0.01), and lower relapse rates (P=0.001) in the donor group. Of note, the survival benefit was most marked in the SR group, while in the HR group, the reduced relapsed rates were offset by the higher nonrelapse mortality (NRM). Two recent meta-analyses, with inclusion of these new studies, have been conducted and demonstrated more pronounced survival benefits for allo-HCT in the SR arm[11,12]. Interestingly, in a systematic review of the same trials, taking into account individual patient data, Gupta *et al.* showed that the improvement in OS in MSD myeloablative allo-HCT was significant only for younger patients (less than 35 years), with an absolute benefit of 10% at 5 years[13]. Table 32.2 summarizes results of the meta-analyses done in this area.

Overall, despite the ambiguity among the results of studies done in this area, most have shown that relapse rates in the allo-HCT arms remain distinctly superior compared to both autologous transplantation as well as conventional chemotherapy (e.g., 63% *versus* 37%, MRC/ECOG trial), suggesting that the conflicting results were due to higher NRM in the HR groups abrogating the OS benefits from allo-HCT [9,10,12,13].

Practice Points

Currently, upfront allo-HCT is the treatment of choice in adult patients with HR (commonly defined by older age >35, elevated WBC count (Table 32.1), recurring cytogenetic abnormalities: t(9;22), t(4;11), complex karyotype, low hypodiploidy, or delayed time to CR1) ALL, with HLA-matched donors. For patients with SR disease, however, the decision for allo-HCT remains controversial; the difficulty of this approach has been identifying SR patients who are unlikely to be cured by chemotherapy alone and for whom allo-HCT would be necessary.

Can Minimal Residual Disease (MRD) Guide Allo-HCT Decisions?

While the above prognostic indicators clearly delineate patients into high and standard risk for relapse, they often lack prognostic precision at the level of the individual patient. In particular, relapses in the SR patient group occur in about 40% to 55% of cases and cannot be predicted by conventional risk factors. In these patients, novel methods for disease assessment such as detection of persistent MRD may help identify appropriate patients for allo-HCT (see Chapters 23 and 24).

Patel *et al.*[14] prospectively analyzed MRD samples following induction, consolidation, and maintenance of 161 patients with non T-lineage, Ph chromosome-negative, ALL subjects treated on the MRC/ECOG trial, and found that MRD status best discriminated outcome after 10 weeks of therapy, when the relative risk of relapse was 8.95-fold higher in MRD-positive patients and the 5-year relapse-free survival was 15% compared to 71% in MRD-negative patients. Similarly, Bruggemann *et al.*[15] for the German Multicenter Study Group for Adult ALL (GMALL) demonstrated that the serial quantification of MRD after induction chemotherapy identified three prognostic subgroups with vastly different 3-year relapse rates ranging from 0% to 94% among 196 SR patients.

In recent years, the GMALL[16], the North Italy Leukemia group (NILG)[17], and the Spanish PETHEMA group[18] (Programa para el Estudio de la Terapéutica en Hemopatía Maligna) have taken MRD use a step further, integrating these results into individualized risk-adapted strategies for allo-HCT with promising outcomes. Gokbuget *et al.*[16] demonstrated that patients with molecular failure (defined as persistent quantifiable MRD positivity within the quantitative range of $\geq 10^{-4}$) after induction/consolidation chemotherapy undergoing allo-HCT in CR1 had significantly improved disease-free survival (DFS) (44% *versus* 11%, $P=0.001$) and OS (54% *versus* 33%, $P=0.06$) compared to those who did not. Within the NILG, Bassan *et al.*[17] performed an MRD-oriented therapy for Ph-negative patients (excluding those with the t(4;11) translocation), and were able to identify a low-risk MRD-

negative population, with bone marrow relapse rates of less than 20%, and DFS nearly 80%, in whom allo-HCT in CR1 was unnecessary. Similarly, a recent publication from the PETHEMA group[18] demonstrated that in HR patients (based on pretreatment characteristics) with rapid MRD clearance, avoiding allo-HCT was safe, with 5-year DFS and OS of 55% and 59%, respectively, from chemotherapy alone. Of note, in all three studies, multivariate analysis showed that the pattern of MRD clearance was the most significant prognostic factor for CR duration and OS, as compared to conventional prognostic risk factors.

Practice Points

These findings taken together suggest that MRD may allow for personalized decision-making among adults with ALL, identifying SR patients with higher risks of relapse where treatment intensification is necessary, and sparing low-risk patients from unnecessary treatment. Well-controlled prospective clinical trials on optimization of standardized techniques, robust quality assurance, and identification of optimal time points for measurement for MRD are, however, necessary before widespread use of MRD-directed therapies can be utilized (see Chapter 24).

Should Pediatric Inspired ALL Regimens Spare Allo-HCT in Young Adults with ALL?

This remains controversial. While the meta-analysis by Gupta *et al.* suggested that patients less than 35 years with a HLA-matched donor (Table 32.2) should be treated with allo-HCT, it is still controversial whether this conclusion can be applied in young adult (AYA) SR patients treated on pediatric protocols. A number of retrospective analyses from large cooperative groups in the United States, as well as in France and the United Kingdom have suggested superior outcomes in young adult patients treated on pediatric protocols[19,20,21]. The limitation of such retrospective analyses, however, has been potential confounding factors, and concerns that the improved outcomes may be due to the pediatric culture of strict adherence to schedule with minimal interruptions rather than due to the actual benefit of more intense chemotherapy regimens. The largest prospective trial assessing the feasibility of a pediatric regimen in AYA patients treated by adult medical hematologists/oncologists is ongoing in North America (C-10403) and will hopefully answer some of these questions. Preliminary data from this study suggest that treatment with a pediatric regimen (C10403) is feasible though clinical outcomes are still being assessed.

Allogeneic HCT for Relapsed/Refractory Adult ALL

Outcomes from Large Cooperative and Multicenter Groups

In patients with primary refractory or relapsed disease, there is usually poor response to subsequent chemotherapy regimens ranging from 40% to 45%[6,22,23], with OS usually less than 10%. Importantly, for patients who respond, various studies have shown that allo-HCT in CR2 offers a better chance of long-term survival (PFS between 25–40%) as compared to chemotherapy and/or autologous transplantation [7,6,23,24] alone. Notably, the outcomes are also much poorer compared to patients transplanted in CR1, underscoring again the importance of identifying poor-risk patients who should be transplanted early in CR1.

Is There a Role for Allo-HCT without Reinduction Chemotherapy in Subjects with "Early" Relapse?

Many patients treated with salvage therapy fail to make it to allo-HCT, either because of refractory disease or due to the toxicities of reinduction chemotherapy precluding allo-HCT [22]. The TRM associated with reinduction chemotherapy may be as high as 20%[22]. One area of debate, therefore, has been whether to proceed directly to allo-HCT if disease tempo allows and an HLA-matched donor is readily available? Duval *et al.*[25] reviewed Center for International Blood and Marrow Transplant Research (CIBMTR) registry results in patients with acute leukemia transplanted in relapse or induction failure, and suggested a number of prognostic markers which might identify patients who would benefit from allo-HCT during relapse, with 3-year OS ranging between 15% and 46%. The nature of the study, however, did not allow for reliable comparison between transplantation in first relapse *versus* chemotherapy. In one of the largest retrospective reviews looking at this issue, Terwey *et al.*[26] demonstrated a 5-year OS rate of 47% in 19 patients with relapsed or refractory disease who received allo-HCT without prior reinduction chemotherapy, a result that was superior to the group that had received prior reinduction chemotherapy (5-year OS: 18%). It should be noted that the patients who went immediately to transplant had very low tumor burden, and such results are not universally shared, with several studies suggesting allo-HCT in CR2 is superior to allo-HCT in refractory disease[27,28].

Practice Points

More prospective data are necessary before any recommendations can be made, and currently, management decisions regarding reinduction chemotherapy *versus* upfront transplant in early relapse will have to be individualized depending on the patient, tempo of the disease, and the availability of donor.

Optimal Conditioning Regimen

Is TBI-Based "Myeloablative" Regimen Necessary in Adult ALL?

Myeloablative conditioning (MAC) regimen for adults with ALL usually has included total body irradiation (TBI) or busulfan. In ALL, the existing large series demonstrated improved PFS and/or OS for TBI-based conditioning regimens [29,30].

These findings together with the ability of TBI-based MAC regimens to eradicate leukemic cells in "sanctuary sites" such as the central nervous system and the testicles have led to TBI + cyclophosphamide as the preferred regimen. The significantly high NRM rates (20–45%) and the long-term effects of TBI-based MAC regimens especially in younger adults has led to the development of alternative non-TBI-based MAC regimens. Table 32.3A shows a number of trials that have reported this strategy. Apart from the traditional busulfan/cyclophosphamide myeloablative conditioning regimens, Daly *et al.*[31], Santarone *et al.*[32], and Kebriaei *et al.*[33] have reported single-institution studies on 29, 44, and 51 subjects, respectively. About two-thirds of the patients were in CR1. These regimens show encouraging rates of PFS and OS, as well as acceptable toxicity profiles, and demonstrate that such reduced toxicity MAC regimens are feasible treatment alternatives to TB-based MAC regimens.

Where is the Role of Reduced Intensity Conditioning (RIC) Regimen in Adult ALL?

The published data for RIC regimen in ALL are less extensive as they are for myeloid neoplasms or low-grade lymphoid malignancies, with no randomized trials comparing RIC to MAC regimens. Nevertheless, there have been two large observational database retrospective registry studies from the European Group of Blood and Marrow Transplantation (EBMT) and CIBMTR [34,35] as well as a number of small single-center prospective studies [36–38] demonstrating the feasibility and efficacy of RIC regimen for adult ALL (Table 32.3B). In patients not in remission, however, RIC regimen appears to be ineffective (see Chapter 27). A study of 22 "HR" adults with ALL , of whom 16 had active disease, had only 4 patients (18%) alive and in CR on follow-up, suggesting a limited role for RIC allo-HCT for ALL not in remission[39].

Practice Point

RIC allo-HCT should be considered for ALL patients in CR1 with anticipated higher NRM, In contrast, for "younger" adults with ALL without comorbidities and higher risks of relapse (e.g., disease in CR2 and beyond), MAC regimens would be the appropriate choice outside of a clinical trial.

Donor Selection: Beyond MSD

Unrelated HLA-Matched Volunteer Donor Transplants

MVD transplants have been previously reserved for patients with "HR" disease due to concerns of potentially increased NRM compared to MSD transplants. Over time, there have been more data suggesting comparable outcomes between MVD and MSD transplants, likely due to improvements in high-resolution HLA typing and better supportive care [29]. Given that almost 40% of adults with ALL in CR1 survive

Table 32.3 Conditioning regimens in adult ALL

(A) "Myeloablative" conditioning regimens without myeloablative doses of TBI in adult ALL

Study and number of subjects	Conditioning regimen	Treatment-related mortality	Relapse rate	Survival
Santarone et al.[32] n=44 CR1, n=27 Ph-negative, n=27	Fludarabine and targeted busulfan (AUC between 5300 and 7500 µM/min)	18% at 2 years	19% at 2 years (CR1) 48% at 2 years (>CR1)	OS 54% at 2 years Relapse-free survival 63% at 2 years (CR1) 34% at 2 years (>CR1)
Daly et al.[31] n=44 CR1, n=32 Ph-negative, n=28	Fludarabine and targeted busulfan (AUC 5000 µM/min) with 400 cGy TBI	13.6% at 100 days post-allo-HCT	16% at 5 years	OS 66% at 5 years DFS 56.7% at 5 years
Kebriaei et al.[33] n=51 CR1, n=30 Ph-negative, n=34	Clofarabine and targeted busulfan (busulfan AUC 5500 µM/min for patients age<60 years and 4000 µM/min for patients age≥60 years	32% at 1 year 25% at 1 year (CR1)	16% at 1 year (CR1) 37% at 1 year (>CR1)	OS: 67% at 1 year 74% at 1 year (CR1) DFS: 54% at 1 year 64% at 1 year (CR1)

(B) Studies with reduced intensity conditioning regimens in adult ALL

Study and number of subjects	Conditioning regimen	Treatment-related mortality	Relapse	Survival
Mohty et al.[34] RIC, n=127 MA, n=449 CR1 RIC, n=105 MA, n=391	Various	29% (MAC) versus 21% (RIC) at 2 years (P=0.03)	31% (MAC) versus 47% (RIC) at 2 years (P<0.001)	DFS: 38% (MAC) versus 32% (RIC) at 2 years (P=0.07) OS: 45% (MAC) versus 48% (RIC) at 2 years (P=0.56)
Marks et al.[35] RIC, n=93 MA, n=1428 Ph-negative – all patients	Various	33% (MAC) versus 32% (RIC) at 3 years (P=0.86)	26% (MAC) versus 35% (RIC) at 2 years (P=0.08)	DFS: 41% (MAC) versus 31% (RIC) at 3 years (P=0.12) OS: 43% (MA) versus 38% (RIC) at 3 years (P=0.39)
Stein et al.[37] n=24 CR1, n=11 Ph-negative, n=14	Fludarabine and melphalan	22% at 2 years	21% at 2 years	OS: 62% at 2 years DFS: 62% at 2 years
Cho et al.[36] n=37 CR1, n=30 Ph-negative, n= 21	Fludarabine and melphalan	18% at 3 years 8% at 3 years (CR1)	36% at 3 years	OS: 64% at 3 years DFS: 63% at 3 years

5 years after MVD transplantation, it is reasonable to consider MVD transplants for "HR" patients in CR1 in the absence of a MSD (see Chapters 7 and 8). Whether this option should be extended to SR patients remains controversial, and is currently being investigated in prospective trials such as the United Kingdom ALL XIV trial. MRD assessment may allow for identification of SR patients with poorer risk disease behavior who may benefit from MVD transplants in CR1.

Cord Blood Transplants (CBT)

The largest data sets for CBT come mainly from registry studies. Feasibility of CBT for ALL was first demonstrated in two large registry studies from the CIBMTR and EBMT. Since then, there have been a number of updated registry as well as single-center studies. Eapen et al.[40] reported on 1525 patients from both groups with acute leukemia and found that leukaemia-free survival in patients after CBT was comparable with that after 8/8 and 7/8 allele-matched

Table 32.4 Cord blood transplants in adult ALL

Study/no. of patients	TRM	Relapse	Survival	Notes
Marks et al.[41] UCB, n=116 8/8 MUD, n=546 7/8 MUD, n=140	42% (UCB) versus 31% (8/8 MUD) versus 39% (7/8 MUD) at 3 years	22% (UCB) versus 25% (8/8 MUD) versus 28% (7/8 MUD) at 3 years	44% (UCB) versus 44% (8/8 MUD) versus 43% (7/8 MUD) at 3 years	Conditioning: myeloablative/various
Ferra et al.[42] UCB, n=62 MUD, n=87	31% (UCB) versus 48% (MUD) at 1 year	29% (UCB) versus 29% (MUD) at 5 years	OS: 33% (UCB) versus 22% (MUD) at 5 years DFS: 22% (UCB) versus 21% (MUD) at 5 years	Myeloablative/various
Tomblyn et al.[44] 1990–2005 cohort UCB, n=51 MRD, n=113	24% (UCB) versus 26% (MSD) at 2 years	Reported as relative risks Similar across all donor types (P=0.33)	OS: 51% (UCB) versus 42% (MSD) at 5 years	Conditioning: myeloablative/TBI based
Bachanova et al.[43] UCB, n=22	27%/3 years	36%/3 years	OS: 50% at 3 years	Conditioning: (reduced intensity conditioning) 200 cGy total body irradiation (day 1) fludarabine 40mg/m^2/day (days 6 through 2) cyclophosphamide 50mg/kg per day intravenously day 6.

Abbreviations: UCB: umbilical cord blood, MSD: matched related donor, MUD: matched unrelated donor.

PBPC or BM transplantation but with higher TRM after CBT than after 8/8 allele-matched PBPC recipients (HR 1.62, 95% CI 1.18–2.23; P=0.003) or BM transplantation (HR 1.69, 95% CI 1.19–2.39; P=0.003). A number of more recent publications from the CIBMTR[41], PETHEMA[42], as well as from the University of Minnesota[43,44] have also compared results using CBT with alternative donor sources, specifically for patients with ALL and showed similar PFS and/or OS (Table 32.4). Although the number of patients in these studies is small; the data are comparable between CBT and MVD allo-HCT.

Haplotype-Matched Transplants

A final option for allo-HCT in patients lacking an HLA-matched donor is an HLA haplotype-matched donor transplant. This, however, requires either T-cell depletion of the graft or modifications in preparative conditioning regimens and immunosuppression, and may be associated with higher incidences of graft failure and slow immune recovery associated with increased infective complications compared to MSD and MVD allo-HCT. In patients with HR ALL, Ciceri

et al. reported a leukemia-free survival (LFS) at 2 years of 13% for those undergoing transplantation in CR1, 30% for those undergoing HCT in second or subsequent remission, and 7% in those undergoing HCT in relapsed "active" disease [45]. Yan et al.[46] described the Chinese experience, comparing HLA-haplotype mismatch transplant (n=79) using their center's protocol, with chemotherapy (n=59) in patients with "SR" ALL and suggested reduced relapse rates and improved DFS for haploidentical HCT. In recent years, the group at John Hopkins developed a novel approach of HLA-haplotype mismatch transplant using post-transplantation cyclophosphamide to eliminate alloreactive T-cells, with encouraging preliminary results [47,48]. The number of patients with ALL included in these studies, however, remains small compared to numbers included in the CBT trials. Results from the clinical trial (BMT CTN1101) that randomizes patients to receive BM grafts from a haploidentical relative or 2 CB units may help determine the most appropriate alternative donor source for patients without matched sibling or unrelated donors.

Novel Agents in the Treatment of ALL and Impact on Allo-HCT

Several novel compounds, including monoclonal antibodies, have been tested as single agents or in combination with chemotherapy for treatment of ALL with promising results[49,50].

Of these agents, inotuzumab, a monoclonal antibody against CD22 and linked to calicheamicin, is furthest along in the line of development and has been used in the setting of relapsed ALL with overall responses of up to 57%[51], but allo-HCT appears to still be necessary for consolidation of treatment response. Importantly, inotuzumab use has been associated with higher risks of veno-occlusive disease (VOD) in patients subsequently undergoing allo-HCT, especially among patients receiving two alkylating agents in their conditioning regimens. [52].These findings are an important reminder for transplanters that with the increased use of novel agents pre-allo-HCT, it is necessary to be aware of the potential impact of these agents on allo-HCT outcomes and measures taken to reduce post-transplantation toxicities.

Blinatumomab, a bispecific anti-CD19/CD3 antibody, is another novel agent that acts by directly recruiting effector T-cells to CD19 expressing ALL cells leading to proliferation of these T-cells and perforin-mediated cell lysis and augmenting the antineoplastic effect of the immune system [53]. The optimal role and use of blinatumomab especially in conjunction with allo-HCT has been investigated in various settings such as the eradication of MRD, salvage therapy in the relapsed/refractory setting, and in the post-allo-HCT relapse setting, with promising results[53–55].

Finally, T-cell redirection towards the CD19 antigen present on leukemic blasts via chimeric antigen receptors (CARs) has been shown to result in dramatic responses in patients with previously refractory ALL[56] (trials are ongoing to further investigate this technology in ALL).

The optimal incorporation of these agents into the treatment algorithm for ALL and the impact of these agents on the outcomes of allo-HCT, however, remain unclear and we await more data and clarification from ongoing phase 3 clinical trials.

Controversies and Expert Opinions

Having reviewed the literature in this field, the authors believe the current evidence clearly shows that allo-HCT provides durable remissions in ALL, albeit balanced against the potential toxicities of the procedure.

For patients in CR1, we currently use standard-risk stratification to guide our decision-making process and Table 32.5 provides guidance for allo-HCT in CR1. We recommend allo-HCT in CR1 for HR patients (commonly defined by older age >35, elevated WBC count (Table 32.1), recurring cytogenetic abnormalities: t(9;22), t(4;11), complex karyotype, low hypodiploidy, or delayed time to CR1), or any standard or high-risk patient with persistent MRD due to poor outcomes with chemotherapy in these patients. Furthermore, for HR patients without available HLA-matched donors, alternative donor transplant (CBT or haplotype matched transplants) is a reasonable option given the generally encouraging outcomes

Table 32.5 Factors influencing decision for allogeneic transplant in adult ALL

Variable	Factors influencing decision of allo-HCT over chemotherapy/AUTO-HCT
Patients' ECOG/comorbidities	Poor performance status and presence of comorbidities will be less likely to favor allo-HCT
Risk factors (see Table 32.1)	Presence of risk factors, e.g. high-risk cytogenetics will favor allo-HCT
Donor	Availability of matched sibling donor will favor allo-HCT If only alternative donors are available, then allo-HCT should be considered only for high-risk disease
Chemotherapy regimen	Use of "adult type" regimen favors allo-HCT, while the use of "pediatric type" regimen favors chemotherapy
Minimal residual "measurable" disease	Persistence of minimal measurable disease at the end of induction and consolidation chemotherapy will favor allo-HCT (see Chapters 23 and 24)

compared with MVD donors. Finally, we recommend using a MAC regimen in younger (<40 years) and fit patients. TBI-based conditioning regimens have been the standard of care in ALL, but results with non-TBI regimens are encouraging, and being increasingly used to avoid the long-term toxicities associated with radiation. RIC regimens are a reasonable option in older adults (defined here >40 years), although prospective data are necessary and ongoing studies by the UK group will be helpful in addressing this issue. In SR patients with MSD, we would recommend allo-HCT based on an estimated low TRM rate. MRD studies have a crucial role in the decision-making process in this situation (see Chapters 23 and 24). Because SR patients with persistent MRD during treatment have a very high expected rate of relapse, we would consider alternative donor transplants. What is unclear are the time points beyond which persistent MRD is considered significant, and we believe results from ongoing trials in the United Kingdom and Germany will help address this issue. Patients with disease beyond CR1 are at high risk for relapse, and should be consolidated as soon as possible with a standard or alternative donor allograft.

The Unknown Territory of MRD in Adult ALL: Controversies Continue

The advent of MRD in the field of ALL is important and will likely affect treatment paradigms in this area. Currently, the optimal treatment strategy utilizing MRD with allo-HCT remains unclear. Some important and unanswered questions include: (1) whether attainment of MRD-negative state prior to transplant is essential, balancing the potential for decreased relapse against the risks of additional therapy to reduce tumor burden; (2) whether conditioning regimens should be intensified with active MRD or de-escalated in the MRD-negative patients; and (3) whether post-transplant immunologic interventions should be considered in MRD-positive patients at the expense of increased TRM and graft-*versus*-host disease. There is a paucity of data currently addressing these issues, and a need for prospective controlled trials to help better answer these questions.

References

1. Kantarjian H, Thomas D, O'Brien S, Cortes J, Giles F, Jeha S, *et al.* Long-term follow-up results of hyperfractionated cyclophosphamide, vincristine, doxorubicin, and dexamethasone (Hyper-CVAD), a dose-intensive regimen, in adult acute lymphocytic leukemia. *Cancer.* 2004;101(12):2788–801. PubMed PMID: 15481055. Epub 2004/10/14. eng.

2. Rowe JM, Buck G, Burnett AK, Chopra R, Wiernik PH, Richards SM, *et al.* Induction therapy for adults with acute lymphoblastic leukemia: results of more than 1500 patients from the international ALL trial: MRC UKALL XII/ECOG E2993. *Blood.* 2005;106(12):3760–7. PubMed PMID: 16105981. Epub 2005/08/18. eng.

3. Weiden PL, Flournoy N, Thomas ED, Prentice R, Fefer A, Buckner CD, *et al.* Antileukemic effect of graft-*versus*-host disease in human recipients of allogeneic-marrow grafts. *The New England Journal of Medicine.* 1979;300(19):1068–73. PubMed PMID: 34792.

4. Oliansky DM, Larson RA, Weisdorf D, Dillon H, Ratko TA, Wall D, *et al.* The role of cytotoxic therapy with hematopoietic stem cell transplantation in the treatment of adult acute lymphoblastic leukemia: update of the 2006 evidence-based review. *Biology of Blood and Marrow Transplantation: Journal of the American Society for Blood and Marrow Transplantation.* 2012;18(1):18–36. e6. PubMed PMID: 21803017.

5. NCCN guidelines for ALL. NCCN Clinical Practice Guidelines in Oncology.

6. Gokbuget N, Stanze D, Beck J, Diedrich H, Horst HA, Huttmann A, *et al.* Outcome of relapsed adult lymphoblastic leukemia depends on response to salvage chemotherapy, prognostic factors, and performance of stem cell transplantation. *Blood.* 2012;120(10):2032–41. PubMed PMID: 22493293.

7. Fielding AK, Richards SM, Chopra R, Lazarus HM, Litzow MR, Buck G, *et al.* Outcome of 609 adults after relapse of acute lymphoblastic leukemia (ALL); an MRC UKALL12/ECOG 2993 study. *Blood.* 2007;109(3):944–50. PubMed PMID: 17032921.

8. Yanada M, Matsuo K, Suzuki T, Naoe T. Allogeneic hematopoietic stem cell transplantation as part of postremission therapy improves survival for adult patients with high-risk acute lymphoblastic leukemia: a metaanalysis. *Cancer.* 2006;106(12):2657–63. PubMed PMID: 16703597. Epub 2006/05/17. eng.

9. Goldstone AH, Richards SM, Lazarus HM, Tallman MS, Buck G, Fielding AK, *et al.* In adults with standard-risk acute lymphoblastic leukemia, the greatest benefit is achieved from a matched sibling allogeneic transplantation in first complete remission, and an autologous transplantation is less effective than conventional consolidation/maintenance chemotherapy in all patients: final results of the International ALL Trial (MRC UKALL XII/ECOG E2993). *Blood.* 2008;111(4):1827–33. PubMed PMID: 18048644. Epub 2007/12/01. eng.

10. Cornelissen JJ, van der Holt B, Verhoef GE, van't Veer MB, van Oers MH, Schouten HC, *et al.* Myeloablative allogeneic *versus* autologous stem cell transplantation in adult patients with acute lymphoblastic leukemia in first remission: a prospective sibling donor *versus* no-donor comparison. *Blood.* 2009;113(6):1375–82. PubMed PMID: 18988865. Epub 2008/11/08. eng.

11. Ram R, Gafter-Gvili A, Vidal L, Paul M, Ben-Bassat I, Shpilberg O, *et al.* Management of adult patients with acute lymphoblastic leukemia in first complete remission: systematic review and meta-analysis. *Cancer.* 116 (14):3447–57. PubMed PMID: 20564092. Epub 2010/06/22. eng.

12. Pidala J, Djulbegovic B, Anasetti C, Kharfan-Dabaja M, Kumar A. Allogeneic hematopoietic cell transplantation for adult acute lymphoblastic leukemia (ALL) in first complete remission. *Cochrane Database of Systematic Reviews.* 2011;10: CD008818. PubMed PMID: 21975786. Epub 2011/10/07. eng.

13. Gupta V, Richards S, Rowe J, Acute Leukemia Stem Cell Transplantation Trialists' Collaborative G. Allogeneic, but not autologous, hematopoietic cell transplantation improves survival only among younger adults with acute lymphoblastic leukemia in first remission: an individual patient data meta-analysis. *Blood.* 2013;121(2):339–50. PubMed PMID: 23165481.

14. Patel B, Rai L, Buck G, Richards SM, Mortuza Y, Mitchell W, *et al.* Minimal residual disease is a significant predictor of treatment failure in non T-lineage adult acute lymphoblastic leukaemia: final results of the international trial UKALL XII/ECOG2993. *British Journal of Haematology.* 2010;148(1):80–9. PubMed PMID: 19863538.

15. Bruggemann M, Raff T, Flohr T, Gokbuget N, Nakao M, Droese J, *et al.* Clinical significance of minimal residual disease quantification in adult patients with standard-risk acute lymphoblastic leukemia. *Blood.* 2006;107(3):1116–23. PubMed PMID: 16195338. Epub 2005/10/01. eng.

16. Gokbuget N, Kneba M, Raff T, Trautmann H, Bartram CR, Arnold R, *et al.* Adult patients with acute lymphoblastic leukemia and molecular failure display a poor prognosis and are candidates for stem cell transplantation and targeted therapies. *Blood.* 2012;120(9):1868–76. PubMed PMID: 22442346.

17. Bassan R, Spinelli O, Oldani E, Intermesoli T, Tosi M, Peruta B, *et al.* Improved risk classification for risk-specific therapy based on the molecular study of minimal residual disease (MRD) in adult acute lymphoblastic leukemia (ALL). *Blood.* 2009;113(18):4153–62. PubMed PMID: 19141862.

18. Ribera JM, Oriol A, Morgades M, Montesinos P, Sarra J, Gonzalez-Campos J, *et al.* Treatment of high-risk

Philadelphia chromosome-negative acute lymphoblastic leukemia in adolescents and adults according to early cytologic response and minimal residual disease after consolidation assessed by flow cytometry: final results of the PETHEMA ALL-AR-03 trial. *Journal of Clinical Oncology: Official Journal of the American Society of Clinical Oncology.* 2014;32(15):1595–604. PubMed PMID: 24752047.

19. Stock W, La M, Sanford B, Bloomfield CD, Vardiman JW, Gaynon P, et al. What determines the outcomes for adolescents and young adults with acute lymphoblastic leukemia treated on cooperative group protocols? A comparison of Children's Cancer Group and Cancer and Leukemia Group B studies. *Blood.* 2008;112(5):1646–54. PubMed PMID: 18502832. Pubmed Central PMCID: 2518876.

20. Boissel N, Auclerc MF, Lheritier V, Perel Y, Thomas X, Leblanc T, et al. Should adolescents with acute lymphoblastic leukemia be treated as old children or young adults? Comparison of the French FRALLE-93 and LALA-94 trials. *Journal of Clinical Oncology: Official Journal of the American Society of Clinical Oncology.* 2003;21(5):774–80. PubMed PMID: 12610173.

21. Ramanujachar R, Richards S, Hann I, Goldstone A, Mitchell C, Vora A, et al. Adolescents with acute lymphoblastic leukaemia: outcome on UK national paediatric (ALL97) and adult (UKALLXII/E2993) trials. *Pediatric blood & Cancer.* 2007;48(3):254–61. PubMed PMID: 16421910.

22. Thomas DA, Kantarjian H, Smith TL, Koller C, Cortes J, O'Brien S, et al. Primary refractory and relapsed adult acute lymphoblastic leukemia: characteristics, treatment results, and prognosis with salvage therapy. *Cancer.* 1999;86(7):1216–30. PubMed PMID: 10506707.

23. Oriol A, Vives S, Hernandez-Rivas JM, Tormo M, Heras I, Rivas C, et al. Outcome after relapse of acute lymphoblastic leukemia in adult patients included in four consecutive risk-adapted trials by the PETHEMA Study Group. *Haematologica.* 2010;95(4):589–96. PubMed PMID:

20145276. Pubmed Central PMCID: 2857188.

24. Tavernier E, Boiron JM, Huguet F, Bradstock K, Vey N, Kovacsovics T, et al. Outcome of treatment after first relapse in adults with acute lymphoblastic leukemia initially treated by the LALA-94 trial. *Leukemia.* 2007;21(9):1907–14. PubMed PMID: 17611565.

25. Duval M, Klein JP, He W, Cahn JY, Cairo M, Camitta BM, et al. Hematopoietic stem-cell transplantation for acute leukemia in relapse or primary induction failure. *Journal of Clinical Oncology: Official Journal of the American Society of Clinical Oncology.* 2010;28(23):3730–8. PubMed PMID: 20625136. Pubmed Central PMCID: 2917308.

26. Terwey TH, Massenkeil G, Tamm I, Hemmati PG, Neuburger S, Martus P, et al. Allogeneic SCT in refractory or relapsed adult ALL is effective without prior reinduction chemotherapy. *Bone Marrow Transplantation.* 2008;42(12):791–8. PubMed PMID: 18711350. Epub 2008/08/20. eng.

27. Doney K, Hagglund H, Leisenring W, Chauncey T, Appelbaum FR, Storb R. Predictive factors for outcome of allogeneic hematopoietic cell transplantation for adult acute lymphoblastic leukemia. *Biology of Blood and Marrow Transplantation: Journal of the American Society for Blood and Marrow Transplantation.* 2003;9(7):472–81. PubMed PMID: 12869961. Epub 2003/07/19. eng.

28. Cornelissen JJ, Carston M, Kollman C, King R, Dekker AW, Lowenberg B, et al. Unrelated marrow transplantation for adult patients with poor-risk acute lymphoblastic leukemia: strong graft-*versus*-leukemia effect and risk factors determining outcome. *Blood.* 2001;97(6):1572–7. PubMed PMID: 11238093. Epub 2001/03/10. eng.

29. Kiehl MG, Kraut L, Schwerdtfeger R, Hertenstein B, Remberger M, Kroeger N, et al. Outcome of allogeneic hematopoietic stem-cell transplantation in adult patients with acute lymphoblastic leukemia: no difference in related compared with unrelated transplant in first complete remission. *Journal of Clinical Oncology: Official Journal of the American Society of*

Clinical Oncology. 2004;22(14):2816–25. PubMed PMID: 15254049.

30. Granados E, de La Camara R, Madero L, Diaz MA, Martin-Regueira P, Steegmann JL, et al. Hematopoietic cell transplantation in acute lymphoblastic leukemia: better long term event-free survival with conditioning regimens containing total body irradiation. *Haematologica.* 2000;85(10):1060–7. PubMed PMID: 11025598.

31. Daly A, Savoie ML, Geddes M, Chaudhry A, Stewart D, Duggan P, et al. Fludarabine, busulfan, antithymocyte globulin, and total body irradiation for pretransplantation conditioning in acute lymphoblastic leukemia: excellent outcomes in all but older patients with comorbidities. *Biology of Blood and Marrow Transplantation: Journal of the American Society for Blood and Marrow Transplantation.* 2012;18(12):1921–6. PubMed PMID: 22842330.

32. Santarone S, Pidala J, Di Nicola M, Field T, Alsina M, Ayala E, et al. Fludarabine and pharmacokinetic-targeted busulfan before allografting for adults with acute lymphoid leukemia. *Biology of Blood and Marrow Transplantation: Journal of the American Society for Blood and Marrow Transplantation.* 2011;17(10):1505–11. PubMed PMID: 21385623.

33. Kebriaei P, Basset R, Ledesma C, Ciurea S, Parmar S, Shpall EJ, et al. Clofarabine combined with busulfan provides excellent disease control in adult patients with acute lymphoblastic leukemia undergoing allogeneic hematopoietic stem cell transplantation. *Biology of Blood and Marrow Transplantation: Journal of the American Society for Blood and Marrow Transplantation.* 2012;18(12):1819–26. PubMed PMID: 22750645.

34. Mohty M, Labopin M, Volin L, Gratwohl A, Socie G, Esteve J, et al. Reduced-intensity *versus* conventional myeloablative conditioning allogeneic stem cell transplantation for patients with acute lymphoblastic leukemia: a retrospective study from the European Group for Blood and Marrow Transplantation. *Blood.* 2010;116(22):4439–43. PubMed PMID: 20716774.

35. Marks DI, Wang T, Perez WS, Antin JH, Copelan E, Gale RP, et al. The outcome of full-intensity and reduced-

intensity conditioning matched sibling or unrelated donor transplantation in adults with Philadelphia chromosome-negative acute lymphoblastic leukemia in first and second complete remission. *Blood.* 2010;116(3):366–74. PubMed PMID: 20404137. Pubmed Central PMCID: 2913452.

36. Cho BS, Lee S, Kim YJ, Chung NG, Eom KS, Kim HJ, *et al.* Reduced-intensity conditioning allogeneic stem cell transplantation is a potential therapeutic approach for adults with high-risk acute lymphoblastic leukemia in remission: results of a prospective phase 2 study. *Leukemia.* 2009;23(10):1763–70. PubMed PMID: 19440217. Epub 2009/05/15. eng.

37. Stein AS, Palmer JM, O'Donnell MR, Kogut NM, Spielberger RT, Slovak ML, *et al.* Reduced-intensity conditioning followed by peripheral blood stem cell transplantation for adult patients with high-risk acute lymphoblastic leukemia. *Biology of Blood and Marrow Transplantation: Journal of the American Society for Blood and Marrow Transplantation.* 2009;15(11):1407–14. PubMed PMID: 19822300. Pubmed Central PMCID: 2795637.

38. Ram R, Storb R, Sandmaier BM, Maloney DG, Woolfrey A, Flowers ME, *et al.* Non-myeloablative conditioning with allogeneic hematopoietic cell transplantation for the treatment of high-risk acute lymphoblastic leukemia. *Haematologica.* 2011;96(8):1113–20. PubMed PMID: 21508120. Epub 2011/04/22. eng.

39. Arnold R, Massenkeil G, Bornhauser M, Ehninger G, Beelen DW, Fauser AA, *et al.* Nonmyeloablative stem cell transplantation in adults with high-risk ALL may be effective in early but not in advanced disease. *Leukemia.* 2002;16(12):2423–8. PubMed PMID: 12454748.

40. Eapen M, Rocha V, Sanz G, Scaradavou A, Zhang MJ, Arcese W, *et al.* Effect of graft source on unrelated donor haemopoietic stem-cell transplantation in adults with acute leukaemia: a retrospective analysis. *Lancet Oncol.* 2010;11(7):653–60. PubMed PMID: 20558104. Epub 2010/06/19. eng.

41. Marks DI, Woo KA, Zhong X, Appelbaum FR, Bachanova V, Barker JN, *et al.* Unrelated umbilical cord blood transplant for adult acute lymphoblastic leukemia in first and second complete remission: a

comparison with allografts from adult unrelated donors. *Haematologica.* 2014;99(2):322–8. PubMed PMID: 24056817. Pubmed Central PMCID: 3912963.

42. Ferra C, Sanz J, de la Camara R, Sanz G, Bermudez A, Valcarcel D, *et al.* Unrelated transplantation for poor-prognosis adult acute lymphoblastic leukemia: long-term outcome analysis and study of the impact of hematopoietic graft source. *Biology of Blood and Marrow Transplantation: Journal of the American Society for Blood and Marrow Transplantation.* 2010;16(7):957–66. PubMed PMID: 20144909.

43. Bachanova V, Verneris MR, DeFor T, Brunstein CG, Weisdorf DJ. Prolonged survival in adults with acute lymphoblastic leukemia after reduced-intensity conditioning with cord blood or sibling donor transplantation. *Blood.* 2009;113(13):2902–5. PubMed PMID: 19179301. Epub 2009/01/31. eng.

44. Tomblyn MB, Arora M, Baker KS, Blazar BR, Brunstein CG, Burns LJ, *et al.* Myeloablative hematopoietic cell transplantation for acute lymphoblastic leukemia: analysis of graft sources and long-term outcome. *Journal of Clinical Oncology: Official Journal of the American Society of Clinical Oncology.* 2009;27(22):3634–41. PubMed PMID: 19581540. Epub 2009/07/08. eng.

45. Ciceri F, Labopin M, Aversa F, Rowe JM, Bunjes D, Lewalle P, *et al.* A survey of fully haploidentical hematopoietic stem cell transplantation in adults with high-risk acute leukemia: a risk factor analysis of outcomes for patients in remission at transplantation. *Blood.* 2008;112(9):3574–81. PubMed PMID: 18606875. Epub 2008/07/09. eng.

46. Yan CH, Jiang Q, Wang J, Xu LP, Liu DH, Jiang H, *et al.* Superior survival of unmanipulated haploidentical hematopoietic stem cell transplantation compared with chemotherapy alone used as post-remission therapy in adults with standard-risk acute lymphoblastic leukemia in first complete remission. *Biology of Blood and Marrow Transplantation: Journal of the American Society for Blood and Marrow Transplantation.* 2014;20(9):1314–21. PubMed PMID: 24747334.

47. Luznik L, BolaÃ±os-Meade J, Zahurak M, Chen AR, Smith BD, Brodsky R, *et al.* High-dose cyclophosphamide as

single-agent, short-course prophylaxis of graft-*versus*-host disease. *Blood.* 2010;115(16):3224–30.

48. Luznik L, O'Donnell PV, Symons HJ, Chen AR, Leffell MS, Zahurak M, *et al.* HLA-haploidentical bone marrow transplantation for hematologic malignancies using nonmyeloablative conditioning and high-dose, posttransplantation cyclophosphamide. *Biology of Blood and Marrow Transplantation: Journal of the American Society for Blood and Marrow Transplantation.* 2008;14(6):641–50. PubMed PMID: S1083-8791(08) 00114-6.

49. Le Jeune C, Thomas X. Antibody-based therapies in B-cell lineage acute lymphoblastic leukaemia. *European Journal of Haematology.* 2015;94(2):99–10. PubMed PMID: 24981395.

50. Kantarjian H, Thomas D, Wayne AS, O'Brien S. Monoclonal antibody-based therapies: a new dawn in the treatment of acute lymphoblastic leukemia. *Journal of Clinical Oncology: Official Journal of the American Society of Clinical Oncology.* 2012;30(31):3876–83. PubMed PMID: 22891271. Pubmed Central PMCID: 3478578.

51. Kantarjian H, Thomas D, Jorgensen J, Jabbour E, Kebriaei P, Rytting M, *et al.* Inotuzumab ozogamicin, an anti-CD22-calecheamicin conjugate, for refractory and relapsed acute lymphocytic leukaemia: a phase 2 study. *Lancet Oncol.* 2012;13(4):403–11. PubMed PMID: 22357140.

52. Kebriaei P, Wilhelm K, Ravandi F, Brandt M, de Lima M, Ciurea S, *et al.* Feasibility of allografting in patients with advanced acute lymphoblastic leukemia after salvage therapy with inotuzumab ozogamicin. *Clinical Lymphoma, Myeloma & Leukemia.* 2013;13(3):296–301. PubMed PMID: 23313065. Pubmed Central PMCID: PMC4102410. Epub 2013/01/15. eng.

53. Topp MS, Gokbuget N, Zugmaier G, Degenhard E, Goebeler ME, Klinger M, *et al.* Long-term follow-up of hematologic relapse-free survival in a phase 2 study of blinatumomab in patients with MRD in B-lineage ALL. *Blood.* 2012;120(26):5185–7. PubMed PMID: 23024237.

54. Topp MS. Anti-CD19 BiTE Blinatumomab induces high complete remission rate and prolongs overall

survival in adult patients with relapsed/refractory B-precursor acute lymphoblastic leukemia (ALL). *American Society of Hematology Annual Meeting.* 2012;670.

55. Schlegel P, Lang P, Zugmaier G, Ebinger M, Kreyenberg H, Witte KE, *et al.* Pediatric posttransplant relapsed/refractory B-precursor acute lymphoblastic leukemia shows durable remission by therapy with the T-cell engaging bispecific antibody blinatumomab. *Haematologica.* 2014;99(7):1212–9. PubMed PMID: 24727818. Pubmed Central PMCID: 4077083.

56. Grupp SA, Kalos M, Barrett D, Aplenc R, Porter DL, Rheingold SR, *et al.* Chimeric antigen receptor-modified T cells for acute lymphoid leukemia. *The New England Journal of Medicine.* 2013;368(16):1509–18. PubMed PMID: 23527958. Pubmed Central PMCID: 4058440.

57. Pui CH, Evans WE. Acute lymphoblastic leukemia. *The New England Journal of Medicine.* 1998;339(9):605–15. PubMed PMID: 9718381. Epub 1998/08/27. eng.

58. Moorman AV, Harrison CJ, Buck GA, Richards SM, Secker-Walker LM, Martineau M, *et al.* Karyotype is an independent prognostic factor in adult acute lymphoblastic leukemia (ALL): analysis of cytogenetic data from patients treated on the Medical Research Council (MRC) UKALLXII/Eastern Cooperative Oncology Group (ECOG) 2993 trial. *Blood.* 2007;109(8):3189–97. PubMed PMID: 17170120. Epub 2006/12/16. eng.

59. Moorman AV, Ensor HM, Richards SM, Chilton L, Schwab C, Kinsey SE, *et al.* Prognostic effect of chromosomal abnormalities in childhood B-cell precursor acute lymphoblastic leukaemia: results from the UK Medical Research Council ALL97/99 randomised trial. *Lancet Oncol.*;11(5):429–38. PubMed PMID: 20409752. Epub 2010/04/23. eng.

60. Marks DI, Paietta EM, Moorman AV, Richards SM, Buck G, DeWald G, *et al.* T-cell acute lymphoblastic leukemia in adults: clinical features, immunophenotype, cytogenetics, and outcome from the large randomized prospective trial (UKALL XII/ECOG 2993). *Blood.* 2009;114(25):5136–45. PubMed PMID: 19828704. Pubmed Central PMCID: 2792210.

61. Orsi C, Bartolozzi B, Messori A, Bosi A. Event-free survival and cost-effectiveness in adult acute lymphoblastic leukaemia in first remission treated with allogeneic transplantation. *Bone Marrow Transplant.* 2007;40(7):643–9. PubMed PMID: 17660839.

Chapter
33

Hematopoietic Cell Transplants for *BCR/ABL Positive* Acute Lymphocytic Leukemia

Netanel A. Horowitz and Jacob M. Rowe

Introduction

Philadelphia chromosome-positive acute lymphoblastic leukemia (Ph$^+$ ALL) is a distinct subgroup comprising 20–30% of adult ALL[1]. The Ph chromosome is a translocation between the *ABL-1* oncogene on the long arm of chromosome 9 and a breakpoint cluster region (*BCR*) on the long arm of chromosome 22, t(9:22), resulting in a fusion gene, *BCR-ABL*, that encodes an oncogenic protein with constitutively active tyrosine kinase activity[2]. However, in contrast to chronic myelogenous leukemia (CML) where the Ph chromosome is often the sole genetic abnormality, in Ph$^+$ ALL, there are many other genetic changes, including copy number abnormalities, epigenetic changes, and mutation downstream of *BCR-ABL* that play an important role in the very aggressive clinical course[3]. The presence of the Ph chromosome in ALL patients is associated with a highly unfavorable prognosis[4]; hence, the recommended consolidation therapy after achieving first complete remission (CR) is allo-HCT from a matched related or unrelated donor. In recent years the introduction of tyrosine kinase inhibitors (TKIs) into the therapy of Ph$^+$ ALL has further improved survival. The aim of this chapter is to review the data regarding HCT (auto- and allo-HCT) in Ph$^+$ ALL, including recent trials introducing TKIs into the overall therapy of the disease. Other controversial areas like the use of MRD as a tool for clinical decision-making will also be considered.

The Need for Allo-HCT in Ph$^+$ ALL

It is widely accepted that a Ph$^+$ ALL patient with a matched related or unrelated donor should undergo allo-HCT as the best postremission therapy. Several studies in the pre-TKI era have demonstrated the benefit of this strategy in terms of prolonged overall survival (OS) and progression-free survival (PFS) relative to chemotherapy alone[5–9]. However, one should bear in mind that these studies describe only patients who actually underwent an allo-HCT, which is why there is an inherent selection bias in these clinical reports. In studies describing patients from diagnosis, the advantage of allo-HCT in the pre-TKI era is more modest. Several factors, including resistant disease, old age, early relapse (prior to allo-HCT), and lack of available donor made this therapy suitable only to a third of Ph$^+$ ALL patients. The largest data series regarding allo-HCT (matched related or unrelated donor) came from the international Eastern Cooperative Oncology Group/Medical Research Council (ECOG/MRC) trial. The 5-year OS was 44%, 36%, and 19% after matched sibling donor (MSD) allo-HCT, matched unrelated donor (MUD) allo-HCT, and chemotherapy alone, respectively. The difference in the outcome between MSD allo-HCT and MUD allo-HCT groups was not statistically significant, but this may be due to the small numbers involved in the analysis and an inherent selection bias. In intention-to-treat analysis for donor-*versus*-no-donor availability, the 5-year OS was better (34% *versus* 25%)[9].

TKI Therapy in Ph$^+$ ALL

Incorporation of TKI Therapy into Ph$^+$ ALL Regimens Improves on Rates of Allo-HCT and Outcomes

Early data regarding combining TKI with Ph$^+$ ALL induction therapy did not demonstrate any benefit. Kebriaei *et al.*[10] from the MD Anderson Cancer Center (MDACC) retrospectively evaluated a large cohort of Ph$^+$ ALL patients who underwent an allo-HCT at first and second CR. The 5-year OS was significantly better for patients transplanted in first CR compared with allo-HCT in advanced disease: 43% *versus* 16%, $P=0.002$. The addition of TKI was not associated with an improved OS in a multivariate analysis. The first analysis from the ECOG/MRC trial conducted in 2007 addressing the same question was also disappointing. The 3-year OS was 26% in the imatinib group relative to 23% in the non-imatinib group[11]. However, a more mature follow-up revealed the critical contribution of adding TKIs to the induction regimen of Ph$^+$ ALL. The CR rate was 92% in the imatinib cohort *versus* 82% in the pre-imatinib cohort ($P=0.004$). The OS at 4 years in the imatinib cohort was 38% *versus* 22% in the pre-imatinib cohort ($P=0.003$; 95% CI 31–45). The main contribution of imatinib was to enable more patients to achieve CR and therefore progress to allo-HCT. In the pre-imatinib cohort, 31% of those starting treatment underwent allo-HCT compared with 46% in the imatinib cohort[12]. Similar data emerged from the Japanese Adult Leukemia Study Group (JALSG). The 3-year OS was 65% using imatinib-based induction followed by allo-HCT, *versus* 44% in those without prior imatinib ($P=0.005$; 95% CI 49–76), with a disease-free-survival (DFS) of 58% *versus* 37% (*P*=0.007; 95% CI, 49–76). The rate of performing allo-HCT was 61%[13].

TKIs: First or Second Generation in Patients with Ph$^+$ ALL?

There is no randomized clinical trial (RCT) comparing imatinib *versus* a second-generation TKI in Ph$^+$ALL. Dasatinib is a second-generation TKI that has a 325-fold greater potency than imatinib and inhibits BCR-ABL and the SRC family kinase as well[14]. In the relapse setting, dasatinib was able to induce rapid hematologic and cytogenetic responses in imatinib-intolerant or resistant patients[15,16]. Using the combination of hyperCVAD and dasatinib resulted in a 2-year OS of 64% in 35 newly diagnosed Ph$^+$ ALL patients. Other clinical trials detailed later in this chapter, examined dasatinib with steroid or "low-dose" chemotherapy regimens in elderly patients and demonstrated higher rates of CR and OS [14,17,18]. Apart from its higher CR and OS rates, dasatinib concentration in the CNS is significantly higher than that of imatinib; therefore, it is has a better clinical activity in cases of CNS leukemia[19,20].

When to Start TKI in Patients with Ph$^+$ ALL?

At the MRC/ECOG Study, patients received 2 phases of induction, followed by intensification before allo-HCT, if they had a donor. Initially in this study, patients received imatinib only after the end of phase 2 of induction (a late imatinib approach) and the subsequent cohort received imatinib after the first phase of induction (an early imatinib approach). Patients who received imatinib earlier had a substantially better OS than those who received later. Similar data have emerged from the German ALL Study[21]. PCR negativity was significantly improved for the patients who received imatinib with induction and continued this uninterrupted until allo-HCT. To conclude, existing data support starting TKI therapy as early as possible.

Older Adults: Can We Omit Chemotherapy from Induction Regimen in the TKI era?

Administering aggressive chemotherapy regimens could be challenging in older Ph$^+$ patients and those with conventional chemotherapy prohibitive comorbidities. Given the high efficacy of TKIs, the idea of achieving CR with reducing or omitting cytoreductive chemotherapy from induction regimens was studied in several clinical trials. An early study by the German Multicenter Study Group for Adult ALL (GMALL) demonstrated that frontline therapy with imatinib resulted in a CR rate of 96% *versus* a significantly lower CR rate of 50% using non-TKI, multiagent, age-adapted chemotherapy regimens[22]. In the GIMEMA (Gruppo Italiano Malattie Ematologiche dell'Adulto) LAL0201 trial, 30 older (defined in this study as >60 years) Ph$^+$ patients were treated

with imatinib, 800 mg daily, and steroids without further chemotherapy. The mean age was 69 years. Twenty-nine patients were evaluable for response and all of them achieved CR. Treatment was well tolerated and no major toxicities occurred. Median survival from diagnosis was 20 months [23]. Rousselot and colleagues[17] demonstrated a 90% CR rate using dasatinib combined with a low-intensity chemotherapy regimen in 22 patients older than 55 years. However, even in studies with a relatively long follow-up, the relapse rate was very high, yielding an OS probability of less than 20%. That being said, the addition of TKI with omission of intensive chemotherapy to induce CR is encouraged in patients who are deemed unfit for intensive chemotherapy.

Younger Adults: Can We Omit Chemotherapy from Induction Regimen in the TKI Era?

The encouraging results obtained in older patients led to other studies implementing a chemotherapy-free strategy in younger Ph$^+$ ALL patients. In the GIMEMA LAL1205 trial, newly diagnosed Ph$^+$ ALL patients, older than 18 years (with no upper age limit) received dasatinib induction therapy for 84 days combined with steroids for the first 32 days and intrathecal chemotherapy. Postremission therapy was not specified. Fifty-three patients were evaluable (median age 53.6 years). The rate of complete hematologic response (CHR) was 92.5% and 10 patients achieved PCR negativity at day 22. The OS and DFS were 69.2% (95% CI 60.7–79.0) and 51.1% (95% CI 44.4–58.7), respectively, at 20 months. During induction, there were no relapses or deaths and the treatment was well tolerated. However, 23 patients relapsed after completing induction and a T315I mutation was detected in 12 of 17 relapsed cases[18]. Despite the remarkable ratio of CR and the safety profile of this potential induction strategy, the long-term outcomes are not yet clear. The heterogeneous therapy that was given subsequent to induction makes this question even more complicated. Long-term data from well-controlled randomized trials are needed before chemotherapy can be reduced or completely omitted from induction regimens in younger adults and older adults fit for chemotherapy.

Cord Blood Unit(s) *versus* HLA-Haplotype-Matched Donor HCT

For cases without availability of a MSD or MRD, alternative donors should be considered. However, limited data exist to support this strategy in Ph$^+$ ALL. Eighty-six ALL (46 adults, only 27 with Ph$^+$ ALL) patients with available MRD assessment data analysis immediately before allo-HCT were prospectively evaluated at the University of Minnesota. Most of the patients (82%) received MA preparative regimen. In multivariate analysis, age, disease status, disease type (precursor B-cell ALL *versus* Ph$^+$ ALL *versus* T-ALL), and time to allo-HCT had no impact on relapse rate. Patients with MRD positivity before CBT had a higher incidence of relapse

(30%) at 2 years and a lower 3-year DFS (30%) compared with those without MRD (relapse rate – 16%; $P=0.05$; DFS 55% $P=0.02$)[24]. MRD was defined using multiparameter flow cytometry.

Another study reported on the outcome of 45 patients with Ph^+ ALL who underwent MA single-unit CBT within the GETH/GITMO Cooperative Group. Median age was 31 years. Thirty-five patients (78%) were in first CR, four (8%) in second CR, and six (14%) in third or subsequent remission; 96% of patients engrafted at a median of 20 days. The incidence of acute grade II–IV graft-*versus*-host disease (GvHD) and chronic GvHD was 31% and 53%, respectively. The TRM was 17% at day +100 and 31% at 5 years. The 5-year relapse, event-free survival (EFS), and OS rates were 31%, 36%, and 44%, respectively[25]. The largest analysis of using cord blood in this difficult clinical scenario has recently been published by a joint initiative of Eurocord, Cord Blood Committee, and the Acute Leukemia Working Party of the European Group for Blood and Marrow Transplantation. Ninety-eight Ph^+ ALL patients received CBT in CR1 (n=79) or CR2 (n=19). MRD was available before CBT. The median age was 38 years and a median follow-up was 36 months. Sixty-three percent of patients received MA preparative regimen and 42% received double-unit CBT. MRD was negative in 39 and positive in 59 patients. Three-year cumulative incidence of nonrelapse mortality was 31%; it was increased in patients older than 35 years ($P=0.02$). Three-year cumulative incidence of relapse was 34%; 45% in MRD-positive and 16% in MRD-negative patients ($P=0.013$; HR: 0.33; 95% CI 0.13–0.79). Leukemia-free survival (LFS) at 3 years was 36%; 27% in MRD-positive and 49% in MRD-negative patients ($P=0.05$), and 41% for CR1 and 14% for CR2 ($P=0.008$; HR: 0.58; 95% CI: 0.34–1.0). Multivariate analysis identified only CR1 as being associated with improved LFS[26]. Taken together, these results suggest that CB should be considered seriously when no other donor source is available, given the poor results of chemotherapy as postinduction therapy.

The role of HLA haplotype mismatch HCT for patients with no available donor is even more elusive, and very limited data related to this issue exist. In a recent study, patients treated between January 2000 and December 2012 were included in the analysis. One hundred and four patients who received conventional chemotherapy were retrospectively compared to 79 patients who were treated with HLA haplotype mismatch HCT. Patients who underwent HLA haplotype mismatch HCT had significantly improved 3-year OS (72.5% *versus* 26.6%; $P<0.001$), 3-year disease free survival (DFS) (63.9% *versus* 21.1%; $P<0.001$), and 3-year relapse (18.7% *versus* 60.5%; $P<0.001$) rates. The nonrelapse mortality (NRM) rate did not differ between patient cohorts (19.2% *versus* 14.4%; $P=0.80$). In multivariate analysis, the only factor associated with improved OS, better DFS, and low risk of relapse was HLA haplotype mismatch HCT[27].

Preparative Regimens: MA Regimen *versus* RIC Regimen

Allo-HCT from a MSD or MUD is the mainstay of postinduction treatment in Ph^+ ALL after achieving CR. In most studies, total body irradiation (TBI) is an integral part of the preparative regimen. In the ECOG/MRC study the preparative regimen was TBI-based MA regimen. If the pretransplant patient's condition allows, then MA regimen is preferred over RIC regimen. Older adults (>45 years) who are candidates for allo-HCT are often not the best candidates for MA regimen. In these cases a RIC allo-HCT that has a lower rate of transplant-related morbidity and mortality might be an alternative compared to no transplant. Several small nonrandomized studies have implemented this strategy and the largest studies are summarized in Table 33.1. The RIC regimens are mainly fludarabine-based, with or without TBI. In a recent retrospective study by the Center for International Blood and Marrow Transplant Research (CIBMTR),

Table 33.1 The largest trials of RIC regimen for *BCR/ABL positive* ALL

Author	Median age (years)	No. of patients	Conditioning regimens	TRM (%)	cGvHD (%)	OS (%)	TKIs post-transplant	Comment
Mohty *et al.*[33]	38	37	Various	28	37	n/a	No	
Bachanova *et al.*[34]	49	14	Flu/Cy/TBI	27	45	n/a	For relapse only	
Ram *et al.*[35][a]	57	25	Flu/TBI	28	44	62 at 3 years	TKIs post-transplant to all patients	The only prospective trial reporting OS
Stein *et al.*[36]	47.5	9	Flu/Mel	22	86	n/a	Some	
Arnold *et al.*[37]	38	11	Flu/Bu +/– ATG	45	46	n/a	No	

[a] In this trial only TKI was given to all patients after CBC recovery.
Abbreviations: Flu – fludarabine; Cy – cyclophosphamide; TBI – total body irradiation; Mel – melphalan; Bu – busulfan; ATG – antithymocyte globulin.

197 adults with Ph$^+$ ALL in first CR were described. Sixty-seven patients receiving RIC regimen were matched with 130 receiving MA regimen for age, donor type, and allo-HCT year. Over 75% received TKI therapy prior to allo-HCT. At a median follow-up of 4.5 years, 1-year treatment-related mortality (TRM) was lower in RIC regimen arm compared with MA arm (13% (95% CI 6−23) *versus* 36% (95% CI 28−44); $P=0.001$), while the 3-year relapse rate was higher in patients who received RIC regimen compared to MA regimen (49% (95% CI 37−61) *versus* 28% (95% CI 20−36) $P=0.058$). The OS did not differ between the cohorts (RIC 39% *versus* 35% $P=0.62$). Interestingly, patients who received TKI therapy prior to allo-HCT and with negative MRD status had a superior OS (55%) compared with patients receiving MA regimen also with a negative MRD status (33%; $P=0.0042$)[28]. In conclusion, based on existing data, RIC preparative regimen is a valid alternative strategy for Ph$^+$ ALL patients ineligible for MA regimen.

Is There a Role of Auto-HCT in ALL?

The UKALL/ECOG 2993 study reported for Ph-negative patients a lower rate of DFS and OS in individuals treated with auto-HCT compared to continued chemotherapy for postinduction therapy. For Ph$^+$ ALL, the CALGB 10001 study reported on 58 patients, 19 of whom underwent auto-HCT and 15 underwent allo-HCT. Induction treatment was based on imatinib plus sequential chemotherapy. The OS (median 6.0 years *versus* not reached) and DFS (median 3.5 *versus* 4.1 years) were similar in the two groups[29]. Ongoing clinical trials are using auto-HCT as consolidation strategy for patients with no available matched donor. For example, at the current NCI (NCT01256398) trial for older patients with Ph$^+$ ALL, patients aged 50–70 years with an HLA-matched related or unrelated donor are assigned to allo-HCT, while patients without an MSD or MUD are assigned to auto-HCT. Patients aged >70 years or who are not transplantation candidates are assigned to alternative chemotherapy. The PETHEMA group uses auto-HCT for young patients without a matched related or unrelated donor (NCT01491763). These studies are recruiting patients and data are expected in the future. Although promising, yet controversial, the latter CALGB 10001 study included a relatively small number of patients; therefore, auto-HCT could be recommended as a post-induction therapy in those cases where donor, e.g., MSD, MUD, CB or haplotype-matched donor, is not available, especially in patients who have reached MRD-negativity as defined by PCR or flow cytometry analysis.

Novel Monoclonal Antibodies and Chimeric Antigen Receptor T-cells

In recent years, novel therapeutic approaches have emerged in ALL and should be considered in Ph$^+$ ALL as well. For example, monoclonal antibodies, such as blinatumomab and inotuzumab have shown significant activity in ALL patients. Blinatumomab enables patient T-cells to recognize malignant B-cells. This antibody has two binding sites: a CD3 site for activating T-cells, and a CD19 site for binding the malignant B-cells. Twenty-one B-ALL patients with MRD persistence or relapse after induction and consolidation therapy were included in a phase 2 study. Blinatumomab administration induced an 80% MRD response rate. Moreover, after a median follow-up of 33 months, the hematologic relapse-free survival of the entire evaluable study cohort of 20 patients was 61% (Kaplan−Meier estimate)[30]. Currently, most blinatumomab ongoing clinical trials are conducted in the relapsed ALL setting. A clinical trial incorporating blinatumomab into the treatment of newly diagnosed Ph$^+$ ALL older patients has been suggested by the NCI (NCT02143414). Inotuzumab ozogamicin is a CD22 monoclonal antibody conjugated to the toxin calecheamicin. Forty-nine relapsed ALL patients were enrolled in a phase 2 clinical trial at the MDACC. Inotuzumab administered as a single-agent therapy resulted in an ORR of 57% and an acceptable toxicity profile[31].

The recently developed chimeric antigen receptor (CAR) T-cell therapy has gained a lot of interest among the hematologic community. In this technique, autologous T-cells are modified to express a receptor capable of recognizing a malignant cell. Recognition of the tumor cell by this specific receptor elicits a signal which can activate the T cell and ultimately lead to elimination of the tumor cell. Thirty relapsed ALL patients were infused with autologous T-cells transuded with a CD19-directed chimeric antigen receptor (CTL019). CR was achieved in 27 patients (90%), 15 of whom had undergone allo-HCT. CTL019 cells proliferated *in-vivo* and were detectable in the blood, CNS, and BM of patients who had a response. Sustained remission was achieved with a 6-month EFS rate of 67% (95% confidence interval [CI], 51 to 88) and an OS rate of 78% (95% CI, 65 to 95)[32]. The novel CAR-T strategy is currently being evaluated in the setting of relapsed and refractory B-ALL and other lymphoid malignancies.

In the future, these exciting new therapies may potentially be incorporated into the frontline setting. Introducing newer monoclonal Abs into remission induction in combination with TKI and with or without chemotherapy will be tested in clinical trials. Furthermore, these novel agents will serve as salvage therapy for primary refractory patients, in which achievement of remission is essential before proceeding to allo-HCT.

Conclusion

1. Patients need to get upfront TKI-based induction and consolidation with CNS prophylaxis or therapy, and TKIs need to be started as early as possible. Existing data suggest that dasatinib may induce a more rapid response and potentially more prolonged OS than imatinib.
2. For patients in first CR, the standard of care at the present time, if they have a matched donor, is to undergo an allo-HCT, even if they are MRD-negative.

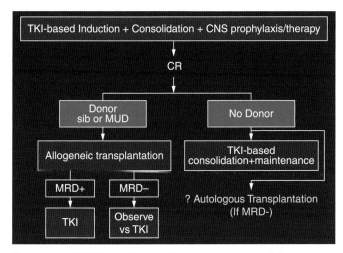

Figure 33.1 *BCR/ABL Positive* **ALL: Suggested Treatment Schema.**
WBC – white blood cell; MRD – minimal residual disease; RIC – reduced intensity conditioning; HCT – hematopoietic cell transplantation; TKI – tyrosine kinase inhibitor; MUD – matched unrelated donor; sib – sibling.

3. Should TKIs be used post-transplant? There is no doubt that patients who are MRD-positive need to continue

with TKIs and for those who are negative the jury is still out; prospective data are awaited, especially for the individuals who are MRD-negative pre- and post-transplant. For patients who do not have a donor, an auto-HCT is reasonable, especially if they have reached MRD negativity.

A suggested treatment schema for Ph+ ALL is given in Figure 33.1.

The future of Ph⁺ ALL treatment is very exciting and many issues need to be tackled. For example, could chemotherapy be excluded from induction for patients who achieve PCR negativity? Can we identify subgroups of patients who may be treated without an allo-HCT, for instance, patients who achieve a very early MRD negativity during induction? The optimal timing and interpretation of MRD results are still unclear. Additionally, the lack of consensus on standardized methodology at least for the more common p190 quantification results in practice and reporting variation. Ongoing efforts are required to improve PCR results comparability in order to use them in real-life practice.

References

1. Moorman AV, Harrison CJ, Buck GA, Richards SM, Secker-Walker LM, Martineau M, *et al.* Karyotype is an independent prognostic factor in adult acute lymphoblastic leukemia (ALL): analysis of cytogenetic data from patients treated on the Medical Research Council (MRC) UKALLXII/ Eastern Cooperative Oncology Group (ECOG) 2993 trial. *Blood.* 2007;109(8):3189–97.

2. Rowley JD. Letter: A new consistent chromosomal abnormality in chronic myelogenous leukaemia identified by quinacrine fluorescence and Giemsa staining. *Nature.* 1973;243(5405):290–3.

3. Hu Y, Liu Y, Pelletier S, Buchdunger E, Warmuth M, Fabbro D, *et al.* Requirement of Src kinases Lyn, Hck and Fgr for BCR-ABL1-induced B-lymphoblastic leukemia but not chronic myeloid leukemia. *Nat Genet.* 2004;36(5):453–61.

4. Larson RA. Management of acute lymphoblastic leukemia in older patients. *Semin Hematol.* 2006;43(2):126–33.

5. Dombret H, Gabert J, Boiron JM, Rigal-Huguet F, Blaise D, Thomas X, *et al.* Outcome of treatment in adults with Philadelphia chromosome-positive acute lymphoblastic leukemia: results of

the prospective multicenter LALA-94 trial. *Blood.* 2002;100(7):2357–66.

6. Forman SJ, O'Donnell MR, Nademanee AP, Snyder DS, Bierman PJ, Schmidt GM, *et al.* Bone marrow transplantation for patients with Philadelphia chromosome-positive acute lymphoblastic leukemia. *Blood.* 1987;70(2):587–8.

7. Chao NJ, Blume KG, Forman SJ, Snyder DS. Long-term follow-up of allogeneic bone marrow recipients for Philadelphia chromosome-positive acute lymphoblastic leukemia. *Blood.* 1995;85(11):3353–4.

8. Barrett AJ, Horowitz MM, Ash RC, Atkinson K, Gale RP, Goldman JM, *et al.* Bone marrow transplantation for Philadelphia chromosome-positive acute lymphoblastic leukemia. *Blood.* 1992;79(11):3067–70.

9. Fielding AK, Rowe JM, Richards SM, Buck G, Moorman AV, Durrant IJ, *et al.* Prospective outcome data on 267 unselected adult patients with Philadelphia chromosome-positive acute lymphoblastic leukemia confirms superiority of allogeneic transplantation over chemotherapy in the pre-imatinib era: results from the International ALL Trial MRC UKALLXII/ECOG2993. *Blood.* 2009;113(19):4489–96.

10. Kebriaei P, Saliba R, Rondon G, Chiattone A, Luthra R, Anderlini P,

et al. Long-term follow-up of allogeneic hematopoietic stem cell transplantation for patients with Philadelphia chromosome-positive acute lymphoblastic leukemia: impact of tyrosine kinase inhibitors on treatment outcomes. *Biol Blood Marrow Transplant.* 2012;18(4):584–92.

11. Fielding AK, Richards SM, Lazarus HM, Litzow MR, Luger SM, Marks DI, *et al.* Does imatinib change the outcome in Philapdelphia chromosome positive acute lymphoblastic leukaemia in adults? Data from the UKALLXII/ ECOG2993 Study. *Blood.* 2007;110(11):10a.

12. Fielding AK, Rowe JM, Buck G, Foroni L, Gerrard G, Litzow MR, *et al.* UKALLXII/ECOG2993: addition of imatinib to a standard treatment regimen enhances long-term outcomes in Philadelphia positive acute lymphoblastic leukemia. *Blood.* 2014;123(6):843–50.

13. Mizuta S, Matsuo K, Maeda T, Yujiri T, Hatta Y, Kimura Y, *et al.* Prognostic factors influencing clinical outcome of allogeneic hematopoietic stem cell transplantation following imatinib-based therapy in BCR-ABL-positive ALL. *Blood Cancer J.* 2012;2(5):e72.

14. O'Hare T, Walters DK, Stoffregen EP, Jia T, Manley PW, Mestan J, *et al.* In

vitro activity of Bcr-Abl inhibitors AMN107 and BMS-354825 against clinically relevant imatinib-resistant Abl kinase domain mutants. *Cancer Res.* 2005;65(11):4500–5.

15. Ottmann O, Dombret H, Martinelli G, Simonsson B, Guilhot F, Larson RA, *et al.* Dasatinib induces rapid hematologic and cytogenetic responses in adult patients with Philadelphia chromosome positive acute lymphoblastic leukemia with resistance or intolerance to imatinib: interim results of a phase 2 study. *Blood.* 2007;110(7):2309–15.

16. Lilly MB, Ottmann OG, Shah NP, Larson RA, Reiffers JJ, Ehninger G, *et al.* Dasatinib 140 mg once daily *versus* 70 mg twice daily in patients with Ph-positive acute lymphoblastic leukemia who failed imatinib: Results from a phase 3 study. *Am J Hematol.* 2010;85(3):164–70.

17. Rousselot P, Coudé MM, Huguet F, Lafage M, Leguay T, Salanoubat C, *et al.* Dasatinib (Sprycel®) and Low intensity chemotherapy for first-line treatment in patients with de novo Philadelphia positive ALL aged 55 and over: final results of the EWALL-Ph-01 Study. *Blood.* 2012;120(21):666a.

18. Foa R, Vitale A, Vignetti M, Meloni G, Guarini A, De Propris MS, *et al.* Dasatinib as first-line treatment for adult patients with Philadelphia chromosome-positive acute lymphoblastic leukemia. *Blood.* 2011;118(25):6521–8.

19. Porkka K, Koskenvesa P, Lundan T, Rimpilainen J, Mustjoki S, Smykla R, *et al.* Dasatinib crosses the blood-brain barrier and is an efficient therapy for central nervous system Philadelphia chromosome-positive leukemia. *Blood.* 2008;112(4):1005–12.

20. Takayama N, Sato N, O'Brien SG, Ikeda Y, Okamoto S. Imatinib mesylate has limited activity against the central nervous system involvement of Philadelphia chromosome-positive acute lymphoblastic leukaemia due to poor penetration into cerebrospinal fluid. *Br J Haematol.* 2002;119(1):106–8.

21. Pfeifer H, Goekbuget N, Völp C, Hüttmann A, Lübbert M, Stuhlmann R, *et al.* Long-term outcome of 335 adult patients receiving different schedules of imatinib and chemotherapy as front-line treatment for Philadelphia-positive acute lymphoblastic leukemia (Ph+ ALL). *Blood.* 2010;116:173

22. Ottmann OG, Wassmann B, Pfeifer H, Giagounidis A, Stelljes M, Duhrsen U, *et al.* Imatinib compared with chemotherapy as front-line treatment of elderly patients with Philadelphia chromosome-positive acute lymphoblastic leukemia (Ph+ALL). *Cancer.* 2007;109(10):2068–76.

23. Vignetti M, Fazi P, Cimino G, Martinelli G, Di Raimondo F, Ferrara F, *et al.* Imatinib plus steroids induces complete remissions and prolonged survival in elderly Philadelphia chromosome-positive patients with acute lymphoblastic leukemia without additional chemotherapy: results of the Gruppo Italiano Malattie Ematologiche dell'Adulto (GIMEMA) LAL0201-B protocol. *Blood.* 2007;109(9):3676–8.

24. Bachanova V, Burke MJ, Yohe S, Cao Q, Sandhu K, Singleton TP, *et al.* Unrelated cord blood transplantation in adult and pediatric acute lymphoblastic leukemia: effect of minimal residual disease on relapse and survival. *Biol Blood Marrow Transplant.* 2012;18(6):963–8.

25. Pinana JL, Sanz J, Picardi A, Ferra C, Martino R, Barba P, *et al.* Umbilical cord blood transplantation from unrelated donors in patients with Philadelphia chromosome-positive acute lymphoblastic leukemia. *Haematologica.* 2014;99(2):378–84.

26. Tucunduva L, Ruggeri A, Sanz G, Furst S, Cornelissen J, Linkesch W, *et al.* Impact of minimal residual disease on outcomes after umbilical cord blood transplantation for adults with Philadelphia-positive acute lymphoblastic leukaemia: an analysis on behalf of Eurocord, Cord Blood Committee and the Acute Leukaemia working party of the European group for Blood and Marrow Transplantation. *Br J Haematol.* 2014;166(5):749–57.

27. Sun YQ, Wang J, Jiang Q, Xu LP, Liu DH, Zhang XH, *et al.* Haploidentical hematopoietic SCT may be superior to conventional consolidation/maintenance chemotherapy as post-remission therapy for high-risk adult ALL. *Bone Marrow Transplant.* 2015;50(1):20–5.

28. Bachanova V, Marks DI, Zhang MJ, Wang H, de Lima M, Aljurf MD, *et al.* Ph+ ALL patients in first complete remission have similar survival after reduced intensity and myeloablative allogeneic transplantation: impact of tyrosine kinase inhibitor and minimal residual disease. *Leukemia.* 2014;28(3):658–65.

29. Wetzler M, Watson D, Stock W, Koval G, Mulkey FA, Hoke EE, *et al.* Autologous transplantation for Philadelphia chromosome-positive acute lymphoblastic leukemia achieves outcomes similar to allogeneic transplantation: results of CALGB Study 10001 (Alliance). *Haematologica.* 2014;99(1):111–5.

30. Topp MS, Gokbuget N, Zugmaier G, Degenhard E, Goebeler ME, Klinger M, *et al.* Long-term follow-up of hematologic relapse-free survival in a phase 2 study of blinatumomab in patients with MRD in B-lineage ALL. *Blood.* 2012;120(26):5185–7.

31. Kantarjian H, Thomas D, Jorgensen J, Jabbour E, Kebriaei P, Rytting M, *et al.* Inotuzumab ozogamicin, an anti-CD22-calecheamicin conjugate, for refractory and relapsed acute lymphocytic leukaemia: a phase 2 study. *Lancet Oncol.* 2012;13(4):403–11.

32. Maude SL, Frey N, Shaw PA, Aplenc R, Barrett DM, Bunin NJ, *et al.* Chimeric antigen receptor T cells for sustained remissions in leukemia. *N Engl J Med.* 2014;371(16):1507–17.

33. Mohty M, Labopin M, Tabrizzi R, Theorin N, Fauser AA, Rambaldi A, *et al.* Reduced intensity conditioning allogeneic stem cell transplantation for adult patients with acute lymphoblastic leukemia: a retrospective study from the European Group for Blood and Marrow Transplantation. *Haematologica.* 2008;93(2):303–6.

34. Bachanova V, Verneris MR, DeFor T, Brunstein CG, Weisdorf DJ. Prolonged survival in adults with acute lymphoblastic leukemia after reduced-intensity conditioning with cord blood or sibling donor transplantation. *Blood.* 2009;113(13):2902–5.

35. Ram R, Storb R, Sandmaier BM, Maloney DG, Woolfrey A, Flowers ME, *et al.* Non-myeloablative conditioning with allogeneic hematopoietic cell

transplantation for the treatment of high-risk acute lymphoblastic leukemia. *Haematologica.* 2011;96(8):1113–20.

36. Stein AS, Palmer JM, O'Donnell MR, Kogut NM, Spielberger RT, Slovak ML, *et al.* Reduced-intensity conditioning followed by peripheral blood stem cell transplantation for adult patients with high-risk acute lymphoblastic leukemia. *Biol Blood Marrow Transplant.* 2009;15(11):1407–14.

37. Arnold R, Massenkeil G, Bornhauser M, Ehninger G, Beelen DW, Fauser AA, *et al.* Nonmyeloablative stem cell transplantation in adults with high-risk ALL may be effective in early but not in advanced disease. *Leukemia.* 2002;16(12):2423–8.

Chapter

34

Hematopoietic Cell Transplants for Acute Myeloid Leukemia: Is There a Best Approach?

Masumi Ueda, Robert Peter Gale, Martin S. Tallman, and Hillard M. Lazarus

Introduction

Advances in diverse areas including supportive care, prevention and therapy of graft-*versus*-host disease (GvHD) and infections, better donor selection, modified pretransplant conditioning regimens, and others have improved outcomes of hematopoietic cell transplants (HCT) in persons with acute myeloid leukemia (AML). Consequently, more such transplants are being carried out (Figure 34.1)[1–3]. Nevertheless, there remains considerable controversy over which persons with AML should receive a transplant, when and how a transplant is best done, who is the best donor, and other issues. These controversies arise from several factors including an incomplete understanding of the complex biology and heterogeneity of AML, an inability to accurately predict survival of patients with AML at the subject-level, and inherent limitations in the conduct of clinical trials. In this chapter, we critically analyze recent data relevant to these issues, discuss the major controversies, and opine on navigating these uncertainties.

Transplant Outcomes and Recent Progress

Data from observational databases such as the European Society for Blood and Marrow Transplantation (EBMT) estimate

58% (95% CI, 55–61%) of persons receiving an HLA-identical sibling donor transplant for AML in 1st remission and 48% (95% CI, 41–55%) of those in 2nd remission are alive 5 years following transplant. Similar figures are reported from the Center for International Blood and Marrow Transplant Research (CIBMTR) (Figure 34.2). For transplants reported to the CIBMTR 2007-10, leukemia-free survival (LFS) at 2 years in persons in 1st remission was 53% (95% CI, 48–59%) for adults <40 years and 51% (95% CI 47–56%) for those >40 years. For persons in 2nd remission comparable outcomes were 60% (95% CI, 52–68%) and 50% (95% CI, 43–57%) (Table 34.1).

Transplant-related mortality (TRM) has decreased over the past 40 years. Data from the CIBMTR in subjects <50 years receiving a transplant from an HLA-identical sibling in 1st remission between 2000 and 2004 had a 50% decrease in TRM compared with those transplanted between 1985 and 1989 (15% *versus* 29%; P<0.001). An even greater reduction in TRM was seen for transplants in 2nd remission (13% *versus* 37%; P<0.001)[4]. There was no difference in relapse risk between these intervals suggesting any improvement in LFS or survival resulted from less TRM and not better leukemia control. This likely reflects

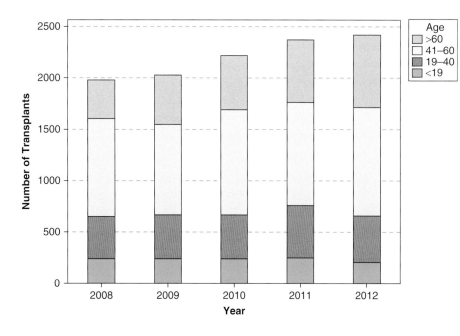

Figure 34.1 Allotransplants for AML in United States 2008–2012 registered with the CIBMTR. These data are preliminary and were obtained from the Statistical Center of the Center for International Blood and Marrow Transplant Research. The analysis has not been reviewed or approved by the Advisory or Scientific Committee of the CIBMTR.

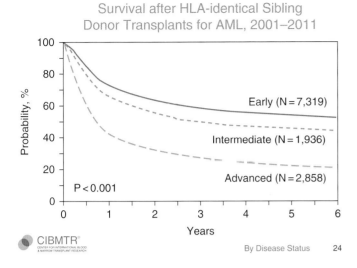

Figure 34.2 Survival after HLA-matched sibling and unrelated transplants for AML reported to the CIBMTR 2001–2011[3].

Graft-*versus*-Leukemia?

Some data from patients with AML receiving allotransplants are consistent with a graft-*versus*-leukemia (GvL) effect including: (1) a lower adjusted relapse risk in persons with acute and chronic GvHD; (2) a higher relapse risk associated with T-cell-depleted grafts; (3) higher relapse risk in recipients of transplants from genetically identical twins; and (4) the ability of donor leukocyte infusions (DLI) to control persistent or recurrent leukemia (see Chapter 25)[7]. Two different mechanisms of GvL, not mutually exclusive, are possible: (1) a nonspecific anti-AML effect associated with acute and/or chronic GvHD; and (2) a specific anti-AML effect. Although there are convincing data supporting the former, there are few if any convincing data supporting a specific immune-mediated anti-leukemia effect[80]. As such, the lower rate of leukemia relapse after allotransplants or DLI is best referred to as a reduction in leukemia relapse risk after an allo-transplant rather than GvL which can be misunderstood as implying a leukemia-specific immune-mediated effect.

Considerable efforts, mostly unsuccessful, have been directed towards increasing a specific GvL effect after transplant without increasing GvHD. Minor histocompatibility antigens (non-HLA antigens) on recipient hematopoietic cells [8] and leukemia-specific antigens such as Wilm tumor antigen (WT1) and proteinase-3 (PR3) were studied as targets for adoptive immune therapy after allotransplants[9,10]. Vaccination of the donor and/or recipient to minor histocompatibility antigens and so-called leukemia-associated antigens to increase anti-AML immunity[11–13], infusion of activated and expanded cytotoxic T-cells[10], adoptive transfer of natural killer (NK) cells[14], and inhibition of negative immune regulatory signals such as CTLA-4[15] are being studied. None of these approaches is convincingly proved to decrease leukemia relapse in randomized trials.

How Do Transplants Compare with Antileukemia Drugs?

Several meta-analyses of trials using donor-*versus*-no-donor comparisons rather than randomization (a poor substitute) report less relapse and better survival in persons <60 years with AML in 1st remission in the transplant cohort[16–18]. This benefit, if any, is limited to persons with intermediate-risk cytogenetics in most studies[19]. Persons with high-risk features who are most in need of an improved outcome did not benefit from a transplant in most studies. Thus, as with many new cancer therapies, allotransplants may be most effective in subjects who need them least, implying disease biology has a greater impact on outcome than therapy. There are other limitations with these types of comparisons including possible selection biases which can operate in the absence of randomization and dropouts in the cohort who have a donor, but who never receive a transplant. However, the most important limitation is the failure to consider the concept of therapy strategy

diverse factors including subject selection, better post-transplant support, and perhaps use of less-intensive pre-transplant conditioning (see below). Similar data are reported from large centers[5].

Despite progress in decreasing TRM, few data indicate less leukemia relapse or improvement in any other outcome. Relapse rates at 2 years post-transplant have increased and LFS has not improved in persons transplanted in 1st remission and 2nd remission reported to the CIBMTR between 1995 and 2010 (Table 34.1). Moreover, use of less-intensive pretransplant conditioning regimens has not convincingly reduced TRM in AML[6] and likely increased relapse rates. Nor is it clear whether targeted busulfan dosing based on pharmacokinetics, improved HLA-matching, increased availability of alternative donors or better selection of transplant recipients has improved LFS or survival.

Table 34.1 Relapse and LFS for AML transplants in the United States between 1995 and 2010 registered with CIBMTR, by years of transplant

| | Relapse at 2 years | | | | | | | | |
| | 1995–1998 | | 1999–2002 | | 2003–2006 | | 2007–2010 | | |
	n	Prob (95% CI)	n	Prob (95% CI)	n	Prob (95% CI)	n	Prob (95% CI)	P-value
CR1 age 18–40	500	15 (12–18)	308	19 (15–23)	411	23 (19–27)	330	29 (24–34)	<0.001
CR1 age 41–60	315	16 (12–20)	321	19 (15–23)	530	23 (20–27)	641	28 (25–32)	<0.001
CR2 age 18–40	169	16 (11–22)	156	22 (15–28)	186	23 (17–29)	137	22 (15–29)	0.38
CR2 age 41–60	110	12 (7–19)	121	24 (17–32)	231	24 (19–30)	211	31 (25–38)	<0.001

| | LFS at 2 years | | | | | | | | |
| | 1995–1998 | | 1999–2002 | | 2003–2006 | | 2007–2010 | | |
	n	Prob (95% CI)	n	Prob (95% CI)	n	Prob (95% CI)	n	Prob (95% CI)	P-value
CR1 age 18–40	500	60 (56–64)	308	58 (53–64)	411	58 (53–63)	330	53 (48–59)	0.37
CR1 age 41–60	315	53 (47–59)	321	49 (44–55)	530	51 (47–56)	641	51 (47–56)	0.80
CR2 age 18–40	169	38 (31–45)%	156	46 (38–54)	186	52 (44–59)	137	60 (52–68)	<0.001
CR2 age 41–60	110	41 (32–50)%	121	45 (36–54)	231	48 (42–55)	211	50 (43–57)	0.44

From M. Pasquini (personal communication).

Table 34.2 Variables in AML transplants

Subject-related	Disease-related	Transplant-related
Age	Etiology	Time to transplant
Comorbidities	Cytogenetics	Graft source
Performance score	Mutations	HLA disparity
	MRD	Graft type
	Disease stage	Young versus old donor age
	Remission duration	Donor–recipient gender match
		CMV state
		CD34 cell dose
		GvHD prophylaxis
		Conditioning regimen
		Post-transplant therapy

Abbreviations: MRD, measurable residual disease; CMV, cytomegalovirus; GvHD, graft-versus-host disease.

which is really early versus late allotransplant in persons failing chemotherapy and not transplant versus no transplant.

Prognostic Variables for Transplant Outcomes

Many subject-, disease-, and transplant-related variables are associated with prognosis after AML transplants (Table 34.2). Most are not prospectively validated. These associations are diverse transplant outcomes such as TRM, GvHD, and relapse.

Combined, their impact may be to affect the balance between these risks which contribute to LFS and survival outcomes. The transplant-specific comorbidity index[20], a weighted scoring system for comorbidities modeled for persons receiving diverse conditioning regimens, is a strong independent predictor of TRM and survival[21]. The EBMT risk score combines age, donor type, interval from diagnosis to transplant, and donor–recipient gender combination to estimate survival[22]. None of these indices is particularly useful to a physician in decision-making on the patient level.

Cytogenetics at diagnosis and at relapse are correlated with relapse risk and survival following transplant[23]. Beyond the usual categories of poor-, intermediate- and favorable-risk, monosomal karyotype (MK) has been recently reported to correlate with an increased relapse risk after allotransplants [24]. Measurable residual disease (MRD) sometimes incorrectly termed minimal residual disease[25], detected before and after transplant, is also correlated with relapse risk[26,27].

Who, if Anyone, Should Receive a Transplant and When?

Risk of relapse and estimated likelihood of cure with conventional therapy are the key variables for deciding whether to consider a transplant in persons with AML. Patients failing to achieve a 1st remission are reasonable candidates for a transplant if their induction chemotherapy was adequate and they are of appropriate age, clinical condition, comorbidity state, and have a suitable donor. However, the situation is far less clear in persons who achieve a remission but then relapse and particularly in patients in 1st remission. Data sometimes considered in making a transplant decision include results of cytogenetic and molecular studies. For example, patients in 1st remission with core-binding factor (CBF)-positive leukemia (t(8;21), inv16, t(16;16)), mutated *NPM-1*/wild-type *FLT3*-ITD, and bi-allelic mutated *CEBPA* with a normal karyotype have a low risk of relapse and are usually not considered for a transplant [23,81]. In contrast, there may be benefit for an allotransplant in persons with a monosomal karyotype or *FLT3*-ITD mutation [24,81]. However, there are no prospective randomized trial data proving patients with unfavorable risk AML benefit from transplant *versus* chemotherapy. Most data are from retrospective analyses and/or observational databases. Recently described mutations, analyzed singly and in combination, may better define risk of relapse in persons with AML [82]. However, it is important to consider these adverse outcome predictors may also operate in transplant recipients similar to poor-risk cytogenetics. The bottom line is just because someone has a poor prognosis with conventional therapy does not mean they should receive a transplant. Controlled and ideally randomized trials are needed to compare LFS and survival as co-primary endpoints. An example of this complexity is persons with concurrent mutations in *NPM-1* and *IDH1* or *IDH2* have longer LFS compared with *NPM-1* mutation without mutated *IDH*[28]. Additionally, in persons with a *FLT3*-ITD mutation, allele level, and ITD insertion site may be associated with transplant outcomes[83,84]. It is likely impossible to conduct randomized trials comparing alternative therapies in these small subsets of persons with AML. The same caveat applies to comparing alternative therapies in persons with mutations in *CEBPA*, *FLT3*, *RUNX1*, *KIT*, *TET-2*, *DNMT3A*[29], *ASXL1*, *PHF6*, and *MLL*[30,31].

Transplants in 1st Remission?

Recently an increasing proportion of persons with AML in 1st remission are receiving allotransplants. Is this reasonable? Two drivers of this trend are the seemingly better outcome of transplants in persons in 1st *versus* 2nd remission (Figure 34.2) and the low rate of 2nd remissions in persons who relapse. However, there are issues with this reasoning. First, the comparison of transplant outcomes in persons in 1st *versus* 2nd remission comes from transplant-based observational databases. Consequently, there is a lack of data on the universe of subjects who could have received a transplant in 1st or 2nd remission but did not. Other biases also operate which cannot be adjusted for in an observational database limited to transplant recipients. For example, in a study of >3000 subjects with AML randomized to subsequent therapies at study-entry only a quarter of subjects randomized to receive an autotransplant did so[85]. There was no benefit of transplants when analyzed on an intent-to-treat basis. The bottom line is even if transplants in 1st remission have a better outcome than transplants in 2nd remission, this is a self-fulfilling prophesy

which does not mean patients with AML should receive a transplant in 1st remission.

The second issue is the notion that the likelihood of achieving a 2nd remission and proceeding to a transplant is small so people should be transplanted in 1st remission. This notion is also flawed. Firstly, some studies report high 2nd remission rates and long LFS in persons with AML who relapse and who have specific favorable prognostic variables such as young age, long 1st remission, and good-risk cytogenetics[32]. Secondly, there are no convincing data proving that attempting to achieve a 2nd remission is better than immediate transplant for many or most people who relapse[32,33]. A recent analysis [34] of >1200 subjects <50 years old with AML who relapsed reported a >50% 2nd remission rate with about 20% 5-year survival. About two-thirds of persons achieving 2nd remission received a transplant; their 5-year survival was about 40%. Better survival after a transplant was reported in subjects with intermediate-risk cytogenetics but not in those with good- or poor-risk cytogenetics. These data again emphasize our difficulty in accurately predicting outcomes in persons with AML, especially at the subject-level, and the fallacy in thinking a benefit of transplants is equally distributed to all risk cohorts. The implication of these data is that delaying transplants until relapse may result in a similar or only slightly different overall outcome to transplants in 1st remission. Admittedly this conclusion is controversial and needs to be confirmed in a prospective study. Unfortunately this is unlikely to be done.

Measurable Residual Disease (MRD)

Data from measurable residual disease (MRD)-testing have become an important variable in therapy decisions in AML. Is this reasonable? Three distinct topics deserve consideration: (1) use of MRD to predict outcome of persons with AML in 1st remission; (2) use of MRD data to select persons with AML in 1st remission who should receive a transplant; and (3) impact of post-transplant MRD data on estimating transplant relapse risk and possibly the consideration of post-transplant therapy such as drugs or immune-mediated interventions.

Data from reports of MRD-testing in persons with AML in 1st remission indicate a correlation with detecting MRD pre-transplant and relapse risk[35,36]. For example, Terwijn *et al.* [37] studied validity of MRD-testing by multiparametric flow cytometry (MFC) as a predictor of relapse risk in adults with AML in a multicenter trial. MRD was tested after two cycles of induction chemotherapy. A positive MRD test was associated with increased relapse risk in multivariate analysis (HR 2.60; 95% CI 1.49–4.55). However, about 30% of subjects who were MRD-positive never relapsed (false positives). Moreover, about one-third of subjects who were MRD-negative relapsed (false negatives). This and several other studies highlight important issues which need to be considered in evaluating MRD-testing in AML such as the method(s) of MRD-testing and the boundary for declaring a test result negative or positive. The most common method of determining MRD in persons with AML uses multiparameter flow cytometry targeting a leukemia antigen phenotype determined at diagnosis in each subject. The target phenotype is not leukemia specific and likely present on normal hematopoietic cells. Results of flow cytometry testing are expressed as a percent positive cells. Various cut-off values are used to define MRD-positive or MRD-negative and there is no consensus between studies. Moreover, use of a binary classifier for a biologic continuum is questionable. Several studies using different MRD detection techniques and different criteria for declaring MRD test-positive or -negative report a greater relapse risk in subjects who are MRD-positive compared with those who are MRD-negative. For example, the detection of *NPM-1*-mutated transcripts in the blood of persons with *NPM-1*-mutated AML (typically considered standard risk) in complete remission after completing post-remission therapy was associated with significantly higher relapse risk compared with persons with no detectable transcripts (hazard ratio 5.09; 95% confidence interval, 2.84, 9.13; $P<0.001$)[91]. This is, of course, not surprising. Analyses of data from several studies of MRD in persons with AML in 1st remission indicate false-positive and false-negative rates each exceeding 30%[37]. This means a physician will frequently mistakenly identify a person as high or low risk for relapse. For example, in the *NPM1* MRD study about one third of MRD-negative subjects relapsed; these are false negatives. More disturbing, about 20% of MRD-postive subjects did not relapse at 5 years. This means basing a transplant decision on results of a positive *NPM1* MRD test using this model results in an unnecessary, potentially fatal, transplant in 1 in every 5 recipients. As we discussed above, even if results of MRD-testing are useful at the cohort level they are of more limited value at the subject level. A further complication in analyzing these data is that most studies allocate rather than randomize subjects who are MRD-positive or -negative to different subsequent therapies. This confounds analyses of predictive value of MRD-testing. Finally, as discussed, the detection of an adverse prognosis is useful only if we have a proved prognosis-altering intervention. The bottom line is results of MRD-testing are not especially accurate in predicting a person's risk of relapse with a C-statistic of only about 0.65–0.80[92] (see Chapters 23 and 24).

Another consideration is the heterogeneity of AML. Results of whole exome or genome sequencing, especially those with deep coverage, indicate each case of AML has a unique mutational fingerprint. Other data indicate multiple, genetically distinct subclones at diagnosis and certainly at relapse. Sometimes, the clone with a *driver* mutation matures morphologically such that at remission we cannot distinguish a person with residual leukemia from one with no residual leukemia cells (if this ever occurs). Given this complexity it is difficult to imagine how results of MRD-testing can help in clinical decision-making save to indicate which persons have many persisting leukemia cells.

Results of MRD-testing in 1st remission have also been used to select subjects to receive a transplant. Buccisano *et al.*[38]

used data from MRD-testing results after consolidation therapy to define low-risk (favorable or intermediate karyotype and MRD-negative after consolidation) and high-risk (unfavorable karyotype, *FLT3*-ITD mutated, or MRD-positive after consolidation) subjects who were assigned to receive an allotransplant and compared with nonconcurrent matched controls. Although relapse was lower and survival longer in the transplant cohort there are many problems with this type of analysis, and results require confirmation in a randomized trial in which high-risk subjects are assigned to receive a transplant or not. A prospective trial of AML therapy in children based on results of MRD-testing also reported better outcome of transplants *versus* chemotherapy in high-risk children[39]. Again, this study is flawed in its statistical design. An ongoing randomized trial (AML19) is investigating whether sequential MRD monitoring in subjects in remission may improve outcomes by carrying out transplants in those with MRD[93].

Finally, do results of MRD-testing post-transplant accurately predict relapse risk? Analysis of the impact of positive post-transplant MRD by fluorescence *in situ* hybridization (FISH) or MFC in 287 subjects with AML showed more relapses in subjects with MRD detected up to 5 years post-transplant[40]. Again, some subjects with MRD did not relapse and others without MRD did. These data indicate substantial rates of false-positive and -negative MRD test results and correlates with probability of relapse, particularly in individuals. One can conclude that MRD-testing is at an early stage in the context of clinical decision-making and should not be used for therapy decisions until reproducible assays are available and until reported associations are validated in randomized trials.

Pretransplant Conditioning Regimens

Cyclophosphamide combined with total body radiation (TBI) or busulfan are the most commonly used high-intensity conditioning regimens for persons with AML receiving an allotransplant. Recently, intravenous busulfan has largely replaced oral busulfan in the cyclophosphamide and busulfan combination. Are any of these regimens better than the others? Analysis of the large observational database of the CIBMTR with > 1200 subjects with AML in 1st remission receiving HLA-identical sibling transplants or HLA-matched unrelated donor transplants compared outcomes with these regimens. The study reported significantly less TRM, less relapse, and better 5-year survival in subjects receiving cyclophosphamide and intravenous busulfan compared with cyclophosphamide and TBI[41]. A prospective cohort study by Bredeson *et al.* in > 1400 mostly AML-subjects reported similar results[42]. In contrast, an observational database study of >1600 subjects with AML reported to the EBMT found similar nonrelapse mortality and survival but slightly more relapses in the cyclophosphamide and intravenous busulfan cohort compared with cyclophosphamide and TBI[43]. There are important technical differences between the CIBMTR and EBMT studies (see Chapter 69). We conclude that cyclophosphamide and intravenous busulfan is at least as good as cyclophosphamide and TBI and may be better.

Reduced Intensity Transplants

Many, perhaps most, persons with AML are inappropriate candidates for a conventional allotransplant because of age, comorbidities, and/or other factors often interacting with intensity of the pretransplant conditioning regimen. Also, as we discussed, considerable data indicate that immune-mediated antileukemia effects linked to GvHD, although not leukemia-specific, operate after transplant. Therefore, intensity of the pretransplant conditioning regimen is only one variable associated with the lower relapse risk of allotransplants compared with chemotherapy. These considerations resulted in the development of less-intensive pretransplant conditioning regimens. Depending on their intensity in the context of bone marrow suppression these regimens are referred to as reduced intensity conditioning (RIC) or non-myeloablative conditioning (another jargon term)[44]. The question is how do the results of these less-intensive regimens compare with conventional regimens and do they decrease TRM? A CIBMTR observational database analysis of >3700 subjects with AML in diverse disease states receiving transplants from HLA-identical siblings, HLA-matched unrelated donors, and HLA-partially or HLA-mismatched unrelated donors addressed this question[6]. Because subjects receiving less-intensive regimens were older and had more comorbidities adjustments were required for comparability. After adjustment, TRM was similar in the cohorts receiving conventional, RIC, or nonmyeloablative conditioning regimens at 3 and 5 years. This is obviously disappointing implying, counter-intuitively, intensity of the pretransplant conditioning regimen is not the predominant determinant of TRM. Subjects receiving less-intensive regimens had a greater relapse risk. Adjusted 5-year survival was similar for the conventional and RIC regimen cohorts and significantly worse in the nonmyeloablative cohort. A second observational database study from the EMBT reported similar results[45]. In a prospective study in subjects with AML in various disease states (most in 1st remission) or with myelodysplastic syndrome (MDS), subjects <50 years were allocated to receive a conventional transplant and those >50 years to receive RIC regimen. Although outcomes were similar these data cannot be used to imply a better outcome for persons >50 years receiving a RIC regimen versus a conventional transplant. A randomized study comparing conventional and RIC transplants was closed because of significantly inferior relapse-free survival in the RIC regimen cohort. Survival was not statistically different[46]. In the aggregate, these data suggest that in comparable patients conventional and RIC regimen transplants result in similar outcomes. Some may interpret these data to favor RIC

regimen transplants since conditioning is less intense and results seem comparable (see Chapter 27).

Types of Grafts

Several types of grafts including bone marrow cells, blood cells, and umbilical cord blood cells are used for AML allotransplants (see Chapter 2). These grafts may be intact or manipulated in-vitro by diverse techniques such as monoclonal antibodies or physical methods to enrich for some cell types such as CD34-positive cells. Grafts may also be depleted of some cell types such as T-cells by positive or negative selection methods (see Chapters 29 and 30). Sometimes graft type is confounded by the degree of donor–recipient HLA matching such as umbilical cord blood cell grafts which are almost always HLA-mismatched with the recipient (see Chapters 59–61). Also, sometimes there is manipulation of the donor before collecting the graft such as giving granulocyte or granulocyte-macrophage colony-stimulating factor (G-CSF and GM-CSF) (see Chapter 10).

Blood cell grafts are commonly used for allotransplants for AML. These grafts are associated with faster bone marrow recovery but more chronic GvHD[43, 47–49]. A randomized trial[49] reported more graft failure with bone marrow grafts but more chronic GvHD with blood cell grafts (see Chapter 19). Other outcomes including survival were similar. Based on these data we favor bone marrow grafts because of the substantial morbidity of chronic GvHD[50]. Interestingly, these are uncommonly used suggesting disagreement with the available data or that issues other than data impact the decision as to which type of graft to use.

Alternative Donors

Most data suggest an HLA-identical sibling is the best donor. However, fewer than 30% of persons with AML considered an appropriate transplant candidate have such a donor. So, who is the best alternative? Inherent to this question is the likelihood that a person who is an "appropriate" transplant candidate for an HLA-identical sibling donor may no longer be appropriate when a transplant from an alternative donor is planned because of an unfavorably altered benefit–risk ratio.

There are several possible alternative donors for an appropriate transplant candidate including: (1) an autotransplant; (2) an HLA-matched or HLA-mismatched unrelated donor; (3) HLA-matched or HLA-mismatched umbilical cord blood cells; and (4) an HLA haplotype matched relative donor and, others. Outcomes of transplants from completely HLA-matched unrelated donors are only slightly inferior to those of transplants from HLA-identical siblings[51–53]. Availability of this type of alternative donor for persons with AML without an HLA-identical sibling donor correlates with race and ethnicity. A recent model based on National Marrow Donor Program (NMDP) data predicted availability of an 8/8 antigen HLA-matched donor for 75% of persons of European descent versus 46% for persons of Middle Eastern or North African descent and only 16–19% for black Americans[54]. Transplants from more discordant HLA-matched unrelated donors have worse outcomes[53,55]. These inferior outcomes are sometimes acceptable in the context of the anticipated outcome of conventional therapy. The issue of alternative donors is discussed in greater detail in Chapter 16.

There are few data on the use of umbilical cord blood cells in adults with AML[56,57]. Recipients of HLA-A, -B, and -DRB1 allele-matched units have low TRM[58]. There is considerable controversy about whether transplants of one or two umbilical cord blood cell units have better outcomes. Studies addressing this question report contradictory conclusions[58–60,86]. A recent study in children and adolescents reported higher risk of GvHD and slower platelet recovery after transplants of two umbilical cord blood cell units[61]. Presently, most data suggest no advantage of transplanting two umbilical cord blood cell units over one. There is consensus that umbilical cord blood grafts are associated with slower bone marrow recovery, less GvHD, more relapses, and worse LFS and survival compared with transplants from HLA-identical siblings or from completely HLA-matched unrelated donors. How results compare with outcomes of transplants from less well HLA-matched unrelated donors is controversial but likely comparable. Again, these worse outcomes are sometimes acceptable in the context of the anticipated outcome of conventional therapy. A recent retrospective analysis of subjects with acute leukemia or myelodysplastic syndrome with pre-transplant MRD showed lower probability of relapse and better survival in subjects receiving an umbilical cord blood cell transplant versus a HLA-matched or –mismatched unrelated donor transplant[94]. These data and others raise the important issue that there may not be a *best* alternative donor for everyone. For example, in a person with a low or no risk of leukemia relapse post-transplant the best donor might be one unlikely to cause GvHD whereas in a person at high relapse risk some degree of GvHD might be desirable. As such the search to determine the best alternative donor for everyone, especially on the subject level, is fruitless.

Another type of alternative donor is a HLA-haplotype-matched relative such as a sibling, parent, or child. The advantage of this approach is donor availability; almost everyone with AML who might be considered for a transplant has such a donor. Several series of HLA-haplotype-matched donor transplants are reported[62,63]. Two major approaches are being studied: (1) manipulation of the graft to prevent GvHD such as CD3/CD19 selection followed by conventional post-transplant immune suppression; and (2) unmodified grafts followed by post-transplant immune suppression with cyclophosphamide. Also, different types of grafts are being studied including blood cells and bone marrow singly or combined. Sometimes blood cell or bone marrow donors receive G- or GM-CSF before the graft is obtained. There are no direct comparisons of these approaches but results seem comparable. Advantages and disadvantages of different alternative donors are shown in Table 34.3. Randomized trials comparing several of these

Table 34.3 Advantages and disadvantages of different alternative donors

	Unrelated donor	Umbilical cord blood	HLA haplotype mismatched relative
Availability	++	+	+++
No marrow recovery	+	+++	++
GvHD	++	+	+++
Infections	+	+++	++
Relapse risk	++	+++	++
LFS	+++	+	++
Survival	+++	++	++

Arbitrary scoring of events and outcomes: +, least likely; +++, most likely.

strategies are in progress such as use of an HLA-matched unrelated donor *versus* a graft of two umbilical cord blood cell units.

T-Cell Depletion

Concepts underlying T-cell depletion and results of clinical trials are reviewed in Chapter 29. Here we focus on data exclusively on studies of T-cell-depletion trials in patients with AML. In-vivo T-cell depletion, a jargon term, using antithymocyte globulin (ATG) or alemtuzumab is associated with less acute and chronic GvHD but similar TRM and increased relapse with worse LFS and survival[64]. Similar conclusions are reported in a large EBMT retrospective analysis of persons with AML receiving HLA-identical sibling donor transplants after RIC regimen[65]. Similar results are also reported using physical techniques for T-cell depletion[66]. Several prospective studies using different types of ATG report a reduction in GvHD. A randomized study using standard GvHD prophylaxis with or without thymoglobulin in subjects receiving conventional HLA-matched unrelated donor bone marrow transplants showed a significant reduction in extensive chronic GvHD (41% *versus* 15%, P=0.01) without an increase in cumulative incidence of relapse[87]. Two multi-center randomized studies of ATG reported lower cumulative incidences of acute and chronic GvHD but no difference in relapse, nonrelapse mortality, or survival after conventional HLA-matched related or unrelated transplants of blood cells [88,89]. A recent randomized ATG study in diverse transplant recipients reported a higher rate of withdrawal of immune suppression at 1 year in the ATG cohort (37% *versus* 16%, P=0.0006) with no differences in risks of relapse or survival [90]. The bottom line is few data supporting using T-cell depletion in persons with AML receiving transplants. In contrast, using ATG seems to decrease GvHD but does not improve LFS or survival. Results of ongoing randomized trials may alter this opinion but this seems unlikely.

Post-Transplant Therapy to Prevent Relapse

A substantial proportion of recipients of allotransplants for AML relapse including about 10–40% of those transplanted in 1st remission, 40–50% of those transplanted in ≥2nd remission[67], and >50% in those transplanted without achieving a 1st remission or with more advanced AML[68]. Other variables correlated with relapse include cytogenetics[69,70], age, preceding myelodysplastic syndrome (MDS)[67], *FLT3*-ITD mutation[71], donor–recipient sex match (female donor with male recipient)[72], donor type, graft type[48], and development of acute and/or chronic GvHD[53].

There were numerous attempts to decrease relapse after transplant in patients with AML including interferon[73], interleukin-2[74], azacitidine[75,76], and tyrosine kinase inhibitors such as sorafenib[77]. Although several phase 1 and 2 studies report favorable outcomes, no intervention is convincingly proved to decrease relapse in this setting (see Chapter 23). Moreover, the large numbers of drugs being tested in this setting suggests none is convincingly effective.

Another approach to preventing relapse after transplant involves vaccines targeting purportedly leukemia-associated or -specific antigens. Examples include vaccination against Wilm tumor (WT1) gene product peptide[78] and HLA-A2 restricted leukemia-associated peptide PR1[79]. These approaches were studied in persons with recurrent AML and are being tested in the post-transplant setting. No approach is convincingly proved to prevent AML relapse in a randomized trial. We think there is no proved benefit for giving post-transplant interventions to decrease relapse after allotransplants for AML and that such interventions should only be done in the context of clinical trials.

Conclusions and Future Directions

Allotransplants have an important role in treating AML. However, this role, like AML itself, is complex and it is often difficult to know on the subject level whether a person should have a transplant and, if yes, when and how? There are improved outcomes of transplants for AML but much results from subject selection and improved supportive care rather than in preventing transplant complications such as GvHD or leukemia relapse. More patients with AML can receive a transplant because of increased donor availability and reduced intensity pretransplant conditioning regimens. However, the dominant question is just because they can receive a transplant, should they? This question and many others are largely unanswered. Moreover, many of these questions are unlikely to be answered because of several reasons including: (1) physicians think they already know the answer (often they do not); (2) difficulty in designing appropriate clinical trials; and (3) failure to consider difference between therapies *versus* comparing therapy strategies and other limitations.

In many seemingly controversial areas we see relatively small differences between competing therapies, the magnitudes of which are greatly overwhelmed by heterogeneity of patients with AML. Namely, differences between patients with AML are typically much greater than differences in the efficacy of therapy alternatives.

References

1. Passweg JR, Baldomero H, Gratwohl A, Bregni M, Cesaro S, Dreger P, et al. The EBMT activity survey: 1990–2010. *Bone Marrow Transplantation.* 2012;47(7):906–23.

2. Passweg JR, Baldomero H, Bregni M, Cesaro S, Dreger P, Duarte RF, et al. Hematopoietic SCT in Europe: data and trends in 2011. *Bone Marrow Transplantation.* 2013;48(9):1161–7.

3. Pasquini MC, Wang Z. Current use and outcome of hematopoietic stem cell transplantation: CIBMTR Summary Slides. 2013.

4. Horan JT, Logan BR, Agovi-Johnson MA, Lazarus HM, Bacigalupo AA, Ballen KK, et al. Reducing the risk for transplantation-related mortality after allogeneic hematopoietic cell transplantation: how much progress has been made? *Journal of Clinical Oncology: Official Journal of the American Society of Clinical Oncology.* 2011;29(7):805–13.

5. Gooley TA, Chien JW, Pergam SA, Hingorani S, Sorror ML, Boeckh M, et al. Reduced mortality after allogeneic hematopoietic-cell transplantation. *The New England Journal of Medicine.* 2010;363(22):2091–101.

6. Luger SM, Ringden O, Zhang MJ, Perez WS, Bishop MR, Bornhauser M, et al. Similar outcomes using myeloablative vs reduced-intensity allogeneic transplant preparative regimens for AML or MDS. *Bone Marrow Transplantation.* 2012;47(2):203–11.

7. Chang YJ, Huang XJ. Donor lymphocyte infusions for relapse after allogeneic transplantation: when, if and for whom? *Blood Reviews.* 2013;27(1):55–62.

8. Bleakley M, Riddell SR. Exploiting T cells specific for human minor histocompatibility antigens for therapy of leukemia. *Immunology and Cell Biology.* 2011;89(3):396–407.

9. Norde WJ, Overes IM, Maas F, Fredrix H, Vos JC, Kester MG, et al. Myeloid leukemic progenitor cells can be specifically targeted by minor histocompatibility antigen LRH-1-reactive cytotoxic T cells. *Blood.* 2009;113(10):2312–23.

10. Warren EH, Fujii N, Akatsuka Y, Chaney CN, Mito JK, Loeb KR, et al. Therapy of relapsed leukemia after allogeneic hematopoietic cell transplantation with T cells specific for minor histocompatibility antigens. *Blood.* 2010;115(19):3869–78.

11. Rezvani K, Yong AS, Mielke S, Savani BN, Musse L, Superata J, et al. Leukemia-associated antigen-specific T-cell responses following combined PR1 and WT1 peptide vaccination in patients with myeloid malignancies. *Blood.* 2008;111(1):236–42.

12. Oka Y, Tsuboi A, Taguchi T, Osaki T, Kyo T, Nakajima H, et al. Induction of WT1 (Wilms' tumor gene)-specific cytotoxic T lymphocytes by WT1 peptide vaccine and the resultant cancer regression. *Proceedings of the National Academy of Sciences of the USA.* 2004;101(38):13885–90.

13. Van Tendeloo VF, Van de Velde A, Van Driessche A, Cools N, Anguille S, Ladell K, et al. Induction of complete and molecular remissions in acute myeloid leukemia by Wilms' tumor 1 antigen-targeted dendritic cell vaccination. *Proceedings of the National Academy of Sciences of the USA.* 2010;107(31):13824–9.

14. Miller JS, Soignier Y, Panoskaltsis-Mortari A, McNearney SA, Yun GH, Fautsch SK, et al. Successful adoptive transfer and in vivo expansion of human haploidentical NK cells in patients with cancer. *Blood.* 2005;105(8):3051–7.

15. Bashey A, Medina B, Corringham S, Pasek M, Carrier E, Vrooman L, et al. CTLA4 blockade with ipilimumab to treat relapse of malignancy after allogeneic hematopoietic cell transplantation. *Blood.* 2009;113(7):1581–8.

16. Yanada M, Matsuo K, Emi N, Naoe T. Efficacy of allogeneic hematopoietic stem cell transplantation depends on cytogenetic risk for acute myeloid leukemia in first disease remission: a metaanalysis. *Cancer.* 2005;103(8):1652–8.

17. Cornelissen JJ, van Putten WL, Verdonck LF, Theobald M, Jacky E, Daenen SM, et al. Results of a HOVON/SAKK donor *versus* no-donor analysis of myeloablative HLA-identical sibling stem cell transplantation in first remission acute myeloid leukemia in young and middle-aged adults: benefits for whom? *Blood.* 2007;109(9):3658–66.

18. Koreth J, Schlenk R, Kopecky KJ, Honda S, Sierra J, Djulbegovic BJ, et al. Allogeneic stem cell transplantation for acute myeloid leukemia in first complete remission: systematic review and meta-analysis of prospective clinical trials. *JAMA: The Journal of the American Medical Association.* 2009;301(22):2349–61.

19. Burnett AK, Wheatley K, Goldstone AH, Stevens RF, Hann IM, Rees JH, et al. The value of allogeneic bone marrow transplant in patients with acute myeloid leukaemia at differing risk of relapse: results of the UK MRC AML 10 trial. *British Journal of Haematology.* 2002;118(2):385–400.

20. Sorror ML, Maris MB, Storb R, Baron F, Sandmaier BM, Maloney DG, et al. Hematopoietic cell transplantation (HCT)-specific comorbidity index: a new tool for risk assessment before allogeneic HCT. *Blood.* 2005;106(8):2912–9.

21. Sorror ML, Sandmaier BM, Storer BE, Maris MB, Baron F, Maloney DG, et al. Comorbidity and disease status based risk stratification of outcomes among patients with acute myeloid leukemia or myelodysplasia receiving allogeneic hematopoietic cell transplantation. *Journal of Clinical Oncology: Official Journal of the American Society of Clinical Oncology.* 2007;25(27):4246–54.

22. Gratwohl A, Stern M, Brand R, Apperley J, Baldomero H, de Witte T, et al. Risk score for outcome after allogeneic hematopoietic stem cell transplantation: a retrospective analysis. *Cancer.* 2009;115(20):4715–26.

23. Armand P, Kim HT, Zhang MJ, Perez WS, Dal Cin PS, Klumpp TR, et al. Classifying cytogenetics in patients with acute myelogenous leukemia in complete remission undergoing allogeneic transplantation: a Center for International Blood and Marrow Transplant Research study. *Biology of Blood and Marrow Transplantation: Journal of the American Society for Blood and Marrow Transplantation.* 2012;18(2):280–8.

24. Cornelissen JJ, Breems D, van Putten WL, Gratwohl AA, Passweg JR, Pabst T, et al. Comparative analysis of the value of allogeneic hematopoietic stem-cell transplantation in acute myeloid leukemia with monosomal karyotype *versus* other cytogenetic risk categories. *Journal of Clinical Oncology: Official Journal of the American Society of Clinical Oncology.* 2012;30(17):2140–6.

25. Goldman JM, Gale RP. What does MRD in leukemia really mean? *Leukemia.* 2014;28(5):1131.

26. Walter RB, Buckley SA, Pagel JM, Wood BL, Storer BE, Sandmaier BM, et al. Significance of minimal residual disease before myeloablative allogeneic hematopoietic cell transplantation for AML in first and second complete remission. *Blood.* 2013;122(10):1813–21.

27. Appelbaum FR. Measurement of minimal residual disease before and after myeloablative hematopoietic cell transplantation for acute leukemia. *Best Practice & Research Clinical Haematology.* 2013;26(3):279–84.

28. Patel JP, Gonen M, Figueroa ME, Fernandez H, Sun Z, Racevskis J, et al. Prognostic relevance of integrated genetic profiling in acute myeloid leukemia. *The New England Journal of Medicine.* 2012;366(12):1079–89.

29. Ley TJ, Ding L, Walter MJ, McLellan MD, Lamprecht T, Larson DE, et al. DNMT3A mutations in acute myeloid leukemia. *The New England Journal of Medicine.* 2010;363(25):2424–33.

30. Allen C, Hills RK, Lamb K, Evans C, Tinsley S, Sellar R, et al. The importance of relative mutant level for evaluating impact on outcome of KIT, FLT3 and CBL mutations in core-binding factor acute myeloid leukemia. *Leukemia.* 2013;27(9):1891–901.

31. Paschka P, Du J, Schlenk RF, Gaidzik VI, Bullinger L, Corbacioglu A, et al. Secondary genetic lesions in acute myeloid leukemia with inv(16) or t(16;16): a study of the German-Austrian AML Study Group (AMLSG). *Blood.* 2013;121(1):170–7.

32. Kurosawa S, Yamaguchi T, Miyawaki S, Uchida N, Sakura T, Kanamori H, et al. Prognostic factors and outcomes of adult patients with acute myeloid leukemia after first relapse. *Haematologica.* 2010;95(11):1857–64.

33. Duval M, Klein JP, He W, Cahn JY, Cairo M, Camitta BM, et al. Hematopoietic stem-cell transplantation for acute leukemia in relapse or primary induction failure. *Journal of Clinical Oncology: Official Journal of the American Society of Clinical Oncology.* 2010;28(23):3730–8.

34. Burnett AK, Goldstone A, Hills RK, Milligan D, Prentice A, Yin J, et al. Curability of patients with acute myeloid leukemia who did not undergo transplantation in first remission. *Journal of Clinical Oncology: Official Journal of the American Society of Clinical Oncology.* 2013;31(10):1293–301.

35. San Miguel JF, Martinez A, Macedo A, Vidriales MB, Lopez-Berges C, Gonzalez M, et al. Immunophenotyping investigation of minimal residual disease is a useful approach for predicting relapse in acute myeloid leukemia patients. *Blood.* 1997;90(6):2465–70.

36. Kern W, Voskova D, Schoch C, Hiddemann W, Schnittger S, Haferlach T. Determination of relapse risk based on assessment of minimal residual disease during complete remission by multiparameter flow cytometry in

unselected patients with acute myeloid leukemia. *Blood.* 2004;104(10):3078–85.

37. Terwijn M, van Putten WL, Kelder A, van der Velden VH, Brooimans RA, Pabst T, *et al.* High prognostic impact of flow cytometric minimal residual disease detection in acute myeloid leukemia: data from the HOVON/SAKK AML 42A study. *Journal of Clinical Oncology: Official Journal of the American Society of Clinical Oncology.* 2013;31(31):3889–97.

38. Buccisano F, Maurillo L, Del Principe MI, Del Poeta G, Sconocchia G, Lo-Coco F, *et al.* Prognostic and therapeutic implications of minimal residual disease detection in acute myeloid leukemia. *Blood.* 2012;119(2):332–41.

39. Rubnitz JE, Inaba H, Dahl G, Ribeiro RC, Bowman WP, Taub J, *et al.* Minimal residual disease-directed therapy for childhood acute myeloid leukaemia: results of the AML02 multicentre trial. *The Lancet Oncology.* 2010;11(6):543–52.

40. Fang M, Storer B, Wood B, Gyurkocza B, Sandmaier BM, Appelbaum FR. Prognostic impact of discordant results from cytogenetics and flow cytometry in patients with acute myeloid leukemia undergoing hematopoietic cell transplantation. *Cancer.* 2012;118(9):2411–9.

41. Copelan EA, Hamilton BK, Avalos B, Ahn KW, Bolwell BJ, Zhu X, *et al.* Better leukemia-free and overall survival in AML in first remission following cyclophosphamide in combination with busulfan compared with TBI. *Blood.* 2013;122(24):3863–70.

42. Bredeson C, LeRademacher J, Kato K, Dipersio JF, Agura E, Devine SM, *et al.* Prospective cohort study comparing intravenous busulfan to total body irradiation in hematopoietic cell transplantation. *Blood.* 2013;122(24):3871–8.

43. Nagler A, Rocha V, Labopin M, Unal A, Ben Othman T, Campos A, *et al.* Allogeneic hematopoietic stem-cell transplantation for acute myeloid leukemia in remission: comparison of intravenous busulfan plus cyclophosphamide (Cy) *versus* total-body irradiation plus Cy as conditioning regimen–a report from the acute leukemia working party of the European group for blood and marrow transplantation. *Journal of Clinical Oncology: Official Journal of the American Society of Clinical Oncology.* 2013;31(28):3549–56.

44. Bacigalupo A, Ballen K, Rizzo D, Giralt S, Lazarus H, Ho V, *et al.* Defining the intensity of conditioning regimens: working definitions. *Biology of Blood and Marrow Transplantation: Journal of the American Society for Blood and Marrow Transplantation.* 2009;15(12):1628–33.

45. Aoudjhane M, Labopin M, Gorin NC, Shimoni A, Ruutu T, Kolb HJ, *et al.* Comparative outcome of reduced intensity and myeloablative conditioning regimen in HLA identical sibling allogeneic haematopoietic stem cell transplantation for patients older than 50 years of age with acute myeloblastic leukaemia: a retrospective survey from the Acute Leukemia Working Party (ALWP) of the European group for Blood and Marrow Transplantation (EBMT). *Leukemia.* 2005;19(12):2304–12.

46. Scott BL, Pasquini MC, Logan B, *et al.* Results of a phase III randomized, multi-center study of allogeneic stem cell transplantation after high versus reduced intensity conditioning in patients with myelodysplastic syndrome or acute myeloid leukemia: Blood and Marrow Transplant Clinical Trials network (BMT CTN) 0901. *Blood.* 2015;126.

47. Bensinger WI, Martin PJ, Storer B, Clift R, Forman SJ, Negrin R, *et al.* Transplantation of bone marrow as compared with peripheral-blood cells from HLA-identical relatives in patients with hematologic cancers. *The New England Journal of Medicine.* 2001;344(3):175–81.

48. Stem Cell Trialists' Collaborative G. Allogeneic peripheral blood stem-cell compared with bone marrow transplantation in the management of hematologic malignancies: an individual patient data meta-analysis of nine randomized trials. *Journal of Clinical Oncology: Official Journal of the American Society of Clinical Oncology.* 2005;23(22):5074–87.

49. Anasetti C, Logan BR, Lee SJ, Waller EK, Weisdorf DJ, Wingard JR, *et al.* Peripheral-blood stem cells *versus* bone marrow from unrelated donors. *The New England Journal of Medicine.* 2012;367(16):1487–96.

50. Appelbaum FR. Pursuing the goal of a donor for everyone in need. *The New England Journal of Medicine.* 2012;367(16):1555–6.

51. Walter RB, Pagel JM, Gooley TA, Petersdorf EW, Sorror ML, Woolfrey AE, *et al.* Comparison of matched unrelated and matched related donor myeloablative hematopoietic cell transplantation for adults with acute myeloid leukemia in first remission. *Leukemia.* 2010;24(7):1276–82.

52. Imahashi N, Suzuki R, Fukuda T, Kakihana K, Kanamori H, Eto T, *et al.* Allogeneic hematopoietic stem cell transplantation for intermediate cytogenetic risk AML in first CR. *Bone Marrow Transplantation.* 2013;48(1):56–62.

53. Gupta V, Tallman MS, He W, Logan BR, Copelan E, Gale RP, *et al.* Comparable survival after HLA-well-matched unrelated or matched sibling donor transplantation for acute myeloid leukemia in first remission with unfavorable cytogenetics at diagnosis. *Blood.* 2010;116(11):1839–48.

54. Gragert L, Eapen M, Williams E, Freeman J, Spellman S, Baitty R, *et al.* HLA match likelihoods for hematopoietic stem-cell grafts in the U.S. registry. *The New England Journal of Medicine.* 2014;371(4):339–48.

55. Lee SJ, Klein J, Haagenson M, Baxter-Lowe LA, Confer DL, Eapen M, *et al.* High-resolution donor-recipient HLA-matching contributes to the success of unrelated donor marrow transplantation. *Blood.* 2007;110(13):4576–83.

56. Barker JN, Scaradavou A, Stevens CE. Combined effect of total nucleated cell dose and HLA match on transplantation outcome in 1061 cord blood recipients with hematologic malignancies. *Blood.* 2010;115(9):1843–9.

57. Eapen M, Klein JP, Sanz GF, Spellman S, Ruggeri A, Anasetti C, *et al.* Effect of donor-recipient HLA matching at HLA A, B, C, and DRB1 on outcomes after umbilical-cord blood transplantation for leukaemia and myelodysplastic syndrome: a retrospective analysis. *The Lancet Oncology.* 2011;12(13):1214–21.

58. Ruggeri A, Sanz G, Bittencourt H, Sanz J, Rambaldi A, Volt F, *et al.* Comparison of outcomes after single or double cord blood transplantation in adults with acute leukemia using

different types of myeloablative conditioning regimen, a retrospective study on behalf of Eurocord and the Acute Leukemia Working Party of EBMT. *Leukemia*. 2014;28(4):779–86.

59. Scaradavou A, Brunstein CG, Eapen M, Le-Rademacher J, Barker JN, Chao N, *et al*. Double unit grafts successfully extend the application of umbilical cord blood transplantation in adults with acute leukemia. *Blood*. 2013;121(5):752–8.

60. Verneris MR, Brunstein CG, Barker J, MacMillan ML, DeFor T, McKenna DH, *et al*. Relapse risk after umbilical cord blood transplantation: enhanced graft-*versus*-leukemia effect in recipients of 2 units. *Blood*. 2009;114(19):4293–9.

61. Wagner JE, Jr., Eapen M, Carter S, Wang Y, Schultz KR, Wall DA, *et al*. One-unit *versus* two-unit cord-blood transplantation for hematologic cancers. *The New England Journal of Medicine*. 2014;371(18):1685–94.

62. Ciceri F, Labopin M, Aversa F, Rowe JM, Bunjes D, Lewalle P, *et al*. A survey of fully haploidentical hematopoietic stem cell transplantation in adults with high-risk acute leukemia: a risk factor analysis of outcomes for patients in remission at transplantation. *Blood*. 2008;112(9):3574–81.

63. Huang XJ, Liu DH, Liu KY, Xu LP, Chen H, Han W, *et al*. Treatment of acute leukemia with unmanipulated HLA-mismatched/haploidentical blood and bone marrow transplantation. *Biology of Blood and Marrow Transplantation: Journal of the American Society for Blood and Marrow Transplantation*. 2009;15(2):257–65.

64. Champlin RE, Passweg JR, Zhang MJ, Rowlings PA, Pelz CJ, Atkinson KA, *et al*. T-cell depletion of bone marrow transplants for leukemia from donors other than HLA-identical siblings: advantage of T-cell antibodies with narrow specificities. *Blood*. 2000;95(12):3996–4003.

65. Baron F, Labopin M, Blaise D, Lopez-Corral L, Vigouroux S, Craddock C, *et al*. Impact of in vivo T-cell depletion on outcome of AML patients in first CR given peripheral blood stem cells and reduced-intensity conditioning allo-SCT from a HLA-identical sibling donor: a report from the Acute Leukemia Working Party of the European Group for Blood and Marrow Transplantation. *Bone Marrow Transplantation*. 2014;49(3):389–96.

66. Bayraktar UD, de Lima M, Saliba RM, Maloy M, Castro-Malaspina HR, Chen J, *et al*. Ex vivo T cell-depleted *versus* unmodified allografts in patients with acute myeloid leukemia in first complete remission. *Biology of Blood and Marrow Transplantation: Journal of the American Society for Blood and Marrow Transplantation*. 2013;19(6):898–903.

67. Pavletic SZ, Kumar S, Mohty M, de Lima M, Foran JM, Pasquini M, *et al*. NCI First International Workshop on the Biology, Prevention, and Treatment of Relapse after Allogeneic Hematopoietic Stem Cell Transplantation: report from the Committee on the Epidemiology and Natural History of Relapse following Allogeneic Cell Transplantation. *Biology of Blood and Marrow Transplantation: Journal of the American Society for Blood and Marrow Transplantation*. 2010;16(7):871–90.

68. Fung HC, Stein A, Slovak M, O'Donnell M R, Snyder DS, Cohen S, *et al*. A long-term follow-up report on allogeneic stem cell transplantation for patients with primary refractory acute myelogenous leukemia: impact of cytogenetic characteristics on transplantation outcome. *Biology of Blood and Marrow Transplantation: Journal of the American Society for Blood and Marrow Transplantation*. 2003;9(12):766–71.

69. Ferrant A, Labopin M, Frassoni F, Prentice HG, Cahn JY, Blaise D, *et al*. Karyotype in acute myeloblastic leukemia: prognostic significance for bone marrow transplantation in first remission: a European Group for Blood and Marrow Transplantation study. Acute Leukemia Working Party of the European Group for Blood and Marrow Transplantation (EBMT). *Blood*. 1997;90(8):2931–8.

70. Tallman MS, Dewald GW, Gandham S, Logan BR, Keating A, Lazarus HM, *et al*. Impact of cytogenetics on outcome of matched unrelated donor hematopoietic stem cell transplantation for acute myeloid leukemia in first or second complete remission. *Blood*. 2007;110(1):409–17.

71. Brunet S, Labopin M, Esteve J, Cornelissen J, Socie G, Iori AP, *et al*. Impact of FLT3 internal tandem duplication on the outcome of related and unrelated hematopoietic transplantation for adult acute myeloid leukemia in first remission: a retrospective analysis. *Journal of Clinical Oncology: Official Journal of the American Society of Clinical Oncology*. 2012;30(7):735–41.

72. Randolph SS, Gooley TA, Warren EH, Appelbaum FR, Riddell SR. Female donors contribute to a selective graft-*versus*-leukemia effect in male recipients of HLA-matched, related hematopoietic stem cell transplants. *Blood*. 2004;103(1):347–52.

73. Goldstone AH, Burnett AK, Wheatley K, Smith AG, Hutchinson RM, Clark RE, *et al*. Attempts to improve treatment outcomes in acute myeloid leukemia (AML) in older patients: the results of the United Kingdom Medical Research Council AML11 trial. *Blood*. 2001;98(5):1302–11.

74. Buyse M, Squifflet P, Lange BJ, Alonzo TA, Larson RA, Kolitz JE, *et al*. Individual patient data meta-analysis of randomized trials evaluating IL-2 monotherapy as remission maintenance therapy in acute myeloid leukemia. *Blood*. 2011;117(26):7007–13.

75. de Lima M, Giralt S, Thall PF, de Padua Silva L, Jones RB, Komanduri K, *et al*. Maintenance therapy with low-dose azacitidine after allogeneic hematopoietic stem cell transplantation for recurrent acute myelogenous leukemia or myelodysplastic syndrome: a dose and schedule finding study. *Cancer*. 2010;116(23):5420–31.

76. Platzbecker U, Wermke M, Radke J, Oelschlaegel U, Seltmann F, Kiani A, *et al*. Azacitidine for treatment of imminent relapse in MDS or AML patients after allogeneic HSCT: results of the RELAZA trial. *Leukemia*. 2012;26(3):381–9.

77. Metzelder SK, Schroeder T, Finck A, Scholl S, Fey M, Gotze K, *et al*. High activity of sorafenib in FLT3-ITD-positive acute myeloid leukemia synergizes with allo-immune effects to induce sustained responses. *Leukemia*. 2012;26(11):2353–9.

78. Keilholz U, Letsch A, Busse A, Asemissen AM, Bauer S, Blau IW, *et al*. A clinical and immunologic phase 2 trial of Wilms tumor gene product 1 (WT1) peptide vaccination in patients

with AML and MDS. *Blood*. 2009;113(26):6541–8.

79. Rezvani K, Yong AS, Mielke S, Jafarpour B, Savani BN, Le RQ, *et al.* Repeated PR1 and WT1 peptide vaccination in Montanide-adjuvant fails to induce sustained high-avidity, epitope-specific CD8+ T cells in myeloid malignancies. *Haematologica*. 2011;96(3):432–40.

80. Gale RP and Fuchs EJ. Is there really a specific graft-versus-leukaemia effect? *Bone Marrow Transplant*. 2016; Nov; 51(11):1413–15.

81. Deol A, Sengsayadeth S, Ahn KW, *et al.* Does FLT 3 mutation impact survival after hematopoietic stem cell transplantation for acute myeloid leukemia? A Center for International Blood and Marrow Transplant Research (CIBMTR) analysis. *Cancer*. 2016;122(19):3005–14.

82. Papaemmanuil E, Gerstung M, Bullinger L, *et al.* Genomic classification and prognosis in acute myeloid leukemia. *New England Journal of Medicine*. 2016;374(23):2209–21.

83. Schlenk RF, Kayser S, Bullinger L, *et al.* Differential impact of allelic ratio and insertion site in FLT3-ITD-positive AML with respect to allogeneic transplantation. *Blood*. 2014;124(23):3441–9.

84. Linch DC, Hills RK, Burnett AK, *et al.* Impact of FLT3(ITD) mutant allele level on relapse risk in intermediate-risk acute myeloid leukemia. *Blood*. 2014;124(2):273–6.

85. Krug U, Berdel WE, Gale RP. Increasing intensity of therapies assigned at diagnosis does not improve survival of adults with acute myeloid leukemia. *Leukemia*. 2016;30(6):1230–6.

86. Sanz J, Gale RP. One or two umbilical cord blood cell units? *Caveat emptor*. *Bone Marrow Transplantation*. In press.

87. Bacigalupo A, Lamparelli T, Barisione G, *et al.* Thymoglobulin prevents chronic graft-versus-host disease, chronic lung dysfunction, and late transplant-related mortality: long-term follow-up of a randomized trial in patients undergoing unrelated donor transplantation. *Biology of Blood and Marrow Transplantation: Journal of the American Society for Blood and Marrow Transplantation*. 2006;12:560–5.

88. Finke J, Bethge WA, Schmoor C, *et al.* Standard graft-versus-host disease prophylaxis with or without anti-T-cell globulin in haematopoietic cell transplantation from matched unrelated donors: a randomised, open-label, multicentre phase 3 trial. *Lancet Oncology*. 2009;10(9):855–64.

89. Kroger N, Solano C, Wolschke C, *et al.* Antilymphocyte globulin for prevention of chronic graft-versus-host-disease. *New England Journal of Medicne*. 2016;374(1):43–53. PMID: 26735993.

90. Walker I, Panzarella T, Couban S, *et al.* Pretreatment with anti-thymocyte globulin versus no anti-thymocyte globulin in patients witih haematological malignancies undergoing haemopoietic cell transplantation from unrelated donors: a randomised, controlled, open-label, phase 3, multicenter trial. *Lancet Oncology*. 2016;17:164–73.

91. Ivey A, Hills RK, Simpson MA, *et al.* Assessment of minimal residual disease in standard-risk AML. *New England Journal of Medicine*. 2016;374(5):422–33.

92. Othus M, Estey E, Gale RP. Assessment of minimal residual disease in standard-risk AML. *New England Journal of Medicine*. 2016;375(6): e9.

93. Adults with acute myeloid leukaemia or high-risk myelodysplastic syndrome (AML 19): a randomized, controlled, open label Phase III trial. Retrieved December 21, 2016, from www.isrctn.com/ISRCTN78449203.

94. Milano F, Gooley T, Wood B, *et al.* Cord-blood transplantation in patients with minimal residual disease. *New England Journal of Medicine*. 2016;375 (10):944–53.

35

Hematopoietic Cell Transplants for Myelodysplastic Syndromes

Natasha Kekre, R. Coleman Lindsley, and John Koreth

Introduction

The myelodysplastic syndromes (MDS) are a group of clonal hematopoietic stem cell disorders characterized by ineffective hematopoiesis, leading to cytopenias and an increased risk of progression to acute myelogenous leukemia (AML). It is mainly a disorder of the elderly population, with a median onset of 65 to 70 years of age. In a recent analysis by Cogle *et al.*, the annual incidence of MDS in the Medicare population was 75 per 100 000 persons, which yields 30 100 new cases in people over the age of 65[1]. The classification of MDS, as defined by the World Health Organization (WHO), is dependent on the number of peripheral blood cytopenias, blast percentage in the blood and bone marrow, and degree of dysplasia seen on bone marrow examination.

Prognostic Stratification in MDS

To create a scoring system that would better predict the overall survival (OS) and risk of transformation to AML for patients diagnosed with MDS, the International MDS Risk Analysis Workshop combined clinical, morphologic, and cytogenetic data to create the International Prognostic Scoring System (IPSS) in the 1990s[2]. This score utilizes percentage of bone marrow blasts, karyotype, and number of cytopenias to determine the risk category and therefore the estimated median overall survival for patients with MDS (Table 35.1). Another prognostic model, the WHO prognostic scoring system (WPSS), includes RBC transfusion dependency as a predictive variable[3]. The widely used IPSS was recently updated to create a revised IPSS (R-IPSS) which included the original risk factors but with more emphasis on degree of cytopenias as well as further characterization of cytogenetics[4]. In both the IPSS and R-IPSS, older age was associated with a worse survival within each risk category. Older MDS patients are also often referred for palliative therapy based partly on comorbidities and performance status, and also on provider bias. Even "fit elderly patients" may be less often referred for allogeneic hematopoietic cell transplant (HCT) due to the misconception that older age precludes HCT[5], even though with reduced intensity conditioning (RIC) regimens, this does not appear to be the case[6]. This may explain why only about 1000 HCTs are conducted per year for MDS in the United States, a small proportion of the new cases diagnosed annually[7].

Nontransplant Treatment Strategies

A discussion of the optimal HCT approach for a patient with MDS requires a clear understanding of non-HCT options. Prior to the development of disease-modifying agents in MDS, the use of hematopoietic growth factors was the mainstay of treatment to improve cytopenias. When compared with patients with a similar IPSS risk who received transfusions alone, patients who received hematopoietic growth factors incurred a survival benefit[8]. The reason for the survival advantage with this approach remains unclear, especially since the risk of progression to AML does not appear to decrease. One explanation is that this could be a reflection of less cytopenia-related consequences like cardiac events and infections and less iron overload due to the avoidance of transfusion in patients who receive hematopoietic growth factors. Unlike hematopoietic growth factors, DNA hypomethylating agents (HMA) have the ability to change the course of MDS. Both azacitidine and decitabine have been shown to be superior to best supportive care (BSC) in patients with MDS. Fenaux *et al.* showed that in patients with intermediate-2 or higher MDS by IPSS, treatment with azacitidine prolonged survival by about 10 months compared to conventional therapy that consisted mainly of best supportive care including transfusions and hematopoietic growth factors, but also included patients receiving cytarabine and induction chemotherapy[9]. Decitabine therapy, in elderly patients who would otherwise only be eligible for BSC, decreased the rate of AML transformation and prolonged progression-free survival in a sizable number of patients with MDS[10]. The addition of DNA hypomethylating agents to the repertoire of non-HCT strategies has thus given clinicians further ammunition against MDS.

The National Cancer Care Network (NCCN) guidelines include both hematopoietic growth factors and HMAs as first-line therapeutic options in patients with low- and intermediate-risk MDS[11]. Other agents recommended by the NCCN include lenalidomide, thalidomide, and immune suppressive therapy such as antithymocyte globulin and cyclosporine, in specific subsets of low- or intermediate-risk MDS. Although the NCCN comments on the early phase data regarding other agents such as anti-TNF receptor fusion

Table 35.1 Risk models in MDS

A. Original International Prognostic Scoring System (IPSS)

Score	Number of peripheral blood cytopenias[a]	Bone marrow blasts (%)	Cytogenetics[b]
0	0 or 1	<5	Good
0.5	2 or 3	5–10	Intermediate
1		–	Poor
1.5		11–20	
2		21–30	

[a] Cytopenias: neutrophils <1.5 × 10^9/L, platelets <100 × 10^9/L, hemoglobin <10 g/dL.
[b] Cytogenetics: good = normal, -Y, del(5q) only, del(20q) only; poor = complex (≥3 abnormalities), or chromosome 7 abnormalities; intermediate = all others.

Score	Risk category	Median overall survival (years)	Median time to 25% AML risk (years)
0	Low	5.7	5.7
0. -1.0	Intermediate-1	3.5	2.7
1.5-2.0	Intermediate-2	1.2	0.95
≥2.5	High	0.4	0.3

B. Revised International Prognostic Scoring System (R-IPSS)

Score	Hemoglobin (g/dL)	Platelets (× 10^9/L)	Neutrophils (× 10^9/L)	Bone marrow blasts (%)	Cytogenetics[a]
0	≥10	≥100	≥ 0.8	≤2	Very good
0.5	–	50–99	< 0.8	–	–
1	8–9.9	<50	–	2.1–4.9	Good
1.5	<8	–	–	–	–
2	–	–	–	5–10	Intermediate
3	–	–	–	>10	Poor
4	–	–	–	–	Very poor

[a] Cytogenetics: very good= -Y, del(11q); good= normal, del(5q), del(12p), del(20q), double including del(5q), intermediate = del(7q), +8, +19, i(17q), any other single or double independent clones; poor = −7, inv(3)/t(3q)/del(3q), double including −7/del(7q), complex with 3 abnormalities; very poor = complex with 3 or more abnormalities.

Score	Risk category	Median overall survival (years)	Median time to 25% AML risk (years)
≤1.5	Very low	8.8	Not reached
2.0–3.0	Low	5.3	10.8
3.5–4.5	Intermediate	3	3.2
5.0–6.0	High	1.6	1.4
>6.0	Very high	0.8	0.73

C. World Health Organization Prognostic Scoring System (WPSS)

Score	WHO category[a]	Transfusion dependence[b]	Cytogenetics[c]
0	RA, RARS, 5q-	No	Good
1	RCMD	Yes	Intermediate
2	RAEB-1	–	Poor
3	RAEB-2	–	–

[a] RA = refractory anemia; RARS=RA with ringed sideroblasts; 5q- = 5q deletion syndrome; RCMD = refractory cytopenia with multilineage dysplasia; RAEB = RA with excess blasts (5–9% in marrow is RAEB-1 and 10–19% in marrow is RAEB-2).
[b] Transfusion dependency is defined as at least one red cell transfusion every 8 weeks over a period of 4 months.
[c] Cytogenetics: good = normal, -Y, del(5q-) only, del(20q-) only; poor = complex (≥3 abnormalities), or chromosome 7 abnormalities; intermediate = all others.

Table 35.1 (cont.)

Score	Risk category	Median overall survival (years)	2-year probability of AML progression (%)
0	Very low	11.8	3
1	Low	5.5	6
2	Intermediate	4	21
3	High	2.2	38
4	Very high	0.75	80

protein and vitamin D analogs, these are not currently recommended therapies for patients with MDS.

Nontransplant Approach *versus* Allo-HCT

The non-HCT options for MDS patients range from best supportive care (BSC) to high-intensity induction chemotherapy; HCT remains the only potentially curative option. There is, however, toxicity associated with HCT which needs to be carefully evaluated *vis-à-vis* non-HCT MDS therapy. Retrospective studies indicate that HCT can be safe in MDS, with a plateau of long-term disease-free survival. Donor-*versus*-no-donor analyses have shown that HCT may provide a survival benefit in selected patients. The robustness of these analyses is limited due to selection bias inherent to retrospective studies. In an effort to improve interpretation of the retrospective literature, decision science has been used to create models to determine which patients would be appropriate for upfront HCT. As HCT outcomes improve, these models continue to be updated. Ultimately however, prospective randomized trials of HCT *versus* non-HCT therapies will be necessary.

The data above offer broad guidelines on HCT utilization, but additional questions remain. Differences in HCT conditioning regimens, for example, are an important factor to consider. This is even more relevant in a disease with an elderly predominance, in whom conditioning intensity is associated with increased morbidity and mortality. Besides the HCT conditioning regimens, there is also debate regarding both pre-and post-HCT therapies for MDS. Role of pre-and post-HCT therapies will need to incorporate recent advances in disease biology, i.e., gene mutations associated with MDS. Recurrent somatic mutations in RNA splicing mechanisms, DNA methylation pathways, multiprotein cohesin complex, and histone modification drive MDS biology and predict outcome. These mutations can identify subsets of patients who do poorly with current therapies. It also raises the question of whether current HCT methodologies can truly abrogate the negative prognostic impact of these novel MDS predictors.

The 2014 NCCN consensus guidelines recommend that if patients with low or intermediate-risk MDS fail non-HCT therapeutic approaches, then HCT should be offered to these patients[11]. They further opine that patients with higher risk MDS who are eligible for HCT and have a donor available should proceed directly to HCT. In part this is because advanced MDS has poor outcomes. In prospective trials, the survival of patients with high-risk MDS after failure of azacitidine has been reported as less than 6 months[12]. In contrast, HCT is the only potentially curative MDS therapy. In a retrospective registry analysis by the European Group for Blood and Marrow Transplantation, patients with intermediate and high-risk MDS had a disease-free survival of approximately 30% at 3 years from HCT, with a plateau in survival observable thereafter[13].

Without randomized control trials, it is still difficult to directly compare HCT and non-HCT strategies. Some would argue that a biologic randomization based on donor-*versus*-no-donor should provide the best available strategy to answer this question. Unfortunately, most donor-*versus*-no-donor analyses are currently retrospective in nature and are inherently fraught with bias as patients are not clearly randomized and followed within their initial assigned arm. Brand *et al.* nicely explain the need for clinical assumptions, which are subjective in nature, in interpreting these data[14]. In a retrospective analysis of patients undergoing allogeneic HCT if a donor was available or treatment with azacitidine if a donor was not available, although there was no significant difference in survival at 1 year, a benefit to HCT was observed at 2 years (HR=0.3; 95% CI 0.1–0.7)[15]. Despite the fact that 41% of patients in the HCT cohort received "myeloablative" conditioning (MAC) regimen, no significant difference in nonrelapse mortality (NRM) was observed between the two groups. This suggests that the concern regarding transplant-related mortality (TRM) may be diffused by longer follow-up, when a survival benefit is seen.

The first prospective trial to compare HCT to non-HCT therapy has only been presented in abstract format at the American Society of Hematology meeting in 2013[16]. Robin *et al.* examined the impact of HCT in MDS patients aged 50 to 70 with intermediate-2 or higher IPSS score, intermediate-1 with prolonged thrombocytopenia, or proliferative chronic myelomonocytic leukemia (CMML). Patients with 10% or fewer blasts in the bone marrow and an available 9 or 10 out of 10 HLA-matched donor received a RIC HCT in the donor arm. Patients with more than 10% blasts in the bone marrow or those without a donor available were analyzed in the no-donor arm. One hundred and twenty-nine patients were analyzed in the donor arm, 70.5% of whom received a HCT. There were no evident clinical or biologic differences between the donor and no-donor arms. Similar to the previous retrospective analysis, an OS benefit with HCT was only observed after 2 years of follow-up from time of HCT (HR=0.068; 95% CI 0.007–0.67). Ongoing prospective randomized analyses are currently underway in the United States and Germany that will hopefully be able to provide additional definitive data (NCT01404741 and NCT02016781).

Decision Models to Address Nontransplant *versus* Allo-HCT Approach: Do We Have an Answer?

Decision analysis can help to quantify the life expectancy benefit of HCT, and assess robustness of the findings in additional sensitivity analyses. Markov decision models have allowed researchers to combine all of the existing literature, including database, retrospective, and prospective cohorts, to help determine the optimal role and timing of HCT for MDS patients.

The decision analysis by Cutler *et al.* evaluated MAC regimen-based allo-HCT for younger MDS patients (under age 60), and demonstrated that quality-adjusted life expectancy was better with upfront HCT for younger MDS patients with higher risk IPSS score at diagnosis (intermediate-2 or higher) [17]. A more recent Markov model used a time-dependent IPSS score that could account for progression of disease in determining the optimal timing of HCT[18]. Although this model also indicated an improvement in outcomes based on upfront HCT for higher risk MDS, it additionally suggested that HCT should be performed even earlier, at progression from low-risk to intermediate-1 IPSS MDS. One criticism of these studies was that the non-HCT comparator groups received only BSC, contrary to the current treatment guidelines for patients with MDS. Another limiting factor of these studies was the younger patient age and MAC regimen, both of which are less common in MDS, which is predominantly a disease of older people. A more recent CIBMTR decision analysis for MDS patients evaluated RIC regimen-based HCT for older MDS patients (age 60–70 years), compared with NCCN-recommended non-HCT therapies based on IPSS risk (BSC and hematopoietic growth factors for lower risk MDS; HMA for higher risk MDS)[19]. This decision analysis, similar to the earlier analysis by Cutler *et al.*, found that older patients with intermediate-2 or higher IPSS score at diagnosis benefit from RIC-based HCT.

A major limitation of decision models is that they are dependent on the underlying cohort outcomes. As an understanding of MDS grows and HCT technology improves, these models may grow obsolete. For instance, none of the existing decision trees use the IPSS-Revised (IPSS-R). One study that

analyzed MDS outcomes in the Italian HCT registry demonstrated that the post-HCT survival was better predicted by the IPSS-R than the IPSS[20]. Using the R-IPSS as opposed to the IPSS changed the risk category of about 65% of patients, with the majority of patients moving to a higher risk category. This suggests that the IPSS-R might be better at discriminating high-risk patients who should be selected for allogeneic HCT.

There are also factors outside of these risk models that might influence the decision to proceed with HCT. For example, there are patients with low-risk MDS who are heavily transfusion dependent, who may benefit from earlier HCT based on quality of life and risk of clinical iron overload. Similarly, MDS patients with severe thrombocytopenia requiring platelet transfusion or neutropenia with frequent infections may derive immediate benefit from cytopenia resolution after HCT. In a decision model that used the WPSS, patients benefited from upfront HCT when there was progression from very low or low risk to intermediate risk, or if intermediate or high risk at diagnosis[18]. The WPSS further delineated a subset of patients with low-risk IPSS who would benefit from upfront HCT, namely those with multilineage dysplasia or transfusion dependency. Conversely, it also found a subset of patients with intermediate-1 IPSS who did not necessarily need upfront HCT, namely those without excess blasts or poor-risk cytogenetics. The decision models created thus far bear significant weight on the decision to transplant, but are clearly not the final answer on this decision-making process.

Allogeneic HCT for MDS

Once the decision is made to proceed with allogeneic HCT, many questions still remain unanswered but must be addressed for practical reasons. The OS of patients undergoing HCT has improved over time despite increased employment of unrelated and cord blood transplants as well as a higher median age of HCT recipients[21]. Importantly, even in patients over the age of 70, allogeneic HCT can be effective [6], and has been deemed safe to perform[22]. The predominance of MDS in elderly patients therefore makes the approach to HCT in these patients an important discussion.

The RIC regimens generally report lower upfront TRM when compared with MAC regimens, but also higher rates of relapse (see Chapter 27). In patients with AML or MDS OS is not significantly different between MAC and RIC regimens, but is lower with non-MAC regimens[23,24]. One study that examined the impact of busulfan dosing in RIC regimens found that perhaps there was a marginal benefit to a higher dose of busulfan in patients with a high risk of clinical relapse after HCT[25]. A randomized controlled trial comparing conditioning intensities in AML and MDS was recently halted early by the Data Safety and Monitoring Board (DSMB), but the results hopefully will better address this important question (NCT01339910).

In addition to conditioning intensity, the use of *in-vivo* T-cell depletion (see Chapter 29), such as antithymocyte globulin (ATG) for graft-*versus*-host disease (GvHD) prophylaxis is controversial. In a CIBMTR analysis, Soiffer *et al.* examined patients with hematologic malignancies who underwent RIC-based HCT with or without *in-vivo* (ATG) T-cell depletion (TCD)[26]. They observed increased relapse and decreased survival with ATG-based TCD. The use of *in-vivo* TCD therefore remains a contentious issue in patients undergoing RIC HCT. In the context of MAC regimen, Finke *et al.* showed that the addition of novel *Fresenius* ATG (F-ATG) to cyclosporine and methotrexate could reduce acute GvHD rates without impacting relapse or survival outcomes[27]. The impact of F-ATG remains to be assessed in RIC-based HCT.

Allogeneic HCT technology continues to evolve, including the broadening of donor choices. Generally with an older MDS patient population comes an older sibling. It has been suggested that survival post-HCT may be better with younger HLA-matched unrelated donors than with older matched siblings in MDS, but this observation needs further verification [28]. Advances in HCT have also allowed for the use of alternative donors, namely HLA-mismatched unrelated, haplotype mismatch, and cord blood transplants to increase the availability of HCT to patients without a suitably HLA-matched donor. It is however still too early to routinely recommend alternative donor HCT for patients with MDS lacking HLA-matched donors. The OS outcomes with alternative donors continue to be inferior to HLA-matched related and unrelated donors. The overall mortality from a 7 out of 8 HLA allele HLA-matched unrelated donor has been shown to be higher than HLA-matched sibling and 8 out of 8 HLA-matched unrelated donors for patients with MDS (RR=1.30; 95% CI 1.01–1.68)[29].

Pretransplant Therapeutic Options

In accordance with the decision models previously described, the NCCN guidelines recommend upfront HCT for patients with higher risk MDS[11]. In aggressive diseases like acute leukemia, it is clear that chemotherapy responsive disease and a low disease burden at HCT are more likely to benefit than those with disease that is refractory to conventional therapy. It is unknown, however, if in MDS, HCT recipients with lower disease burden (e.g., low percentage of bone marrow blasts) will similarly do better. From the general principle however, it would be reasonable to consider reducing the burden of MDS with HMA therapy prior to HCT. This remains an ongoing area of interest but its benefit remains to be shown in a prospective fashion.

In a recent retrospective analysis that compared HCT outcomes in patients with MDS who received HMA therapy prior to HCT *versus* those who did not, there was no difference in survival in those receiving HMA therapy[30]. Although a small early phase study, this does suggest that there is at the very least no increased toxicity from HMA therapy as a bridge to HCT. In fact, this study suggests that patients with a bone marrow blast count over 5% who received HMA treatment had lower nonrelapse mortality than those who did not receive pre-HCT therapy. In a larger cohort of 265 patients, of which 58% were intermediate-2 or higher by IPSS score, there was no difference in 3-year overall or disease-free survival in patients who received azacitidine, induction chemotherapy, or combination therapy with azacitidine and chemotherapy prior to HCT[31]. The majority of patients in this study received a RIC regimen. Although not statistically significant, there was a trend toward better survival in patients who received azacitidine alone than in those who received chemotherapy alone or combination therapy (3-year overall survival 55%, 48%, and 32% respectively, $P = 0.07$). This benefit with HMA therapy compared with chemotherapy prior to HCT has been even more evident in patients receiving myeloablative conditioning[32]. Not surprisingly, these studies suggest that if trying to reduce disease burden prior to HCT, the best approach is likely HMA therapy as it is better tolerated when compared to higher intensity chemotherapy.

Post-Transplant Therapeutic Options to Prevent Morphologic Relapse: Is There a Standard?

Post-transplantation MDS relapse remains a major concern [20]. The OS in patients who relapse after HCT has been reported to be around 6 months[33]. There is an interest in post-HCT strategies to reduce MDS relapse after HCT (see Chapters 23 and 65). Immune suppression withdrawal as well as donor lymphocyte infusion (DLI) are modalities to enhance the graft-*versus*-leukemia (GvL) effect of HCT, usually in an effort to treat disease relapse. Azacitidine in combination with DLI has resulted in durable remissions as a rescue therapy for relapsed MDS after HCT[34]. There are now ongoing efforts to prevent morphologic relapse by adding preemptive MDS therapy based on minimal residual disease assessment or using it as routine maintenance therapy after HCT.

Minimal residual disease (see Chapter 24) can be difficult to measure in MDS as there are not always clear FISH or flow cytometry markers for early disease relapse. Instead, falling donor chimerism can be used as a surrogate for early relapse. This preemptive strategy was attempted by Platzbecker *et al.* in an effort to prevent morphologic relapse in patients with a CD34-specific donor chimerism that fell below 80%[35]. Twenty patients were treated with azacitidine for up to four cycles for falling chimerism. Half of the patients had recovery of chimerism and no relapse. Eventually, 65% of patients experienced relapse, but treatment with azacitidine was thought to delay this (median time to relapse was 231 days). Although preemptive azacitidine had acceptable toxicity in this study, it is difficult to know if it improved relapse rates given the lack of a control arm. In the patients with recovery of chimerism and no relapse, it is unclear if these patients would have ever relapsed regardless of intervention. In addition, relapse was still very prevalent in this study, arguing against any benefit to this preemptive strategy.

Another approach that has been adopted in clinic is maintenance therapy after HCT. The ideal maintenance drug would be one that has minimal toxicity as this would need to be given soon after HCT, a time in which patients are vulnerable to HCT-related complications. The drug would need to be effective against the disease, but not impair the graft-*versus*-tumor effect that is anticipated with HCT. Azacitidine has been a potential maintenance strategy that remains in study at present. In a dose and schedule finding study, toxicity with azacitidine after HCT resulted in an acceptable toxicity profile, with reversible thrombocytopenia being the dose-limiting factor [36]. In fact, it has been suggested that azacitidine may enhance the graft-*versus*-tumor effect of HCT by inducing a cytotoxic T-cell response to tumor antigens, while decreasing the rate of GvHD by increasing T-regulatory cells which establish tolerance to the graft after HCT[37].

More novel strategies to improve relapse rates after HCT consist of immune manipulation, namely a vaccine strategy. In this approach, the beneficial graft-*versus*-tumor response that is afforded by HCT is amplified by immunization with irradiated, autologous GM-CSF secreting blast cells early after HCT. Reactions similar to those seen in vaccine trials for non-HCT solid tumor patients were observed post-HCT[38]. This phase 1 study identified leukemia cell vaccine post-HCT to be safe and suggested long-term remission in some patients. Larger randomized trials are needed to test for possible improvement in MDS relapse rates with post-HCT strategies. Currently, there is no standard to prevent morphologic relapse after allogeneic HCT due to lack of randomized controlled trials.

Genetic Alterations in MDS: Changing the Paradigm of Transplantation

Recent studies have characterized the landscape of recurrent somatic point mutations in MDS in large, heterogeneous cohorts[39,40]. Common recurrent mutations affect genes involved in a broad range of core biologic processes, such as RNA splicing (*SF3B1*, *SRSF2*, *U2AF1*, *ZRSR2*), epigenome regulation via DNA methylation (*TET2*, *DNMT3A*) or histone modification (*EZH2*, *ASXL*), transcriptional regulation (*RUNX1*, *GATA2*, *CEBPA*), chromatin cohesion (*STAG2*), cellular signaling (*NRAS*, *KRAS*, *CBL*, *PTPN11*), DNA damage response (*TP53*), and others (*BCOR*, *SETBP1*). At least one somatic mutation can be identified in 80–90% of MDS cases, with most cases having multiple mutations in distinct pathways. Importantly, many studies have identified close associations between specific mutations and distinct clinicopathologic phenotypes. For example, mutations in *SF3B1* are associated with the presence of ring sideroblasts and mutations in *SRSF2*, *TET2*, and *ASXL1* are enriched in diseases with marked myelomonocytic differentiation.

In addition to the gross chromosomal alterations already integrated into current risk models, recent studies have revealed a central role for specific point mutations in driving clinical MDS outcomes. For example, in a study that analyzed over 400 bone marrow samples from patients with MDS, a multivariate Cox regression model identified five molecular abnormalities that retained independent prognostic significance: *TP53* (HR for death from any cause, 2.48; 95% CI 1.60–3.84), *EZH2* (HR=2.13; 95% CI 1.36–3.33), *ETV6* (HR=2.04; 95% CI 1.08–3.86), *RUNX1* (HR 1.47; 95% CI 1.01–2.15), and *ASXL1* (HR= 1.38; 95% CI 1.00–1.89)[41]. The presence of one of these prognostic mutations enabled further prognostic stratification beyond conventional variables. In a different study that focused on patients with lower risk MDS, it was demonstrated that those who have an *EZH2* mutation may actually have a poorer OS (HR=2.90; 95% CI 1.85–4.52)[42]. These studies suggest that inclusion of molecular genetic variables into future risk models may more accurately stratify MDS patients into clinically conforming subgroups.

Molecular aberrations observed in MDS have yet to be incorporated formally into MDS classification schema or consensus treatment recommendations. In part, this is due to the interpretive challenges associated with clinical sequencing data. For example, mutation allele fraction provides information about the proportion of hematopoietic cells that harbor a specific alteration. When a mutation initiates development of a clonal myeloid disease, it is present in all neoplastic cells and is typically detectable at a high allele fraction. However, through genetic diversification and selection, MDS can acquire additional mutations and undergo a process of clonal evolution [43]. By definition, disease cure is only attainable through eradication of the founder clone and all subclones, although subclonally directed therapies may be of limited utility. Subclonal mutations that are observed at a low allele fraction could still be clinically relevant since they may mediate relapse, progression of disease, or symptomatic cytopenias (Figure 35.1). The relative prognostic value of co-occurring mutations present at disparate allele fractions is likely context-dependent and remains to be systematically studied.

An increasingly refined understanding of MDS genetics may be of particularly high significance to clinical HCT by identifying novel, molecularly defined subgroups that benefit

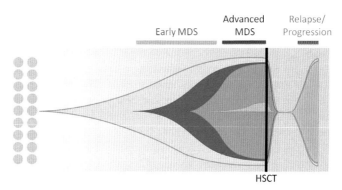

Figure 35.1 Clonal evolution of MDS.

from HCT. In a single-institution study, Bejar *et al.* demonstrated that regardless of IPSS-R or cytogenetics, MDS patients with *TP53*, *DNMT3A*, or *TET2* mutations had markedly worse post-HCT survival and relapse outcomes than patients without these mutations[44]. Another independent predictor of poor outcomes with HCT has been monosomal karyotype. In one study that analyzed over 1000 patients with MDS who underwent HCT, the presence of a monosomal karyotype increased the rates of relapse and mortality even after assessing for IPSS and 5-group cytogenetic risk profile[45]. In an Italian registry study of 519 allografted MDS patients, those with monosomal karyotype had a 5-year OS of only 10% and a cumulative incidence of relapse of 49%, significantly worse than those without monosomal karyotype[20].

Although the traditional approach has been to offer upfront HCT for hematologic malignancies with poor prognosis, it remains to be determined whether conventional HCT strategies offer a survival benefit for MDS patients with high-risk mutations. Indeed, patients with *TP53* mutations for instance may require alternative therapies to improve outcomes with or without HCT. Identification of these disease-driving genetic alterations may additionally define novel therapeutic vulnerabilities that could be targeted by new treatment approaches. With continued biologic investigation and drug development, application of novel therapeutics to pre-HCT strategies to reduce disease burden or post-HCT strategies to prevent relapse may transform our approach to HCT in MDS.

Practice Points

The MDS represent a disease spectrum ranging from patients with low disease burden requiring occasional transfusions to advanced disease with survival worse than *de novo* AML. The currently prevalent risk models, namely the IPSS and R-IPSS, often dictate the approach to treatment for MDS patients. Intermediate- to high-risk IPSS patients are generally offered early HCT, largely based on decision models utilizing cohort data to determine quality-adjusted life expectancy benefit, with emerging prospective randomized trial data supporting this consensus. There remains controversy over how to perform HCT in these patients, including conditioning regimen intensity, the use of alternative donors, and whether *in-vivo* T-cell depletion is needed, continue to be issues that are debated. Generally, HCT is from a matched adult related or unrelated donor, and most commonly with a RIC regimen for older patients, and MAC regimens for younger MDS patients.

In the era of DNA hypomethylating agents as well as newer experimental drugs and combination therapies that are entering clinical trials at present, it is unclear how to intercalate these strategies with a curative HCT approach. Patients who fail these therapies should be offered HCT. In patients offered upfront HCT, there is no good evidence to routinely recommend pre-HCT therapy to reduce the burden of disease prior to HCT, but in practical terms, it is often utilized to control disease while a donor search is undertaken, with data suggesting that

azacitidine use in this context does not impair HCT outcomes. The current standard of care remains to use HCT for higher risk disease and to consider a DNA HMA as a bridge to HCT. For the near future, incorporating data on MDS mutations into treatment decision-making will be a major focus.

There is not yet clear evidence of benefit to post-HCT interventions to prevent relapse. However, it is uncertain if HCT alone can abrogate the negative impact of high-risk mutations, such as *TP53*-mutated MDS, for example. Trials of novel post-HCT interventions targeted at patients with a particularly high risk of relapse after HCT will be a clinical priority in the future. For now, it is important to remember that the morbidity and mortality associated with HCT means that this decision needs to be tailored to the individual patient. Nevertheless, potentially curative HCT should not be excluded based merely on older patient age or provider bias. Early referral for HCT, a comprehensive assessment of disease, patient and donor factors, and a collaborative discussion of HCT risks and benefits offer the potential to improve outcomes in MDS patients even today.

Controversies in Allo-HCT for MDS

Controversy #1: When to Transplant: Is There a Role for Allo-HCT Earlier in MDS (e.g., low-/int-1 IPSS)?

Proponents: MDS is a neoplastic bone marrow disorder that impairs patient survival even in lower risk disease (low- and int-1 IPSS MDS), and with propensity to progress to higher risk disease (int-2 and high-risk MDS) and secondary AML. Allo-HCT is the only curative modality, but the therapeutic GvL effect is limited, and relapse remains a major risk after transplantation in higher risk MDS. Conceptually, deploying allo-HCT earlier in MDS may enhance cure rates, providing treatment toxicity can be controlled. Empirically, there are also data from a decision model to support allo-HCT in lower risk MDS.

Opponents: Allo-HCT can be curative in MDS, but also has significant upfront toxicities (e.g., GvHD, infection) with impaired quality of life. Evidence of improved cure rates with early allo-HCT in MDS is controversial at best, albeit based on a limited sampling that is prone to selection bias. Nonetheless, most decision analyses do not support early allo-HCT in lower risk MDS, suggesting that close monitoring for MDS progression is the preferred approach in such cases.

Our take: In our opinion, IPSS-based models do not fully capture MDS risk, and recently described genomic mutations represent powerful and independent drivers of MDS biology and outcomes. MDS patients with poor-risk mutations (e.g. *DNMT3A*, *ASXL1*) and worse anticipated outcomes could be considered for transplantation earlier in their disease course. Systematically capturing allo-HCT outcomes of such patients will be vital to determine whether or not transplantation can improve their survival.

Controversy #2: Whom to Transplant: Is There a Role for Allo-HCT in Very-High-Risk MDS (e.g., Monosomal Karyotype, *TP53* Mutation)?

Proponents: The presence of very-high-risk mutations (e.g., MK+, *TP53* mutation) predicts impaired MDS outcomes and poor survival with nontransplantation therapies. However, after allo-HCT, some patients, even those with very-high-risk MDS mutations, enjoy extended survivals and appear to be cured. Further, as discussed above, there is a rationale for deploying allo-HCT earlier in the disease course (e.g., low/int-1 IPSS MDS) in such patients, reduce early relapse risk, and maximize time for GvL effect.

Opponents: Allo-HCT does not appear to abrogate the negative survival impact of very-poor-risk MDS mutations described above. Such patients are unlikely to benefit from transplantation, but are equally if not more likely, to experience treatment toxicity. Therefore, such patients could be excluded from allo-HCT on the basis of its lack of efficacy.

Our take: We recognize impaired outcomes associated with very-poor-risk MDS mutations that appear to be incompletely ameliorated by allo-HCT, although these data are currently limited. We also recognize that reduced intensity conditioning (RIC) allo-HCT is commonly utilized in MDS that is critically dependent on a timely GvL effect, due to limited tumor debulking from conditioning chemotherapy. Deploying allo-HCT later in the MDS course (int-2, high-risk IPSS), when blast counts are often higher, may also not be optimal. Outside of a clinical trial, we therefore favor attempting early intervention (e.g., low/int-1 IPSS MDS) with higher intensity conditioning (e.g., near-ablative or myeloablative reduced toxicity conditioning regimens). It remains to be determined, however, whether such enhanced allo-HCT maneuvers actually improve outcomes.

References

1. Cogle CR, Craig BM, Rollison DE, List AF. Incidence of the myelodysplastic syndromes using a novel claims-based algorithm: high number of uncaptured cases by cancer registries. *Blood.* 2011;117(26):7121–5.

2. Greenberg P, Cox C, LeBeau MM, Fenaux P, Morel P, Sanz G, et al. International scoring system for evaluating prognosis in myelodysplastic syndromes. *Blood.* 1997;89(6):2079–88.

3. Malcovati L, Germing U, Kuendgen A, Della Porta MG, Pascutto C, Invernizzi R, et al. Time-dependent prognostic scoring system for predicting survival and leukemic evolution in myelodysplastic syndromes. *Journal of Clinical Oncology: Official Journal of the American Society of Clinical Oncology.* 2007;25(23):3503–10.

4. Greenberg PL, Tuechler H, Schanz J, Sanz G, Garcia-Manero G, Sole F, et al. Revised international prognostic scoring system for myelodysplastic syndromes. *Blood.* 2012;120(12):2454–65.

5. Estey E, de Lima M, Tibes R, Pierce S, Kantarjian H, Champlin R, et al. Prospective feasibility analysis of reduced-intensity conditioning (RIC) regimens for hematopoietic stem cell transplantation (HCT) in elderly patients with acute myeloid leukemia (AML) and high-risk myelodysplastic syndrome (MDS). *Blood.* 2007;109(4):1395–400.

6. McClune BL, Weisdorf DJ, Pedersen TL, Tunes da Silva G, Tallman MS, Sierra J, et al. Effect of age on outcome of reduced-intensity hematopoietic cell transplantation for older patients with acute myeloid leukemia in first complete remission or with myelodysplastic syndrome. *Journal of Clinical Oncology: Official Journal of the American Society of Clinical Oncology.* 2010;28(11):1878–87.

7. Pasquini MC, Wang Z. Current use and outcome of hematopoietic stem cell transplantation: CIBMTR Summary Slides. Updated 2013. Available from: www.cibmtr.org.

8. Park S, Grabar S, Kelaidi C, Beyne-Rauzy O, Picard F, Bardet V, et al. Predictive factors of response and survival in myelodysplastic syndrome treated with erythropoietin and G-CSF: the GFM experience. *Blood.* 2008;111(2):574–82.

9. Fenaux P, Mufti GJ, Hellstrom-Lindberg E, Santini V, Finelli C, Giagounidis A, et al. Efficacy of azacitidine compared with that of conventional care regimens in the treatment of higher-risk myelodysplastic syndromes: a randomised, open-label, phase III study. *The Lancet Oncology.* 2009;10(3):223–32.

10. Lubbert M, Suciu S, Baila L, Ruter BH, Platzbecker U, Giagounidis A, et al. Low-dose decitabine *versus* best supportive care in elderly patients with intermediate- or high-risk myelodysplastic syndrome (MDS) ineligible for intensive chemotherapy: final results of the randomized phase III study of the European Organisation for Research and Treatment of Cancer Leukemia Group and the German MDS Study Group. *Journal of Clinical Oncology: Official Journal of the American Society of Clinical Oncology.* 2011;29(15):1987–96.

11. Greenberg PL, Attar E, Bennett JM, Bloomfield CD, De Castro CM, Deeg HJ, et al. NCCN Clinical Practice Guidelines in Oncology: myelodysplastic syndromes. *Journal of the National Comprehensive Cancer Network: JNCCN.* 2011;9(1):30–56.

12. Prebet T, Gore SD, Esterni B, Gardin C, Itzykson R, Thepot S, et al. Outcome of high-risk myelodysplastic syndrome after azacitidine treatment failure. *Journal of Clinical Oncology: Official Journal of the American Society of Clinical Oncology.* 2011;29(24):3322–7.

13. de Witte T, Hermans J, Vossen J, Bacigalupo A, Meloni G, Jacobsen N, et al. Haematopoietic stem cell transplantation for patients with myelo-dysplastic syndromes and secondary acute myeloid leukaemias: a report on behalf of the Chronic Leukaemia Working Party of the European Group for Blood and Marrow Transplantation (EBMT). *British Journal of Haematology.* 2000;110(3):620–30.

14. Brand R, Putter H, van Biezen A, Niederwieser D, Martino R, Mufti G, et al.

Comparison of allogeneic stem cell transplantation and non-transplant approaches in elderly patients with advanced myelodysplastic syndrome: optimal statistical approaches and a critical appraisal of clinical results using non-randomized data. *PLoS One.* 2013;8(10):e74368.

15. Platzbecker U, Schetelig J, Finke J, Trenschel R, Scott BL, Kobbe G, et al. Allogeneic hematopoietic cell transplantation in patients age 60-70 years with de novo high-risk myelodysplastic syndrome or secondary acute myelogenous leukemia: comparison with patients lacking donors who received azacitidine. *Biology of Blood and Marrow Transplantation: Journal of the American Society for Blood and Marrow Transplantation.* 2012;18(9):1415–21.

16. Robin M, Porcher R, Ades L, Raffoux E, Michallet M, Francois S, et al. Outcome of patients with IPSS intermediate (int) or high risk myelodysplastic syndrome (MDS) according to donor availability: a multicenter prospective non interventional study for the SFGM-TC and GFM. *Blood.* 2013;122(301).

17. Cutler CS, Lee SJ, Greenberg P, Deeg HJ, Perez WS, Anasetti C, et al. A decision analysis of allogeneic bone marrow transplantation for the myelodysplastic syndromes: delayed transplantation for low-risk myelodysplasia is associated with improved outcome. *Blood.* 2004;104(2):579–85.

18. Alessandrino EP, Porta MG, Malcovati L, Jackson CH, Pascutto C, Bacigalupo A, et al. Optimal timing of allogeneic hematopoietic stem cell transplantation in patients with myelodysplastic syndrome. *American Journal of Hematology.* 2013;88(7):581–8.

19. Koreth J, Pidala J, Perez WS, Deeg HJ, Garcia-Manero G, Malcovati L, et al. Role of reduced-intensity conditioning allogeneic hematopoietic stem-cell transplantation in older patients with de novo myelodysplastic syndromes: an international collaborative decision analysis. *Journal of Clinical Oncology: Official Journal of the American Society of Clinical Oncology.* 2013;31(21):2662–70.

20. Della Porta MG, Alessandrino EP, Bacigalupo A, van Lint MT, Malcovati L, Pascutto C, et al. Predictive factors for the outcome of allogeneic transplantation in patients with MDS stratified according to the revised IPSS-R. *Blood.* 2014;123(15):2333–42.

21. Hahn T, McCarthy PL, Jr., Hassebroek A, Bredeson C, Gajewski JL, Hale GA, et al. Significant improvement in survival after allogeneic hematopoietic cell transplantation during a period of significantly increased use, older recipient age, and use of unrelated donors. *Journal of Clinical Oncology: Official Journal of the American Society of Clinical Oncology.* 2013;31(19):2437–49.

22. Brunner AM, Kim HT, Coughlin E, Alyea EP, 3rd, Armand P, Ballen KK, et al. Outcomes in patients age 70 or older undergoing allogeneic hematopoietic stem cell transplantation for hematologic malignancies. *Biology of Blood and Marrow Transplantation: Journal of the American Society for Blood and Marrow Transplantation.* 2013;19(9):1374–80.

23. Luger SM, Ringden O, Zhang MJ, Perez WS, Bishop MR, Bornhauser M, et al. Similar outcomes using myeloablative vs reduced-intensity allogeneic transplant preparative regimens for AML or MDS. *Bone Marrow Transplantation.* 2012;47(2):203–11.

24. Martino R, de Wreede L, Fiocco M, van Biezen A, von dem Borne PA, Hamladji RM, et al. Comparison of conditioning regimens of various intensities for allogeneic hematopoietic SCT using HLA-identical sibling donors in AML and MDS with <10% BM blasts: a report from EBMT. *Bone Marrow Transplantation.* 2013;48(6):761–70.

25. Chen YB, Coughlin E, Kennedy KF, Alyea EP, Armand P, Attar EC, et al. Busulfan dose intensity and outcomes in reduced-intensity allogeneic peripheral blood stem cell transplantation for myelodysplastic syndrome or acute myeloid leukemia. *Biology of Blood and Marrow Transplantation: Journal of the American Society for Blood and Marrow Transplantation.* 2013;19(6):981–7.

26. Soiffer RJ, Lerademacher J, Ho V, Kan F, Artz A, Champlin RE, et al. Impact of immune modulation with anti-T-cell antibodies on the outcome of reduced-intensity allogeneic hematopoietic stem cell transplantation for hematologic malignancies. *Blood.* 2011;117(25):6963–70.

27. Finke J, Bethge WA, Schmoor C, Ottinger HD, Stelljes M, Zander AR, et al. Standard graft-*versus*-host disease prophylaxis with or without anti-T-cell globulin in haematopoietic cell transplantation from matched unrelated donors: a randomised, open-label, multicentre phase 3 trial. *The Lancet Oncology.* 2009;10(9):855–64.

28. Kroger N, Zabelina T, de Wreede L, Berger J, Alchalby H, van Biezen A, et al. Allogeneic stem cell transplantation for older advanced MDS patients: improved survival with young unrelated donor in comparison with HLA-identical siblings. *Leukemia.* 2013;27(3):604–9.

29. Saber W, Cutler CS, Nakamura R, Zhang MJ, Atallah E, Rizzo JD, et al. Impact of donor source on hematopoietic cell transplantation outcomes for patients with myelodysplastic syndromes (MDS). *Blood.* 2013;122(11):1974–82.

30. Kim Y, Kim IH, Kim HJ, Park S, Lee KH, Kim SJ, et al. Multicenter study evaluating the impact of hypomethylating agents as bridging therapy to hematopoietic stem cell transplantation in myelodysplastic syndromes. *International Journal of Hematology.* 2014;99(5):635–43.

31. Damaj G, Duhamel A, Robin M, Beguin Y, Michallet M, Mohty M, et al. Impact of azacitidine before allogeneic stem-cell transplantation for myelodysplastic syndromes: a study by the Societe Francaise de Greffe de Moelle et de Therapie-Cellulaire and the Groupe-Francophone des Myelodysplasies. *Journal of Clinical Oncology: Official Journal of the American Society of Clinical Oncology.* 2012;30(36):4533–40.

32. Gerds AT, Gooley TA, Estey EH, Appelbaum FR, Deeg HJ, Scott BL. Pretransplantation therapy with azacitidine vs induction chemotherapy and post-transplantation outcome in patients with MDS. *Biology of Blood and Marrow Transplantation: Journal of the American Society for Blood and Marrow Transplantation.* 2012;18(8):1211–8.

33. Pollyea DA, Artz AS, Stock W, Daugherty C, Godley L, Odenike OM, et al. Outcomes of patients with AML and MDS who relapse or progress after reduced intensity allogeneic hematopoietic cell transplantation. *Bone Marrow Transplantation.* 2007;40(11):1027–32.

34. Schroeder T, Czibere A, Platzbecker U, Bug G, Uharek L, Luft T, et al. Azacitidine and donor lymphocyte infusions as first salvage therapy for relapse of AML or MDS after allogeneic stem cell transplantation. *Leukemia*. 2013;27(6):1229–35.

35. Platzbecker U, Wermke M, Radke J, Oelschlaegel U, Seltmann F, Kiani A, et al. Azacitidine for treatment of imminent relapse in MDS or AML patients after allogeneic HCT: results of the RELAZA trial. *Leukemia*. 2012;26(3):381–9.

36. de Lima M, Giralt S, Thall PF, de Padua Silva L, Jones RB, Komanduri K, et al. Maintenance therapy with low-dose azacitidine after allogeneic hematopoietic stem cell transplantation for recurrent acute myelogenous leukemia or myelodysplastic syndrome: a dose and schedule finding study. *Cancer*. 2010;116(23):5420–31.

37. Goodyear OC, Dennis M, Jilani NY, Loke J, Siddique S, Ryan G, et al. Azacitidine augments expansion of regulatory T cells after allogeneic stem cell transplantation in patients with acute myeloid leukemia (AML). *Blood*. 2012;119(14):3361–9.

38. Ho VT, Vanneman M, Kim H, Sasada T, Kang YJ, Pasek M, et al. Biologic activity of irradiated, autologous, GM-CSF-secreting leukemia cell vaccines early after allogeneic stem cell transplantation. *Proceedings of the National Academy of Sciences of the United States of America*. 2009;106(37):15825–30.

39. Haferlach T, Nagata Y, Grossmann V, Okuno Y, Bacher U, Nagae G, et al. Landscape of genetic lesions in 944 patients with myelodysplastic syndromes. *Leukemia*. 2014;28(2):241–7.

40. Papaemmanuil E, Gerstung M, Malcovati L, Tauro S, Gundem G, Van Loo P, et al. Clinical and biological implications of driver mutations in myelodysplastic syndromes. *Blood*. 2013;122(22):3616–27; quiz 99.

41. Bejar R, Stevenson K, Abdel-Wahab O, Galili N, Nilsson B, Garcia-Manero G, et al. Clinical effect of point mutations in myelodysplastic syndromes. *The New England Journal of Medicine*. 2011;364(26):2496–506.

42. Bejar R, Stevenson KE, Caughey BA, Abdel-Wahab O, Steensma DP, Galili N, et al. Validation of a prognostic model and the impact of mutations in patients with lower-risk myelodysplastic syndromes. *Journal of Clinical Oncology: Official Journal of the American Society of Clinical Oncology*. 2012;30(27):3376–82.

43. Bejar R. Prognostic models in myelodysplastic syndromes. *Hematology/the Education Program of the American Society of Hematology American Society of Hematology Education Program*. 2013;2013:504–10.

44. Bejar R, Stevenson KE, Caughey B, Lindsley RC, Mar BG, Stojanov P, et al. Somatic mutations predict poor outcome in patients with myelodysplastic syndrome after hematopoietic stem-cell transplantation. *Journal of Clinical Oncology: Official Journal of the American Society of Clinical Oncology*. 2014;32(25):2691–8.

45. Deeg HJ, Scott BL, Fang M, Shulman HM, Gyurkocza B, Myerson D, et al. Five-group cytogenetic risk classification, monosomal karyotype, and outcome after hematopoietic cell transplantation for MDS or acute leukemia evolving from MDS. *Blood*. 2012;120(7):1398–408.

Hematopoietic Cell Transplants for Chronic Myeloid Leukemia: Still a Role for Allogeneic Transplant?

Andrew J. Innes and Jane F. Apperley

Introduction

The role of allogeneic haematopoietic cell transplantation (HCT) was established more than 30 years ago following the observation that transplantation from a syngeneic donor was capable of eradicating Philadelphia-positive cells responsible for chronic myeloid leukemia (CML)[1]. Subsequent data demonstrating HLA-matched sibling donor HCT as an effective treatment for CML rapidly established this as the standard of care for eligible patients through the 1980s and 1990s[2]. The use of HLA-matched volunteer unrelated donors (VUD), in order to improve accessibility to HCT for those without an HLA-matched sibling, was initially hampered by high transplant-related mortality (TRM)[3]. Gradually, with improved conditioning regimens, better supportive care, and the introduction of T-cell depletion (TCD), the outcome for VUD-HCT improved and now rivals that of sibling HCT[4]. Understanding that the graft-*versus* leukemic effect is the cornerstone of cure in CML[5,6,7] led to the development of reduced intensity conditioning regimens (RIC)[8,9], often with early preemptive donor lymphocyte infusions (DLI)[10]. While this improved accessibility to HCT for those who would have been deemed unfit for conventional myeloablative conditioning (MAC) regimens, the necessity for heavy TCD resulted in high post-transplant relapse rates[9] and their use remains controversial.

The pioneering work in HCT for CML formed the basis upon which much of current transplant practice across all hematological malignancies is based. However, the advent of the tyrosine kinase inhibitors (TKIs) has completely revolutionized the management of CML[11]. Despite their success, TKIs are neither universally effective nor tolerable, and there remains a group for whom HCT offers a feasible alternative. This review will focus on the role of HCT for CML in the 21st century, with particular attention paid to indications for transplant, transplant outcome, and some of the most controversial issues in current practice.

Frontline Therapy for Newly Diagnosed CML Patients: Is Cure Possible?

CML is a triphasic disease characterized by a natural history of a chronic phase (CP) which may last many years before ultimately progressing to accelerated (AP) and blast phase (BP) which, left untreated, is universally fatal. Early treatment strategies including arsenic, busulfan, splenic irradiation, or hydroxycarbamide controlled the symptoms of the disease but did little to alter its natural course[12]. HCT was the first and remains the only treatment capable of curing CML. However, the TKIs, while also providing symptom control have had a significant impact on survival, particularly in CP which accounts for the majority of new presentations. Eight-year follow-up data from the seminal International Randomized Study of Interferon and STI571 (IRIS) show an estimated 8-year overall survival (OS) of 85% with 92% estimated freedom from progression to AP/BP and two separate studies have now shown that life expectancy of CML patients in the TKI era is essentially indistinguishable from normal controls [13,14,15]. It is this success that has secured the position of the TKIs as first-line agents of choice in a newly presenting CP patient with CML.

Since the introduction of the TKIs, the European Leukemia Net (ELN) has established criteria for assessing response and predicting long-term outcome[16]. These definitions establish response in three categories, haematologic, cytogenetic, and molecular, and require that complete hematologic response (CHR), complete cytogenetic response (CCyR), and major molecular response (MMR) be achieved within defined timescales. Achieving the required responses in a timely fashion identifies optimal responders, while slow or absent response identifies 'warning' and 'failure' groups in whom alternative treatments should be considered. The most recent guideline incorporates the findings by several groups that failure to achieve a 10-fold reduction in BCR-ABL1 transcripts by 3 months, defined by a real-time quantitative reverse transcription polymerase chain reaction (RQ-PCR) of less than 10% on the international scale, is associated with a relatively poor outcome[17–19]. The addition of this assessment at an early time point serves to give early warning of patients likely to fare poorly, and for whom HCT should be considered and discussed early in their treatment course.

Second-generation TKIs (2GTKI) appear even more effective than imatinib in frontline therapy. Dasatinib and Nilotinib achieve MMRs at 4 years of 76% and 73–76% respectively compared to 63% and 56% for imatinib in the respective

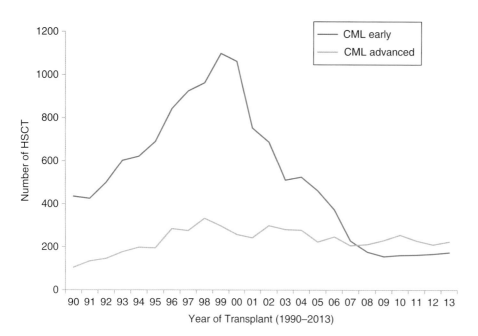

Figure 36.1 Number of allogeneic HCT by year from 1990 to 2013 from the EBMT Transplant Registry. Courtesy of Helen Baldomero, EBMT Transplant Activity Survey Office.

trials[20,21]. Bosutinib has also been used in first-line setting and again appears to show superiority to imatinib with early follow-up data reporting MMR of 59% *versus* 49% at 24 months[22]. Because of the excellent response and survival rates of those treated with TKIs, it is unsurprising that the goal of curing CML with HCT has now been replaced with that of achieving a deep and durable remission with an oral therapy. Most recently considerable attention has been focused on the ability to discontinue imatinib in a relatively small proportion of patients who achieved sustained RQ-PCR negativity. A few studies, in which imatinib was discontinued in patients who had been RQ-PCR-negative for at least 2 years, showed that 40% could remain off treatment indefinitely[23,24] providing close molecular monitoring is maintained. Further analysis from one of these groups suggests that approximately one-third of patients treated with imatinib from diagnosis will achieve sufficiently deep molecular responses to become eligible for a trial of stopping therapy [24]. If 40% of these patients maintain molecular remission without TKI, in essence, this means that overall perhaps as many as 15% of patients will experience an "operational cure"[25] but of course 85% will not. In fact the 15% of excellent responders are balanced by the same proportion of patients who will fail TKI therapy completely because of resistance and/ intolerance. For this group of patients allogeneic HCT remains a valuable rescue strategy.

Current Controversies in HCT for CML

Allogeneic HCT was the standard of care for CML for more than 20 years. Early transplant outcome, although offering the only prospect of long-term survival at the time, suffered from high transplant mortality. Long-term follow-up data from transplants undertaken in the 1980s and early 1990s reported

a 20-year OS of 40%, 20%, and 10% for CP, AP, and BP, respectively, with early TRM approaching 40%[26,27]. Those transplanted in first CP at our institution between 2000 and 2010 had a 3-year OS of 74%[28], reflecting improvements in conditioning regimens and supportive care. Impressively, reports from the German CML study IV showed a 3-year OS in excess of 90% with 100-day TRM of 8%[29].

Many of the dilemmas of HCT in CML, such as choice of conditioning regimen, use of TCD, choice of alternative donor, and graft source, are common to all hematologic malignancies. However, the most controversial issue of patient selection has been more radically challenged in CML in the last 15 years than in any other disease. HCT has clearly been displaced from first-line treatment and is now reserved for those failing multiple TKIs or with more advanced phase CML. While at the peak of transplantation for CML in the 1990s the vast majority of those undergoing HCT were CP patients; the proportions are changing, and now an increasing percentage of those undergoing the procedure have advanced phase disease (Figure 36.1), making the procedures more complex to plan and orchestrate.

Controversies in Current Indications for HCT in CML
Chronic Phase CML and Controversies
Identifying High-risk Patients

While prolonged follow-up from the IRIS study showed that imatinib can induce durable remissions in the long term, at 8 years of follow-up more than 40% of patients had discontinued treatment either as a result of failing to achieve an optimal response or because of intolerable side effects on the drug [13]. Similar patterns are seen irrespective of the choice of first-line agent, with only 68% of patients remaining on dasatinib at 4 years in the DASISION study [20], and

57–69% on nilotinib in ENESTnd [21]. Treatment failure may result from the emergence of clones harboring mutations in the tyrosine kinase domain, or may result without evidence of such a mutation. Mutational analysis is therefore a key investigation to guide management and maximize the opportunities for TKI success in a patient developing resistance[30]. In some cases, mutations may confer resistance to one or other TKI, and switching to an alternative agent may result in disease control; however, others such as the T315I mutation confer resistance to multiple agents[31]. Until recently the presence of a T315I mutation, associated with resistance to all first and second-generation TKIs, was a strong indication for HCT[32]; however now, ponatinib, a third-generation TKI, has good activity against this mutation. Even in the presence of this mutation MMR can be achieved in up to 56% of patients[33], although long-term durability of response and safety of ponatinib have not yet been demonstrated. In the remainder of imatinib-resistant/intolerant patients, 2GTKI may offer an effective strategy, with up to 50% achieving CCyR[34,35]. However, again, long-term follow-up from both phase II/III studies of dasatinib and nilotinib in this setting show the majority of patients discontinue treatment for one reason or another. By 6 years, approximately 70% of patients have discontinued their first choice 2GTKI [34,35], suggesting that many patients require multiple changes in treatment strategy. Importantly, at any time while off therapy or on ineffective therapy each individual patient remains at risk of disease progression and the tragedy observed in recent years is that these patients are frequently only referred for transplant after this has occurred. Our goal must therefore be to identify this group of patients, destined to "fail" TKIs, whether through resistance, intolerance, or both, as early as possible in their disease course and instigate a change in their treatment strategy to salvage their response.

It has recently become apparent that early response to TKIs is predictive of long-term outcome. Failure to achieve a RQ-PCR <10% at 3 months of first or second-line therapy now identifies a group of patients with poorer survival [18,19,36]. Although a highly valuable observation, the group failing to achieve this response clearly contains a mixture of patients, because their overall survival is still superior to historical cohorts treated with busulfan, hydroxycarbamide, and interferon, demonstrating that they do still gain survival advantage from TKIs. Of course some of this heterogeneity will be explained by temporary dose cessation, dose reduction, and possible nonadherence to therapy in the early weeks of treatment. However, rigorous monitoring, attention to compliance with therapy, and a willingness to change treatment early should allow the majority of patients with inherently poor prognosis on TKI therapy to be identified within a year of diagnosis, and to be referred for transplant before disease progression (Figure 36.2).

Existing risk stratification systems, developed in the pre-TKI-era, continue to be of value in prognostication. The Sokal risk score, despite being developed in the mid-1990s, continues to be relevant in the TKI era: low-risk patients treated with imatinib or nilotinib progress infrequently[21] while high-risk patients require extremely close observation. Timely escalation through TKIs is particularly important in these high-risk individuals, because they are at greatest risk of early disease progression. Given the inferior outcome of those transplants beyond first CP, every effort must be made to identify patients necessitating transplant before they progress, but while still giving them every opportunity to respond to TKIs. Even in Sokal high-risk patients the 3-month PCR result still remains the strongest predictor of outcome, and while we can assume that more low-risk than high-risk patients will achieve a BCR-ABL1 PCR <10% at 3 months of treatment, those high-risk patients who do have equal long-term outcome irrespective of their presenting Sokal risk score. So while high Sokal risk patients may still achieve the excellent long-term outcome associated with BCR-ABL1 <10% at 3 months, clinicians need a heightened awareness that if these patients do not respond, they are at high risk of early disease progression and alternative strategies must be employed promptly in order to avoid progression beyond first chronic phase (CP1).

The impact of patient age at diagnosis is increasingly controversial. Historically the Sokal score associated increasing age with increasing risk[37]; however, emerging data challenge that dogma, even suggesting that the opposite may be true. One retrospective analysis showed adolescents and young adults (aged 15–29 years) have significantly lower response rates (CCyR, MMR, and CMR) to first-line TKI than their older counterparts (aged over 30 years)[38]. Data from the recent German CML IV indicate that younger CML patients present with more aggressive disease (larger spleen size, more frequent symptoms of organomegaly, higher white blood count, higher percentage of peripheral blasts, and lower hemoglobin levels), and have lower probability of achieving BCR-ABL1 <10% at 3 months, although in this study there was no difference in response rate, probability of progression, or OS [39]. While we await more data on the outcome of adolescents and young adults we should remain vigilant that these patients may pose a higher risk of treatment failure and progression, also bearing in mind that the predicted outcome with HCT for young patients remains very positive.

Accelerated- and Blast- Phase CML and Focus on Controversies

Blast crisis is considered a direct result of persistent BCR-ABL1 activity, resulting in DNA damage, impaired DNA damage repair and chromosomal instability, typically leading to clonal evolution[40]. While the advent of the TKIs has completely changed the landscape in terms of long-term outcome and survival in CP disease, the same cannot be said of AP and BP. The median survival in BP in the TKI era has risen only modestly from 3–4 months in the pre-TKI era to 7–11 months with the introduction of these agents [40] and attempts to treat BP with TKI alone are essentially futile: A recent report on 98 patients presenting in BP of CML in China demonstrated that treatment with the TKIs alone

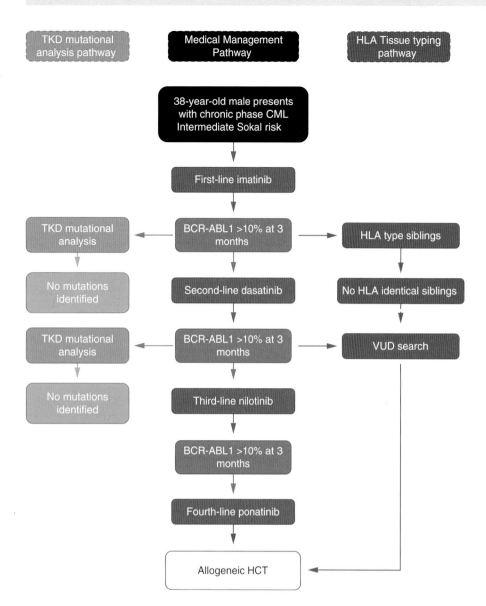

Figure 36.2 Placement of allogeneic HCT within an example treatment algorithm for a new patient presenting with CML in blast phase within our institute. Prompt aggressive treatment should aim to achieve a second chronic phase and move swiftly to allogeneic HCT.

offered only a 10% 4-year OS. Consolidation with HCT, however, significantly improved outcome, with a 4-year OS of 47% [41]. It is therefore in this context that HCT offers the only realistic prospect of long-term survival, and remains the standard of care for eligible patients (Figure 36.3).

A retrospective analysis of 449 patients transplanted for advanced phase disease (BP, AP, second chronic phase (CP2)) from the Center for International Blood and Marrow Transplant Research (CIBMTR) provides some of the most recent published outcomes on these high-risk patients[42]. Several important points are drawn from these data. Firstly, transplantation in the blast phase continues to be associated with a dismal long-term outlook, with a 3-year OS of 14%. The prior use of imatinib on those transplanted in frank BP had no impact. Those transplanted in AP or those who can be returned to chronic phase prior to transplant (CP2) had a more favorable outlook with a 3-year OS of 43% and 36%, respectively. Clearly this supports the notion that every effort

must be made to return BP patients to CP2 prior to HCT, but also raises the question of how this should be achieved. The TKIs are capable of inducing a transient remission in BP. Imatinib alone is superior to chemotherapy alone in inducing a remission (55% *versus* 29%) when compared to traditional cytarabine-based regimens, and is associated with lower toxicity rates[43]. Second-generation TKIs show similar rates of hematological remission and no significant superiority to imatinib has been demonstrated to date [40]. While early studies of imatinib combined with combination chemotherapy did hint at higher remission rates[44,45], these studies were small, and failed to convince many of the superiority of this approach to imatinib alone [40]. The combination of dasatinib and FLAG-Ida chemotherapy regimen shows promise in a small group of patients from our institution with all patients returning to CP2 prior to HCT[46], and this continues to be our approach, but the relative rarity of this patient population prevents the generation of large-scale data sets.

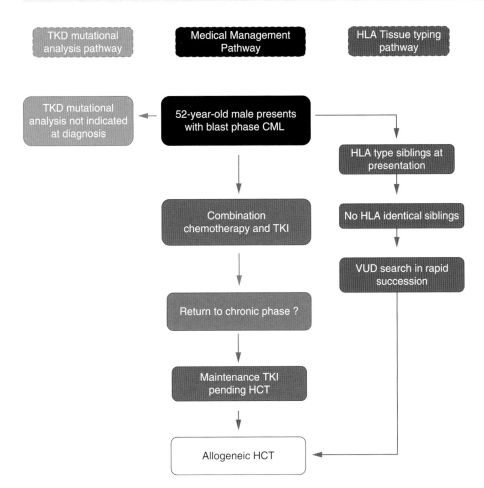

Figure 36.3 Placement of allogeneic HCT within an example treatment algorithm for a new patient presenting with CML in chronic phase within our institute. Patients failing to achieve BCR-ABL <10% at 3 months are predicted to fare poorly, and should rapidly escalate through treatment options, and proceed to HCT as required. This algorithm allows those with the poorest risk disease to proceed to allogeneic HCT within 1 year of diagnosis.

Intriguingly, despite the aggressive nature of BP, the most frequent cause of death post-HCT is not in fact progressive disease. These patients suffer extremely high TRM, 46% and 54% at 1 and 3 years respectively, if transplanted in BP [42]. These figures are slightly lower for those transplanted in CP2, (33% and 39% at 1 and 3 years, respectively) but still considerably higher than the 8% 1-year TRM seen in those transplanted in CP1 in the German data set [29]. The reasons for this are unclear. It may be that the higher TRM results from the use of pretransplant chemotherapy, drug toxicity or atypical/fungal infections resulting from prolonged immunosuppression, but this is purely speculative. Registry data may be able to provide circumstantial evidence that pretransplant chemotherapy contributes to the TRM if those treated with imatinib alone (rather than in combination with or instead of chemotherapy) had superior OS. However, it would be difficult to conclude that the differences did not result from the status of the disease (i.e., those treated with imatinib alone may have had "better" or less aggressive disease than those who were treated with chemotherapy). For all these reasons, although we all can agree that return to CP2 offers the best prospect of long-term survival, there is no clear consensus on the optimal way to achieve this status.

Accelerated phase disease (compared to BP) consists of a heterogeneous mix of patients: some with disease on the brink of transformation to very aggressive BP, others in early transition from CP, with eminently salvageable disease. This is confounded by the fact that AP was defined in a pre-TKI era where loss of response to therapy would constitute progression to AP, whereas now it would most likely simply trigger a change of TKI. While for those in the transition between CP and AP, a TKI-based regimen may well suffice, those on the more aggressive end of the spectrum, rapidly heading toward BP require prompt aggressive therapy in order to offer long-term survival.

The tyrosine kinase inhibitors are capable of inducing a remission in some AP patients, but the duration of remission remains less clear. For those progressing to AP while on treatment, who should be considered as a separate entity from those presenting in AP, second-generation agents can achieve CCyR in 70% at 24 months[47], but many would still feel uneasy about withholding transplantation in these circumstances because of the inherently higher risk of loss of response.

Jiang and et al.[48] attempted to develop a risk stratification system in order to identify those patients in whom HCT offered no advantage over imatinib. Three independent risk factors were identified (CML duration >12 months, hemoglobin <100 g/L, and peripheral blood blasts >5%). For low-risk patients (with no risk factors) HCT conferred no advantage over imatinib (6-year OS 81% *versus* 100%), but these patients constituted less than a third of AP patients. The outcome for high-risk patients (two or three risk factors) who did not receive HCT was poor (5-year OS 18% *versus* 100%). Recent data from patients presenting in AP suggested that first- and second-generation TKIs could induce MMR in 63–76%, and offer a 3-year OS of 87–95%[49]. It is likely that those who present in AP, rather than develop AP on treatment, are at a much earlier disease stage at the time of intervention. Those progressing to AP while on treatment may well have developed tyrosine kinase domain mutation, which typically occurs after selective pressure is exerted by a TKI. Importantly, while these mutations may confer resistance to one or more TKI, their presence has little or no impact on the efficacy of HCT because it relies on a graft-*versus*-leukemia effect (see Chapters 25 and 65) not TK inhibition to exert disease control. For this reason those developing AP on treatment are much less likely to respond to TKI and any response is likely to be transient, whereas HCT is eminently capable of regaining disease control.

Despite the encouraging data from those presenting in AP treated with TKIs, this still remains a controversial issue. Unlike in CP, we do not know whether failure to achieve a BCR-ABL1 <10% within 3 months signals a poor outcome, nor whether achieving this target confers the same probability of long-term survival (mainly because of lack of long-term follow-up in AP studies). This uneasiness combined with the well-described inferior outcome associated with progression to blast phase makes the prospect of withholding HCT in eligible AP patients with a suitable donor unnerving.

Prediction of Allotransplant Risk in the TKI Era

The European Group for Blood and Marrow Transplantation (EBMT) developed a risk scoring system in the 1990s when CML was the commonest indication for allogeneic HCT[50]. The data set of more than 3000 patients bases predictions on five variables (Table 36.1) with predicted 5-year OS varying between 20% and 72% in high- to low-risk groups, respectively. The score was subsequently independently validated across hematological malignancies based on a data set of more than 56000 transplants by CIBMTR[51], and remains the most useful predictor of outcome in current practice. While these data were accumulated in the pre-TKI era, a recent reanalysis of EBMT data confirms its ongoing prognostic value. The retrospective analysis sought to validate the score by reviewing the outcome of more than 5500 patients transplanted for CML between 2000 and 2011[52]. Overall, similar 5-year OS and progression-free survivals (PFS) were seen in TKI-treated (OS 59% and PFS 42%) compared to TKI naïve (OS 61% and PFS 46%) transplant recipients. Independent analysis of time to transplant demonstrated that while diagnosis to transplant time of greater than 12 months remained a predictor of outcome in those who did not receive a TKI prior to transplantation, this was no longer the case in the TKI-treated cohort.

Table 36.1 EBMT risk score

Risk factor	Category	Score
Donor type	HLA-identical sibling	0
	Matched unrelated donor	1
Disease stage	1st chronic phase	0
	Accelerated phase	1
	Blast crisis	2
Age of recipient	<20 years	0
	20–40 years	1
	>40 years	2
Gender combination	All except:	0
	Male recipient/female donor	1
Time from diagnosis to transplant	<12 months	0
	>12 months	1

Risk score	Probability of outcome at 5 years (%)		
	LFS	OS	TRM
0	60	72	20
1	60	70	23
2	47	62	31
3	37	48	46
4	35	40	51
5	19	18	71
6	16	22	73

LFS: leukemia-free survival; OS: overall survival; TRM: transplant-related mortality.
Data from Gratwohl *et al.*[51].

This is difficult to fully understand; however, it could be speculated that even in those resistant to TKI (and especially those intolerant rather than resistant), the drugs do continue to have some effect in delaying the natural progression of the disease, which would otherwise be responsible for the worsening outcome with increasing time to transplantation. However, the data set may have been confounded by patients transplanted in the very early TKI era, who, despite responding well to TKI, underwent HCT because of a lack of long-term outcome data at the time. In this manner, "good risk" patients responding to TKI may take longer than 12 months to reach transplant, confounding the analysis. Given that the poor outcome in those with prolonged time to transplant from the original data set was attributable to high TRM rather than disease relapse, it seems to difficult to understand how TKI therapy could impact on this and it would seem more likely that there are confounders in the data.

In addition to the EBMT score, which focuses on the recipient age, disease characteristic, and donor–recipient match, it has been shown that comorbidities at the time of transplant impact significantly on transplant outcome[53]. The HCT comorbidity index (HCT-CI) has been used to predict nonrelapse mortality and OS across multiple hematological malignancies[53,54,55] (see Chapter 4). This tool has been validated in CML patients, and many of those included in the validation had received TKIs, justifying its use in current transplant risk assessment. Within our institution we have validated the use of the HCT-CI for predicting outcome of CML patients in the TKI era, and furthermore identified that C-reactive protein (CRP) is an independent predictor of outcome[56]. CRP>10 mg/L at the time of initiating conditioning independently predicts poor outcome. While the identification of these parameters indicating inferior outcome may have value in prognostication, it remains unclear if it is possible to modify the risk by optimizing the parameters. *If a patient's CRP is raised on admission, should we delay transplant in order to investigate and treat a biomarker in an otherwise well patient?* Perhaps we should in light of the fact that TRM poses a more imminent threat than relapse in the highest risk patients in HCT for CML; however, no data exist to corroborate the fact that reducing the CRP or indeed managing any comorbidity influences outcome.

Impact of TKIs on Allotransplant Outcome in Current Practice

It is now almost inevitable that CML patients coming to HCT will have received prior TKI therapy. While many of the early studies supported the idea that TKI therapy *per se* did not negatively impact on outcome[57,58,59], these data were frequently confounded; often this was because the non-TKI group was a historical comparator rather than

contemporaneously transplanted patients or because the reason for choice of using TKI or not was rarely given, making it uncertain if the two groups are truly comparable. More recent data do, however, reiterate the findings of these early reports. As discussed, the retrospective reanalysis of the large EBMT data set risk data seems to suggest that TKI prior to HCT does not negatively impact on outcome [52]. Additionally Saussele and colleagues presented some interesting data from the transplanted cohort of patients in the German CML VI study in 2010 [29]. In 56 patients transplanted in CP, either because of patient choice or imatinib failure, the 3-year probability of OS was 91% with an 8% TRM. In a matched paired analysis 106 patients not undergoing HCT were compared to those transplanted and similar overall survival was observed (96% *versus* 92%, respectively). Patients who elected to undergo HCT rather than continuing imatinib treatment (n=19) had survival similar to those who proceeded to transplantation because of imatinib failure (n=37) (3-year OS of 88% and 94%, respectively) supporting the notion that prolonged prior use of imatinib does not negatively impact on transplant outcome, while also demonstrating that both approaches have excellent outcomes. As expected, in advanced phase disease the outcome was poorer with a 3-year OS of 59% in the 28 patients transplanted.

Implication of General Transplant Controversies in CML

Just as the number of transplants fell following the widespread introduction of the TKIs, so too did the number of publications upon which to base clinical practice (Figure 36.4). Data generated from HCT in CML over the past 40 years have informed the principles of HCT across all malignancies. Had

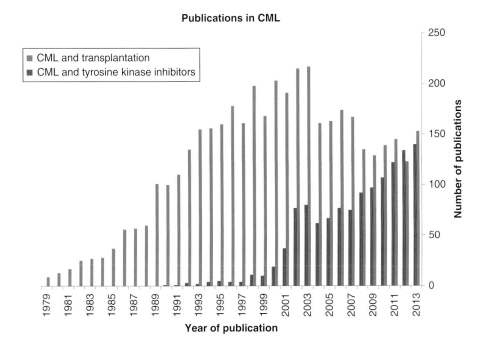

Publications in CML

- CML and transplantation
- CML and tyrosine kinase inhibitors

Year of publication

Number of publications

Figure 36.4 Pubmed citations by year; search terms "CML and transplantation" and "CML and tyrosine kinase inhibitor."

that momentum continued, it is likely that we may have had more clear answers to some of the most important questions: What is the optimal choice of conditioning regimen? What is the optimal choice of hematopoietic graft source? When and how should TCD be used? Sadly, however, over the last 5 years there have been relatively few reports directly addressing transplant outcome, and as a result many key questions remain largely unanswered.

What is the Optimal "Intensity" of Conditioning Regimen?

Traditional conditioning regimes for HCT in CML (see Chapter 27) were often irradiation based with additional cyclophosphamide or other cytotoxic agent[28]. For many centers these regimens still remain the standard of care. However, following better understanding of the graft-*versus*-leukemia effect, and its importance in HCT for CML, RIC regimens were developed in attempts to reduce the TRM. Comparison of outcome following RIC and MAC regimen protocols is always plagued by discrepancies between the two groups, confounded by the fact that frequently the reason for regimen choice is not specified. Warlick *et al.*[60] reported CIBMTR data on RIC HCT in 2012, with the aim of ascertaining whether increasing age was associated with inferior outcome. In this group of 306 patients increased aged was neither associated with increased TRM (18%, 20%, and 13% for 40–49, 50–59, and over 60 years, respectively) nor significantly inferior 3-year OS (54%, 52%, and 41%). Here imatinib use was associated with improved survival (56% *versus* 37%), but in the context of noncontemporaneous transplants. While these data support the use of RIC regimens in older patients who may otherwise be unsuitable for HCT, the lower than expected OS and high relapse rates would generally discourage the use of RIC regimens in those fit enough to tolerate MAC particularly for high-risk disease, which comprises an increasing percentage of transplants in current practice. In contrast to MAC regimens, where concern needs to be focused on TRM and OS (because nonsurvivors most frequently succumb to nonrelapse causes), attention should be drawn to leukemia-free survival (LFS) in outcome assessment of RIC regimen, where low TRM rates can be predicted but so too can high relapse rates. With this in mind, longer-term LFS data are awaited before truly informed decisions on intermediate- and low-risk patients can be made. The use of RIC regimens necessitates that particular attention should be paid to achieving full donor chimerism, a prerequisite for eradicating *BCR-ABL1 positive* cells, with careful BCR-ABL1 monitoring and prompt management of post-transplant relapse[61].

Optimal Choice of Hematopoietic Cell Source: Peripheral Blood *versus* Bone Marrow?

Peripheral blood hematopoietic cells (PBHC) have largely replaced bone marrow (BM) as the favored hematopoietic cell source, partly because they offer faster engraftment, and partly reflecting donor choice. A randomized controlled trial of BM *versus* PBHC published in 2012 reported higher rates of chronic graft-*versus*-host disease with PBHC (53% *versus* 41%) but marginally higher rates of graft failure with BM (9% *versus* 3%)[62]. There was no impact on OS or PFS. While this study included, but was not limited to CML patients, the findings are particularly pertinent to those with CML. Up to 50% of patients transplanted for CP CML will subsequently develop molecular relapse necessitating DLI (see Chapter 25), particularly if RIC regimen is employed[63]. Importantly, active chronic graft-*versus*-host disease may preclude the use of DLI, making management of relapse more difficult. For this reason, and particularly if RIC regimens or T-cell-depleted methods (see Chapter 29) are to be employed, it could be argued that BM should remain the first choice over PBHC. Data investigating the outcome of those receiving DLI for relapse following transplantation found that in CP patients, the choice of hematopoietic cell source did not influence the outcome post-DLI; however, in advanced phase, patients who had received PBHC had an inferior post-DLI survival, again favoring the use of BM in patients in whom there is concern about subsequent relapse[64]. Interestingly, longer term follow-up data from patients undergoing HCT in the United States between 2000 and 2008 showed that transplantation of *PBHC* for those in first CP was associated with higher rates of NRM and, consequently, lower rates of survival, which again would favor the use of BM in CP patients too[65]. The survival differences were no longer evident in transplant for disease beyond CP2, therefore it would seem that BM offers no benefit over PBHC in this group of high-risk patients; however, cumulation of the accrued data suggests a cautious approach would continue to favor BM.

T-Cell Depletion: Yes or No in CML?

Almost 30 years since the observation that TCD reduces the incidence and severity of GvHD at the expense of higher relapse risk [5], controversy persists over who and how to T-cell deplete (see Chapters 29 and 30). Particularly problematic in CML is that those at highest risk of NRM are those with highest risk of disease, i.e., those beyond CP1. At our institution we routinely use TCD in recipients of unrelated or mismatched donors transplanted in CP1 and although there are some reports of good outcome with sibling transplants, particularly in combination with DLI[66], we do not routinely carry out TCD in these patients. For those with advanced phase disease, the choice is based on an assessment of TRM *versus* relapse risk. In worldwide practice, the choice to T-cell deplete or not is typically institute or physician dependent, and unfortunately there are little recent data addressing the problems. Socié *et al.*[67] reported from their randomized open-label phase 3 trial that the use of rabbit antithymocyte globulin (ATG) was capable of reducing GvHD risk without increasing relapse risk in recipients of unrelated transplant following

MAC regimen. While these data cannot be interpreted as definitive, and should not be extrapolated to sibling nor RIC regimens, they remain encouraging that dissociation of the benefits from the risks of TCD are possible.

Post-Transplant Issues and Management of Post-HCT Relapse

The monitoring of minimal residual disease was pioneered in CML (see Chapters by 23 and 24). Reliable criteria exist defining molecular relapse (MR) which are highly predictive of progressive disease[68]. Molecular relapse following HCT for CML is common, and occurs in up to 50% of chronic phase patients[69]. In the pre-TKI era, DLI was the mainstay of treatment [5]. Escalating dose DLI is safe for use in recipients of sibling, VUD[70], and even HLA-mismatched-VUD[71] HCT providing sufficient time has elapsed from the transplant procedure. It can restore remission in 70–80% of those receiving it, and subsequent relapse is rare[72]. It does, however, require that cells are available from the original donor, and is inadvisable in the presence of active chronic GvHD. Much of the DLI data were accumulated in the pre-TKI era and its ongoing validity remains to be seen. It has recently been suggested that as a result of transplantation now being reserved for biologically poorer risk disease, DLI may not be as efficacious as it was in the pre-TKI era[73] and that TKIs may provide the best approach to post-HCT relapse management. However, these conclusions were drawn on an extremely small data set, and in practical terms most patients coming to transplant in the 21st century have already developed resistance or intolerance to multiple TKI making their use futile in the resistant and difficult in the intolerant. In our patients, DLI remains the first-line treatment choice at relapse and continues to be effective.

It is, however, true that the relative proportion of patients transplanted in AP or BP is rising, and much of the data accumulated in the use of DLI came from patients transplanted in CP1. While DLI still appears to be an effective strategy in these more aggressive stages, often their relapses occur early, within the first 6 to 9 months when the use of DLI may be contraindicated because of the high risk of GvHD. Combinations of DLI and TKI have recently been reported but the numbers are small and benefits over their individual uses unclear[41].

Conclusions

No cancer has undergone such remarkable changes to its management in the last two decades as CML. The TKIs have revolutionized its management and displaced HCT from first-line therapy. However, HCT remains a viable treatment option for many CML patients, and with increasingly complex patients undergoing HCT, physicians face increasingly complex decisions about their management. The vast transplant evidence base built in the pre-TKI era provides an important resource upon which these decisions can be made going forward; however caution must be exerted in data extrapolation. The patient population undergoing transplantation for CML in the 21st century is very different to those transplanted in the decade before, and while much effort has been made to validate the pre-TKI data in contemporary patient cohorts, this remains an ongoing challenge. A number of questions remain unanswered, and given the relative reduction in transplant procedures for CML, collaborative studies are likely to hold the best prospect of answering these. Ultimately as CML physicians, we are immensely thankful to be able to offer many CML patients a near normal life expectancy with TKIs, but for some, transplantation continues to be the best option, and we remain focused on optimizing patient selection and minimizing transplant risk in the 21st century.

Acknowledgments

We are extremely grateful to the EBMT Transplant Activity Survey office, and in particular Helen Baldomero and Alois Gratwohl for the data in Figure 36.1.

References

1. Fefer A, Cheever MA, Thomas ED, Boyd C, Ramberg R, Glucksburg H, et al. Disappearance of Ph1-positive cells in four patients with chronic granulocytic leukemia after chemotherapy, irradiation and marrow transplantation from an identical twin. N Engl J Med. 1979;300:333–7.

2. Goldman JM, Apperley JF, Jones LM, Marcus R, Goolden A, Batchelor R, et al. Bone marrow transplantation for patients with chronic myeloid leukaemia. N Eng J Med. 1986;314:202–7.

3. Goldman JM, Mackinnon S. Bone marrow transplantation for chronic myeloid leukaemia using matched unrelated donors. Bone Marrow Transplant. 1989;Suppl 4:38–9.

4. Goldman JM, Majhail NS, Klein JP, Wang Z, Sobocinski KA, Arora M, et al Relapse and late mortality in 5-year survivors of myeloablative allogeneic hematopoietic cell transplantation for chronic myeloid leukemia in first chronic phase. J Clin Oncol. 2010;28:1888–95.

5. Apperley JF, Jones L, Hale G, Waldmann H, Hows J, Rombos Y, et al. Bone marrow transplantation for patients with chronic myeloid leukaemia: T-cell depletion with Campath-1 reduces the incidence of graft-versus-host disease but may increase the risk of leukaemic relapse. Bone Marrow Transplant. 1986;1:53–66.

6. Kolb HJ, Mittermüller J, Clemm C, Holler E, Ledderose G, Brehm G et al. Donor leukocyte transfusions for treatment of recurrent chronic myelogenous leukemia in marrow transplant patients. Blood. 1990;76:2462–5.

7. Kolb HJ, Schattenberg A, Goldman JM, Hertenstein B, Jacobsen N, Arcese W et al. Graft-versus-leukemia effect of donor lymphocyte transfusions in

marrow grafted patients. *Blood*. 1995;86:2041–50.

8. Or R, Shapira MY, Resnick I, Amar A, Ackerstein A, Samuel S et al. Nonmyeloablative allogeneic stem cell transplantation for the treatment of chronic myeloid leukemia in first chronic phase. *Blood*. 2003;101:441–5.

9. Crawley C, Szydlo R, Lalancette M, Bacigalupo A, Lange A, Brune M, et al. Outcomes of reduced-intensity transplantation for chronic myeloid leukemia: an analysis of prognostic factors from the Chronic Leukemia Working Party of the EBMT. *Blood*. 2005;106:2969–76.

10. Kebriaei P, Detry MA, Giralt S, Carrasco-Yalan A, Anagnostopoulos A, Couriel D, et al. Long-term follow-up of allogeneic hematopoietic stem-cell transplantation with reduced-intensity conditioning for patients with chronic myeloid leukemia. *Blood*. 2007;110:3456–62.

11. Druker BJ1, Talpaz M, Resta DJ, Peng B, Buchdunger E, Ford JM, et al. Efficacy and safety of a specific inhibitor of the BCR-ABL tyrosine kinase in chronic myeloid leukemia. *N Engl J Med*. 2001;344:1031–7.

12. Goldman JM. Chronic myeloid leukemia: a historical perspective. *Semin Hematol*. 2010;47: 302–11.

13. Deininger M, O'Brien SG, Guilhot F, Goldman JM, Hochhaus A, Hughes TP et al. International randomized study of interferon vs STI571 (IRIS) 8-year follow up: sustained survival and low risk for progression or events in patients with newly diagnosed chronic myeloid leukemia in chronic phase treated with imatinib [abstract]. *Blood (ASH Annual Meeting Abstracts)*. 2009;114:Abstract 1126.

14. Sasaki K, Strom S, O'Brien S. Relative survival in patients with chronic-phase chronic myeloid leukaemia in the tyrosine-kinase inhibitor era: analysis of patient data from six prospective clinical trials. *Lancet Haem*. 2015;2:186–93.

15. Bower H, Bjorkholm M, Dickman P, Hoglund M, Lambert P, Andersson TML. Life expectancy of patients with chronic myeloid leukemia approaches the life expectancy of the general population. *JCO*. 2016;34:2851–7.

16. Baccarani M, Saglio G, Goldman J, Hochhaus A, Simonsson B, Appelbaum F, et al. European LeukemiaNet. Evolving concepts in the management of chronic myeloid leukemia: recommendations from an expert panel on behalf of the European LeukemiaNet. *Blood* 2006;108: 1809–1820.

17. Baccarani M, Deininger MW, Rosti G, Hochhaus A, Soverini S, Apperley JF, et al. European LeukemiaNet recommendations for the management of chronic myeloid leukemia: 2013. *Blood*. 2013;122:872–84.

18. Hanfstein B, Müller MC, Hehlmann R, Erben P, Lauseker M, Fabarius A, et al. Early molecular and cytogenetic response is predictive for long-term progression-free and overall survival in chronic myeloid leukemia (CML). *Leukemia*. 2012;26:2096–102.

19. Marin D, Ibrahim AR, Lucas C, Gerrard G, Wang L, Szydlo RM, et al. Assessment of BCR-ABL1 transcript levels at 3 months is the only requirement for predicting outcome for patients with chronic myeloid leukemia treated with tyrosine kinase inhibitors. *J Clin Oncol*. 2012;30:232–8.

20. Cortes JE, Hochhaus A, Kim D, Shah NP, Mayer J, Rowlings P, et al. Four-year (yr) follow-up of patients (pts) with newly diagnosed chronic myeloid leukemia in chronic phase (CML-CP) receiving dasatinib or imatinib: efficacy based on early response. *Blood (ASH Annual Meeting Abstracts)*. 2013; 122: Abstract 653.

21. Saglio G, Hochhaus A, Hughes TP, Clark RE, Nakamae H, Kim D, et al. ENESTnd update: nilotinib (NIL) vs imatinib (IM) in patients (pts) with newly diagnosed chronic myeloid leukemia in chronic phase (CML-CP) and the impact of early molecular response (EMR) and Sokal risk at diagnosis on long-term outcomes. *Blood (ASH Annual Meeting Abstracts)*. 2013; 122:Abstract 632.

22. Brümmendorf TH, Cortes JE, de Souza CA, Guilhot F, Duvillié L, Pavlov D, et al. Bosutinib *versus* imatinib in newly diagnosed chronic-phase chronic myeloid leukaemia: results from the 24-month follow-up of the BELA trial. *Br J Haematol*. 2014;Sep 8. doi: 10.1111/bjh.13108. [Epub ahead of print]

23. Mahon FX, Réa D, Guilhot J, Guilhot F, Huguet F, Nicolini F, et al. Discontinuation of imatinib in patients with chronic myeloid leukaemia who have maintained complete molecular remission for at least 2 years: the prospective, multicentre Stop Imatinib (STIM) trial. *Lancet Oncol*. 2010;11:1029–35.

24. Ross DM, Branford S, Seymour JF, Schwarer AP, Arthur C, Yeung DT, et al. Safety and efficacy of imatinib cessation for CML patients with stable undetectable minimal residual disease: results from the TWISTER study. *Blood*. 2013;122:515–22.

25. Goldman J, Gordon M. Why do chronic myelogenous leukemia stem cells survive allogeneic stem cell transplantation or imatinib: does it really matter? *Leuk Lymphoma*. 2006;47:1–7.

26. Gratwohl A, Brand R, Apperley J, C Crawley, T Ruutu, P Corradini, et al. Allogeneic hematopoietic stem cell transplantation for chronic myeloid leukemia in Europe 2006: transplant activity, long-term data and current results. An analysis by the Chronic Leukemia Working Party of the European Group for Blood and Marrow Transplantation (EBMT). *Haematologica*. 2006;91:513–21.

27. Gratwohl A, Heim D. Current role of stem cell transplantation in chronic myeloid leukaemia. *Best Pract Res Clin Haematol*. 2009;22:431–43.

28. Pavlu J, Szydlo RM, Goldman JM, Apperley JF. Three decades of transplantation for chronic myeloid leukemia: what have we learned? *Blood*. 2011;117:755–63.

29. Saussele S, Lauseker M, Gratwohl A, Beelen DW, Bunjes D, Schwerdtfeger R, et al. Allogeneic hematopoietic stem cell transplantation (allo SCT) for chronic myeloid leukemia in the imatinib era: evaluation of its impact within a subgroup of the randomized German CML Study IV. *Blood*. 2010;115:1880–5.

30. Soverini S, Hochhaus A, Nicolini FE, Gruber F, Lange T, Saglio G, et al. BCR-ABL kinase domain mutation analysis in chronic myeloid leukemia patients treated with tyrosine kinase inhibitors: recommendations from an expert panel on behalf of European LeukemiaNet. *Blood*. 2011;118:1208–15.

31. Ernst T, La Rosée P, Müller MC, Hochhaus A. BCR-ABL mutations in chronic myeloid leukemia. *Hematol Oncol Clin North Am*. 2011;25: 997–1008.

32. Nicolini FE1, Basak GW, Soverini S, Martinelli G, Mauro MJ, Müller MC, et al. Allogeneic stem cell transplantation for patients harboring T315I BCR-ABL mutated leukemias. Blood. 2011;118:5697–700.

33. Cortes JE, Kim DW, Pinilla-Ibarz J, le Coutre P, Paquette R, Chuah C, et al. A phase 2 trial of ponatinib in Philadelphia chromosome-positive leukemias. N Engl J Med. 2013;369:1783–96.

34. Shah NP, Guilhot F, Cortes JE, Schiffer CA, le Coutre P, Brümmendorf TH, et al. Long-term outcome with dasatinib after imatinib failure in chronic-phase chronic myeloid leukemia: follow-up of a phase 3 study. Blood. 2014;123:2317–24.

35. Giles FJ, le Coutre PD, Pinilla-Ibarz J, Larson RA, Gattermann N, Ottmann OG et al. Nilotinib in imatinib-resistant or imatinib-intolerant patients with chronic myeloid leukemia in chronic phase: 48-month follow-up results of a phase II study. Leukemia. 2013;27:107–12.

36. Kim DD, Lee H, Kamel-Reid S, Lipton JH. BCR-ABL1 transcript at 3 months predicts long-term outcomes following second generation tyrosine kinase inhibitor therapy in the patients with chronic myeloid leukaemia in chronic phase who failed Imatinib. Br J Haematol. 2013;160:630–9.

37. Sokal JE, Cox EB, Baccarani M, Tura S, Gomez GA, Robertson JE, et al. Prognostic discrimination in "good-risk" chronic granulocytic leukemia. Blood. 1984;63:789–99.

38. Pemmaraju N, Kantarjian H, Shan J, Jabbour E, Quintas-Cardama A, Verstovsek S, et al. Analysis of outcomes in adolescents and young adults with chronic myelogenous leukemia treated with upfront tyrosine kinase inhibitor therapy. Haematologica. 2012;97:1029–35.

39. Kalmanti L, Saussele S, Lauseker M, Proetel U, Müller MC, Hanfstein B, et al. Younger patients with chronic myeloid leukemia do well in spite of poor prognostic indicators: results from the randomized CML study IV. Ann Hematol. 2014;93:71–80.

40. Hehlmann R. How I treat CML blast crisis. Blood. 2012;120:737–47.

41. Jiang H, Xu LP, Liu DH, Liu KY, Chen SS, Jiang B, et al. Allogeneic hematopoietic SCT in combination with tyrosine kinase inhibitor treatment compared with TKI treatment alone in CML blast crisis. Bone Marrow Transplant. 2014;49:1146–54.

42. Khoury HJ, Kukreja M, Goldman JM, Wang T, Halter J, Arora M, et al. Prognostic factors for outcomes in allogeneic transplantation for CML in the imatinib era: a CIBMTR analysis. Bone Marrow Transplant. 2012,47.010–6.

43. Kantarjian HM, Cortes J, OíBrien S, Giles FJ, Albitar M, Rios MB et al. Imatinib mesylate (STI571) therapy for Philadelphia chromosome-positive chronic myelogenous leukemia in blast phase. Blood. 2002;99:3547–53.

44. Fruehauf S, Topaly J, Buss EC, et al. Imatinib combined with mitoxantrone/etoposide and cytarabine is an effective induction therapy for patients with chronic myeloid leukemia in myeloid blast crisis. Cancer. 2007;109:1543–9.

45. Oki Y, Kantarjian HM, Gharibyan V, et al. Phase II study of low-dose decitabine in combination with imatinib mesylate in patients with accelerated or myeloid blastic phase of chronic myelogenous leukemia. Cancer. 2007;109:899–906.

46. Milojkovic D, Ibrahim A, Reid A, Foroni L, Apperley J, Marin D. Efficacy of combining dasatinib and FLAG-IDA for patients with chronic myeloid leukemia in blastic transformation. Haematologica. 2012;97:473–4.

47. Hochhaus A, Giles F, Apperley J, Ossenkoppele G, Wang J, Gallagher NJ, et al. Nilotinib in chronic myeloid leukemia patients in accelerated phase (cml-ap) with imatinib resistance or intolerance: 24-month follow-up results of a phase 2 study. Haematologica 2009;94(Suppl 2):256 (abstract 0631).

48. Jiang Q, Xu LP, Liu DH, Liu KY, Chen SS, Jiang B, et al Imatinib mesylate versus allogeneic hematopoietic stem cell transplantation for patients with chronic myelogenous leukemia in the accelerated phase. Blood. 2011;117:3032–40.

49. Ohanian M, Kantarjian HM, Quintas-Cardama A, Jabbour E, Abruzzo L, Verstovsek S, et al. Tyrosine kinase inhibitors as initial therapy for patients with chronic myeloid leukemia in accelerated phase. Clin Lymphoma Myeloma Leuk. 2014;14:155–62.

50. Gratwohl A, Hermans J, Goldman JM, Arcese W, Carreras E, Devergie A, et al. Risk assessment for patients with chronic myeloid leukaemia before allogeneic blood or marrow transplantation. Chronic Leukemia Working Party of the European Group for Blood and Marrow Transplantation. Lancet. 1998;352:1087–92.

51. Gratwohl A, Stern M, Brand R, Apperley J, Baldomero H, de Witte T, et al. Risk score for outcome after allogeneic hematopoietic stem cell transplantation: a retrospective analysis. Cancer. 2009;115:4715–26.

52. Milojkovic D,Szydlo D, Hoek J, Beelen D, Hamladji R, Kyrcz-Krzemien S, et al. Prognostic significance of EBMT score for chronic myeloid leukaemia patients in the era of tyrosine kinase inhibitor therapy: a retrospective study from the chronic malignancy working party of the european group for blood and marrow transplantation (EBMT). Bone Marrow Transplant. 2014;49:S34–5.

53. Sorror ML, Maris MB, Storb R, Baron F, Sandmaier BM, Maloney DG, et al. Hematopoietic cell transplantation (HCT)-specific comorbidity index: a new tool for risk assessment before allogeneic HCT. Blood 2005;106:2912–9.

54. Sorror M, Storer B, Sandmaier BM, Maloney DG, Chauncey TR, Langston A, et al. Hematopoietic cell transplantation-comorbidity index and Karnofsky performance status are independent predictors of morbidity and mortality after allogeneic nonmyeloablative hematopoietic cell transplantation. Cancer. 2008;112:1992–2001.

55. Zipperer E, Pelz D, Nachtkamp K, Kuendgen A, Strupp C, Gattermann N, et al. The hematopoietic stem cell transplantation comorbidity index is of prognostic relevance for patients with myelodysplastic syndrome. Haematologica. 2009;94:729–32.

56. Pavlů J, Kew AK, Taylor-Roberts B, Auner HW, Marin D, Olavarria E et al. Optimizing patient selection for myeloablative allogeneic hematopoietic cell transplantation in chronic myeloid leukemia in chronic phase. Blood. 2010;115:4018–20.

57. Zaucha JM, Prejzner W, Giebel S, Gooley TA, Szatkowski D, Kałwak K, et al. Imatinib therapy prior to myeloablative allogeneic stem cell

transplantation. *Bone Marrow Transplant.* 2005;36:417–24.

58. Deininger M, Schleuning M, Greinix H, Sayer HG, Fischer T, Martinez J, *et al.* The effect of prior exposure to imatinib on transplant-related mortality. *Haematologica.* 2006;91:452–9.

59. Lee SJ, Kukreja M, Wang T, Giralt SA, Szer J, Arora M, *et al.* Impact of prior imatinib mesylate on the outcome of hematopoietic cell transplantation for chronic myeloid leukemia. *Blood.* 2008;112:3500–7.

60. Warlick E, Ahn KW, Pedersen TL, Artz A, de Lima M, Pulsipher M, *et al.* Reduced intensity conditioning is superior to nonmyeloablative conditioning for older chronic myelogenous leukemia patients undergoing hematopoietic cell transplant during the tyrosine kinase inhibitor era. *Blood.* 2012;119:4083–90.

61. Uzunel M, Mattsson J, Brune M, Johansson JE, Aschan J, Ringdén O. *et al.* Kinetics of minimal residual disease and chimerism in patients with chronic myeloid leukemia after nonmyeloablative conditioning and allogeneic stem cell transplantation. *Blood.* 2003;101:469–72.

62. Anasetti C, Logan BR, Lee SJ, Waller EK, Weisdorf DJ, Wingard JR, *et al.* Peripheral-blood stem cells *versus* bone marrow from unrelated donors. *N Engl J Med.* 2012;367:1487–96.

63. Krejci M, Mayer J, Doubek M, Brychtova Y, Pospisil Z, Racil Z, *et al.* Clinical outcomes and direct hospital costs of reduced-intensity allogeneic

transplantation in chronic myeloid leukemia. *Bone Marrow Transplant.* 2006;38:483–91.

64. Basak GW, de Wreede LC, van Biezen A, Wiktor-Jedrzejczak W, Halaburda K, Schmid C *et al.* Donor lymphocyte infusions for the treatment of chronic myeloid leukemia relapse following peripheral blood or bone marrow stem cell transplantation. *Bone Marrow Transplant.* 2013;48:837–42.

65. Eapen M, Logan BR, Appelbaum F, Antin A, Anasetti C, Couriel DR, *et al.* Long-term survival after transplantation of unrelated donor peripheral blood or bone marrow hematopoietic cells for hematologic malignancy. *Biol Blood Marrow Transplant.* 2015;21:55–9.

66. Sehn LH1, Alyea EP, Weller E, Canning C, Lee S, Ritz J, *et al.* Comparative outcomes of T-cell-depleted and non-T-cell-depleted allogeneic bone marrow transplantation for chronic myelogenous leukemia: impact of donor lymphocyte infusion. *J Clin Oncol.* 1999;17:561–8.

67. Socié G, Schmoor C, Bethge WA, Ottinger HD, Stelljes M, Zander AR, *et al.* Chronic graft-*versus*-host disease: long-term results from a randomized trial on graft-*versus*-host disease prophylaxis with or without anti-T-cell globulin ATG-Fresenius. *Blood.* 2011;117:6375–82.

68. Lin F, van Rhee F, Goldman JM, Cross NC. Kinetics of increasing BCR-ABL transcript numbers in chronic myeloid leukemia patients who relapse after

bone marrow transplantation. *Blood.* 1996;87:4473–8.

69. Krejci M, Mayer J, Doubek M, Brychtova Y, Pospisil Z, Racil Z, *et al.* Clinical outcomes and direct hospital costs of reduced-intensity allogeneic transplantation in chronic myeloid leukemia. *Bone Marrow Transplant.* 2006;38:483–91.

70. Dazzi F, Szydlo RM, Craddock C, Cross NC, Kaeda J, Chase A, *et al.* Comparison of single-dose and escalating-dose regimens of donor lymphocyte infusion for relapse after allografting for chronic myeloid leukemia. *Blood.* 2000;95:67–71.

71. Innes AJ, Beattie R, Sergeant R, Damaj G, Foroni L, Marin D, *et al.* Escalating-dose HLA-mismatched DLI is safe for the treatment of leukaemia relapse following alemtuzumab-based myeloablative allo-SCT. *Bone Marrow Transplant.* 2013;48:1324–8.

72. Innes AJ, Lurkins J, Szydlo R, Guerra A, Milojkovic D, Pavlu J *et al.* The majority of patients receiving donor lymphocyte infusions for relapsed chronic myeloid leukemia remain PCR positive despite maintaining long-term remission. *Blood.* 2011:118: Abstract 4103.

73. Zeidner JF1, Zahurak M, Rosner GL, Gocke CD, Jones RJ, Smith BD. The evolution of treatment strategies for patients with chronic myeloid leukemia relapsing after allogeneic bone marrow transplant: can tyrosine kinase inhibitors replace donor lymphocyte infusions? *Leuk Lymphoma.* 2015;56:128–34.

Allogeneic Hematopoietic Cell Transplants for *BCR/ABL Negative* Myeloproliferative Neoplasms

Nicolaus Kröger

Introduction

The term myelofibrosis (MF) refers to primary myelofibrosis (PMF) which is a hematopoietic stem cell-derived hematologic disorder characterized by a clonal proliferation of multiple cell elements, especially the megakaryocytes. This proliferation is accompanied by an increased secretion of different cytokines with a secondary intramedullary fibrosis, osteosclerosis, angiogenesis, and extramedullary hematopoiesis[1]. Additionally, MF may develop as a late evolution of two other myeloproliferative neoplasms: polycythemia vera (post-PV MF) and essential thrombocythemia (post-ET MF)[2]. The life expectancy of patients with PMF is variable and the median survival is 69 months (95% CI 61–76). Causes of death are: transformation to acute myelogenous leukemia (AML) (31%), progression without acute transformation (19%), thrombosis and cardiovascular complications (14%), infection (10%) or bleeding (5%), portal hypertension (4%), and other less common causes (14%)[3].

Prognostic Stratification for PMF

A recent study established the International Prognostic Scoring System (IPSS) for PMF which employs five prognostic variables: age >65 years, constitutional symptoms related to disease, hemoglobin (Hb) <10 g/dL, white blood cell (WBC) count >25×10^9/L, and the presence of circulating blasts. Median survival in the low-risk category (no risk factor) was 135 months, intermediate-1 risk category (one risk factor) 95 months, intermediate-2 risk category (two risk factors) 48 months, and high-risk category 27 months. The IPSS is a powerful risk stratification tool to estimate the life expectancy of PMF patients at diagnosis. To track change of prognosis due to acquisition of new risk factors over time, IWG-MRT introduced the dynamic IPSS (DIPSS)[4], which includes the same variables used in IPSS but applies more weight on the acquisition of anemia. Recently, several other IPSS independent risk factors such as unfavorable cytogenetics (+8, −7/7q-, i(17q), inv(3), −5/5q-, 12p- or 11q23 rearrangement, median survival approximately 40 months)[5], and transfusion dependency (median survival approximately 20 months)[6] were identified and combined with DIPSS to result in the "DIPSSplus" stratification system[7]. The systems are increasingly used in the

daily praxis to advise PMF patients about their individualized risk status and guide therapy decisions (see Table 37.1). More recently it has been found that molecular mutations can also be used as a prognostic model for survival[8]. PMF can be cured with successful allogeneic hematopoietic cell transplant (allo-HCT)[9]. The applicability of allo-HCT is however limited due to the associated treatment-related mortality (TRM).

Nontransplant Strategies for PMF

Conventional therapies for treatment of PMF/MF include the use of hematopoietic growth factors such as erythropoietin, androgens, immune-modulating drugs, interferon-alpha, cytoreductive agents, and nonpharmacologic options such as blood transfusion, spleen irradiation, and splenectomy. None of these approaches have been shown to prolong patient survival.

JAK2V617F mutation is an acquired point mutation in the pseudo-kinase domain of *the Janus kinase-2* which confers a constitutive JAK2 pathway activation with resulting growth factor-independent proliferation of myeloid precursors[10,11].

JAK inhibitors are compounds developed for the treatment of myeloproliferative neoplasm. Ruxolitinib is the first JAK inhibitor approved by the US Food and Drug Administration (FDA) for use in patients with intermediate- or high-risk MF (primary MF, post-PV/ET-MF) and in Europe for symptomatic MF patients with splenomegaly, regardless of the IPSS risk classification. Ruxolitinib, a JAK1/ JAK2 inhibitor, showed early and sustained clinical benefits in patients with intermediate-2 and high-risk MF, including spleen size reduction and improvement of constitutional symptoms in a phase 1/2 trial (INCB18424-251) and the phase 3 trials COMFORT-I and COMFORT-II[12–14]. A survival benefit with ruxolitinib was shown in the COMFORT-I analysis and in a 3-year follow-up of the COMFORT-II study [15,16] and also more recently according to DIPSS[17].

Allogeneic Hematopoietic Cell Transplant for PMF

Allo-HCT Statistics and Myeloablative Conditioning *versus* Reduced Intensity Conditioning

The published experience in allo-HCT for myelofibrosis is summarized in Table 37.2. In the late 1980s and the early

Table 37.1 Prognostic scoring systems for PMF

IPSS[3]				
Clinical feature	**Points**	**Prognostic category**	**Points**	**Median survival (months)**
Age >65 years	1	Low	0	135
Constitutional symptoms1	1	Intermediate-1	1	95
Hb <10 g/dL	2	Intermediate-2	2	48
WBC count >25 × 10⁹/L	1	High	≥3	27
Peripheral blasts ≥1%	1	Low	0	135
DIPSS[4]				
Clinical feature	**Points**	**Prognostic category**	**Points**	**Median survival (months)**
Age >65 years	1	Low	0	Not reached
Constitutional symptoms[a]	1	Intermediate-1	1–2	170
Hb <10 g/dL	2	Intermediate-2	3–4	48
WBC count >25 × 10⁹/l	1	High	5–6	18
Peripheral blasts ≥1%	1			
DIPSS –Plus[7]				
Clinical feature	**Points**	**Prognostic category**	**Points**	**Median survival (months)**
DIPSS-low	0	Low	0	185
DIPSS-int-1	1	Intermediate-1	1	78
DIPSS-int-2	2	Intermediate-2	2–3	35
DIPSS-high	1	High	4–6	16
PLUS				
Unfavorable karyotype[b]	1			
Transfusion dependence	1			
Platelet <100000/μL	1			

[a] Constitutional symptoms: weight loss >10% of the baseline value in the year preceding PMF diagnosis and/or unexplained fever or excessive sweats persisting for more than 1 months.
[b] Unfavorable karyotype: complex karyotype or single or two abnormalities including +8, -7/7q-, i(17q), -5/5q-,12p-, inv(3), or 11q23 rearrangement.

1990s the feasibility of allo-HCT for MF could be shown in small reports[18,19]. One multicenter European-American report was published in the late 1990s and described a retrospective study with larger cohort in which allo-HCT was performed using myeloablative conditioning (MAC) regimens in relatively young patients (median age 42 years). Nonrelapse mortality (NRM) was 27% and the incidence of graft failure was 9%. The median overall survival (OS) and progression-free survival (PFS) reached 47% and 39% at 5 years[20]. Another important study from the Fred Hutchinson Cancer Center in Seattle was first published in 2003 and updated 5 years later to include 104 patients most of whom received allo-HCT after MAC regimens. In this study, NRM at 5 years of 34% and OS at 7 years of 61% were reported[9,21]. A TBI-based study resulted in a high-risk NRM of 48% and a 2-year OS of 41%[22].

Since MF is a disease of elderly, the need was urgent to improve the tolerability of allo-HCT and enable more patients with advanced age to benefit from this treatment modality. The evidence of graft-*versus*-leukemia effect was already available through documented responses to donor lymphocyte infusion (DLI) after failure of allo-HCT[23,24]. This justified the use of reduced intensity conditioning (RIC) in the setting of allo-HCT for MF. Small pilot reports could confirm that RIC can reduce NRM without jeopardizing engraftment [25–28]. Larger clinical trials were published thereafter but the only prospective study with a large sample size was conducted by the European Group of Blood and Marrow Transplantation (EBMT) and published in 2009 after including 103 patients. The median age was 55 years and the NRM at 1 year was only 16%. Cumulative incidence of relapse was 22% at 3 years. The

Table 37.2 Selected trials of allogeneic hematopoietic cell transplant in myelofibrosis

Author	No. of patients	Conditioning regimen	Median age	Transplant-related mortality at 1 year	Overall survival
MAC regimen					
Guardiola et al. 1999[20]	55	TBI-based (n=35), various (n=20)	42	27%	39% (at 5 years)
Deeg et al. 2003[21]	56	Busulfan-based (n=44), TBI-based (n=12)	43	20%	31% (at 5 years)
Kerbauy et al. 2007[9]	104	TBI-based (n=15), busulfan-based (n=80), reduced intensity (n=9)	49	34% (at 5 years)	61% (at 7 years)
Daly et al. 2003[22]	25	TBI-based		48%	41% (at 2 years)
RIC conditioning					
Hessling et al. 2002[25]	3	Busulfan/fludarabine	51	0%	100% (at 1 year)
Devine et al. 2002[26]	4	Melphalan/fludarabine	56	0%	100% (at 1 year)
Rondelli et al. 2005[27]	21	Various	54	10%	85% (at 2.5 years)
Kröger et al. 2005[28]	21	Busulfan/fludarabine	53	16%	84% (at 3 years)
Bacigalupo et al. 2010 [32]	46	Thiotepa-based	51	24% (at 5 years)	45% (at 5 years)
Kröger et al. 2009[29]	103	Busulfan/fludarabine	55	16%	67% (at 5 years)
Gupta et al. 2014[33]	233	Various	55	24% (at 5 years)	47% (at 5 years)
Rondelli et al. 2014[31]	66	Melphalan/fludarabine	56	22% (sibling) 59% (unrelated donor)	75% (sibling) 32% (unrelated donor)
MAC regimen + RIC					
Stewart et al. 2010[34]	51	Different	49	32%	45% (at 5 years)
Ballen et al. 2010[35]	170 (sibling)	Different	45	18% at day 100	100% (at 16 months)
	117 (MUD)		47	35% at day 100	67% (at 5 years)
	33 (alternative related)		40	19% at day 100	44 % (at 3 years)
Robin et al. 2011[36]	147	Different	53	16%	37% (5 years)
Patriarca et al. 2008[42]	100	Different	49	43% (at 3 years)	42% (at 3 years)
Gupta et al. 2009[37]	46	Different	47 (MAC regimen) 54 (RIC)	48% MAC regimen 27% RIC	48% MAC regimen (at 3 years) 68% RIC
Abelsson et al. 2012[38]	92	Different	46 (MAC regimen) 55 (RIC)	32% STD (at 2 years) 24% RIC (at 2 years)	49% MAC regimen (at 5 years) 59% RIC (at 5 years)
Ditschkowsky et al. 2012[39]	76	Different	50.5	36% (at 5 years)	53% (at 5 years)
Nivison-Smith et al. 2012[41]	57	Different	47	25% (at 1 years)	58% (at 5 years)
Scott et al. 2012[40]	170	Different	51.5	34% (at 5 years)	57% (at 5 years)

PFS and OS at 5 years were 51% and 67%, respectively. Advanced age and HLA-mismatched donor were independent predictive factors for reduced OS[29]. The study was updated recently after a median follow-up of 60 months and published in abstract form. Eight-year OS was 65% with a stable plateau after 5.3 years follow-up. The 5-year DFS was 40% and 5-year cumulative incidence of relapse/progression was 28% with 3-year NRM of 21%[30]. The prospective study of the Myeloproliferative Disorder Research Consortium included 66 patients with PMF or post-ET/PV MF who received a melphalan/fludarabine-based RIC regimen followed by HLA-identical sibling or unrelated donor cell transplantation. While the OS of the sibling transplantation was 75%, the survival of the unrelated donor grafts was only 32% due to a higher nonrelapse mortality (59% *versus* 22%)[31].

Other studies using RIC or MAC regimens confirmed the curative effect of allo-HCT irrespectively of the intensity of the conditioning regimen[32–42]. It could be speculated that reduction of NRM achieved using RIC regimens may be offset by the theoretical increased risk of relapse. Unfortunately, there is to date no prospective comparison between MAC and RIC regimens in PMF. However, a retrospective comparison could not show any statistically significant difference in outcome or relapse incidence[37].

Prevention and Treatment of Relapse

The efficacy of relapse prevention and treatment has improved in recent years due to the employment of minimal residual disease (MRD) monitoring strategies (see Chapters 23 and 24). Using sensitive assays to monitor JAK2V617F mutation – detectable in 60% of patients with MPN – after allo-HCT, MRD and molecular relapse could be treated early using DLIs in lower doses resulting in no or less severe graft-*versus*-host disease (GvHD)[43]. Recently, more mutations and molecular markers such as MPLW515L/K, TET2, ASXL-1, or CALR have been discovered in Ph-neg MPN[44–46]. The possibility to use those markers for MRD analysis in MF should be elucidated in future studies. Even those patients who did not respond to DLI or could not receive DLI for different reasons, a second allo-HCT resulted in a 2-year OS of 70%[47] (see Chapters 25, 26, and 65).

Timing of Transplantation: Limitations and Recommendations

According to the published recommendations of the European LeukemiaNet (ELN) it seems justified to offer allo-HCT to eligible patients with PMF whose median survival is expected to be less than 5 years with nontransplant strategies (described above). This typically includes patients with intermediate-2 risk and high-risk groups according to IPSS or DIPSS and those with transfusion dependency or unfavorable cytogenetic[48]. Retrospective studies from Germany and the United States have shown that allo-HCT for low-risk disease

Table 37.3 Allogeneic HCT for MPN transformed to acute leukemia

Author	No. of patients	TRM	Relapse	3-year OS
Alchalby et al. 2014 [50]	46	28%	47%	33%
Lussana et al. 2014 [52]	57 (transformed from ET or PV)	29%	53%	28%
Cahu et al. 2014[51]	60	22%	68%	18%

according to IPSS or DIPSS resulted in a long-term survival of more than 80%[40,49] but the inherent therapy-related mortality and the long-term survival of low-risk disease patients without transplantation argues against a general recommendation for allo-HCT in those patients. For intermediate-1 patients the transplant indication should be determined according to individual risk factors, mainly in younger patients. It is possible that besides DIPSS, molecular markers may help in the future to identify patients with intermediate-1 risk who will benefit from allo-HCT. If the disease is transformed to acute leukemia, results of conventional therapy are poor. Even transplantation of patients with transformed acute leukemia resulted in worse outcome but some patients can be cured by allo-HCT. The EBMT reports a 3-year OS of 33%[50], the Societe Française de Greffe de Moelle et de Therapie Cellulaire (SFGM-TC) reported a 3-year OS of 18%[51], while patients with PV/ET who transformed to AML achieved a 28% OS after allo-HCT within an EBMT study[52]. In all studies achievement of complete remission prior to transplantation resulted in an improved outcome. In all studies the major treatment failure was a high incidence of relapse (see Table 37.3).

Specific Considerations and Controversies Related to Outcomes After allo-HCT

Disease-Specific Factors

The status of the disease determined either by the Lille score or by IPSS/DIPSS influenced the outcome of transplantation in the majority of studies[29,35,36,39,40]. The more advanced the disease was classified, the shorter was the OS. Other disease-specific factors such as spleen size[32], cytogenetics[20], JAK2V617F mutation[53], CALR mutation[54], circulating CD34+ cells[55], and transfusion dependency[32] have not been confirmed by the majority of studies or still need confirmation by others.

Age of the Subject

Age as a risk factor for outcome after transplantation has been reported by several investigators[20,21,29,49]. Here, apart from being a risk factor within the IPSS and DIPSS classification, age *per se* has been shown to be an independent risk factor. Other patient-related factors were constitutional symptoms[49], lower performance status[35], and higher comorbidity score[56]. Despite the strong effect of age on outcome after transplantation "older patients" with PMF can be transplanted successfully[57].

Type of Donor: Does It Matter in PMF

While in acute leukemia and MDS the transplant results of HLA-identical sibling and fully matched unrelated donor are similar, few studies in PMF reported worse outcome after unrelated donor cell transplantation[31,32]. Mismatched unrelated donor cell transplantation resulted in inferior outcome in most of the studies[29,36,49]. Alternative donor source such as cord blood resulted in a higher risk of graft failure (20%) and survival of 44% at 2 years, which cannot be regarded as an equivalent alternative to HLA-matched unrelated allo-HCT[58].

The Role of Splenectomy Prior to Allo-HCT

The role of splenectomy before allo-HCT remains controversial[29,35,40]. However, nearly all studies showed faster engraftment for patients who received splenectomy prior to transplantation[20,29,59]. The high morbidity and mortality in case of splenectomy prior to transplantation has to be taken into account. A procedure-related mortality of about 7% has been reported[60]. A more recent available option to reduce spleen size prior to transplantation is the use of JAK inhibition[61].

Effect of Bone Marrow Fibrosis on Allo-HCT Outcomes

Bone marrow fibrosis is a hallmark of primary or post-ET/PV myelofibrosis[62]. The fibrogenesis is not completely understood and probably caused by cytokines such as platelet-derived growth factor (PDGF), beta-fibroblast-derived growth factor (βFGF), or transforming growth factor β (TGF-β) secreted from clonal megakaryocytes and/or clonal monocyte/histiocyte proliferation[63–65].

Fibrosis grade correlates with other clinical parameters such as hemoglobin, myeloblasts, LDH, and spleen size[66] and some studies found a correlation between grade of fibrosis and survival[66–68]. However, some studies did not find an effect on survival regarding grading of fibrosis [49,69–71]. Overall, bone marrow fibrosis is not included in any of the currently used risk classifications (Lille score, Cervantes Score, IPSS, DIPSS, and DIPSS plus). Bone marrow fibrosis regression after allo-HCT has been reported[72] and in some cases after treatment with interferon-alpha[73], pomalidomide[74], and more recently after ruxolitinib[75]. A recent study showed that rapid bone marrow fibrosis regression on day +100 after reduced allo-HCT resulted in a favorable survival independently of IPSS

risk score at transplantation. In contrast patients with persistent grade 2 or 3 fibrosis at day +100 were more likely to be transfusion-dependent regarding red blood cells ($P=0.014$) or platelets ($P=0.018$)[76].

JAK Signal Inhibition for Myelofibrosis

JAK Inhibition

The discovery of MPN-associated molecular markers (especially JAK2V617F) resulted in numerous efforts to develop efficient targeted therapies hoping to alter disease process. JAK2 inhibitors were developed, tested clinically, and found to alleviate some disease-related symptoms. The first JAK inhibition that was approved for treatment of myelofibrosis was the JAK1/2 inhibitor ruxolitinib (INCBO18424) in the United States and Europe.

Ruxolitinib (INCB018424): Is There a Survival Benefit?

This drug is a JAK1 and JAK2 inhibitor which has already completed two phase 3 clinical trials. By using a dose of 15 mg twice daily a significant reduction of splenomegaly and constitutional symptoms can be reached in about 50% of patients. Responses could be reached also in JAK2-unmutated patients and correlated well with reduction of serum inflammatory cytokines. Worsening of anemia or reversible thrombocytopenia are the main toxic effects. In the COMFORT-I trial patients were randomized to start the drug at a dose of 15 mg or 20 mg orally twice a day depending on baseline platelet count against placebo. At week 24 the proportion of patients with ≥50% improvement in splenomegaly was 45.9% *versus* 5.3%[77]. The COMFORT-II trial, on the other hand, randomized ruxolitinib against best available therapy and included 219 patients. Again, reduction of the spleen volume of ≥35% from baseline at 48 weeks of therapy was reached in 28.5% of patients compared with 0% in the control arm[78]. A survival benefit was seen in the COMFORT-I and COMFORT-II study. Long-term studies of the initial phase 2 study showed that intermediate-2 and high-risk patients showed a survival benefit in comparison to a historical control, and the discontinuation rate at 1, 2, and 3 years was 24%, 36%, and 46%, respectively. Furthermore, patients with significant (>50%) spleen size reduction had prolonged survival whereas there was only moderate, if any, reduction in JAK2 allelic burden; recent data reported some regression of bone marrow fibrosis after ruxolitinib treatment[75]. Other JAK1 or JAK2 inhibitors are currently being tested in clinical trials and are not approved as yet.

JAK2 Inhibitors Before Allo-HCT: Is It Safe?

Reduction of spleen size, improving constitutional symptoms, and reduction of proinflammatory state and cytokine

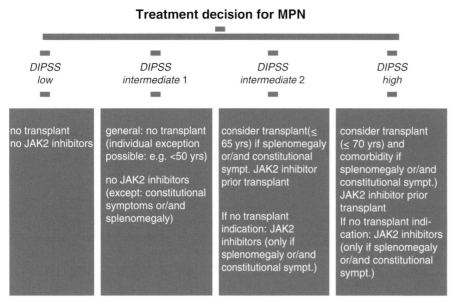

Treatment decision for MPN

Figure 37.1 Treatment decision for MPN

DIPSS low	DIPSS intermediate 1	DIPSS intermediate 2	DIPSS high
no transplant no JAK2 inhibitors	general: no transplant (individual exception possible: e.g. <50 yrs) no JAK2 inhibitors (except: constitutional symptoms or/and splenomegaly)	consider transplant(≤ 65 yrs) if splenomegaly or/and constitutional sympt. JAK2 inhibitor prior transplant If no transplant indication: JAK2 inhibitors (only if splenomegaly or/and constitutional sympt.)	consider transplant (≤ 70 yrs) and comorbidity if splenomegaly or/and constitutional sympt.) JAK2 inhibitor prior transplant If no transplant indication: JAK2 inhibitors (only if splenomegaly or/and constitutional sympt.)

dysregulation prior to transplantation as the major benefits of JAK inhibitors might improve outcome after transplantation. These benefits are seen regardless of JAK2 mutational status. Reduction of spleen size may improve engraftment and graft function. Constitutional symptoms at time of transplantation have been shown to be a major risk factor for survival after allo-HCT[49]. Therefore it seems reasonable to use JAK2 inhibitors prior to transplantation. In addition, down-regulation of inflammatory cytokines (IL-6, IL-1ra, MIP-1β, TNF-α, and CRP) and modulation of T-cell response seen with JAK inhibitor use may reduce the incidence of GvHD after transplant, a significant cause of morbidity and mortality[79]. The few available data mainly suggest feasibility without significant withdrawal symptoms[61,80]. However, because one prospective study reported complications on withdrawal of ruxolitinib, including cardiogenic shock, tumor lysis syndrome, and severe GvHD[81], more data and studies are needed before a valid conclusion can be drawn.

Practice Points

The management of patients with MF has improved in the last decade. A growing experience in allo-HCT as the only curative treatment accumulated over time and new promising novel therapies were developed for the palliative application. Through the improved understanding and prediction of the natural history of the disease it is now possible to estimate the life expectancy of every patient individually and at every time point after diagnosis. Asymptomatic patients corresponding to a low or intermediate IPSS risk score should be offered a "watch and wait" strategy if there are no constitutional symptoms or splenomegaly. When symptoms warrant treatment, medical therapy can be initiated and the approach should be symptom-oriented. It should, however, be kept in mind that palliative therapy may change

blood counts and reduce systemic complaints without altering the disease process. Those patients should be carefully monitored for acquisition of new risk factors and for disease acceleration. JAK2 inhibitor therapy can also be offered to symptomatic patients and the main goal of therapy should be alleviating symptoms and maintaining quality of life. Patients with limited life expectancy who are otherwise in good condition and have a suitable donor should be offered allo-HCT through at an experienced transplant center. Some of those patients (allo-HCT candidates) may already have exhausting symptoms and may be offered medical therapy prior to transplantation. It may be possible that reduction of disease burden or improving the general condition before allo-HCT may positively influence its outcome. Early data using ruxolitinib before transplantation in order to reduce spleen size and constitutional symptoms have shown feasibility and did not negatively affect outcome of transplantation[61,80]. But, on the other hand, it is now too early to exclude that some of those medications may negatively interfere with allo-HCT outcome and cardiac toxicity and tumor lysis syndrome have been reported[81]. This issue is currently the subject of clinical trials (NCT 01795677). A potential algorithm is listed in Figure 37.1.

Conclusion

Overall improvement in management of allo-HCT for myelofibrosis has increased the number of the procedure which remains the only curative treatment approach. By harnessing the major effect of JAK inhibitors such as spleen size reduction and improvement of constitutional symptoms before transplantation further reduction of treatment-related complications is likely which will result in an improved survival.

References

1. Tefferi A. Pathogenesis of myelofibrosis with myeloid metaplasia. *J Clin Oncol.* 2005;23(33):8520–30.

2. Mesa RA, Verstovsek S, Cervantes F, Barosi G, Reilly JT, Dupriez B, *et al.* Primary myelofibrosis (PMF), post polycythemia vera myelofibrosis (post-PV MF), post essential thrombocythemia myelofibrosis (post-ET MF), blast phase PMF (PMF-BP): Consensus on terminology by the international working group for myelofibrosis research and treatment (IWG-MRT). *Leuk Res.* 2007;31(6):737–40.

3. Cervantes F, Dupriez B, Pereira A, Passamont F, Reilly JT, Morra E, *et al.* New prognostic scoring system for primary myelofibrosis based on a study of the International Working Group for Myelofibrosis Research and Treatment. *Blood.* 2009;113(13):2895–901.

4. Passamonti F, Cervantes F, Vannucchi AM, Morra E, Rumi E, Pereira A, *et al.* A dynamic prognostic model to predict survival in primary myelofibrosis: a study by the IWG-MRT (International Working Group for Myeloproliferative Neoplasms Research and Treatment). *Blood.* 2010;115(9):1703–08.

5. Caramazza D, Begna KH, Gangat N, Vaidya R, Siragusa S, Van Dyke DL, *et al.* Refined cytogenetic-risk categorization for overall and leukemia-free survival in primary myelofibrosis: a single center study of 433 patients. *Leukemia.* 2011;25(1):82–8.

6. Tefferi A, Siragusa S, Hussein K, Schwager SM, Hanson CA, Pardanani A, *et al.* Transfusion-dependency at presentation and its acquisition in the first year of diagnosis are both equally detrimental for survival in primary myelofibrosis—prognostic relevance is independent of IPSS or karyotype. *Am J Hematol.* 2010;85(1):14–7.

7. Gangat N, Caramazza D, Vaidya R, George G, Begna K, Schwager S, *et al.* DIPSS plus: a refined Dynamic International Prognostic Scoring System for primary myelofibrosis that incorporates prognostic information from karyotype, platelet count, and transfusion status. *J Clin Oncol.* 2011;29(4):392–7.

8. Guglielmelli P, Lasho TL, Rotunno G, Score J, Mannarelli C, Pancrazzi A, *et al.* The number of prognostically detrimental mutations and prognosis in primary myelofibrosis: an international study of 797 patients. *Leukemia.* 2014;28(9):1804–10.

9. Kerbauy DM, Gooley TA, Sale GE, Flowers ME, Doney KC, Georges GE, *et al.* Hematopoietic cell transplantation as curative therapy for idiopathic myelofibrosis, advanced polycythemia vera, and essential thrombocythemia. *Biol Blood Marrow Transplant.* 2007;13(3):355–65.

10. Kralovics R, Passamonti F, Buser AS, Teo SS, Tiedt R, Passweg JR, *et al.* A gain-of-function mutation of JAK2 in myeloproliferative disorders. *N Engl J Med.* 2005;352(17):1779–90.

11. James C, Ugo V, Le Couedic JP, Staerk J, Delhommeau F, Lacout C, *et al.* A unique clonal JAK2 mutation leading to constitutive signaling causes polycythaemia vera. *Nature.* 2005;434(7037):1144–8.

12. Verstovsek S, Kantarjian H, Mesa R, Pardanani AD, Cortes-Franco J, Thomas DA, *et al.* Safety and efficacy of INCB018424, a JAK1 and JAK2 inhibitor, in myelofibrosis. *N Eng J Med.* 2010;363(12):1117–27.

13. Harrison C, Kiladjian JJ, Al-Ali HK, Gisslinger H, Waltzman R, Stabovskaya V, *et al.* JAK inhibition with ruxolitinib *versus* best available therapy for myelofibrosis. *N Eng J Med.* 2012;366(9):787–98.

14. Verstovsek S, Mesa RA, Gotlib JR, Levy RS, Gupta V, DiPersio JF, *et al.* A double-blind, placebo-controlled trial of ruxolitinib for myelofibrosis. *N Eng J Med.* 2012;366(9):799–807.

15. Cervantes F, Vannucchi AM, Kiladjian JJ, Al-Ali HK, Sirulnik A, Stalbovskaya V, *et al.* Three-year efficacy, safety, and survival findings from COMFORT-II, a phase 3 study comparing ruxolitinib with best available therapy for myelofibrosis. *Blood* 2013;122(25):4057–3.

16. Verstovsek S, Mesa RA, Gotlib J, Levy RS, Gupta V, DiPersio JF, *et al.* Efficacy, safety and survival with ruxolitinib treatment in patients with myelofibrosis: results of a median 2-year follow-up of COMFORT-I. *Haematologica.* 2013;98(12):1865–71.

17. Passamonti F, Maffioli M, Cervantes F, Vannucchi AM, Morra E, Barbui T, et al. Impact of ruxolitinib on the natural history of primary myelofibrosis: a comparison of the DIPSS and the COMFORT-2 cohorts. *Blood.* 2014;123(12):1833–5.

18. Dokal I, Jones L, Deenmamode M, Lewis SM, Goldman JM. Allogeneic bone marrow transplantation for primary myelofibrosis. *Br J Haematol.* 1989;71(1):158–60.

19. Creemers, GJ, Lowenberg B, Hagenbeek A. Allogeneic bone marrow transplantation for primary myelofibrosis. *Br J Haematol.* 1992;82(4):772–3.

20. Guardiola P, Anderson JE, Bandini G, Cervantes F, Runde V, Arcese W, *et al.* Allogeneic stem cell transplantation for agnogenic myeloid metaplasia: a European Group for Blood and Marrow Transplantation, Société Française de Greffe de Moelle, Gruppo Italiano per il Trapianto del Midollo Osseo, and Fred Hutchinson Cancer Research Center Collaborative Study. *Blood.* 1999;93(9):2831–8.

21. Deeg HJ, Gooley TA, Flowers ME, Sale GE, Slattery JT, Anasetti C, *et al.* Allogeneic hematopoietic stem cell transplantation for myelofibrosis. *Blood.* 2003;102(12):3912–18.

22. Daly A, Song K, Nevill T, Nantel S, Toze C, Hogge D, *et al.* Stem cell transplantation for myelofibrosis: a report from two Canadian centers. *Bone Marrow Transplant.* 2003;32(1):35–40.

23. Byrne JL, Beshti H, Clark D, Ellis I, Haynes AP, Das-Gupta E, *et al.* Induction of remission after donor leucocyte infusion for the treatment of relapsed chronic idiopathic myelofibrosis following allogeneic transplantation: evidence for a 'graft vs. myelofibrosis' effect. *Br J Haematol.* 2000;108(2):430–3.

24. Cervantes F, Rovira M, Urbano-Ispizua A, Rozman M, Carreras E, Montserrat E. Complete remission of idiopathic myelofibrosis following donor lymphocyte infusion after failure of allogeneic transplantation: demonstration of a graft-*versus*-myelofibrosis effect. *Bone Marrow Transplant.* 2000;26(6):697–9.

25. Hessling J, Kröger N, Werner M, Zabelina T, Hansen A, Kordes U, *et al.* Dose-reduced conditioning regimen followed by allogeneic stem cell transplantation in patients with myelofibrosis with myeloid metaplasia. *Br J Haematol.* 2002;119(3):769–72.

26. Devine SM, Hoffman R, Verma A, Shah R, Bradlow BA, Stock W, et al. Allogeneic blood cell transplantation following reduced-intensity conditioning is effective therapy for older patients with myelofibrosis with myeloid metaplasia. *Blood.* 2002;99(6):2255–8.

27. Rondelli D, Barosi G, Bacigalupo A, Prchal U, Alessandrino EP, Spivak JL, et al. Allogeneic hematopoietic stem-cell transplantation with reduced-intensity conditioning in intermediate- or high-risk patients with myelofibrosis with myeloid metaplasia. *Blood.* 2005;105(10):4115–9.

28. Kröger N, Zabelina T, Schieder H, Panse J, Ayuk F, Stute N, et al. Pilot study of reduced-intensity conditioning followed by allogeneic stem cell transplantation from related and unrelated donors in patients with myelofibrosis. *Br J Haematol.* 2005;128(5):690–7.

29. Kröger N, Holler E, Kobbe G, Bornhäuser M, Schwerdtfeger R, Baurmann H, et al. Allogeneic stem cell transplantation after reduced-intensity conditioning in patients with myelofibrosis: a prospective, multicenter study of the Chronic Leukemia Working Party of the European Group for Blood and Marrow Transplantation. *Blood.* 2009;114(26):5264–70.

30. Alchalby H, Zabelina T, Wolff D, Kobbe G, Bornhäuser M, Baurmann H, et al. Long Term Follow-up of the Prospective Multicenter Study of reduced-Intensity Allogeneic Stem Cell Transplantation for Primary or Post ET/PV Myelofibrosis. *Blood (ASH Annual Meeting Abstracts).* 2011;118: Abstract 1019.

31. Rondelli D, Goldberg J, Isola L, Price LS, Shore TB, Boyer M, et al. MPD-RC 101 prospective study of reduced intensity allogeneic hematopoietic stem cell transplantation in patients with myelofibrosis. *Blood.* 2014;124(7):1183–91.

32. Bacigalupo A, Soraru M, Dominietto A, Pozzi S, Geroldi S, Van Lint MT, et al. Allogeneic hemopoietic SCT for patients with primary myelofibrosis: a predictive transplant score based on transfusion requirement, spleen, and donor type. *Bone Marrow Transplant.* 2010;45(3): 458–63.

33. Gupta V, Malone AK, Hari PN, Ahn KW, Hu ZH, Gale RP, et al. Reduced-intensity hematopoietic cell transplantation for patients with primary myelofibrosis: a cohort analysis from the center for international blood and marrow transplant research. *Biol Blood Marrow Transplant.* 2014;20(1): 89–97.

34. Stewart WA, Pearce R, Kirkland KE, Bloor A, Thomson K, Apperley J, et al. The role of allogeneic SCT in primary myelofibrosis: a British Society for Blood and Marrow Transplantation study. *Bone Marrow Transplant.* 2010;45(11):1587–93.

35. Ballen KK, Shrestha A, Sobocinski KA, Zhang MJ, Bashey A, Bolwell BJ, et al. Outcome of transplantation for myelofibrosis. *Biol Blood Marrow Transplant.* 2010;16(3):358–67.

36. Robin M, Tabrizi R, Mohty M, Furst S, Michallet M, Bay JO, et al. Allogeneic haematopoietic stem cell transplantation for myelofibrosis: a report of the Société Française de Greffe de Moelle et de Thérapie Cellulaire (SFGM-TC). *Br J Haematol.* 2011;152(3):331–9.

37. Gupta V, Kröger N, Aschan J, Xu W, Leber B, Dalley C, et al. A retrospective comparison of conventional intensity conditioning and reduced-intensity conditioning for allogeneic hematopoietic cell transplantation in myelofibrosis. *Bone Marrow Transplant.* 2009;44(5):317–20.

38. Abelsson J, Merup M, Birgegard G, Weis Bjerrum O, Brinch L, Brune M, et al. The outcome of allo-HSCT for 92 patients with myelofibrosis in the Nordic countries. *Bone Marrow Transplant.* 2012;47(3):380–6.

39. Ditschkowski M, Elmaagacli AH, Trenschel R, Gromke T, Steckel NK, Koldehoff M, et al. Dynamic International Prognostic Scoring scores, pre-transplant therapy and chronic graft-*versus*-host disease determine outcome after allogeneic hematopoietic stem cell transplantation for myelofibrosis. *Haematologica.* 2012;97(10):1574–81.

40. Scott BL, Gooley TA, Sorror ML, Rezvani AR, Linenberger ML, Grim J, et al. The Dynamic International Prognostic Scoring System for myelofibrosis predicts outcomes after hematopoietic cell transplantation. *Blood.* 2012;119(11): 2657–64.

41. Nivison-Smith I, Dodds AJ, Butler J, Bradstock KF, Ma DD, Simpson JM, et al. Allogeneic hematopoietic cell transplantation for chronic myelofibrosis in Australia and New Zealand: older recipients receiving myeloablative conditioning at increased mortality risk. *Biol Blood Marrow Transplant.* 2012;18(2):302–8.

42. Patriarca F, Bacigalupo A, Sperotto A, Isola M, Soldano F, Bruno B, et al. Allogeneic hematopoietic stem cell transplantation in myelofibrosis: the 20-year experience of the Gruppo Italiano Trapianto di Midollo Osseo (GITMO). *Haematologica.* 2008;93(10):1514–22.

43. Kröger N, Alchalby H, Klyuchnikov E, Badbaran A, Hildebrandt Y, Ayuk F, et al. JAK2-V617F-triggered preemptive and salvage adoptive immunotherapy with donor-lymphocyte infusion in patients with myelofibrosis after allogeneic stem cell transplantation. *Blood.* 2009;113(8):1866–8.

44. Vainchenker W, Delhommeau F, Constantinescu SN, Bernard OA. New mutations of myeloproliferative neoplasms. *Blood.* 2011;118(7):1723–35.

45. Klampfl T, Gisslinger H, Harutyunyan AS, Nivarthi H, Rumi E, Milosevic JD, et al. Somatic mutations of calreticulin in myeloproliferative neoplasms. *N Engl J Med.* 2013;369(25):2379–90.

46. Nangalia J, Massie CE, Baxter EJ, Nice FL, Gundem G, Wedge DC, et al. Somatic CALR mutations in myeloproliferative neoplasms with nonmutated JAK2. *N Engl J Med.* 2013;369(25):2391–405.

47. Klyuchnikov E, Holler E, Bornhäuser M, Kobbe G, Nagler A, Shimoni A, et al. Donor lymphocyte infusions and second transplantation as salvage treatment for relapsed myelofibrosis after reduced-intensity allografting. *Br J Haematol.* 2012;159(2):172–81.

48. Barbui T, Barosi G, Birgegard G, Cervantes F, Finazzi G, Griesshammer M, et al. Philadelphia-negative classical myeloproliferative neoplasms: critical concepts and management recommendations from European LeukemiaNet. *J Clin Oncol.* 2011;29(6):761–70.

49. Alchalby H, Yunus DR, Zabelina T, Kobbe G, Holler E, Bornhäuser M, et al. Risk models predicting survival after reduced-intensity transplantation for myelofibrosis. *Br J Haematol.* 2012;157(1):75–85.

50. Alchalby H, Zabelina T, Stübig T, van Biezen A, Bornhäuser M, Di Bartolomeo M, et al. Allogeneic stem cell transplantation for myelofibrosis with leukemic transformation: a study from the Myeloproliferative Neoplasm Subcommittee of the CMWP of the European Group for Blood and Marrow Transplantation. *Biol Blood Marrow Transplant.* 2014;20(2):279–81.

51. Cahu X, Chevallier P, Clavert A, Suarez F, Michallet M, Vincent L, et al. Allo-SCT for Philadelphia-negative myeloproliferativer neoplasms in blast phase: a study from the Societe Française de Greffe de Moelle et de Therapie Cellulaire (SFGM-TC). *Bone Marrow Transplant.* 2014;49(6):756–60.

52. Lussana F, Rimbaldi A, Finazzi MC, van Biezen A, Scholten M, Oldani E, et al. Allogeneic hematopoietic stem cell transplantation in patients with polycythemia vera or essential thrombocythemia transformed to myelofibrosis or acute myeloid leukemia: a report from the MPN Subcommittee of the Chronic Malignancies Working Party of the European Group for Blood and Marrow Transplantation. *Haematologica.* 2014;99(5):916–21.

53. Alchalby H, Badbaran A, Zabelina T, Kobbe G, Hahn J, Wolff D, et al. Impact of JAK2V617F mutation status, alelle burden, and clearance after allogeneic stem cell transplantation for myelofibrosis. *Blood.* 2010;116(18):3572–81.

54. Panagiota V, Thol F, Markus B, Fehse B, Alchalby H, Badbaran A, et al. Prognostic effect of calreticulin mutations in patients with myelofibrosis after allogeneic hematopoietic stem cell transplantation. *Leukemia.* 2014;28(7):1552–5.

55. Alchalby H, Lioznov M, Fritzsche-Friedland U, Badbaran A, Zabelina T, Bacher U, et al. Circulating CD34(+) cells as prognostic and follow-up marker in patients with myelofibrosis undergoing allo-SCT. *Bone Marrow Transplant.* 2012;47(1):143–5.

56. Kerbauy DM, Gooley TA, Sale GE, Flowers ME, Doney KC, Georges GE, et al. Hematopoietic cell transplantation as curative therapy for idiopathic myelofibrosis, advanced polycythemia very, and essential thrombocythemia. *Biol Blood Marrow Transplant.* 2007;13(3):355–65.

57. Samuelson S, Sandmaier BM, Heslop HE, Popat U, Carrum G, Champlin RE, et al. Allogeneic haematopoietic cell transplantation for myelofibrosis in 30 patients 60–78 years of age. *Br J Haematol.* 2011;153(1):76–82.

58. Robin M, Giannotti F, Deconinck E, Mohty M, Michallet M, Sanz G, et al. Unrelated cord blood transplantation for patients with primary or secondary myelofibrosis. *Biol Blood Marrow Transplant.* 2014;20(11):1841–6.

59. Ciurea SO, Sadegi B, Wilbur A, Alagiozian-Angelova V, Gaitonde S, Dobogai LC, et al. Effects of extensive splenomegaly in patients with myelofibrosis undergoing a reduced intensity allogeneic stem cell transplantation. *Br J Haematol.* 2008;141(1):80–3.

60. Mesa RA, Nagorney DS, Schwager S, Allred J, Tefferi A. Palliative goals, patient selection, and perioperative platelet management: outcomes and lessons from 3 decades of splenectomy for myelofibrosis with myeloid metaplasia at the Mayo Clinic. *Cancer.* 2006;107(2):361–70.

61. Stübig T, Alchalby H, Ditschkowski M, Wolf D, Wulf G, Zabelina T, et al. JAK inhibition with ruxolitinib as pretreatment for allogeneic stem cell transplantation in primary or post-ET/PV myelofibrosis. *Leukemia.* 2014;28(8):1736–8.

62. Tefferi A, Constantinescu SN. Introduction to 'A special spotlight review series on BCR-ABL-negative myeloproliferative neoplasms'. *Leukemia.* 2008;22(1):3–13.

63. Tefferi A. Myelofibrosis with myeloid metaplasia. *N Engl J Med.* 2000;342(17):1255–66.

64. Chagraoui H, Komura E, Tulliez M, Giraudier S, Vainchenker W, Wendling F. Prominent role of TGF-beta 1 in thrombopoietin-induced myelofibrosis in mice. *Blood.* 2002;100(10):3495–503.

65. Le Bousse-Kerdilès MC, Martyré MC, Samson M. Cellular and molecular mechanisms underlying bone marrow and liver fibrosis: a review. *Eur Cytokine Netw.* 2008;19(2):69–80.

66. Thiele J, Kvasnicka HM. Grade of bone marrow fibrosis is associated with relevant hematological findings– a clinicopathological study on 865 patients with chronic idiopathic myelofibrosis. *Ann Hematol.* 2006;85(4):226–32.

67. Barosi G, Rosti V, Bonetti E, Campanelli R, Carolei A, Catarsi P, et al. Evidence that prefibrotic myelofibrosis is aligned along a clinical and biological continuum featuring primary myelofibrosis. *PLOS One.* 2012;7:e35631

68. Gianelli U, Vener C, Bossi A, et al. The European Consensus on grading of bone marrow fibrosis allows a better prognostication of patients with primary myelofibrosis. *Mod Pathol.* 2012;25(9):1193–202.

69. Nazha A, Estrov Z, Cortes J, Bueso-Ramos CE, Kantarjian H, Verstovsek S. Prognostic implications and clinical characteristics associated with bone marrow fibrosis. *Leuk Lymphoma.* 2013;54(11):2537–9.

70. Strasser-Weippl K, Steurer M, Kees M, Agustin F, Tzankov A, Dirnhofer S, et al. Age and hemoglobin level emerge as most important clinical prognostic parameters in patients with osteomyelofibrosis: introduction of a simplified prognostic score. *Leuk Lymphoma.* 2006;47(3):441–50.

71. Anger B, Seidler R, Haug U, Popp C, Heimpel H. Idiopathic myelofibrosis: a retrospective study of 103 patients. *Haematologica.* 1990;75(3): 226–34.

72. Thiele J, Kvasnicka HM, Dietrich H, Stein G, Hann M, Kaminski A, et al. Dynamics of bone marrow changes in patients with chronic idiopathic myelofibrosis following allogeneic stem cell transplantation. *Histol Histopathol.* 2005;20(3):879–89.

73. Silver RT, Vadris K, Goldman JJ. Recombinant interferon-α may retard progression of early primary myelofibrosis: a preliminary report. *Blood.* 2011;117(24):6669–72.

74. Tefferi A, Verstovsek S, Barosi G, Passamonti F, Roboz GJ, Gisslinger H, et al. Pomalidomide is active in the treatment of anemia associated with myelofibrosis. *J Clin Oncol.* 2009;27(27):4563–9.

75. Kvasnicka HM, Thiele J, Bueso-Ramos CE, Hou K, Cortes JE, Kantarjian HM, et al. Exploratory analysis of the effect of ruxolitinib on bone marrow morphology in patients with myelofibrosis. (ASCO Annual Meeting Abstract). *J Clin Oncol.* 2013;31(15):7030.

76. Kröger N, Zabelina T, Alchalby H, Stübig T, Wolschke C, Ayuk F, et al.

Dynamic of bone marrow fibrosis regression predicts survival after allogeneic stem cell transplantation for myelofibrosis. *Biol Blood Marrow Transplant*. 2014;20(6):812–5.

77. Verstovsek S, Mesa RA, Gotlib JR, Levy RS, Gupta V, DiPersio JF, *et al*. Results of COMFORT-I, a randomized double-blind phase III trial of JAK1/2 inhibitor INCB18424 (424) *versus* placebo (PB) for patients with myelofibrosis (MF) (ASCO Annual Meeting Abstract). *J Clin Oncol*. 2011;29(15):6500.

78. Harrison CN, Kiladijan H, Al-Ali HK, Gisslinger H, Waltzman RJ, Stalbovskaya V, *et al*. Results of a randomized study of the JAK inhibitor INC424 compared with best available therapy (BAT) in primary myelofibrosis (PMF), post-polycythemia vera-myelofibrosis (PPV-MF) or post-essential thrombocythemia myelofibrosis (PET-MF). (ASCO Annual Meeting Abstract). *J Clin Oncol*. 2011;29(15): LBA6501.

79. Spoerl S, Mathew NR, Bscheider M, Schmitt-Graeff A, Chen S, Mueller T, *et al*. Activity of therapeutic JAK ½ blockade in graft-*versus*-host disease. *Blood*. 2014;123(24):3832–42.

80. Jaekel N, Behre G, Behning A, Wickenhauser C, Lange T, Niederwieser D, *et al*. Allogeneic hematopoietic cell transplantation for myelofibrosis in patients pretreated with the JAK1 and JAK2 inhibitor ruxolitinib. *Bone Marrow Transplant*. 2014;49(2):179–84.

81. Robin M, Francois S, Huynh A, Cassimat B, Bay JO, Cornillon J, *et al*. Ruxolitinib before allogeneic hematopoietic stem cell transplantation (HSCT) in patients with myelofibrosis: a preliminary descriptive report of the JAK ALLO study, a phase II trial sponsored by Goelams-FIM in collaboration with the Sfgmtc. *Blood*. 2013;122(21):abstract 306.

Chapter

38

Hematopoietic Cell Transplants for Hodgkin Lymphoma

Paolo F. Caimi

Introduction

Hodgkin lymphoma (HL) has high rates of response and cure after first-line therapy[1]. However, relapsed or refractory disease is encountered in approximately 10% of early stage and up to 30% of advanced stage patients with HL[2]. High-dose chemotherapy (HDT) followed by autologous hematopoietic cell transplant (HCT) is an established therapy for chemotherapy-sensitive HL, providing an opportunity of cure. There is no clear consensus on what salvage regimen is superior and whether there is a standard conditioning regimen. Other transplantation strategies, including first-line intensification with autologous HCT (auto-HCT), use of tandem auto-HCT, and allogeneic hematopoietic cell transplant have been studied with varied results in advanced patients with high-risk features for relapse and relapsed HL. It is still unclear whether graft-*versus*-lymphoma effect is relevant in HL. The introduction of brentuximab has allowed more patients to successfully receive allogeneic HCT.

Historical Perspective

Carella *et al.* reported the initial study of auto-HCT with 50 subjects with relapsed/refractory HL[3]. Disease status and treatment history were diverse: 25 patients did not receive salvage therapy before transplant (7 patients in first relapse and 18 patients with disease refractory to first-line therapy) and among the 25 patients that had salvage therapy, 12 had resistant disease. High-dose chemotherapy included cyclophosphamide, $3\,g/m^2$ per day for 2 days, etoposide $300\,mg/m^2$ per day for 2 days, and carmustine (BCNU) $300\,mg/m^2$ per day for 2 days. Overall response rate (ORR) was 80%, with 24 patients (48%) achieving a complete remission (CR). Complete responses were achieved in all patient groups, although those with chemotherapy-resistant disease had a lower rate of CR. Hematologic toxicity was predominant, with profound neutropenia and thrombocytopenia lasting a median of 16 and 18 days, respectively. All patients experienced febrile neutropenia requiring antibiotics, nausea, vomiting, and elevated liver enzymes. Four patients had carmustine-induced lung toxicity and two patients died as a result of the transplant. This initial report demonstrated the activity of autologous HCT in relapsed HL, and set the stage for subsequent prospective studies.

European Randomized Controlled Trials: Auto-HCT as the Standard of Care in Relapsed Setting

The establishment of auto-HCT as the standard of care for patients with relapsed HL came out of two prospective randomized studies. The first study, conducted by the British National Lymphoma Investigation (BNLI)[4] included relapsed or refractory HL patients after first-line chemotherapy. Subjects were randomized to receive up to three cycles of miniBEAM (carmustine $60\,mg/m^2$; etoposide $300\,mg/m^2$; cytarabine $800\,mg/m^2$; and melphalan $30\,mg/m^2$) or BEAM (carmustine $300\,mg/m^2$; etoposide $800\,mg/m^2$; cytarabine $1600\,mg/m^2$; and melphalan $140\,mg/m^2$) followed by HCT. This trial was closed early and included only 40 patients, after superior results were observed in the BEAM-HCT group. Complete remission rates were 15% after miniBEAM and 42% after BEAM-HCT ($P=0.06$), whereas 3-year event-free survival (EFS) was 10% and 53%, respectively ($P=0.025$). Overall survival was not statistically different, although it must be noted that at the time of reporting, 4 of 11 surviving miniBEAM subjects had received subsequent salvage with HCT. This first randomized trial demonstrated the superiority of HDT-HCT over conventional salvage chemotherapy, although it did not clarify whether the benefit was to any specific subgroup of HL patients[5]. A second, larger randomized study of HDT-HCT was conducted by the German Hodgkin Study Group (GHSG), and included 161 patients with relapsed HL[6]. Initial salvage was done with Dexa-BEAM (dexamethasone, carmustine $60\,mg/m^2$; etoposide $1000\,mg/m^2$; cytarabine $800\,mg/m^2$; and melphalan $20\,mg/m^2$). Patients who had a CR or partial response (PR) after salvage were randomized to receive two additional cycles of Dexa-BEAM or to receive myeloablative BEAM doses followed by HCT. Supportive care for HCT included the use of granulocyte colony-stimulating factor starting on the day of hematopoietic cell infusion. At a median follow-up of 39 months, freedom from treatment failure (FFTF) was superior in the transplant arm (55% *versus* 34%, $P=0.019$)[5]. The benefit of HDT-HCT occurred regardless of the time of relapse, although patients with late relapses appeared to have further improvements of FFTF. Overall survival was not different between treatment arms. Patients with multiple relapses did not benefit from HDT-HCT[6]. This trial established HDT-HCT as standard therapy for patients with chemosensitive disease. However, the high rates of toxicity and treatment-related mortality associated with Dexa-BEAM suggest its intensity was too high for use in salvage without hematopoietic cell support, and may have biased the results towards a benefit of HDT-HCT. Patients with disease refractory to first-line therapy were not included. The absence of OS improvement was most likely related to subsequent salvage with HDT-HCT in patients randomized to standard therapy, but long-term effects, in particular the development of secondary malignancies, could affect the lack of survival benefit for HDT-HCT. In conclusion, the trials conducted by BNLI and GHSG established HDT-HCT as standard therapy for patients with chemosensitive disease based on EFS and FFTF benefit. The role of HDT-HCT in patients with refractory disease or those with multiple relapses was not established through these studies, and will be explored in a separate section.

Is There One Superior Conditioning Regimen for Autologous Transplant in HL?

In addition to BEAM-type regimen, several conditioning regimens have been studied and reported (Table 38.1), but no direct or randomized comparisons have been done[2]. Regimens include: CBV (cyclophosphamide, etoposide, and carmustine)[3,7]; melphalan and etoposide[8]; CBVP (cyclophosphamide, infusional etoposide, carmustine, and cisplatin) [9]; CCV (cyclophosphamide, lomustine, and etoposide)[10]; high-dose melphalan[11]; and total lymphoid irradiation followed by etoposide and cyclophosphamide[12]. More recently, a new regimen including bendamustine, etoposide, cytarabine, and melphalan (BeEAM) has been reported as safe conditioning regimen for relapsed HL and NHLs[13]. The significant variability regarding the inclusion of patients with refractory disease and use of pretransplant radiation therapy make comparisons between conditioning regimens difficult. Moreover, the simultaneous progress in supportive care of transplant patients impedes adopting clear conclusions regarding differences in the tolerability of regimens used in different decades.

Is There a Role of Autologous Transplant in Subjects with Primary Refractory HL?

Subjects who never achieve remission with first-line chemotherapy and those who experience relapse less than 3 months after achieving CR have an extremely poor prognosis. As mentioned before, the initial randomized trials of autologous HCT for relapsed HL did not include these patients[4,6]. Two separate retrospective analyses examined the use of HDT-HCT in this patient population. André *et al.* compared the outcomes of 86 refractory or early relapsed HL patients who received HCT with 258 matched controls treated without transplant [14]. Six patients (7%) did not receive second-line salvage before HCT. The most commonly used conditioning regimens were BEAM and CBV. The 5-year OS and EFS for transplanted

patients were 35% and 25%, respectively. When compared with nontransplanted controls, 6-year OS did not reach statistical difference (38% *versus* 29%, $P=0.056$). Pretransplantation status of disease after salvage chemotherapy was the only parameter associated with poor survival. Investigators from the Autologous Blood and Marrow Transplant Registry (ABMTR) reported on the outcomes of HCT for a cohort of 122 HL patients who never achieved CR[15]. Forty-two percent of patients did not receive salvage before proceeding to HCT. Fifty percent of patients achieved CR and 16% achieved PR. Mortality at 100 days after autologous HCT was 12%. Three-year OS and PFS were 50% and 38%, respectively. Since these patients had not achieved CR at the time of HCT, chemosensitivity (in this patient population only) was defined as the presence of any response. The presence of B-symptoms and lower Karnofsky performance scores (KPS) were associated with decreased survival. Although the patient populations studied in these two reports were disparate, both represent the subgroup of patients with poorest prognosis and validate the use of HCT as salvage strategy, albeit with worse outcomes than patients who truly have chemosensitive disease. Patients with any response to salvage regimen (nonprogressive disease or less than PR in this patient population *versus* progressive disease), absence of symptoms, and better performance status are most likely to benefit from autologous HCT; however, caution is advised due to higher than usual post-transplant day-100 mortality.

Treatment Intensification Strategies in Primary Refractory and Subgroup of Patients with Relapsed HL: Is It Worth a Try or Not?

It was the recognition that BEAM-type conditioning regimens do not always work in certain subgroups of patients with relapsed HL which led to research for more intense approaches surrounding autologous HCT. The intensification strategies include: (1) augmented dose mobilization regimens (2); additional chemotherapy between hematopoietic cell mobilization and HDT; and (3) tandem HCT[2,16].

High-Intensity Conditioning Regimens

A retrospective analysis compared 60 patients conditioned with busulfan, melphalan, and thiotepa (BuMelTt) with 40 patients treated with other regimens[17]. After a median follow-up of 4.3 years, 5-year OS and PFS were 73% and 66% for patients treated with BuMelTt compared with 44% and 37% with other regimens, respectively ($P=0.05$ and 0.03, respectively). Nonrelapse mortality was comparable among groups. Mucositis was more common with BuMelTt. The effect of conditioning regimen intensity on the outcomes of patients with "poor-risk" relapsed HL was recently investigated by researchers from MD Anderson Cancer Center[18]. Poor risk was defined as patients with primary induction failure, relapse within 12 months of completion of first-line therapy,

Table 38.1 Conditioning regimens for autologous hematopoietic cell transplantation in Hodgkin lymphoma

Reference	Regimen	n	Agents	CR (%)	Progression endpoint (%)		TRM (%)	Comments
Carella et al. 1988 [3]	CBV	50	Cyclophosphamide 6g/m² Etoposide 600mg/m² Carmustine 300mg/m²	48	n/a	n/a	4	• Included patients with refractory disease
Linch et al. 1993[4]	BEAM	20	Carmustine 300mg/m² Etoposide 800mg/m² Cytarabine 1600mg/m² Melphalan 140mg/m²	42	3-y EFS	53	10	• Initial randomized trial of HCT versus chemotherapy • No OS benefit observed • Early closure secondary to poor accrual • Patients randomized to chemotherapy subsequently were salvaged with HCT
	miniBEAM (no HCT control)	20	Carmustine 60mg/m² Etoposide 300mg/m²; Cytarabine 800mg/m²; Melphalan 30mg/m²	15		10	0	
Schmitz et al. 2002 [6]	BEAM	61	Carmustine 300mg/m² Etoposide 1200mg/m² Cytarabine 1600mg/m² Melphalan 140mg/m²	85	3-y FFTF	55	8	• Larger randomized study • FFTF benefit observed only on chemosensitive patients • Dexa-BEAM was associated with high rate of hematologic toxicity • Cytarabine dose was decreased to 600mg/m² because of toxicity
	Dexa-BEAM (no HCT control)	56	Dexamethasone (8mg every 8h orally, days 1–10) Carmustine 60mg/m² Etoposide 1000mg/m² Cytarabine 600–800mg/m² Melphalan 20mg/m²	70		34	12	
Crump et al. 1993 [8]	Melphalan–Etoposide	73	Etoposide 60mg/kg Melphalan 160mg/m²	75	4-y DFS	38.6	9.6	• Included 16 refractory patients and 57 relapsed patients • Pretransplant salvage given to all patients • 40 patients received post-transplant extended field radiation to areas of bulky disease • Patients transplanted in CR had 4-year DFS of 68% versus 26% for those transplanted with persistent disease • Most common toxicity was mucositis
Reece et al. 1999[9]	CBVP	68	Cyclophosphamide 7.2g/m² Etoposide 2400mg/m² Carmustine 500mg/m² Cisplatin 150mg/m²	n/a	PFS**	50	7	• Etoposide was given in continuous infusion • Pulmonary toxicity (grade I–IV) occurred in 21% of patients

Table 38.1 *(cont.)*

Reference	Regimen	n	Agents	CR (%)	Progression endpoint (%)	TRM (%)	Comments
Stuart et al. 2001[10]	CCV	59	Cyclophosphamide 100mg/kg Etoposide 60mg/kg Lomustine (CCNU) 2–15mg/kg	n/a	3-year EFS 52	8.5	• 34 patients (62.7%) developed post-transplant interstitial pneumonitis • Thoracic XRT appeared to increase risk of interstitial pneumonitis
Stewart et al. 2000 [11]	HDM	46	Melphalan 200mg/m² b	n/a	5-year EFS 52	0	• Included 21 patients who received dose-intensive cyclophosphamide, etoposide, and cisplatin (DICEP) after mobilization and prior to HDM • 2-year EFS for patients receiving DICEP was 72% *versus* 48% for those not receiving this salvage (P=0.096) • No early treatment mortality was observed, long-term-data not available
Moskowitz et al. 2001 [12]	TLI-CE	2	Total lymphoid irradiation, 1800 cGy Cyclophosphamide 4.5g/m² Etoposide 1g/m²		3-year EFS 68	3.6 c	• Radiation naïve patients were given TLI. Separate arm in protocol gave CBV to patients previously irradiated (not shown)
Visani et al. 2013[13]	BeEAM	43	Bendamustine 320–400mg/m² Etoposide 800mg/m² Cytarabine 1600mg/m² Melphalan 140mg/m²	72 a,b	3-year PFS 75	0 c	• Gastrointestinal toxicity and mucositis were the most common nonhematologic toxicities

a Interval not specified, median follow-up was 5.1 years.
b One patient received 140mg/m² and one patient 160mg/m².
c Early transplant-related mortality only, no long-term data available.
d Continued complete remission 41 months after HCT.
EFS: event-free survival; FFTF: freedom from treatment failure; DFS: disease-free-survival; TRM: transplant-related mortality; NRM: nonrelapse mortality; XRT: radiation therapy.

extranodal relapse, or disease refractory to salvage therapy. Forty-eight percent of patients had primary induction failure. Induction regimens included busulfan–melphalan (BuMel) (n=39), gemcitabine–busulfan–melphalan (GemBuMel) (n=84), or BEAM-type regimen (n=57). The CR rates after BuMel, GemBuMel, and BEAM were 58%, 74%, and 56%, respectively ($P=0.16$). GemBuMel had superior EFS and OS than BuMel and BEAM combined. These data suggest that the patient population described above ("poor risk") may benefit from more intense conditioning regimens than BEAM-type regimen, and set the basis for future prospective studies.

"Double Intensity" Salvage Regimen and Post-CD34+ Cell Mobilization Therapy

Data from University of Calgary

Investigators from Calgary evaluated a "double intensity" salvage regimen[19], DICEP (cyclophosphamide $1.75\,g/m^2$, etoposide $350\,mg/m^2$, and cisplatin $35\,mg/m^2$, given on days 1–3) followed by G-CSF and hematopoietic cell collection. Conditioning for HCT was done with high-dose melphalan ($200\,mg/m^2$). Seventy-three patients with refractory or relapsed HL were included. Mobilization was successful in 97.3% of cases, with a median CD34+ cell dose of $15.6 \times 10^6/kg$. Overall response to DICEP was 86%, although CR was observed in only 18% of cases. After median follow-up of 56 months, 5-year PFS and OS were 61% and 80%, respectively. Hematologic toxicity was frequent and one treatment-related death occurred. This treatment approach represents an integrated, high-intensity strategy comprising salvage, mobilization, and HDT-HCT; however, additional research is needed to determine more optimal regimens to be used, in light of the low rates of complete remission after DICEP.

Data from German Hodgkin Study Group

The GHSG evaluated the use of additional therapy between salvage and HCT[20,21]. Patients were treated with two cycles of salvage chemotherapy, followed by high-dose cyclophosphamide ($4\,g/m^2$) and G-CSF prior to hematopoietic cell collection. Subsequent post-mobilization treatment included high-dose methotrexate ($8\,g/m^2$), vincristine ($1.4\,mg/m^2$), and etoposide ($2\,g/m^2$), proceeding 3 weeks later to BEAM conditioning and HCT. After initial reports suggested feasibility and tolerability of this sequential approach[20], a randomized trial compared it against DHAP followed directly by BEAM and HCT[21]. This randomized study included 281 HL patients with early (27%), late (57%), or multiple relapses (7%); 241 patients responding to initial salvage with DHAP proceeded to randomization. Response rates, OS, and FFTF were not different among treatment arms. Sequential therapy was associated with longer treatment duration and higher rates of toxicity. The inclusion of patients of all risks may have accounted for the lack of benefit of sequential strategy and future studies could investigate its use in very high-risk patients such as those with refractory disease and early relapse.

Tandem Autologous HCT in HL

Data from City of Hope

Researchers from the City of Hope Comprehensive Cancer Center presented the results of two sequential HCT procedures (tandem HCT) in patients with refractory HL (61%) or with relapsed disease with an additional poor prognosis factor (39%)[22]. The first HCT was done with melphalan conditioning ($150\,mg/m^2$), followed by a second HCT with total body irradiation (TBI) (1200 cGy) or carmustine ($450\,mg/m^2$), etoposide ($60\,mg/kg$), and cyclophosphamide ($100\,mg/kg$). Forty-six patients were included, but five (11%) could not receive the second HCT because of insufficient hematopoietic cell collection (n=4) or consent withdrawal (n=1). Seven patients received additional radiation to residual bulky disease. After median follow-up of 5.3 years, 5-year OS, PFS, and freedom from progression were 54%, 49%, and 55%, respectively. Mortality at day 100 was 4%.

Data from Groupe d'Etude des Lymphomes de l'Adulte

A prospective study conducted by the Groupe d'Etude des Lymphomes de l'Adulte (GELA) used a risk-adapted approach for the selection of tandem HCT[23]. Patients with standard-risk relapsed HL received a single HCT, whereas those with high-risk relapse (refractory disease, relapse <12 months, advanced stage at relapse or relapse in prior radiation field) were given tandem HCT. First conditioning was done with CBV and mitoxantrone ($30\,mg/m^2$). The second HCT was done 45 to 90 days later with TBI (1200 cGy), cytarabine ($6\,g/m^2$), and melphalan ($140\,mg/m^2$) conditioning. Busulfan ($4\,mg/kg$ per day for 4 days) was substituted for TBI in patients with prior radiation. Post-transplant involved field radiation therapy (IFRT) was given to involved nodal sites or residual lesions larger than 5 cm. One hundred and fifty patients were enrolled – 137 presented response to salvage chemotherapy and progressed to first HCT (71 refractory patients and 66 patients with unfavorable relapse) and 105 received a second HCT. After a median follow-up of 51 months, 5-year OS and FFTF for patients assigned to tandem HCT were 57% and 46%, respectively. Treatment-related mortality for "poor-risk" patients was 4%. In conclusion, this prospective study demonstrated the feasibility and activity of tandem HCT for high-risk relapsed HL patients, although further studies are needed to define the optimal regimens as well as the appropriate patient selection criteria.

What Is the Role of Radiation Therapy before or after Autologous HCT?

Retrospective studies evaluating the use of IFRT in the setting of HCT have reported a benefit in local disease control and improved PFS and decreased relapse, but few have reported an improvement in OS. Biswas et al. analyzed 62 HL patients treated with HCT[24]. Thirty-three (53%) received IFRT up to 6 months after HCT (median 2 months). Median IFRT dose was 30.6 Gy (range 6.0–44.2 Gy). There were no standardized criteria for selection, although IFRT was given to patients with bulky recurrence or residual disease after salvage. Estimated 3-year OS was 69.6% for the IFRT group and 40% for the non-IFRT group (*P*=0.05). The pattern of relapse was different, with irradiated patients failing in distant sites. Researchers from Emory University conducted a case–control study including 46 patients treated with IFRT in the setting of HCT and 46 matched controls treated with HCT alone[25]. Thirty-eight patients received IFRT less than 2 months before HCT and eight patients had IFRT up to 2 months after transplant. Patients who received IFRT were more likely to have bulky disease at relapse (63% *versus* 13%, *P* < 0.001). Use of IFRT did not result in improved OS or disease-free-survival (DFS). Patients with nonbulky disease receiving IFRT had superior DFS to those with nonbulky disease without IFRT as well as patients with bulky relapse that were irradiated. In a retrospective analysis of 100 HCT patients[26], 24 had IFRT before or after transplant. The effect of IFRT on EFS and OS was not statistically significant for the whole cohort, but in patients with stage I–III at relapse, radiation resulted in improved freedom-from-relapse (FFR) (100% *versus* 67%, *P*=0.04) with trends towards improved OS and EFS. Irradiated patients with stage I–III and no prior IFRT had improved FFR (100% *versus* 51%, *P*=0.03), OS (90% *versus* 50%, *P*=0.04), and EFS (90% *versus* 43%, *P*=0.05). These studies illustrate the variability in the available data regarding use of IFRT before or after HCT. Their retrospective nature, use of different endpoints, timing, and radiation dose as well as variability in the indications for radiation impede making general conclusions regarding the benefit of IFRT. From the available data, IFRT provides a benefit in disease control and may improve PFS, and should be considered for patients with localized persistent disease after salvage chemotherapy. Further research should clarify the optimal timing for IFRT in HCT as well as clarify the subgroup of patients most likely to benefit from this intervention.

Autologous HCT Failures: What is the Next Step?

Approximately 40–50% of chemosensitive HL patients treated with HCT will subsequently relapse, whereas up to three-quarters of refractory patients will have disease recurrence after HCT[16]. Median survival in this situation is less than 2 years[27]. Early relapse (i.e., less than 6 to 12 months after HCT), poor ECOG performance status, advanced stage, and bulky relapse have been associated with worse outcomes[28].

There is no standard treatment for HL patients relapsed after autologous HCT. Outside of a clinical trial, alternatives include salvage chemotherapy without transplant or an allogeneic HCT (allo-HCT). Retrospective analyses published in the 1990s showed that myeloablative conditioning regimens are associated with high rates of nonrelapse mortality (NRM) [29,30]. A report from the European Group for Blood and Marrow Transplantation (EBMT) showed "myeloablative" conditioning regimen-based allo-HCT resulted in a 4-year procedure-related mortality of 51.7%, with a 4-year OS of 24.7%[31]. The outcomes of allo-HCT were inferior for HL compared to other lymphomas, and there was a continuous pattern of relapse, raising the question of whether graft-*versus*-lymphoma (GvL) effect occurs in HL[32] (see Chapters 26 and 65).

What Is the Optimal Reduced Intensity Conditioning Regimen for Allogeneic HCT in Autologous HCT Failures?

The introduction of reduced intensity conditioning (RIC) regimens with decreased transplant-related mortality (TRM) has increased the applicability of allo-HCT for relapsed HL (see Chapter 27). A retrospective study evaluated the outcomes of 185 HL patients referred for allo-HCT with RIC regimen [33] according to donor availability (available donor=122; no donor available=63). Two-year PFS and OS were better for patients with an available donor (2-year PFS: 39.3% *versus* 14.2%, *P* < 0.001; 2-year OS: 66% *versus* 42%, *P* < 0.001). Patients who received allo-HCT in CR had better OS, PFS, and lower risk of relapse, again highlighting the importance of chemosensitivity in the outcomes of HL. Sureda *et al.* on behalf of EBMT compared the outcomes of 168 HL patients undergoing allo-HCT with RIC (n=89) or "myeloablative" conditioning regimens (n=79)[34]. Regimens containing total body irradiation (≥ 8 Gy) or high-dose busulfan (16 mg/kg total dose) were considered myeloablative. Three-month and one-year NRM rates were 15% and 23%, respectively, for RIC, and 28% and 46%, respectively, for myeloablative conditioning regimens (*P*=0.001). Overall survival was superior with RIC regimen (hazard ratio (HR) 2.05; 95% CI 1.27–3.29; *P*=0.04). In patients who received allo-HCT after autologous HCT, risk of relapse was not different among conditioning strategies, but RIC regimen resulted in superior OS. Nevertheless, the long-term outcomes were still disappointing, with a 5-year OS for RIC allo-HCT of 28%.

Several prospective trials have evaluated the addition of melphalan to fludarabine in RIC regimens for HL. A study reported by Peggs *et al.* included 49 relapsed HL patients, 44 (90%) after autologous HCT[35]. Conditioning included fludarabine 30 mg/m^2 from day T-7 through T-3, melphalan 140 mg/m^2 on day T-2, and alemtuzumab (*in-vivo* T-cell depletion) (see Chapters 12, 29, and 30). Patients with progressive disease and absence of graft-*versus*-host disease (GvHD) 3 months after transplant were given donor lymphocyte infusions (DLI) every 3 months (see Chapter 25). Thirty-one patients received grafts from an HLA-matched donor and 18 from a matched unrelated donor (MUD). After 2 years, NRM was 16.3%, higher for subjects receiving MUD grafts.

Estimated 4-year OS and PFS were 55.7% and 39%, respectively. Sixteen patients were given DLI, with 9 (56%) presenting disease response. This study presented initial evidence that graft-*versus*-lymphoma can be observed in HL when RIC regimen with *in-vivo* T-cell depletion is used. Anderlini *et al.* reported the experience at MD Anderson Cancer Center with two RIC regimens for HL[36]. Fourteen patients received fludarabine ($25\,mg/m^2$ intravenously daily for 5 days) and cyclophosphamide ($1\,g/m^2$ daily for 3 days) with antithymocyte globulin (ATG) used for patients receiving MUD grafts. After high rates of relapse were observed, the regimen was intensified by substituting melphalan ($70\,mg/m^2$ daily for 2 days) for cyclophosphamide (n=26). Transplant-related mortality (TRM) after 100 days was 5%, and the cumulative incidence of TRM at 18 months was 22%. Estimated 18-month OS was superior for fludarabine–melphalan (73% *versus* 39%, $P=0.03$) and there was a trend for superior PFS as well.

A larger prospective study of fludarabine and melphalan conditioning was recently reported by investigators from the GEL/TAMO[37]. The conditioning regimen included fludarabine ($150\,mg/m^2$) and melphalan ($140\,mg/m^2$), with ATG given for GvHD prophylaxis of patients receiving MUD grafts. Ninety-two patients were enrolled; 86% had received a prior autologous HCT. Donor sources were HLA-matched siblings (n=55, 70%) and MUD (n=23, 30%). Nonrelapse mortality was 8% at 100 days and 15% at 1 year. Four-year OS and PFS were 43% and 24%, respectively. These results show the safety and tolerability of fludarabine and melphalan as RIC regimen for allo-HCT in HL. Disease relapse remains the main limitation of this therapeutic approach. The results of a more intensified RIC regimen consisting of gemcitabine ($800\,mg/m^2$ once), fludarabine ($33\,mg/m^2 \times 4$ doses), and melphalan ($70\,mg/m^2 \times 2$ doses) were recently reported[38]. The cumulative incidence of TRM was 15%; nine patients had pulmonary toxicity, three were grade 4–5. These early results indicate additional intensification strategies are feasible in RIC-based allo-HCT.

What Is the Optimal Hematopoietic Cell Source for Allo-HCT in HL?

Investigators from the Center for International Blood and Marrow Transplant Research (CIBMTR) reported on the outcomes of 143 RIC allo-HCT receiving grafts from unrelated donors[39]. TRM at 100 days and 2 years was 15% and 33%, respectively, and 2-year OS and PFS were 37% and 20%, respectively. Several additional retrospective analyses of RIC allo-HCT have not found a difference in outcomes between patients receiving grafts from HLA-matched related donors (MRD) or HLA MUDs[32]. In the phase 2 trial conducted by GEL/TAMO[37], OS and PFS were not affected by donor source. These studies indicate MUD grafts should be considered a valid alternative for relapsed HL patients who lack HLA-matched sibling donor (see Chapters 7 and 8).

The use of alternative donor sources has been evaluated retrospectively. An initial report comparing the outcomes of RIC allo-HCT[40] showed OS was comparable between MRD (n=38), MUD (n=24), and HLA-haplotype mismatch HCT (n=28). Recipients of HLA-haplotype mismatch HCT had lower rates of NRM and decreased risk of relapse. A recent comparison of 92 HL patients treated with RIC allo-HCT included 58 HLA-matched grafts and 38 HLA-haplotype mismatch grafts[41]. Chemosensitive patients (i.e., those undergoing transplant in CR or PR) had better PFS when receiving a HLA-haplotype mismatch HCT. It is possible that there is increased GvL with HLA-haplotype mismatch HCT, although the benefit in PFS will need to be confirmed in larger prospective studies (see Chapter 59). If relapse prevention is confirmed, the increasing expertise in modern HLA-haplotype mismatch HCT across transplant centers may make them the graft source of choice in relapsed HL.

The outcomes of allo-HCT using cord blood (CB) have not been consistent (see Chapter 60). Majhail *et al.* compared the outcomes of 9 HL patients receiving CB transplant (CBT) and 12 receiving MRD grafts[42]. Incidence of acute GvHD was 33% in both groups, whereas chronic GvHD was 11% for CBT and 33% for MRD ($P=0.24$). After 17 and 24 months of follow-up in CBT and MRD cohorts, respectively, 2-year PFS were comparable (CBT=25%; MRD=20%); there were no differences in OS. A retrospective study from the French Society of Bone Marrow Transplantation and Cellular Therapy (SFGM-TC) included 191 patients, of whom 17 (9%) were CBTs[43]. In multivariate analysis, use of CBTs was associated with worse OS than other graft sources (HR=3.49; 95% CI 1.26–9.63; $P=0.016$), while MRD and MUD transplants had similar OS. These contradictory results highlight the need for further prospective studies investigating the use of CB for treatment of relapsed HL. As already discussed, in light of early data suggesting improved PFS, it is possible HLA-haplotype mismatch family donors may be a preferable alternative graft source.

Donor Lymphocyte Infusions: When and Under Which Conditions Does It Work Best?

The use of donor lymphocyte infusions (DLI) for treatment of persistent disease after allo-HCT is debated. Peggs *et al.* initially reported DLI could induce responses in HL patients who had prior RIC allo-HCT with *in-vivo* T-cell depletion using alemtuzumab[35]. The occurrence of GvHD correlated with clinical responses. In a follow-up study, the same group reported the outcomes of 76 patients treated with RIC allo-HCT, 45 of whom received DLI for relapsed disease (n=24) or mixed chimerism (n=24)[44]. DLI-related mortality was 7% at 3 years, and GvHD requiring immunosuppression occurred in 54% and 23% of those receiving DLI for relapse or mixed chimerism, respectively. Development of GvHD was associated with decreased relapse (4-year cumulative incidence of relapse 22% *versus* 53%, $P=0.0188$), indicating the presence of graft-*versus*-lymphoma effect. Four-year survival from relapse was 59% for patients receiving DLI. Other investigators have reported DLI results with responses between 30% and 40%[43,45], but a survival benefit has been observed consistently. Based on these data, DLI is an alternative for patients who relapse after allo-HCT and who have limited complications after this procedure, in particular absence of GvHD and serious infectious complications (see Chapter 25 for details on prophylactic *versus* preemptive *versus* therapeutic DLI).

Transplantation in the Era of Targeted Therapy for Hodgkin Lymphoma: the Changing Landscape

The introduction of novel agents with activity against HL (i.e., brentuximab vedotin, HDAC inhibitors, mTOR inhibitors, lenalidomide) represents a significant expansion of the armamentarium available for treatment of Hodgkin lymphoma patients. The antibody–drug conjugate brentuximab vedotin (BV), in particular, has been shown to have remarkable single-agent activity in HL patients relapsed after HCT[46], leading to FDA approval in 2011.

What Is the Role of Allogeneic Transplant in Patients Who Have Received Salvage with BV After Failure of Autologous HCT?

The use of RIC allo-HCT in patients salvaged with BV has been limited to patient series. Chen *et al.* reported the outcomes of 21 patients salvaged with BV followed by RIC allo-HCT with fludarabine and melphalan and compared them with 23 historic controls that were treated with the same conditioning without prior BV salvage[47]. The majority of patients (38/44) had undergone prior autologous HCT. Transplantation in CR was more common in the BV group. The 2-year PFS was 59.6% for BV-treated patients *versus* and 26.1% for subjects salvaged without BV prior to allo-HCT. Saliba Rima *et al.* reported the outcomes after allo-HCT RIC with gemcitabine, fludarabine, and melphalan conditioning according to prior BV treatment[38]. Complete response prior to allo-HCT was 79% for BV-treated patients and 46% for BV-naïve subjects. After a median follow-up of 18 months, actuarial estimates for OS and PFS were 69% and 55%, respectively. These very early data indicate allo-HCT outcomes may significantly improve as a result of novel targeted salvage strategies.

On the other hand, there are emerging data indicating a subgroup of patients treated with BV will have sustained remissions without subsequent therapy[48]. Moreover, a recent study showed that retreatment with BV can result in high response rates[49], allowing for postponement or avoidance of allo-HCT[48]. It is possible that combinations of chemotherapy, BV, and possibly other agents will result in higher rates of long-term remissions or responses in relapses after initial BV. A major focus of future studies will be to clarify the role of allo-HCT in the era of highly effective and well-tolerated targeted agents.

What Will Be the Role of Autologous HCT in Subjects Treated with Brentuximab Vedotin in First or Second Line?

The remarkable activity of BV against HL has led to investigation of its use in first-line and as salvage prior to autologous HCT. A recent phase 1 trial in previously untreated HL patients found the combination of BV with adriamycin, bleomycin, vinblastine and dacarbazine (ABVD) to be associated with an unacceptable rate of pulmonary toxicity; in the same trial, the combination of BV with adriamycin, vinblastine and dacarbazine (AVD) produced high rates of CR (96%) without associated pulmonary complications. A large multicenter randomized trial comparing BV plus AVD *versus* ABVD will determine the role of BV in first-line therapy for HL.

Use of BV as part of salvage therapy of HL prior to autologous HCT has also been reported. A recent retrospective study by investigators from the University of Washington included 15 HL patients with disease refractory to platinum-containing regimens[50]. Treatment with BV achieved FDG PET negativity in 8/15 (53%) patients, with responses observed in patients that had at least achieved stable disease after platinum-containing chemotherapy. Responding patients proceeded to autologous HCT, with seven remaining free of progression after a median of 18.5 months follow-up after transplant. A phase 2 trial conducted at the City of Hope Medical Center is evaluating single-agent BV as first salvage for patients with HL relapsed or refractory to first-line therapy (www.clinicaltrials.gov #NCT01393717). Investigators from Memorial Sloan-Kettering Cancer Center are conducting a study of FDG PET adaptive therapy with BV used as initial salvage for relapsed HL (www.clinicaltrials.gov #NCT01508312). Patients with negative PET after two cycles proceed to HCT while those with persistent disease will receive augmented ifosfamide, carboplatin and etoposide (ICE) salvage. Because of the good tolerability of BV, several ongoing trials are investigating its use in combination with cytotoxic agents such as gemcitabine (www.clinicaltrials.gov #NCT01780662), bendamustine (www.clinicaltrials.gov #NCT01874054), and ICE (www.clinicaltrials.gov #NCT02227199).

The use of BV in earlier lines of therapy for HL will give rise to two important questions for patients who subsequently relapse. First, what is the optimal salvage for patients who relapse after a BV-containing regimen? If retreatment with BV can result in high response rates in patients relapsed after allo-HCT, it is likely that this will extend to earlier lines of therapy. Salvage regimens including BV in combination with other agents will need to be evaluated through further research studies. And second, what is the role of autologous HCT after first relapse if BV is effective in this setting? Current studies are examining the feasibility and efficacy of strategies that include BV and HCT, but separate research will have to clarify whether HCT is necessary if a remission is achieved through BV-containing regimens. This reevaluation of HCT will require large, well-planned studies to generate interpretable results.

Controversies

The use of autologous HCT in the treatment of HL has been well studied over the last three decades. Autologous HCT is a well-established standard for patients with chemosensitive relapse, although its benefit is only based on disease progression endpoints and not on OS benefit. The evidence for conventional autologous HCT with BEAM type conditioning regimens in patients with "high or poor-risk" relapsed and primary refractory HL is less conclusive. The use of high-intensity conditioning regimens and other intensification strategies prior to autologous HCT may benefit certain "high or poor-risk" relapsed HL patients, but evidence of their benefit is limited and affected significantly by patient selection criteria. Further research studies using risk- and therapy-adapted criteria for high-intensity strategies may clarify whether these treatments are beneficial for this subgroup of patients.

The evidence supporting the use of allo-HCT for HL patients who relapse after autologous HCT is more recent.

Myeloablative conditioning regimens should not be used, as they are associated with high toxicity with limited survival benefit. Only after RIC regimens were introduced was a graft-*versus* Hodgkin effect demonstrated, but long-term survival after RIC allo-HCT for HL remains very poor. Future research will need to clarify whether moderate intensification of RIC regimens can improve outcomes. Recent results with HLA-haplotype mismatch HCT suggest this graft source may improve disease control in relapsed HL, but the data are limited and maturing. Studies will be needed to determine if a higher rate of disease control with HLA-haplotype mismatch HCT is real and whether it supersedes higher rates of NRM. The introduction of BV represents a major advance in the treatment of HL. Very early results suggest allo-HCT may have improved outcomes after BV salvage. This is possibly because of increased disease control and improved patient performance status after BV, given its favorable toxicity profile. Autologous HCT is also feasible when BV is used in first relapse. However, given the high activity of BV against HL, the possibility of retreatment with BV, and expected enhanced disease control when used in combination with other agents may allow for avoidance or delay of allo-HCT as well as HCT. Future studies will need to clarify the correct indications and timing of hematopoietic cell transplantation in the era of targeted therapy for HL.

References

1. Townsend W, Linch D. Hodgkin's lymphoma in adults. *Lancet* 2012;380(9844):836–847.

2. Kuruvilla J, Keating A, Crump M. How I treat relapsed and refractory Hodgkin lymphoma. *Blood* 2011;117(16):4208–4217.

3. Carella AM, Congiu AM, Gaozza E, Mazza P, Ricci P, Visani G, et al. High-dose chemotherapy with autologous bone marrow transplantation in 50 advanced resistant Hodgkin's disease patients: an Italian study group report. *J Clin Oncol* 1988;6(9):1411–1416.

4. Linch DC, Winfield D, Goldstone AH, Moir D, Hancock B, McMillan A, et al. Dose intensification with autologous bone-marrow transplantation in relapsed and resistant Hodgkin's disease: results of a BNLI randomised trial. *Lancet* 1993;341(8852):1051–1054.

5. Carella AM. Role of hematopoietic stem cell transplantation in relapsed/refractory Hodgkin lymphoma. *Mediterr J Hematol Infect Dis* 2012;4(1): e2012059.

6. Schmitz N, Pfistner B, Sextro M, Sieber M, Carella AM, Haenel M, et al.

Aggressive conventional chemotherapy compared with high-dose chemotherapy with autologous haemopoietic stem-cell transplantation for relapsed chemosensitive Hodgkin's disease: a randomised trial. *Lancet* 2002;359(9323):2065–2071.

7. Bierman PJ, Bagin RG, Jagannath S, Vose JM, Spitzer G, Kessinger A, et al. High dose chemotherapy followed by autologous hematopoietic rescue in Hodgkin's disease: long-term follow-up in 128 patients. *Ann Oncol* 1993;4(9):767–773.

8. Crump M, Smith AM, Brandwein J, Couture F, Sherret H, Sutton DM, et al. High-dose etoposide and melphalan, and autologous bone marrow transplantation for patients with advanced Hodgkin's disease: importance of disease status at transplant. *J Clin Oncol* 1993;11(4):704–711.

9. Reece DE, Nevill TJ, Sayegh A, Spinelli JJ, Brockington DA, Barnett MJ, et al. Regimen-related toxicity and non-relapse mortality with high-dose cyclophosphamide, carmustine (BCNU) and etoposide (VP16-213) (CBV) and CBV plus cisplatin (CBVP) followed by autologous stem cell

transplantation in patients with Hodgkin's disease. *Bone Marrow Transplant* 1999;23(11):1131–1138.

10. Stuart MJ, Chao NS, Horning SJ, Wong RM, Negrin RS, Johnston LJ, et al. Efficacy and toxicity of a CCNU-containing high-dose chemotherapy regimen followed by autologous hematopoietic cell transplantation in relapsed or refractory Hodgkin's disease. *Biol Blood Marrow Transplant* 2001;7(10):552–560.

11. Stewart DA, Guo D, Gluck S, Morris D, Chaudhry A, deMetz C, et al. Double high-dose therapy for Hodgkin's disease with dose-intensive cyclophosphamide, etoposide, and cisplatin (DICEP) prior to high-dose melphalan and autologous stem cell transplantation. *Bone Marrow Transplant* 2000;26(4):383–388.

12. Moskowitz CH, Nimer SD, Zelenetz AD, Trippett T, Hedrick EE, Filippa DA, et al. A 2-step comprehensive high-dose chemoradiotherapy second-line program for relapsed and refractory Hodgkin disease: analysis by intent to treat and development of a prognostic model. *Blood* 2001;97(3):616–623.

13. Visani G, Stefani PM, Capria S, Malerba L, Galieni P, Gaudio F, Specchia G, et al. Bendamustine, etoposide,

cytarabine and melphalan (BEEAM) followed by autologous stem cell transplantation produce a 3-year progression-free survival of 75% in heavily pre-treated Hodgkin and non-Hodgkin lymphoma. *Blood* 2013;122(21):2134.

14. Andre M, Henry-Amar M, Pico JL, Brice P, Blaise D, Kuentz M, et al. Comparison of high-dose therapy and autologous stem-cell transplantation with conventional therapy for Hodgkin's disease induction failure: a case-control study. Societe Francaise de Greffe de Moelle. *J Clin Oncol* 1999;17(1):222–229.

15. Lazarus HM, Rowlings PA, Zhang MJ, Vose JM, Armitage JO, Bierman PJ, et al. Autotransplants for Hodgkin's disease in patients never achieving remission: a report from the Autologous Blood and Marrow Transplant Registry. *J Clin Oncol* 1999;17(2):534–545.

16. Hertzberg M. Relapsed/refractory Hodgkin lymphoma: what is the best salvage therapy and do we need RIC-alloSCT? *Hematol Oncol Clin North Am* 2014;28(1):123–147.

17. Bains T, Chen AI, Lemieux A, Hayes-Lattin BM, Leis JF, Dibb W, et al. Improved outcome with busulfan, melphalan and thiotepa conditioning in autologous hematopoietic stem cell transplant for relapsed/refractory Hodgkin lymphoma. *Leuk Lymphoma* 2014;55(3):583–587.

18. Nieto Y, Popat U, Anderlini P, Valdez B, Andersson B, Liu P, et al. Autologous stem cell transplantation for refractory or poor-risk relapsed Hodgkin's lymphoma: effect of the specific high-dose chemotherapy regimen on outcome. *Biol Blood Marrow Transplant* 2013;19(3):410–417.

19. Shafey M, Duan Q, Russell J, Duggan P, Balogh A, Stewart DA. Double high-dose therapy with dose-intensive cyclophosphamide, etoposide, cisplatin (DICEP) followed by high-dose melphalan and autologous stem cell transplantation for relapsed/refractory Hodgkin lymphoma. *Leuk Lymphoma* 2012;53(4):596–602.

20. Josting A, Sieniawski M, Glossmann JP, Staak O, Nogova L, Peters N, et al. High-dose sequential chemotherapy followed by autologous stem cell transplantation in relapsed and refractory aggressive non-Hodgkin's lymphoma: results of a multicenter phase II study. *Ann Oncol* 2005;16(8):1359–1365.

21. Josting A, Muller H, Borchmann P, Baars JW, Metzner B, Dohner H, et al. Dose intensity of chemotherapy in patients with relapsed Hodgkin's lymphoma. *J Clin Oncol* 2010;28(34):5074–5080.

22. Fung HC, Stiff P, Schriber J, Toor A, Smith E, Rodriguez T, et al. Tandem autologous stem cell transplantation for patients with primary refractory or poor risk recurrent Hodgkin lymphoma. *Biol Blood Marrow Transplant* 2007;13(5):594–600.

23. Morschhauser F, Brice P, Ferme C, Divine M, Salles G, Bouabdallah R, et al. Risk-adapted salvage treatment with single or tandem autologous stem-cell transplantation for first relapse/refractory Hodgkin's lymphoma: results of the prospective multicenter H96 trial by the GELA/SFGM study group. *J Clin Oncol* 2008;26(36):5980–5987.

24. Biswas T, Culakova E, Friedberg JW, Kelly JL, Dhakal S, Liesveld J, et al. Involved field radiation therapy following high dose chemotherapy and autologous stem cell transplant benefits local control and survival in refractory or recurrent Hodgkin lymphoma. *Radiother Oncol* 2012;103(3):367–372.

25. Kahn S, Flowers C, Xu Z, Esiashvili N. Does the addition of involved field radiotherapy to high-dose chemotherapy and stem cell transplantation improve outcomes for patients with relapsed/refractory Hodgkin lymphoma? *Int J Radiat Oncol Biol Phys* 2011;81(1):175–180.

26. Poen JC, Hoppe RT, Horning SJ. High-dose therapy and autologous bone marrow transplantation for relapsed/refractory Hodgkin's disease: the impact of involved field radiotherapy on patterns of failure and survival. *Int J Radiat Oncol Biol Phys* 1996;36(1):3–12.

27. von Tresckow B, Muller H, Eichenauer DA, Glossmann JP, Josting A, Boll B, et al. Outcome and risk factors of patients with Hodgkin Lymphoma who relapse or progress after autologous stem cell transplant. *Leuk Lymphoma* 2014;55(8):1922–1924.

28. Martinez C, Canals C, Sarina B, Alessandrino EP, Karakasis D, Pulsoni A, et al. Identification of prognostic factors predicting outcome in Hodgkin's lymphoma patients relapsing after autologous stem cell transplantation. *Ann Oncol* 2013;24(9):2430–2434.

29. Gajewski JL, Phillips GL, Sobocinski KA, Armitage JO, Gale RP, Champlin RE, et al. Bone marrow transplants from HLA-identical siblings in advanced Hodgkin's disease. *J Clin Oncol* 1996;14(2):572–578.

30. Milpied N, Fielding AK, Pearce RM, Ernst P, Goldstone AH. Allogeneic bone marrow transplant is not better than autologous transplant for patients with relapsed Hodgkin's disease. European Group for Blood and Bone Marrow Transplantation. *J Clin Oncol* 1996;14(4):1291–1296.

31. Peniket AJ, Ruiz de Elvira MC, Taghipour G, Cordonnier C, Gluckman E, de Witte T, et al. An EBMT registry matched study of allogeneic stem cell transplants for lymphoma: allogeneic transplantation is associated with a lower relapse rate but a higher procedure-related mortality rate than autologous transplantation. *Bone Marrow Transplant* 2003;31(8):667–678.

32. Kharfan-Dabaja MA, Hamadani M, Sibai H, Savani BN. Managing Hodgkin lymphoma relapsing after autologous hematopoietic cell transplantation: a not-so-good cancer after all! *Bone Marrow Transplant* 2014;49(5):599–606.

33. Sarina B, Castagna L, Farina L, Patriarca F, Benedetti F, Carella AM, et al. Allogeneic transplantation improves the overall and progression-free survival of Hodgkin lymphoma patients relapsing after autologous transplantation: a retrospective study based on the time of HLA typing and donor availability. *Blood* 2010;115(18):3671–3677.

34. Sureda A, Robinson S, Canals C, Carella AM, Boogaerts MA, Caballero D, et al. Reduced-intensity conditioning compared with conventional allogeneic stem-cell transplantation in relapsed or refractory Hodgkin's lymphoma: an analysis from the Lymphoma Working Party of the European Group for Blood and Marrow Transplantation. *J Clin Oncol* 2008;26(3):455–462.

35. Peggs KS, Hunter A, Chopra R, Parker A, Mahendra P, Milligan D, et al.

Clinical evidence of a graft-*versus*-Hodgkin's-lymphoma effect after reduced-intensity allogeneic transplantation. *Lancet* 2005;365(9475):1934–1941.

36. Anderlini P, Saliba R, Acholonu S, Okoroji GJ, Donato M, Giralt S, *et al*. Reduced-intensity allogeneic stem cell transplantation in relapsed and refractory Hodgkin's disease: low transplant-related mortality and impact of intensity of conditioning regimen. *Bone Marrow Transplant* 2005;35(10):943–951.

37. Sureda A, Canals C, Arranz R, Caballero D, Ribera JM, Brune M, *et al*. Allogeneic stem cell transplantation after reduced intensity conditioning in patients with relapsed or refractory Hodgkin's lymphoma. Results of the HDR-ALLO study — a prospective clinical trial by the Grupo Espanol de Linfomas/Trasplante de Medula Osea (GEL/TAMO) and the Lymphoma Working Party of the European Group for Blood and Marrow Transplantation. *Haematologica* 2012;97(2):310–317.

38. Anderlini P, Saliba RM, Ledesma C, Chancoco CM, Alexander T, Alousi A, Hosing CM, *et al*. Reduced-intensity conditioning (RIC) and allogeneic stem cell transplantation (allo-SCT) for relapsed/refractory Hodgkin lymphoma (HL) in the brentuximab vedotin era: Favorable overall and progression-free survival (OS/PFS) with low transplant-related mortality (TRM). *Blood* 2013;122(21):410.

39. Devetten MP, Hari PN, Carreras J, Logan BR, van Besien K, Bredeson CN, *et al*. Unrelated donor reduced-intensity allogeneic hematopoietic stem cell transplantation for relapsed and refractory Hodgkin lymphoma. *Biol Blood Marrow Transplant* 2009;15(1):109–117.

40. Burroughs LM, O'Donnell PV, Sandmaier BM, Storer BE, Luznik L, Symons HJ, *et al*. Comparison of outcomes of HLA-matched related, unrelated, or HLA-haploidentical related hematopoietic cell transplantation following nonmyeloablative conditioning for relapsed or refractory Hodgkin lymphoma. *Biol Blood Marrow Transplant* 2008;14(11):1279–1287.

41. Castagna L, Bramanti S, Furst S, Sarina B, El-Cheikh J, Granata A, *et al*. Lower relapse and better PFS among chemosensitive patients undergoing allogeneic transplantation by haploidentical compared with HLA-identical donor: results on a cohort of 94 patients with Hodgkin's lymphoma. *Blood* 2013;122(21):2144.

42. Majhail NS, Weisdorf DJ, Wagner JE, Defor TE, Brunstein CG, Burns LJ. Comparable results of umbilical cord blood and HLA-matched sibling donor hematopoietic stem cell transplantation after reduced-intensity preparative regimen for advanced Hodgkin lymphoma. *Blood* 2006;107(9):3804–3807.

43. Marcais A, Porcher R, Robin M, Mohty M, Michalet M, Blaise D, *et al*. Impact of disease status and stem cell source on the results of reduced intensity conditioning transplant for Hodgkin's lymphoma: a retrospective study from the French Society of Bone Marrow Transplantation and Cellular Therapy (SFGM-TC). *Haematologica* 2013;98(9):1467–1475.

44. Peggs KS, Kayani I, Edwards N, Kottaridis P, Goldstone AH, Linch DC, *et al*. Donor lymphocyte infusions modulate relapse risk in mixed chimeras and induce durable salvage in relapsed patients after T-cell-depleted

allogeneic transplantation for Hodgkin's lymphoma. *J Clin Oncol* 2011;29(8):971–978.

45. Anderlini P, Saliba R, Acholonu S, Okoroji GJ, Ledesma C, Andersson BS, *et al*. Donor leukocyte infusions in recurrent Hodgkin lymphoma following allogeneic stem cell transplant: 10-year experience at the M. D. Anderson Cancer Center. *Leuk Lymphoma* 2012;53(6):1239–1241.

46. Younes A, Gopal AK, Smith SE, Ansell SM, Rosenblatt JD, Savage KJ, *et al*. Results of a pivotal phase II study of brentuximab vedotin for patients with relapsed or refractory Hodgkin's lymphoma. *J Clin Oncol* 2012;30(18):2183–2189.

47. Chen R, Palmer JM, Tsai NC, Thomas SH, Siddiqi T, Popplewell L, *et al*. Brentuximab vedotin is associated with improved progression-free survival after allogeneic transplantation for hodgkin lymphoma. *Biol Blood Marrow Transplant* 2014;20(11):1864–1868.

48. Younes A. Brentuximab vedotin for the treatment of patients with Hodgkin lymphoma. *Hematol Oncol Clin North Am* 2014;28(1):27–32.

49. Bartlett NL, Chen R, Fanale MA, Brice P, Gopal A, Smith SE, *et al*. Retreatment with brentuximab vedotin in patients with CD30-positive hematologic malignancies. *J Hematol Oncol* 2014;7:24.

50. Onishi M, Graf SA, Holmberg L, Behnia S, Shustov AR, Schiavo K, *et al*. Brentuximab vedotin administered to platinum-refractory, transplant-naive Hodgkin lymphoma patients can increase the proportion achieving FDG PET negative status. *Hematol Oncol* 2015;33(4):187–91.

39 Hematopoietic Cell Transplants for Chronic Lymphocytic Leukemia: Changing Landscape?

Alex F. Herrera and Edwin P. Alyea

Introduction

Chronic lymphocytic leukemia (CLL), including small lymphocytic lymphoma (SLL), is one of the most common lymphoid neoplasms in persons of European descent. CLL is most common in older persons, with a median age at diagnosis of 70 years. CLL is incurable with current therapies, but the disease is often slowly progressive and may not require treatment. Some patients have a more aggressive disease course requiring treatment – poor prognostic factors in CLL are summarized in Table 39.1[1]. Autologous hematopoietic cell transplant (auto-HCT) can produce complete remissions and improve progression-free survival (PFS) in some persons with CLL but remissions are typically brief and there are no convincing data of survival benefit. Conventional or myeloablative conditioning (MAC) regimen allogeneic hematopoietic cell transplants (allo-HCT) can result in improvement in long-term survival but there is substantial transplant-related mortality (TRM). Reduced intensity conditioning (RIC) allows allo-HCT in older persons, produces durable remissions, and has less TRM. However, relapse remains an important cause of treatment failure. There are several newer therapies for CLL, including ibrutinib and idelalisib. Their introduction raises important questions about the role of allo-HCT in CLL. In this chapter we summarize transplant data (auto-HCT and allo-HCT), discuss selected new drugs and

Table 39.1 Prognostic factors associated with poor outcomes after conventional chemotherapy in CLL

17p deletion

11q deletion

ZAP-70 positivity

Unmutated IGVH

CD38 expression

TP53 mutation

Purine-analog refractoriness

strategies, and will attempt to address important controversies evolving around the treatment of CLL.

Autologous Hematopoietic Cell Transplant in CLL

In persons with relapsed/refractory or poor-risk (cytogenetically defined) CLL at diagnosis, high-dose chemotherapy and radiation followed by an auto-HCT produced responses but remissions were typically brief. Although PFS may improve, there are no convincing data of a survival benefit[2–5]. Auto-HCT have also been used as *consolidation* therapy for high-risk (cytogenetically defined) CLL patients in first remission. A Medical Research Council (MRC) pilot study reported 5-year PFS and survival rates of 52% (95% CI 33–70%) and 78% (95% CI 57–98%) with most subjects achieving a molecular remission[6]. A retrospective risk-matched analysis reported a survival benefit for auto-HCT over conventional therapy in previously untreated subjects (HR 0.39, 95% CI 0.16–0.92; $P = 0.03$)[7].

Upfront auto-HCT consolidation for CLL was studied in two large European randomized trials, which reported longer PFS but no survival benefit was seen with auto-HCT. In the first study of patients with previously untreated Binet stage B or C CLL, estimated 3-year PFS was 80% (95% CI 69–92%) after an auto-HCT *versus* 35% (95% CI 23.9–52.4%) in controls. However, 3-year survival was 96% (95% CI 90–100%) *versus* 98% (95% CI 94–100%). No differences in PFS or survival after auto-HCT *versus* observation were detected in persons not achieving complete remission after upfront therapy according to the 1996 NCI-WG criteria[8,9]. Similarly, the second study of subjects in remission according to the 1996 NCI-WG criteria[8] after first- or second-line therapy reported improved 5-year freedom from relapse and PFS (42% for auto-HCT, 24% for observation, $P < 0.001$) in subjects randomized to receive an auto-HCT *versus* observation but no difference in 5-year survival (86% for auto-HCT, range 77–94%; 84% for observation, range 75–93%; $P = 0.77$)[10]. Despite improved PFS, auto-HCT was associated with poorer net quality of life compared to observation[11]. Finally, a retrospective risk-matched analysis compared subjects in the fludarabine, cyclophosphamide, and rituximab (FCR) arm of the GCLLSG CLL8 trial to subjects receiving an *in-vitro*-purged auto-HCT in the

CLL3 study. There was a PFS benefit with auto-HCT (median, 6.2 years *versus* 4.3 years; $P = 0.009$) but no 4-year survival benefit (86%, 95% CI 80–93% *versus* 90%, 95% CI 84–95%; $P = 0.39$)[12]. In summary, these studies show that auto-HCT in first remission is associated with better PFS, but with comparable survival and poorer quality of life.

Auto-HCT results in occasional long remissions but leukemia cells in the graft and persisting in the recipient (probably both) limit efficacy. Based on the lack of survival benefit observed, we do not recommend auto-HCT in CLL in any disease state outside of a clinical trial.

Myeloablative Allogeneic Hematopoietic Cell Transplant in CLL

Myeloablative or conventional allo-HCT can cure CLL but are associated with high TRM. Data from early studies were encouraging[13–16], but these results are difficult to compare with current outcomes with reduced intensity conditioning (RIC) because of differences in subject selection, HLA typing, graft sources, supportive care, and other factors. Because of substantial TRM, conventional allo-HCT is not recommended for most persons with CLL. However, higher intensity preparative regimens may be considered in selected persons with CLL.

Graft-*versus* Anti-CLL Effect: Does It Exist?

There is direct and indirect evidence supporting a graft-*versus*-leukemia (G*v*L) effect after allo-HCT for CLL. Indirect evidence for a G*v*L effect is the decreased relapses seen over time after allo-HCT compared to the continuous pattern of relapse seen after standard therapy or auto-HCT[13,15,16]. Additional indirect evidence for a G*v*L effect is the association between G*v*HD and reduced relapse risk and the increased relapse risk after T-cell depleted grafts. In one series chronic G*v*HD was strongly associated with a lower relapse risk (relapse 6%, CI 0–23%, compared to 48%, CI 10–79%, in patients without chronic G*v*HD, $P = 0.02$)[16]. Similarly, a European Bone Marrow Transplant Group (EBMT) study of RIC allo-HCT reported chronic G*v*HD was correlated with fewer relapses[17]. Clinical trials of alemtuzumab to decrease G*v*HD are associated with a continuous risk of relapse rather than the plateau as reported in most allo-HCT studies[2,18]. The strongest direct evidence of a G*v*L effect in CLL are remissions induced by donor lymphocyte infusion (DLI; see Chapter 25)[2,17]. Clearance of MRD (measured by MRD flow cytometry or allele-specific IgH qPCR) after decreasing post-transplant immune suppression or after DLI is additional evidence for a G*v*L effect[19]. G*v*L effects appear to be independent of high-risk genetic features[18–20]. For example, acute and chronic G*v*HD were associated with a lower risk of relapse or progression (RR 0.2, CI 0.06–0.63, $P = 0.006$) compared to patients who did not develop G*v*HD in a cohort of patients with 17p deletion[18].

Reduced Intensity Allogeneic Hematopoietic Cell Transplant in CLL

RIC and nonmyeloablative (NMA) allotransplants result in durable remission to similar conventional MAC allo-HCT with decreased TRM. RIC and NMA conditioning regimens facilitate transplants in older persons with CLL, which constitutes the majority of CLL patients. Table 39.2 summarizes several retrospective and prospective studies of RIC or NMA allo-HCT for CLL. In one of the largest series, 82 subjects with advanced CLL underwent NMA allo-HCT, resulting in a 5-year PFS of 39%, overall survival of 50%, and cumulative incidence of relapse (CIR) of 38%[20]. In another study of 76 high-risk subjects who received a RIC allo-HCT, 5-year PFS was 43% (CI 31–55%), overall survival was 63% (CI 51–73%), CIR was 40%, and NRM was 23%. When analyzed by year of transplant, relapse was 26% and NRM was 10% in subjects transplanted between 2004 and 2009[21,22]. The GCLLSG CLL3X trial prospectively studied 90 poor-risk CLL subjects with fludarabine and cyclophosphamide conditioning, along with antithymocyte globulin (ATG) for unrelated donors. Poor risk was defined as early relapse or refractoriness to purine-analog-containing therapy, relapse after auto-HCT, or progressive disease with 11qdel, 17pdel, or unmutated IGHV – 4-year survival was 65% (CI 53–74%), relapse 40% (CI 26–45%), and NRM 23% (CI 9–41%)[19]. Overall, RIC allo-HCT is associated with durable remissions with a plateau in survival curves and less TRM than conventional allo-HCT. Use of RIC regimen has expanded allo-HCT access to a larger population of older persons with CLL and is an attractive and potentially curative option for persons with relapsed/refractory CLL. One group devised a prognostic model for PFS in their RIC allo-HCT cohort. Variables in the model included: disease status at transplant, LDH, comorbidities, and blood lymphocyte count. The model successfully stratified subjects into cohorts with a 5-year PFS ranging from 83% to 6%. The model also predicted survival and relapse risks[22]. This model is currently being validated in a larger Center for International Blood and Marrow Transplant Research (CIBMTR) cohort.

The long-term remissions observed after RIC/NMA conditioning in the absence of high-dose therapy are further evidence that G*v*L is the driver of the curative potential of allotransplants.

Selection of RIC and NMA Regimen for Allo-HCT in CLL

A number of preparative RIC and NMA (see Chapter 27) allo-HCT regimens have been studied in CLL. Studied regimens include fludarabine and low-dose TBI, busulfan and fludarabine, fludarabine and melphalan, and fludarabine and cyclophosphamide. Rituximab, ATG, and alemtuzumab have been added to regimens with no clear impact on outcomes. A new regimen of rituximab, fludarabine, and bendamustine was studied and appears to be associated with low rates of G*v*HD

Table 39.2 Reduced intensity conditioning allogeneic HCT for CLL

Reference	n	Age in years (range)	Prior treatment, when applicable – median number of prior regimens (range)	Donor	Conditioning (most common)	NRM	Relapse	Gr II-IV acute GvHD	Chronic GvHD	Survival
Dreger et al. 2003 [17]	77	54 (30–66)	3 (0–8)	81% related 19% unrelated	Mixed	18% (1 year)	31% (2 years)	34%	58% total	OS 72% EFS 56%
Schetelig et al. 2003 [32]	30	50 (12–63)	33% fludarabine refractory; 3 (0–8)	50% related 50% unrelated	Bu-Flu-ATG	15% (2 years)	60% not in CR (2 years median fu)	56%	85% total 21% extensive	OS 72% PFS 67%
Delgado et al. 2006 [33]	41	54 (37–67)	31% fludarabine refractory; 3 (1–6)	58% related 42% unrelated	Flu Mel + alemtuzumab	26% (2 years)	29% (2 years)	41% total Gr I-IV	33% total 5% extensive	OS 51% PFS 45% (2 years)
Sorror et al. 2008 [20]	82	56 (42–72)	87% fludarabine refractory; 77% with ≥ 3 prior regimens	63% related 37% unrelated	Flu TBI (2 Gy)	23% (5 years)	38% (5 years)	55% in related 66% in unrelated	Extensive: 39% related 53% unrelated	OS 50% PFS 39% (5 years)
Dreger et al. 2010 [19]	90	53 (27–65)	47% purine-analog refractory; 4 (1–11)	40% related 45% unrelated 15% unknown	Flu Cy (+ ATG for unrelated donors)	23% (6 years)	46% (6 years)	45%	73% total 55% extensive (2 years)	OS 53% EFS 38% (6 years)
Khouri et al. 2011 [34]	86	58 (36–70)	83% purine-analog refractory	50% related 50% unrelated	Flu Cy-R	17% (1 year)	39% (3 years)	37%	56% extensive (5 years)	OS 51%, PFS 36% (5 years)
Brown et al. 2013 [22]	76	55 (36–73)	4 (1–9)	37% related 63% unrelated	BuFu	16% at 5 years (9.5% from 2004 to 2009)	40% at 5 years (26% from 2004–2009)	30%	65% total (2 years)	OS 63%, PFS 43% (5 years)
Khouri et al. 2014 [23]	15	59 (30–70) (entire cohort)	3 (1–7) [entire cohort]	54% related 46% unrelated (entire cohort}	BFR	9% (1 year) (entire cohort)	16%, 26 months median follow-up (entire cohort)	11% (entire cohort)	26% extensive (2 years) (entire cohort)	OS 91% PFS 77% (2 years) (includes FL and CLL)

OS – overall survival, PFS – progression-free survival, Bu – busulfan, FL – follicular lymphoma, Flu – fludarabine, Fu – follow-up, Cy – cyclophosphamide, R – rituximab, BFR – bendamustine, fludarabine, and rituximab.

and favorable survival[23]. No studies have compared RIC or NMA regimens, and the current data are derived primarily from single-center or single-arm studies. Regimens are generally selected based on institutional experience. At this time, there is no evidence to support selecting one regimen above another. A cooperative group study evaluating the addition of rituximab to conditioning followed by maintenance is ongoing.

Comparison Between RIC and MAC Allo-HCT Regimens in CLL

Studies have compared outcomes of conventional *versus* RIC allo-HCTs regimens, demonstrating lower TRM but higher relapse rates with RIC regimen. A retrospective EBMT registry population-matched analysis compared conventional allo-HCT to RIC regimen transplants. There was significantly less TRM (HR 0.4, CI 0.18–0.9, P=0.03) but an increased relapse risk (HR 2.65, CI 0.98–7.12, P =0.054) after RIC allo-HCT with no difference in EFS or survival[24]. Similarly, a retrospective analysis comparing conventional MAC and RIC regimens in British Columbia reported a higher probability of CR (OR 6; P = 0.02) and lower risk of progression (OR = 0.1; P = 0.04) but a trend towards higher NRM (OR = 7; P = 0.06) after conventional transplants with no significant difference in survival[25]. In an interesting analysis of this cohort, no difference was demonstrated in OS between patients with CLL relapse after allo-HCT compared to patients who did not relapse[25]. This suggests that patients could be rescued even after allo-HCT relapse. A much larger CIBMTR analysis comparing conventional MAC and RIC regimen transplants from HLA-identical siblings reported higher TRM and fewer relapses with conventional MAC allo-HCT. Improved survival was seen after conventional transplants before 2001 (before RIC regimen was widely used) and superior survival with RIC allo-HCT was observed thereafter[26]. In summary, although relapse risk may be higher after RIC allo-HCT there is less TRM and similar survival compared to conventional MAC allotransplants.

High-Risk CLL and Allo-HCT

Allo-HCT may overcome the adverse prognostic impact of clinical, molecular, and genetic markers. Consequently, some experts believe these data justify early allo-HCT in persons with high-risk CLL, particularly those with del(17p). Several studies report favorable allo-HCT outcomes in persons with high-risk CLL, independent of the presence of poor-risk cytogenetic abnormalities[18–20,27] (Figure 39.1). In an EBMT analysis of patients with del(17p) who underwent allo-HCT, 3-year PFS, survival, and relapse were 37% (CI 22–52%), 44% (CI 28–60%), and 34% (95% CI 20–48%), respectively, comparable to historical survival and relapse rates[18]. In the CLL3X study, various cytogenetic abnormalities, including del(11q) and/or del(17p), and mutations in

TP53, SF3B1, and/or NOTCH1 did not negatively impact outcomes[18,28]. However, other studies have demonstrated poorer outcomes after allo-HCT in patients with del(17p) or del(11q)[25,29]. Unmutated IGVH[27,30], ZAP-70 positivity [31], and CD38-positivity[20] do not appear to adversely impact allo-HCT outcomes. Finally, in the CLL3X study and other studies, fludarabine-refractoriness was not associated with a worse transplant outcome[19,32]. Overall, in most studies, traditional adverse prognostic factors do not appear to be associated with outcomes after allo-HCT for CLL.

Targeted Agents in CLL: Does Allo-HCT Have a Role?

There has been a dramatic shift in the therapeutic landscape of advanced CLL, which raises questions regarding the role and timing of allo-HCT in CLL. It is expected that most persons with CLL considered for a transplant will have received these new drugs. It remains to be seen how these agents will be incorporated into practice and how to position their use in the context of a potentially curative strategy of allo-HCT

Several novel agents have demonstrated promise in clinical trials, including ibrutinib, venetoclax, and idelalisib, which have both been FDA-approved for treatment of CLL (Table 39.3). Ibrutinib, a potent inhibitor of Bruton tyrosine kinase (BTK) – an important kinase in the B-cell receptor (BCR) signaling pathway (Figure 39.2) – is FDA-approved for the treatment of persons with CLL who failed ≥1 prior therapy and in a frontline setting for patients with 17p deletion[35–37]. In the relapsed/refractory setting, about one-third of patients treated in trials of ibrutinib had a 17p deletion, and response rates were favorable with an ORR of approximately 70%. PFS and OS were shorter in patients with 17p-deletion than other patients. Enhanced BCR signaling has been demonstrated in CLL[38–40], and PI3K is a key BCR pathway mediator that impacts CLL cell survival, chemokine networks, and microenvironment interactions[41–43]. Venetoclax (formerly ABT-199) is a BCL2 homology 3 domain (BH3)-mimetic that is approved for patients with 17p deletion who have failed one prior therapy. In patients with high-risk relapsed or refractory CLL, venetoclax resulted in an ORR of 79%, with 20% of patients achieving a CR. Idelalisib is an oral inhibitor of PI3Kδ that is also effective in treating advanced CLL and is approved for patients who have failed at least two prior systemic therapies[44,45]. However, despite these advances, CRs are uncommon in persons treated with these novel agents. There is a continuing pattern of relapse and the duration of responses observed remains unclear. Biomarkers predicting relapse after response to these agents should be studied and may help determine candidacy for allo-HCT. There are no data to suggest that these novel drugs will eliminate a role for allo-HCT in the treatment of CLL.

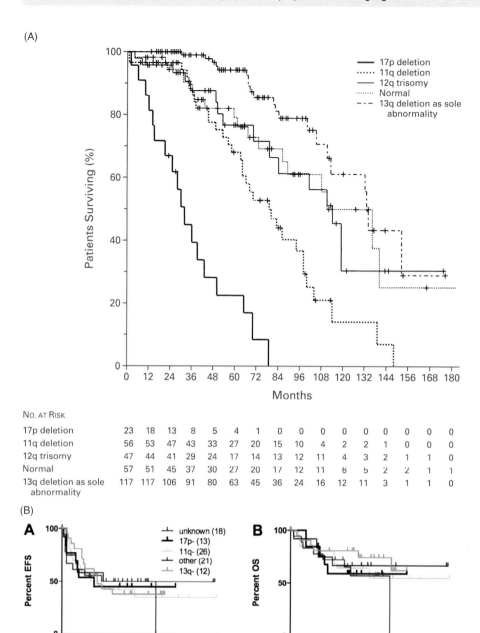

Figure 39.1 (A) Survival among CLL patients with cytogenetic abnormalities and (B) survival and event-free survival among CLL patients with cytogenetic abnormalities after allogeneic HCT.

Chimeric Antigen Receptor-Modified T-Cells for CLL

Chimeric antigen receptor-modified T-cells (CAR T-cells) are one of many novel immune therapies for CLL. CAR T-cells are T-cells with virally tranduced T-cell receptors specific for CD19, an antigen on normal B-cells[48,49].CAR T-cells have produced remissions in persons with advanced CLL, including some patients who have relapsed after an allo-HCT. CAR T-cells directed against ROR1, present on most CLL cells but not normal B-cells, are also being studied.

Newer monoclonal antibodies, such as obinutuzumab[50], drugs targeting the CLL microenvironment (BMS-936564/ MDX-1338), bispecific T-cell engaging (BiTE®) antibodies specific for B-cell antigens, and many other immune therapies are also being developed for treatment of CLL.

Controversies and Future Directions

New FDA-Approved Agents and Allo-HCT in CLL

A critical question facing transplant physicians is how to incorporate these novel agents into CLL therapy[29]. Despite the responses observed thus far, there is a continuing pattern

Table 39.3 Trials of novel agents for relapsed refractory CLL

Reference	n	Age in years (range)	Prior treatment; median number of prior regimens (range)	High-risk features	Dose	Response rate	Median duration of response/PFS	Relapse	Survival	High-risk outcomes
Ibrutinib										
Advani et al. 2012 [35]	16	65 (41–82)	3 (1–10) (entire cohort)	NR	Ph 1 dose escalation	69% ORR 12.5% CR 56.5% PR 19% SD 12.5% NE	13.6 months PFS (entire cohort)	NR	NR	NR
Byrd et al. 2013 [37]	85	66 (37–82)	4 (1–12)	33% 17p del 36% 11q del	60% 420mg daily 40% 840mg daily	71% ORR 2% CR 69% PR 18% PR+L	NR	13% (26 months)	OS 83% PFS 75% (26 months)	17p del: ORR 68% OS 70% PFS 57% (26 months)
Byrd et al. 2014 [36]	195	67 (30–86)	3 (1–12); 45% purine-analog refractory	32% 17p del 32% 11q del	420mg daily	63% ORR 43% PR 20% PR+L 32% SD	DOR: not reached	NR	OS 90% (1 year) PFS 88% (6 months)	17p del: PFS 83% (6 months)
Idelalisib										
Brown et al. 2014 [44]	54	63 (37–82)	5 (2–14)	24% 17p del/p53 mut 28% 11q del 17% NOTCH1	Ph 1 dose escalation	72% ORR 39% PR 33% PR+L	16.2 months DOR 15.8 months PFS	NR	NR	17p del: ORR 54%
Furman et al. 2014 [45]	110	71 (48–90)	3 (1–12)	42% 17p del/p53 mut	Rituximab with maintenance Idelalisib: 150mg daily 300mg after PD	81% ORR 81% PR	PFS: not reached	NR	OS 92% (1 year) PFS 93% (24 weeks)	NR
ABT-199										
Seymour et al. 2014 [46]	105	66 (36–86)	4 (1–11)	28% 17p del	Ph 1 dose escalation	77% ORR 23% CR 54% PR	DOR: not reached 18 months PFS	21%	400mg or higher: PFS 59% (2 year)	17p del: ORR 79%
Ma et al. 2014 [47]	45	69 (50–88)	2 (1–5)	20% 17p del	ABT-199: Ph 1 dose escalation Rituximab: 375mg/m² × 3 weeks, 500mg/m² monthly × 5 months	84% ORR 36% CR 48% PR	NR	11%	NR	NR

NR – not reported, PFS – progression-free survival, OS – overall survival, ORR – overall response rate, CR – complete response, PR – partial remission, PD – progressive disease, DOR – duration of response, Ph – phase, del – deletion.

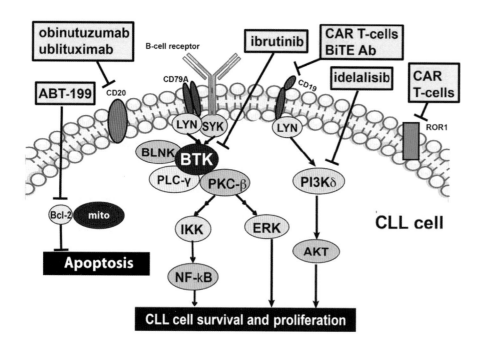

Figure 39.2 Novel therapeutic targets in CLL and their sites of action in the CLL cell. CAR, chimeric antigen receptor; Mito, mitochondria; Bcl-2, B-cell lymphoma-2; BLNK, B-cell linker protein; BTK, Bruton's tyrosine kinase; ERK, extracellular-signal-regulated kinase; IKK, inhibitor of NF-κB kinase; NFKB, nuclear factor kappa B; PKC, protein kinase C; PI3K, phosphatidylinositide 3-kinase; PLC, phospholipase C; ROR1, receptor-tyrosine-kinase-like orphan receptor 1.

of relapse after treatment and there is no evidence that the targeted therapies are curative. Data about the depth of response, MRD, or clonal evolution after treatment with targeted agents are lacking, though resistance mechanisms are emerging[51]. New drug combinations and the addition of these agents to upfront therapy are under study, and it is possible that these strategies will result in deeper remissions that may impact long-term survival. Another unanswered question is the sequencing of these novel treatments, as there have not been studies comparing them against one another.

In 2007, EBMT published a consensus statement regarding indications for allo-HCT in persons with high-risk CLL: (1) nonresponse or early relapse within 12 months of purine analog therapy; (2) relapse within 24 months after achievement of response with purine analog-based combination therapy or auto-HCT; and (3) patients with p53 abnormalities requiring treatment[52]. Although still applicable, these criteria require reconsideration in the context of novel, targeted therapies for CLL. Because of the poor outcomes in persons with del(17p) with conventional therapy, many are considered for an early allo-HCT. However, several new drugs seem effective in persons with del(17p), challenging this concept. Allo-transplant is associated with considerable risks and there may be effective salvage therapy for these patients. Nevertheless, complete remissions with ibrutinib or idelalisib are few. Estimated 26-month PFS was 57% for del(17p) patients in the ibrutinib study with the longest follow-up, suggesting a significant proportion of these patients will relapse[37]. At this time, there is no consensus whether an early allo-HCT is appropriate in persons with del (17p); more data are needed and preference of subsequent therapy after relapse is highly dependent on the treating physician.

The timing of allo-HCT in persons with del(11q) and/or del(17p) with relapsed or refractory CLL, and/or fludarabine refractory patients is also controversial. Many will achieve a remission with one of the novel agents, but then several questions arise: (1) Should an allo-HCT be considered? (2) If proceeding with allo-HCT, how long or deep a remission should be targeted beforehand? (3) When should these medications be discontinued prior to allo-HCT? (4) Should they be given after allo-HCT? (5) If a recipient relapses should he/she be retreated with the same agents? and (6) How should the novel agents and immune therapy be sequenced after transplant relapse?

The concept of using ibrutinib or idelalisib post-transplant is enticing. Both are B-cell receptor pathway inhibitors, and since B cells may contribute to the pathogenesis of chronic GvHD (see Chapter 19), this approach might reduce relapse and chronic GvHD. Clinical trials of ibrutinib in chronic GvHD are ongoing.

Although the novel agents are promising, few persons achieve a CR and remission may not be durable. Consequently, there remains an important role for allo-HCT in treating high-risk CLL. Patients who meet the EBMT criteria, even in the setting of response to a targeted agent, should still be referred for consideration of allo-HCT.

Minimal Residual Disease Monitoring and Implications in CLL

The role of minimal residual disease (MRD) assessment after allo-HCT continues to be studied. MRD negativity in CLL is defined as <1 CLL cell per 10000 blood or marrow leukocytes in an asymptomatic patient (see Chapter 24). Oligotide-specific quantitative PCR (qPCR) and multicolor

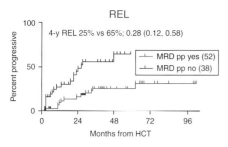

Figure 39.3 Survival and relapse after MRD monitoring in patients treated on the CLL3X study. Patients treated at centers where MRD monitoring was performed had improved event-free survival and decreased relapse risk.

flow cytometry are used most commonly for MRD evaluation. A novel MRD assessment method, ClonoSIGHT (Sequenta, Inc.), uses PCR and high-throughput sequencing to determine a leukemia "clonotype" and assess the relative frequency of CLL sequences in blood and bone marrow samples[53].

The presence of MRD after allo-HCT for CLL is associated with outcomes[18,52,53]. Early MRD status after allo-HCT for CLL is an unreliable marker of disease course, but MRD status at 1 year, and potentially as early as 6 months after allo-HCT, is predictive of subsequent relapse and LFS. In the CLL3X study, MRD-negativity 1 year after a RIC allo-HCT correlated strongly with a lower incidence of relapse (HR=0.037, CI 0.008–0.18; P <0.0001)[19]. Nearly one-half of subjects became MRD-negative only after decreased post-transplant immune suppression, infusion of donor lymphocytes (see Chapter 25), and/or onset of chronic GvHD. Similar data are reported from a small Italian study[54]. Likewise, MRD positivity detected by ClonoSIGHT 1-year post-transplant correlated with relapse and LFS in a small series. In MRD studies to date, MRD clearance has been highly correlated with the development of GvHD[19,54,55].

Detection of MRD after an allo-HCT may present an opportunity for preemptive immune-related interventions. The CLL3X study did not prespecify defined preemptive immune modulation for MRD-positive subjects, but those prospectively monitored for MRD had a significantly lower risk of relapse (HR=0.28, CI 0.12–0.58; P, not reported; Figure 39.3). More studies of prospective MRD monitoring with preemptive immune modulation, hopefully randomized and blinded, are needed to test this strategy. Until this issue is resolved, MRD-testing is not recommended outside of the setting of a clinical trial.

Novel Approaches to Prevent Relapse Following Allo-HCT

Relapse is the leading cause of treatment failure after allo-HCT for CLL especially after RIC and NMA regimens. Developing improved methods of preventing and treating relapse are critical for improving outcomes. Potential peri- or post-transplant interventions comprise chemotherapy and immune therapy, including antibodies, adoptive cellular therapies, immune checkpoint inhibitors, and anti-CLL vaccines.

Autologous CLL cell vaccination with irradiated CLL cells mixed with irradiated GM-CSF-secreting bystander cells was studied at the Dana-Farber Cancer Institute. Subjects had similar rates of GvHD as contemporaneous controls and 13 subjects are in continuous CR with an estimated 2-year PFS of 82% (CI 54–94%) and survival of 88% (CI 59–97%). Correlative studies confirmed that reconstituting donor CD8+ T-cells generated CLL-specific responses with enhanced cytokine secretion[56]. This approach continues to be studied in an ongoing clinical trial. Studies to identify tumor neoantigens using next-generation sequencing of somatic mutations is under study and may lead to better vaccines[57].

Donor chimerism at 30 and 100 days post-RIC allo-HCT is associated with relapse in CLL[26,58]. Chimerism-based intervention may provide an opportunity to decrease relapse risk and initial results are promising[58].

CAR T-cells have induced responses in persons with advanced CLL failing an allo-HCT[48,49]. Trials of CD19 CAR T-cells to prevent relapse after allo-HCT for CLL are in progress. Other possible approaches to preventing or treating post-transplant relapse include antibody therapy with traditional or novel monoclonal antibodies or BiTE antibodies specific for B-cell antigens. Blinatumomab, a BiTE specific for CD19 on CLL cells and CD3 on T-cells, is being studied as treatment for relapsed B-cell malignancies after allo-HCT.

Immune checkpoint inhibitors have been used to treat relapse after allo-HCT[59] and merit further study in CLL. CLL cells and T-cells in the CLL microenvironment express the immune checkpoint antibody PD-1 which dampens immune responses[58,60]. Antibodies to PD-1 or its ligand PD-L1 are active in hematologic neoplasms[61,62]. A trial evaluating PD-1 inhibition to prevent relapse after auto-HCT for diffuse large B-cell lymphoma reported promising results (see Chapter 43)[63].

Conclusion

Although the therapeutic landscape in CLL is changing rapidly with the introduction of novel targeted therapies, allo-HCT remains an important therapy option for persons with high-risk or relapsed/refractory disease with curative potential. RIC allo-HCT results in long-term remissions, possibly overcoming clinical and genetic poor prognostic factors with less toxicity than conventional MAC regimen. MRD monitoring and MRD-based interventions are potentially powerful tools for decreasing relapse, but require further study. Novel approaches to preventing CLL relapse after allo-HCT are needed. New drugs such as ibrutinib and idelalisib are active in advanced CLL but there are few data regarding remission duration or cure. Determining how novel agents and transplants should be integrated in the treatment of high-risk or relapsed/refractory CLL is of critical importance.

References

1. Dohner H, Stilgenbauer S, Benner A, Leupolt E, Krober A, Bullinger L, et al. Genomic aberrations and survival in chronic lymphocytic leukemia. The New England Journal of Medicine. 2000;343(26):1910–6. PubMed PMID: 11136261.

2. Gribben JG, Zahrieh D, Stephans K, Bartlett-Pandite L, Alyea EP, Fisher DC, et al. Autologous and allogeneic stem cell transplantations for poor-risk chronic lymphocytic leukemia. Blood. 2005;106(13):4389–96. PubMed PMID: 16131571. Pubmed Central PMCID: 1895235.

3. Jantunen E, Itala M, Siitonen T, Juvonen E, Koivunen E, Koistinen P, et al. Autologous stem cell transplantation in patients with chronic lymphocytic leukaemia: the Finnish experience. Bone Marrow Transplantation. 2006;37(12):1093–8. PubMed PMID: 16699533.

4. Pavletic ZS, Bierman PJ, Vose JM, Bishop MR, Wu CD, Pierson JL, et al. High incidence of relapse after autologous stem-cell transplantation for B-cell chronic lymphocytic leukemia or small lymphocytic lymphoma. Annals of Oncology : Official Journal of the European Society for Medical Oncology/ ESMO. 1998;9(9):1023–6. PubMed PMID: 9818078.

5. Rabinowe SN, Soiffer RJ, Gribben JG, Daley H, Freedman AS, Daley J, et al. Autologous and allogeneic bone marrow transplantation for poor prognosis patients with B-cell chronic lymphocytic leukemia. Blood. 1993;82(4):1366–76. PubMed PMID: 7688995.

6. Milligan DW, Fernandes S, Dasgupta R, Davies FE, Matutes E, Fegan CD, et al. Results of the MRC pilot study show autografting for younger patients with chronic lymphocytic leukemia is safe and achieves a high percentage of molecular responses. Blood. 2005;105(1):397–404. PubMed PMID: 15117764.

7. Dreger P, Stilgenbauer S, Benner A, Ritgen M, Krober A, Kneba M, et al. The prognostic impact of autologous stem cell transplantation in patients with chronic lymphocytic leukemia: a risk-matched analysis based on the VH gene mutational status. Blood. 2004;103(7):2850–8. PubMed PMID: 14670929.

8. Cheson BD, Bennett JM, Grever M, Kay N, Keating MJ, O'Brien S, et al. National Cancer Institute-sponsored Working Group guidelines for chronic lymphocytic leukemia: revised guidelines for diagnosis and treatment. Blood. 1996;87(12):4990–7. PubMed PMID: 8652811.

9. Sutton L, Chevret S, Tournilhac O, Divine M, Leblond V, Corront B, et al. Autologous stem cell transplantation as a first-line treatment strategy for chronic lymphocytic leukemia: a multicenter, randomized, controlled trial from the SFGM-TC and GFLLC. Blood. 2011;117(23):6109–19. PubMed PMID: 21406717.

10. Michallet M, Dreger P, Sutton L, Brand R, Richards S, van Os M, et al. Autologous hematopoietic stem cell transplantation in chronic lymphocytic leukemia: results of European intergroup randomized trial comparing autografting versus observation. Blood. 2011;117(5):1516–21. PubMed PMID: 21106985.

11. de Wreede LC, Watson M, van Os M, Milligan D, van Gelder M, Michallet M, et al. Improved relapse-free survival after autologous stem cell transplantation does not translate into better quality of life in chronic lymphocytic leukemia: lessons from the randomized European Society for Blood and Marrow Transplantation-Intergroup study. American Journal of Hematology. 2014;89(2):174–80. PubMed PMID: 24123244.

12. Dreger P, Dohner H, McClanahan F, Busch R, Ritgen M, Greinix H, et al. Early autologous stem cell transplantation for chronic lymphocytic leukemia: long-term follow-up of the German CLL Study Group CLL3 trial. Blood. 2012;119(21):4851–9. PubMed PMID: 22490331.

13. Michallet M, Archimbaud E, Bandini G, Rowlings PA, Deeg HJ, Gahrton G, et al. HLA-identical sibling bone marrow transplantation in younger patients with chronic lymphocytic leukemia. European Group for Blood and Marrow Transplantation and the International Bone Marrow Transplant Registry. Annals of Internal Medicine. 1996;124(3):311–5. PubMed PMID: 8554226.

14. Pavletic ZS, Arrowsmith ER, Bierman PJ, Goodman SA, Vose JM, Tarantolo SR, et al. Outcome of allogeneic stem

cell transplantation for B cell chronic lymphocytic leukemia. Bone Marrow Transplantation. 2000;25(7):717–22. PubMed PMID: 10745256.

15. Doney KC, Chauncey T, Appelbaum FR, Seattle Bone Marrow Transplant T. Allogeneic related donor hematopoietic stem cell transplantation for treatment of chronic lymphocytic leukemia. Bone Marrow Transplantation. 2002;29(10):817–23. PubMed PMID: 12058231.

16. Toze CL, Galal A, Barnett MJ, Shepherd JD, Conneally EA, Hogge DE, et al. Myeloablative allografting for chronic lymphocytic leukemia: evidence for a potent graft-versus-leukemia effect associated with graft-versus-host disease. Bone Marrow Transplantation. 2005;36(9):825–30. PubMed PMID: 16151430.

17. Dreger P, Brand R, Hansz J, Milligan D, Corradini P, Finke J, et al. Treatment-related mortality and graft-versus-leukemia activity after allogeneic stem cell transplantation for chronic lymphocytic leukemia using intensity-reduced conditioning. Leukemia. 2003;17(5):841–8. PubMed PMID: 12750695.

18. Schetelig J, van Biezen A, Brand R, Caballero D, Martino R, Itala M, et al. Allogeneic hematopoietic stem-cell transplantation for chronic lymphocytic leukemia with 17p deletion: a retrospective European Group for Blood and Marrow Transplantation analysis. Journal of Clinical Oncology: Official Journal of the American Society of Clinical Oncology. 2008;26(31):5094–100. PubMed PMID: 18711173.

19. Dreger P, Dohner H, Ritgen M, Bottcher S, Busch R, Dietrich S, et al. Allogeneic stem cell transplantation provides durable disease control in poor-risk chronic lymphocytic leukemia: long-term clinical and MRD results of the German CLL Study Group CLL3X trial. Blood. 2010;116(14):2438–47. PubMed PMID: 20595516.

20. Sorror ML, Storer BE, Sandmaier BM, Maris M, Shizuru J, Maziarz R, et al. Five-year follow-up of patients with advanced chronic lymphocytic leukemia treated with allogeneic hematopoietic cell transplantation after nonmyeloablative conditioning. Journal of Clinical Oncology: Official Journal of

the American Society of Clinical Oncology. 2008;26(30):4912–20. PubMed PMID: 18794548. Pubmed Central PMCID: 2652085.

21. Brown JR, Kim HT, Li S, Stephans K, Fisher DC, Cutler C, et al. Predictors of improved progression-free survival after nonmyeloablative allogeneic stem cell transplantation for advanced chronic lymphocytic leukemia. *Biology of Blood and Marrow Transplantation: Journal of the American Society for Blood and Marrow Transplantation.* 2006;12(10):1056–64. PubMed PMID: 17084369.

22. Brown JR, Kim HT, Armand P, Cutler C, Fisher DC, Ho V, et al. Long-term follow-up of reduced-intensity allogeneic stem cell transplantation for chronic lymphocytic leukemia: prognostic model to predict outcome. *Leukemia.* 2013;27(2):362–9. PubMed PMID: 22955330. Pubmed Central PMCID: 3519975.

23. Khouri IF, Wei W, Korbling M, Turturro F, Ahmed S, Alousi A, et al. BFR (bendamustine, fludarabine, and rituximab) allogeneic conditioning for chronic lymphocytic leukemia/lymphoma: reduced myelosuppression and GVHD. *Blood.* 2014;124(14):2306–12. PubMed PMID: 25145344. Pubmed Central PMCID: 4260365.

24. Dreger P, Brand R, Milligan D, Corradini P, Finke J, Lambertenghi Deliliers G, et al. Reduced-intensity conditioning lowers treatment-related mortality of allogeneic stem cell transplantation for chronic lymphocytic leukemia: a population-matched analysis. *Leukemia.* 2005;19(6):1029–33. PubMed PMID: 15830011.

25. Toze CL, Dalal CB, Nevill TJ, Gillan TL, Abou Mourad YR, Barnett MJ, et al. Allogeneic haematopoietic stem cell transplantation for chronic lymphocytic leukaemia: outcome in a 20-year cohort. *British Journal of Haematology.* 2012;158(2):174–85. PubMed PMID: 22640008.

26. Sobecks RM, Leis JF, Gale RP, Ahn KW, Zhu X, Sabloff M, et al. Outcomes of human leukocyte antigen-matched sibling donor hematopoietic cell transplantation in chronic lymphocytic leukemia: myeloablative *versus* reduced-intensity conditioning regimens. *Biology of Blood and Marrow Transplantation: Journal of the*

American Society for Blood and Marrow Transplantation. 2014;20(9):1390–8. PubMed PMID: 24880021. Pubmed Central PMCID: 4174349.

27. Caballero D, Garcia-Marco JA, Martino R, Mateos V, Ribera JM, Sarra J, et al. Allogeneic transplant with reduced intensity conditioning regimens may overcome the poor prognosis of B-cell chronic lymphocytic leukemia with unmutated immunoglobulin variable heavy-chain gene and chromosomal abnormalities (11q- and 17p-). *Clinical Cancer Research: An Official Journal of the American Association for Cancer Research.* 2005;11(21):7757–63. PubMed PMID: 16278397.

28. Dreger P, Schnaiter A, Zenz T, Bottcher S, Rossi M, Paschka P, et al. TP53, SF3B1, and NOTCH1 mutations and outcome of allotransplantation for chronic lymphocytic leukemia: six-year follow-up of the GCLLSG CLL3X trial. *Blood.* 2013;121(16):3284–8. PubMed PMID: 23435461.

29. Chavez JC, Kharfan-Dabaja MA, Kim J, Yue B, Dalia S, Pinilla-Ibarz J, et al. Genomic aberrations deletion 11q and deletion 17p independently predict for worse progression-free and overall survival after allogeneic hematopoietic cell transplantation for chronic lymphocytic leukemia. *Leukemia Research.* 2014;38(10):1165–72. PubMed PMID: 24889511.

30. Moreno C, Villamor N, Colomer D, Esteve J, Martino R, Nomdedeu J, et al. Allogeneic stem-cell transplantation may overcome the adverse prognosis of unmutated VH gene in patients with chronic lymphocytic leukemia. *Journal of Clinical Oncology: Official Journal of the American Society of Clinical Oncology.* 2005;23(15):3433–8. PubMed PMID: 15809449.

31. Khouri IF, Saliba RM, Admirand J, O'Brien S, Lee MS, Korbling M, et al. Graft-*versus*-leukaemia effect after non-myeloablative haematopoietic transplantation can overcome the unfavourable expression of ZAP-70 in refractory chronic lymphocytic leukaemia. *British Journal of Haematology.* 2007;137(4):355–63. PubMed PMID: 17456058.

32. Schetelig J, Thiede C, Bornhauser M, Schwerdtfeger R, Kiehl M, Beyer J, et al. Evidence of a graft-*versus*-leukemia effect in chronic lymphocytic leukemia

after reduced-intensity conditioning and allogeneic stem-cell transplantation: the Cooperative German Transplant Study Group. *Journal of Clinical Oncology: Official Journal of the American Society of Clinical Oncology.* 2003;21(14):2747–53. PubMed PMID: 12860954.

33. Delgado J, Thomson K, Russell N, Ewing J, Stewart W, Cook G, et al. Results of alemtuzumab-based reduced-intensity allogeneic transplantation for chronic lymphocytic leukemia: a British Society of Blood and Marrow Transplantation Study. *Blood.* 2006;107(4):1724–30. PubMed PMID: 16239425.

34. Khouri IF, Bassett R, Poindexter N, O'Brien S, Bueso-Ramos CE, Hsu Y, et al. Nonmyeloablative allogeneic stem cell transplantation in relapsed/refractory chronic lymphocytic leukemia: long-term follow-up, prognostic factors, and effect of human leukocyte histocompatibility antigen subtype on outcome. *Cancer.* 2011;117(20):4679–88. PubMed PMID: 21455998.

35. Advani RH, Buggy JJ, Sharman JP, Smith SM, Boyd TE, Grant B, et al. Bruton tyrosine kinase inhibitor ibrutinib (PCI-32765) has significant activity in patients with relapsed/refractory B-cell malignancies. *Journal of Clinical Oncology: Official Journal of the American Society of Clinical Oncology.* 2013;31(1):88–94. PubMed PMID: 23045577.

36. Byrd JC, Brown JR, O'Brien S, Barrientos JC, Kay NE, Reddy NM, et al. Ibrutinib *versus* ofatumumab in previously treated chronic lymphoid leukemia. *The New England Journal of Medicine.* 2014;371(3):213–23. PubMed PMID: 24881631.

37. Byrd JC, Furman RR, Coutre SE, Flinn IW, Burger JA, Blum KA, et al. Targeting BTK with ibrutinib in relapsed chronic lymphocytic leukemia. *The New England Journal of Medicine.* 2013;369(1):32–42. PubMed PMID: 23782158. Pubmed Central PMCID: 3772525.

38. de Rooij MF, Kuil A, Geest CR, Eldering E, Chang BY, Buggy JJ, et al. The clinically active BTK inhibitor PCI-32765 targets B-cell receptor- and chemokine-controlled adhesion and migration in chronic lymphocytic

leukemia. *Blood*. 2012;119(11):2590–4. PubMed PMID: 22279054.

39. Herman SE, Gordon AL, Hertlein E, Ramanunni A, Zhang X, Jaglowski S, *et al.* Bruton tyrosine kinase represents a promising therapeutic target for treatment of chronic lymphocytic leukemia and is effectively targeted by PCI-32765. *Blood*. 2011;117(23):6287–96. PubMed PMID: 21422473. Pubmed Central PMCID: 3122947.

40. Ponader S, Chen SS, Buggy JJ, Balakrishnan K, Gandhi V, Wierda WG, *et al.* The Bruton tyrosine kinase inhibitor PCI-32765 thwarts chronic lymphocytic leukemia cell survival and tissue homing in vitro and in vivo. *Blood*. 2012;119(5):1182–9. PubMed PMID: 22180443.

41. Cuni S, Perez-Aciego P, Perez-Chacon G, Vargas JA, Sanchez A, Martin-Saavedra FM, *et al.* A sustained activation of PI3K/NF-kappaB pathway is critical for the survival of chronic lymphocytic leukemia B cells. *Leukemia*. 2004;18(8):1391–400. PubMed PMID: 15175625.

42. Hoellenriegel J, Meadows SA, Sivina M, Wierda WG, Kantarjian H, Keating MJ, *et al.* The phosphoinositide 3'-kinase delta inhibitor, CAL-101, inhibits B-cell receptor signaling and chemokine networks in chronic lymphocytic leukemia. *Blood*. 2011;118(13):3603–12. PubMed PMID: 21803855.

43. Longo PG, Laurenti L, Gobessi S, Sica S, Leone G, Efremov DG. The Akt/Mcl-1 pathway plays a prominent role in mediating antiapoptotic signals downstream of the B-cell receptor in chronic lymphocytic leukemia B cells. *Blood*. 2008;111(2):846–55. PubMed PMID: 17928528.

44. Brown JR, Byrd JC, Coutre SE, Benson DM, Flinn IW, Wagner-Johnston ND, *et al.* Idelalisib, an inhibitor of phosphatidylinositol 3-kinase p110delta, for relapsed/refractory chronic lymphocytic leukemia. *Blood*. 2014;123(22):3390–7. PubMed PMID: 24615777.

45. Furman RR, Sharman JP, Coutre SE, Cheson BD, Pagel JM, Hillmen P, *et al.* Idelalisib and rituximab in relapsed chronic lymphocytic leukemia. *The New England Journal of Medicine*. 2014;370(11):997–1007. PubMed PMID: 24450857.

46. Seymour JF, Davids MS, Pagel JM, *et al.*, editors. ABT-199 (GDC-0199) in Relapsed/Refractory (R/R) Chronic Lymphocytic Leukemia (CLL) and Small Lymphocytic Lymphoma (SLL): High Complete Response Rate and Durable Disease Control, American Society of Clinical Oncology Annual Meeting, 2014.

47. Ma S, Seymour JF, Brander D, *et al.*, editors. ABT-199 (GDC-0199) Combined with Rituximab in Patients with Relapsed/Refractory Chronic Lymphocytic Leukemia: Interim Results of a Phase 1b Study. American Society of Clinical Oncology Annual Meeting, 2014.

48. Cruz CR, Micklethwaite KP, Savoldo B, Ramos CA, Lam S, Ku S, *et al.* Infusion of donor-derived CD19-redirected virus-specific T cells for B-cell malignancies relapsed after allogeneic stem cell transplant: a phase 1 study. *Blood*. 2013;24:122(17):2965–73. PubMed PMID: 24030379. Pubmed Central PMCID: 3811171.

49. Kochenderfer JN, Dudley ME, Feldman SA, Wilson WH, Spaner DE, Maric I, *et al.* B-cell depletion and remissions of malignancy along with cytokine-associated toxicity in a clinical trial of anti-CD19 chimeric-antigen-receptor transduced T cells. *Blood*. 2012;119(12):2709–20. PubMed PMID: 22160384. Pubmed Central PMCID: 3327450.

50. Goede V, Fischer K, Busch R, Engelke A, Eichhorst B, Wendtner CM, *et al.* Obinutuzumab plus chlorambucil in patients with CLL and coexisting conditions. *The New England Journal of Medicine*. 2014;370(12):1101–10. PubMed PMID: 24401022.

51. Woyach JA, Johnson AJ. Targeted therapies in CLL: mechanisms of resistance and strategies for management. *Blood*. 2015;126(4):471–7. PubMed PMID: 26065659.

52. Dreger P, Corradini P, Kimby E, Michallet M, Milligan D, Schetelig J, *et al.* Indications for allogeneic stem cell transplantation in chronic lymphocytic leukemia: the EBMT transplant consensus. *Leukemia*. 2007;21(1):12–7. PubMed PMID: 17109028.

53. Logan AC, Zhang B, Narasimhan B, Carlton V, Zheng J, Moorhead M, *et al.* Minimal residual disease quantification using consensus primers and high-throughput IGH sequencing predicts post-transplant relapse in chronic lymphocytic leukemia. *Leukemia*. 2013;27(8):1659–65. PubMed PMID: 23419792. Pubmed Central PMCID: 3740398.

54. Farina L, Carniti C, Dodero A, Vendramin A, Raganato A, Spina F, *et al.* Qualitative and quantitative polymerase chain reaction monitoring of minimal residual disease in relapsed chronic lymphocytic leukemia: early assessment can predict long-term outcome after reduced intensity allogeneic transplantation. *Haematologica*. 2009;94(5):654–62. PubMed PMID: 19377072. Pubmed Central PMCID: 2675677.

55. Moreno C, Villamor N, Colomer D, Esteve J, Gine E, Muntanola A, *et al.* Clinical significance of minimal residual disease, as assessed by different techniques, after stem cell transplantation for chronic lymphocytic leukemia. *Blood*. 2006;107(11):4563–9. PubMed PMID: 16449533.

56. Burkhardt UE, Hainz U, Stevenson K, Goldstein NR, Pasek M, Naito M, *et al.* Autologous CLL cell vaccination early after transplant induces leukemia-specific T cells. *The Journal of Clinical Investigation*. 2013;123(9):3756–65. PubMed PMID. 23912587. Pubmed Central PMCID: 3754265.

57. Rajasagi M, Shukla SA, Fritsch EF, Keskin DB, DeLuca D, Carmona E, *et al.* Systematic identification of personal tumor-specific neoantigens in chronic lymphocytic leukemia. *Blood*. 2014;124(3):453–62. PubMed PMID: 24891321.

58. Richardson SE, Khan I, Rawstron A, Sudak J, Edwards N, Verfuerth S, *et al.* Risk-stratified adoptive cellular therapy following allogeneic hematopoietic stem cell transplantation for advanced chronic lymphocytic leukaemia. *British Journal of Haematology*. 2013;160(5):640–8. PubMed PMID: 23293871.

59. Bashey A, Medina B, Corringham S, Pasek M, Carrier E, Vrooman L, *et al.* CTLA4 blockade with ipilimumab to treat relapse of malignancy after allogeneic hematopoietic cell transplantation. *Blood*. 2009;113(7):1581–8. PubMed PMID: 18974373. Pubmed Central PMCID: 2644086.

60. Xerri L, Chetaille B, Serriari N, Attias C, Guillaume Y, Arnoulet C, *et al.* Programmed death 1 is a marker of angioimmunoblastic T-cell lymphoma and B-cell small lymphocytic

lymphoma/chronic lymphocytic leukemia. *Human Pathology.* 2008;39(7):1050–8. PubMed PMID: 18479731.

61. Ansell SM, Lesokhin AM, Borrello I, Halwani A, Scott EC, Gutierrez M, *et al.* PD-1 blockade with nivolumab in relapsed or refractory Hodgkin's lymphoma. *The New England Journal of Medicine.* 2015;372(4):311–9. PubMed PMID: 25482239.

62. Westin JR, Chu F, Zhang M, Fayad LE, Kwak LW, Fowler N, *et al.* Safety and activity of PD1 blockade by pidilizumab in combination with rituximab in patients with relapsed follicular lymphoma: a single group, open-label, phase 2 trial. *The Lancet Oncology.* 2014;15(1):69–77. PubMcd PMID: 24332512. Pubmed Central PMCID: 3922714.

63. Armand P, Nagler A, Weller EA, Devine SM, Avigan DE, Chen YB, *et al.* Disabling immune tolerance by programmed death-1 blockade with pidilizumab after autologous hematopoietic stem-cell transplantation for diffuse large B-cell lymphoma: results of an international phase II trial. *Journal of Clinical Oncology: Official Journal of the American Society of Clinical Oncology.* 2013;31(33):4199–206. PubMed PMID: 24127452.

Hematopoietic Cell Transplants for Waldenström Macroglobulinemia

Veronika Bachanova, Robert Frank Cornell, and Linda J. Burns

Introduction

The consensus panel recommendations from the Second International Workshop on Waldenström's macroglobulinemia (WM) redefined WM as a distinct clinicopathologic entity characterized by bone marrow involved by lymphoplasmacytic lymphoma (LPL) and IgM monoclonal gammopathy[1]. Central to the diagnosis of this indolent non-Hodgkin lymphoma (NHL) is the demonstration of >10% marrow infiltration with clonal small lymphocytes expressing pan-B markers CD19, CD20, and CD79a and lacking CD10 and BCL6. In contrast to IgM multiple myeloma, immunoglobulin localization is on the cell surface and cells express CD45[2]. These clonal B-lymphoplasmacytic cells are arrested after germinal center somatic hypermutation prior to plasma cell terminal differentiation[3]. In addition to the bone marrow, the liver and lymphatics may become infiltrated. WM accounts for only 5% of non-Hodgkin lymphomas, although the incidence may be declining[4,5]. The disease is considered incurable in most cases; however, recent surveillance, epidemiology and end results (SEER) data demonstrate improved survival with 5- and 10-year rates of 78% and 68%, respectively[6].

WM is a rare disease, with an incidence of 0.5 cases per 100 000 population, with a median age at diagnosis of 64 years (SEER data). Disease presentations in WM can be highly variable; a third of patients may be asymptomatic at diagnosis. The most common presenting symptom is fatigue, often related to anemia. Hepcidin is produced by lymphoplasmacytic cells of WM patients, and is thought to contribute to the pathophysiology of the underlying anemia[7]. When WM progresses, it can manifest as constitutional symptoms (20%), low blood counts (20%), adenopathy (15%), splenomegaly (15%), and hepatomegaly (20%). Monoclonal protein accumulation can cause peripheral neuropathy, headache, visual changes, dizziness, delirium, ataxia, parasthesias, and stupor (or even coma) in severe cases[8]. Hyperviscosity symptoms manifest in approximately one-quarter of patients, occurring when the serum viscosity exceeds 4.0 cP and the serum pentameric IgM paraprotein IgM level is greater than 4–5 g/dL[9]. Coexisting conditions to be considered include cryoglobulinemia[10], antimyelin-associated glycoprotein[11], autoimmune hemolytic anemia[9,12], and light chain (AL) amyloidosis.

Genetics and Epigenetics in WM

Whole exome sequencing has identified WM-specific genetic alterations including a single nucleotide somatic mutation of the myeloid differentiation primary response gene 88 (MYD88^{L265P}) on chromosome 3[13]. This mutation occurs in almost 90% of patients with WM and is rare in other B-cell disorders with overlapping features. MYD88 promotes cell growth via Bruton's tyrosine kinase and interleukin-1 receptor associated kinase; mutational analysis is clinically available via polymerase chain reaction (PCR) assays and can be used to confirm the diagnosis[13]. In addition, WHIM-like mutation of chemokine receptor type 4 (CXCR4) is present in approximately one- third of WM patients and correlates with disease aggressiveness, including hypogammaglobulinemia, recurrent infections, and hyperviscosity syndrome. The specific type of CXCR4 mutation (frameshift or nonsense) in combination with the MYD88 mutation can predict disease phenotype and resistance to alkylators and ibrutinib[13]. The most common cytogenetic abnormality is deletion of chromosome 6q; however, it is unclear if this abnormality has prognostic implications[14,15]. Micro-RNA aberrations and hypoacetylated histones may also drive WM pathogenesis. WM tumor cells present with a unique micro-RNA (miRNA) signature compared with their normal counterparts. Among deregulated miRNAs that are overexpressed in WM, miRNA-155 appears to act as an oncogenic miRNA with loss of function leading to inhibition of WM tumor cell growth[16]; miRNA-9* modulates the histone acetylation status in WM cells, and may be responsible for the up-regulation of acetyl histone H3 and H4[17].

Prognostic Factors

The International Prognostic Scoring System for WM (IPSSWM) has been developed as an easily applied clinical tool to predict survival outcomes of an individual patient, enabling a risk-adapted therapeutic approach in WM[18]. The IPSSWM utilizes five readily available clinical and laboratory features that stratify patients treated with first-line therapy into three risk groups (Table 40.1). The utility of this robust staging system was confirmed in patients receiving rituximab-based first-line regimens; furthermore, the addition of an elevated

Table 40.1 The International Prognostic Scoring System for Waldenström Macroglobulinemia (IPSSWM)[18]

Variable prior to treatment initiation	Points
Age >65 years	1
Hemoglobin ≤11.5 g/dL	1
Platelet count ≤100 × 10^9/L	1
β2-microglobulin >3 mg/dL	1
Monoclonal IgM concentration >7.0 g/dL	1

Stratum	Score	Median survival in months
Low	0 or 1 (except age)	142.5
Intermediate	Age or 2	98.6
High	≥3	43.5

Table 40.2 Novel therapeutic agents used in Phase 1 or 2 clinical trials for Waldenström macroglobulinemia

Agent	Mechanism of action
Rituximab	Anti CD20 monoclonal antibody
131I-tositumomab	Anti-CD20 radiolabeled monoclonal antibody
Alemtuzumab	Anti-CD52 monoclonal antibody
Thalidomide	Immunomodulatory
Lenalidomide	Immunomodulatory
Everolimus	Mammalian target of rapamycin (mTOR) inhibitor
Bortezomib	Proteasome inhibitor
Sildenafil citrate	Phosphodiesterase-5 inhibitor
Enzastaurin	Protein kinase C inhibitor
Panobinostat	Histone deacetylase inhibitor
Perifosin	Akt inhibitor

serum lactate dehydrogenase (LDH) to the IPSSWM identified a subset of high-risk patients with a median overall survival (OS) of less than 3 years[19].

Therapy for WM
First-Line Therapy for WM

Since WM is an indolent lymphoma, many patients are asymptomatic and can be managed with a watch and wait approach. Indications for treatment include constitutional symptoms, progressive cytopenias, bulky organomegaly, or IgM-associated symptoms[20]. When symptoms of hyperviscosity are present, plasmapheresis should be instituted urgently followed by systemic therapy to lower the IgM protein level. There is no standard initial treatment regimen for patients requiring chemotherapy, but first-line therapies are associated with overall high response rates. Therapy choice is based on patient age, comorbidities, presenting symptoms, and disease burden. The consensus panel of the International Workshop on WM concluded that individualized approaches to first-line therapy are necessary given the lack of evidence favoring any particular treatment option[21].

A non-stem cell toxic regimen should be selected in patients who may eventually require hematopoietic cell transplantation (HCT). Potential stem cell toxins such as chlorambucil and fludarabine also carry with them a risk of secondary malignancies, including myelodysplastic syndrome and acute myelogenous leukemia[22,23]. In a very large study of 400 patients with WM, patients were randomized to therapy with chlorambucil or fludarabine. Fludarabine demonstrated a higher overall response rate (ORR) compared with chlorambucil (48% *versus* 39%, respectively) with significantly fewer secondary malignancies (3.7% *versus* 21%)[24]. Since the disease is most common in older adults who may have multiple comorbidities and often relatively low disease burden, the use of rituximab alone or in combination with cyclophosphamide/

dexamethasone (DRC) provides a durable response[21]. The ORR with rituximab alone ranges between 25 and 45%[25–27]. Patients with heavy disease burden requiring therapy that induces a rapid response may respond well to the combination of bortezomib with rituximab with or without dexamethasone (BDR)[28]. As upfront therapy, BDR has demonstrated an ORR of 85% with a median progression-free survival (PFS) of 42 months[29].

The combination of bendamustine and rituximab (BR) is well tolerated and has demonstrated an ORR of 80%. Thalidomide in combination with rituximab and dexamethasone (R-TD) resulted in an ORR of 72%[30]. Lenalidomide at an oral dose of 25 mg daily resulted in excessive anemia; however, lower doses maybe safe and effective[31,32].

Treatment for Relapsed/Refractory Disease and Novel Agents

Similar to upfront chemotherapy for WM, there is no standard approach for relapsed/refractory disease. Patients should be considered for clinical trials when possible. In the transplant eligible, careful selection of hematopoietic progenitor cell sparing regimens is important. Therapeutic choices include combinations of chemotherapy, immunotherapy, proteasome inhibitors, nucleoside analogs, and alkylating agents [21,28,33,34]. Novel drugs being studied in WM include ibrutinib (a Bruton's tyrosine kinase inhibitor), perifosine (an alkylophospholipid targeting protein kinase B, or Akt), enzastaurin (an oral serine/threonine kinase inhibitor targeting protein kinase C and PI$_3$K/AKT pathways), everolimus (a mammalian target of rapamycin [mTOR] inhibitor)[35], panobinostat (a histone deacetylase inhibitor), and alemtuzumab (an anti-CD52 monoclonal antibody) (Table 40.2). However, disease responses are transient and often only

Table 40.3 Summary of autologous hematopoietic cell transplantation for Waldenström macroglobulinemia

Site/center	Disease status	No. of patients	Median age, years (range)	DFS, 5-year (%)	OS, 5-year (%)	TRM, 1-year (%)	Relapse (%)	Follow-up (years)	Reference
CIBMTR	Relapsed	10	51 (30–76)	65[a]	70[a]	11[b]	24[a]	5.4	Anagnostopoulos et al. 2006 [38]
UK Registry	Relapsed	9	50 (38–58)	43[c]	73[c]	0	NA	3.6	Gilleece et al. 2008 [39]
France	Relapsed	32	56	NA	58	12.5	56	3.7	Dhedin et al. 2007 [40]
EBMTR	Relapsed	158	53 (21–70)	40	68	4; 8[a]	52	4.2	Kyriakou et al. 2010 [41]
France	1st remission	12	49 (39–61)	50	100	0	50	5.7	Dreger et al. 2007 [42]
Italy	1st remission	5	53 (41–66)	100	100	0	0	5.5	Caravita et al. 2009 [43]

[a] 3-year.
[b] 100 days.
[c] 4-year.

Abbreviations: CIBMTR = Center for International Blood and Marrow Transplantation Registry; DFCI = Dana-Farber Cancer Institute; DFS = disease-free-survival; EBMTR = European Group for Blood and Marrow Transplantation; NA = not available; OS = overall survival; TRM = treatment-related mortality.

partial. Some mutations, such as the WHIM-like CXCR4 mutations, harbor resistance to ibrutinib[36] and can serve as a prognostic marker to recommend transplant therapy at an early time point.

WM patients with high-risk disease and lack of complete response to initial standard chemoimmunotherapy and younger patients with relapsed WM in overall good health should be considered for autologous or allogeneic HCT.

Hematopoietic Cell Transplantation for WM

Autologous HCT for WM

Several clinical studies have examined the safety and efficacy of high-dose chemotherapy followed by autologous (auto-HCT) in patients with high-risk WM[37–45] (Table 40.3). Twenty-four previously published cases, reviewed by Anagnostopoulos et al.[37,45], included heavily pretreated patients treated with a variety of conditioning regimens, including intravenous melphalan 200 mg/m^2, thiotepa/busulfan/cyclophosphamide, or cyclophosphamide (Cy) with total body irradiation (TBI). These regimens were relatively well tolerated with low treatment-related mortality (TRM), manageable non-hematologic toxicities, and 5-year survivals approaching 70%. A Center for International Blood and Marrow Transplant Research (CIBMTR) analysis of patients undergoing HCT between 1986 and 2002 has been reported [38]. Within the entire cohort of 36 patients, 10 with a median age 56 years received high-dose chemotherapy followed by auto-HCT. The 3-year OS was 70% and PFS was 65%, with a TRM and relapse rate of 11% and 29%, respectively. Durable responses beyond 5 years observed in

several patients suggest that auto-HCT can be very effective in patients with relapsed WM. The British Society of Blood and Marrow Transplantation registry data included nine auto-HCT recipients; there was no TRM and an encouraging 4-year PFS of 43% and OS of 73%[39]. The French updated their transplant experience in WM and reported 54 cases from 18 institutions; 32 patients received auto-HCT with either carmustine (BCNU), etoposide, cytarabine arabinoside, and melphalan (BEAM) or melphalan and TBI conditioning[40]. TRM was 12.5% with a median event-free survival of 32 months. Three- and 5-year survivals were 77% and 58%, respectively. The largest study to date of auto-HCT analyzed 158 adults with WM reported to the European Marrow and Blood Transplant Registry (EBMTR) between 1991 and 2005[41]. At the time of transplant, 93% of patients had chemosensitive disease and most were within 2 years of initial diagnosis. Almost half of patients received BEAM and a third received TBI-based conditioning. The TRM was only 3.8% and at 2 years, 68% of patients were alive; PFS was 61% at 3 years and 39% at 5 years, suggesting no plateau in the survival curves. Progression was observed in 45% of patients at a median of 1.3 years from transplantation. The achievement of complete response (CR) or very good partial response (VGPR), confirmed by negative immunofixation (IF) within 6 months post-HCT, was associated with improved survival. The primary factor impacting TRM was poor performance status at time of transplant. OS was significantly worse with >3 lines of prior therapy, chemoresistance, male sex, and age over 50 years. The incidence of secondary malignancies, particularly myelodysplastic syndrome, was 8.4% at 5 years.

Table 40.4 Summary of allogeneic hematopoietic cell transplant for Waldenström macroglobulinemia

Site/ center	No. of patients	MAC regimen/ RIC (%)	Median age, years (range)	DFS, 5-year (%)	OS, 5-year (%)	TRM, 1-year (%)	Relapse (%)	Follow-up (years)	Reference
France	10	NA	46	60	60	40	0	1.5	Tournilhac et al. 2003 [46]
CIBMTR	26	81/19	51 (30–76)	31	46[a]	40[a]	29[a]	5.4	Anagnostopoulos et al. 2006[38]
France	46	34/12	NA	NA	46	40	NA	NA	Meniane et al. 2007 [48]
UK Registry	9	100/0	49 (39–56)	44[b]	56[b]	44	NA	2.6	Gilleece et al. 2008 [39]
FHCRC	13	0/100	NA	60	31	NA	46	NA	Maloney et al. 2008 [49]
France	25	45/55	48 (24–64)	58	67	25	25	5.3	Garnier et al. 2010 [50]
EBMTR	86	43/57	49 (23–64)	56 versus 49[c]	49 versus 64[c]	33 versus 23[a,c]	11 versus 26[a,c]	3	Kyriakou et al. 2010 [41]
Summary	215		48–51 (30–76)	31–60	31–67	23–44	0–29	1.5–5.3	

[a] 3-year.
[b] 4-year.
[c] MAC regimen versus RIC.
Abbreviations: CIBMTR = Center for International Blood and Marrow Transplantation Registry; DFS = disease-free-survival; EBMTR = European Group for Blood and Marrow Transplantation; FHCRC = Fred Hutchinson Cancer Research Center; MAC regimen/RIC = myeloablative conditioning/reduced intensity conditioning; NA = not available; OS = overall survival; TRM = treatment-related mortality.

Auto-HCT as Initial Therapy

Given the success of chemotherapy followed by auto-HCT as part of first-line management of multiple myeloma, investigators tested this approach in WM. In a study by Dreger and Schmitz, 12 patients were treated with dexamethasone plus BEAM mobilization followed by a conditioning regimen of TBI/high-dose Cy, and then rescued with grafts purged by B-cell-negative or CD34-positive selection[42]. Only two of nine patients were negative for presence of disease by IF; six positive patients subsequently relapsed at a median time of 69 months. A second study by Caravita et al. piloted a treatment strategy combining rituximab, Cy, hydroxydoxorubicin, vincristine, and prednisone (R-CHOP) followed by Cy mobilization and upfront consolidation with auto-HCT using high-dose melphalan conditioning[43]. At a median follow-up of 66 months, all five patients maintained a stable partial remission. These small pilot series demonstrated the efficacy of auto-HCT as part of first-line therapy; however, the follow-up times were short and number of patients small, therefore auto-HCT in this setting remains investigational and should be performed only in the context of well-designed prospective clinical trials for high-risk WM patients. The selection of patients for auto-HCT is critically important due to the long median survival of this malignancy that must be weighed against the risk of developing post-transplant secondary malignancies and late transplant-related toxicities. This modality is best used for patients with relapsed but chemosensitive WM before they receive more than three chemotherapy regimens. The choice of conditioning does not appear to affect outcomes; however, the use of BEAM or melphalan plus TBI has been associated with responses lasting more than 4 to 5 years.

Allogeneic HCT for WM

Similar to other NHL, allogeneic (allo-HCT) may offer curative potential in WM. Compared with auto-HCT or chemotherapy alone, it yields lower relapse rates and favorable lymphoma-free survival. Recent series and selected trials in WM are summarized in Table 40.4.

Myeloablative Conditioning Allogeneic HCT

Early single-institution series included multiply relapsed patients and used myeloablative conditioning (MAC) regimens. In the French experience, 10 patients with advanced WM underwent a TBI-based conditioning regimen followed by an HLA-identical sibling donor transplant. At a median follow-up of 1.5 years, six patients were alive, two without relapse, while four had died from transplant complications between 3 and 18 months post-transplant[46]. In a report from Canada, four of five patients achieved a partial remission with evidence of delayed decline of IgM levels over 6 months post-transplant without any subsequent therapy[47]. These observations suggested evidence of a graft-*versus*-WM effect. A CIBMTR report included 26 allo-HCT recipients with advanced WM[45]. Almost 50% were resistant to prior salvage chemotherapy; 52% received TBI-based MAC regimens and 19% a reduced intensity conditioning (RIC) regimen. Results demonstrated unacceptably high TRM (40%) after MAC regimen and an approximate 30% relapse rate. At a median follow-up of 5 years, 3-year OS and PFS were 46% and 31%, respectively. The French reported 46 patients in whom two-thirds received MAC regimen HCT; 1-year TRM was 40% and 5-year OS 46%, suggestive of promising long-term disease control [48]. These data demonstrate that extended survival after allo-HCT is possible even in advanced WM; however, MAC regimen carries with it a very high mortality and should be used sparingly only in selected young patients with limited prior therapy.

Reduced Intensity Allo-HCT

Reducing the conditioning regimen intensity prior to allo-HCT can decrease toxicity while allowing engraftment and a subsequent graft-*versus*-lymphoma (GvL) effect. Hence, elderly patients and those with pretransplant comorbidities can be considered for RIC allo-HCT. Maloney *et al.* collected data on 13 patients who underwent allo-HCT with RIC regimen consisting of fludarabine and low-dose TBI (2 Gy)[49]. An ORR of 91% and PFS and OS rates of 60% suggested favorable long-term outcomes. Similarly promising were the results from the British registry on nine WM patients that reported 4-year DFS and OS of 44% and 56%, respectively[39]. In 2010, Garnier *et al.* updated the French registry data by including WM patients who received RIC HCT[50]. The median age among the 25 patients undergoing RIC allo-HCT was 48 years. The median number of lines of prior therapies was 3% and 44% of patients had chemorefractory disease prior to transplant. The ORR of the entire group was 92% and half were complete responses. Five-year OS and PFS were 67% and 58%, respectively. Notably, only one relapse occurred >3 years after transplant suggesting that durable remissions can be attained even in heavily pretreated WM.

The EBMTR series, the largest published analysis to date, compared outcomes based on conditioning regimen intensity for 86 patients with advanced WM treated with allo-HCT[41]. Most patients received fludarabine-based RIC regimen (n=49) and *in-vivo* or *ex-vivo* T-cell depleted grafts (n=51); eight patients had failed prior auto-HCT, and almost 70% of WM patients had chemosensitive disease at the time of allo-HCT. The median time to response was 6 months, and 15 patients achieved a CR confirmed by IF. VGPR, PR, and stable disease were observed in 13, 17, and 6 patients, respectively. TRM was modestly reduced with RIC (23%) compared to MAC regimen (33%). The relapse rate at 3 years was 25% for RIC and 11% for MAC regimen. Although a third of patients were high risk according to the IPSSWM staging system and expected to have an estimated survival of 3 years, OS was 75% at a median

follow-up of 50 months. The estimated 5-year OS and PFS rates were 62% and 56%, respectively, with no difference in either outcome based on conditioning intensity. It is important to note that median age in this series was 39 years (MAC regimen cohort) and 46 years (RIC cohort), respectively, which is much lower than the median age of WM patients in general. Patients with poor performance status at the time of HCT had significantly inferior PFS.

What is the Evidence for a Graft-*versus*-WM Effect Following Allo-HCT?

Current data indicate there is a robust graft-*versus*-tumor effect in this disease. The Seattle group demonstrated that patients who developed extensive chronic graft-*versus*-host disease (GvHD) had longer survival and protection from relapse[49]. These results were confirmed in the EBMTR series, where results from a landmark analysis at 6 months showed that chronic GvHD significantly reduced disease progression (P=0.03) and tendency to improved PFS[41]. The observation that alemtuzumab and T-cell depletion increased the relapse rate after HCT provides additional evidence for a beneficial T-cell mediated graft-*versus*-tumor effect[39]. Another line of evidence comes from an analysis of EBMTR data on donor lymphocyte infusion (DLI)[41]. Twenty-one patients received DLI, six for mixed chimerism and fourteen for persistent or relapsed disease post-allo-HCT. The ORR to DLI was 80% (CR (n=7), PR (n=4)), with only two patients failing to respond. Importantly, the OS and DFS survival curves of patients treated with allo-HCT reached a plateau over time, in contrast to the outcomes from auto-HCT, where late relapses continued to occur. In aggregate, evidence suggests that a potent graft-*versus*-WM effect may offer protection from relapse for selected patients.

Future Directions

Research in WM must continue to focus on developing genetic and molecular tools to allow for more precise disease stratification, particularly the early identification of those patients with short survival and genetic resistance to chemotherapy. Testing for MYD88 and CXCR4 mutations is becoming available in clinical practice, and may provide additional benefit in risk stratification. Given the relapsing nature of WM and advanced median age, clinical trials should include quality of life measures and an evaluation of the economic impact of therapy. Innovations in supportive care and advances in management of GvHD after allo-HCT may lead to safer allograft transplants and offer greater hope for more WM patients.

Controversies in Incorporating HCT into a Treatment Algorithm

Due to the lack of comparative studies, clinical recommendations regarding incorporating HCT into a treatment algorithm are largely based on opinions of experts and WM study groups

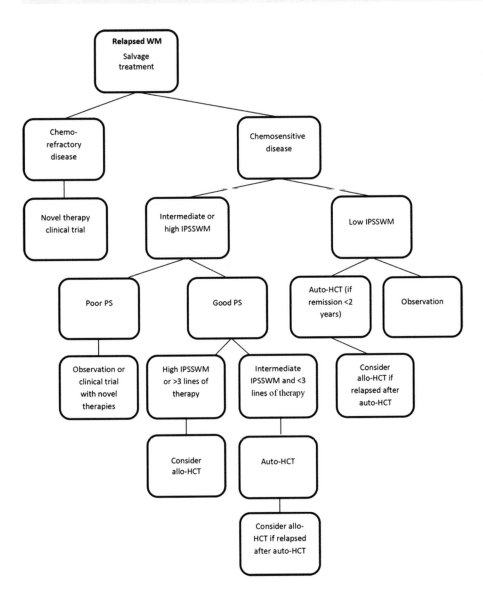

Figure 40.1 Algorithm for management of relapse Waldenström macroglobulinemia WM=Waldenström macroglobulinemia, IPSSWM=International Prognostic Score for Waldenstrom Macroglobulinemia, PS=performance score, HCT=hematopoietic cell transplantation, auto=autologous, allo=allogeneic.

[8,21,51]. The first controversial area concerns auto-HCT: What is the appropriate timing and indication for auto-HCT for WM? (Figure 40.1) Auto-HCT should be considered for recurrent chemotherapy-sensitive WM, particularly in individuals with intermediate or high IPPSWM score or short PFS after initial chemotherapy. Auto-HCT is well tolerated with low TRM; therefore, age should not be a barrier to auto-HCT. However, the timing of auto-HCT is critical in WM. Patients with chemoresistant disease and more than three prior regimens will likely not derive benefit from auto-HCT. We recommend limiting or avoiding the use of nucleoside analogs and alkylating agents in transplant-eligible patients due to higher risks of mobilization failure and second malignancies. Auto-HCT could be carefully considered for consolidation in first remission in patients with very high-risk WM, but only in the setting of a clinical trial.

Which patients with WM should be considered for allo-HCT (Figure 40.1)? Outcomes of allo-HCT for WM are comparable to those with indolent lymphoma and proper patient selection leads to 45–65% long-term disease-free survival. Younger, healthy patients with short duration of first response and very high-risk IPSSWM scores and high LDH could be considered for allo-HCT with curative intent. In addition, patients with good performance status, chemosensitive disease, and limited comorbidities can benefit from allograft even if they have relapsed after multiple lines of therapy and/or prior autograft. Increasing experience with RIC regimens extends the benefit of allo-HCT to older patients and those with comorbidities, thus offering the possibility of prolonged PFS to many patients with otherwise poor outcomes with chemotherapy. Both RIC and MAC regimens can be considered for allo-HCT; the choice should be guided by the patient's age, disease status, and comorbidities.

The authors declare no conflict of interest in the writing of this chapter.

References

1. Treon SP, Patterson CJ, Munshi NC, Anderson KC. Proceedings of the Seventh International Workshop on Waldenstrom Macroglobulinemia. *Clin Lymphoma Myeloma Leuk* 2013;13(2):181–183.

2. Gertz MA. Waldenstrom macroglobulinemia: 2013 update on diagnosis, risk stratification, and management. *Am J Hematol* 2013;88(8):703–711.

3. Sahota SS, Forconi F, Ottensmeier CH, Provan D, Oscier DG, Hamblin TJ, *et al.* Typical Waldenstrom macroglobulinemia is derived from a B-cell arrested after cessation of somatic mutation but prior to isotype switch events. *Blood* 2002;100(4):1505–1507.

4. Morton LM, Wang SS, Devesa SS, Hartge P, Weisenburger DD, Linet MS. Lymphoma incidence patterns by WHO subtype in the United States, 1992-2001. *Blood* 2006 Jan 1;107(1):265-276.

5. Boise LH, Kaufman JL, Heffner LT, Shah NN, Lechowicz MJ, Lonial S, *et al.* Changing epidemiology and improved survival in patients with Waldenstrom macroglobulinemia: review of surveillance, epidemiology, and end results (SEER) data. *Blood* 2013;122(21):3135–3135.

6. Castillo JJ, Olszewski AJ, Cronin AM, Hunter ZR, Treon SP. Survival trends in Waldenstrom macroglobulinemia: an analysis of the Surveillance, Epidemiology and End Results database. *Blood* 2014;123(25):3999–4000.

7. Ciccarelli BT, Patterson CJ, Hunter ZR, Hanzis C, Ioakimidis L, Manning R, *et al.* Hepcidin is produced by lymphoplasmacytic cells and is associated with anemia in Waldenstrom's macroglobulinemia. *Clin Lymphoma Myeloma Leuk* 2011;11(1):160–163.

8. Ansell SM, Kyle RA, Reeder CB, Fonseca R, Mikhael JR, Morice WG, *et al.* Diagnosis and management of Waldenstrom macroglobulinemia: Mayo stratification of macroglobulinemia and risk-adapted therapy (mSMART) guidelines. *Mayo Clin Proc* 2010;85(9):824–833.

9. Garcia-Sanz R, Montoto S, Torrequebrada A, de Coca AG, Petit J, Sureda A, *et al.* Waldenstrom macroglobulinaemia: presenting features and outcome in a series with 217 cases. *Br J Haematol* 2001;115(3):575–582.

10. Michael AB, Lawes M, Kamalarajan M, Huissoon A, Pratt G. Cryoglobulinaemia as an acute presentation of Waldenstrom's macroglobulinaemia. *Br J Haematol* 2004;124(5):565.

11. Nobile-Orazio E, Marmiroli P, Baldini L, Spagnol G, Barbieri S, Moggio M, *et al.* Peripheral neuropathy in macroglobulinemia: incidence and antigen-specificity of M proteins. *Neurology* 1987;37(9):1506–1514.

12. Mauro FR, Foa R, Cerretti R, Giannarelli D, Coluzzi S, Mandelli F, *et al.* Autoimmune hemolytic anemia in chronic lymphocytic leukemia: clinical, therapeutic, and prognostic features. *Blood* 2000;95(9):2786–2792.

13. Treon SP, Cao Y, Xu L, Yang G, Liu X, Hunter ZR. Somatic mutations in MYD88 and CXCR4 are determinants of clinical presentation and overall survival in Waldenstrom macroglobulinemia. *Blood* 2014;123(18):2791–2796.

14. Ocio EM, Schop RFJ, Gonzalez B, Van Wier SA, Hernandez-Rivas JM, Gutierrez NC, *et al.* 6q deletion in Waldenström macroglobulinemia is associated with features of adverse prognosis. *Br J Haematol* 2007;136(1):80–86.

15. Nguyen-Khac F, Lambert J, Chapiro E, Grelier A, Mould S, Barin C, *et al.* Chromosomal aberrations and their prognostic value in a series of 174 untreated patients with Waldenström's macroglobulinemia. *Haematologica* 2013;98(4):649–654.

16. Sacco A, Zhang Y, Maiso P, Manier S, Rossi G, Treon SP, *et al.* microRNA aberrations in Waldenstrom macroglobulinemia. *Clin Lymphoma Myeloma Leuk* 2013;13(2):205–207.

17. Roccaro AM, Sacco A, Jia X, Azab AK, Maiso P, Ngo HT, *et al.* microRNA-dependent modulation of histone acetylation in Waldenstrom macroglobulinemia. *Blood* 2010;116(9):1506–1514.

18. Morel P, Duhamel A, Gobbi P, Dimopoulos MA, Dhodapkar MV, McCoy J, *et al.* International prognostic scoring system for Waldenström macroglobulinemia. *Blood* 2009;113(18):4163–4170.

19. Kastritis E, Zervas K, Repoussis P, Michali E, Katodrytou E, Zomas A, *et al.* Prognostication in young and old patients with Waldenstrom's macroglobulinemia: importance of the International Prognostic Scoring System and of serum lactate dehydrogenase. *Clin Lymphoma Myeloma* 2009;9(1):50–52.

20. Kyle RA, Treon SP, Alexanian R, Barlogie B, Bjorkholm M, Dhodapkar M, *et al.* Prognostic markers and criteria to initiate therapy in Waldenstrom's macroglobulinemia: consensus panel recommendations from the Second International Workshop on Waldenstrom's Macroglobulinemia. *Semin Oncol* 2003;30(2):116–120.

21. Dimopoulos M, Kastritis E, Owen RG, Kyle RA, Landgren O, Morra E, *et al.* Treatment recommendations for patients with Waldenström macroglobulinemia (WM) and related disorders: IWWM-7 consensus *Blood* 2014;124(9):1404–1411.

22. Ricci F, Tedeschi A, Montillo M, Morra E. Therapy-related myeloid neoplasms in chronic lymphocytic leukemia and Waldenstrom's macroglobulinemia. *Mediterr J Hematol Infect Dis* 2011;3(1): e2011031.

23. Cornell RF, Palmer J. Adult acute leukemia. *Dis Mon* 2012;58(4):219–238.

24. Leblond V, Johnson S, Chevret S, Copplestone A, Rule S, Tournilhac O, *et al.* Results of a randomized trial of chlorambucil versus fludarabine for patients with untreated Waldenström macroglobulinemia, marginal zone lymphoma, or lymphoplasmacytic lymphoma. *J Clin Oncol* 2013;31(3):301–307.

25. Dimopoulos MA, Alexanian R, Gika D, Anagnostopoulos A, Zervas C, Zomas A, *et al.* Treatment of Waldenstrom's macroglobulinemia with rituximab: prognostic factors for response and progression. *Leuk Lymphoma* 2004;45(10):2057–2061.

26. Gertz MA, Rue M, Blood E, Kaminer LS, Vesole DH, Greipp PR. Multicenter phase 2 trial of rituximab for Waldenstrom macroglobulinemia (WM): an Eastern Cooperative Oncology Group Study (E3A98). *Leuk Lymphoma* 2004;45(10):2047–2055.

27. Treon SP, Emmanouilides C, Kimby E, Kelliher A, Preffer F, Branagan AR, et al. Extended rituximab therapy in Waldenstrom's macroglobulinemia. Ann Oncol 2005;16(1):132–138.

28. Ghobrial IM, Xie W, Padmanabhan S, Badros A, Rourke M, Leduc R, et al. Phase II trial of weekly bortezomib in combination with rituximab in untreated patients with Waldenström Macroglobulinemia. Am J Hematol 2010;85(9):670–674.

29. Dimopoulos MA, Garcia-Sanz R, Gavriatopoulou M, Morel P, Kyrtsonis MC, Michalis E, et al. Primary therapy of Waldenstrom macroglobulinemia (WM) with weekly bortezomib, low-dose dexamethasone, and rituximab (BDR): long-term results of a phase 2 study of the European Myeloma Network (EMN). Blood 2013;122(19):3276–3282.

30. Treon SP, Soumerai JD, Branagan AR, Hunter ZR, Patterson CJ, Ioakimidis L, et al. Thalidomide and rituximab in Waldenstrom macroglobulinemia. Blood 2008;112(12):4452–4457.

31. Treon SP, Soumerai JD, Branagan AR, Hunter ZR, Patterson CJ, Ioakimidis L, et al. Lenalidomide and rituximab in Waldenstrom's macroglobulinemia. Clin Cancer Res 2009;15(1):355–360.

32. Rosenthal AC, Dueck AC, Gano K, Ansell SM, Conley C, Nowakowski GS, et al. A Phase 2 Study of lenalidomide, rituximab, cyclophosphamide and dexamethasone (LR-CD) for untreated low grade non-Hodgkin lymphoma requiring therapy: Waldenström's macroglobulinemia cohort results. Blood 2013;122(21):4352.

33. Chen CI, Kouroukis CT, White D, Voralia M, Stadtmauer E, Stewart AK, et al. Bortezomib is active in patients with untreated or relapsed Waldenstrom's macroglobulinemia: a phase II study of the National Cancer Institute of Canada Clinical Trials Group. J Clin Oncol 2007;25(12):1570–1575.

34. Treon SP, Hanzis C, Tripsas C, Ioakimidis L, Patterson CJ, Manning RJ, et al. Bendamustine therapy in patients with relapsed or refractory Waldenstrom's macroglobulinemia. Clin Lymphoma Myeloma Leuk 2011;11(1):133–135.

35. Ghobrial IM, Witzig TE, Gertz M, LaPlant B, Hayman S, Camoriano J, et al. Long-term results of the phase II trial of the oral mTOR inhibitor everolimus (RAD001) in relapsed or refractory Waldenstrom Macroglobulinemia. Am J Hematol 2014;89(3):237–242.

36. Tripsas CK, Yang G, Cao Y, Xu L, Hunter Z, Cropper SJ, et al. A prospective multicenter study of the bruton's tyrosine kinase inhibitor ibrutinib in patients with relapsed or refractory Waldenstrom's macroglobulinemia. Blood 2013;122(21):251–251.

37. Anagnostopoulos A, Dimopoulos MA, Aleman A, Weber D, Alexanian R, Champlin R, et al. High-dose chemotherapy followed by stem cell transplantation in patients with resistant Waldenstrom's macroglobulinemia. Bone Marrow Transplant 2001;27(10):1027–1029.

38. Anagnostopoulos A, Hari PN, Pérez WS, Ballen K, Bashey A, Bredeson CN, et al. Autologous or Allogeneic Stem Cell Transplantation in Patients with Waldenstrom's Macroglobulinemia. Biology of Blood and Marrow Transplantation 2006;12(8):845–854.

39. Gilleece MH, Pearce R, Linch DC, Wilson M, Towlson K, Mackinnon S, et al. The outcome of haemopoietic stem cell transplantation in the treatment of lymphoplasmacytic lymphoma in the UK: a British Society Bone Marrow Transplantation study. Hematology 2008;13(2):119–127.

40. Dhedin N, Tabrizi R, Bulabois PE, Le Gouill S, Coiteux V, Dartigeas C, et al. Hematopoietic stem cell transplantation (HSCT) in Waldenstrom macroglobulinemia (Wm): update of the French experience in 54 cases. ASH Annual Meeting Abstracts 2007;110(11):3015.

41. Kyriakou C, Canals C, Sibon D, Cahn JY, Kazmi M, Arcese W, et al. High-dose therapy and autologous stem-cell transplantation in Waldenström macroglobulinemia: The Lymphoma Working Party of the European Group for Blood and Marrow Transplantation. J Clin Oncol 2010;28(13):2227–2232.

42. Dreger P, Schmitz N. Autologous stem cell transplantation as part of first-line treatment of Waldenstrom's macroglobulinemia. Biol Blood Marrow Transplant 2007;13(5):623–624.

43. Caravita T, Siniscalchi A, Tendas A, Cupelli L, Dentamaro T, Natale G, et al. High-dose therapy with autologous PBSC transplantation in the front-line treatment of Waldenstrom's macroglobulinemia. Bone Marrow Transplant 2009;43(7):587–588.

44. Munshi NC, Barlogie B. Role for high-dose therapy with autologous hematopoietic stem cell support in Waldenstrom's macroglobulinemia. Semin Oncol 2003;30(2):282.

45. Anagnostopoulos A, Aleman A, Giralt S. Autologous and allogeneic stem cell transplantation in Waldenstrom's macroglobulinemia: review of the literature and future directions. Semin Oncol 2003;30(2):286–290.

46. Tournilhac O, Leblond V, Tabrizi R, Gressin R, Senecal D, Milpied N, et al. Transplantation in Waldenstrom's macroglobulinemia: the French experience. Semin Oncol 2003;30(2):291–296.

47. Stakiw J, Kim DH, Kuruvilla J, Gupta V, Messner H, Lipton JH. Evidence of graft-versus-Waldenstrom's macroglobulinaemia effect after allogeneic stem cell transplantation: a single centre experience. Bone Marrow Transplant 2007;40(4):369–372.

48. Meniane JC, El-Cheikh J, Faucher C, Furst S, Bouabdallah R, Blaise D, et al. Long-term graft-versus-Waldenstrom macroglobulinemia effect following reduced intensity conditioning allogeneic stem cell transplantation. Bone Marrow Transplant 2007;40(2):175–177.

49. Maloney D. Allogeneic transplantation following nonmyeloablative conditioning for aggressive lymphoma. Bone Marrow Transplant 2008;42(Suppl 1):S35–S36.

50. Garnier A, Robin M, Larosa F, Golmard JL, Le Gouill S, Coiteux V, et al. Allogeneic hematopoietic stem cell transplantation allows long-term complete remission and curability in high-risk Waldenstrom's macroglobulinemia. Results of a retrospective analysis of the Societe Francaise de Greffe de Moelle et de Therapie Cellulaire. Haematologica 2010;95(6):950–955.

51. Owen RG, Pratt G, Auer RL, Flatley R, Kyriakou C, Lunn MP, et al. Guidelines on the diagnosis and management of Waldenstrom macroglobulinaemia. Br J Haematol 2014;165(3):316–333.

41

Hematopoietic Cell Transplants for Indolent Lymphomas

Vijaya R. Bhatt, James O. Armitage, and R. Gregory Bociek

Is Transplantation Still a Reasonable Option for Indolent Lymphomas in the Chemoimmunotherapy and Molecular Era?

The therapeutic landscape has changed dramatically since the first trials demonstrated the benefit of autologous or allogeneic hematopoietic cell transplant in indolent lymphoma. Long-term outcomes for patients with indolent lymphoma have improved significantly from the addition of concurrent and/or consolidative and maintenance monoclonal antibody therapy to chemotherapy in the setting of upfront or relapsed disease, including prolongation of survival in many trials[1–6]. Newer chemoimmunotherapy regimens with less toxicity are at minimum likely noninferior to older regimens and are increasingly being used as frontline therapy[7,8]. The approval of newer therapies such as idelalisib offer additional choices that while noncurative, are likely to be less toxic options for this patient population. In this context, one could ask what the role of high-dose therapy and autologous (HDT and auto-HCT) and/or allogeneic (allo-HCT) transplant are for indolent lymphomas in the modern chemoimmunotherapy era. It is, however, important to remember in the context of this illness that approximately 10% of untreated follicular lymphoma (FL) patients are refractory to rituximab-based chemotherapy, and nearly one-third relapse within 3 years[2,9]. This chapter will review recent data to try to place the value of HCT in a more recent context, and pose some contemporary questions through the process.

HDT and Auto-HCT for FL in First Remission

Compared to conventional therapy, HDT and auto-HCT in first remission improves progression-free survival (PFS) without any significant improvement in overall survival (OS) in FL (Table 41.1). The *German Low Grade Lymphoma Study Group trial* (n=240)[10], *French Groupe Ouest Est des Leucémies et Autres Maladies du Sang trial* (n=172)[11], and *Groupe d'Etude des Lymphomes de l'Adulte trial* (n=401)[12] all demonstrated a significant improvement in PFS at 5 to 7 years with HDT and auto-HCT compared to conventional chemotherapy. However, no OS advantage was demonstrable in any of these trials. This likely reflects in part the effectiveness of salvage "rescue" therapy at first relapse, offsetting OS advantage in this

setting. In the French trial, an 18% actuarial risk of secondary malignancies at 5 years' post-auto-HCT may also have contributed to the lack of a survival advantage[11].

The addition of rituximab to induction and in transplant strategies has essentially confirmed the same results in the modern frontline transplant setting[13–16]. The *Gruppo Italiano Trapianto di Midollo Osseo* was a randomized trial evaluating the role of upfront HDT and auto-HCT in the rituximab era in high-risk FL patients (n=134). Rituximab supplemented HDT and auto-HCT, compared to R-CHOP, resulted in a higher complete remission rate (85% *versus* 62%, $P < 0.001$), higher molecular remission (80% *versus* 44% of evaluable patients, $P < 0.002$) and longer 4-year event-free survival (EFS) (61% *versus* 28%, $P < 0.001$) but no difference in OS (81% *versus* 80%, $P=0.96$). Seventy-one percent of patients, who relapsed after R-CHOP, were able to go on to HDT and auto-HCT with a complete remission rate of 85% and 3-year EFS of 68%[14]. In a Cochrane review and other meta-analyses, the same outcomes were seen, and in addition there was no measurable difference between control and intervention groups with respect to treatment-related mortality (TRM) or secondary malignancies[13,15,16].

Practice Point

Given the results of randomized trials that include pre- and post-rituximab era strategies, the absence of an OS advantage continues to mitigate against upfront auto-HCT in FL.

HDT and Auto-HCT for Relapsed or Refractory FL

Table 41.2 summarizes older results of HDT and auto-HCT for FL in relapse. A retrospective European Blood and Marrow Transplant registry (EBMTR) study compared long-term outcome of FL who underwent HDT and auto-HCT in first complete remission (n=131) or in primary refractory, partial remission, or relapsed setting (n=562). Five-year NRM was 9%, whereas PFS and OS of the entire cohort were 31% and 52% respectively at 10 years. A multivariate analysis demonstrated age <45 years ($P=0.003$) and auto-HCT in first complete remission ($P < 0.001$) to be predictive of longer PFS, whereas age ≥ 45 years ($P < 0.001$), chemoresistant disease

Table 41.1 Upfront autologous hematopoietic cell transplantation in follicular lymphoma

Authors	n	Characteristics	Treatment arms	Induction therapy	Subsequent therapy	PFS/EFS	OS
Lenz et al. 2004[10]	240	≤60 years in CR1/PR1	Auto-HCT versus chemo	4–6 cycles of CHOP or MCP	Dexa-BEAM mobilization followed by Cy/TBI and auto-HCT versus 2 additional cycles of chemotherapy followed by interferon maintenance	64% versus 33% at 5 years, P < 0.0001	Not mature (84% at 5 years for the entire cohort)
Deconinck et al. 2005 [11]	172	≤60 years in CR1/PR1 (patients who responded to DHAP were also transplanted)	Auto-HCT versus chemo	2–3 cycles of VCAP versus 6 cycles of CHVP and interferon	Ifosfamide, methotrexate, and etoposide followed by Cy/TBI and purged auto-HCT versus CHVP and interferon maintenance for a year	60% versus 48% at 5 years, P=0.05	84% versus 78% at 5 years, P=0.49
Sebban et al. 2006 [12]	401	≤60 years	Auto-HCT versus chemo	4 cycles of CHOP versus 6 monthly courses of CHVP and interferon	Cyclophosphamide and etoposide mobilization followed by Cy/etoposide/TBI and auto-HCT versus 6 courses of CHVP plus interferon maintenance for a year	38% versus 28% at 7 years, P=0.11	76% versus 71% at 7 years, P=0.53
Ladetto et al. 2008 [14]	134	≤60 years	Auto-HCT versus chemo	2 cycles of APO versus 6 cycles of CHOP followed by 4 doses of rituximab	High-dose etoposide, then 2 rituximab courses, then high-dose cyclophosphamide, and in-vivo purging with 2 doses of rituximab, followed by high-dose mitoxantrone and melphalan prior to auto-HCT versus none	61% versus 28% at 4 years, P < 0.001	81% versus 80% at 4 years, P=0.96

APO = doxorubicin, vincristine, prednisone; auto-HCT = autologous hematopoietic cell transplant; BEAM = carmustine, etoposide, cytarabine, and melphalan; CHOP = cyclophosphamide, doxorubicin, vincristine, and prednisone; CHVP = cyclophosphamide, doxorubicin, teniposide, and prednisone; CR1 = first complete remission; Cy/TBI = cyclophosphamide/total body irradiation; EFS = event-free survival; n = number; MCP = mitoxantrone, chlorambucil, and prednisolone; OS = overall survival; PFS = progression-free survival; PR1 = first partial remission; VCAP = cyclophosphamide, high-dose doxorubicin, prednisone, and vincristine.

Table 41.2 Autologous hematopoietic cell transplantation in relapsed or refractory follicular lymphoma

Author	n	Characteristics	Treatment arms	Salvage induction	Subsequent therapy	PFS/EFS	OS
Schouten et al. 2003 [19]	140	Relapsed, <65 years	Purged versus unpurged auto-HCT versus chemo	3 cycles of CHOP for auto-HCT arms versus 6 cycles of CHOP	Cy/TBI prior to purged or unpurged auto-HCT versus none	55% versus 58% versus 26% at 2 years (P=0.0037)	77% versus 71% versus 46% at 4 years (P=0.079)
Montoto et al. 2007 [17]	693	First remission, relapsed or refractory, <65 years	Auto-HCT in CR1 versus in responses other than CR1	Not reported	TBI (58%) or chemotherapy-based conditioning (BEAM/BEAC/others) (42%) followed by purged (45%) or unpurged auto-HCT	39% versus 26% at 15 years	60% versus 44% at 15 years
Vose et al. 2008[21]	248	Relapsed or refractory, <67 years	Auto-HCT	Not reported	Cy/TBI, BEAM, BEAC, rituximab-BEAM followed by unpurged auto-HCT	44% at 5 years	63% at 5 years
Le Gouill et al. 2011 [20]	175	Relapsed or refractory after rituximab-based induction, <75 years	Auto-HCT versus chemo	Various (cytarabine, cyclophosphamide, anthracycline, and fludarabine-based) with rituximab (64%)	Cy/TBI or BEAM (76%) versus none	73% versus 39% at 3 years (P=0.005).	92% versus 63% at 3 years (P=0.0003)

Auto-HCT = autologous hematopoietic cell transplantation; BEAC = carmustine, etoposide, cytarabine, cyclophosphamide; BEAM = carmustine, etoposide, cytarabine, and melphalan; CHOP = cyclophosphamide, doxorubicin, vincristine, and prednisone; CR1 = first complete remission; Cy/TBI = cyclophosphamide/total body irradiation; EFS = event-free survival; N = number; OS = overall survival; PFS = progression-free survival.

(P<0.001), use of bone marrow plus peripheral blood hematopoietic cells (P=0.007), and total body irradiation (TBI)-containing regimens (P=0.004) were predictive of shorter OS. A plateau in PFS curve observed with a long follow-up suggested the curative possibility of HDT and auto-HCT in a proportion of patients. Age ≥ 45 years (P < 0.001), refractory disease (P <0.001) and TBI-containing regimens (P=0.04) predicted worse NRM. At 7 years, second malignancy and secondary myeloid neoplasm were seen in 9% and 5.7% of patients respectively. Approximately 85% of secondary myeloid neoplasms were associated with the use of TBI[17]. In fact, the use of TBI is considered as one of the most important risk factors for therapy-related myeloid neoplasms[18]. The EBMTR study, although conducted in the pre-rituximab era, confirmed that auto-HCT in the relapse or refractory setting offers OS benefit similar to first complete remission[17].

Several additional studies including the randomized European CUP (random treatment assignments to chemotherapy alone *versus* HDT and auto-HCT with Unpurged, or Purged treatment groups) trial[19] have demonstrated excellent long-term outcomes in relapsed FL patients using HDT and auto-HCT[19–21]. Although accrual to the CUP trial was shorter than anticipated and survival was a secondary endpoint, mature data did eventually demonstrate an OS advantage to the transplanted group. A study at the University of Nebraska Medical Center highlighted prior exposure to ≥ 3 chemotherapy regimens, histologic grade of FL 3, and a high-risk FLIPI score at the time of HDT and auto-HCT to be associated with worse PFS and OS[21]. In at least two trials, patients with prior exposure to rituximab had excellent outcomes with HDT and auto-HCT at the time of relapse suggesting no adverse impact of prior exposure to rituximab[20] (unlike the CORAL study in relapsed diffuse large B-cell lymphoma)[22].

Practice Points

Given these considerations and collective data, it is our preferred approach to offer a non-TBI-based conditioning regimen with HDT and auto-HCT to "fit" chemosensitive patients in first relapse with the understanding that virtually all patients will have received prior rituximab, either as part of initial therapy, at salvage, or both. For the rare patients, without exposure to rituximab as part of recue therapy, we would generally offer 1–2 rituximab infusions pretransplant.

Additional Considerations in the Rituximab Era for Auto-HCT

Given the inferior outcomes for patients with prior rituximab exposure in the CORAL study[22], some additional modern rituximab-based data are worth consideration. A retrospective review of outcomes at relapse for patients enrolled in the GELA/GOELEMS FL 2000 trial demonstrated that the use of rituximab during induction did not affect EFS or OS for FL patients undergoing HDT and auto-HCT at relapse[20].

Similarly Kothari *et al.* published a single-center retrospective study of 70 patients undergoing HDT and auto-HCT demonstrating no difference in PFS or OS when comparing patients who received rituximab (single agent or in combination with chemotherapy) as a treatment line prior to transplant *versus* those who did not[23]. A large retrospective analysis by the National Comprehensive Cancer Network (NCCN) looked at the effects of prior rituximab in both the autologous-HCT (n=136) and allogeneic-HCT (n=48) setting. Though not directly compared to a cohort of rituximab-unexposed patients, the TRM, PFS, and OS for both groups appears comparable to data from the pre-rituximab era[24]. A retrospective analysis from Alberta demonstrated inferior PFS (Hazard ratio (HR) =2.04) and OS (HR=4.3) for patients undergoing auto-HCT who had not been exposed to rituximab within 6 months of transplant[25].

Practice Points

Therefore, it seems reasonable to conclude that the use of HDT and auto-HCT still offers a reasonable benefit in the rituximab era, though patients deemed refractory to rituximab may do less well with HDT and auto-HCT[26]. Conditioning regimens employing radioimmunotherapy (see Chapter 28) have shown feasibility and outcomes comparable to regimens using chemotherapy alone [27,28], but a lack of controlled trials precludes the ability to directly compare results to strategies employing rituximab.

The Role of Rituximab in Graft Purging

Graft purging has been investigated with a goal to improve outcomes[19,29,30]. In what is likely the best known pre-rituximab era purging study, the CUP trial randomized 140 patients with relapsed FL to chemotherapy alone *versus* chemotherapy followed by auto-HCT with purged or unpurged marrow harvests[19]. Bone marrow hematopoietic cells were purged *in-vitro* with anti-B-cell monoclonal antibodies and rabbit complement. The trial was not powered for the effect of purging as a primary endpoint and was unable to show any clinical benefit to this strategy.

In a modern proof-of-principle study by Arcaini *et al.*, 64 patients with advanced relapsed/refractory FL underwent rituximab-based immunochemotherapy followed by *in-vivo* purging and peripheral blood progenitor cell mobilization with high-dose cytarabine and rituximab[30]. For patients with evidence of a bcl-2 rearrangement in the marrow at baseline, a molecular remission rate of 87% was achieved following immunochemotherapy and all hematopoietic cell harvests were polymerase chain reaction (PCR) negative. Five-year OS and PFS were 94% and 59% respectively. Not surprisingly the attainment of molecular remission in the marrow after transplant predicted for prolonged disease control rates but the lack of a control group precludes the ability to determine whether or not these outcomes are simply a surrogate for disease sensitivity overall rather than the specific effects of purging.

The Role of Rituximab Consolidation/Maintenance after Auto-HCT

As rituximab maintenance prolongs PFS in the setting of conventional dose chemotherapy, the same potential for at least a PFS benefit might exist with the use of rituximab as a consolidative/maintenance therapy after HDT and auto-HCT. In a prospective phase II study, high-risk advanced stage relapsed FL patients (n=23) underwent in-vivo graft purging with single-dose rituximab and post-auto-HCT rituximab maintenance (two 4-week cycles of rituximab $375\,mg/m^2$ at weeks 8 and 24 post-auto-HCT). These patients had not received prior rituximab. This trial reported a 5-year PFS and OS of 59% and 78%, respectively. The time to progression with this strategy was significantly longer than the most recent therapy (P <0.001). Molecular remission after auto-HCT was associated with a prolonged PFS (P=0.001) but without prolongation of OS[31]. Another study confirmed an improvement in molecular remission with a single 4-week course of rituximab after auto-HCT in FL patients treated without rituximab-based induction[32].

For patients who fail to attain a complete remission after HDT and auto-HCT, it would seem possible that rituximab could also prolong time to progression for this group. In a phase II study, FL patients (n=39) with clinical or molecular residual disease detectable 3 months after auto-HCT underwent four weekly courses of rituximab. Rituximab use resulted in a response rate of >70%, frequently durable, in patients with both clinical and molecular residual disease. Molecular remission was associated with excellent disease control, and molecular relapse preceded clinical relapse by ≥12 months [33]. Again in the absence of a control group it is difficult to ascertain the true benefit of this strategy. A recent randomized trial from the EBMT utilized a very elegant 2 × 2 factorial design to simultaneously look at the effect of rituximab in-vivo purging and rituximab maintenance. This trial failed to show any benefit to in-vivo purging prior to harvest, but did show an improvement in PFS (10-year PFS 54% versus 37%, P=0.012) for patients randomized to maintenance rituximab after auto-HCT[34].

Practice Point

Contrary to experts in some centers, we do not currently recommend maintenance rituximab post-auto-HCT in low-grade lymphomas.

Allo-HCT for FL (Table 41.1)

Although auto-HCT continues to be supportable by reasonable evidence in the rituximab era, disease progression/relapse continues to be the most common reason for the failure of auto-HCT. Allo-HCT has consistently been associated with a lower

probability of relapse presumably principally because of the putative graft-versus-lymphoma effect, but is also consistently associated with a higher probability of TRM, in general offsetting any survival gain that could result from the reduction in relapse. The biologic need to have a donor precludes the ability to perform conventional randomized trials. Nonetheless many investigators believe that allo-HCT does offer curative potential for patients with indolent lymphomas. This section will look at the outcomes of allo-HCT in indolent lymphoma with a view towards more recent comparisons of auto-HCT with allo-HCT and comparisons of "myeloablative conditioning regimens" (MAC regimen) with less-intense myelotoxic conditioning regimens (see Chapters 2 and 27).

Conditioning Regimen Intensity in Allo-HCT

Although the history of allo-HCT is rooted in the concept of MAC regimen, the past few decades have seen maturing data using reduced intensity conditioning (RIC) or nonmyeloablative conditioning (NMC) regimens with the hope of reducing TRM and toxicity. However, a large CIBMTR study (n=208) of RIC versus MAC regimen allo-HCT in FL resulted in similar TRM (28% versus 25%, P=0.60), PFS (55% versus 67%, P=0.07), and OS (62% versus 71%, P=0.15) at 3 years. Karnofsky performance status ≥90% and chemosensitive disease was associated with lower TRM and higher OS and PFS. However, RIC allo-HCT was associated with a nearly three-fold increased relative risk of disease progression in a multivariate analysis but it is worth noting that the RIC regimen cohort were a median of 7 years older than the MAC regimen cohort[35].

A trial of 73 patients with various indolent histology lymphomas or myeloma using matched related or unrelated donors and fludarabine/cyclophosphamide conditioning demonstrated a 14% incidence of grade II–IV acute graft-versus-host disease (GvHD) and a clear plateau in relapse at 25% for FL subjects. All relapses appear to have occurred early but 3-year NRM was 19% likely demonstrating the ongoing risks associated with chronic GvHD and late infections[36]. Other trials using the same regimen have demonstrated a similar incidence of disease progression and a lower 3-year TRM (9% in CALGB 109901)[37]. The fludarabine, cyclophosphamide, and rituximab (FCR) regimen as described by Khouri et al. has produced a 12-year PFS of 72% in 47 patients with relapsed FL[38]. Other published RIC/NMC regimens with data showing good long-term outcomes include fludarabine/low-dose TBI[39] and fludarabine/busulfan/^{90}yttrium tiuxetan [40]. RIC/NMC allo-HCT can be carried out with good outcomes in appropriately selected patients with NHL who have failed prior auto-HCT[41].

It is important to note that the median age of patients in the above studies was in the range of 51–55 years. This suggests that RIC/NMC regimens are clearly feasible in older and to some extent less fit patients, and as such, have expanded to some extent the patient population eligible for allo-HCT.

Table 41.3 Autologous *versus* allogeneic hematopoietic cell transplant in follicular lymphoma

Author	n	Characteristics	Treatment arms	Common regimens	NRM	PFS/EFS	OS
van Besien *et al.* 2003 [44]	904	<65 years for allo-HCT and <72 years for auto-HCT	Unpurged *versus* Purged auto-HCT *versus* allo-HCT	Various	8% *versus* 14% *versus* 30% at 5 years	31% *versus* 39% *versus* 45% at 5 years	55% *versus* 62% *versus* 51% at 5 years
Ingram *et al.* 2008 [45]	126	Relapsed, <60 years for allo-HCT and <75 years for auto-HCT	Auto-HCT *versus* allo-HCT	BEAM *versus* BEAM-alemtuzumab	2% *versus* 20% at 1 year	56% *versus* 58% at 3 years	67% *versus* 69% at 3 years
Tomblyn *et al.* 2011 [46]	30	Relapsed chemosensitive, <67 years	Auto-HCT *versus* RIC allo-HCT	Cy and rituximab mobilization, then CBV or Cy/etoposide/TBI for auto-HCT *versus* FCR for allo-HCT	21% *versus* 0% at 3 years	63% *versus* 86% at 3 years	73% *versus* 100% at 3 years
Robinson *et al.* 2013 [50]	875	Beyond first CR or PR	Auto-HCT *versus* RIC allo-HCT	BEAM (auto-HCT) Various Fludarabine-based regimens for allo-HCT	5% *versus* 22% at 3 years	48% *versus* 57% at 5 years	72% *versus* 67% at 5 years
Evens *et al.* 2013[24]	135	Relapsed or refractory after rituximab-based induction, ≤70 years	Auto-HCT	CBV, BEAM or TBI-based	1% at day 100, and 3% at 1 year	57% at 3 years	87% at 3 years
	49	Relapsed or refractory after rituximab-based induction, <65 years	Allo-HCT: MRD 63%, MUD 37%	Flu/Mel (31%), TBI-based (29%), Bu/Flu (23%)	6% at day 100, and 24% at 1 year	52% at 3 years	61% at 3 years

Auto-HCT = autologous hematopoietic cell transplant; allo-HCT = allogeneic hematopoietic cell transplant; BEAM = carmustine, etoposide, cytarabine, and melphalan; Bu/Flu = busulfan/fludarabine; CBV = cyclophosphamide, bis-chloro-ethylnitrosourea (BCNU), and etoposide; CR1 = first complete remission; Cy/TBI = cyclophosphamide/total body irradiation; EFS = event-free survival; FCR = fludarabine, cyclophosphamide, and rituximab; Flu/Mel = fludarabine/melphalan; n = number; NRM = nonrelapse mortality; OS = overall survival; PFS = progression-free survival; PR1 = first partial remission; RIC= reduced intensity conditioning regimen; TBI = total body irradiation.

Nonetheless, careful selection of potential candidates remains crucial since most of the TRM is associated with GvHD and post-allo-HCT infections. Although RIC/NMC regimens appear to be associated with less direct regimen-related toxicity, there may also be some loss of disease control associated with the reduction in the "intensity" of the preparative regimen. Regardless of outcome data, it appears that RIC allo-HCT has become the preferred strategy over myeloablative allo-HCT as evidenced by a steady increase in the proportion of RIC allo-HCT from <10% in 1997 to >80% in 2002 in the CIBMTR study[35].

Perhaps the best of both elements of transplant could be combined by using an initial chemotherapy intense auto-HCT followed in time by RIC allo-HCT (tandem auto/allotransplant) which would combine therapy but separate to a large extent the toxicity of each component over time. This strategy is clearly feasible[42,43]. Crochiollo *et al.*[43] have demonstrated very encouraging results in a small trial of selected patients but cost considerations and a lack of high-level comparative trials makes comparison with other strategies extremely difficult.

Practice Point

Our approach is to offer auto-HCT in first relapse for chemosensitive patients, reserving RIC allo-HCT for "fit" patients in whom disease control can be obtained again after failure of auto-HCT.

Comparing Auto-HCT and Allo-HCT

A few observational studies have compared the results of auto-HCT and allo-HCT (Table 41.3). In an International Bone Marrow Transplant Registry/Autologous Blood and Marrow Transplant Registry study of FL patients (n=904), allo-HCT, compared to purged and unpurged auto-HCT, resulted in higher 5-year TRM (30% *versus* 14% *versus* 8%), lower 5-year relapse risk (21% *versus* 43% *versus* 58%), and comparable OS (51% *versus* 62% *versus* 55%). In multivariate analysis, the OS was higher with purged *versus* unpurged auto-HCT, lower during the first 6 months, and similar after 6 months in allo-HCT *versus* unpurged auto-HCT. Age >40 years, poor performance status, elevated lactate dehydrogenase, time interval from diagnosis to HCT of >1 year, chemoresistant disease, HCT after first remission or first relapse, and year of HCT predicted worse OS. Additionally, involvement of bone marrow at HCT was a predictor of higher relapse risk, and the use of TBI-based conditioning was a predictor of lower relapse and higher TRM[44]. High TRM with allo-HCT, offsetting the benefit of lower relapse, has been observed in other studies also[24,45]. High TRM frequently results in similar or even lower OS with allo-HCT, compared to auto-HCT

[24,44,45]. Allo-HCT patients, although frequently younger, are more likely to have unfavorable characteristics such as chemoresistant disease, multiple prior therapies, advanced stage, and bone marrow involvement at the time of transplant[24,44,45].

A Blood and Marrow Transplant Clinical Trials Network trial (n=30) attempted to prospectively compare the outcomes of auto-HCT and RIC allo-HCT in relapsed chemosensitive FL using *sibling donor* availability to select treatment strategy. Unfortunately, the trial was prematurely closed because of slow accrual. Compared to auto-HCT, RIC allo-HCT resulted in lower TRM (0 *versus* 21%), similar relapse risk (14% *versus* 15%), higher PFS (86% *versus* 63%), and higher OS (100% *versus* 73%) at 3 years. Although a definite conclusion cannot be made from this study, the study suggests that the outcome of RIC allo-HCT may be similar to auto-HCT in carefully selected patients[46].

Practice Point

The authors believe that auto-HCT is a reasonable first option at chemosensitive relapse, i.e., prioritize autografts first given the higher risk of treatment-related morbidity and mortality associated with chronic G*v*HD. Further, patients who have progression after auto-HCT still may be candidates for allo-HCT.

T-Cell Depletion in Allo-HCT for FL

While RIC regimen reduces the direct toxicity of conditioning regimen, G*v*HD continues to contribute to a high TRM. The strategy of TCD in allo-HCT (see Chapter 29) has been investigated to maintain the curative potential of allo-HCT, while reducing toxicity and TRM. In a study by Delgado *et al.*, the outcomes of RIC matched sibling allo-HCT with or without TCD (using alemtuzumab or antithymocyte globulin for TCD) was investigated in relapsed FL patients (n=164) with prior rituximab use in 44%. The incidence of grade II–IV acute G*v*HD (17% *versus* 31%, P=0.04) and chronic G*v*HD (33% *versus* 73%, p<.01) was significantly lower in the TCD cohort with no difference in NRM at a median follow-up of about 3 years. The 3-year probability of relapse was higher (28% *versus* 14%, P=0.05) and the PFS inferior (52% *versus* 67%, P=0.01) in the TCD cohort but there was no difference in OS (74% *versus* 74%). Not surprisingly, donor lymphocyte infusion (DLI) was utilized significantly more in the TCD cohort (33% *versus* 7%, P=0.001), thus suggesting that relapses can be salvaged with DLI[47]. This study demonstrated that TCD method does not improve OS in matched sibling allo-HCT.

The method of TCD has been explored in other studies with both matched related and unrelated donors. In a retrospective study, among 126 patients with advanced stage relapsed FL, BEAM (carmustine, etoposide, cytarabine, and melphalan)-alemtuzumab allo-HCT as compared to BEAM auto-HCT resulted in a higher 1-year NRM (20% *versus* 2%, P=0.001) and lower 3-year relapse (20% *versus* 43%, P=0.01)

but similar 3-year disease-free survival (DFS) (58% *versus* 56%, P=0.90) and OS (69% *versus* 67%, P=0.99). A plateau in survival curves, crossing of survival curves over time, as well as achievement of remission with DLI suggested favorable outcomes with the TCD allo-HCT cohort as compared to the auto-HCT cohort[45]. A subsequent analysis of these data with longer follow-up continued to demonstrate a lower incidence of relapse (31% *versus* 55%) and what appears to be a continued plateau in the allo-HCT group. However, the duration of follow-up and number of patients makes the future demonstration of a survival advantage unlikely even though the curves cross in favor of the allo-HCT group at approximately 4 years[48]. In a prospective study of 82 relapsed FL patients, T-cell depleted RIC allo-HCT using alemtuzumab resulted in a 4-year NRM of 15% and 4-year PFS and OS of 76%. Of 19 patients, who relapsed after allo-HCT, 25 DLIs were administered to 13 patients leading to a reinduction of remission in 77% of patients, the majority of which (90%) were durable. Additionally, 1–4 DLIs were administered to 28 patients with mixed chimerism resulting in full donor chimerism in approximately 60% of patients. The use of DLI in patients with mixed chimerism was associated with a significant decline in the relapse rate (P=0.03)[49].

Practice Points

Although the role of T-cell-depleted RIC allo-HCT remains to be established, these studies indicate a useful role of DLI (see Chapter 25) in patients relapsing after allo-HCT. Patients relapsing after allo-HCT do not have many therapeutic options; hence DLI may be an attractive strategy.

Controversies in Indolent Lymphoma Transplantation

As the landscape of therapy for indolent lymphomas evolves and the number of treatment options expands it can become more difficult for clinicians to understand how and where each of these therapies may belong for an individual patient. For example, is it better to defer a higher risk therapy such as allo-HCT (that may potentially prolong the survival of, or cure a patient with an indolent lymphoma) in favor of a less toxic therapy that may not be associated with a survival advantage or chance of cure but is much easier for a patient to take? The risk of deferral must be measured against the likelihood of being able to attain a future remission thus still allowing allo-HCT to have a reasonable chance of success. These difficult choices are unfortunately going to be part of our uncertainties likely for decades given the rapid increase in new therapies and inability to realistically place each of these into a perfect context utilizing large randomized trials that include the use of transplantation as part of the therapy.

Perhaps the most commonly considered question in transplantation is the consideration of timing of transplantation. Based on existing evidence, some of which was discussed in this review, we feel that for the majority of chemosensitive relapsed patients, especially those with a long first remission, auto-HCT is most appropriately considered at the time of first relapse. The risk/benefit and associated reported survival gains at first relapse seem to merit strongest consideration here in our opinion. One could also rightly ask whether allo-HCT should be favored at first relapse given this might be the best chance to offer curative therapy for a patient. With imperfect data we feel that the probability of treatment-related mortality at this point in the patient's illness outweighs the benefit and our preference is to reserve early use of allogeneic hematopoietic cell transplant for patients with obvious biologic insensitivity to chemoimmunotherapy (e.g., primary refractory or very short remission duration patients). The assessment of fitness for allogeneic transplant has to involve age, performance status, comorbidities, and donor type, and there has to be an implicit understanding of the risk–benefit for the patient as well as a good understanding of what it means to live with chronic GvHD and other potential post-transplant complications. This takes a tremendous amount of time and commitment to the process and is not an easy discussion for many patients to understand in a way that can be measured or quantified. We often have repeated discussions with patients and also offer them discussions with patients who have undergone allo-HCT to help the process as much as possible.

The question of intensity of regimen again is fraught with an absence of prospective studies and although RIC regimens may be associated with a higher probability of relapse, this would be a standard approach for patients who have had prior auto-HCT, and for most patients that undergo allo-HCT as a first transplant, reserving full-intensity regimens for very young fit patients who may need more disease control pre-transplant. Unfortunately there will very likely never be meaningful properly powered prospective studies that can address some of the former issues. The choice of regimen for either auto-HCT or allo-HCT we feel remains institutional based on experience with specific regimens and an absence of any data suggesting a "best" regimen in any particular setting for indolent lymphomas specifically.

A comprehensive list of planned/ongoing/completed trials in transplant for indolent lymphoma is beyond the scope of this article but includes a randomized phase 2 trial of bendamustine as a substitute for carmustine in the BEAM (carmustine, etoposide, cytarabine, melphalan) regimen (BeAM versus BEAM, NCT02278796) for patients with relapsed non-Hodgkin lymphoma including follicular lymphoma. This may offer slightly less nausea and pulmonary complications in the setting of auto-HCT for follicular lymphoma. A phase 3 randomized trial comparing BEAM to ^{90}Y ibritumomab tiuxetan is being conducted in relapsed follicular lymphoma (NCT01827605) to compare toxicity and progression-free survival of each regimen. Post-transplant maintenance therapy, modeled on the benefit of maintenance therapy after auto-HCT for multiple myeloma, is an attractive area of investigation since so many newer therapies are oral and/or relatively

nonmyelosuppressive. We are in the process of completing a phase 1–2 trial of post-transplant lenalidomide for high-risk lymphomas including relapsed/refractory indolent lymphomas (NCT01035463). Other examples include a phase 2 trial of bortezomib and vorinostat after auto-HCT (NCT00992446), and a phase 2 trial of rituximab and sargramostim (GM-CSF) for two 4-week courses beginning 49–70 days post-auto-HCT is being investigated in relapsed follicular lymphoma (NCT00521014). As initial therapy for patients with advanced stage high tumor burden follicular lymphoma the *Groupe Ouest Est d'Etude des Leucémies et Autres Maladies du Sang* (GOELAMS) have recently completed a randomized trial of CHVP (cyclophosphamide, doxorubicin, teniposide, and prednisone) for six cycles followed by CHVP every 2 months for 1 year with concomitant subcutaneous interferon α-2b three times per week for 18 months *versus* VCAP (vindesine, cyclophosphamide, doxorubicin, prednisone, and vincristine) for two to three cycles followed by one course of IMVP16 (ifosfamide, methotrexate, and etoposide) followed by cyclophosphamide/TBI/auto-HCT (NCT00696735).

Planned/ongoing/recently completed trials relevant to allo-HCT include a number of tandem transplant trials (auto-HCT followed by allo-HCT), the combination of high-dose rituximab with fludarabine and cyclophosphamide (BMT CTN 0701, NCT00912223) as a conditioning regimen for follicular lymphoma/allo-HCT. Trials evaluating the ability of rituximab to attenuate GvHD are also of interest; however, we recently closed such a trial at our institution after observing what we felt was a high incidence of clinically severe BK associated hemorrhagic cystitis when used in conjunction with ATG as part of the conditioning regimen for unrelated donor transplants (NCT01044745).

Conclusion

Advances in the field of transplantation such as the availability of high-resolution molecular typing and improved supportive care (e.g., improved antimicrobial prophylaxis and therapy, additional mobilization agents) have likely contributed to some extent to improved outcomes of both auto-HCT and allo-HCT. Meanwhile, improvements in conventional chemotherapy including the use of chemoimmunotherapy plus maintenance or consolidative monoclonal antibody therapy have improved upfront outcomes for patients who require therapy for indolent lymphomas. Nevertheless, patients with indolent lymphomas continue to experience relapses after primary therapy and in the relapsed/refractory setting we feel there is still a well-defined benefit from auto-HCT. Allo-HCT, although associated with lower relapse rates than auto-HCT, has similar OS because of higher TRM from GvHD. The utilization of RIC/NMC allo-HCT, while having reduced TRM and expanded access to allo-HCT to older and less fit patients, has not necessarily improved OS compared to myeloablative allo-HCT. However, we still feel that present-day data support the possibility of cure for some patients who can undergo stem

Table 41.4 Allogeneic hematopoietic cell transplant in relapsed or refractory follicular lymphoma

Author	n	Characteristics	Treatment arms	Common regimens	NRM	PFS/EFS	OS
Hari et al. 2008[35]	208	≤70 years	RIC versus "myeloablative" allo-HCT	Flu or TBI-based versus Cy/TBI, Bu/Cy, or TBI	28% versus 25% at 3 years	55% versus 67% at 3 years	62% versus 71% at 3 years
Thomson et al. 2010 [49]	82	≤65 years	T-cell depleted RIC allo-HCT	Flu/Mel and alemtuzumab	15% at 4 years	76% at 4 years	76% at 4 years
Delgado et al. 2011 [47]	164	Relapsed, 44% prior rituximab use, <65 years	ATG versus alemtuzumab versus No T-cell depletion	Flu with alkylating agent (Mel, Bu, or Cy); also ATG and alemtuzumab in respective arms	18% versus 18% versus 17% at 3 years (P=NS)	55% versus 44% versus 67% at 3 years (P=0.015)	70% versus 68% versus 74% (P=NS)
Cohen et al. 2012 [42]	27	Relapsed, <65 years	Tandem auto-HCT and NMA MRD allo-HCT	Cy mobilization, BEAM or BEAC and auto-HCT. Then Cy/Flu prior to allo-HCT	4% at 3 years	96% at 3 years	96% at 3 years

Allo-HCT = allogeneic hematopoietic cell transplant; ATG = antithymocyte globulin; BEAC = carmustine, etoposide, cytarabine, cyclophosphamide; BEAM = carmustine, etoposide, cytarabine, and melphalan; Bu/Cy = busulfan/ cyclophosphamide; Bu/Flu = busulfan/fludarabine; Cy/Flu = cyclophosphamide/fludarabine; Cy/TBI = cyclophosphamide/total body irradiation; EFS = event-free survival; Flu/Mel = fludarabine/melphalan; n = number; NS = nonsignificant; NMA MRD = nonmyeloablative matched related donor; NRM = nonrelapse mortality; OS = overall survival; PFS = progression-free survival; RIC = reduced intensity conditioning regimen; TBI = total body irradiation.

cell transplantation. The benefit of other therapeutic strategies such as rituximab maintenance post-transplant, graft purging, radioimmunotherapy-based conditioning, and TCD remain unclear because of a lack of high-level data. Relapse continues to remain a major problem in transplanted patients. Although DLI with or without additional therapy may offer disease control in some patients who relapse after allo-HCT, continued research to understand the value of preemptive therapy based on minimal residual disease, as well as the continued development of new therapies with novel mechanisms of action that may be utilized as part of the transplant process, are clearly needed.

References

1. Marcus R, Imrie K, Solal-Celigny P, Catalano JV, Dmoszynska A, Raposo JC, et al. Phase III study of R-CVP compared with cyclophosphamide, vincristine, and prednisone alone in patients with previously untreated advanced follicular lymphoma. J Clin Oncol. 2008;26(28):4579–86.

2. Hiddemann W, Kneba M, Dreyling M, Schmitz N, Lengfelder E, Schmits R, et al. Frontline therapy with rituximab added to the combination of cyclophosphamide, doxorubicin, vincristine, and prednisone (CHOP) significantly improves the outcome for patients with advanced-stage follicular lymphoma compared with therapy with CHOP alone: results of a prospective randomized study of the German Low-Grade Lymphoma Study Group. Blood. 2005;106(12):3725–32.

3. Forstpointner R, Dreyling M, Repp R, Hermann S, Hanel A, Metzner B, et al. The addition of rituximab to a combination of fludarabine, cyclophosphamide, mitoxantrone (FCM) significantly increases the response rate and prolongs survival as compared with FCM alone in patients with relapsed and refractory follicular and mantle cell lymphomas: results of a prospective randomized study of the German Low-Grade Lymphoma Study Group. Blood. 2004;104(10):3064–71.

4. van Oers MH, Klasa R, Marcus RE, Wolf M, Kimby E, Gascoyne RD, et al. Rituximab maintenance improves clinical outcome of relapsed/resistant follicular non-Hodgkin lymphoma in patients both with and without rituximab during induction: results of a prospective randomized phase 3 intergroup trial. Blood. 2006;108(10):3295–301.

5. Salles G, Seymour JF, Offner F, Lopez-Guillermo A, Belada D, Xerri L, et al. Rituximab maintenance for 2 years in patients with high tumour burden follicular lymphoma responding to rituximab plus chemotherapy (PRIMA): a phase 3, randomised controlled trial. Lancet. 2011;377(9759):42–51.

6. Morschhauser F, Radford J, Van Hoof A, Vitolo U, Soubeyran P, Tilly H, et al. Phase III trial of consolidation therapy with yttrium-90-ibritumomab tiuxetan compared with no additional therapy after first remission in advanced follicular lymphoma. J Clin Oncol. 2008;26(32):5156–64.

7. Rummel MJ, Niederle N, Maschmeyer G, Banat GA, von Grunhagen U, Losem C, et al. Bendamustine plus rituximab versus CHOP plus rituximab as first-line treatment for patients with indolent and mantle-cell lymphomas: an open-label, multicentre, randomised, phase 3 non-inferiority trial. Lancet. 2013;381(9873):1203–10.

8. Flinn IW, van der Jagt R, Kahl BS, Wood P, Hawkins TE, Macdonald D, et al. Randomized trial of bendamustine-rituximab or R-CHOP/R-CVP in first-line treatment of indolent NHL or MCL: the BRIGHT study. Blood. 2014;123(19):2944–52.

9. Federico M, Luminari S, Dondi A, Tucci A, Vitolo U, Rigacci L, et al. R-CVP versus R-CHOP versus R-FM

for the initial treatment of patients with advanced-stage follicular lymphoma: results of the FOLL05 trial conducted by the Fondazione Italiana Linfomi. *J Clin Oncol.* 2013;31(12):1506–13.

10. Lenz G, Dreyling M, Schiegnitz E, Forstpointner R, Wandt H, Freund M, *et al.* Myeloablative radiochemotherapy followed by autologous stem cell transplantation in first remission prolongs progression-free survival in follicular lymphoma: results of a prospective, randomized trial of the German Low-Grade Lymphoma Study Group. *Blood.* 2004;104(9):2667–74.

11. Deconinck E, Foussard C, Milpied N, Bertrand P, Michenet P, Cornillet-LeFebvre P, *et al.* High-dose therapy followed by autologous purged stem-cell transplantation and doxorubicin-based chemotherapy in patients with advanced follicular lymphoma: a randomized multicenter study by GOELAMS. *Blood.* 2005;105(10):3817–23.

12. Sebban C, Mounier N, Brousse N, Belanger C, Brice P, Haioun C, *et al.* Standard chemotherapy with interferon compared with CHOP followed by high-dose therapy with autologous stem cell transplantation in untreated patients with advanced follicular lymphoma: the GELF-94 randomized study from the Groupe d'Etude des Lymphomes de l'Adulte (GELA). *Blood.* 2006;108(8):2540–4.

13. Al Khabori M, de Almeida JR, Guyatt GH, Kuruvilla J, Crump M. Autologous stem cell transplantation in follicular lymphoma: a systematic review and meta-analysis. *J Natl Cancer Inst.* 2012;104(1):18–28.

14. Ladetto M, De Marco F, Benedetti F, Vitolo U, Patti C, Rambaldi A, *et al.* Prospective, multicenter randomized GITMO/IIL trial comparing intensive (R-HDS) *versus* conventional (CHOP-R) chemoimmunotherapy in high-risk follicular lymphoma at diagnosis: the superior disease control of R-HDS does not translate into an overall survival advantage. *Blood.* 2008;111(8):4004–13.

15. Schaaf M, Reiser M, Borchmann P, Engert A, Skoetz N. High-dose therapy with autologous stem cell transplantation *versus* chemotherapy or immuno-chemotherapy for follicular lymphoma in adults. *Cochrane Database Syst Rev.* 2012;1:CD007678.

16. Wang B, Ren C, Zhang W, Ma X, Xia B, Sheng Z. Intensified therapy followed by autologous stem-cell transplantation *versus* conventional therapy as first-line treatment of follicular lymphoma: a meta-analysis. *Hematol Oncol.* 2013;31(1):29–33.

17. Montoto S, Canals C, Rohatiner AZ, Taghipour G, Sureda A, Schmitz N, *et al.* Long-term follow-up of high-dose treatment with autologous haematopoietic progenitor cell support in 693 patients with follicular lymphoma: an EBMT registry study. *Leukemia.* 2007;21(11):2324–31.

18. Akhtari M, Bhatt VR, Tandra PK, Krishnamurthy J, Horstman H, Dreessen A, *et al.* Therapy-related myeloid neoplasms after autologous hematopoietic stem cell transplantation in lymphoma patients. *Cancer Biol Ther.* 2013 1;14(12):1077–88.

19. Schouten HC, Qian W, Kvaloy S, Porcellini A, Hagberg H, Johnsen HE, *et al.* High-dose therapy improves progression-free survival and survival in relapsed follicular non-Hodgkin's lymphoma: results from the randomized European CUP trial. *J Clin Oncol.* 2003;21(21):3918–27.

20. Le Gouill S, De Guibert S, Planche L, Brice P, Dupuis J, Cartron G, *et al.* Impact of the use of autologous stem cell transplantation at first relapse both in naive and previously rituximab exposed follicular lymphoma patients treated in the GELA/GOELAMS FL2000 study. *Haematologica.* 2011;96(8):1128–35.

21. Vose JM, Bierman PJ, Loberiza FR, Lynch JC, Bociek GR, Weisenburger DD, *et al.* Long-term outcomes of autologous stem cell transplantation for follicular non-Hodgkin lymphoma: effect of histological grade and Follicular International Prognostic Index. *Biol Blood Marrow Transplant.* 2008;14(1):36–42.

22. Gisselbrecht C, Glass B, Mounier N, Singh Gill D, Linch DC, Trneny M, *et al.* Salvage regimens with autologous transplantation for relapsed large B-cell lymphoma in the rituximab era. *J Clin Oncol.* 2010;28(27):4184–90.

23. Kothari J, Peggs KS, Bird A, Thomson KJ, Morris E, Virchis AE, *et al.* Autologous stem cell transplantation for follicular lymphoma is of most benefit early in the disease course and can result in durable remissions,

irrespective of prior rituximab exposure. *Br J Haematol.* 2014;165(3):334–40.

24. Evens AM, Vanderplas A, LaCasce AS, Crosby AL, Nademanee AP, Kaminski MS, *et al.* Stem cell transplantation for follicular lymphoma relapsed/refractory after prior rituximab: a comprehensive analysis from the NCCN lymphoma outcomes project. *Cancer.* 2013;119(20):3662–71.

25. Peters AC, Duan Q, Russell JA, Duggan P, Owen C, Stewart DA. Durable event-free survival following autologous stem cell transplant for relapsed or refractory follicular lymphoma: positive impact of recent rituximab exposure and low-risk Follicular Lymphoma International Prognostic Index score. *Leuk Lymphoma.* 2011;52(11):2124–9.

26. Phipps C, Gopal AK, Storer BE, Cassaday RD, Press OW, Till BG, *et al.* Autologous transplant for relapsed follicular lymphoma: impact of pre-transplant rituximab sensitivity. *Leuk Lymphoma.* 2014;17:1–5.

27. Gopal AK, Gooley TA, Rajendran JG, Pagel JM, Fisher DR, Maloney DG, *et al.* Mycloablative I-131-tositumomab with escalating doses of fludarabine and autologous hematopoietic transplantation for adults age >/= 60 years with B cell lymphoma. *Biol Blood Marrow Transplant.* 2014;20(6):770–5.

28. Decaudin D, Mounier N, Tilly H, Ribrag V, Ghesquières H, Bouabdallah K, *et al.* 90Y Ibritumomab tiuxetan (zevalin) combined with BEAM (Z-BEAM) conditioning regimen plus autologous stem cell transplantation in relapsed or refractory low-grade CD20-positive B-cell lymphoma. A GELA phase II prospective study. *Clin Lymphoma Myeloma Leuk.* 2011;11(2):212–8.

29. Brown JR, Feng Y, Gribben JG, Neuberg D, Fisher DC, Mauch P, *et al.* Long-term survival after autologous bone marrow transplantation for follicular lymphoma in first remission. *Biol Blood Marrow Transplant.* 2007;13(9):1057–65.

30. Arcaini L, Montanari F, Alessandrino EP, Tucci A, Brusamolino E, Gargantini L, *et al.* Immunochemotherapy with in vivo purging and autotransplant induces long clinical and molecular remission in advanced relapsed and

refractory follicular lymphoma. *Ann Oncol.* 2008;19(7):1331–5.

31. Hicks LK, Woods A, Buckstein R, Mangel J, Pennell N, Zhang L, et al. Rituximab purging and maintenance combined with auto-SCT: long-term molecular remissions and prolonged hypogammaglobulinemia in relapsed follicular lymphoma. *Bone Marrow Transplant.* 2009;43(9):701–8.

32. Brugger W, Hirsch J, Grunebach F, Repp R, Brossart P, Vogel W, et al. Rituximab consolidation after high-dose chemotherapy and autologous blood stem cell transplantation in follicular and mantle cell lymphoma: a prospective, multicenter phase II study. *Ann Oncol.* 2004;15(11):1691–8.

33. Morschhauser F, Recher C, Milpied N, Gressin R, Salles G, Brice P, et al. A 4-weekly course of rituximab is safe and improves tumor control for patients with minimal residual disease persisting 3 months after autologous hematopoietic stem-cell transplantation: results of a prospective multicenter phase II study in patients with follicular lymphoma. *Ann Oncol.* 2012;23(10):2687–95.

34. Pettengell R, Schmitz N, Gisselbrecht C, Smith G, Patton WN, Metzner B, et al. Rituximab purging and/or maintenance in patients undergoing autologous transplantation for relapsed follicular lymphoma: a prospective randomized trial from the Lymphoma Working Party of the European Group for Blood and Marrow Transplantation. *J Clin Oncol.* 2013;31(13):1624–30.

35. Hari P, Carreras J, Zhang MJ, Gale RP, Bolwell BJ, Bredeson CN, et al. Allogeneic transplants in follicular lymphoma: higher risk of disease progression after reduced-intensity compared to myeloablative conditioning. *Biol Blood Marrow Transplant.* 2008;14(2):236–45.

36. Auer RL, MacDougall F, Oakervee HE, Taussig D, Davies JK, Syndercombe-Court D, et al. T-cell replete fludarabine/cyclophosphamide reduced intensity allogeneic stem cell transplantation for lymphoid malignancies. *Br J Haematol.* 2012;157(5):580–5.

37. Shea T, Johnson J, Westervelt P, Farag S, McCarty J, Bashey A, et al. Reduced-intensity allogeneic transplantation provides high event-free and overall survival in patients with advanced indolent B cell malignancies: CALGB 109901. *Biol Blood Marrow Transplant.* 2011;17(9):1395–403.

38. Khouri IF, Champlin RE. Nonmyeloablative allogeneic stem cell transplantation for non-hodgkin lymphoma. *Cancer J.* 2012;18(5):457–62.

39. Mortensen BK, Petersen SL, Kornblit B, Andersen PK, Braendstrup P, Andersen NS, et al. Single-institution long-term outcomes for patients receiving nonmyeloablative conditioning hematopoeitic cell transplantation for chronic lymphocytic leukemia and follicular lymphoma. *Eur J Haematol.* 2012;89(2):151–9.

40. Abou-Nassar KE, Stevenson KE, Antin JH, McDermott K, Ho VT, Cutler CS, et al. (90)Y-ibritumomab tiuxetan followed by reduced-intensity conditioning and allo-SCT in patients with advanced follicular lymphoma. *Bone Marrow Transplant.* 2011;46(12):1503–9.

41. Freytes CO, Zhang MJ, Carreras J, Burns LJ, Gale RP, Isola L, et al. Outcome of lower-intensity allogeneic transplantation in non-Hodgkin lymphoma after autologous transplantation failure. *Biol Blood Marrow Transplant.* 2012;18(8):1255–64.

42. Cohen S, Kiss T, Lachance S, Roy DC, Sauvageau G, Busque L, et al. Tandem autologous-allogeneic nonmyeloablative sibling transplantation in relapsed follicular lymphoma leads to impressive progression-free survival with minimal toxicity. *Biol Blood Marrow Transplant.* 2012;18(6):951–7.

43. Crocchiolo R, Castagna L, Furst S, El-Cheikh J, Faucher C, Oudin C, et al. Tandem autologous-allo-SCT is feasible in patients with high-risk relapsed non-Hodgkin's lymphoma. *Bone Marrow Transplant.* 2013;48(2):249–52.

44. van Besien K, Loberiza FR, Jr., Bajorunaite R, Armitage JO, Bashey A, Burns LJ, et al. Comparison of autologous and allogeneic hematopoietic stem cell transplantation for follicular lymphoma. *Blood.* 2003;102(10):3521–9.

45. Ingram W, Devereux S, Das-Gupta EP, Russell NH, Haynes AP, Byrne JL, et al. Outcome of BEAM-autologous and BEAM-alemtuzumab allogeneic transplantation in relapsed advanced stage follicular lymphoma. *Br J Haematol.* 2008;141(2):235–43.

46. Tomblyn MR, Ewell M, Bredeson C, Kahl BS, Goodman SA, Horowitz MM, et al. Autologous *versus* reduced-intensity allogeneic hematopoietic cell transplantation for patients with chemosensitive follicular non-Hodgkin lymphoma beyond first complete response or first partial response. *Biol Blood Marrow Transplant.* 2011;17(7):1051–7.

47. Delgado J, Canals C, Attal M, Thomson K, Campos A, Martino R, et al. The role of in vivo T-cell depletion on reduced-intensity conditioning allogeneic stem cell transplantation from HLA-identical siblings in patients with follicular lymphoma. *Leukemia.* 2011;25(3):551–5.

48. Noriega V, Kaur H, Devereux S, Byrne J, Marcus R, Haynes A, et al. Long-term follow-up of BEAM-autologous and BEAM-alemtuzumab allogeneic stem cell transplantation in relapsed advanced stage follicular lymphoma. *Leuk Res.* 2014;38(7):737–43.

49. Thomson KJ, Morris EC, Milligan D, Parker AN, Hunter AE, Cook G, et al. T-cell-depleted reduced-intensity transplantation followed by donor leukocyte infusions to promote graft-*versus*-lymphoma activity results in excellent long-term survival in patients with multiply relapsed follicular lymphoma. *J Clin Oncol.* 2010;28(23):3695–700.

50. Robinson SP, Canals C, Luang JJ, Tilly H, Crawley C, Cahn JY, et al. The outcome of reduced intensity allogeneic stem cell transplantation and autologous stem cell transplantation when performed as a first transplant strategy in relapsed follicular lymphoma: an analysis from the Lymphoma Working Party of the EBMT. *Bone Marrow Transplant.* 2013;48(11):1409–14.

Chapter

42

Hematopoietic Cell Transplants for Mantle Cell Lymphoma

Sai Ravi Pingali and Timothy S. Fenske

Introduction

Mantle cell lymphoma (MCL) is a distinct subtype of B-cell non-Hodgkin lymphoma (NHL) characterized by the t(11;14)(q13;32) translocation, which results in cyclin D1 overexpression[1,2]. Typical immunophenotypic features include expression of CD5, CD19, CD20, CD79a, cyclin D1, SOX11, and FMC7, with a lack of CD10 and CD23. MCL accounts for approximately 3–6% of all NHL, possibly with some geographic variation. There has been an increase in incidence over the last two decades[3–6]. The median age for MCL is 63–68 years with a 3:1 male predominance[6–8]. MCL is twice as common in Caucasians compared to African Americans[6].

Up to 75% of patients present with advanced stage (III–IV) disease and 90% will have extranodal disease, with involvement of the gastrointestinal tract and bone marrow; peripheral blood involvement is common[6,9,10]. While localized presentation of MCL can occur, this is relatively rare[6,11]. Patients presenting with apparent stage I/II disease should therefore undergo CT or PET scan, and bone marrow biopsy to confirm early stage disease, as the management of early and advanced stage disease differs. MCL is a heterogeneous disease with morphologic and biologic variants that define a spectrum of disease. On one end of the spectrum is "indolent" MCL, which may not need any treatment for several years. On the other end of the spectrum is the blastoid variant of MCL, which follows a highly aggressive course. The MCL international prognostic index (or "MIPI score"), which is based on age, performance status, lactate dehydrogenase (LDH), and leukocyte count, classifies MCL into three prognostic groups: low-, intermediate-, and high-risk groups. These groups have 5-year OS rates of 83%, 63%, and 34%, respectively[12,13]. The MIPI score has been validated across several studies, and is a robust predictor of prognosis irrespective of treatment strategy used. Gene expression profile signature, complex karyotype, and especially proliferation index (as measured by Ki-67 staining) also provide important prognostic information[14–19]. However, the practical utility of these markers is limited by a lack of consistent scoring of Ki-67 staining between pathologists, and lack of routine availability of gene expression profiling in clinical practice[20]. Routine chromosome analysis, while providing prognostic information according to one study, is not always performed on the initial diagnostic material. As a result, although several robust and promising prognostic tools have been developed in MCL, there is a lack of consensus on how to best use these tools to select treatment for individual patients in routine clinical practice.

Over the past two decades the median overall survival (OS) of patients with MCL has improved significantly. However, MCL continues to have a less favorable prognosis when compared to other B-cell NHL subtypes, and remains incurable with conventional chemotherapy approaches[21]. Recent advances in the understanding of the basic biology of MCL has led to the approval of several novel agents or "targeted" therapies such as bortezomib, lenalidomide, and ibrutinib for relapsed and refractory MCL. Several other agents look promising and are in various stages of development for MCL. Incorporation of these targeted therapies into treatment strategies is expected to further improve prognosis, especially in elderly patients who are not candidates for intensive treatment approaches. However, despite this considerable progress, MCL remains a challenging clinical problem with most patients experiencing repeated relapses and ultimately succumbing to the disease. As a result, hematopoietic cell transplantation (HCT) continues to be a commonly used and important tool in managing MCL. Currently, there is a lack of consensus regarding optimal frontline therapy as well as regarding indications for autologous HCT, allogeneic HCT, and maintenance therapy following induction therapy and transplant. Treatment strategies need to be tailored depending on patient factors such age, comorbidity profile, performance status (PS), MIPI score, and disease burden. In this chapter we discuss the current state of the art in the management of MCL, with an emphasis on the continued important role of autologous and allogeneic HCT, even in this era of multiple new and novel agents.

Frontline Therapy

There is no standard frontline therapy for MCL. In general, more aggressive approaches (often including upfront HCT) designed to produce long first remissions are utilized in "younger fit" patients, while older and/or less fit patients are treated with more conservative nontransplant approaches designed to minimize toxicity. With intensive treatment approaches, a median progression-free survival (PFS) of 5–10 years can reasonably be expected in chemosensitive, younger "fit" patients. Because the majority of MCL patients are over age 60–65 at diagnosis, many patients will not be candidates for intensive approaches. However, all treatment choices must be weighed against toxicities and with higher expected PFS comes a higher risk of toxicity. For determining appropriate frontline therapy, it is useful to separate patients into "younger fit," "older fit or younger unfit," and "frail" categories.

Younger Fit Patients

Patients <60–65 years of age with good PS and no significant comorbidities should be considered for more intensive induction chemotherapy, potentially followed by consolidation with HCT (in most cases, autologous HCT). It is accepted that rituximab generally improves the response to frontline therapy, as was demonstrated by the German Low Grade Lymphoma Study Group, who compared the combination of cyclophosphamide, doxorubicin, vincristine, and prednisone (CHOP) and rituximab with CHOP (R-CHOP) as first-line therapy for advanced stage MCL. In this study, there was a superior ORR (94% versus 75%), CR rate (34% versus 7%), and time to treatment failure (TTF) (21 versus 7 months) in favor of R-CHOP[22]. While this study did not show an OS benefit in favor of R-CHOP, a retrospective study from MD Anderson Cancer Center and a meta-analysis of three randomized trials showed improved OS (hazard ratio of 0.6) associated with rituximab-containing frontline therapy[23,24]. However, we do not recommend R-CHOP for younger fit patients for the reasons described below.

High-dose cytarabine is highly active in MCL including patients who are refractory to CHOP therapy. Lefrere et al. reported an 81% CR and 89% ORR with addition of 2–3 cycles of DHAP (dexamethasone, high-dose cytarabine (AraC), and cisplatin) in patients who had partial response or less after four cycles of CHOP[25]. Similarly van't Veer et al. reported a doubling of CR from 15% with three cycles of R-CHOP to 29% with the addition of a single cycle of high-dose AraC before auto-HCT[26].

The Nordic MCL2 study was a phase 2 study using an augmented CHOP regimen (maxi-CHOP) alternating with high-dose cytarabine every 3 weeks. Rituximab was given from cycle 4 to 6 and consolidated with BEAM (carmustine, etoposide, AraC, melphalan) or BEAC (carmustine, etoposide, AraC, cylcophosphamide) and auto-HCT. This approach yielded an ORR of 96% and CR rate of 54%. The median PFS was 7.4 years with a 58% 10-year OS[27]. Recently, Hermine et al. presented results from a large randomized study which compared 6 courses of R-CHOP (arm A) versus alternating courses of 3 × R-CHOP and 3 × R-DHAP (arm B) in patients <65 years, with all patients then proceeding to auto-HCT. Conditioning was Cytoxan + 12 Gy TBI for patients in arm A and 10 Gy TBI, AraC, and melphalan for patients in arm B. After auto-HCT, the ORR and CR were similar in both groups; however, median TTF was significantly longer in the

R-CHOP/R-DHAP group (9.1 years versus 3.9 years). At a median follow-up of 6.1 years, median OS did not differ significantly between the two arms. Treatment-related mortality was only 3.4% in each arm[28].

R-hyperCVAD (rituximab, hyperfractionated cyclophosphamide, vincristine, doxorubicin, and dexamethasone) alternating with R-Mtx/AraC (rituximab, high-dose methotrexate (Mtx)/cytarabine) is another commonly used induction regimen in MCL for patients <65 years age. Investigators from MD Anderson reported a phase 2 single-institution study with R-hyperCVAD and R-Mtx/AraC therapy without subsequent auto-HCT consolidation. The ORR was 97% and CR was 87%. At median follow-up of 13.4 years, median FFS was 4.8 years without a plateau in the curve. Median OS was 10.7 years[29]. However, the treatment dropout rate was high at 29% particularly from toxicity related to the R-Mtx/AraC part of the treatment. In addition, in retrospect, this study was relatively enriched for low MIPI patients, which would be predicted to enhance the results[29]. Two subsequent multicenter studies, using the same regimen, confirmed high rates of ORR and CR, but with very high treatment dropout rates of 39% and 63%, respectively[30,31]. In addition the treatment-related mortality (TRM) was 8–10%, which is actually significantly higher than the rate of TRM with auto-HCT currently[29,30]. In these multicenter studies (which are likely more reflective of routine practice than a single-institution study), the very poor treatment completion rate was likely from the Mtx/araC component since using only the R-hyperCVAD component repeatedly, without the Mtx/araC component (referred to as "modified hyperCVAD"), has much more modest toxicity[32,33].

Recently, a US SWOG/Intergroup study was designed as a randomized phase II comparison of R-hyperCVAD-Mtx/AraC induction followed by consolidation with auto-HCT versus R-bendamustine followed by auto-HCT for patients <65 years age with untreated MCL. Unfortunately, this study was closed early into accrual due to an unacceptably high incidence of failed peripheral blood hematopoietic cell collection in the R-hyperCVAD-Mtx/AraC arm[121].

For younger fit patients, we recommend induction therapy with a rituximab/chemotherapy combination that includes high-dose AraC. We feel that either the Nordic MCL-2 regimen or R-CHOP alternating with R-DHAP accomplishes this while maintaining a low toxicity profile relative to other regimens. The Nordic MCL-2 regimen has the added benefit of avoiding cisplatin and is also feasible to be completely administered in an outpatient setting.

Older Fit Patients and Young Patients Not Fit for Transplantation

Treatment strategies for older (over 60–65 years of age) fit patients and young patients ineligible for transplantation are similar. Select older patients with no significant comorbidities can be considered for auto-HCT. A study from the European Society for Blood and Marrow Transplantation (EBMT)

Table 42.1 Phase II/III prospective trials for transplant-ineligible MCL patients

Study	Patients	Regimen(s)	ORR	CR	OS	PFS in months
Kluin-Nelemans et al.[40]	485	Induction: R-CHOP versus R-FC	86%	40%	4 years 62%	28
		Maintenance: R versus IFN-α	78%	34%	4 years 47%	26
Lenz et al.[22]	112	CHOP	75%	7%	2 years 76%	14
		R-CHOP	94%	34%	2 years 76%	21
Rummel et al.[35]	94	R-CHOP	91%	30%	Median OS not reached	21
		BR	93%	40%	Median OS not reached	35
Herold et al.[96]	90	MCP	63%	15%	4 years 52%	18
		R-MCP	71%	32%	4 years 56%	20
Smith et al.[97]	50	R-CHOP + yttrium-90-ibritumomab tiuxetan	64%	46%	5 years 73%	31
Houot et al.[98]	39	R-PAD + chlorambucil	79%	59%	2 years 69%	26
Ruan et al.[99]	36	R-CHOP + bortezomib	82%	36%	3 years 82%	18
Visco et al.[39]	20	R-BAC	100%	95%	2 years 100%	2 years 95%
Robak et al. [122]	487	RCHOP versus	89%	42%	4 years 54%	14
		VR-CAP	92%	53%	4 years 64%	25
Ruan et al. [123]	38	R-Lenalidomide	92%	64%	2 years 97%	2 years 85%

R-CHOP = rituximab, cyclophosphamide, doxorubicin, vincristine, and prednisone; R-FC = rituximab, fludarabine, and cyclophosphamide; IFN = α-interferon-alpha; BR = bendamustine, rituximab; R-MCP = rituximab, mitoxantrone, chlorambucil, and prednisolone; R-PAD = rituximab, bortezomib, doxorubicin, and dexamethasone; R-BAC = rituximab, bendamustine, and AraC; ORR = overall response rate; CR = complete response; OS = overall survival; PFS = progression-free survival.

compared outcomes of patients ≥65 years with patients <65 years age with auto-HCT. Despite patients >65 years receiving more therapy pretransplant and few patients being in complete remission prior to transplant, the rates of OS, PFS, and TRM were similar for the two groups. This study suggests auto-HCT is feasible and safe in patients ≥65 years and that similar benefits can be expected compared to patients <65 years of age. Therefore, age alone should not be a criterion to preclude auto-HCT[34].

However, despite our ability to increasingly offer HCT to older patients, the fact remains that many patients over age 60–65 will not be good candidates for HCT due to comorbidities and frailty. For such patients, the overall treatment strategy involves the use of an effective induction regimen with a tolerable side effect profile, potentially followed by maintenance therapy, given in the hope of prolonging the remission duration. Recommended induction for such patients is chemoimmunotherapy, most commonly R-CHOP or R-bendamustine (BR) as summarized in Table 42.1. Rummel et al. published a randomized, noninferiority study of BR versus R-CHOP in untreated indolent and MCL patients. Looking specifically at the subset of MCL patients, the median PFS was 35 months for BR versus 21 months for R-CHOP. Additionally BR was better tolerated compared to R-CHOP with significantly lower risk of peripheral neuropathy, alopecia, and hematologic toxicities[35]. The BRIGHT study also compared the safety and efficacy of BR with R-CHOP or R-CVP as first-line treatment for indolent NHL or MCL. While PFS for the MCL subset was not reported in this study, MCL patients showed higher CR of 50% versus 27% in favor of the BR arm[36]. Treatment with BR was associated with significantly better quality of life compared to the R-CHOP/R-CVP arm[37].

A recent international randomized trial of 487 transplant-ineligible MCL patients evaluated R-CHOP versus VR-CAP (R-CHOP with bortezomib replacing vincristine) as frontline therapy. Outcomes were superior in the VR-CAP arm with median PFS of 25 versus 14 months in the R-CHOP arm[38]. Of note, no maintenance therapy was used in either arm of this study.

A small (n=40) phase 2 study with rituximab, AraC, and bendamustine (RBAC) for frontline and relapsed refractory MCL showed excellent results. In the 20 previously untreated patients, an ORR of 100% and CR rate of 95% was reported, with a 2-year PFS of 95%. This regimen was also highly active against relapsed/refractory disease with an ORR of 80%, CR rate of 70%, and PFS of 70% at 2 years. However, the treatment drop out rate was about 15% and grade 3–4 thrombocytopenia was the most common toxicity[39].

Another recent small (n=38) phase 2 study used rituximab plus lenalidomide as initial treatment for mantle cell lymphoma. Although a small study with relatively short follow up, this low-intensity regimen was remarkably active with a 92% ORR, 64% CR rate, and 2-year PFS of 85%.

Role of Maintenance Therapy in Elderly Patients

The European MCL network conducted a randomized phase 3 trial in elderly patients not eligible for AUTO-HCT. The study aimed to compare induction with R-CHOP versus R-FC (rituximab, fludarabine, and cyclophosphamide), with a second randomization comparing maintenance rituximab versus interferon-α. ORR was superior with R-CHOP at 87% versus 78%, and CR rate was similar in both groups at 34% versus 40% (P = 0.10). Four-year OS was 62% with R-CHOP compared to 47% with R-FC. Patients who received maintenance rituximab after R-CHOP therapy had significantly better 4-year OS compared to the interferon-α arm (87% versus 63%, P = 0.005)[40].

The Wisconsin Oncology Network (WON) conducted a phase 2 study with modified hyperCVAD induction therapy followed by rituximab maintenance for 2 years in a patient group with median age of 62 years. ORR and CR with induction therapy were 77% and 64%, respectively. At a median follow-up of 62 months median OS is 70 months, with 62% of patients alive at 5 years, which is comparable to outcomes with more intensive treatment strategies[33].

For elderly fit patients and young "unfit" patients we recommend induction with BR, R-CHOP, or VR-CAP followed by maintenance rituximab. BR and VR-CAP each appear to be superior to R-CHOP; however, it remains unclear whether maintenance rituximab has the same benefit following BR or VR-CAP as was seen following R-CHOP.

Frail Patients

There are relatively limited options for very elderly or frail patients with MCL. Asymptomatic patients with low disease burden can be observed and treatment can be deferred until symptoms develop[41]. Oral chlorambucil as a single agent, chlorambucil in combination with rituximab, or rituximab with low-dose bendamustine, or rituximab with lenalidomide are also good options[42,43]. Alternatively, single-agent rituximab given weekly for 4 weeks, which has an ORR of 27%, can be considered[123]. In contrast to the results seen in follicular lymphoma, extended therapy with rituximab does not improve response rate, PFS, or duration of response[44]. Ibrutinib, while very active in the relapsed and refractory setting, has not yet been tested as first-line therapy in MCL.

Should Consolidation of First Remission with Auto-HCT Be Pursued in all Transplant-Eligible Patients?

The European mantle cell lymphoma (EMCL) network trial is the only randomized study evaluating consolidation with auto-HCT following frontline therapy for MCL. In that study, patients received CHOP-like therapy followed by auto-HCT versus maintenance therapy with interferon-α. There was significant improvement in PFS with auto-HCT compared to the

interferon-α arm (39 versus 17 months, P = 0.0108). This, however, did not quite translate into an OS advantage (83% versus 77% at 3 years P = 0.18) most likely related to the crossover design of the study, and also to use of total body irradiation (TBI) based preparative regimen which is associated with higher TRM than chemotherapy conditioning regimens[45]. Although not a prospective trial, a meta-analysis by Hoster et al. confirmed an advantage of auto-HCT in first remission for younger patients, with superior median OS of 90 months versus 54 months in favor of auto-HCT[46]. Additionally, in a recent Center for International Blood and Marrow Transplant Research (CIBMTR) study evaluating timing of transplant in MCL, looking specifically at all chemosensitive patients who underwent auto-HCT, multivariate analysis revealed a survival benefit (from the time of diagnosis) in favor of early auto-HCT[47].

Although studies with hyperCVAD and Mtx/AraC without auto-HCT consolidation show comparable outcomes with R-AraC-based regimens followed by auto-HCT, toxicity and treatment drop out rates are significantly higher with a full course of R-hyperCVAD alternating with R-M/A. A retrospective study with 167 patients comparing first-line therapy outcomes for R-hyperCVAD with auto-HCT, R-hyperCVAD without auto-HCT, and R-CHOP with auto-HCT showed a 3-year PFS of 55%, 58%, and 56%, respectively. Three-year PFS was significantly lower with R-CHOP without auto-HCT at 18%. Toxicity rates were higher for the R-hyperCVAD group with or without auto-HCT[48]. Collectively, several groups have now reported that intensive chemotherapy followed by auto-HCT can lead to favorable outcomes, including ORR of over 90% and median PFS in the 4–8-year range, and median OS as high as 7–10 years. How much auto-HCT specifically contributes to these outcomes, versus other components of therapy, and whether similar outcomes could be achieved using alternatives to auto-HCT (such as maintenance therapies) are issues which need to be addressed with prospective clinical trials.

At this time, given the collective available data on outcomes with auto-HCT consolidation (Table 42.2), the now relatively low TRM of <5% using non-TBI-based preparative regimens [49], and the relative lack of mature data on how to incorporate novel agents, maintenance therapy, or MRD into the management of younger fit patients with newly diagnosed MCL, we feel that younger fit patients are best served with consolidative auto-HCT in first remission. Particularly in patients achieving CR prior to transplant, this approach leads to excellent outcomes, with a median PFS in the 9-year range[47].

Can Maintenance Therapy Replace Auto-HCT?

There are evolving data on the role of rituximab maintenance after frontline therapy without subsequent auto-HCT. However, to date, there are no randomized studies comparing auto-HCT versus maintenance therapy after induction with rituximab and H-AraC-based regimens. Rituximab is known to induce molecular remission in patients who have recurrent

Table 42.2 Studies with first-line intensive chemotherapy and consolidative autologous HCT for MCL

Study	Patients	Regimen(s)	ORR	CR	OS[c]	PFS[d]
Hermine et al. [28]	455	R-CHOP + auto-HCT	98%	63%	6.8 years	3.8 years
		R-CHOP/R-DHAP + auto-HCT	97%	61%	NR	7.3 years
Eskelund et al. [27]	160	R-Maxi-CHOP + H-AraC + auto-HCT	96%	54%	58% at 10 years	7.4 years
Dreyling et al. [45]	122	R-CHOP + auto-HCT	98%	81%	83% at 3 years	3.3 years
		R-CHOP + IFN-α	99%	37%	77% at 3 years	1.4 years
van't Veer et al. [26]	87	R-CHOP + H-AraC + auto-HCT	70%	64%	66% at 4 years	36% at 4 years
Damon et al. [91]	77	R-CHOP + Mtx + H-AraC/VP16 + auto-HCT	88%	69%	64% at 5 years	56% at 5 years
Delarue et al. [92]	60	R-CHOP/R-DHAP + auto-HCT	100%	96%	75% at 5 years	6.9 years
Gressin et al. [93]	26	R-VADC	73%	46%	62% at 3 years	4.8 years
Fenske et al. [47]	249[a]	Chemo + auto-HCT	NA	NA	61% at 5 years	52% at 5 years
	132[b]	Chemo + auto-HCT	NA	NA	44% at 5 years	29% at 5 years
Vandenberghe et al. [94]	195	Chemo + auto-HCT	NA	NA	50% at 5 years	33% at 5 years
Touzeau et al. [95]	396	H-AraC-based regimen + auto-HCT	97%	77%	83% at 3 years	67% at 3 years

[a] Early cohort-transplantation performed in first PR or CR with no more than two prior lines of chemotherapy.
[b] Late cohort-transplantation performed in the remaining patients.
[c] Median OS where follow-up duration is not specified.
[d] Median PFS where follow-up duration is not specified.
R-CHOP = rituximab, cyclophosphamide, doxorubicin, vincristine, and prednisone; R-DHAP = rituximab, dexamethasone, AraC, and cisplatin; H-AraC = high-dose AraC; IFN-α = interferon-alpha; R-hyperCVAD = rituximab, hyperfractionated cyclophosphamide, vincristine, doxorubicin, and dexamethasone; R-VADC = rituximab, vincristine, doxorubicin, dexamethasone, and chlorambucil; auto-HCT = autologous hematopoietic cell transplant; ORR = overall response rate; CR = complete response; OS = overall survival; PFS = progression-free survival; NA = not available.

minimal residual disease after auto-HCT[50,51]. Maintenance rituximab was studied in frontline therapy by the Eastern Cooperative Oncology Group study (E1405) in which patients received rituximab, bortezomib, modified hyperCVAD (VcR-CVAD) induction. and maintenance rituximab (MR) for 2 years. Transplant-eligible patients had an option of receiving auto-HCT instead of MR. However, the decision to pursue auto-HCT was at the discretion of the treating physician and was not a randomization. For the entire group, the ORR was 95% and CR was 68%. At a median follow-up of 4.5 years, 3-year PFS was 72% and OS was 88%. There was no significant difference between the MR and auto-HCT groups in terms of outcomes or toxicities[32]. Longer follow-up and further studies with randomization are needed to confirm these findings.

Owing to insufficient data, at this time we do not recommend maintenance rituximab as a substitute for consolidation with auto-HCT. We do, however, strongly encourage further study of this question with prospective randomized trials, as it may be possible to identify a subset of MCL patients, such as those who achieve MRD-negative remission with induction therapy, for whom maintenance therapy could produce outcomes equal to auto-HCT.

Should Patients Receive Maintenance Therapy after Auto-HCT?

The role of rituximab maintenance after auto-HCT has been investigated in recent studies. Dietrich et al. compared outcomes of patients treated on a phase 2 trial with rituximab maintenance post-auto-HCT for 2 years with patients who did not receive any maintenance during the same time period. At a median follow-up of 56 months, PFS (65% versus 90% P = 0.014) was significantly improved with maintenance therapy; however, OS (84% versus 90% P = 0.51) was not significantly different[52]. This potential benefit of 3 years of maintenance rituximab has been evaluated prospectively in a phase 3 randomized European trial in patients receiving auto-HCT after four cycles of R-DHAP. Patients were randomized to either 3 years of maintenance rituximab (375 mg/m² every two months) versus observation. The final analysis of this study was presented at ASH 2016, and showed improved 4-year PFS and OS. This will likely establish maintenance rituximab after auto-HCT for MCL as a new standard of care[53]. It should be pointed out that the induction therapy used in this study (R-DHAP × 4) is not commonly used in the USA.

At this time, due to a lack of survival benefit, significant cost, and potential for long-term hypogammaglobulinemia, we do not feel that the routine application of maintenance rituximab therapy following auto-HCT should be considered standard of care outside of a clinical trial. Rather, as was done in the Nordic MCL-2 study, we prefer monitoring patients closely for relapse using MRD, and then treating these MRD relapses preemptively with rituximab[27]. This approach has a high success rate of converting patients back to an MRD-negative state and overall considerably reduces the amount of post-transplant rituximab needed.

What is the Ideal Conditioning Regimen for Auto-HCT?

BEAM, BEAC, CBV, and TBI-based regimens are the most commonly used preparative regimens for auto-HCT. The use of TBI-based preparative regimens has significantly declined over the last decade due to short-term and long-term toxicities associated with total body radiation. A retrospective study of MCL patients (still only presented in abstract form) from the EBMT comparing TBI- versus non-TBI-based regimens showed a decrease in relapse rate in patients receiving TBI-based auto-HCT in PR. There was also a trend towards improved disease-free-survival for the patients in PR who received TBI[54]. In a recent comparison of patients treated on the Nordic MCL2, HOVON 45, and European MCL Younger trials, there was also a trend towards decreased PFS in patients transplanted in PR1 on the MCL Younger trial, in which patients received TBI. However, there were also differences in the total doses of H-AraC given in these studies which might account for the difference as well[55].

In a recent study from the CIBMTR, outcomes for patients who underwent auto-HCT in first remission were analyzed. Nearly 80% of these patients received non-TBI conditioning. For patients transplanted in CR1 (with one line of therapy), CR1 (with two lines of therapy), or PR1, 5-year PFS was 70%, 56%, and 30%, respectively. Patients failing to achieve CR with 1 or 2 lines of therapy may therefore benefit from an approach other than a standard BEAM auto-HCT[47].

The Nordic MCL3 study evaluated the role of radioimmunotherapy with 90Y-ibritumomab-tiuxetan added to BEAM/BEAC in non-CR patients before transplant. Improved outcomes were not seen with the addition of 90Y-ibritumomab-tiuxetan. The authors concluded that intensification of the preparative regimen may be too late in the course of treatment to improve outcomes[56].

For patients going to auto-HCT in first CR, we recommend non-TBI conditioning such as BEAM. For patients who have not achieved CR prior to transplant, we recommend second-line therapy (including H-AraC if not already given) in hopes of achieving CR prior to auto-HCT. If CR is still not achieved after two lines of therapy, the optimal conditioning regimen is unclear. However, a standard BEAM auto-HCT produces inferior results. Outcomes for such patients may be improved with TBI conditioning. Alternatively, such patients may be better served with allo-HCT (either in first response or later in the disease course) depending on patient age, comorbidity profile, and donor availability.

Relapsed/Refractory Patients Eligible for Transplantation

Decisions regarding treatment of a patient with relapsed/refractory MCL depend on patient factors (age, performance status, comorbidity profile), which determine whether the patient is eligible for HCT. In addition disease factors (chemosensitivity, disease burden) and donor availability need to be considered.

For younger patients eligible for transplantation, auto-HCT can be considered for chemosensitive patients who have not received auto-HCT previously. Such patients undergoing auto-HCT later in the disease course can achieve remissions lasting 2–4 years. Allo-HCT is also an option for such patients and, while having a higher risk of TRM, showed a trend towards lower relapse[47]. The decision regarding allo-HCT versus auto-HCT for such patients needs to be based on perceived risk/aggressiveness of the lymphoma, patient age, comorbidity profile, and donor availability. For patients with relapsed disease after auto-HCT, or with chemoresistant disease, allo-HCT should be considered.

Major studies reporting outcomes of allo-SCT are summarized in Table 42.3.

In 1999, Khouri et al. reported a series of 16 patients with MCL treated with myeloablative allo-HCT, demonstrating that durable remissions were possible and that a graft-versus-lymphoma effect could be achieved in MCL[57]. In an attempt to reduce treatment-related mortality, reduced intensity conditioning regimens (RIC) were developed which rely more on the graft-versus-lymphoma (GvL) effect to achieve long-term disease control[57,58]. Allo-HCT with RIC regimens for relapsed/refractory MCL can achieve long-term remission with acceptable TRM[23,59](see Table 42.3).

For patients who relapse after an auto-HCT, the only option with a significant chance for long-term remission is an allo-HCT. An EBMT registry study evaluating outcomes and prognostic factors of MCL patients relapsing after auto-HCT showed remission duration after auto-HCT was the only significant factor, which impacted outcomes with allo-HCT. Two-year OS after allo-HCT was 46%. A second auto-HCT for patients relapsing after auto-HCT did not provide long-term remission[60]. Le Gouill et al. reported a multicenter retrospective study looking at outcomes of RIC allo-HCT for patients with relapsed disease after auto-HCT. At a median follow-up of 24 months, EFS was 50% and OS 53% and TRM was 32%[61]. A CIBMTR study looking at outcomes of allo-HCT in patients relapsing after auto-HCT also reported some durable responses, with a 5-year PFS of 20% and 5-year OS of 37%[62].

For patients with chemoresistant disease, allo-HCT may still offer benefit. Hamadani et al. reported results of allo-HCT for chemorefractory MCL with myeloablative and RIC regimens. The results were similar with TRM, relapse, PFS, and OS of 43%, 32%, 25%, and 30% with RIC compared to 47%, 33%, 20%, and 25% with myeloablative conditioning regimens, respectively[63].

Based on the above data, for patients with relapsed/refractory MCL, we recommend allo-HCT, with RIC regimen for patients with prior auto-HCT or those who are chemoresistant. For those with chemosensitive disease and no prior auto-HCT, auto-HCT or allo-HCT can be considered. For those patients,

Table 42.3 Studies summarizing allogeneic HCT in MCL

Study	Regimen	TRM	Relapse	PFS	OS	Follow-up duration
Maris et al.[59]	Flu/TBI	24%	9%	60%	65%	2 years
Tam et al.[23]	FCR	9% (1 year)	NA	46%	53%	6 years
Cook et al.[100]	Flu/Mel +/− Ale Flu/Bu +/− Ale	21%	65%	14%	37%	5 years
Hari et al.[62]	RIC/MAC	46%	34%	20%	37%	5 years
Le Gouill et al.[61]	RIC	32%	NA	50%	53%	2 years
Hamadani et al.[101][a]	RIC	43%	32%	25%	30%	3 years
	MAC	47%	33%	20%	25%	3 years
Fenske et al.[47]	RIC (early)[b]	25%	15%	55%	62%	5 years
	RIC (late)[c]	17%	38%	24%	31%	5 years
Kruger et al.[76]	MAC	NA	NA	68%	73%	2.8 years
Dietrich et al.[60]	RIC	30%	33%	NA	46%	2 years

[a] Study retricted to chemoresistant patients.
[b] Early cohort-transplantation performed in first PR or CR with no more than two prior lines of chemotherapy.
[c] Late cohort-transplantation performed in the remaining chemosensitive patients.
RIC = reduced intensity conditioning; MAC = myeloablative conditioning regimen; Flu = fludarabine; Mel = melphalan; Ale = alemtuzumab; TBI = total body irradiation; FCR = fludarabine; cyclophosphamide, and rituximab; TRM = treatment-related mortality; PFS = progression-free survival; OS = overall survival.

Table 42.4 Summary of outcomes with regimens for relapsed/refractory MCL

Study	Patients	Regimen(s)	ORR	CR	PFS
Forstpointner et al.[102]	47	R-FCM + R maintenance	58%	29%	45% at 2 years
		R-FCM	79%	20%	9% at 2 years
Robinson et al.[103]	12	BR	92%	59%	23 months
Rummel et al.[104]	16	BR	75%	50%	18 months
Thomas et al.[105]	16	FC +/− R	75%	56%	11 months
Kouroukis et al.[106]	36	G + bortezomib	60%	NA	11.4 months
Hitz et al.[107]	18	Single agent G	28%	5%	8 months
Garbo et al.[108]	16	R-GM	47%	20%	Median PFS not reached at 10 months
Rodriguez et al.[109]	14	R-GOx	85%	64%	45% at 1 years
Morschhauser et al.[110]	18	GDP	44%	NA	8.5 months

R-FCM = rituximab, fludarabine, cyclophosphamide, mitoxantrone; BR = bendamustine-rituximab; FCR = fludarabine, cyclophosphamide, rituximab; G = gemcitabine; R-GM =rituximab, gemcitabine, mitoxantrone; R = GOx-rituximab, gemcitabine, oxaliplatin; GDP = gemcitabine, dexamethasone, cisplatin; ORR = overall response rate; CR = complete response; PFS = progression-free survival.

choice of transplant depends on perceived aggressiveness of the lymphoma, donor availability, patient comorbidity profile, performance status, and chemosensitivity. In terms of long-term disease control allo-HCT appears to be a superior choice but at the cost of more treatment-related mortality risk up front.

Relapsed/Refractory Patients Ineligible for Transplantation

Patients with relapsed/refractory disease who are not candidates for transplantation should be considered for clinical trials. If the duration of remission was several years with the first line of therapy, the same regimen can be considered again, if there are no concerns of dose-limiting or cumulative toxicities. Alternatively any regimen listed in Table 42.1 or Table 42.4 can be considered, as well as various new or novel agents (see below, and Table 42.5).

Small Molecule Targeted Therapies

With better understanding of signaling pathways involved in MCL, treatment approaches have been developed to target

Table 42.5 Summary of outcomes with various novel agents in MCL

Regimens	ORR	CR	OS	PFS
Proteosome inhibitors[68,106,111–113]	29–81%	8–44%	23–38 months	2–12 months
Immunomodulatory agents (Imids)[69,70,114–116]	28–73%	8–36%	19–24 months	4–12 months
mTOR-inhibitors[66,67,117–119]	6–59%	2–19%	10–29 months	3–9 months
Ibrutinib[65]	68%	21%	1.5 years 58%	13.9 months
yttrium-90-ibritumomab tiuxetan[71]	31%	16%	21 months	6 months
Obinutuzumab[120]	27%	13%	NA	2.7 months
Idelalisib[72]	40%	5%	NA	3.7 months
Abexinostat[73]	27%	NA	NA	4 months
ABT-199[74]	100%	0%	NA	NA

ORR = overall response rate; CR = complete response; NA =not available; OS = overall survival; PFS = progression.

dysregulated pathways[64]. Table 42.5 summarizes the activity of various targeted therapies studied in phase 2 trials. Some of these agents are now being incorporated into frontline therapies in clinical trials that are in early stages.

Ibrutinib is an oral Bruton's tyrosine kinase inhibitor, which acts by inducing apoptosis, inhibiting cell adhesion and cellular migration. A multicenter phase 2 study by Wang *et al.* in 111 patients with relapsed/refractory MCL showed an excellent ORR of 68% with a CR rate of 21%. Within responding patients, the median duration of response was 17.5 months, with a PFS of 13.9 months, and an OS that was not reached[65]. Side effects from therapy included mild fatigue, nausea, and diarrhea. Grade 3–4 or more hematologic toxicities were seen in less than 20% of patients.

Mammalian target of rapamycin (mTOR) inhibitors, such as temsirolimus and everolimus, are active in MCL. They act on the PI3 kinase/Akt/mTOR signaling pathway, which is dysregulated in a third of human cancers. A phase 3 open-label randomized trial comparing the activity of temsirolimus *versus* investigator's choice in relapsed/refractory MCL showed a significantly better PFS in the temsirolimus arm (4.8 *versus* 1.9 months). However, PFS of all regimens was quite modest as was ORR at 22%[66]. Studies with everolimus also have shown similar response rates and PFS[67] (see Table 42.5).

The proteosome inhibitor bortezomib has been shown to have activity as a single agent or in combination with immunochemotherapy in multiple phase 2 studies. As a single agent bortezomib has an ORR of 33%[68]. However, the ORR of bortezomib in combination with chemotherapy is more favorable (see Table 42.5).

The immunomodulatory agent lenolidamide, as single agent (ORR 28–35%) and in combination with rituximab (ORR 57%), has significant activity in relapsed/refractory MCL with a favorable toxicity profile[69,70]. This regimen is a particularly attractive option for elderly or frail patients with relapsed or refractory MCL.

Radioimmunotherapy (RIT) with yttrium-90-ibritumomab tiuxetan as a single agent has a modest activity with a 31% ORR, a 16% CR rate, and a median PFS of 6 months. RIT can therefore be used in select patients with relapsed/refractory MCL[71]. RIT is not recommended in patients with significant bone marrow involvement or significant underlying cytopenias.

Numerous other agents have also shown promise in relapsed and refractory MCL in recent clinical trials. Idelalisib, an oral phosphatidylinositol-3-kinase δ (PI3Kδ) inhibitor produced an ORR of 40% and CR rate of 5% in heavily pretreated patients with an acceptable toxicity profile of diarrhea, pyrexia, fatigue, and rash[72]. Preliminary results with the histone deacetylase inhibitor abexinostat and BCL-2 inhibitor (ABT-199) are also encouraging in patients with relapsed or refractory MCL (see Table 42.5)[73,74].

Future Directions and Areas of Uncertainty

The rapidly growing armamentarium of small molecule targeted therapies, though exciting, has raised several questions. As more targeted or novel agents become available, the question arises as to whether incorporation of these agents earlier in the disease course might preclude the need for consolidation therapy with transplantation. At this time, we feel it would be premature to abandon the use of consolidative auto-HCT in lieu of early incorporation of targeted therapies, outside of a clinical trial. Another important question is whether new/novel agents can be incorporated early to help improve response prior to, or following, auto-HCT. Minimal residual disease analysis could potentially be used to guide such therapy. Evaluation of such approaches would provide excellent questions for randomized clinical trials.

Is a Risk-Adapted Approach an Option?

There are several available tools (such as MIPI score, proliferation index, blastoid histology, post-treatment PET scan, or MRD analysis), which could theoretically be used to target patients at high risk for relapse. Such patients could then undergo risk-adapted (i.e., more intensified) treatment approaches. For example, patients with the "blastoid variant" or high MIPI score, and/or high Ki-67 index could be treated with allo-HCT as opposed to auto-HCT in first remission. While such an approach might seem attractive on the surface, currently there are no data showing improved long-term outcomes with such risk-adapted approaches[75]. In addition, targeting such patients for early allo-HCT may simply expose some patients to additional risk without improving outcomes. Findings from two prospective multicentered studies (OSHO # 074 and OSHO# 60) showed similar outcomes with allo-HCT consolidation in the frontline *versus* the relapsed setting[76]. A recent analysis by the CIBMTR, which showed similar outcomes in patients receiving auto-HCT *versus* allo-HCT early in the course of disease, also argues against upfront allo-HCT[47]. However, these studies were not stratified based on prognostic factors. Similarly, for patients with low-risk disease, there are no data to indicate that therapy de-escalation (e.g., omission of auto-HCT) can be performed without compromising outcomes.

Given these findings, at this time we feel it is preferred that, outside of a clinical trial, treatment of MCL patients not be risk-adapted. There may be exceptional patients with particularly high-risk disease for whom the risk of an upfront allo-HCT may be justified. However, there is no consensus on how to identify such patients currently. We therefore feel that it is preferable whenever possible to enroll high-risk patients in clinical trials to evaluate novel approaches.

Special Circumstances
Indolent MCL

While the majority of patients with MCL will have an aggressive clinical course, up to 10% of patients follow an indolent clinical course[77]. Usually these patients present with non-nodal disease, splenomegaly, and leukemic phase. Prognostic factors at diagnosis will often be favorable, with a low proliferation rate, normal LDH, and low MIPI score. These patients have a better prognosis compared to the typical MCL patient[78,79]. This variant of MCL also has a different gene expression profile with hypermutated immunoglobulin genes, noncomplex cytogenetics, and is typically SOX11 negative[80,81]. However, SOX11 negativity in MCL does not reliably predict indolent behavior[82]. Currently there are no reliable histopathologic tools in routine practice to diagnose indolent MCL; this distinction still requires careful clinicopathologic correlation by the treating

physician. Patients with asymptomatic indolent disease can be initially observed (often for several years) without any apparent impact on OS[83]. Treatment is eventually recommended once there is evidence of disease progression or development of symptoms, as outlined earlier in the chapter.

Blastoid Variant MCL

There are several histomorphologic variants of MCL, such as classic, pleomorphic, and blastoid variants[84]. Most of these variants do not have prognostic relevance. The blastoid variant, however, does carry a less favorable prognosis and is associated with specific clinical features. Patients with blastoid MCL usually have aggressive disease with a high proliferation index. CNS involvement is more frequently seen at diagnosis and at relapse hence diagnostic evaluation of cerebrospinal fluid is recommended[85–88]. High-risk cytogenetics with chromosome 17 abnormalities and p53 deletion is seen in 56% of cases[89]. Such patients have a poor prognosis with a median OS of 14.5 months and even patients with localized disease should be treated aggressively, given the high incidence of systemic relapse[90]. Interestingly, however, in the 10-year update of hyperCVAD for patients with MCL, outcomes were not inferior for the patients with the blastoid variant[29]. It therefore may be possible to overcome the adverse prognosis associated with the blastoid variant with an aggressive treatment program.

For patients with blastoid variant MCL, we recommend aggressive therapy using a regimen that includes agents (like H-AraC) with good CNS penetration, followed by consolidation with HCT in transplant-eligible patients. Whether auto-HCT or allo-HCT is superior for such patients is not known.

Conclusions

MCL is a relatively rare form of NHL, which represents a spectrum of disease, ranging from indolent to highly aggressive forms. Given this heterogeneity, combined with variable patients factors (age, frailty, comorbidity), the treatment for MCL has to be individualized. Patients should undergo transplant evaluation early in the disease course. Though multiple treatment options are available for frontline and relapsed disease, the relative paucity of published prospective randomized trials makes clinical decision-making a challenge. We present an algorithm (Figure 42.1A,B) to summarize our recommended treatment approach.

Disclosures

Dr. Fenske discloses that he has received honoraria for consulting from Celgene, Pharmacyclics, and Janssen. These companies produce products that are mentioned in this article.

(A)

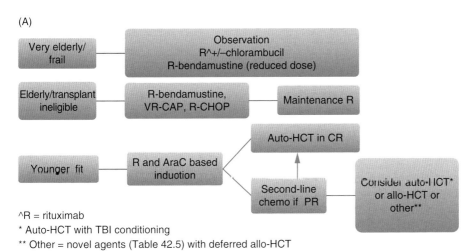

^R = rituximab
* Auto-HCT with TBI conditioning
** Other = novel agents (Table 42.5) with deferred allo-HCT

(B)

Elderly frail	R^ alone, R-chlorambucil, R-bendamustine (reduced dose), or novel agents	
Elderly/transplant ineligible	R-bendamustine, R-CHOP, VR-CAP, or novel agents	? Maintenance R
Younger ·fit	R-hyperCVAD or R-ICE or R-CHOP or R-bendamustine	auto-HCT or allo-HCT@

^R = rituximab
@Consolidation with allo-HCT if previously received auto-HCT or if chemoresistant; for chemosensitive patients with no prior auto-HCT, auto-HCT or allo-HCT are options

Figure 42.1. (A) Treatment options for newly diagnosed MCL. (B) Treatment options for relapsed MCL.

References

1. Harris NL, Jaffe ES, Stein H, *et al.* A revised European-American classification of lymphoid neoplasms: a proposal from the International Lymphoma Study Group. *Blood.* 1994;84: 1361–1392.

2. Swerdlow SH, Williams ME. From centrocytic to mantle cell lymphoma: a clinicopathologic and molecular review of 3 decades. *Hum Pathol.* 2002;33: 7–20.

3. van Leeuwen MT, Turner JJ, Joske DJ, *et al.* Lymphoid neoplasm incidence by WHO subtype in Australia 1982-2006. *Int J Cancer.* 2014;135(9): 2146–2156.

4. Project TN-HsLC. A clinical evaluation of the International Lymphoma Study Group classification of non-Hodgkin's lymphoma. The Non-Hodgkin's Lymphoma Classification Project. *Blood.* 1997;89: 3909-3918.

5. Ohshima K, Suzumiya J, Sato K, Kanda M, Haraoka S, Kikuchi M. B-cell lymphoma of 708 cases in Japan: incidence rates and clinical prognosis according to the REAL classification. *Cancer Lett.* 1999;135: 73–81.

6. Zhou Y, Wang H, Fang W, *et al.* Incidence trends of mantle cell lymphoma in the United States between 1992 and 2004. *Cancer.* 2008;113: 791–798.

7. Argatoff LH, Connors JM, Klasa RJ, Horsman DE, Gascoyne RD. Mantle cell lymphoma: a clinicopathologic study of 80 cases. *Blood.* 1997;89: 2067–2078.

8. Bosch F, Lopez-Guillermo A, Campo E, *et al.* Mantle cell lymphoma: presenting features, response to therapy, and prognostic factors. *Cancer.* 1998;82: 567–575.

9. Romaguera JE, Medeiros LJ, Hagemeister FB, *et al.* Frequency of gastrointestinal involvement and its clinical significance in mantle cell lymphoma. *Cancer.* 2003;97: 586–591.

10. Dreyling M, Hiddemann W. Current treatment standards and emerging strategies in mantle cell lymphoma. *Hematology Am Soc Hematol Educ Program.* 2009:542–551.

11. Leitch HA, Gascoyne RD, Chhanabhai M, Voss NJ, Klasa R, Connors JM. Limited-stage mantle-cell lymphoma. *Ann Oncol.* 2003;14: 1555–1561.

12. Hoster E, Dreyling M, Klapper W, *et al.* A new prognostic index (MIPI) for patients with advanced-stage mantle cell lymphoma. *Blood.* 2008;111: 558–565.

13. Hoster E, Klapper W, Hermine O, *et al.* Confirmation of the mantle-cell lymphoma International Prognostic Index in randomized trials of the European Mantle-Cell Lymphoma Network. *J Clin Oncol.* 2014;32: 1338–1346.

14. Royo C, Salaverria I, Hartmann EM, Rosenwald A, Campo E, Bea S. The complex landscape of genetic alterations in mantle cell lymphoma. *Semin Cancer Biol.* 2011;21: 322–334.

15. Rosenwald A, Wright G, Wiestner A, *et al.* The proliferation gene expression signature is a quantitative integrator of oncogenic events that predicts survival in mantle cell lymphoma. *Cancer Cell.* 2003;3: 185–197.

16. Jares P, Campo E. Advances in the understanding of mantle cell lymphoma. *Br J Haematol.* 2008;142: 149–165.

17. Klapper W, Hoster E, Determann O, *et al.* Ki-67 as a prognostic marker in mantle cell lymphoma-consensus guidelines of the pathology panel of the European MCL Network. *J Hematop.* 2009;2: 103–111.

18. Cohen JB, Ruppert AS, Heerema NA, *et al.* Complex Karyotype (CK) Is Associated with a Shortened Progression-Free Survival (PFS) in Patients (pts) with Newly Diagnosed Mantle Cell Lymphoma (MCL). *ASH Annual Meeting Abstracts.* 2012.

19. Espinet B, Salaverria I, Bea S, *et al.* Incidence and prognostic impact of secondary cytogenetic aberrations in a series of 145 patients with mantle cell lymphoma. *Genes Chromosomes Cancer.* 2010;49: 439–451.

20. Dreyling M, Thieblemont C, Gallamini A, *et al.* ESMO Consensus conferences: guidelines on malignant lymphoma. part 2: marginal zone lymphoma, mantle cell lymphoma, peripheral T-cell lymphoma. *Ann Oncol.* 2013;24: 857–877.

21. Herrmann A, Hoster E, Zwingers T, *et al.* Improvement of overall survival in advanced stage mantle cell lymphoma. *J Clin Oncol.* 2009;27: 511–518.

22. Lenz G, Dreyling M, Hoster E, *et al.* Immunochemotherapy with rituximab and cyclophosphamide, doxorubicin, vincristine, and prednisone significantly improves response and time to treatment failure, but not long-term outcome in patients with previously untreated mantle cell lymphoma: results of a prospective randomized trial of the German Low Grade Lymphoma Study Group (GLSG). *J Clin Oncol.* 2005;23: 1984–1992.

23. Tam CS, Bassett R, Ledesma C, *et al.* Mature results of the M. D. Anderson Cancer Center risk-adapted transplantation strategy in mantle cell lymphoma. *Blood.* 2009;113: 4144–4152.

24. Schulz H, Bohlius JF, Trelle S, *et al.* Immunochemotherapy with rituximab and overall survival in patients with indolent or mantle cell lymphoma: a systematic review and meta-analysis. *J Natl Cancer Inst.* 2007;99: 706–714.

25. Lefrere F, Delmer A, Suzan F, *et al.* Sequential chemotherapy by CHOP and DHAP regimens followed by high-dose therapy with stem cell transplantation induces a high rate of complete response and improves event-free survival in mantle cell lymphoma: a prospective study. *Leukemia.* 2002;16: 587–593.

26. van 't Veer MB, de Jong D, MacKenzie M, *et al.* High-dose Ara-C and beam with autograft rescue in R-CHOP responsive mantle cell lymphoma patients. *Br J Haematol.* 2009;144: 524–530.

27. Eskelund CW, Kolstad A, Jerkeman M, *et al.* 15-year follow-up of the Second Nordic Mantle Cell Lymphoma trial (MCL2): prolonged remissions without survival plateau. *Br J Haematol.* 2016; July 5. doi: 10.1111/bjh.14241.

28. Hermine O, Hoster E, Walewski J, *et al.* Addition of high-dose cytarabine to immunochemotherapy before autologous stem-cell transplantation in patients aged 65 years or younger with mantle cell lymphoma (MCL Younger): a randomised, open-label, phase 3 trial of the European Mantle Cell Lymphoma Network. *Lancet.* 2016; Aug 6;388(10044):565–75. doi: 10.1016/S0140-6736(16)00739-X.

29. Chihara D, Cheah CY, Westin JR, *et al.* Rituximab plus hyper-CVAD alternating with MTX/Ara-C in patients with newly diagnosed mantle cell lymphoma: 15-year follow-up of a phase II study from the MD Anderson Cancer Center. *Br J Haematol.* 2016 Jan;172(1):80–8. doi: 10.1111/bjh.13796.

30. Bernstein SH, Epner E, Unger JM, *et al.* A phase II multicenter trial of hyperCVAD MTX/Ara-C and rituximab in patients with previously untreated mantle cell lymphoma; SWOG 0213. *Ann Oncol.* 2013;24: 1587–1593.

31. Merli F, Luminari S, Ilariucci F, *et al.* Rituximab plus HyperCVAD alternating with high dose cytarabine and methotrexate for the initial treatment of patients with mantle cell lymphoma, a multicentre trial from Gruppo Italiano Studio Linfomi. *Br J Haematol.* 2012;156: 346–353.

32. Chang JE, Li H, Smith MR, *et al.* Phase 2 study of VcR-CVAD with maintenance rituximab for untreated mantle cell lymphoma: an Eastern Cooperative Oncology Group study (E1405). *Blood.* 2014;123: 1665–1673.

33. Kenkre VP, Long WL, Eickhoff JC, *et al.* Maintenance rituximab following induction chemo-immunotherapy for mantle cell lymphoma: long-term follow-up of a pilot study from the Wisconsin Oncology Network. *Leuk Lymphoma.* 2011;52: 1675–1680.

34. Jantunen E, Canals C, Attal M, *et al.* Autologous stem-cell transplantation in patients with mantle cell lymphoma beyond 65 years of age: a study from the European Group for Blood and Marrow Transplantation (EBMT). *Ann Oncol.* 2012;23: 166–171.

35. Rummel MJ, Niederle N, Maschmeyer G, *et al.* Bendamustine plus rituximab *versus* CHOP plus rituximab as first-line treatment for patients with indolent and mantle-cell lymphomas: an open-label, multicentre, randomised, phase 3 non-inferiority trial. *Lancet.* 2013;381: 1203–1210.

36. Flinn IW, van der Jagt R, Kahl BS, *et al.* Randomized trial of bendamustine-rituximab or R-CHOP/R-CVP in first-line treatment of indolent NHL or MCL: the BRIGHT study. *Blood.* 2014;123: 2944–2952.

37. Burke JM, Van der Jagt RH, Kahl BS, *et al.* Differences in quality of life between bendamustine plus rituximab compared with standard first-line treatments in patients with previously untreated advanced indolent non-Hodgkin's lymphoma or mantle cell lymphoma. *ASH Annual Meeting Abstracts.* 2012;120: 155.

38. Cavalli F, Rooney B, Pei L, Van De Velde H, Robak T. Investigators aobotL. Randomized phase 3 study of rituximab, cyclophosphamide, doxorubicin, and prednisone plus vincristine (R-CHOP) or bortezomib (VR-CAP) in newly diagnosed mantle cell lymphoma (MCL) patients (pts) ineligible for bone marrow transplantation (BMT). *ASCO Meeting Abstracts.* 2014;8500.

39. Visco C, Finotto S, Zambello R, *et al.* Combination of rituximab, bendamustine, and cytarabine for patients with mantle-cell non-Hodgkin lymphoma ineligible for intensive regimens or autologous transplantation. *J Clin Oncol.* 2013;31: 1442–1449.

40. Kluin-Nelemans HC, Hoster E, Hermine O, *et al.* Treatment of older patients with mantle-cell lymphoma. *N Engl J Med.* 2012;367: 520–531.

41. Martin P, Smith M, Till B. Management of mantle cell lymphoma in the elderly. *Best Pract Res Clin Haematol.* 2012;25: 221–231.

42. Weidmann E, Neumann A, Fauth F, *et al.* Phase II study of bendamustine in combination with rituximab as first-line treatment in patients 80 years or older with aggressive B-cell lymphomas. *Ann Oncol.* 2011;22: 1839–1844.

43. Ghielmini M, Zucca E. How I treat mantle cell lymphoma. *Blood.* 2009;114: 1469–1476.

44. Ghielmini M, Schmitz SF, Cogliatti S, *et al.* Effect of single-agent rituximab given at the standard schedule or as prolonged treatment in patients with mantle cell lymphoma: a study of the Swiss Group for Clinical Cancer Research (SAKK). *J Clin Oncol.* 2005;23: 705–711.

45. Dreyling M, Lenz G, Hoster E, *et al.* Early consolidation by myeloablative radiochemotherapy followed by autologous stem cell transplantation in first remission significantly prolongs progression-free survival in mantle-cell lymphoma: results of a prospective randomized trial of the European MCL Network. *Blood.* 2005;105: 2677–2684.

46. Hoster E, Metzner B, Forstpointner R, *et al.* Autologous stem cell transplantation and addition of rituximab independently prolong response duration in advanced stage mantle cell lymphoma. *Blood.* 2009;114: 880.

47. Fenske TS, Zhang MJ, Carreras J, *et al.* Autologous or reduced-intensity conditioning allogeneic hematopoietic cell transplantation for chemotherapy-sensitive mantle-cell lymphoma: analysis of transplantation timing and modality. *J Clin Oncol.* 2014;32: 273–281.

48. LaCasce AS, Vandergrift JL, Rodriguez MA, *et al.* Comparative outcome of initial therapy for younger patients with mantle cell lymphoma: an analysis from the NCCN NHL Database. *Blood.* 2012;119: 2093–2099.

49. Geisler CH, Kolstad A, Laurell A, *et al.* Long-term progression-free survival of mantle cell lymphoma after intensive front-line immunochemotherapy with in vivo-purged stem cell rescue: a nonrandomized phase 2 multicenter study by the Nordic Lymphoma Group. *Blood.* 2008;112: 2687–2693.

50. Ladetto M, Magni M, Pagliano G, *et al.* Rituximab induces effective clearance of minimal residual disease in molecular relapses of mantle cell lymphoma. *Biol Blood Marrow Transplant.* 2006;12: 1270–1276.

51. Andersen NS, Pedersen LB, Laurell A, *et al.* Pre-emptive treatment with rituximab of molecular relapse after autologous stem cell transplantation in mantle cell lymphoma. *J Clin Oncol.* 2009;27: 4365–4370.

52. Dietrich S, Weidle J, Rieger M, *et al.* Rituximab maintenance therapy after autologous stem cell transplantation prolongs progression-free survival in patients with mantle cell lymphoma. *Leukemia.* 2014;28: 708–709.

53. Le Gouill S, Thieblemont G, Oberic L, *et al.* Maintenance after autologous stem cell transplantation prolongs survival in younger patients with mantle cell lymphoma: final results of randomized phase 3 LyMa trial of the Lysa/Goelams group. *ASH Annual Meeting Abstracts*, 2016 [Abstract 145].

54. Rubio Marie T, Boumendil A, Luan JJ, *et al.* Is there still a place for total body irradiation (TBI) in the conditioning regimen of autologous stem cell transplantation in mantle cell lymphoma?: a retrospective study from the Lymphoma Working Party of the EBMT. *ASH Annual Meeting Abstracts.* 2010;116:688.

55. Hoster E, Christian H Geisler, Jeanette K Doorduijn, *et al.* Role of high-dose cytarabine and total body irradiation conditioning before autologous stem cell transplantation in mantle cell lymphoma: a comparison of nordic MCL2, HOVON 45, and European MCL Younger Trials. *Blood.* 2013;122: 3367.

56. Kolstad A, Laurell A, Jerkeman M, *et al.* Nordic MCL3 study: 90Y-ibritumomab-tiuxetan added to BEAM/C in non-CR patients before transplant in mantle cell lymphoma. *Blood.* 2014;123: 2953–2959.

57. Khouri IF, Lee MS, Romaguera J, *et al.* Allogeneic hematopoietic transplantation for mantle-cell lymphoma: molecular remissions and evidence of graft-*versus*-malignancy. *Ann Oncol.* 1999;10: 1293–1299.

58. Khouri IF, Lee MS, Saliba RM, *et al.* Nonablative allogeneic stem-cell transplantation for advanced/recurrent mantle-cell lymphoma. *J Clin Oncol.* 2003;21: 4407–4412.

59. Maris MB, Sandmaier BM, Storer BE, *et al.* Allogeneic hematopoietic cell transplantation after fludarabine and 2 Gy total body irradiation for relapsed and refractory mantle cell lymphoma. *Blood.* 2004;104: 3535–3542.

60. Dietrich S, Boumendil A, Finel H, *et al.* Outcome and prognostic factors in patients with mantle-cell lymphoma relapsing after autologous stem-cell transplantation: a retrospective study of the European Group for Blood and Marrow Transplantation (EBMT). *Ann Oncol.* 2014;25: 1053–1058.

61. Le Gouill S, Kroger N, Dhedin N, *et al.* Reduced-intensity conditioning allogeneic stem cell transplantation for relapsed/refractory mantle cell lymphoma: a multicenter experience. *Ann Oncol.* 2012;23: 2695–2703.

62. Hari PN, Maloney DG, Carreras J, *et al.* Allogeneic transplantation (AlloHCT) for patients with mantle cell lymphoma (MCL) progressing after autologous transplantation (AutoHCT). on behalf of the writing committee, Center for International Blood & Marrow Transplant Research (CIBMTR), Medical College of Wisconsin, Milwaukee, WI 11th International Conference on Malignant Lymphoma. Lugano, Switzerland. *Ann Oncol* 2011;Suppl 4:Abstract 038.

63. Hamadani M, Saber W, Ahn KW, *et al.* Allogeneic hematopoietic cell transplantation for chemotherapy-unresponsive mantle cell lymphoma: a cohort analysis from the center for international blood and marrow transplant research. *Biol Blood Marrow Transplant.* 2013;19: 625–631.

64. Perez-Galan P, Dreyling M, Wiestner A. Mantle cell lymphoma: biology, pathogenesis, and the molecular basis of treatment in the genomic era. *Blood.* 2011;117: 26–38.

65. Wang ML, Rule S, Martin P, *et al.* Targeting BTK with ibrutinib in relapsed or refractory mantle-cell lymphoma. *N Engl J Med.* 2013;369: 507–516.

66. Hess G, Herbrecht R, Romaguera J, *et al.* Phase III study to evaluate temsirolimus compared with investigator's choice therapy for the treatment of relapsed or refractory mantle cell lymphoma. *J Clin Oncol.* 2009;27: 3822–3829.

67. Renner C, Zinzani PL, Gressin R, *et al.* A multicenter phase II trial (SAKK 36/ 06) of single-agent everolimus (RAD001) in patients with relapsed or refractory mantle cell lymphoma. *Haematologica.* 2012;97: 1085–1091.

68. Goy A, Bernstein SH, Kahl BS, *et al.* Bortezomib in patients with relapsed or refractory mantle cell lymphoma: updated time-to-event analyses of the multicenter phase 2 PINNACLE study. *Ann Oncol.* 2009;20: 520–525.

69. Goy A, Sinha R, Williams ME, *et al.* Single-agent lenalidomide in patients with mantle-cell lymphoma who relapsed or progressed after or were refractory to bortezomib: phase II MCL-001 (EMERGE) study. *J Clin Oncol.* 2013;31: 3688–3695.

70. Wang M, Fayad L, Wagner-Bartak N, *et al.* Lenalidomide in combination with rituximab for patients with relapsed or refractory mantle-cell lymphoma: a phase 1/2 clinical trial. *Lancet Oncol.* 2012;13: 716–723.

71. Wang M, Oki Y, Pro B, *et al.* Phase II study of yttrium-90-ibritumomab tiuxetan in patients with relapsed or refractory mantle cell lymphoma. *J Clin Oncol.* 2009;27: 5213–5218.

72. Kahl BS, Spurgeon SE, Furman RR, *et al.* A phase 1 study of the PI3Kdelta inhibitor idelalisib in patients with relapsed/refractory mantle cell lymphoma (MCL). *Blood.* 2014;123: 3398–3405.

73. Evens AM, Vose JM, Harb W, *et al.* A Phase II multicenter study of the histone deacetylase inhibitor (HDACi) abexinostat (PCI-24781) in relapsed/ refractory follicular lymphoma (FL) and mantle cell lymphoma (MCL). *ASH Annual Meeting Abstracts.* 2012;120: 55.

74. Davids MS, Seymour JF, Gerecitano JF, *et al.* The single-agent Bcl-2 inhibitor ABT-199 (GDC-0199) in patients with relapsed/refractory (R/R) non-Hodgkin lymphoma (NHL): responses observed in all mantle cell lymphoma (MCL) patients. *Blood.* 2013;122(21)1789.

75. Robinson S, Dreger P, Caballero D, *et al.* The EBMT/EMCL consensus project on the role of autologous and allogeneic stem cell transplantation in mantle cell lymphoma. *Leukemia.* 2015;29(2):464–473.

76. Kruger WH, Hirt C, Basara N, *et al.* Allogeneic stem cell transplantation for mantle cell lymphoma-final report from the prospective trials of the East German Study Group Haematology/ Oncology (OSHO). *Ann Hematol.* 2014;93(9): 1587–1597.

77. Dreyling M. Mantle cell lymphoma: biology, clinical presentation, and therapeutic approaches. *Am Soc Clin Oncol Educ Book.* 2014: 191–198.

78. Tiemann M, Schrader C, Klapper W, *et al.* Histopathology, cell proliferation indices and clinical outcome in 304 patients with mantle cell lymphoma (MCL): a clinicopathological study from the European MCL Network. *Br J Haematol.* 2005;131: 29–38.

79. Jares P, Colomer D, Campo E. Genetic and molecular pathogenesis of mantle cell lymphoma: perspectives for new targeted therapeutics. *Nat Rev Cancer.* 2007;7: 750–762.

80. Fernàndez V, Salamero O, Espinet B, *et al.* Genomic and gene expression profiling defines indolent forms of mantle cell lymphoma. *Cancer Res.* 2010;70: 1408–1418.

81. Ondrejka SL, Lai R, Smith SD, Hsi ED. Indolent mantle cell leukemia: a clinicopathological variant characterized by isolated lymphocytosis, interstitial bone marrow involvement, kappa light chain restriction, and good prognosis. *Haematologica.* 2011;96: 1121–1127.

82. Nygren L, Baumgartner Wennerholm S, Klimkowska M, Christensson B, Kimby E, Sander B. Prognostic role of SOX11 in a population-based cohort of mantle cell lymphoma. *Blood.* 2012;119: 4215–4223.

83. Martin P, Chadburn A, Christos P, *et al.* Outcome of deferred initial therapy in mantle-cell lymphoma. *J Clin Oncol.* 2009;27: 1209–1213.

84. Swerdlow SH. *WHO Classification of Tumours of Haematopoietic and Lymphoid Tissues.* Lyon: World Health Organization, 2008.

85. Cheah CY, George A, Gine E, *et al.* Central nervous system involvement in mantle cell lymphoma: clinical features, prognostic factors and outcomes from the European Mantle Cell Lymphoma Network. *Ann Oncol.* 2013;24: 2119–2123.

86. Conconi A, Franceschetti S, Lobetti-Bodoni C, *et al.* Risk factors of central nervous system relapse in mantle cell lymphoma. *Leuk Lymphoma.* 2013;54: 1908–1914.

87. Ferrer A, Bosch F, Villamor N, *et al.* Central nervous system involvement in mantle cell lymphoma. *Ann Oncol.* 2008;19: 135–141.

88. Vose JM. Mantle cell lymphoma: 2012 update on diagnosis, risk-stratification, and clinical management. *Am J Hematol.* 2012;87: 604–609.

89. Schlette E, Lai R, Onciu M, Doherty D, Bueso-Ramos C, Medeiros LJ. Leukemic mantle cell lymphoma: clinical and pathologic spectrum of twenty-three cases. *Mod Pathol.* 2001;14: 1133–1140.

90. Bernard M, Tsang RW, Le LW, *et al.* Limited-stage mantle cell lymphoma: treatment outcomes at the Princess Margaret Hospital. *Leuk Lymphoma.* 2013;54: 261–267.

91. Damon LE, Johnson JL, Niedzwiecki D, *et al.* Immunochemotherapy and autologous stem-cell transplantation for untreated patients with mantle-cell lymphoma: CALGB 59909. *J Clin Oncol.* 2009;27: 6101–6108.

92. Delarue R, Haioun C, Ribrag V, *et al.* CHOP and DHAP plus rituximab followed by autologous stem cell transplantation in mantle cell lymphoma: a phase 2 study from the Groupe d'Etude des Lymphomes de l'Adulte. *Blood.* 2013;121: 48–53.

93. Gressin R, Caulet-Maugendre S, Deconinck E, *et al.* Evaluation of the (R) VAD+C regimen for the treatment of newly diagnosed mantle cell lymphoma. Combined results of two prospective phase II trials from the French GOELAMS group. *Haematologica.* 2010;95: 1350–1357.

94. Vandenberghe E, Ruiz de Elvira C, Loberiza FR, *et al.* Outcome of autologous transplantation for mantle cell lymphoma: a study by the European Blood and Bone Marrow Transplant and Autologous Blood and Marrow Transplant Registries. *Br J Haematol.* 2003;120: 793–800.

95. Touzeau C, Leux C, Bouabdallah R, *et al.* Autologous stem cell transplantation in mantle cell lymphoma: a report from the SFGM-TC. *Ann Hematol.* 2014;93: 233–242.

96. Herold M, Haas A, Srock S, *et al.* Rituximab added to first-line mitoxantrone, chlorambucil, and prednisolone chemotherapy followed by interferon maintenance prolongs survival in patients with advanced follicular lymphoma: an East German Study Group Hematology and Oncology Study. *J Clin Oncol.* 2007;25: 1986–1992.

97. Smith MR, Li H, Gordon L, *et al.* Phase II study of rituximab plus cyclophosphamide, doxorubicin, vincristine, and prednisone immunochemotherapy followed by yttrium-90-ibritumomab tiuxetan in untreated mantle-cell lymphoma: Eastern Cooperative Oncology Group Study E1499. *J Clin Oncol.* 2012;30: 3119–3126.

98. Houot R, Le Gouill S, Ojeda Uribe M, *et al.* Combination of rituximab, bortezomib, doxorubicin, dexamethasone and chlorambucil (RiPAD+C) as first-line therapy for elderly mantle cell lymphoma patients: results of a phase II trial from the GOELAMS. *Ann Oncol.* 2012;23: 1555–1561.

99. Ruan J, Gregory SA, Christos P, *et al.* Long-term follow-up of R-CHOP with bevacizumab as initial therapy for mantle cell lymphoma: clinical and correlative results. *Clin Lymphoma Myeloma Leuk.* 2014;14: 107–113.

100. Cook G, Smith GM, Kirkland K, *et al.* Outcome following reduced-intensity allogeneic stem cell transplantation (RIC AlloSCT) for relapsed and refractory mantle cell lymphoma (MCL): a study of the British Society for Blood and Marrow Transplantation. *Biol Blood Marrow Transplant.* 2010;16: 1419–1427.

101. Hamadani M, Saber W, Ahn KW, *et al.* Allogeneic hematopoietic cell transplantation for chemotherapy-unresponsive mantle cell lymphoma: a cohort analysis from the Center for International Blood and Marrow Transplant Research. *Biol Blood Marrow Transplant.* 2013;19: 625–631.

102. Forstpointner R, Unterhalt M, Dreyling M, *et al.* Maintenance therapy with rituximab leads to a significant prolongation of response duration after salvage therapy with a combination of rituximab, fludarabine, cyclophosphamide, and mitoxantrone (R-FCM) in patients with recurring and refractory follicular and mantle cell lymphomas: Results of a prospective randomized study of the German Low Grade Lymphoma Study Group (GLSG). *Blood.* 2006;108: 4003–4008.

103. Robinson KS, Williams ME, van der Jagt RH, *et al.* Phase II multicenter study of bendamustine plus rituximab in patients with relapsed indolent B-cell and mantle cell non-Hodgkin's lymphoma. *J Clin Oncol.* 2008;26: 4473–4479.

104. Rummel MJ, Al-Batran SE, Kim SZ, *et al.* Bendamustine plus rituximab is effective and has a favorable toxicity profile in the treatment of mantle cell and low-grade non-Hodgkin's lymphoma. *J Clin Oncol.* 2005;23: 3383–3389.

105. Thomas DW, Owen RG, Johnson SA, *et al.* Superior quality and duration of responses among patients with mantle-cell lymphoma treated with fludarabine and cyclophosphamide with or without rituximab compared with prior responses to CHOP. *Leuk Lymphoma.* 2005;46: 549–552.

106. Kouroukis CT, Fernandez LA, Crump M, *et al.* A phase II study of bortezomib and gemcitabine in relapsed mantle cell lymphoma from the National Cancer Institute of Canada Clinical Trials Group (IND 172). *Leuk Lymphoma.* 2011;52: 394–399.

107. Hitz F, Martinelli G, Zucca E, *et al.* A multicentre phase II trial of gemcitabine for the treatment of patients with newly diagnosed, relapsed or chemotherapy resistant mantle cell lymphoma: SAKK 36/03. *Hematol Oncol.* 2009;27: 154–159.

108. Garbo LE, Flynn PJ, MacRae MA, Rauch MA, Wang Y, Kolibaba KS. Results of a Phase II trial of gemcitabine, mitoxantrone, and rituximab in relapsed or refractory mantle cell lymphoma. *Invest New Drugs.* 2009;27: 476–481.

109. Rodriguez J, Gutierrez A, Palacios A, *et al.* Rituximab, gemcitabine and oxaliplatin: an effective regimen in patients with refractory and relapsing mantle cell lymphoma. *Leuk Lymphoma.* 2007;48: 2172–2178.

110. Morschhauser F, Depil S, Jourdan E, *et al.* Phase II study of gemcitabine-dexamethasone with or without cisplatin in relapsed or refractory mantle cell lymphoma. *Ann Oncol.* 2007;18: 370–375.

111. Lamm W, Kaufmann H, Raderer M, *et al.* Bortezomib combined with rituximab and dexamethasone is an active regimen for patients with relapsed and chemotherapy-refractory mantle cell lymphoma. *Haematologica.* 2011;96: 1008–1014.

112. Friedberg JW, Vose JM, Kelly JL, *et al.* The combination of bendamustine, bortezomib, and rituximab for patients with relapsed/refractory indolent and mantle cell non-Hodgkin lymphoma. *Blood.* 2011;117: 2807–2812.

113. Baiocchi RA, Alinari L, Lustberg ME, *et al.* Phase 2 trial of rituximab and bortezomib in patients with relapsed or refractory mantle cell and follicular lymphoma. *Cancer.* 2011;117: 2442–2451.

114. Zinzani PL, Vose JM, Czuczman MS, *et al.* Long-term follow-up of lenalidomide in relapsed/refractory mantle cell lymphoma: subset analysis of the NHL-003 study. *Ann Oncol.* 2013;24: 2892–2897.

115. Zaja F, De Luca S, Vitolo U, *et al.* Salvage treatment with lenalidomide and dexamethasone in relapsed/refractory mantle cell lymphoma: clinical results and effects on microenvironment and neo-angiogenic biomarkers. *Haematologica.* 2012;97: 416–422.

116. Ruan J, Martin P, Coleman M, *et al.* Durable responses with the metronomic rituximab and thalidomide plus prednisone, etoposide, procarbazine, and cyclophosphamide regimen in elderly patients with recurrent mantle cell lymphoma. *Cancer.* 2010;116: 2655–2664.

117. Witzig TE, Geyer SM, Ghobrial I, *et al.* Phase II trial of single-agent temsirolimus (CCI-779) for relapsed mantle cell lymphoma. *J Clin Oncol.* 2005;23: 5347–5356.

118. Ansell SM, Tang H, Kurtin PJ, *et al.* Temsirolimus and rituximab in patients with relapsed or refractory mantle cell lymphoma: a phase 2 study. *Lancet Oncol.* 2011;12: 361–368.

119. Ansell SM, Inwards DJ, Rowland KM, Jr., *et al.* Low-dose, single-agent

temsirolimus for relapsed mantle cell lymphoma: a phase 2 trial in the North Central Cancer Treatment Group. *Cancer*. 2008;113: 508–514.

120. Morschhauser FA, Cartron G, Thieblemont C, *et al*. Obinutuzumab (GA101) monotherapy in relapsed/ refractory diffuse large B-cell lymphoma or mantle-cell lymphoma:

results from the phase II GAUGUIN study. *J Clin Oncol*. 2013;31: 2912–2919.

121. Chen RW, Hongli L, Bernstein SH, Rimsza LM, Foreman SJ, Constine L, *et al*. BR but not R-HCVAD is a feasible induction prior to ASCT in frontline MCL: Results of SWOG study 1106. *Br J Haematol*; in press.

122. Robak T, Huang H, Jin J, Zhu J, Liu T, Samoilova O, *et al*. Bortezomib-based

therapy for newly diagnosed mantle-cell lymphoma. *N Engl J Med*. 2015;372(10):944–53.

123. Ruan J, Martin P, Shah B, Chuster SJ, Smith SM, Furman RR, *et al*. Lenalidomide plus rituximab as initial treatment for mantle-cell lymphoma. *N Engl J Med*. 2015;373(19):1835–44.

Hematopoietic Cell Transplants for Aggressive B-Cell Lymphomas

Lori S. Muffly and Sonali M. Smith

Introduction

Aggressive B-cell lymphomas include a number of well-defined clinicopathologic and other emerging entities, including diffuse large B-cell lymphoma (DLBCL), Burkitt lymphoma (BL), B-cell lymphoma intermediate between DLBCL and BL (BCLU), and transformed lymphomas. Among these diseases, DLBCL is both the most common and the prototype of aggressive B-cell lymphomas and has been the best studied in terms of hematopoietic cell transplant (HCT). DLBCL accounts for 30% of all new lymphoma diagnoses in North America. With the advent of rituximab added to anthracycline-based chemotherapy, cure rates have substantially improved and, depending on clinical and biologic features, 50–95% of patients can expect long-term disease control[1]. The wide range likely reflects the current understanding that DLBCL comprises at least two genetically distinct subtypes (germinal center and nongerminal center) based on the "cell-of-origin" model, and that there are additional cytogenetic and molecular "hits" conferring negative clinical consequences. This includes the discovery that 5–7% of DLBCL (and a higher percentage of BCLU) harbor both MYC and BCL2 rearrangements (also called "double-hit lymphomas", or DHL), and that up to one-third of patients have protein overexpression of MYC and BCL2, again reducing the cure rates with standard frontline approaches.

While frontline management of DLBCL has seen great improvements, patients with relapsed or refractory aggressive lymphomas fare more poorly. The most established approach for relapsed disease is with autologous (auto-HCT; Table 43.1) or allogeneic hematopoietic cell transplant (allo-HCT), both of which retain important roles in the overall management of DLBCL. The use of auto-HCT remains the standard of care for relapsed chemosensitive DLBCL; however, the observed outcomes with salvage auto-HCT are less robust in the current era, and there is controversy over its true benefit. Allo-HCT is typically reserved for relapse after auto-HCT or for those with chemorefractory disease, but the precise timing and optimal patient selection of allo-HCT remain areas of debate. This chapter reviews the current state of HCT for DLBCL. Special populations such as DHL, DLBCL arising from follicular lymphoma, and BL are briefly discussed. Current controversies in the field are highlighted, and recommendations are proposed.

Autologous Hematopoietic Cell Transplantation for Diffuse Large B-Cell Lymphoma

Auto-HCT for Relapsed/Refractory DLBCL

Historically, auto-HCT became the standard of care for relapsed chemosensitive aggressive lymphomas when the Parma group demonstrated an approximate 20% survival advantage to auto-HCT over standard DHAP (dexamethasone, cisplatin, cytarabine) salvage in a randomized setting[2]. Response rates (84% *versus* 44%), event-free survival (EFS; 46% *versus* 12%, $P=0.001$), and OS (53% *versus* 32%, $P=0.038$) all significantly favored auto-HCT. Although practice is changing, several study limitations are worth noting. First, only 58% of 215 patients had chemosensitive disease and could be randomized. Second, patients over age 60 years and those with marrow involvement were excluded. In addition, the Parma study was conducted prior to routine rituximab incorporation into frontline and salvage regimens, calling into question whether the results are still relevant. Unfortunately, since the Parma report, there have been no prospective randomized trials comparing auto-HCT *versus* nontransplant salvage, making the true impact of auto-HCT in the current era difficult to define.

While not directly addressing the superiority of auto-HCT over nontransplant approaches, there are now three large-scale prospective trials and several registry studies that are informative and support the continued benefit of auto-HCT, albeit arguably in a smaller proportion of patients. The CORAL (Collaborative Trial in Relapsed Aggressive Lymphoma) study was designed to compare the efficacy and mobilization rates of two chemoimmunotherapy salvage regimens, and to secondarily evaluate the role of maintenance rituximab after auto-HCT[3]. The CORAL study randomized 400 DLBCL patients with relapse or incomplete response to CHOP (cyclophosphamide, doxorubicin, vincristine, prednisone) or rituximab-CHOP (R-CHOP) to either R-DHAP or R-ICE (rituximab, ifosfamide, carboplatin, etoposide) followed by auto-HCT with BEAM (carmustine, etoposide, cytarabine, melphalan) conditioning[4]. While overall response rates and 3-year outcomes were similar, R-DHAP was associated with more severe

Table 43.1 Auto-HCT studies in DLBCL

Setting	Study design	Reference	n	Treatment	PFS/DFS/EFS	OS	Comments
PR/CR1	RCT	Haioun et al. (2000)	236 aaIPI high/int or high-risk in CR after induction	Chemo consolidation (control) versus CBV/auto-HCT	8-year DFS: 39% (control) versus 55% (HCT); P=0.02	8-year OS: 49% (control) versus 64% (HCT); P=0.04	-Pre-rituximab era -Prospective trial retrospectively analyzed on basis of aaIPI
		Gisselbrecht et al. (2002)	370 aaIPI high/int or high-risk, 61% DLBCL	ACVBP × 4 + chemo consolidation (control) versus CVEP × 3 + BEAM/auto-HCT	5-year EFS: 51% (control) versus 39% (HCT); P=0.09	5-year OS: 60% (control) versus 46% (HCT); P=0.006	-Pre-rituximab era -Less-intense induction in HCT arm may have biased results
		Kaiser et al. (2002)	312 aaIPI high/int or high-risk, 60% DLBCL	CHOEP × 5 + IFRT (control) versus CHOEP × 3 + BEAM/auto-HCT +IFRT	3-year EFS: 49% (control) versus 59% (HCT); P=0.22	3-year OS: 63% (control) versus 62% (HCT); P=0.68	-Pre-rituximab era
		Martelli et al. (2003)	150 aaIPI high/int or high-risk, 76% DLBCL	MACOPB × 12 weeks (control) versus MACOPB × 8 weeks + BEAC/auto-HCT	5-year PFS: 49% (control) versus 61% (HCT); P=0.21	5-year OS: 65% (control) versus 64% (HCT); P=0.95	-Pre-rituximab era -40% in HCT arm did not undergo HCT
		Milpied et al. (2004)	197 aaIPI low or low/int or high/int, 76% DLBCL	CHOP × 8 (control) versus CEEP × 2 + MC + BEAM/auto-HCT	5-year EFS: 37% (control) versus 55% (HCT); P=0.037	5-year OS: 56% (control) versus 71% (HCT); P=0.076	-Pre-rituximab era -Significant OS benefit with HCT in aaIPI high/int group -aaIPI high-risk excluded
		Vitolo et al. (2005)	126 aaIPI high/int or high-risk, 100% DLBCL	MegaCEOP × 4–8 (control) versus HDS + HDT/auto-HCT	5-year EFS: 48% (control) versus 45% (HCT); P=0.56	6-year OS: 63% (control) versus 49% (HCT); P=0.06	-Pre-rituximab era -Entirely different induction chemotx between groups
		Betticher et al. (2006)	136 aaIPI low/int to high, 73% DLBCL	CHOP× 6–8 (control) versus 5 phase chemo (SHiDo) + HDT/auto-HCT	3-year EFS: 33% (control) versus 39% (HCT); P=0.67	3-year OS: 46% (control) versus 53% (HCT); P=0.48	-Pre-rituximab era -Trial closed early after interim analysis detected no difference between arms
		Stiff et al. (2013)	370 enrolled; 253 aaIPI high/int or high-risk randomized	(R)CHOP × 8 (control) versus (R)CHOP × 6 + HDT/auto-HCT	2-year PFS: 55% (control) versus 69% (HCT); P=0.005	2-year OS: 71% (control) versus 74% (HCT); P=0.30	-47% received R-CHOP -Significant PFS and OS benefit in high-risk patients treated with HCT
Relapsed/ refractory	RCT	Philip et al. (1995)	215 enrolled in 1st/ 2nd relapse; 109 chemosensitive randomized	DHAP × 2→ DHAP × 4 (control) versus BEAC/auto-HCT	5-year EFS: 12% (control) versus 46% (HCT); P=0.001	5-year OS: 32% (control) versus 53% (HCT); P=0.038	-Pre-rituximab era -Results only apply to chemosensitive patients; refractory patients were excluded from randomization

Table 43.1 (*cont.*)

Setting	Study design	Reference	n	Treatment	PFS/DFS/EFS	OS	Comments
		Gisselbrecht *et al.* (2010)	400 enrolled; 206 in PR/CR received HDT/auto-HCT	R-ICE × 3 + BEAM/auto-HCT *versus* R-DHAP × 3 + BEAM/auto-HCT	3-year EFS: 31% 3-year PFS: 37% 3-year PFS with HCT: 53%	3-year OS: 49%	-No differences seen between R-ICE and R-DHAP -Only chemosensitive patients underwent HCT -Prior rituximab, early relapse, aaIPI affected outcomes
		Vose *et al.* (2013)	224 in PR1 or PR2/CR2 after salvage	R-BEAM *versus* B-BEAM	2-year PFS 49% (R-BEAM) *versus* 48% (B-BEAM); *P*= 0.94	2-year OS: 66% (R-BEAM) *versus* 61% (B-BEAM); *P*= 0.38	-Improved outcomes in CR2 relative to PR1/PR2 -More mucositis with B-BEAM; otherwise no differences seen between arms
Single-arm Phase II		Armand *et al.* (2013)	72 without progression following auto-HCT	3 cycles of pidilizumab maintenance post-auto-HCT	16-month PFS: 72%	16-month OS: 85%	-Responses seen in post-auto-HCT PET-positive patients (CR 34%, ORR 51%) -No autoimmune toxicity or TRM

Abbreviations: PR, partial response; CR, complete response; RCT, randomized controlled trial; aaIPI, age-adjusted International Prognostic Index; PFS, progression-free survival; DFS, disease-free survival; EFS, event-free survival; OS, overall survival; CBV, cyclophosphamide, carmustine, etoposide; DLBCL, diffuse large B-cell lymphoma; HCT, hematopoietic stem cell transplant; ACVBP, doxorubicin, cyclophosphamide, vindesine, bleomycin, prednisone; R-CHOP, rituximab, cyclophosphamide, doxorubicin, vincristine, prednisone; CHOEP, cyclophosphamide, doxorubicin, vincristine, etoposide, prednisone; BEAM, carmustine, etoposide, cytarabine, melphalan; IFRT, involved-field radiation therapy; MACOP-B, methotrexate, doxorubicin, cyclophosphamide, vincristine, prednisone, bleomycin; BEAC, carmustine, etoposide, cytarabine, cyclophosphamide; CEEP+MC, cyclophosphamide, epirubicin, vindesine, prednisolone, methotrexate, cytarabine; CEOP, cyclophosphamide, etoposide, vincristine, prednisone; SHiDo, sequential high dose chemotherapy ; DHAP, dexamethasone, high-dose cytarabine, cisplatin; RICE, rituximab, ifosfamide, carboplatin, etoposide; B-BEAM, bexxar, carmustine, etoposide, cytarabine, melphalan.

hematologic toxicity and greater renal toxicity. Importantly, and similarly to the Parma trial, only half of the enrolled population achieved a response to salvage treatment and were able to undergo auto-HCT; these patients had a 3-year PFS of 53% (by intention-to-treat), with no survival differences between the R-ICE and R-DHAP arms.

Although not powered for subset analysis, the CORAL investigators had stratified all initially enrolled patients by type of frontline therapy (R-CHOP *versus* CHOP) and time to relapse after frontline therapy (less than *versus* greater than 12 months), both of which emerged as significant prognostic factors. Patients who both relapsed within 12 months *and* had received rituximab in the frontline setting had the worst outcome, with only 50% response rates to salvage therapy and 3-year PFS of 23%. Those responding to salvage and able to undergo auto-HCT (n=68) had a better 3-year PFS of 39% relative to patients who did not receive transplantation (n= 119) where 3-year PFS was only 14%. Since rituximab-containing treatment is now the standard of care for frontline

DLBCL, many have interpreted these results as negative for patients with early relapse following R-CHOP-like regimens.

Two other prospective trials have compared chemoimmunotherapy salvage regimens with auto-HCT consolidation in relapsed DLBCL. The NCIC Clinical Trials Group LY.12 study randomized 619 patients to either R-GDP (gemcitabine, dexamethasone, cisplatin) or R-DHAP[5]. Similar to the CORAL findings, response rates and clinical outcomes did not differ based on salvage regimen. R-GDP was administered outpatient and had fewer grade 3 and 4 adverse events and better quality of life parameters. Regardless of salvage regimen, 4-year EFS and OS were 26% and 39%, respectively; outcomes for patients undergoing auto-HCT were slightly better with approximate 40% long-term EFS. Importantly, 70% of patients in the NCIC-CTG LY.12 trial had either primary refractory disease or had relapsed within 12 months of initial diagnosis. A second trial comparing salvage regimens was based on the premise that novel anti-CD20 antibodies may be superior to rituximab in relapsed patients. This study, recently presented in preliminary form, randomized patients to either R-DHAP or ofatumumab-DHAP prior to auto-HCT. There were no differences by salvage regimen, and long-term PFS was only 26% for all patients[6].

An emerging theme in these trials is that time to relapse after initial treatment may be an important prognostic factor; however, none of these trials were powered to specifically address this issue. The CIBMTR performed a large analysis to evaluate auto-HCT in DLBCL patients with early versus late relapse[7]. There was no significant difference in 3-year PFS between patients undergoing HCT with early relapse (relapse within 12 months of diagnosis) versus late relapse (44% versus 52%, $P=0.10$) as long as chemosensitivity could be demonstrated. Further, patients with primary refractory disease (primary induction failure) were often effectively salvaged with auto-HCT, with comparable PFS and OS to the early relapse cohort. This analysis highlights the ongoing utility of auto-HCT in relapsed DLBCL independent of time to relapse, although there is a selection bias since patients with chemorefractory disease and thus unable to undergo auto-HCT are not included. The outcomes of these patients are dismal; the British Colombia Cancer Agency found that the median survival for relapsed DLBCL patients unable to undergo transplant was only 4 months[8]. While not direct comparisons, it is clear that transplant has yet to be routinely replaced by another approach.

Controversy #1: Does Salvage Autologous Hematopoietic Cell Transplantation Retain a Role in Relapsed DLBCL in the Current Era?

As frontline treatment has evolved and improved, the management of relapsed DLBCL has become more challenging, with several lines of evidence that salvage auto-HCT may be less beneficial. In particular, the publication of the CORAL results showing very poor outcomes for early relapse after rituximab-based induction chemoimmunotherapy were sobering and challenged the role of auto-HCT. The aforementioned studies suggest that patients with relapsed DLBCL after chemoimmunotherapy may have a worse biology undermining the ability of high-dose chemotherapy to overcome drug resistance. However, it is also clear that chemosensitivity to second-line regimens is the most important predictor of outcome after auto-HCT, perhaps independent of time to relapse. The above-mentioned CIBMTR analysis reported that the early rituximab failure (ERF) cohort had a higher risk of treatment failure (progression/relapse or death) (RR 2.08; $P < 0.001$) and overall mortality (RR 3.75; $P < 0.001$) within the first 9 months after autologous HCT. However, for patients surviving beyond 9 months, there were no differences between early and late rituximab failures. In addition, the 3-year PFS of 44% far exceeds outcomes for patients not undergoing transplant[9]. In our practice, we routinely consider auto-HCT for relapsed and refractory DLBCL if chemosensitivity to second-line therapy is demonstrated.

Auto-HCT as First Remission Consolidation

Most reports of auto-HCT for DLBCL as first remission consolidation are from the pre-rituximab era. Several randomized phase 3 studies in the 1980s and 1990s did not show superiority of auto-HCT consolidation[10–13], but this was mainly because the margin of benefit for low-risk patients was negligible. However, a retrospective analysis focused solely on patients with high-intermediate or high-risk disease by aaIPI did find a significant advantage in favor of auto-HCT relative to chemotherapy (8-year DFS 55% versus 39%, $P=0.02$; 8-year OS 64% versus 49%, $P=0.04$)[14]. The benefit of consolidative auto-HCT for higher risk patients was subsequently supported in some studies[15,16], but not in others[17,18].

More recently, the US/Canadian intergroup trial S9704 readdressed the value of consolidative auto-HCT in high-risk aggressive lymphomas in rituximab-treated patients[19]. Two hundred and fifty-three patients with aaIPI high-intermediate or high-risk aggressive lymphoma in first PR/CR following CHOP or R-CHOP were randomized to receive additional cycles of induction chemotherapy (control group) or high-dose therapy and auto-HCT (transplantation group). Two-year PFS favored transplantation (69%) relative to the control group (55%) (hazard ratio (HR) in control group 1.72; 95% CI 1.18–2.51). Two-year OS did not significantly differ between the study groups (74% versus 71%, HR 1.26; 95% CI 0.82–1.94), possibly because a large proportion (47%) of those who relapsed or progressed in the control group subsequently underwent auto-HCT. Interestingly, exploratory analyses demonstrated a significant interaction between treatment and aaIPI risk group (high-intermediate versus high-risk) for both PFS and OS, suggesting that auto-HCT may preferentially benefit those with high-risk disease.

The most recent update to the American Society for Blood and Marrow Transplantation (ASBMT) evidence-based review on the role of HCT in DLBCL published in 2011 recommended against the use of first-line auto-HCT for any IPI risk group[20]. In contrast, the 2014 NCCN (National Comprehensive Cancer Network) non-Hodgkin lymphoma panel lists consolidative auto-HCT as an option for high-risk patients. Whether early transplantation as part of frontline strategy should be offered to those with high-risk DLBCL, defined by high-risk clinical and/or biologic features, remains an unresolved question in the field.

Controversy #2: Should Auto-HCT Be Used to Consolidate First-Line Remission in DLBCL?

The intergroup study S9704 randomized patients with high-risk aggressive lymphomas, defined by the IPI, achieving either a CR or PR to CHOP (with or without rituximab) to consolidative auto-HCT versus completion of anthracycline-based therapy. High risk was defined as high-intermediate- or high-risk IPI and patients with both B- and T-cell histologies, including primary mediastinal B-cell lymphoma, were included. The benefit of consolidative auto-HCT was limited to the 88 patients with high-risk IPI, accounting for one-third of all initially enrolled patients. Although the benefit persisted in a subset analysis restricted to B-cell histologies, there are several caveats to the study that limit wide applicability, mainly related to the lack of biologic information and lack of PET scans for response assessment. In addition, the study was not powered to detect survival differences for this high-risk subset, and many questions remain about patient selection at an individual level. For these reasons, we do not routinely offer auto-HCT consolidation in DLBCL.

Improving Outcomes of Auto-HCT: Conditioning, Maintenance, Novel Agents, and Approaches

Owing to its favorable tolerability and efficacy, BEAM (carmustine, etoposide, cytarabine, melphalan) is the most commonly used auto-HCT conditioning regimen for DLBCL, while total body irradiation (TBI)-based regimens are used infrequently[21]. Attempts to improve upon outcomes with alternative chemotherapy regimens have resulted in similar efficacy with increased toxicity[22]. Radioimmunotherapy (RIT), which is generally well tolerated and results in bone marrow suppression, has been combined with BEAM in order to potentially improve disease control without compromising tolerability. A small randomized study evaluating standard dose yttrium-90-ibritumomab tiuxetan in combination with BEAM (Z-BEAM) versus BEAM alone found no significant difference in 2-year PFS between the arms (59% versus 37%, P=0.2), with a borderline 2-year OS advantage in favor of Z-BEAM (91% versus 62%, P=0.05)[23]. A larger, phase 3 randomized study conducted by the Blood and Marrow Transplant Clinical Trials Network evaluating standard dose iodine-131–tositumomab in combination with BEAM (B-BEAM) versus rituximab plus BEAM (R-BEAM) similarly showed no significant benefit in the RIT arm (2-year PFS 48.6% versus 47.9%, P=0.94; 2-year OS 65.6% versus 61%, P=0.38)[24]. Although dose escalation of RIT has been attempted[25], it is unclear whether this strategy would be tolerable or more efficacious than BEAM alone in a randomized study.

The use of maintenance therapy after auto-HCT remains investigational. The previously mentioned CORAL trial included a second randomization evaluating post-HCT maintenance rituximab delivered every 2 months for 1 year following HCT[26]. Maintenance offered no significant benefit over observation, and was associated with a 15% increase in reported serious adverse events, primarily infectious. Subgroup analysis demonstrated that relative to men, women receiving maintenance rituximab had improved survival. This may be secondary to higher rituximab clearance in men resulting in decreased exposure, and requires prospective confirmation.

Immune manipulation following auto-HCT has also been tested as a consolidation/maintenance strategy. In prospective, randomized studies, T-cell up-regulation by IL-2 at varying doses and in combination with γ-IFN and cyclosporine following auto-HCT was not associated with improved PFS or OS[27,28]. Most recently, enhancement of antitumor immunity through immune checkpoint blockade is being tested. A phase 2 study of antiprogrammed death-1 (PD-1) antibody, pidilizumab, following auto-HCT in relapsed and refractory DLBCL patients found an encouraging 18-month PFS of 69%, and this strategy is now being tested in a randomized trial[29].

Many agents, most of which are targeted and/or otherwise specifically active in B cell malignancies, are now being tested in all phases of the peritransplant period, including lenalidomide, bortezomib, and vorinostat. Newer agents targeting the B-cell receptor pathway, such as Bruton's tyrosine kinase (BTK) inhibitors and phosphoinositide 3-kinase (PI3K) inhibitors are being studied in relapsed DLBCL and will likely be evaluated as a bridge to HCT and/or as post-HCT consolidation/maintenance. Higher affinity anti-CD20 monoclonal antibodies such as obinotuzumab, and antibody–drug conjugates targeting B-cell antigens such as CD22 are being tested in a range of B-cell malignancies. Targeted cellular therapies such as chimeric antigen receptor T-cell (CAR T-cells) show great promise and may eventually displace HCT as a less toxic cellular therapeutic strategy.

Controversy #3: Should Maintenance Therapy Be Routinely Incorporated after Auto-HCT?

The CORAL study clearly established that routine post-auto-HCT rituximab offers no significant advantage in progression-free or overall survival. While the potential benefit in women is enticing, the study was not powered to test gender-based differences. In addition, increased post-auto-HCT toxicity in the form of cytopenias and infections must be considered. For these reasons, we do not use post-transplant maintenance after auto-HCT in relapsed aggressive lymphomas.

Allogeneic Hematopoietic Cell Transplantation for Diffuse Large B-Cell Lymphoma

Allo-HCT Following Failed Auto-HCT

Relative to auto-HCT, allo-HCT theoretically offers improved disease control as a result of graft-versus-lymphoma (GvL) effects, at the expense of greater toxicity and nonrelapse mortality (NRM). Although the GvL effect in DLBCL has been debated, disease response to withdrawal of post-transplant immunosuppression and to donor lymphocyte infusion (DLI) support a GvL effect in DLBCL, albeit likely less robust than in indolent NHL[30,31].

In clinical practice, allo-HCT for DLBCL is most frequently reserved as third-line therapy in the setting of relapse after auto-HCT. The Italian GITMO group and the European Group for Blood and Marrow Transplantation (EBMT) separately evaluated outcomes of DLBCL patients allografted following failed auto-HCT. In the GITMO analysis, only 19% of 884 relapsing or progressing after auto-HCT actually received an allo-HCT[32]. With 2-year median follow-up, nonrelapse mortality (NRM), PFS, and OS for those undergoing allo-HCT were 28%, 32%, and 39%, respectively, with disease response prior to allo-HCT significantly associated with PFS and OS in multivariate analyses. The EBMT registry study evaluated outcomes in 101 DLBCL patients receiving allo-HCT after auto-HCT relapse, and found 3-year NRM, PFS, and OS to be 28.2% (95% CI 20–39%), 41.7% (95% CI 32–52%), and 53.8% (95% CI 4464%), respectively[33]. In multivariate analysis, relapse within 1 year of auto-HCT was significantly associated with both increased NRM and reduced PFS. The CIBMTR evaluated the efficacy and toxicity of both myeloablative and reduced intensity allo-HCT after prior failed auto-HCT, and unfortunately found that the NRM remained high irrespective of regimen intensity; however, higher Karnofsky performance score, longer time between the auto-HCT and allo-HCT, TBI-based preparative regimen, and disease status at transplantation impacted outcomes, and approximately 20% of patients had long-term survival[34,35]. Taken together, allo-HCT after failed auto-HCT will be successful in approximately one-third of patients able to undergo transplant with varying outcomes depending on remission duration following auto-HCT and chemosensitivity prior to allo-HCT.

Allo-HCT for High-Risk and/or Refractory DLBCL

The poor results with auto-HCT for high-risk populations (e.g., patients with early relapse after R-CHOP, high aaIPI, poor-risk biologic features, primary refractory disease) may prompt consideration of allo-HCT earlier in the disease course for certain DLBCL patients. While there are no prospective comparative data, retrospective comparisons of auto-HCT *versus* allo-HCT as salvage for relapsed DLBCL have found either similar overall outcomes, or favor auto-HCT due to increased NRM from allo-HCT[36,37]. These studies are substantially limited by uncontrolled differences in patient populations due to selection bias: usually the inclusion of more chemorefractory disease, more lines of treatment, and more high-risk features in the allo-HCT cohorts.

Recently, the German group reported outcomes of a prospective study of allo-HCT for relapsed/refractory aggressive lymphoma[38]. The majority of the 84 patients enrolled had refractory lymphoma. Patients received a transplant conditioning regimen of fludarabine, busulfan, and cyclophosphamide, and were randomized to receive post-transplant rituximab *versus* observation. Post-transplant rituximab did not influence outcomes or rates of graft-*versus*-host disease (GvHD). Regardless, transplant outcomes were impressive, with 1-year PFS and OS of 45% and 52%, respectively, with a median follow-up of 4 years. Further, although high-risk patients (defined by early relapse or primary refractory disease) fared worse, 1-year OS was still over 30–40% for these high-risk

populations. Given the otherwise dismal outcomes of refractory DLBCL, early HLA typing should be considered for patients considered to be at high risk for failure with conventional salvage therapy.

Role of Conditioning Regimen Intensity

The largest study to compare allo-HCT outcomes for DLBCL following differing conditioning regimen intensity was recently published[39]. In this Center for International Blood and Marrow Transplant Research (CIBMTR) analysis of 396 recipients of allo-HCT for DLBCL between 2000 and 2009, 5-year NRM was higher with myeloablative (MAC) than reduced intensity (RIC) and nonmyeloablative (NMAC) conditioning regimens (56% *versus* 47% *versus* 36%; $P=0.007$). Five-year relapse/progression was lower in MAC regimen than in RIC/NMAC (26% *versus* 38% *versus* 40%; $P=0.031$); 5-year PFS (15–25%) and OS (18–26%) did not significantly differ between conditioning regimen cohorts. As expected, relative to the NMAC/RIC cohorts, recipients of MAC regimen tended to be younger, have more resistant disease, and were less likely to have had a prior auto-HCT. Although there is clearly room for improvement, these results confirm the curative potential of allo-HCT in advanced DLBCL. Additionally, for younger patients with aggressive disease, MAC regimens appear to result in greater disease control. Conversely, for less fit patients, or perhaps those with less-advanced disease, RIC/NRM regimens are associated with lower NRM and may lead to long-term lymphoma-free survival.

Controversy #4: When Should Allo-HCT Be Used in Relapsed Aggressive Lymphomas?

The true impact of allo-HCT in DLBCL is difficult to evaluate, mainly because the vast majority of patients have either refractory disease, relapsed after prior auto-HCT, or are otherwise higher risk as compared to patients routinely undergoing auto-HCT. As elegantly discussed in detail elsewhere[40] we acknowledge that allo-HCT applies to a minority of patients with DLBCL and is associated with high nonrelapse mortality. Nevertheless, relapse is consistently lower with allo-HCT as compared to reported outcomes with auto-HCT and the evidence of a graft-*versus*-lymphoma (GvL) effect is encouraging. In addition, approximately one-third of patients have long-term disease control despite the numerous adverse features described in detail above. For these reasons, we consider allo-HCT for selected individuals with appropriate stem cell donors and very high-risk disease, and for patients with chemosensitive disease after a failed auto-HCT. In addition, as our ability to risk-stratify DLBCL into biologic subsets is refined, there may be patients less likely to benefit from auto-HCT and more likely to require a potent GvL effect for optimal disease control. Allo-HCT remains an important tool for relapsed and refractory DLBCL, and we anticipate that improvements in risk stratification will better identify patients most likely to benefit.

Transplantation for Aggressive B-Cell NHL: Special Patient Populations

Burkitt Lymphoma

Burkitt lymphoma (BL) is an uncommon, highly aggressive B-cell NHL, characterized by *MYC* gene translocations and a propensity for extranodal involvement. BL is more common in children, presents at a median age of 45 years in adults, and is less common in the elderly. BL may be differentiated from the subset of DLBCL with *MYC* rearrangement by pathologic and cytogenetic evaluation. The entity "B-cell lymphoma, unclassifiable, with features intermediate between DLBCL and BL (BCLU)" has replaced the older term "atypical BL," and describes cases without typical morphologic or immunophenotypic features of BL. BCLU and DLBCL harboring translocations in both *MYC* and *BCL2* (and/or *BCL6*) are addressed below.

The contemporary treatment of BL with short, dose-intensive multiagent rituximab-containing chemotherapy regimens and aggressive CNS prophylaxis results in CR and OS rates of 80–90% in adults[41,42]. Limited studies have evaluated the role of high-dose chemotherapy/auto-HCT consolidation in BL, and many were performed prior to the routine separation of BCLU. In a small prospective study conducted by the Dutch–Belgian Hematolo-Oncology Cooperative Group (HOVON), patients with BL or Burkitt-like lymphoma (n=27) received two cycles of intensive induction followed by consolidation with BEAM and auto-HCT[43]. CR and 5-year OS were both 81%. The outcome of consolidative transplantation for BL was also addressed in a recent CIBMTR registry study[44]. This study represents the largest report of transplantation in BL, describing all transplant outcomes reported to the CIBMTR between 1985 and 2007. Patients in CR1 undergoing consolidative auto-HCT (n=48) or allo-HCT (n=30) had a 5-year OS of 83% and 53%, respectively. The authors conclude that given these data, auto-HCT in CR1 does not appear to be inferior, but is unlikely to offer an additional advantage over current dose-intense chemotherapy regimens. Allo-HCT in CR1 resulted in high NRM (23%) and inferior OS, and is not recommended.

Relapsed or refractory BL patients are often considered for salvage HCT. The CIBMTR BL transplant analysis included 57 and 80 relapsed/refractory patients undergoing auto-HCT or allo-HCT, respectively[44]. Those receiving allo-HCT tended to be younger, but were more heavily pretreated and more likely to have chemoresistant disease. Survival rates with auto-HCT and allo-HCT were comparable (5-year OS 31% *versus* 20%), again with the caveat that important biases make a true comparison impossible. Five-year NRM was higher and relapse was slightly lower following allo-HCT relative to auto-HCT (5-year NRM allo-HCT *versus* auto-HCT: 30% *versus*

12%; relapse allo-HCT *versus* auto-HCT: 51% *versus* 61%). Relapsed or primary refractory patients not in CR at the time of transplant fared the worst, with long-term survival rates of 22% and 12% with auto-HCT and allo-HCT, respectively. Thus, while HCT may have a role in relapsed/refractory BL, long-term results are suboptimal.

"Double-Hit" B-Cell Lymphoma

There is increasing recognition that a subset of aggressive B-cell lymphoma patients harboring genetic translocations in *MYC* and *BCL2* and/or *BCL6* (or MYC and BCL2 and/or BCL6 protein overexpression) have poor outcomes following conventional R-CHOP therapy. A proportion of these patients have pathologic features consistent with typical DLBCL; the remainder fit the WHO criteria for BCLU. When both *MYC* and *BCL2* (or *BCL6*) are rearranged, these malignancies are commonly referred to as "double-hit" lymphoma (DHL), and are characterized by an aggressive disease course.

The optimal initial therapy for DHL is not currently known; however, outcomes with R-CHOP are insufficient. For example, in a large series of DLBCL patients treated with R-CHOP in British Columbia, 5-year PFS and OS for DHL patients were significantly inferior relative to those without double-hit features (18% and 27% for DHL *versus* 65% and 71% for non-DHL)[45]. More recently, several retrospective reports suggest a superior outcome with DA-R-EPOCH and other augmented regimens[46–48]. The role of consolidative transplant is controversial, with some of these previously referenced reports suggesting a benefit and others showing no impact on outcome as long as a complete remission to induction chemotherapy was attained. The largest, and only multicenter, series evaluated outcome by initial regimen and response to treatment for 311 patients with DHL; notably, roughly half of these patients had DLBCL and half had BCLU[48]. The authors report significant improvement in PFS with augmented initial regimens (including DA-EPOCH-R, R-hyperCVAD, and others) as compared to R-CHOP. One of the most important predictors of outcome was complete response to treatment, and neither consolidative auto-HCT nor allo-HCT further improved outcome in this series. A smaller, single-institution series similarly found that HCT consolidation for patients achieving CR to initial treatment did not further improve outcomes[49].

In contrast to non-DHL, relapsed DHL is not effectively salvaged with R-chemotherapy and auto-HCT. The CORAL investigators retrospectively evaluated outcomes for *MYC*+ patients (mostly double hit) enrolled on the CORAL study who received either R-ICE or R-DHAP and BEAM auto-HCT[50]. Relative to *MYC*− patients, 4-year PFS and OS were significantly lower in *MYC*+ patients (4-year PFS, 18% *versus* 42%, P=0.0322; 4-year OS 29% *versus* 62%, P=0.0113). Salvage regimen (R-ICE *versus* R-DHAP) did not significantly impact outcomes for *MYC*+ patients. Collectively, these reports confirm the negative prognostic impact of DHL, and support the prioritization of future study for this high-risk biologic subtype in both frontline and relapsed/refractory settings.

DLBCL Transformed from Follicular Lymphoma

Histologic transformation of follicular lymphoma to DLBCL occurs at a rate of 3% per year after initial diagnosis, and is typically associated with a poor outcome[51]. Although there is no standard of care for DLBCL arising from follicular lymphoma, most patients will receive a conventional rituximab-containing chemotherapy regimen, and some will undergo consolidative auto-HCT or allo-HCT. The role of consolidative transplantation for transformed follicular lymphoma in the rituximab era was the focus of a recent retrospective report by the Canadian Blood and Marrow Transplant Group[52]. Although 5-year survival rates were not significantly different across groups (46% allo-HCT *versus* 55% auto-HCT *versus* 40% R-chemo, $P = 0.12$), multivariate analysis showed a significant OS advantage favoring auto-HCT consolidation (HR 0.13; 95% CI 0.05–0.34; $P < 0.001$). A report from the CIBMTR evaluating transplant outcomes for DLBCL transformed from follicular lymphoma found a trend towards increasing use of allo-HCT in this population, but more favorable outcomes in those receiving auto-HCT as compared to allo-HCT (5-year PFS and OS for auto-HCT and allo-HCT 35% and 50% *versus* 18% and 22%, respectively)[53] with the worse outcomes for allo-HCT attributed to the unusually high 1-year NRM of 41% in this cohort. Although some caution is required in interpreting retrospective analyses, the data continue to support the consideration of auto-HCT for most patients.

Summary: Controversies in Transplantation for Aggressive B-Cell NHL

There are a number of unresolved issues that complicate the use of HCT in aggressive B-cell lymphomas. First, DLBCL is increasingly understood to harbor molecular heterogeneity which directly impacts prognosis. This includes not only the dichotomy of DLBCL into germinal center and nongerminal center subtypes, but also the growing appreciation of dual *MYC* and *BCL2* translocations in unselected DLBCL, the mutational landscape of DLBCL, and the possibility that dual MYC and BCL2 protein overexpression represents unique biologic entities independent of the genetic rearrangements. Given these sources of heterogeneity, interpretation of the literature is difficult and likely heavily influenced by the subsets. Second, very few of the studies included functional imaging such as PET, which offers a more sensitive means of establishing response. This is likely very important when evaluating the impact of transplant on patients in CR *versus* PR, for example. Finally, improved histologic assessment and identification of BCLU *versus* DLBCL *versus* BL (for example) is still being refined and probably affects interpretation of the earlier studies that included a mixture of aggressive histologies.

Nevertheless, both auto-HCT and allo-HCT retain important roles in the overall management of patients with aggressive lymphomas. We consider auto-HCT to be the standard of care for chemosensitive, relapsed aggressive lymphomas. Patients with chemoresistance, high-risk biologic features, and requiring multiple lines of therapy to enter remission should be considered for allo-HCT. New immune approaches promise to impact the role and utility of HCT in lymphomas, and may either enhance or supplant transplant.

References

1. Sehn LH, Berry B, Chhanabhai M, Fitzgerald C, Gill K, Hoskins P, et al. The revised International Prognostic Index (R-IPI) is a better predictor of outcome than the standard IPI for patients with diffuse large B-cell lymphoma treated with R-CHOP. *Blood*. 2007;109(5):1857–61.

2. Philip T, Guglielmi C, Hagenbeek A, Somers R, Van der Lelie H, Bron D, et al. Autologous bone marrow transplantation as compared with salvage chemotherapy in relapses of chemotherapy-sensitive non-Hodgkin's lymphoma. *The New England Journal of Medicine*. 1995;333(23):1540–5.

3. Gisselbrecht C, Glass B, Mounier N, Singh Gill D, Linch DC, Trneny M, et al. Salvage regimens with autologous transplantation for relapsed large B-cell lymphoma in the rituximab era. *Journal of Clinical Oncology: Official Journal of the American Society of Clinical Oncology*. 2010;28(27):4184–90.

4. Gisselbrecht C, Schmitz N, Mounier N, Ma D, Trneny M, Hagberg H, et al. R-ICE *versus* R-DHAP in relapsed patients with CD20 diffuse large B-cell lymphoma (DLBCL) followed by stem cell transplantation and maintenance treatment with rituximab or not: first interim analysis on 200 patients. CORAL Study. *Blood*. 2007;110(Abstract 517).

5. Crump M, Kuruvilla J, Couban S, MacDonald DA, Kukreti V, Kouroukis CT, et al. Randomized comparison of gemcitabine, dexamethasone, and cisplatin *versus* dexamethasone, cytarabine, and cisplatin chemotherapy before autologous stem-cell transplantation for relapsed and refractory aggressive lymphomas: NCIC-CTG LY.12. *Journal of Clinical Oncology: Official Journal of the American Society of Clinical Oncology*. 2014;32(31):3490–6.

6. Van Imhoff GW, McMillan A, Matasar MJ, Radford J, Ardeshna KM, Kuliczkowski L, et al. Ofatumumab *Versus* Rituximab Salvage Chemoimmunotherapy in Relapsed or Refractory Diffuse Large B-Cell Lymphoma: The Orcharrd Study (OMB110928) *Blood*. 2014;124(630 abstract).

7. Hamadani M, Hari PN, Zhang Y, Carreras J, Akpek G, Aljurf MD, et al. Early failure of frontline rituximab-containing chemo-immunotherapy in diffuse large B cell lymphoma does not predict futility of autologous hematopoietic cell transplantation. *Biology of Blood and Marrow Transplantation: Journal of the American Society for Blood and Marrow Transplantation*. 2014;20(11):1729–36.

8. Kansara RR, Savage KJ, Villa D, Shenkier T, Gerrie AS, Klasa R, et al. Outcome in unselected patients with relapsed/refractory diffuse large B-cell lymphoma (DLBCL) following R-CHOP when stem cell transplantation is not feasible. *Blood*. 2014;124(Abstract 3069).

9. Colosia A, Njue A, Trask PC, Olivares R, Khan S, Abbe A, et al. Clinical efficacy and safety in relapsed/refractory diffuse large b-cell lymphoma: a systematic literature review. *Clinical Lymphoma, Myeloma & Leukemia*. 2014;14(5):343–55 e6.

10. Gisselbrecht C, Lepage E, Molina T, Quesnel B, Fillet G, Lederlin P, et al. Shortened first-line high-dose chemotherapy for patients with poor-prognosis aggressive lymphoma. *Journal of Clinical Oncology: Official Journal of the American Society of Clinical Oncology*. 2002;20(10):2472–9.

11. Kaiser U, Uebelacker I, Abel U, Birkmann J, Trumper L, Schmalenberg H, et al. Randomized study to evaluate the use of high-dose therapy as part of primary treatment for "aggressive" lymphoma. *Journal of Clinical Oncology: Official Journal of the American Society of Clinical Oncology*. 2002;20(22):4413–9.

12. Martelli M, Gherlinzoni F, De Renzo A, Zinzani PL, De Vivo A, Cantonetti M, et al. Early autologous stem-cell transplantation *versus* conventional chemotherapy as front-line therapy in high-risk, aggressive non-Hodgkin's lymphoma: an Italian multicenter randomized trial. *Journal of Clinical Oncology: Official Journal of the American Society of Clinical Oncology*. 2003;21(7):1255–62.

13. Haioun C, Lepage E, Gisselbrecht C, Bastion Y, Coiffier B, Brice P, et al. Benefit of autologous bone marrow transplantation over sequential chemotherapy in poor-risk aggressive non-Hodgkin's lymphoma: updated results of the prospective study LNH87-2. Groupe d'Etude des Lymphomes de l'Adulte. *Journal of Clinical Oncology: Official Journal of the American Society of Clinical Oncology*. 1997;15(3):1131–7.

14. Haioun C, Lepage E, Gisselbrecht C, Salles G, Coiffier B, Brice P, et al. Survival benefit of high-dose therapy in poor-risk aggressive non-Hodgkin's lymphoma: final analysis of the prospective LNH87-2 protocol–a groupe d'Etude des lymphomes de l'Adulte study. *Journal of Clinical Oncology: Official Journal of the American Society of Clinical Oncology*. 2000;18(16):3025–30.

15. Milpied N, Deconinck E, Gaillard F, Delwail V, Foussard C, Berthou C, et al. Initial treatment of aggressive lymphoma with high-dose chemotherapy and autologous stem-cell support. *The New England Journal of Medicine*. 2004;350(13):1287–95.

16. Greb A, Bohlius J, Trelle S, Schiefer D, De Souza CA, Gisselbrecht C, et al. High-dose chemotherapy with autologous stem cell support in first-line treatment of aggressive non-Hodgkin lymphoma - results of a comprehensive meta-analysis. *Cancer Treatment Reviews*. 2007;33(4):338–46.

17. Vitolo U, Liberati AM, Cabras MG, Federico M, Angelucci E, Baldini L, et al. High dose sequential chemotherapy with autologous transplantation *versus* dose-dense chemotherapy MegaCEOP as first line treatment in poor-prognosis diffuse large cell lymphoma: an "Intergruppo Italiano Linfomi" randomized trial. *Haematologica*. 2005;90(6):793–801.

18. Betticher DC, Martinelli G, Radford JA, Kaufmann M, Dyer MJ, Kaiser U, et al. Sequential high dose chemotherapy as initial treatment for aggressive sub-types of non-Hodgkin lymphoma: results of the international randomized phase III trial (MISTRAL). *Annals of Oncology: Official Journal of the European Society for Medical Oncology/ ESMO*. 2006;17(10):1546–52.

19. Stiff PJ, Unger JM, Cook JR, Constine LS, Couban S, Stewart DA, et al. Autologous transplantation as consolidation for aggressive non-Hodgkin's lymphoma. *The New England Journal of Medicine*. 2013;369(18):1681–90.

20. Oliansky DM, Czuczman M, Fisher RI, Irwin FD, Lazarus HM, Omel J, et al. The role of cytotoxic therapy with hematopoietic stem cell transplantation in the treatment of diffuse large B cell lymphoma: update of the 2001 evidence-based review. *Biology of Blood and Marrow Transplantation: Journal of the American Society for Blood and Marrow Transplantation*. 2011;17(1):20–47 e30.

21. McCarthy PL, Jr., Hahn T, Hassebroek A, Bredeson C, Gajewski J, Hale G, et al. Trends in use of and survival after autologous hematopoietic cell transplantation in North America, 1995–2005: significant improvement in survival for lymphoma and myeloma during a period of increasing recipient age. *Biology of Blood and Marrow Transplantation: Journal of the American Society for Blood and Marrow Transplantation*. 2013;19(7):1116–23.

22. Kim JE, Lee DH, Yoo C, Kim S, Kim SW, Lee JS, et al. BEAM or BuCyE high-dose chemotherapy followed by autologous stem cell transplantation in non-Hodgkin's lymphoma patients: a single center comparative analysis of efficacy and toxicity. *Leukemia Research*. 2011;35(2):183–7.

23. Shimoni A, Avivi I, Rowe JM, Yeshurun M, Levi I, Or R, et al. A randomized study comparing yttrium-90 ibritumomab tiuxetan (Zevalin) and high-dose BEAM chemotherapy *versus* BEAM alone as the conditioning regimen before autologous stem cell transplantation in patients with aggressive lymphoma. *Cancer*. 2012;118(19):4706–14.

24. Vose JM, Carter S, Burns LJ, Ayala E, Press OW, Moskowitz CH, et al. Phase III randomized study of rituximab/ carmustine, etoposide, cytarabine, and melphalan (BEAM) compared with iodine-131 tositumomab/BEAM with autologous hematopoietic cell transplantation for relapsed diffuse large B-cell lymphoma: results from the BMT CTN 0401 trial. *Journal of Clinical Oncology: Official Journal of the American Society of Clinical Oncology*. 2013;31(13):1662–8.

25. Winter JN, Inwards DJ, Spies S, Wiseman G, Patton D, Erwin W, et al. Yttrium-90 ibritumomab tiuxetan doses calculated to deliver up to 15 Gy to critical organs may be safely combined with high-dose BEAM and autologous transplantation in relapsed or refractory B-cell non-Hodgkin's lymphoma. *Journal of Clinical Oncology: Official Journal of the American Society of Clinical Oncology*. 2009;27(10):1653–9.

26. Gisselbrecht C, Schmitz N, Mounier N, Singh Gill D, Linch DC, Trneny M, et al. Rituximab maintenance therapy after autologous stem-cell transplantation in patients with relapsed CD20(+) diffuse large B-cell lymphoma: final analysis of the collaborative trial in relapsed aggressive lymphoma. *Journal of Clinical*

Oncology: *Official Journal of the American Society of Clinical Oncology.* 2012;30(36):4462–9.

27. Bolanos-Meade J, Garrett-Mayer E, Luznik L, Anders V, Webb J, Fuchs EJ, *et al.* Induction of autologous graft-*versus*-host disease: results of a randomized prospective clinical trial in patients with poor risk lymphoma. *Biology of Blood and Marrow Transplantation: Journal of the American Society for Blood and Marrow Transplantation.* 2007;13(10):1185–91.

28. Thompson JA, Fisher RI, Leblanc M, Forman SJ, Press OW, Unger JM, *et al.* Total body irradiation, etoposide, cyclophosphamide, and autologous peripheral blood stem-cell transplantation followed by randomization to therapy with interleukin-2 *versus* observation for patients with non-Hodgkin lymphoma: results of a phase 3 randomized trial by the Southwest Oncology Group (SWOG 9438). *Blood.* 2008;111(8):4048–54.

29. Armand P, Nagler A, Weller EA, Devine SM, Avigan DE, Chen YB, *et al.* Disabling immune tolerance by programmed death-1 blockade with pidilizumab after autologous hematopoietic stem-cell transplantation for diffuse large B-cell lymphoma: results of an international phase II trial. *Journal of Clinical Oncology: Official Journal of the American Society of Clinical Oncology.* 2013;31(33):4199–206.

30. van Besien KW, de Lima M, Giralt SA, Moore DF, Jr., Khouri IF, Rondon G, *et al.* Management of lymphoma recurrence after allogeneic transplantation: the relevance of graft-*versus*-lymphoma effect. *Bone Marrow Transplantation.* 1997;19(10):977–82.

31. Bishop MR, Dean RM, Steinberg SM, Odom J, Pavletic SZ, Chow C, *et al.* Clinical evidence of a graft-*versus*-lymphoma effect against relapsed diffuse large B-cell lymphoma after allogeneic hematopoietic stem-cell transplantation. *Annals of Oncology: Official Journal of the European Society for Medical Oncology/ESMO.* 2008;19(11):1935–40.

32. Rigacci L, Puccini B, Dodero A, Iacopino P, Castagna L, Bramanti S, *et al.* Allogeneic hematopoietic stem cell transplantation in patients with diffuse large B cell lymphoma relapsed after autologous stem cell transplantation: a GITMO study. *Annals of Hematology.* 2012;91(6):931–9.

33. van Kampen RJ, Canals C, Schouten HC, Nagler A, Thomson KJ, Vernant JP, *et al.* Allogeneic stem-cell transplantation as salvage therapy for patients with diffuse large B-cell non-Hodgkin's lymphoma relapsing after an autologous stem-cell transplantation: an analysis of the European Group for Blood and Marrow Transplantation Registry. *Journal of Clinical Oncology: Official Journal of the American Society of Clinical Oncology.* 2011;29(10):1342–8.

34. Freytes CO, Loberiza FR, Rizzo JD, Bashey A, Bredeson CN, Cairo MS, *et al.* Myeloablative allogeneic hematopoietic stem cell transplantation in patients who experience relapse after autologous stem cell transplantation for lymphoma: a report of the International Bone Marrow Transplant Registry. *Blood.* 2004;104(12):3797–803.

35. Freytes CO, Zhang MJ, Carreras J, Burns LJ, Gale RP, Isola L, *et al.* Outcome of lower-intensity allogeneic transplantation in non-Hodgkin lymphoma after autologous transplantation failure. *Biology of Blood and Marrow Transplantation: Journal of the American Society for Blood and Marrow Transplantation.* 2012;18(8):1255–64.

36. Peniket AJ, Ruiz de Elvira MC, Taghipour G, Cordonnier C, Gluckman E, de Witte T, *et al.* An EBMT registry matched study of allogeneic stem cell transplants for lymphoma: allogeneic transplantation is associated with a lower relapse rate but a higher procedure-related mortality rate than autologous transplantation. *Bone Marrow Transplantation.* 2003;31(8):667–78.

37. Lazarus HM, Zhang MJ, Carreras J, Hayes-Lattin BM, Ataergin AS, Bitran JD, *et al.* A comparison of HLA-identical sibling allogeneic *versus* autologous transplantation for diffuse large B cell lymphoma: a report from the CIBMTR. *Biology of Blood and Marrow Transplantation: Journal of the American Society for Blood and Marrow Transplantation.* 2010;16(1):35–45.

38. Glass B, Hasenkamp J, Wulf G, Dreger P, Pfreundschuh M, Gramatzki M, *et al.* Rituximab after lymphoma-directed conditioning and allogeneic stem-cell transplantation for relapsed and refractory aggressive non-Hodgkin lymphoma (DSHNHL R3): an open-label, randomised, phase 2 trial. *The Lancet Oncology.* 2014;15(7):757–66.

39. Bacher U, Klyuchnikov E, Le-Rademacher J, Carreras J, Armand P, Bishop MR, *et al.* Conditioning regimens for allotransplants for diffuse large B-cell lymphoma: myeloablative or reduced intensity? *Blood.* 2012;120(20):4256–62.

40. Klyuchnikov E, Bacher U, Kroll T, Shea TC, Lazarus HM, Bredeson C, *et al.* Allogeneic hematopoietic cell transplantation for diffuse large B cell lymphoma: who, when and how? *Bone Marrow Transplantation.* 2014;49(1):1–7.

41. Rizzieri DA, Johnson JL, Byrd JC, Lozanski G, Blum KA, Powell BL, *et al.* Improved efficacy using rituximab and brief duration, high intensity chemotherapy with filgrastim support for Burkitt or aggressive lymphomas: cancer and Leukemia Group B study 10 002. *British Journal of Haematology.* 2014;165(1):102–11.

42. Hoelzer D, Walewski J, Dohner H, Schmid M, Hiddemann W, Baumann A, *et al.* Substantially improved outcome of adult Burkitt non-Hodgkin lymphoma and leukemia patients with rituximab and a short-intensive chemotherapy; report of a large prospective multicenter trial. *ASH Annual Meeting Abstracts.* 2012;120(21):667.

43. van Imhoff GW, van der Holt B, MacKenzie MA, Ossenkoppele GJ, Wijermans PW, Kramer MH, *et al.* Short intensive sequential therapy followed by autologous stem cell transplantation in adult Burkitt, Burkitt-like and lymphoblastic lymphoma. *Leukemia.* 2005;19(6):945–52.

44. Maramattom LV, Hari PN, Burns LJ, Carreras J, Arcese W, Cairo MS, *et al.* Autologous and allogeneic transplantation for burkitt lymphoma outcomes and changes in utilization: a report from the center for international blood and marrow transplant research. *Biology of Blood and Marrow Transplantation: Journal of the American Society for Blood and Marrow Transplantation.* 2013;19(2):173–9.

45. Johnson NA, Slack GW, Savage KJ, Connors JM, Ben-Neriah S, Rogic S,

et al. Concurrent expression of MYC and BCL2 in diffuse large B-cell lymphoma treated with rituximab plus cyclophosphamide, doxorubicin, vincristine, and prednisone. *Journal of Clinical Oncology: Official Journal of the American Society of Clinical Oncology.* 2012;30(28):3452–9.

46. Oki Y, Noorani M, Lin P, Davis RE, Neelapu SS, Ma L, *et al.* Double hit lymphoma: the MD Anderson Cancer Center clinical experience. *British Journal of Haematology.* 2014;166(6):891–901.

47. Gandi M, Petrich AM, Cassaday RD, Press OW, Shah K, Whyman J, *et al.* Impact of induction regimen and consolidative stem cell transplantation in patients with double hit lymphoma (DHL): a large multicenter retrospective analysis. *Blood.* 2014;124(15):2354–61.

48. Petrich AM, Gandhi M, Jovanovic B, Castillo JJ, Rajguru S, Yang DT, *et al.*

Impact of induction regimen and stem cell transplantation on outcomes in double-hit lymphoma: a multicenter retrospective analysis. *Blood.* 2014;124(15):2354–61.

49. Oki Y, Noorani M, Lin P, Davis RE, Neelapu SS, Ma L, *et al.* Double hit lymphoma: the MD Anderson Cancer Center clinical experience. *British Journal of Haematology.* 2014;166(6):891–901.

50. Cuccuini W, Briere J, Mounier N, Voelker HU, Rosenwald A, Sundstrom C, *et al.* MYC+ diffuse large B-cell lymphoma is not salvaged by classical R-ICE or R-DHAP followed by BEAM plus autologous stem cell transplantation. *Blood.* 2012;119(20):4619–24.

51. Al-Tourah AJ, Gill KK, Chhanabhai M, Hoskins PJ, Klasa RJ, Savage KJ, *et al.* Population-based analysis of incidence and outcome of transformed

non-Hodgkin's lymphoma. *Journal of Clinical Oncology: Official Journal of the American Society of Clinical Oncology.* 2008;26(32):5165–9.

52. Villa D, Crump M, Panzarella T, Savage KJ, Toze CL, Stewart DA, *et al.* Autologous and allogeneic stem-cell transplantation for transformed follicular lymphoma: a report of the Canadian blood and marrow transplant group. *Journal of Clinical Oncology: Official Journal of the American Society of Clinical Oncology.* 2013;31(9):1164–71.

53. Wirk B, Fenske TS, Hamadani M, Zhang MJ, Hu ZH, Akpek G, *et al.* Outcomes of hematopoietic cell transplantation for diffuse large B cell lymphoma transformed from follicular lymphoma. *Biology of Blood and Marrow Transplantation: Journal of the American Society for Blood and Marrow Transplantation.* 2014;20(7):951–9.

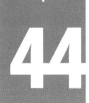

Chapter

44

Hematopoietic Cell Transplants for T-Cell Lymphomas

Francesco d'Amore, Thomas Relander, Grete F. Lauritzsen, Esa Jantunen, Susanna Mannisto, Peter Meyer, Fredrik Ellin, Martin Bjerregård Pedersen, and Helle Toldbod, Members of the NLG-T-Cell Working Group

Introduction

Peripheral T-cell lymphomas (PTCL) comprise a variety of rare malignancies derived from mature (post-thymic) T-cells and NK cells accounting for 10–15% of all non-Hodgkin's lymphomas worldwide. Clinically, most entities are systemic and aggressive diseases with overall poor prognosis and unsatisfactory response to classical treatments. The biology and pathophysiology of PTCL is complex and to a large extent still poorly characterized. The currently applied classification of PTCL from the World Health Organization [1] relies on a combination of morphologic, immunophenotypic, genetic, and clinical features, and attempts to correlate disease entities with normal cellular counterparts.

The most common histopathologic subtypes are PTCL, not otherwise specified (PTCL-NOS), angioimmunoblastic T-cell lymphoma (AITL), and anaplastic large cell lymphoma (ALCL), with or without expression of the fusion protein nucleophosmin-anaplastic lymphoma kinase (ALK) [2]. These subtypes have a predominantly nodal presentation. Other entities are more frequently extranodal and comprise: extranodal NK/T-cell lymphoma, nasal type (NKTCL), enteropathy-associated T-cell lymphoma (EATL), hepatosplenic T-cell lymphoma (HSTCL), and subcutaneous panniculitis-like T-cell lymphoma (SPTCL). Most commonly, PTCL occurs in middle-aged to elderly patients and with prognostically unfavorable clinical characteristics, such as advanced clinical stage, B-symptoms, and elevated LDH [3]. Conventionally treated PTCL have a poorer outcome than aggressive B-cell lymphomas [4]. Since the original report by Falini et al. [5], anaplastic large cell lymphoma, alk-positive (ALCL ALK+) has been regarded as having a more favorable prognosis than its ALK-negative counterpart [5,6]. However, part of this difference could be due to a skewed distribution of clinical prognostic factors, particularly age (younger age in ALK-positive cases) [7–10], but recent reports have described biologically defined ALK-negative subgroups where the DUSP22 rearranged have similar outcome to the ALK-positives [11,12]. In the near future, the distinction between ALK-negative and ALK-positive and how to treat them, might need reconsideration. The present review will only focus on systemic PTCL, i.e., primary cutaneous or leukemic entities will not be covered in this chapter.

Conventional Chemotherapy with CHOP Regimen

In PTCL, with the exception of ALCL ALK+, the outcome observed with a standard regimen of cyclophosphamide, hydroxydaunorubicin, vincristine, and prednisone (CHOP) has been modest. Although initially leading to encouraging ORR of 60–70%, standard CHOP/CHOP-like regimens are frequently characterized by subsequent relapses, overall survival (OS) rates at 5 years in the range of 25–35%, and even lower progression-free survival (PFS) values [13]. Therefore, an intensification of standard CHOP chemotherapy by either shortening the chemotherapy intervals, increasing its dose, and/or adding other drugs has been attempted.

Should Etoposide Be Added to CHOP Backbone in PTCL?

The German High-grade Non-Hodgkin Lymphoma Study Group (DSHNHL) reported a retrospective subset analysis on 320 mostly nodal PTCL patients included in eight prospective DSHNHL trials [14]. Patients under the age of 60 years and with a normal LDH had a significantly improved outcome with CHOP plus etoposide (CHOEP) as compared to CHOP alone (3-year EFS: 75.4% versus 51%); however, no significant impact on OS was found. A majority of the patients in that series (60%) had either ALCL ALK+ or anaplastic large cell lymphoma, alk-negative (ALCL ALK−). The greatest benefit of adding etoposide was seen in the ALCL ALK+ group. Furthermore, toxicity was a limiting factor for CHOEP given in patients aged over 60 years. Previously, another prospectively conducted phase 2 study from the German group had shown good outcome results after the addition of etoposide to a CHOP backbone in the VACPE regimen (vincristine, doxorubicin, cyclophosphamide, prednisone, etoposide). Five-year OS and event-free survival (EFS) values were 62% and 48%, respectively [15]. Recently, a large registry-based study from the Swedish Lymphoma Group also demonstrated significant superior PFS in patients ≤60 years treated with CHOEP versus CHOP (HR= 0.49) [10].

What About Other Regimens Besides CHOP +/− Etoposide in PTCL?

A retrospective analysis described the experience at MD Anderson Cancer Center with the management of treatment-naïve PTCL within the period 1996–2002. Outcome data for the CHOP regimen were compared with more intensive regimens such as HyperCVAD (cyclophosphamide, mesna, doxorubicin, vincristine, prednisone, methotrexate, cytarabine), Hyper-CHOP, and a schedule alternating three regimens: ASHAP (doxorubicin, methylprednisolone, high-dose cytarabine, cisplatin), M-BACOS (methotrexate, bleomycin, doxorubicin, cyclophosphamide, vincristine, methylprednisolone), and MINE (mesna, ifosfamide, mitoxantrone, etoposide) [16]. There was no significant difference in 3-year OS between patients treated with CHOP and the intensive regimens: (i) 62% *versus* 56%, respectively, for all PTCL including ALCL, and (ii) 43% *versus* 49%, respectively, after the exclusion of ALCL. The same authors reported the results obtained with a modification of the HyperCVAD regimen using liposomal doxorubicin in a PTCL cohort lacking ALCL ALK+ cases [17]. Preliminary results in 38 patients showed a high ORR of 87%, but the CR rate was similar (59%) to that obtained in their previous study.

Sung *et al.* investigated the impact of CEOP-B (cyclophosphamide, epirubicin, vincristine, prednisone, and bleomycin) on PTCL. In a patient cohort characterized by a low-risk profile (38% IPI 0 or 1), the authors reported a 5-year OS and PFS of 49% and 30%, respectively [18]. Based on piloting observations of high single-agent activity in PTCL, gemcitabine has been investigated as single agent or as part of combination regimens in both previously untreated and recurrent disease [19,20]. In the frontline setting, the intensive CHOP-EG (cyclophosphamide, doxorubicin, vincristine, prednisone, etoposide, gemcitabine) regimen was feasible in 26 patients with PTCL [21]. At a median follow-up of 1 year, 77% of the patients were alive; however, the median EFS was only 7 months, suggesting that remissions were not durable. A cisplatin, etoposide, gemcitabine, and high-dose methylprednisolone (PEGS) regimen was investigated in both newly diagnosed and relapsed PTCL patients in a recent phase 2 SWOG trial [22]. In newly diagnosed patients, the study revealed a disappointing ORR of 39% and a 2-year PFS of only 14%.

In summary, anthracycline-void regimens have so far failed to demonstrate their superiority as a standard chemotherapy backbone alternative to CHOP/CHOEP. An exception seems to be the NKTCL that has a unique place in the context of PTCL, since it is sensitive to L-asparaginase-containing regimens such as SMILE (dexamethasone, methotrexate, ifosfamide, L-asparaginase, etoposide) and AspaMetDex (L-asparaginase, methotrexate, dexamethasone) and local radiotherapy [23,24]. Anthracycline-based regimens (CHOP or CHOP-like) are not effective in this subtype [25], which is much more frequent in Asians than Caucasians.

Hematopoietic Cell Transplant

Auto-HCT in PTCL

First-Line Treatment with Auto-HCT: Does It Make Sense in PTCL?

So far, the role of upfront auto-HCT in PTCL has not been investigated in a randomized trial. The impact of this consolidation approach on the outcome of chemosensitive disease compared to conventional chemotherapy alone remains therefore unclear. However, since 2000 there have been an increasing number of phase 2 trials evaluating upfront auto-HCT in PTCL [26–29]. ALCL ALK+ patients and patients with stage I disease of other peripheral T-cell lymphomas have often been excluded from upfront auto-HCT studies due to their superior outcome with conventional regimens compared to the other common PTCL subtypes.

Some reports focus exclusively on single subtypes, e.g., AITL [30–32], EATL [33,34], NKTCL [35], ALCL [36], or PTCL-NOS [37]. Overall, 3- and 5-year OS and EFS were fairly high, ranging from 40–50% to over 80%. This may partly be due, at least in some of the studies, to the inclusion of ALCL cases, but also to the fact that retrospective analyses are often limited to responding cases with a satisfactory pretransplant status. Therefore, the problem of primary refractory or early relapsing disease in PTCL is not always sufficiently highlighted in retrospective reports. The impact of auto-HCT in previously untreated systemic PTCL is best evaluated by prospective, PTCL-restricted clinical trials. Table 44.1 summarizes those reported so far. Some of them have specific features that make their comparison with other studies difficult [29,38,39].

The study of Corradini *et al.* [29] was characterized by a long accrual period and a heterogeneous induction schedule. Two different types of induction + conditioning regimens were given: one (n=32) consisting of two courses of APO, (doxorubicin, vincristine, prednisone) and two courses of DHAP (cisplatin, cytarabine, dexamethasone) followed by high-dose sequential chemotherapy with cyclophosphamide, cytarabine, cisplatin, and etoposide, consolidated by high-dose mitoxantrone, melphalan, and auto-HCT; the other (n=30) scheduling MACOP-B for 8 weeks followed by a 3-day course of mitoxantrone and high-dose cytarabine followed by BEAM and auto-HCT. The ORR was 72%. At a median follow-up of 76 months, the estimated 12-year DFS was 55%, and 12-year OS and S were 34% and 30%, respectively. Pretransplant CR was a strong indicator for long-term outcome.

Rodriguez *et al.* reported the experience of the GEL-TAMO group [26] in a small series of PTCL patients (n=26) with low median age (44 years), high-risk profile at presentation, and a positive gallium scan. All patients received three courses of high-dose CHOP (cyclophosphamide $2\,g/m^2$, doxorubicin $90\,mg/m^2$) followed by a new gallium scan. If scan-negative, patients received another course of high-dose CHOP followed by hematopoietic progenitor and stem cell (HPSC) collection and auto-HCT with BEAM conditioning (n=12). Those with persistent scan-positivity received two courses of IFE

Table 44.1 Prospective clinical trials on upfront auto-HCT in PTCL from 2005 to 2014

Study	n	n reaching auto-HCT	Median age (years)	Regimen	Conditioning regimen	CR(%) before/after allo-HCT	Median follow-up (months)	OS (%)
Corradini et al. 2006 [29]	62	46	43	APO/DHAP/ MACOP-B/Cy +VP16	Mitoxantrone + melphalan	76/89	76	34 (12-year OS)
Rodríguez et al. 2007 [67]	26	19	44	MegaCHOP/ IFE	BEAM	–/89	27	73 (3-year OS)
Mercadal et al. 2008 [39]	41	17	47	CHOP/ESHAP	BEAM/BEAC	49/51	34.8	39 (4-year OS)
Reimer et al. 2009 [27]	83	55	47	CHOP	Cy + TBI	73/87.3	33	48 (3-year OS)
d'Amore et al. 2012 [28]	160	115	57	CHOP/ CHOEP-14	BEAM/BEAC	51/78	60.5	51 (5-year OS)

(ifosfamide $10 g/m^2$ days 1–3 and etoposide $150 mg/m^2/12$ h days 1–3) followed by auto-HCT if a new gallium scan showed PR or CR (n=7). At a median follow-up of 35 months, 3-year OS and PFS were 73% and 53%, respectively. There was no treatment-related mortality (TRM).

A GELCAB trial reported by Mercadal et al. [39] was characterized by a particularly low percentage of patients undergoing auto-HCT, i.e., 17 of 41 patients (41%). In this study, induction therapy consisted of three courses of high-dose CHOP alternating with three courses of ESHAP (etoposide, cisplatin, cytarabine, and prednisone). Primary failures were seen in 17 patients (41%) and a further seven patients did not make it to transplant due to mobilization failure (n=3), severe toxicity (n=2), early relapse prior to auto-HCT (n=1), and patient decision (n=1). At a median follow-up of 3.2 years there was a reported 4-year OS and PFS of 39% and 30%, respectively.

The two studies that are most homogeneous and comparable are also the two largest ones [27,28]. The German study by Reimer et al. [27] reported on 83 patients treated initially with four courses of CHOP-21, restaged and supplemented by two further courses, if not in CR. If in PR/CR, patients received 1–2 courses with either Dexa-BEAM (dexamethasone, carmustine, etoposide, cytarabine, and melphalan) or ESHAP followed by auto-HCT with total body irradiation and high-dose cyclophosphamide as conditioning regimen. After induction treatment, 32 patients were in CR and 33 in PR (ORR 79%). Of these 65 patients, 55 (66% of the entire cohort) underwent auto-HCT. At a median follow-up of 33 months, 3-year OS, PFS, and DFS were 48%, 38%, and 55%, respectively. The 3-year OS for the 55 transplanted patients was 71%. For the 28 not-transplanted ones, the 3-year OS value was only 11%.

Recently, the Nordic group published the final results of a large phase 2 trial (NLG-T-01), where 6 courses of bi-weekly CHOEP were followed by auto-HCT in chemosensitive patients [28]. The ORR rate was 82% with 51% of the patients

achieving a CR. At a median follow-up of 4.5 years the three included nodal PTCL entities had an estimated 5-year OS and PFS of 70% and 61% (ALCL ALK–), 52% and 49% (AITL), and 47% and 38% (PTCL-NOS).

On the basis of the Nordic phase 2 trial and the retrospective analysis of the German trials with CHOP versus CHOEP in lymphomas of aggressive histology, a dose-dense CHOEP/ EPOCH schedule followed by auto-HCT in chemosensitive and transplant-eligible patients represents at present one of the most evidence-based approaches adoptable outside of a clinical trial. In a recent large population-based registry study from the Swedish Lymphoma Group, an intention-to-treat analysis in 252 nodal PTCL and EATL patients (excluding ALCL ALK+) found upfront auto-HCT associated with a significantly superior OS and PFS compared with patients treated without auto-HCT [10].

In EATL, recent reports indicate that for patients sufficiently fit to tolerate more aggressive chemotherapy regimens than standard CHOP, outcome can be significantly improved. For example, 26 patients treated with a regimen including ifosfamide, vincristine, epirubicin, and methotrexate followed by auto-HCT had a 5-year OS and PFS of 60% and 52%, respectively [40].

Early Relapse and Refractory PTCL: An Unsolved Problem

Prospective studies have shown that early treatment failures remain an unsolved problem and novel induction strategies are needed. Ongoing collaborative phase 3 studies currently investigate the impact of new drugs given in combination with CHOP on the frequency of primary refractory disease and, in responding patients, on duration of responses. For example, in a collaborative effort, Nordic and German lymphoma groups have recently conducted such a phase 3 trial testing the addition of the anti-CD52 antibody alemtuzumab to six courses

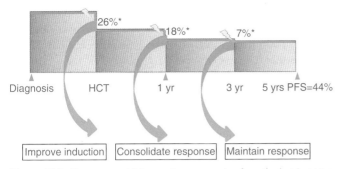

Figure 44.1. Response and failure patterns emerging from the first-line HCT trials run in PTCL and corresponding interventional strategies to improve outcomes. The % implies patients from the original study cohort experiencing relapse/progression at the different time points: [1] 26% up to autotransplant, [2] 18% after autotransplant but within the first 2 years post-transplant, and [3] 7% after the first 2 years post-autotransplant.

of an intensified CHOP induction schedule. In this study, patients up to 60 years received consolidation with auto-HCT. A final analysis of this phase 3 trial will be performed in 2015 (ACT-2) and 2017 (ACT-1). From the unique features of the NLG-T-01 trial, i.e., large cohort and long median follow-up, a pattern of response/failure in the first-line setting of PTCL was observed [28]. Some cases are treatment refractory (approximately 20% of the patients), and do not reach the consolidation step. In other instances, relapses occur early after auto-HCT, in primarily chemosensitive patients. In these patients, residual minor disease activity after auto-HCT is a likely explanation for treatment failure and should be challenged by novel post-transplant consolidation and/or maintenance strategies. The response and failure patterns emerging from the clinical experience of the upfront auto-HCT trials in PTCL are illustrated in Figure 44.1.

Auto-HCT in Relapsed/Refractory PTCL: Are We Sure That One Size Fits All?

Patients with relapsed aggressive lymphoma are considered candidates for auto-HCT since the Parma study showed superior results of auto-HCT consolidation after salvage chemotherapy over salvage chemotherapy alone [41]. Auto-HCT has therefore been an accepted standard approach for aggressive histologies of both B- and T-cell phenotype. A substantial number of retrospective single-institution series on auto-HCT preformed in relapsed PTCL patients have been reported. Most series consist of small patient cohorts, further challenged by the presence of several PTCL subtypes, including ALCL [32,42,43]. Owing to the heterogeneous nature of these patient cohorts, no firm and unequivocal conclusions can be drawn. However, in general, outcome of the patients transplanted after a relapse seems to be comparable with the results obtained in patients with relapsed or refractory diffuse large B-cell lymphoma [44]. The best prognosis is found in patients with ALCL. The fraction of ALK-positive cases among ALCL patients is rarely reported in these retrospective series. According to a number of reports, an additional important factor, in terms of favorable long-term outcome, is the achievement of CR prior

to auto-HCT, reflecting tumor chemosensitivity [29,45]. In ALCL, auto-HCT may be useful as rescue therapy in patients with partial remission after primary induction therapy [46] or at relapse [42]. In a retrospective registry study on patients transplanted in first PR or who had primary refractory disease, 51% were alive and in remission at a median follow-up of 3 years; TRM rate was 11% [46]. In patients with ALCL ALK−, treatment outcome with conventional chemotherapy is worse than in ALCL ALK+. The same seems to hold true for auto-HCT, where the post-transplant relapse rate seems to be high when auto HCT is performed in relapsing/refractory patients [37]. In a study including 16 cases of systemic ALCL ALK−, 13 of them relapsed after auto-HCT with a median PFS of only 3 months [43]. These observations suggest that auto-HCT might be preferable in first CR or PR in patients with systemic ALCL ALK−. Results in patients with PTCL-NOS have in general been less promising than in patients with ALCL [29,47,48]. In a Canadian study of relapsed or refractory patients, 3-year OS was 35% and EFS 23% [47]. In a retrospective study by Schetelig et al., a total of 29 AITL patients were included. Of these, 52% had experienced at least one relapse. OS was 44% and EFS 37% at 5 years, respectively [31]. Limited data are available on the use of auto-HCT in the more rare subtypes of systemic PTCL. Results of auto-HCT have been reported in patients with NKTCL transplanted at relapse in Asian patients. An apparent survival advantage was demonstrated compared with historical controls [35,49].

Allogeneic Hematopoietic Cell Transplant (Allo-HCT)
Allo-HCT as First-Line Treatment for PTC: Do We Know?

Allo-HCT is a potentially curative option for patients affected by PTCL. However, limited small single center data are available on the feasibility and efficacy of allo-HCT in patients with PTCL [50]. The first prospective phase 2 results demonstrated sustained responses in relapsed/refractory PTCL patients, suggesting the existence of a possible "graft-versus-T-cell lymphoma" effect [51,52]. The NRM was low, supporting the feasibility of a reduced intensity conditioning (RIC) allo-HCT even in heavily pretreated patients. Retrospective and registry-based analyses also confirmed that allo-HCT can yield long-term responses in relapsed/refractory PTCL [53–55]. In extranodal subtypes data are anecdotal, but generally supportive of the feasibility and efficacy of allo-HCT. In a recently reported prospective trial performed in treatment-naïve PTCL patients, after an induction phase with intensive chemoimmunotherapy, responding patients were randomized to auto- or allo-HCT based on the availability of an HLA-identical sibling or matched unrelated donor [56]. Owing to limited sample size it was not possible to identify a superiority of any of the two approaches; however, allo- and auto-HCT patients had a 4-year PFS of 69% and 70%, respectively. Recently, Voss et al. reported the Memorial Sloan-Kettering experience in HSTCL with encouraging responses to the more intense regimens of

ICE (ifosfamide, carboplatin, etoposide) or IVAC (ifosfamide, cytarabine, etoposide) followed by HCT, mostly allogeneic [57]. For rare leukemic forms of PTCL, allo-HCT might also be considered as a part of first-line treatment [58,59].

Allo-HCT in Relapsed/Refractory PTCL: Yes or No?

Using a standard allo-HCT approach, Utsunomiya *et al.* [59] observed not only relatively high treatment-related mortality (4/10 patients), but also promising outcome in patients with adult T-cell leukemia/lymphoma (ATLL). This observation is of interest, especially with regard to the poor outcome reported after auto-HCT in this leukemic PTCL subtype [58,60]. Promising results have also been reported in children and adolescents with relapsed ALCL [61]. A clear graft-*versus*-lymphoma (GvL) effect is present in adult systemic PTCL treated with RIC allo-HCT. Corradini *et al.* reported data on 17 patients with relapsed or refractory PTCL undergoing RIC allo-HCT [51]. After a median follow-up of 28 months, 14 of the 17 patients were alive. The estimated 3-year OS and PFS rates were 81% and 46%, respectively. The TRM rate was 6%. In fact, some additional reports suggest that RIC allografting might represent an efficacious option in relapsed PTCL [55,62,63]. In terms of toxicity, RIC allo-HCT seems clearly more attractive than a standard allo-HCT approach. As an example, a retrospective registry analysis of 18 relapsed/refractory lymphoma patients who received full-intensity allo-HCT revealed that eight patients died from causes not related to lymphoma relapse [64].

Controversies in HCT for PTCL: Upfront or at Relapse? Auto-HCT *versus* Allo-HCT?

Since 2000 there have been an increasing number of phase 2 trials evaluating upfront auto-HCT in PTCL [26–28,65]. ALCL ALK+ patients have characteristically been excluded due to their superior outcome with conventional regimens. The largest of these studies supports the impression of a beneficial effect of upfront auto-HCT in chemosensitive patients, particularly for the nodal subtypes and EATL [27,28]. Hence, a dose-dense CHOEP/EPOCH schedule followed by auto-HCT in chemosensitive and transplant-eligible patients currently represents the most evidence-based upfront approach for these subtypes. This approach has been included in internationally recognized recommendations such as the NCCN and ESMO guidelines. The upfront experience with allo-HCT is still scarce and has primarily been retrospectively investigated [66]. Small phase 2 trials have suggested the presence of a substantial GvL effect [51,67–68], but toxicity remains a concern. A phase 3 trial from the German Study Group on Aggressive non-Hodgkin Lymphomas (DSHNHL 2006-1A; EudraCT Number: 2007-001052-39) comparing upfront auto- and allo-HCT has recently been prematurely closed after a planned interim futility analysis. Therefore, the evidence for the use of upfront allo-HCT in the most common PTCL subtypes is still insufficient and further testing within

clinical trials is warranted. For patients with relapsed/refractory PTCL (with or without previous auto-HCT), who respond to reinduction therapy, consolidation with allo-HCT is a preferable and potentially curative strategy.

Conclusion and Perspectives

In conclusion, auto-HCT is a feasible treatment option in patients with PTCL and currently represents, in the absence of randomized trials, a commonly accepted and recommended consolidation in the first-line treatment of eligible patients with both nodal and extranodal PTCL subtypes. However, additional prospective data improving our knowledge on long-term outcome with regard to auto-HCT *versus* conventional (CHOP-like) therapy as a part of first-line treatment are needed. Although difficult to perform, the optimal option would be a randomized trial comparing induction therapy with and without auto-HCT consolidation. Like in the aggressive B-cell setting, auto-HCT may also be efficacious in relapsed patients responsive to reinduction chemotherapy. With regard to allo-HCT, this modality should be considered at relapse in transplant-eligible patients including those who failed a prior autograft. Also in the allo-HCT setting the outcome benefit seems most evident in chemosensitive patients. Based on the existing evidence, a RIC-allo-HCT should be preferred to a myeloablative approach in order to reduce NRM. The role of allo-HCT in the upfront setting is still unclear; upfront allo-HCT should therefore be primarily performed within prospective clinical trials.

Practice Points

- Dose-dense CHOEP/EPOCH schedule followed by auto-HCT in chemosensitive and transplant-eligible patients currently represents the most evidence-based upfront approach particularly for the nodal subtypes and EATL, and excluding ALCL ALK+ (Table 44.1) [27,28].
- The evidence for the use of upfront allo-HCT in the most common PTCL subtypes is still insufficient and further testing within clinical trials is warranted.
- For rare leukemic forms of PTCL, allo-HCT might also be considered as a part of first-line treatment [58,59].
- Like in the aggressive B-cell setting, auto-HCT may also be efficacious in relapsed patients responsive to reinduction chemotherapy, particularly persons with ALCL.
- For patients with relapsed/refractory PTCL (with or without previous auto-HCT) who respond to reinduction therapy consolidation with RIC-based allo-HCT is a preferable (excluding ALCL ALK+; where auto-HCT would be preferred and ALCL ALK− if without failure of previous auto-HCT) and potentially curative strategy.

Acknowedgment

The authors wish to thank Ms Malene Møller Staal for secretarial assistance during the preparation of the manuscript.

References

1. Swerdlow SH, Campo E, Harris NL, Jaffe ES, Pileri SA, Stein H, et al., Editors. *WHO Classification of Tumours of Haematopoietic and Lymphoid Tissue*, 4th Edition. WHO; 2008.

2. Vose J, Armitage J, Weisenburger D. International peripheral T-cell and natural killer/T-cell lymphoma study: pathology findings and clinical outcomes. *J Clin Oncol* 2008;26(25):4124−30.

3. Foss FM, Zinzani PL, Vose JM, Gascoyne RD, Rosen ST, Tobinai K. Peripheral T-cell lymphoma. *Blood* 2011;117(25):6756−67.

4. Gisselbrecht C, Gaulard P, Lepage E, Coiffier B, Briere J, Haioun C, et al. Prognostic significance of T-cell phenotype in aggressive non-Hodgkin's lymphomas. Groupe d'Etudes des Lymphomes de l'Adulte (GELA). *Blood* 1998;92(1):76−82.

5. Falini B, Pileri S, Zinzani PL, Carbone A, Zagonel V, Wolf-Peeters C, et al. ALK+ lymphoma: clinico-pathological findings and outcome. *Blood* 1999;93(8):2697−706.

6. Savage KJ, Harris NL, Vose JM, Ullrich F, Jaffe ES, Connors JM, et al. ALK- anaplastic large-cell lymphoma is clinically and immunophenotypically different from both ALK+ ALCL and peripheral T-cell lymphoma, not otherwise specified: report from the International Peripheral T-Cell Lymphoma Project. *Blood* 2008;111(12):5496−504.

7. Sibon D, Fournier M, Briere J, Lamant L, Haioun C, Coiffier B, et al. Long-term outcome of adults with systemic anaplastic large-cell lymphoma treated within the Groupe d'Etude des Lymphomes de l'Adulte trials. *J Clin Oncol* 2012;30(32):3939−46.

8. Suzuki R, Kagami Y, Takeuchi K, Kami M, Okamoto M, Ichinohasama R, et al. Prognostic significance of CD56 expression for ALK-positive and ALK-negative anaplastic large-cell lymphoma of T/null cell phenotype. *Blood* 2000;96(9):2993−3000.

9. Pedersen MB, Hamilton-Dutoit SJ, Bendix K, Moller MB, Norgaard P, Johansen P, et al. Evaluation of clinical trial eligibility and prognostic indices in a population-based cohort of systemic peripheral T-cell lymphomas from the Danish Lymphoma Registry. *Hematol Oncol* 2015;33(4):120−8.

10. Ellin F, Landstrom J, Jerkeman M, Relander T. Real-world data on prognostic factors and treatment in peripheral T-cell lymphomas: a study from the Swedish Lymphoma Registry. *Blood* 2014;124(10):1570−7.

11. Parrilla Castellar ER, Jaffe ES, Said JW, Swerdlow SH, Ketterling RP, Knudson RA, et al. ALK-negative anaplastic large cell lymphoma is a genetically heterogeneous disease with widely disparate clinical outcomes. *Blood* 2014;124(9):1473−80.

12. Feldman AL, Dogan A, Smith DI, Law ME, Ansell SM, Johnson SH, et al. Discovery of recurrent t(6;7)(p25.3; q32.3) translocations in ALK-negative anaplastic large cell lymphomas by massively parallel genomic sequencing. *Blood* 2011;117(3):915−9.

13. Abouyabis AN, Shenoy PJ, Sinha R, Flowers CR, Lechowicz MJ. A systematic review and meta-analysis of front-line anthracycline-based chemotherapy regimens for peripheral T-cell lymphoma. *ISRN Hematol* 2011;2011:623924. doi: 10.5402/2011/ 623924. Epub;%2011 Jun 16.:623924.

14. Schmitz N, Trumper L, Ziepert M, Nickelsen M, Ho AD, Metzner B, et al. Treatment and prognosis of mature T-cell and NK-cell lymphoma: an analysis of patients with T-cell lymphoma treated in studies of the German High-Grade Non-Hodgkin Lymphoma Study Group. *Blood* 2010;116(18):3418−25.

15. Karakas T, Bergmann L, Stutte HJ, Jager E, Knuth A, Weidmann E, et al. Peripheral T-cell lymphomas respond well to vincristine, adriamycin, cyclophosphamide, prednisone and etoposide (VACPE) and have a similar outcome as high-grade B-cell lymphomas. *Leuk Lymphoma* 1996;24(1–2):121–9.

16. Escalon MP, Liu NS, Yang Y, Hess M, Walker PL, Smith TL, et al. Prognostic factors and treatment of patients with T-cell non-Hodgkin lymphoma: the M. D. Anderson Cancer Center experience. *Cancer* 2005;103(10):2091–8.

17. Chihara D, Pro B, Loghavi S, Miranda RN, Medeiros LJ, Fanale MA, et al. *Phase II study of HCVIDD/MA in patients with newly diagnosed peripheral T-cell lymphoma. Br J Haematol.* 2015;171(4):509−16.

18. Sung HJ, Kim SJ, Seo HY, Sul HR, Choi JG, Choi IK, et al. Prospective analysis of treatment outcome and prognostic factors in patients with T-cell lymphomas treated by CEOP-B: single institutional study. *Br J Haematol* 2006;134(1):45–53.

19. Zinzani PL, Venturini F, Stefoni V, Fina M, Pellegrini C, Derenzini E, et al. Gemcitabine as single agent in pretreated T-cell lymphoma patients: evaluation of the long-term outcome. *Ann Oncol* 2010;21(4):860−3.

20. Zinzani PL, Baliva G, Magagnoli M, Bendandi M, Modugno G, Gherlinzoni F, et al. Gemcitabine treatment in pretreated cutaneous T-cell lymphoma: experience in 44 patients. *J Clin Oncol* 2000;18(13):2603−6.

21. Kim JG, Sohn SK, Chae YS, Kim DH, Baek JH, Lee KB, et al. CHOP plus etoposide and gemcitabine (CHOP-EG) as front-line chemotherapy for patients with peripheral T cell lymphomas. *Cancer Chemother Pharmacol* 2006;58(1):35–9.

22. Mahadevan D, Unger JM, Spier CM, Persky DO, Young F, LeBlanc M, et al. Phase 2 trial of combined cisplatin, etoposide, gemcitabine, and methylprednisolone (PEGS) in peripheral T-cell non-Hodgkin lymphoma: Southwest Oncology Group Study S0350. *Cancer* 2013;119(2):371–9.

23. Kwong YL, Kim WS, Lim ST, Kim SJ, Tang T, Tse E, et al. SMILE for natural killer/T-cell lymphoma: analysis of safety and efficacy from the Asia Lymphoma Study Group. *Blood* 2012;120(15):2973–80.

24. Jaccard A, Gachard N, Marin B, Rogez S, Audrain M, Suarez F, et al. Efficacy of L-asparaginase with methotrexate and dexamethasone (AspaMetDex regimen) in patients with refractory or relapsing extranodal NK/T-cell lymphoma, a phase 2 study. *Blood* 2011;117(6):1834–9.

25. Kim WS, Song SY, Ahn YC, Ko YH, Baek CH, Kim DY, et al. CHOP followed by involved field radiation: is it optimal for localized nasal natural killer/T-cell lymphoma? *Ann Oncol* 2001;12(3):349–52.

26. Rodriguez J, Conde E, Gutierrez A, Arranz R, Leon A, Marin J, et al. Frontline autologous stem cell

transplantation in high-risk peripheral T-cell lymphoma: a prospective study from The Gel-Tamo Study Group. *Eur J Haematol* 2007;79(1):32–8.

27. Reimer P, Rudiger T, Geissinger E, Weissinger F, Nerl C, Schmitz N, et al. Autologous stem-cell transplantation as first-line therapy in peripheral T-cell lymphomas: results of a prospective multicenter study. *J Clin Oncol* 2009;27(1):106–13.

28. d'Amore F, Relander T, Lauritzsen GF, Jantunen E, Hagberg H, Anderson H, et al. Up-front autologous stem-cell transplantation in peripheral T-cell lymphoma: NLG-T-01. *J Clin Oncol* 2012;30(25):3093–9.

29. Corradini P, Tarella C, Zallio F, Dodero A, Zanni M, Valagussa P, et al. Long-term follow-up of patients with peripheral T-cell lymphomas treated up-front with high-dose chemotherapy followed by autologous stem cell transplantation. *Leukemia* 2006;20(9):1533–8.

30. Kyriakou C, Canals C, Goldstone A, Caballero D, Metzner B, Kobbe G, et al. High-dose therapy and autologous stem-cell transplantation in angioimmunoblastic lymphoma: complete remission at transplantation is the major determinant of Outcome-Lymphoma Working Party of the European Group for Blood and Marrow Transplantation. *J Clin Oncol* 2008;26(2):218–24.

31. Schetelig J, Fetscher S, Reichle A, Berdel WE, Beguin Y, Brunet S, et al. Long-term disease-free survival in patients with angioimmunoblastic T-cell lymphoma after high-dose chemotherapy and autologous stem cell transplantation. *Haematologica* 2003;88(11):1272–8.

32. Rodriguez J, Conde E, Gutierrez A, Arranz R, Gandarillas M, Leon A, et al. Prolonged survival of patients with angioimmunoblastic T-cell lymphoma after high-dose chemotherapy and autologous stem cell transplantation: the GELTAMO experience. *Eur J Haematol* 2007;78(4):290–6.

33. Jantunen E, Juvonen E, Wiklund T, Putkonen M, Nousiainen T. High-dose therapy supported by autologous stem cell transplantation in patients with enteropathy-associated T-cell lymphoma. *Leuk Lymphoma* 2003;44(12):2163–4.

34. Jantunen E, Boumendil A, Finel H, Luan JJ, Johnson P, Rambaldi A, et al. Autologous stem cell transplantation for enteropathy-associated T-cell lymphoma: a retrospective study by the EBMT. *Blood* 2013;121(13):2529–32.

35. Au WY, Lie AK, Liang R, Kwong YL, Yau CC, Cheung MM, et al. Autologous stem cell transplantation for nasal NK/T-cell lymphoma: a progress report on its value. *Ann Oncol* 2003;14(11):1673–6.

36. Deconinck E, Lamy T, Foussard C, Gaillard F, Delwail V, Colombat P, et al. Autologous stem cell transplantation for anaplastic large-cell lymphomas: results of a prospective trial. *Br J Haematol* 2000;109(4):736–42.

37. Jagasia M, Morgan D, Goodman S, Hamilton K, Kinney M, Shyr Y, et al. Histology impacts the outcome of peripheral T-cell lymphomas after high dose chemotherapy and stem cell transplant. *Leuk Lymphoma* 2004;45(11):2261–7.

38. Rodriguez J, Conde E, Gutierrez A, Arranz R, Leon A, Marin J, et al. Frontline autologous stem cell transplantation in high-risk peripheral T-cell lymphoma: a prospective study from The Gel-Tamo Study Group. *Eur J Haematol* 2007;79(1):32–8.

39. Mercadal S, Briones J, Xicoy B, Pedro C, Escoda L, Estany C, et al. Intensive chemotherapy (high-dose CHOP/ESHAP regimen) followed by autologous stem-cell transplantation in previously untreated patients with peripheral T-cell lymphoma. *Ann Oncol* 2008;19(5):958–63.

40. Sieniawski M, Angamuthu N, Boyd K, Chasty R, Davies J, Forsyth P, et al. Evaluation of enteropathy-associated T-cell lymphoma comparing standard therapies with a novel regimen including autologous stem cell transplantation. *Blood* 2010;115(18):3664–70.

41. Philip T, Guglielmi C, Hagenbeek A, Somers R, Van der Lelie H, Bron D, et al. Autologous bone marrow transplantation as compared with salvage chemotherapy in relapses of chemotherapy-sensitive non-Hodgkin's lymphoma. *N Engl J Med* 1995;333(23):1540–5.

42. Fanin R, Ruiz de Elvira MC, Sperotto A, Baccarani M, Goldstone A. Autologous stem cell transplantation for T and null

cell CD30-positive anaplastic large cell lymphoma: analysis of 64 adult and paediatric cases reported to the European Group for Blood and Marrow Transplantation (EBMT). *Bone Marrow Transplant* 1999;23(5):437–42.

43. Zamkoff KW, Matulis MD, Mehta AC, Beaty MW, Hutchison RE, Gentile TC. High-dose therapy and autologous stem cell transplant does not result in long-term disease-free survival in patients with recurrent chemotherapy-sensitive ALK-negative anaplastic large-cell lymphoma. *Bone Marrow Transplant* 2004;33(6):635–8.

44. Kewalramani T, Zelenetz AD, Teruya-Feldstein J, Hamlin P, Yahalom J, Horwitz S, et al. Autologous transplantation for relapsed or primary refractory peripheral T-cell lymphoma. *Br J Haematol* 2006;134(2):202–7.

45. Kim MK, Kim S, Lee SS, Sym SJ, Lee DH, Jang S, et al. High-dose chemotherapy and autologous stem cell transplantation for peripheral T-cell lymphoma: complete response at transplant predicts survival. *Ann Hematol* 2007;86(6):435–42.

46. Rodriguez J, Caballero MD, Gutierrez A, Gandarillas M, Sierra J, Lopez-Guillermo A, et al. High dose chemotherapy and autologous stem cell transplantation in patients with peripheral T-cell lymphoma not achieving complete response after induction chemotherapy. The GEL-TAMO experience. *Haematologica* 2003;88(12):1372–7.

47. Song KW, Mollee P, Keating A, Crump M. Autologous stem cell transplant for relapsed and refractory peripheral T-cell lymphoma: variable outcome according to pathological subtype. *Br J Haematol* 2003;120(6):978–85.

48. Jantunen E, Itala M, Juvonen E, Leppa S, Keskinen L, Vasala K, et al. Autologous stem cell transplantation in elderly (>60 years) patients with non-Hodgkin's lymphoma: a nation-wide analysis. *Bone Marrow Transplant* 2006;37(4):367–72.

49. Kwong YL, Anderson BO, Advani R, Kim WS, Levine AM, Lim ST. Management of T-cell and natural-killer-cell neoplasms in Asia: consensus statement from the Asian Oncology Summit 2009. *Lancet Oncol* 2009;10(11):1093–101.

50. Loirat M, Chevallier P, Leux C, Moreau A, Bossard C, Guillaume T, et al. Upfront allogeneic-stem cell transplantation for patients with non-localized untreated peripheral T-cell lymphoma: an intention-to-treat analysis from a single center. *Ann Oncol* 2015;26(2):386–92.

51. Corradini P, Dodero A, Zallio F, Caracciolo D, Casini M, Bregni M, et al. Graft-*versus*-lymphoma effect in relapsed peripheral T-cell non-Hodgkin's lymphomas after reduced-intensity conditioning followed by allogeneic transplantation of hematopoietic cells. *J Clin Oncol* 2004;22(11):2172–6.

52. Dodero A, Spina F, Narni F, Patriarca F, Cavattoni I, Benedetti F, et al. Allogeneic transplantation following a reduced-intensity conditioning regimen in relapsed/refractory peripheral T-cell lymphomas: long-term remissions and response to donor lymphocyte infusions support the role of a graft-*versus*-lymphoma effect. *Leukemia* 2012;26(3):520–6.

53. Kim SW, Tanimoto TE, Hirabayashi N, Goto S, Kami M, Yoshioka S, et al. Myeloablative allogeneic hematopoietic stem cell transplantation for non-Hodgkin lymphoma: a nationwide survey in Japan. *Blood* 2006;108(1):382–9.

54. Le GS, Milpied N, Buzyn A, De Latour RP, Vernant JP, Mohty M, et al. Graft-*versus*-lymphoma effect for aggressive T-cell lymphomas in adults: a study by the Societe Francaise de Greffe de Moelle et de Therapie Cellulaire. *J Clin Oncol* 2008;26(14):2264–71.

55. Smith SM, Burns LJ, van BK, Leradamacher J, He W, Fenske TS, et al. Hematopoietic cell transplantation for systemic mature T-cell non-Hodgkin lymphoma. *J Clin Oncol* 2013;31(25):3100–9.

56. Corradini P, Vitolo U, Rambaldi A, Miceli R, Patriarca F, Gallamini A, et al. Intensified chemo-immunotherapy with or without stem cell transplantation in newly diagnosed patients with peripheral T-cell lymphoma. *Leukemia* 2014;28(9):1885–91.

57. Voss MH, Lunning MA, Maragulia JC, Papadopoulos EB, Goldberg J, Zelenetz AD, et al. Intensive induction chemotherapy followed by early high-dose therapy and hematopoietic stem cell transplantation results in improved outcome for patients with hepatosplenic T-cell lymphoma: a single institution experience. *Clin Lymphoma Myeloma Leuk* 2013;13(1):8–14.

58. Bazarbachi A, Cwynarski K, Boumendil A, Finel H, Fields P, Raj K, et al. Outcome of patients with HTLV-1-associated adult T-cell leukemia/lymphoma after SCT: a retrospective study by the EBMT LWP. *Bone Marrow Transplant* 2014;49(10):1266–8.

59. Utsunomiya A, Miyazaki Y, Takatsuka Y, Hanada S, Uozumi K, Yashiki S, et al. Improved outcome of adult T cell leukemia/lymphoma with allogeneic hematopoietic stem cell transplantation. *Bone Marrow Transplant* 2001;27(1):15–20.

60. Tsukasaki K, Maeda T, Arimura K, Taguchi J, Fukushima T, Miyazaki Y, et al. Poor outcome of autologous stem cell transplantation for adult T cell leukemia/lymphoma: a case report and review of the literature. *Bone Marrow Transplant* 1999;23(1):87–9.

61. Woessmann W, Peters C, Lenhard M, Burkhardt B, Sykora KW, Dilloo D, et al. Allogeneic haematopoietic stem cell transplantation in relapsed or refractory anaplastic large cell lymphoma of children and adolescents–a Berlin-Frankfurt-Munster group report. *Br J Haematol* 2006;133(2):176–82.

62. Wulf GG, Hasenkamp J, Jung W, Chapuy B, Truemper L, Glass B. Reduced intensity conditioning and allogeneic stem cell transplantation after salvage therapy integrating alemtuzumab for patients with relapsed peripheral T-cell non-Hodgkin's lymphoma. *Bone Marrow Transplant* 2005;36(3):271–3.

63. Jacobsen ED, Kim HT, Ho VT, Cutler CS, Koreth J, Fisher DC, et al. A large single-center experience with allogeneic stem-cell transplantation for peripheral T-cell non-Hodgkin lymphoma and advanced mycosis fungoides/Sezary syndrome. *Ann Oncol* 2011;22(7):1608–13.

64. Feyler S, Prince HM, Pearce R, Towlson K, Nivison-Smith I, Schey S, et al. The role of high-dose therapy and stem cell rescue in the management of T-cell malignant lymphomas: a BSBMT and ABMTRR study. *Bone Marrow Transplant* 2007;40(5):443–50.

65. Corradini P, Dodero A, Farina L, Fanin R, Patriarca F, Miceli R, et al. Allogeneic stem cell transplantation following reduced-intensity conditioning can induce durable clinical and molecular remissions in relapsed lymphomas: pretransplant disease status and histotype heavily influence outcome. *Leukemia* 2007;21(11):2316–23.

66. Corradini P, Vitolo U, Rambaldi A, Miceli R, Patriarca F, Gallamini A, et al. Intensified chemo-immunotherapy with or without stem cell transplantation in newly diagnosed patients with peripheral T-cell lymphoma. *Leukemia* 2014;28(9):1885–91.

67. Rodriguez J, Conde E, Gutierrez A, Arranz R, Leon A, Marin J, et al. The results of consolidation with autologous stem-cell transplantation in patients with peripheral T-cell lymphoma (PTCL) in first complete remission: the Spanish Lymphoma and Autologous Transplantation Group experience. *Ann Oncol* 2007;18(4):652–7.

68. Kyriakou C, Canals C, Finke J, Kobbe G, Harousseau JL, Kolb HJ, et al. Allogeneic stem cell transplantation is able to induce long-term remissions in angioimmunoblastic T-cell lymphoma: a retrospective study from the lymphoma working party of the European group for blood and marrow transplantation. *J Clin Oncol* 2009;27(24):3951–8.

Chapter

45

Hematopoietic Cell Transplants for Central Nervous System Lymphomas

Andy I. Chen and Richard T. Maziarz

Introduction

Non-Hodgkin lymphoma (NHL) can involve the central nervous system (CNS) either as primary CNS lymphoma (PCNSL) or as secondary CNS lymphoma (CNSL). PCNSL is limited to the CNS and is a rare entity, constituting less than 5% of all NHLs and of all brain tumors. In contrast, secondary CNSL is a complication of systemic lymphoma, either at diagnosis or relapse. Owing to the rarity of both PCNSL and secondary CNSL, there are limited prospective or randomized data to guide management, and both entities were historically associated with poor survival. However, with time more effective strategies have emerged with improved clinical outcomes.

PCNSL

Presentation, Pathogenesis, and Evaluation

PCNSL can occur throughout the neural axis including the brain parenchyma, leptomeninges, cranial nerves, spinal cord, and intraocular space. The clinical manifestation typically reflects the location of the disease. The majority of patients will have focal neurologic deficits or cognitive/neuropsychiatric symptoms. In addition, signs and symptoms related to mass effect such as headaches, visual changes, and seizures are not uncommon.

The vast majority of PCNSL are CD20+ diffuse large B-cell lymphomas (DLBCL), and PCNSL is recognized as a distinct subtype of DLBCL in the World Health Organization classification. Although PCNSL typically expresses an activated B-cell (ABC) phenotype on immunohistochemistry (CD10−, BCL6+, MUM1+) [1], it does not fit either germinal center (GCB) or ABC type gene expression profiles (GEP) of conventional systemic DLBCL [2,3]. By GEP, MYC and JAK/STAT pathways are activated in PCNSL [2,3]. In addition, mutations of MYD88 which activate the toll-like receptor pathway are the most frequent mutations identified in PCNSL [4]. Cell adhesion pathways are also aberrantly expressed in PCNSL [3], and the chemokines CXCL12 and CXCL13 may explain in part the tropism of PCNSL to the CNS microenvironment [5]. On histology PCNSL demonstrates angiotropism (tumor growth in close proximity to blood vessels), suggesting local disruption of the blood–brain barrier. Rarely, other types of lymphomas can present with isolated CNS disease, such as peripheral T-cell lymphoma and marginal zone lymphoma and should be differentiated from typical PCNSL.

Brain MRI is a key first step in diagnostic evaluation (Figure 45.1). CNSL is typically supratentorial and can appear as single or multiple masses. By MRI CNSL are generally T1 hypointense, T2 iso- to hypointense, enhancing with contrast and diffusion restricted. On CT, CNSL appears as a hyperdense enhancing mass. If PCNSL is suspected, steroids should be avoided, unless there is significant mass effect. Treatment with steroids can lead to nondiagnostic biopsies, delaying definitive diagnosis and treatment. Diagnosis can often be ascertained by flow cytometry and cytology of cerebrospinal fluid (CSF), although lumbar puncture should be avoided if there is significant tumor mass effect due to risk of herniation. A slit lamp eye exam is recommended, as up to 15% of patients will have intraocular involvement which warrants management stratifications. If the CSF and eye exams are nondiagnostic, then stereotactic needle biopsy is preferred over surgery, as resection of tumor bulk does not improve outcome in PCNSL. Standard work-up of PCNSL also includes HIV testing and an evaluation for systemic lymphoma. Although there is not a widely accepted standardized test, assessing baseline cognitive function is also crucial.

Immunodeficiency is a significant risk factor for the development of CNS lymphoma. In HIV disease, PCNSL is an AIDS defining illness and is associated with advanced AIDS with a very low CD4+ T-cell count. AIDS-associated CNS lymphoma is typically of the immunoblastic DLBCL type and is linked to Epstein–Barr Virus (EBV). The incidence of AIDS-associated PCNSL has decreased in the highly active antiretroviral therapy (HAART) era. PCNSL can also occur in the setting of congenital immunodeficiencies or as a manifestation of post-transplant lymphoproliferative disorder (PTLD) following solid organ transplantation.

Prognostic Models

The prognosis of PCNSL is largely dependent on age and performance status at presentation. In the Memorial Sloan Kettering Cancer Center (MSKCC) model based solely on these two factors, patients younger than 50 had a median overall survival (OS) of 8 years, while patients older than 50 with a poor performance status (Karnofsky <70) had a

(A)

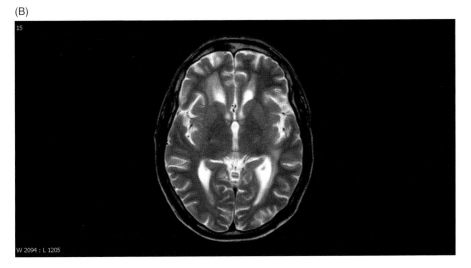

(B)

Figure 45.1 Comparison of brain MRI axial T2-weighted images of PCNSL at relapse (A) and 6 months after auto-HCT (B).

median OS of only 1 year [6]. In addition to age and performance status, the International Extranodal Lymphoma Study Group (IELSG) model also includes serum lactate dehydrogenase (LDH), CSF protein concentration, and involvement by lymphoma of deep brain structures (periventricular regions, basal ganglia, brainstem, cerebellum); using this model, the 2-year OS ranged from 80% for 0–1 risk factors to 15% for 4–5 risk factors [7]. Older fit patients should not be excluded from standard induction therapy, as a recent CALGB study of intensive immunochemotherapy has reported similar outcomes between patients younger and older than 60 years [8].

Treatment

Systemic high-dose methotrexate (HD Mtx) is the backbone of induction chemotherapy for PCNSL. The optimal dose of HD Mtx is uncertain, but doses ≥ 3 g/m^2 are associated with improved survival [9]. Because of the blood–brain barrier, many standard chemotherapeutic agents for lymphomas, for example doxorubicin in R-CHOP, do not sufficiently penetrate the CNS and are not recommended. In a large retrospective

analysis, treatment with a HD Mtx regimen was the only therapy-related factor associated with improved survival [10]. In a prospective phase 2 multicenter study, HD Mtx as a single agent in induction and maintenance resulted in a CR in half of patients, and 40% of those achieving a CR remained in remission at 7 years [11].

As the majority of patients with PCNSL still relapse after HD Mtx alone, additional therapeutic agents have been combined with HD Mtx. In a randomized phase 2 trial by the IELSG, the addition of cytarabine to HD Mtx improved the CR rate from 18% to 46% and the overall response rate from 40% to 69% [12]. The CALGB 50202 study combined rituximab and temozolamide with HD Mtx during induction (R-MT), followed by consolidation with cytarabine and etoposide [8]. This strategy yielded a CR rate of 66% and 4-year PFS of 47% and OS of 65%. A phase 2 single-institution study by MSKCC added procarbazine, vincristine, and rituximab to HD Mtx (R-MPV) followed by radiation, resulting in a median PFS of 3 years and median OS of 6 years [13]. A multicenter three-arm phase 3 study sponsored by the IELSG has been initiated comparing the addition of rituximab and/or thiotepa to HD

Table 45.1 Frontline auto-HCT for PCNSL

Reference	n(CR)	Regimen	Neurotoxicity	NRM	PFS	OS
Abrey et al. 2003 [18]	14[8]	BEAM	0	7%	43% (3 years)	60% (3 years)
Colombat et al. 2006 [19]	17(NR)	BEAM + WBRT	13%	6%	46% (4 years)	64% (4 years)
Montemurro et al. 2006 [23]	16[12]	BuT ± WBRT	39%	13%	61% (2 years)	61% (2 years)
Kasenda et al. 2012 [22] – from Illerhaus [20–21]	34[12]	BT ± WBRT	9%	0%	79% (5 years)	82% (5 years)
Rubenstein et al. 2013 [8]	44	Non-HCT protocol (R-MT + EA)	0	2%	47% (4 years)	65% (4 years)

Studies of consolidative auto-HCT for PCNSL with non-HCT CALGB 50202 as comparator. n: number; CR: number in CR entering HCT; NR: not reported; NRM: nonrelapse mortality; BEAM: BCNU/etoposide/cytarabine/melphalan; WBRT: whole brain radiotherapy; BuT: busulfan/thiotepa; BT: BCNU/thiotepa; R-MT: rituximab/methotrexate/temozolamide; EA: etoposide/cytarabine.

Mtx/cytarabine as induction (MA versus R-MA versus R-MATt; NCT01011920).

The addition of intrathecal chemotherapy to HD Mtx is controversial, as intrathecal methotrexate did not improve outcomes in a retrospective analysis [14]. A longstanding controversy in lymphoma is whether prophylactic or therapeutic intrathecal therapy in the CSF, presumably directed at the leptomeninges, has any benefit on disease in the brain parenchyma. Some CNS treatment protocols include intrathecal therapy only if there is leptomeningeal involvement, although other groups omit intrathecal therapy entirely regardless of CSF status. However, intraventricular immunochemotherapy with rituximab via an Ommaya reservoir is effective for relapsed PCNSL in both the leptomeninges and parenchyma [15]. Studies of intraventricular rituximab as part of frontline therapy have not been reported to date.

Although responses were relatively short and associated with significant toxicity, radiation was the original mainstay of treatment of PCNSL, and it is still frequently used as consolidation or salvage therapy. A combined modality approach of HD Mtx induction followed by whole brain radiotherapy (WBRT) is effective but can cause severe neurotoxicity, particularly in older (≥60) adults [16]. A large randomized phase 3 study of HD Mtx-based induction with or without WBRT has found no benefit in median survival (32 versus 37 months) from combined modality therapy, suggesting that WBRT could be reserved for relapse [17]. Although WBRT doubled the incidence of clinical neurotoxicity, it did improve median PFS (18 versus 12 months), so there continues to be interest in consolidation WBRT, particularly in those at lower risk of neurotoxicity. Reducing the dose of WBRT in combined modality therapy can reduce neurotoxicity [13], and this approach is being tested in a randomized study by the RTOG (NCT01399372).

Consolidative Transplant

To improve the outcomes in PCNSL, several studies have incorporated consolidative auto-HCT (Table 45.1; [8,18–23]). These reports suggest that high-dose therapy is active in PCNSL without significant neurotoxicity or treatment-related mortality. Impressive results have been seen with consolidative auto-HCT from the German group with PFS and OS >70% at 5 years [22]. Despite the caveats of a nonrandomized transplant series, these results are superior to any multicenter nontransplant study. Two multicenter randomized trials are underway to determine whether frontline consolidative auto-HCT is beneficial in PCNSL. The IELSG study comparing different induction regimens has a second randomization in responders to standard dose WBRT versus auto-HCT with BCNU/thiotepa conditioning (NCT01011920). In the United States, the CALGB/Alliance group is comparing nonablative etoposide/cytarabine consolidation versus high-dose BCNU/thiotepa conditioned auto-HCT (NCT01511562). The IELSG and Alliance studies are powered for 2-year PFS/failure-free survival (FFS) as the primary objective, with OS as a secondary objective. The results of these two randomized studies are expected to clarify the role of frontline consolidative auto-HCT in PCNSL.

Preparative Regimen for Auto-HCT

The optimal high-dose regimen for PCNSL has not been defined. Busulfan and thiotepa both penetrate the brain very well with CSF levels >80% plasma concentration [24,25]. BCNU, cytarabine, cyclophosphamide, and etoposide also cross the blood–brain barrier to a lesser extent [26]. The standard systemic lymphoma conditioning regimen of BCNU/etoposide/cytarabine/melphalan (BEAM) appears to be suboptimal [18]. Thus, both randomized studies of consolidative auto-HCT are utilizing the BCNU/thiotepa preparative regimen [20]. The French thiotepa/busulfan/cyclophosphamide (TbuC) regimen is also active in relapsed PCNSL (Table 45.2) [27]. A recent phase 2 study of adding rituximab to this regimen reported a remarkable 2-year PFS of 84% in a heterogeneous population of CNSL (including primary, secondary, frontline, and relapsed) [28]. There are no prospective studies comparing conditioning regimens in CNSL, and retrospective comparative analyses through the CIBMTR and European Group for Blood and Marrow Transplantation (EBMT) registries have not been pursued due to limited

Table 45.2 Auto-HCT for relapsed CNSL (PCNSL or secondary CNSL)

Reference	n(CR)	Regimen	NRM	Neurotoxicity	PFS	OS
Soussain *et al.* 2001 [38]	22, PCNSL[8]	TBuC	5%	32%	53% (3 years)	60% (3 years)
Soussain *et al.* 2008 [27]	27, PCNSL[12]	TBuC	0	18%	58% (2 years)	69% (2 years)
Cote *et al.* 2012 [35]	16, PCNSL16, secondary(18 total)	TBuC	3%	3%	93% (1 year)	90% (1 year)
Korfel *et al.* 2013 [36]	24, secondary[7]	BTE	0%	4%	58% (2 years)	68% (2 years)
Williams *et al.* 1994 [39]	62, secondary[45]	Varied	9% if CR 29% CNSact	NR	42% (5 years) if CR 9% (6 years) CNSact	NR
Maziarz *et al.* 2013 [37]	150, secondary(95)	Varied	5% (1 year)	NR	46% if CR (3 years) 19% if CNSact (3 years)	58% if CR (3 years) 31% if CNSact (3 years)

Studies of auto-HCT for relapsed CNSL.
n: number; CR: number in CR entering HCT; NRM: nonrelapse mortality; TBuC: thiotepa/busulfan/cyclophosphamide; BTE: BCNU/thiotepa/etoposide; NR: not reported; CNSact: active CNS disease entering HCT.

numbers of non-thiotepa-based cases. Across studies, BCNU/thiotepa appears less toxic than TBuC, but the patient population differed significantly making comparisons difficult, as BCNU/thiotepa was studied as frontline but TBuC in relapse. Of note, thiotepa has been affected by manufacturing shortages in the United States, stimulating interest in non-thiotepa-based regimens due to the expense of drug acquisition.

Secondary CNSL

Secondary CNSL at Diagnosis

Secondary CNSL is a dreaded complication of systemic lymphoma. Patients who present simultaneously with CNS and systemic disease pose a therapeutic challenge. There are no prospective studies or large multicenter retrospective series to inform management of these patients; thus, consensus expert opinion largely guides management. Typical approaches include alternating cycles of anthracycline-based chemotherapy with dose-escalated methotrexate (e.g., R-CHOP/HD Mtx or R-hyperCVAD/MtxAraC). The randomized studies of consolidative auto-HCT in the R-CHOP era excluded patients with active CNS, so the role of transplant in this population is undefined.

CNS Prophylaxis in Certain Groups of Subjects with "DLBCL"

The role of CNS prophylaxis to prevent secondary CNSL is controversial, as no randomized study in the R-CHOP era has shown a benefit in preventing leptomeningeal or parenchymal relapse. Relapse in the CNS occurs in <5% of DLBCL cases treated with R-CHOP, but patients with multiple sites of extranodal disease, a high serum lactate dehydrogenase, and a poor performance status have a >30% risk for developing secondary CNSL[29]. A CNS IPI has been proposed for risk of CNS relapse in DLBCL treated with R-CHOP which incorporates the IPI risk factors plus kidney/adrenal involvement[30].

Patients with ≥ 4 risk factors have a 10% risk of CNS relapse in this model. Lymphomas with a MYC gene rearrangement also have an increased risk of CNS disease. Although often considered in "high-risk" patients, intrathecal methotrexate prophylaxis did not reduce the incidence of CNS relapse (parenchymal or leptomeningeal) in the German RICOVER-60 trial in patients treated with R-CHOP, even when analysis was restricted to high-risk patients [29]. Similarly, there was no benefit from CNS prophylaxis in the randomized SWOG 8516 study in the pre-rituximab era [31]. In the pre-rituximab era, consolidation with two cycles of systemic HD Mtx did show benefit in a randomized study [32]. A more recent retrospective series has reported that adding cycles of HD Mtx for CNS prophylaxis to R-CHOP is effective in systemic DLBCL at high risk for CNS disease with only a 3% CNS relapse rate [33].

Relapsed CNSL

Auto-HCT is effective for chemosensitive relapsed PCNSL and selected secondary CNSL (Table 45.2)[27,34–39]. A prospective multicenter phase 2 trial reported a median PFS of 41 months and median OS of 58 months in patients who completed salvage therapy and auto-HCT with thiotepa/busulfan/cyclophosphamide conditioning [27]. Chemosensitivity to salvage therapy is important, as those with refractory PCNSL to salvage had inferior survival compared to chemosensitive patients after auto-HCT (median OS 18 months *versus* not reached). However, patients with PCNSL who achieved a first CR with HD Mtx induction can have an excellent response to retreatment with salvage HD Mtx without transplant, suggesting that auto-HCT may not be necessary at first relapse for this subgroup [40].

Relapsed secondary CNSL has a dismal prognosis with median survival of only 7 months [34]. An international retrospective analysis has found that the greatest predictor for survival in relapsed secondary CNSL was auto-HCT (1-year OS 62% *versus* 25%) [41]. However, only a third of patients were able to undergo auto-HCT, highlighting the need for better salvage therapies prior to transplant or allogeneic HCT in patients with negative CNS disease. In the only prospective treatment trial of salvage therapy and auto-HCT in relapsed secondary CNSL, 80% of patients were able to proceed to auto-HCT after combination salvage with HD Mtx/ifosfamide and cytarabine/thiotepa [36]. Of those undergoing auto-HCT, 58% remained in remission at 2 years.

Two registry analyses have found that disease status at transplant was the most critical factor of outcome for relapsed secondary CNSL [37,39]. In the larger, contemporary CIBMTR analysis, 3-year PFS was 19% in patients with active CNSL entering auto-HCT compared to 46% in those who were

in CR at time of transplant (Figure 45.2) [37]. In a CIBMTR case–control analysis, the outcomes of patients with relapsed secondary CNSL who were in CR entering auto-HCT was similar to relapsed systemic NHL without CNS disease (Figure 45.3) [37]. Although achieving CR before auto-HCT is an important goal, caution is necessary when combining WBRT with auto-HCT because of the risk of severe neurotoxicity, particularly in older adults. Also, smaller prospective studies with thiotepa-based conditioning have reported durable remissions in patients not in CR entering HCT [35,36].

Controversies and Future Directions

Frontline Consolidative Auto-HCT for PCNSL

Two randomized studies are currently underway examining the role of frontline consolidative auto-HCT for PCNSL. Off protocol, we would recommend upfront auto-HCT in fit patients who do not achieve a complete response to intensive induction but have chemosensitive disease. We would also consider upfront auto-HCT in fit patients who were induced with only HD Mtx, as opposed to an augmented combination regimen (e.g., R-MPV, R-MT, R-MA).

Auto-HCT Preparative Regimen

BEAM is likely not adequate as a transplant conditioning regimen for CNS lymphoma, but there are no comparative studies with other transplant regimens. The CIBMTR and EBMT have not pursued a registry analysis of optimal transplant conditioning for PCNSL, and no randomized studies are underway. In the CIBMTR study of auto-HCT for secondary CNSL, conditioning regimen was not a significant factor for survival, but there were very few non-thiotepa cases [37]. Based on phase 2 results and CNS penetration, our recommendation is to use thiotepa/busulfan/cyclophosphamide for CNS lymphoma, as this regimen contains both thiotepa and busulfan which cross into the CNS significantly

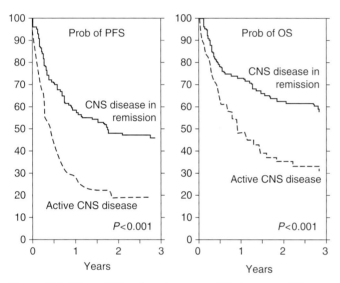

Figure 45.2 PFS and OS for relapsed secondary CNSL in patients with active disease entering auto-HCT (dashed line) compared to those in CR at the time of auto-HCT (solid line). Adapted from [36], used with permission.

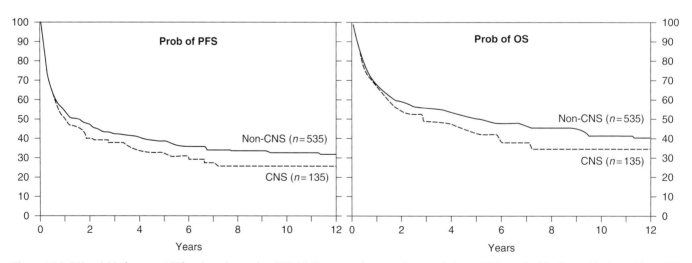

Figure 45.3 PFS and OS after auto-HCT for relapsed secondary CNSL (CNS) compared to control group of relapsed NHL matched for disease histology without CNS involvement (Non-CNS). *P-value* was nonsignificant for PFS and OS. Adapted from [36], used with permission.

better than other high-dose therapy agents. BCNU/thiotepa is a reasonable alternative, and a busulfan-containing regimen is recommended if thiotepa is not available.

Allogeneic HCT

There is a paucity of data on allogeneic HCT in PCNSL or secondary CNSL, and there are no prospective clinical trials exploring this strategy. Few cases have been reported to the central transplant registries, and the published literature is limited [42,43]. As donor lymphocytes circulate to the CNS, a graft-*versus*-lymphoma effect would presumably be active in CNSL. Graft-*versus*-host disease (GvHD) has been reported in the CNS as a complication of allogeneic transplant for other malignancies [44]. Given the very limited data, our recommendation is to reserve allogeneic transplant to fit patients with excellent disease control who fail hematopoietic progenitor cell mobilization or relapse after auto-HCT.

Disease Status and Transplant

Although small prospective series suggest chemosensitivity may be adequate [35,36], large registry series have found that active disease entering HCT is strongly associated with poor outcome in secondary CNSL [37,39]. So, our approach is to attempt an alternative rescue regimen or radiation prior to transplant in secondary CNSL with residual disease after first rescue regimen. However, there are no large registry series in PCNSL, and chemosensitivity – rather than CR status – appears to be sufficient for success of auto-HCT in PCNSL [21,27].

Intrathecal Prophylaxis of Secondary CNSL

In the R-CHOP era, isolated CNS relapse of DLBCL is rare, and intrathecal methotrexate is ineffective as CNS prophylaxis. However, patients with a poor performance status, multiple extranodal sites, and an elevated LDH at diagnosis are still at significant risk of CNS relapse. Our approach is to incorporate 2–3 cycles of systemic HD Mtx with R-CHOP in fit patients who are at high risk for secondary CNSL to prevent both leptomeningeal and parenchymal disease. Intrathecal prophylaxis is also recommended in subjects with "double- or triple-hit" lymphomas with c-myc rearrangements by FISH.

Rituximab

Although there can be local disruption at sites of tumor, rituximab has poor penetration across the blood–brain barrier with CSF levels <1% of systemic concentrations [28]. However, phase 2 studies support adding systemic rituximab to HD Mtx in PCNSL, and this is our recommendation until results from the randomized IELSG study become available. In addition, intraventricular rituximab could supplant systemic administration during induction, given the effectiveness of intraventricular rituximab in

relapsed/refractory disease – both parenchymal and leptomeningeal [15]. In this CALGB study, rituximab (25 mg) was given twice weekly in conjunction with weekly methotrexate via Ommaya.

Novel Imaging Techniques

MRI has been the standard for imaging CNSL. In challenging diagnostic cases, advanced MRI techniques such as dynamic contrast enhanced perfusion and diffusion-weighted imaging can help distinguish PCNSL from glioblastomas barrier [45]. Brain FDG PET imaging can be complementary to MRI in assessing treatment response to identify patients who would benefit from further therapy, analogous to the role of PET *versus* CT in systemic lymphoma [46,47].

Novel Therapies

Although auto-HCT is effective in CNSL, many patients with CNSL are not candidates for high-dose therapy because of age, comorbidities, fitness, or disease control. Studies of novel therapies in NHL typically exclude patients with active CNS disease. Some – but not all – small molecule targeted agents such as lenalidomide and ibrutinib can cross the blood–brain barrier and presumably would be active in CNSL. Since MYD88 mutations are frequently identified in PCNSL, there is currently interest in exploring BTK-inhibitors for PCNSL, as ibrutinib is effective in Waldenstroms macroglobulinemia with mutated MYD88 [48]. As more small molecule targeted agents are developed for systemic NHL, these new therapies may increase the armamentarium against CNSL.

Chimeric Antigen Receptor T (CAR T) Cells

Finally, CAR T-cell therapy has attracted great attention due to impressive responses in relapsed/refractory pre-B-ALL and CLL. Studies are now planned of this approach in systemic DLBCL. Of interest to CNSL, CAR T-cells cross into the CNS and are able to persist in the CSF for months [49]. It is conceivable that based upon these observations that trials will emerge for patients with PCNSL and secondary CNSL in the future.

Conclusion

Auto-HCT is effective for CNSL. In PCNSL, phase 2 studies have reported impressive outcomes with frontline auto-HCT, and randomized studies are underway to confirm these benefit. Consolidative auto-HCT is a reasonable option for these patients, preferably on a clinical trial. In relapsed PCNSL, phase 2 and retrospective data have shown that auto-HCT can lead to durable remissions and is recommended in chemosensitive fit patients. Based largely on retrospective and registry data, auto-HCT is also recommended for relapsed secondary CNSL, where disease status entering transplant is crucial for success.

References

1. Camilleri-Broet S, Criniere E, Broet P, Delwail V, Mokhtari K, Moreau A, et al. A uniform activated B-cell-like immunophenotype might explain the poor prognosis of primary central nervous system lymphomas: analysis of 83 cases. *Blood*. 2006;107(1):190–6.

2. Rubenstein JL, Fridlyand J, Shen A, Aldape K, Ginzinger D, Batchelor T, et al. Gene expression and angiotropism in primary CNS lymphoma. *Blood*. 2006;107(9):3716–23.

3. Sung CO, Kim SC, Karnan S, Karube K, Shin HJ, Nam DH, et al. Genomic profiling combined with gene expression profiling in primary central nervous system lymphoma. *Blood*. 2011;117(4):1291–300.

4. Montesinos-Rongen M, Schmitz R, Brunn A, Gesk S, Richter J, Hong K, et al. Mutations of CARD11 but not TNFAIP3 may activate the NF-kappaB pathway in primary CNS lymphoma. *Acta Neuropathologica*. 2010;120(4):529–35.

5. Fischer L, Korfel A, Pfeiffer S, Kiewe P, Volk HD, Cakiroglu H, et al. CXCL13 and CXCL12 in central nervous system lymphoma patients. *Clinical Cancer Research: An Official Journal of the American Association for Cancer Research*. 2009;15(19):5968–73.

6. Abrey LE, Ben-Porat L, Panageas KS, Yahalom J, Berkey B, Curran W, et al. Primary central nervous system lymphoma: the Memorial Sloan-Kettering Cancer Center prognostic model. *Journal of Clinical Oncology: Official Journal of the American Society of Clinical Oncology*. 2006;24(36):5711–5.

7. Ferreri AJ, Blay JY, Reni M, Pasini F, Spina M, Ambrosetti A, et al. Prognostic scoring system for primary CNS lymphomas: the International Extranodal Lymphoma Study Group experience. *Journal of Clinical Oncology: Official Journal of the American Society of Clinical Oncology*. 2003;21(2):266–72.

8. Rubenstein JL, Hsi ED, Johnson JL, Jung SH, Nakashima MO, Grant B, et al. Intensive chemotherapy and immunotherapy in patients with newly diagnosed primary CNS lymphoma: CALGB 50202 (Alliance 50202). *Journal of Clinical Oncology: Official Journal of the American Society of Clinical Oncology*. 2013;31(25):3061–8.

9. Reni M, Ferreri AJ, Guha-Thakurta N, Blay JY, Dell'Oro S, Biron P, et al. Clinical relevance of consolidation radiotherapy and other main therapeutic issues in primary central nervous system lymphomas treated with upfront high-dose methotrexate. *International Journal of Radiation Oncology, Biology, Physics*. 2001;51(2):419–25.

10. Blay JY, Conroy T, Chevreau C, Thyss A, Quesnel N, Eghbali H, et al. High-dose methotrexate for the treatment of primary cerebral lymphomas: analysis of survival and late neurologic toxicity in a retrospective series. *Journal of Clinical Oncology: Official Journal of the American Society of Clinical Oncology*. 1998;16(3):864–71.

11. Gerstner ER, Carson KA, Grossman SA, Batchelor TT. Long-term outcome in PCNSL patients treated with high-dose methotrexate and deferred radiation. *Neurology*. 2008;70(5):401–2.

12. Ferreri AJ, Reni M, Foppoli M, Martelli M, Pangalis GA, Frezzato M, et al. High-dose cytarabine plus high-dose methotrexate versus high-dose methotrexate alone in patients with primary CNS lymphoma: a randomised phase 2 trial. *Lancet*. 2009;374(9700):1512–20.

13. Morris PG, Correa DD, Yahalom J, Raizer JJ, Schiff D, Grant B, et al. Rituximab, methotrexate, procarbazine, and vincristine followed by consolidation reduced-dose whole-brain radiotherapy and cytarabine in newly diagnosed primary CNS lymphoma: final results and long-term outcome. *Journal of Clinical Oncology: Official Journal of the American Society of Clinical Oncology*. 2013;31(31):3971–9.

14. Khan RB, Shi W, Thaler HT, DeAngelis LM, Abrey LE. Is intrathecal methotrexate necessary in the treatment of primary CNS lymphoma? *Journal of Neuro-Oncology*. 2002;58(2):175–8.

15. Rubenstein JL, Li J, Chen L, Advani R, Drappatz J, Gerstner E, et al. Multicenter phase 1 trial of intraventricular immunochemotherapy in recurrent CNS lymphoma. *Blood*. 2013;121(5):745–51.

16. DeAngelis LM, Seiferheld W, Schold SC, Fisher B, Schultz CJ, Radiation Therapy Oncology Group S. Combination chemotherapy and radiotherapy for primary central nervous system lymphoma: Radiation Therapy Oncology Group Study 93-10. *Journal of Clinical Oncology: Official Journal of the American Society of Clinical Oncology*. 2002;20(24):4643–8.

17. Thiel E, Korfel A, Martus P, Kanz L, Griesinger F, Rauch M, et al. High-dose methotrexate with or without whole brain radiotherapy for primary CNS lymphoma (G-PCNSL-SG-1): a phase 3, randomised, non-inferiority trial. *The Lancet Oncology*. 2010;11(11):1036–47.

18. Abrey LE, Moskowitz CH, Mason WP, Crump M, Stewart D, Forsyth P, et al. Intensive methotrexate and cytarabine followed by high-dose chemotherapy with autologous stem-cell rescue in patients with newly diagnosed primary CNS lymphoma: an intent-to-treat analysis. *Journal of Clinical Oncology: Official Journal of the American Society of Clinical Oncology*. 2003;21(22):4151–6.

19. Colombat P, Lemevel A, Bertrand P, Delwail V, Rachieru P, Brion A, et al. High-dose chemotherapy with autologous stem cell transplantation as first-line therapy for primary CNS lymphoma in patients younger than 60 years: a multicenter phase II study of the GOELAMS group. *Bone Marrow Transplantation*. 2006;38(6):417–20.

20. Illerhaus G, Marks R, Ihorst G, Guttenberger R, Ostertag C, Derigs G, et al. High-dose chemotherapy with autologous stem-cell transplantation and hyperfractionated radiotherapy as first-line treatment of primary CNS lymphoma. *Journal of Clinical Oncology: Official Journal of the American Society of Clinical Oncology*. 2006;24(24):3865–70.

21. Illerhaus G, Muller F, Feuerhake F, Schafer AO, Ostertag C, Finke J. High-dose chemotherapy and autologous stem-cell transplantation without consolidating radiotherapy as first-line treatment for primary lymphoma of the central nervous system. *Haematologica*. 2008;93(1):147–8.

22. Kasenda B, Schorb E, Fritsch K, Finke J, Illerhaus G. Prognosis after high-dose chemotherapy followed by autologous stem-cell transplantation as first-line treatment in primary CNS lymphoma–a long-term follow-up study. *Annals of Oncology: Official Journal of the*

European Society for Medical Oncology/ESMO. 2012;23(10):2670–5.

23. Montemurro M, Kiefer T, Schuler F, Al-Ali HK, Wolf HH, Herbst R, et al. Primary central nervous system lymphoma treated with high-dose methotrexate, high-dose busulfan/thiotepa, autologous stem-cell transplantation and response-adapted whole-brain radiotherapy: results of the multicenter Ostdeutsche Studiengruppe Hamato-Onkologie OSHO-53 phase II study. *Annals of Oncology: Official Journal of the European Society for Medical Oncology/ESMO.* 2007;18(4):665–71.

24. Hassan M, Ehrsson H, Smedmyr B, Totterman T, Wallin I, Oberg G, et al. Cerebrospinal fluid and plasma concentrations of busulfan during high-dose therapy. *Bone Marrow Transplantation.* 1989;4(1):113–4.

25. Heideman RL, Cole DE, Balis F, Sato J, Reaman GH, Packer RJ, et al. Phase I and pharmacokinetic evaluation of thiotepa in the cerebrospinal fluid and plasma of pediatric patients: evidence for dose-dependent plasma clearance of thiotepa. *Cancer Research.* 1989;49(3):736–41.

26. Wiebe VJ, Smith BR, DeGregorio MW, Rappeport JM. Pharmacology of agents used in bone marrow transplant conditioning regimens. *Critical Reviews in Oncology/Hematology.* 1992;13(3):241–70.

27. Soussain C, Hoang-Xuan K, Taillandier L, Fourme E, Choquet S, Witz F, et al. Intensive chemotherapy followed by hematopoietic stem-cell rescue for refractory and recurrent primary CNS and intraocular lymphoma: Societe Francaise de Greffe de Moelle Osseuse-Therapie Cellulaire. *Journal of Clinical Oncology: Official Journal of the American Society of Clinical Oncology.* 2008;26(15):2512–8.

28. Chen YB, Batchelor T, Li S, Hochberg E, Brezina M, Jones S, et al. Phase 2 trial of high-dose rituximab with high-dose cytarabine mobilization therapy and high-dose thiotepa, busulfan, and cyclophosphamide autologous stem cell transplantation in patients with central nervous system involvement by non-Hodgkin lymphoma. *Cancer.* 2015;121(2):226–33.

29. Boehme V, Schmitz N, Zeynalova S, Loeffler M, Pfreundschuh M. CNS events in elderly patients with aggressive lymphoma treated with modern chemotherapy (CHOP-14) with or without rituximab: an analysis of patients treated in the RICOVER-60 trial of the German High-Grade Non-Hodgkin Lymphoma Study Group (DSHNHL). *Blood.* 2009;113(17):3896–902.

30. Schmitz N, Zeynalova S, Nickelsen M, Kansara R, Villa D, Sehn LH, et al. CNS international prognostic index: A risk model for CNS relapse in patients with diffuse large B-cell lymphoma treated with R-CHOP. *Journal of Clinical Oncology: Official Journal of the American Society of Clinical Oncology.* 2016;34(26):3150–6.

31. Bernstein SH, Unger JM, Leblanc M, Friedberg J, Miller TP, Fisher RI. Natural history of CNS relapse in patients with aggressive non-Hodgkin's lymphoma: a 20-year follow-up analysis of SWOG 8516 – the Southwest Oncology Group. *Journal of Clinical Oncology: Official Journal of the American Society of Clinical Oncology.* 2009;27(1):114–9.

32. Tilly H, Lepage E, Coiffier B, Blanc M, Herbrecht R, Bosly A, et al. Intensive conventional chemotherapy (ACVBP regimen) compared with standard CHOP for poor-prognosis aggressive non-Hodgkin lymphoma. *Blood.* 2003;102(13):4284–9.

33. Abramson JS, Hellmann M, Barnes JA, Hammerman P, Toomey C, Takvorian T, et al. Intravenous methotrexate as central nervous system (CNS) prophylaxis is associated with a low risk of CNS recurrence in high-risk patients with diffuse large B-cell lymphoma. *Cancer.* 2010;116(18):4283–90.

34. Bromberg JE, Doorduijn JK, Illerhaus G, Jahnke K, Korfel A, Fischer L, et al. Central nervous system recurrence of systemic lymphoma in the era of stem cell transplantation: an International Primary Central Nervous System Lymphoma Study Group project. *Haematologica.* 2013;98(5):808–13.

35. Cote GM, Hochberg EP, Muzikansky A, Hochberg FH, Drappatz J, McAfee SL, et al. Autologous stem cell transplantation with thiotepa, busulfan, and cyclophosphamide (TBC) conditioning in patients with CNS involvement by non-Hodgkin lymphoma. *Biology of Blood and Marrow Transplantation: Journal of the American Society for Blood and Marrow Transplantation.* 2012;18(1):76–83.

36. Korfel A, Elter T, Thiel E, Hanel M, Mohle R, Schroers R, et al. Phase II study of central nervous system (CNS)-directed chemotherapy including high-dose chemotherapy with autologous stem cell transplantation for CNS relapse of aggressive lymphomas. *Haematologica.* 2013;98(3):364–70.

37. Maziarz RT, Wang Z, Zhang MJ, Bolwell BJ, Chen AI, Fenske TS, et al. Autologous haematopoietic cell transplantation for non-Hodgkin lymphoma with secondary CNS involvement. *British Journal of Haematology.* 2013;162(5):648–56.

38. Soussain C, Suzan F, Hoang-Xuan K, Cassoux N, Levy V, Azar N, et al. Results of intensive chemotherapy followed by hematopoietic stem-cell rescue in 22 patients with refractory or recurrent primary CNS lymphoma or intraocular lymphoma. *Journal of Clinical Oncology: Official Journal of the American Society of Clinical Oncology.* 2001;19(3):742–9.

39. Williams CD, Pearce R, Taghipour G, Green ES, Philip T, Goldstone AH. Autologous bone marrow transplantation for patients with non-Hodgkin's lymphoma and CNS involvement: those transplanted with active CNS disease have a poor outcome–a report by the European Bone Marrow Transplant Lymphoma Registry. *Journal of Clinical Oncology: Official Journal of the American Society of Clinical Oncology.* 1994;12(11):2415–22.

40. Plotkin SR, Betensky RA, Hochberg FH, Grossman SA, Lesser GJ, Nabors LB, et al. Treatment of relapsed central nervous system lymphoma with high-dose methotrexate. *Clinical Cancer Research: An Official Journal of the American Association for Cancer Research.* 2004;10(17):5643–6.

41. Doolittle ND, Abrey LE, Shenkier TN, Tali S, Bromberg JE, Neuwelt EA, et al. Brain parenchyma involvement as isolated central nervous system relapse of systemic non-Hodgkin lymphoma: an International Primary CNS Lymphoma Collaborative Group report. *Blood.* 2008;111(3):1085–93.

42. Lotze C, Schuler F, Kruger WH, Hirt C, Kirsch M, Vogelgesang S, et al. Combined immunoradiotherapy induces long-term remission of CNS relapse of peripheral, diffuse, large-cell lymphoma after allogeneic stem cell

transplantation: case study. *Neuro-oncology*. 2005;7(4):508–10.

43. Varadi G, Or R, Kapelushnik J, Naparstek E, Nagler A, Brautbar C, *et al*. Graft-*versus*-lymphoma effect after allogeneic peripheral blood stem cell transplantation for primary central nervous system lymphoma. *Leukemia & Lymphoma*. 1999;34(1–2):185–90.

44. Saad AG, Alyea EP, 3rd, Wen PY, Degirolami U, Kesari S. Graft-*versus*-host disease of the CNS after allogeneic bone marrow transplantation. *Journal of Clinical Oncology: Official Journal of the American Society of Clinical Oncology*. 2009;27(30):e147–9.

45. Kickingereder P, Wiestler B, Sahm F, Heiland S, Roethke M, Schlemmer HP, *et al*. Primary central nervous system lymphoma and atypical glioblastoma: multiparametric differentiation by using diffusion-, perfusion-, and susceptibility-weighted MR imaging. *Radiology*. 2014;272(3):843–50.

46. Maza S, Buchert R, Brenner W, Munz DL, Thiel E, Korfel A, *et al*. Brain and whole-body FDG-PET in diagnosis, treatment monitoring and long-term follow-up of primary CNS lymphoma. *Radiology and Oncology*. 2013;47(2):103–10.

47. Kasenda B, Haug V, Schorb E, Fritsch K, Finke J, Mix M, *et al*. 18F-FDG PET is an independent outcome predictor in primary central nervous system lymphoma. *Journal of Nuclear Medicine: Official Publication, Society of Nuclear Medicine*. 2013;54(2):184–91.

48. Treon SP, Cao Y, Xu L, Yang G, Liu X, Hunter ZR. Somatic mutations in MYD88 and CXCR4 are determinants of clinical presentation and overall survival in Waldenstrom macroglobulinemia. *Blood*. 2014;123(18):2791–6.

49. Grupp SA, Kalos M, Barrett D, Aplenc R, Porter DL, Rheingold SR, *et al*. Chimeric antigen receptor-modified T cells for acute lymphoid leukemia. *The New England Journal of Medicine*. 2013;368(16):1509–18.

Chapter

46

Autologous Hematopoietic Cell Transplants for Plasma Cell Myeloma: One, Two, or None?

Jesus F. San Miguel, Juan J. Lahuerta, Laura Rosiñol,
María Victoria Mateos, and Joan Bladé

Introduction

Multiple myeloma (MM) is the most common malignant plasma cell disorder with an incidence of 4–5 new cases per 100 000 individuals/year. Since Blokhin *et al.* published in 1958 the clinical experience with sarcolysin (melphalan) in neoplastic diseases[1], including activity in multiple myeloma, no other antimyeloma effective drug was discovered in the subsequent 40 years. In fact, the combination of melphalan and prednisone introduced by Bergsagel and Alexanian[2] in the 1960s remained as the standard of care until recently, since more complex chemotherapy combinations, such as VCMP, VBMCP, VBAD, and VAD (vincristine, doxorubicin, and dexamethasone), resulted in small increases in the overall response rate (RR) without significant differences in survival, as demonstrated in a large meta-analysis including over 6000 patients[3]. In fact, the only major step forward in myeloma treatment, until the recent development of drugs with novel mechanism of action, such as thalidomide, as the first immunomodulatory agent[4], and bortezomib, as the first proteasome inhibitor[5], was the use of high-dose melphalan followed by autograft for young myeloma patients[6]. In this transplant setting it was recognized early on that long-term use of melphalan was associated with a detrimental effect on hematopoietic cell (HC) collection, and alkylator-free regimens, such as VAD, (vincristine, adriamycin, dexamethasone), soon gained popularity as debulking regimes before autologous hematopoietic cell transplant (auto-HCT)[7]. In order to maintain the responses obtained following auto-HCT the concept of maintenance therapy was introduced, and interferon (+/− prednisone) was adopted as standard maintenance although the survival benefit was limited with about a median of 6 months gain[8]. Altogether, the above indicates that the philosophy of "induction→auto-HCT→maintenance" was already introduced at the end of the 1990s. Although in most European studies, the cut-off age for eligibility for auto-HCT was 65 years, outside the context of clinical trials auto-HCT is an option up to the age of 70, if the patient is in good clinical condition[9]. In most US transplant centers there is no specific age exclusion for auto-HCT, though for patients over age 70, a reduced melphalan dose is commonly used but the benefit is questionable.

In this article we will first briefly review (1) the results of randomized trials comparing auto-HCT *versus* chemotherapy that represented the basis for myeloma being the most common indication for auto-HCT in North America and Europe. Subsequently, we will try to answer the following questions: (2) What are the optimal induction regimens? (3) Does auto-HCT upgrade the depth of response in the era of new induction regimens or not, and what is the best high-dose regimen? (4) What is the role of consolidation and maintenance after auto-HCT? (see Chapter 47); and finally (5) What is the role of single, tandem, and delayed auto-HCT?

Autologous HCT *versus* Conventional Chemotherapy: The Basis for the Expanded Use of Auto-HCT

Eight randomized trials[10–17] have compared auto-HCT, usually based on melphalan 200 mg/m^2 (MEL200) followed by auto-HCT *versus* conventional chemotherapy. In all but one the auto-HCT was associated with a significant increase in complete or very good partial response (CR/VGPR), as well as in event-free survival (EFS), but there was a significant prolongation in overall survival (OS) in only three of them.

The studies conducted by the French (IFM90)[10] and English (MRC VII)[13] groups as well as in the Italian M97G trial[18] were the three positive ones in terms of OS and provided evidence for survivorship beyond 10 years from auto-HCT in at least a subset of patients. By contrast, in the US study (SWOG 9321)[11], the French MAG91 study[15], and the Spanish PETHEMA-94[12] trials, although they confirmed the benefit of auto-HCT in terms of response and EFS, auto-HCT did not result in a significant longer OS as compared to conventional chemotherapy (Table 46.1). These discrepancies can be, at least in part, explained by: (1) differences in the studies' design (the Spanish study only randomized patients responding to initial therapy while, in the others, randomization was performed upfront), (2) differences in the conditioning regimens, and (3) differences in the intensity and duration of the chemotherapy arm (the dose of alkylating agents and steroids was higher in the SWOG and Spanish trials, which may explain why OS for conventionally treated patients was longer in these two studies as compared to the

Table 46.1 Randomized trials comparing autologous hematopoietic cell transplant *versus* conventional chemotherapy

Reference	Trial	Patients	CR(%)		EFS (months)		OS (months)	
			Auto-HCT	CT	Auto-HCT	CT	Auto-HCT	CT
Attal,NEJM 1996;335:9–97	IFM90	200	22 $P<0.001$	5	28 $P=0.01$	18	57 $P=0.03$	37
Fermand, Blood 1998;92:3131–6	MAG-90[a]	185	18 NA	5	39 NA	13	64 $P=0.9$	64
Seregen, Blood 2003;101:2144–51	HOVON	261	29 $P=0.002$	13	21 NS	22	50 NS	47
Child, NEJM 2003;348:1875–83	MRC VII	401	44 $P<0.001$	9	31 $P<0.001$	20	55 $P=0.04$	42
Palumbo, Blood 2004;104:3052–7	IMMSG	194	25[b] $P=0.05$	8[b]	28 $P<0.0001$	16	NR, 3-year 77% $P=0.0005$	43
Fermand, JCO 2005;23:9227–33	MAG-91	190	36 NA	20	25 $P=0.07$	19	48/47 NS	47
Blade, Blood 2005;106:3755–59[a]	PETHEMA	185	30 $P=0.002$	11	42 NS	34	67 NS	65
Barlogie, JCO 2006;24:929–36	USIG-9321	516	17 NS	15	25 NS	21	58 NS	53

[a] Nonstandard study, + significant benefits for high-dose therapy regimens.
[b] % of near complete remissions.
Auto-HCT: autologous hematopoietic cell transplant , CT: chemotherapy, NA: data not available, NS: no statistically significant, NR: not reached.

IFM and MRC trials). In spite of these controversial results, auto-HCT was assumed as the standard of care for younger patients in multiple myeloma, mainly based on the benefit in terms of response rate and EFS[19].

A large study of long follow-up, which included studies from European and US cooperative groups and institutions and pooled data from more than 10000 MM patients diagnosed between 1982 and 2002[20], showed an important significant reduction in risk of death among patients treated with auto-HCT compared to those who received standard chemotherapy. In parallel, long follow-up of population-based studies has detected a clear increase in MM survival associated with the introduction of auto-HCT in the therapeutic armamentarium of MM[21].

Practice Points

In aggregate, the long-term results show a survival superiority of auto-HCT *versus* conventional chemotherapy and accordingly auto-HCT represents a landmark in the therapeutic history of MM.

What are the Optimal Induction Regimens Prior to Auto-HCT?

Prior to initiation of HCs collection, patients receive induction therapy for 3–6 cycles, with the intent of disease debulking, and improvement in the end-organ damage that was the reason for initiation of therapy. Until recently the combination of vincristine, doxorubicin, and dexamethasone (VAD) has been the gold standard as a preparatory regimen for young newly diagnosed MM candidates for auto-HCT[7], with partial response (PR) rates ranging between 52% and 63%, and CR rates between 3% and 13%. However, novel drug combinations are superior to VAD or VAD-like regimens for initial tumor reduction. Thus, three randomized trials[22–24] have compared thalidomide (T)-based regimens (TAD, T+VAD, or cyclophosphamide (C)TD) *versus* VAD as initial therapy in transplant-eligible patients, and have shown superiority for the triplets of thalidomide combinations with approximately 80% > PR, including 10–20% CR (Table 46.2). By contrast the efficacy of thalidomide plus dexamethasone is in the range of that of VAD. In studies evaluating bortezomib (Bz) combination therapy, data from a French randomized trial comparing BzD *versus* VAD, and the HOVON trial comparing BzAD (PAD) *versus* VAD showed superiority to Bz regimens with >80% PR and 10–30% CR. The Italian[25] and Spanish[26] groups have reported that the triplet BzTD (VTD) is significantly superior to TD both before and after transplant and this triple combination appears to be also superior to BzDd (Table 46.2). Moreover, VTD was not only associated with higher responses but also with a significant prolongation in PFS, reaching a median of 56 months in the Spanish study. Another effective debulking regimen widely used is BzCD (VCD or CyBorD); however, it is probably slightly inferior to VTD as it has been recently shown in a French prospective trial [27] that showed a higher rate of VGPR: 70% *versus* 60% for

Table 46.2 Response obtained with novel induction regimens in randomized trials

Reference	Regimen	Patients	Response	
			>PR (%)	CR+ nCR (%)
Rajkumar, JCO 2008;26(13):2171–7	TD versus D	470	63 versus 46	7.7 versus 2.6
Lokhorst, Blood 2010;115:1113–20	TAD versus VAD	400	72 versus 54	7 versus 3
Zervas, Ann Oncol 2007;18:1369–75	T+VAD versus VAD	230	81 versus 66	
Morgan, Clin Cancer Res 2013;19:6030–8	CTD versus CVAD	254	87 versus 75	19 versus 9
Harousseau, JCO 2010;28:4621–9	BzDx versus VA	486	82 versus 65	15 versus 7
Cavo, Lancet, 2010;376:2075–85	BzTD versus TD	256	94 versus 79	32 versus 12
Rosiñol, Blood 2012;120:1589–96	BzTD/TD/QBz	173	80/66/78	30/20/6
Sonnoveld, JCO 2012;30:2946–55	BzAD versus VAD	300	83 versus 59	5 versus 1
Rajkumar, Lancet 2010;11:29–37	LD versus Len-d	485	82 versus 71	4 versus 2
Zonder, Blood 2010;116:5838–41	LD versus D	198	85 versus 71	22 versus 4

Bz: bortezomib, T: thalidomide, D: dexamethasone, d: dexamethasone low doses, L: lenalidomide, C: cyclophosphamide, V: vincristine, A: adriamycin (doxorubicin), Q: chemotherapy, nCR: near complete response; PR: partial response.

VTD, respectively. These results have been confirmed in a retrospective trial conducted by the Italian group[38]. Regarding lenalidomide (L), two large randomized[28,29] studies have shown that the majority of patients (>85%) respond to LD induction, but probably a minimum of six cycles would be required to achieve a substantial number of CR. Recent data using BzLD (VRD) indicate that most patients (>90%) achieve at least PR with over 20% stringent CR (sCR) [27]. Moreover, a randomized trial comparing BzLD versus Ld, presented by Durie at the ASH 2015 meeting (Abstr 25) has shown a highly significant superiority for the triplet combination in terms of CR rate (15.7% versus 8.4%) PFS (43 versus 30 months) and OS (75 versus 64 months).

A recent meta-analysis of four European randomized trials (IFM, HOVON/GMMG, PETHEMA/GEM and GIMEMA), including 1572 patients[30], supports the use of Bz-containing regimens as induction therapy before auto-HCT. Bortezomib-based regimens were superior to non-bortezomib-based regimens in terms of response rate, EFS, and OS. Thus, CR rate pretransplant was 14% versus 4% and the CR rate post-transplant was 26% versus 14% for bortezomib-based and non-bortezomib-based regimens, respectively. The PFS was 35.9 months versus 28.6 months (P<0.001) and the 3-year OS was 79% versus 74% (P=0.04) (median not reached) in favor of the Bz-based regimens.

It should be noted also that the achievement of high-quality responses when using Bz-containing regimens are related to dose intensity and duration of the induction. Thus, the CR rate with PAD at reduced doses of Bz was only 11% versus 24% in a trial with PAD at a standard dose[31]. In addition, the CR rate in the Spanish study with six induction cycles of VTD is 35% versus only 19% in the Italian study[32] with three induction cycles. In fact, 60% of the patients who achieved CR in the Spanish trial achieved it beyond the first three cycles.

Similar efficacy, if not higher, has been reported in pilot studies for the combination of carfilzomib (second-generation proteasome inhibitor) with lenalidomide plus dexamethasone, with up to 50% CR rate[33]. The combination of carfilzomib with thalidomide and dexamethasone has also been tested with promising results[34].

Two-, Three- or Four-Drug Therapy Combinations as Induction Therapy in MM?

While there has been considerable controversy about whether a doublet regimen (BzD, LD, TD) or a triplet regimen (VTD, VRD, VCD, PAD) should be used for induction, most investigators now agree that triplets are more effective than doublets since they induce a higher VGPR/CR rate before auto-HCT and this is associated with improved survival. This does not necessarily mean that if patients do not achieve a VGPR following induction the treatment should be changed before proceeding to transplant (with the exception of those that achieve <PR, which should be considered as primary refractory and may benefit from a rescue regimen prior to high-dose melphalan). In any event, one should choose the induction regimen with the highest likelihood of achieving a VGPR or better. In this context it should be noted that in the PETHEMA/GEM05MENOS65 study[26] our initial observation that VTD induced higher CR rates as compared to TD and VBMCP/VBAD/Bz can now also be expanded to a higher proportion of minimal residual disease (MRD) negative cases before auto-HCT (unpublished data).

Four-drug combinations have also been investigated. However, the results of the EVOLUTION study[35] comparing VDCR versus VDR versus VDC, a phase 2 trial testing the efficacy of VTD plus cyclophosphamide, or the CYCLONE study[36], investigating the combination of carfilzomib,

Table 46.3 Response before and after autologous hematopoietic cell transplant in randomized trials

Reference	Regimen	% Complete responses and near CR	
		Pre auto-HCT	Post first auto-HCT
Cavo, Lancet 2010;376:2075–85	TD	5	38
Rosiñol, Blood 2012;120:1589–96	TD	14	24
Lokhorst, Blood 2010;115:1113–20	TAD	4	31
Harousseau, JCO 2010;28:4621–9	BzD	15	35
Cavo , Lancet 2010;376:2075–85	BzTD	19	55
Rosiñol, Blood 2012;120:1589–96	BzTD	35	46
Sonneveld, JCO 2012;30:2946–55	BzAD	11	30

cyclophosphamide, thalidomide, and dexamethasone, have been disappointing, with an increased toxicity with no significant benefit in response rate.

Regarding the influence of novel drugs on HC collection, thalidomide or bortezomib combinations did not affect stem cell collection or post-transplant blood counts recovery. For lenalidomide, initial reports indicated a decrease in CD34+ cells harvested[37], but if collection is performed after no more than 3–4 cycles, the numbers of HCs are adequate for one or two transplants.

In summary, the current results show that with triple combinations such as VTD or VRD >90% of MM patients will respond and at least a third will achieve CR after 4–6 cycles being at an optimal situation for auto-HCT. Similar results can be achieved when BzD is associated with cyclophosphamide or doxorubicin but the depth of response may be a bit lower. In fact, as mentioned above, a recent meta-analysis[38] comparing VTD *versus* VCD showed a significantly higher CR/nCR (34% *versus* 6%, P=0.002) as well as higher VGPR or better (62% *versus* 27%, P<0.001) with VTD. In addition, the superiority of carfilzomib-dexamethasone over bortezomib-dexamethasone in relapsing patients would support the investigation of carfilzomib-lenalidomide-dexamethasone as an alternative to VRD or VTD. Finally, monoclonal antibodies, particularly anti CD38, such as daratumumab are showing impressive efficacy in the relapsed setting in combination with either bortezomib or lenalidomide. Accordingly, we can hyphothesize that a cuadruplet combination with anti CD38 plus VRD or Carfilzomib-RD may become the optimal induction regimen.

Practice Points

Taking all this information together at present we recommend 4–6 cycles of induction (with HC collected after cycle 3 or 4) with a triplet that includes a proteasome inhibitor plus an immunomodulatory drug (IMiD) and dexamethasone; we would keep the alkylator for use at high dose in the conditioning regimen. In the near future anti CD38 would probably be added in the induction schemes. It should be emphasized that

prolonged induction may result in difficulties of collecting adequate numbers of hematopoietic progenitor cells.

Does Auto-HCT Upgrade the Depth of Response in the Era of New Induction Regimens: Is It Possible to Optimize the Conditioning Regimen?

In the setting of novel agents it is important to define whether or not auto-HCT enhances the response rates obtained with these new induction regimens. Table 46.3 summarizes the CR or near CR rates before and after transplant in randomized studies using novel agents as induction therapy[22,26,30,39,40]. All of them consistently showed an increase in CR following auto-HCT (Table 46.3). These data suggest that induction with novel agents and auto-HCT are complementary rather than alternative treatment approaches. Moreover, in the PETHEMA/ GEM05MENOS65 trial we have investigated the MRD kinetics before and after auto-HCT. Minimal residual disease (MRD)-negative rates increased 2.7-, 1.6-, and 1.5-fold in patients randomized to TD, VBMCP/VBAD/Bz, and VTD, respectively, suggesting that even in more effective combinations (e.g., VTD) MEL200 was able to eradicate MRD among a substantial proportion of patients that were already in CR after induction (unpublished data).

The next question is the possibility of optimizing the conditioning regimen used prior to auto-HCT. MEL200 is considered the gold standard conditioning regimen. The IFM randomized trial[41] confirmed that patients receiving MEL200 displayed a better median OS as compared to patients treated with melphalan 140 mg/m^2 in combination with TBI (65% *versus* 45% survival at 45 months). Other studies using intensification of the melphalan doses or addition of alkylating agents have not demonstrated significant improvement either in terms of response rate or in outcome. The exception to this latter statement are the data recently reported by the Spanish group[42] showing that although the combination of oral busulfan and melphalan (BuMel) was equivalent to MEL200 in terms of PFS during the first 2 years, subsequently the survival curves separated with a significant long-term benefit for the BuMel arm (PFS: 41 *versus* 31 months, *P*=0.009). This may be due to the potential effect of busulfan on myeloma progenitor cells. However, this trial was stopped because BuMel with oral busulfan resulted in an unacceptable toxicity with a high incidence of veno-occlusive disease (VOD) and transplant-related mortality (TRM). With the use of intravenous busulfan the incidence of VOD is drastically reduced and a randomized trial by the Spanish group is ongoing in order to confirm these results. Several pilot studies are investigating the addition of bortezomib to melphalan using different doses and schedules. In a phase 1 trial investigating the bortezomib dose (1–1.6 mg/m^2) and sequence (24 hours before or 24 hours after melphalan administration), the combination of MEL200 along with the aforementioned bortezomib dose and schedule resulted in a PR rate or better of 93%, with a toxicity profile and engraftment kinetics similar to that observed in an historical control receiving MEL200 alone[43]. The IFM group used bortezomib on days −6, −3, 1, and 4 along with MEL200 on day −2 in 35 patients with high-risk MM, and the results on engraftment and response were encouraging[44]. The results of these studies suggest that bortezomib can enhance the antitumor effect of melphalan, probably through the inhibition of DNA repair after melphalan-induced damage[45,46].

Finally, we should also emphasize that there are strategies to improve safety and maximize the effectiveness of melphalan, such as the use of a less toxic propylene glycol-free preparation, or by tailoring drug delivery to the individual patient, through knowledge of its pharmacokinetics and pharmacogenomics[47].

Practice Points

Current data indicate that induction with novel agents and auto-HCT are complementary rather than alternative treatment approaches, and that there is probably still room for improvement in the efficacy of conditioning regimens.

What is the Role of Consolidation and Maintenance after Auto-HCT?

Consolidation Therapy

Consolidation is a short treatment given after auto-HCT aiming to improve response or to induce deeper responses; while maintenance treatment (see Chapter 47) is given for a prolonged period of time to maintain response achieved following therapy. The Arkansas group was the first to demonstrate the efficacy of consolidation and maintenance therapies through their four consecutive total therapy programs with up to 50% long-term survivors[48]. More recently, Ladetto *et al.*[49] have shown that the use of four consolidation cycles of VTD (bortezomib, thalidomide, and dexamethasone), in patients in >VGPR after auto-HCT, increases the CR rate from 15% to 49%, and molecular remissions from 3% after

auto-HCT to 18% after VTD, a figure so far only reported with allogeneic transplant. The Italian randomized trial[32] that compares VTD *versus* TD both as induction and consolidation, in patients undergoing double auto-HCT, has also confirmed the efficacy of consolidation (the quality of the response improved in 55% of patients, with 5 log reduction in tumor burden by RQ-PCR). VTD upgraded the CR rate postconsolidation by 30% as compared with 16% with TD, with a 3-year PFS of 60% *versus* 48%. Moreover, the superior PFS with VTD over TD consolidation was maintained across poor prognosis subgroups (t(4;14) and/or del(17q), del(13q), β$_2$-M, LDH, International Staging System (ISS)).

Maintenance Therapy

Regarding maintenance (see Chapter 47), interferon and/or prednisone showed a median survival prolongation of around 6 months, but due to the toxicity they have been abandoned [8,50]. The availability of novel agents, particularly those in oral formulations (thalidomide and lenalidomide), has renewed the concept of maintenance in an attempt to prolong the duration of the responses after transplant. Seven randomized trials[22,23,51–55] have demonstrated a superiority of thalidomide maintenance (with or without prednisone) *versus* no maintenance or prednisone or interferon in terms of PFS; although in original publications only the two oldest trials showed improvements in OS[51,54], and in one trial concern was raised about whether the continuous use of thalidomide may induce more resistant relapses[23]. Nevertheless, when these studies were reanalyzed after longer follow-up, it was generally found that maintenance with thalidomide also improves survival[23,48,52,56,57], and meta-analyses of these trials[58–62] have confirmed that thalidomide prolongs PFS and OS with HR values of 0.6 and 0.8, respectively (approximately 6 months of benefit). However, the benefit of thalidomide maintenance for patients who are already in CR was not clear and results in those with poor cytogenetic profile are contradictory[23,52]. Additionally, the high dropout rate due to intolerance to thalidomide, mainly as a result of polyneuropathy, limits the applicability of this treatment.

As far as lenalidomide maintenance is concerned, two large randomized trials, one conducted by the IFM[63] and the other by the CALGB[64] groups, have investigated the role of lenalidomide maintenance. The first conclusion is that the tolerability is much better than with thalidomide. In addition, a highly significant benefit in terms of PFS has been reported for lenalidomide maintenance with respect to control arms in both trials (46 months *versus* 27 months in CALGB trial and 41 *versus* 23 months in IFM trial), and this translated into an OS advantage in the American but not in the French trial. A third Italian randomized trial[65] has explored the value of lenalidomide maintenance after induction with four cycles of lenalidomide–dexametasone followed by intensification with either six courses of lenalidomide, melphalan, and prednisone or melphalan 200 mg/m^2 (MEL200) supported

Table 46.4 Tandem *versus* single autologous transplants randomized trials

Reference	Trial	Patients	Median EFS (months)		Median OS (months)	
			Tandem	Single	Tandem	Single
Attal, N Engl J Med 2003;349:2495–502	IFM94	399	30 P=0.03	25	58 P=0.01	48
Fermand, Haematologica 2005;90:40	MAG95	227	34 NS	31	75 NS	57
Cavo, JCO 2007;25:2434–41	Bologna 96	321	35 P=0.001	23	75 NS	65
Goldschmidt , Haematologica 2005;90:38	GMMG-HD2	261	29 NS	25	77 NS	72
Einsele, Haematologica 2005;90:131	DSMM1	198	36 NS	43	NR NS	NR

NS: nonsignificant.

with auto-HCT. In a landmark analysis, lenalidomide maintenance was associated with a significant prolongation both in PFS (43 *versus* 18 months) and OS (4 years: 80% *versus* 62%). Maintenance with lenalidomide is associated with an increased risk of secondary malignancies; however this is outweighed by the survival benefit[66]. In recent meta-analysis of the three trials a significant benefit in OS was confirmed (62% *versus* 50% at 7 years) for patients receiving maintenance therapy, with an estimated 2.5 year increase in median survival; nevertheless patients with stage III or high-risk cytogenetics did not benefit from lenalidomide maintenance in terms of OS (unpublished data).

Bortezomib has been tested as maintenance therapy in two randomized trials. The HOVON-65 study[67,68], after induction with either PAD (bortezomib, doxorubicin, dexamethasone) or VAD (vincristine, doxorubicin, dexamethasone) followed by MEL200 with auto-HCT and maintenance with bortezomib in the PAD arm or thalidomide in the VAD arm, showed a significantly longer PFS and OS for patients treated with bortezomib. Although the results of bortezomib *versus* thalidomide maintenance in the HOVON-65 study cannot be isolated from induction, the increase of CR rate during maintenance with bortezomib (12%) or thalidomide (11%) was similar and a landmark analysis from start of maintenance for PFS did not show a significant difference between thalidomide and bortezomib maintenances. In the PETHEMA/GEM05MENOS65 trial[69], after auto-HCT, maintenance with bortezomib-thalidomide showed a significantly longer PFS (78% at 2 years) compared with thalidomide (63%) or interferon (49%), but without differences in OS.

Practice Points

Lenalidomide maintenance prolongs survival in transplanted patients providing, so far, the best results; nevertheless it could be speculated that the outcome could probably be improved by combination with low-dose corticosteroids or proteasome inhibitors in this setting.

Single, Tandem, or Auto-HCT Upfront or at Relapse?

Tandem Transplants

To improve the limited antitumor efficacy of available therapeutic agents in the era of conventional chemotherapy, The Arkansas group investigated the capacity of tandem auto-HCT to improve the outcome of myeloma patients. The first Total Therapy study[70] was based on a series of alternative induction treatments and two consecutive auto-HCT conditioning with MEL200 (tandem transplants), or MEL200→auto-HCT with a second allogeneic transplant if a HLA-match donor was available, followed by interferon maintenance. The tandem auto-HCT approach gained many adepts in subsequent years, and became almost standard of care in some centers until the introduction of novel agents and the possibility of efficient consolidation schemes. The analysis of accumulated experience tandem auto-HCT yields contradictory results. In a Cochrane systematic review of controlled studies[71] from 1995 to 2011, including five randomized trials[72–76] enrolling 1406 patients in total (Table 46.4), the median EFS prolongation with respect to a single auto-HCT ranged between 3 and 12 months in four of the five trials, while OS was statistically significantly improved in one trial only. A formal meta-analysis has not been possible due to the high clinical and methodologic heterogeneity between the trials examined. These results were not significantly different from those of a previous meta-analysis of six randomized trials[77], according to which patients treated with tandem auto-HCT *versus* single auto-HCT did not have longer OS (HR=0.94) or EFS (HR=0.86). Nevertheless, this latter meta-analysis has been criticized [78–80] because it included a randomized trial that used two cycles of attenuated nonablative doses of melphalan[81], as well as one retracted trial[82]; if these two latter trials are excluded, the EFS becomes longer in patients treated with

Table 46.5 Phase 3 trials comparing tandem HDT/AUTO-HCT *versus* HDT/AUTO-HCT followed by dose-reduced allograft

Reference	Trial	Patients	Median EFS/PFS (months) or % at years EFS/PFS		Median OS (months) or % at years OS	
			Tandem auto-HCT	AUTO-HCT/ allo-RIC	Tandem auto-HCT	Auto-HCT/ allo-RIC
Garban, Blood 2006;107:3474–80	IFM99-03	284	35 NS	32	42 P=0.07	35
Bruno, N Engl J Med 2007;356:1110–20	ITALIAN	162	29 P=0.02	35	54 P=0.01	80
Rosiñol, Blood 2008;112:3591–3	GEM2000	110	31 P=0.08	NR	58 NS	NR
Lokhorst, Blood 2012;119:6219-25	HOVON_50	260	6-year, 28% NS	6-year, 22%	6-year, 55% NS	6-year, 55%
Krishnan, Lancet Oncol 2011;12:1195–203	BMT CTN 0102	625	3-year, 46% NS	3-year, 43%	3-year, 80% NS	3-year, 77%
Gahrton, Blood 2013;121:5055–63	EBMT-NMAM2000	357	12 P=0.02	22	60 P=0.0002	82

NS, nonsignificant; NR, not reached.

tandem auto-HCT. Moreover, the results of the IFM trial[72] also indicated that tandem auto-HCT may be of differential benefit for distinct cohorts of patients; thus, it was more valuable in patients younger than 60 years, and those who have had a suboptimal response to a single transplant ($\leq$VGPR patients: 11% 7-year OS in single auto-HCT arm *versus* 43% in tandem auto-HCT arm, P=0.001). These results were confirmed by the Bologna 96 randomized trial[73], in which, although globally a second auto-HCT prolonged EFS but failed to prolong OS, those patients in $\leq$VGPR achieved both longer EFS (42 *versus* 22 months) and OS (7-year OS 60% *versus* 47%) with the tandem as compared with single auto-HCT.

As mentioned above the use of tandem auto-HCT has decreased in the last decade due to the apparent similar benefit that could be obtained upon using consolidation therapy with novel agents. Nevertheless, the value of tandem auto-HCT needs to be revisited in the era of novel agents. Thus, the BMT CTN 0702 trial comparing tandem auto-HCT *versus* single plus consolidation with VRD *versus* only single, including lenalidomide maintenance (for 3 years) in the three arms, has been completed and awaits results. Moreover, the recent information derived from a meta-analysis [39], including patients from the French, Italian, German, Dutch, and Spanish Cooperative Groups, suggests that patients with high-risk cytogenetics benefit more from tandem auto-HCT and that this procedure may, at least in part, abrogate the adverse prognosis of t(4;14) and deletion 17p. A second transplant at late relapse is being increasingly used, provided that the duration of the response to first transplant has lasted for at least 2 years. This consideration would support the collection of sufficient cells for multiple transplants at the time of initial harvest.

Practice Points

The role of tandem auto-HCT needs to be revisited in the era of novel agents, through randomized trials focusing on both patients with high- and standard-risk cytogenetics.

Tandem Auto-HCT and Allogeneic Transplantation

Six clinical trials[83–88] (Table 46.5) have compared double auto-HCT *versus* auto-HCT followed by an allogeneic HCT (allo-HCT) using reduced intensity conditioning regimens (RIC). Only two out of the six studies (GIMEMA and EBMT) showed a significant prolongation in PFS and OS with this approach. Differences in patient characteristics, graft-*versus*-host disease (GvHD) prophylaxis, and conditioning regimens could contribute to these discrepant results. Two meta-analyses[89,90] and a systematic review[91] confirm that although the allo therapeutic approach improves response rates compared to tandem auto-HCT, the mortality associated with the procedure neutralizes the potential benefits of a higher anti-tumor effect. It has been argued that evaluation of the efficacy of allotransplant should be done in the long term. Accordingly, a recent long-term follow-up analysis of the NMAM200 EBMT trial[84] (which did not show statistical differences in survival at the initial analysis), now shows, after a median follow-up of 7 years, a significant survival benefit for patients allocated to the auto-HCT/allo-HCT arm (at 96 months: PFS 22% *versus* 12%, OS 49% *versus* 36%). By contrast, the analysis of the HOVON-50 randomized trial[92] has failed to show improvement of tandem auto-HCT/allo-HCT as compared to single auto-HCT followed by thalidomide maintenance therapy even after a median follow-up of 90 months. Moreover, unfortunately, a high proportion of patients developed extramedullary relapses without bone marrow involvement, indicating that although the disease may be under control in the bone marrow milieu, extramedullary spread may occur. In any event, about 10–15% of patients undergoing an allogeneic transplant are cured.

Allogeneic Transplants as Rescue Therapy

Allogeneic HCT remains the only curative therapeutic approach in MM. However, it is associated with a high TRM of up to 15–40% and high morbidity, mainly due to chronic GvHD. In order to decrease TRM, different RIC regimens, mainly based on fludarabine and melphalan or fludarabine plus radiotherapy (2 Gy), have been introduced. The TRM decreases to 10–20% but this is associated with a higher incidence of relapses[93]. Accordingly, upfront allogeneic transplant should be performed only in the context of clinical trials in carefully defined patient populations.

With regard to the use of allo-HCT as rescue therapy[94,95], this can be an attractive option for patients having an early relapse after receiving an optimized induction regimen plus auto-HCT, particularly if they have high-risk cytogenetics. But, in any case a prerequisite is to obtain a CR or VGPR before the allotransplant since most patients with active disease will not benefit from this procedure. These transplants should be performed by experienced groups and within controlled clinical trials.

Practice Points

We do not recommend the use of allogeneic transplant upfront outside of clinical trials, and these should be restricted to high-risk patients. Nevertheless, the role of allo-HCT should be revisited in the era of novel drugs through integrated investigative programs.

Early or Delayed Auto-HCT

The timing of auto-HCT is now being challenged by the efficacy of continuous treatment with novel agents. Some investigators, particularly US based, consider that upfront transplants are challenged by the optimal results obtained with "long-term" treatment with novel agent combinations (i.e., bortezomib–lenalidomide–dexamethasone) and they propose to reserve the auto-HCT for the time of relapse[96,97]. In order to clarify this debate, several groups are testing these two alternatives through randomized trials. Data derived from the E4A03 clinical trial[98] investigating the use of lenalidomide with either high-dose or low-dose dexamethasone have shown that the patients who proceeded to auto-HCT achieved a superior OS compared to those who continued on primary therapy (3-year OS: 94% versus 78%). However, this was a retrospective subanalysis with potential bias. A recent preliminary report[99] pooled data from 791 patients enrolled in two alike prospective phase 3 randomized Italian trials[65,100] for newly diagnosed MM patients under 65 years, both using the same lenalidomide-dexamethasone induction followed by MEL200→ auto-HCT (early transplant) versus six cycles of conventional chemotherapy (melphalan or

cyclophosphamide) plus lenalidomide and steroids and, followed by lenalidomide-based regimens or placebo as maintenance. In both trials, patients assigned to the nontransplant arm were allowed to receive auto-HCT at relapse (delayed transplant). Early auto-HCT improved PFS1 (3-year rate: 59% versus 35%, $P < 0.001$) and PFS2 (3-year rate: 77% versus 68%, $P = 0.01$), and marginally OS (4-year rate: 83% versus 72%, $P = 0.09$) in comparison with delayed auto-HCT at relapse. At the ASH 2015 meeting (Abstr 391) Attal has presented the French data corresponding to the IFM/DFCI 2009 trial comparing early versus late transplant. The initial results indicate a significant benefit for early transplant in terms of VGPR (88% versus 78%) and PFS (43 versus 34 months) although no yet significant differences have been observed for OS.

Although current data favor the use of frontline auto-HCT even in the novel agent era, the final answer will come from the confirmation of the above-mentioned Italian and IFM/DFCI-2009 trials that seek to address the question of timing of transplant (early versus late) for patients receiving lenalidomide, bortezomib, and dexamethasone based induction in a prospective fashion.

Practice Points

Until the results from randomized trials become available we consider that upfront auto-HCT should remain as the standard of care based on the following arguments: (1) the patient at the initial phases of the disease is more fit (both physically and psychologically) to tolerate intensive and repetitive therapies; (2) auto-HCT is associated with a long treatment-free interval and excellent quality of life; (3) auto-HCT is no more expensive than the cost of novel agents; and (4) we know that relapses after auto-HCT are sensitive to rescue with novel agents, but we don't know the opposite scenario: how efficient MEL200 will be after long-term exposure to novel agents? Until this is answered through the randomized trials we should not embark our patients on uncontrolled alternative therapeutic approaches, unless the patient is reluctant to proceed to an upfront auto-HCT.

More Controversies in MM

Controversy #1: What Is the Role of Auto-HCT in the Era of Conventional Chemotherapy?

Although some of the trials comparing auto-HCT versus chemotherapy showed only differences in response rate and PFS, but not in OS, long-term follow-up analysis has consolidated auto-HCT as standard of care for patients with MM aged <65–70 years.

Controversy #2: What Are the Optimal Induction Regimens for Auto-HCT?

At present we recommend 4–6 cycles of induction based on a triplet that includes a proteasome inhibitor plus an IMiD and dexamethasone; we do not use alkylators to avoid HC damage and because high-dose melphalan will be included in the conditioning regimen for auto-HCT.

Controversy #3: Does Auto-HCT Upgrade the Depth of Response in the Era of New Induction Regimens? Is It Possible to Optimize the Conditioning Regimen?

Current data indicate that induction with novel agents and auto-HCT are complementary rather than alternative treatment approaches since HDT upgrades the quality of the response and prolongs PFS. Moreover, there is probably still room for improvement on the efficacy of conditioning regimens (through the addition of bortezomib or busulfan to melphalan).

Controversy #4: What Is the Role of Consolidation and Maintenance After Auto-HCT?

Consolidation improves CR rate and PFS. Lenalidomide maintenance prolongs PFS and OS in transplanted patients, and so far is the preferred maintenance option; nevertheless it could be speculated that the outcome will probably be improved by its combination with low-dose corticosteroids or proteasome inhibitors (see Chapter 47).

Controversy #5: One or Two Auto-HCT?

We do not recommend tandem auto-HCT outside of clinical trials with the potential exception of patients with "high-risk cytogenetics." Nevertheless, the role of tandem auto-HCT needs to be revisited in the era of novel agents, through randomized trials focusing on both patients with high and standard risk.

Controversy #6: What Is the Role of Tandem Auto-HCT→Allo-HCT?

We do not recommend the use of allo-HCT upfront outside of clinical trials, and these trials should be restricted to "high-risk" patients. Nevertheless, the role of allo-transplant should be revisited in the era of novel drugs through integrated investigative programs.

Controversy #7: Early or Delayed Autologous Transplant?

Until consolidated results from randomized trials become available we consider that upfront auto-HCT should remain as the standard of care.

Acknowledgments

This study was supported by the Cooperative Research Thematic Network grants RD12/0036/0058 and RD12/0036/0046 of the Red de Cancer (Cancer Network of Excellence); Instituto de Salud Carlos III, Spain, Instituto de Salud Carlos III/Subdirección General de Investigación Sanitaria (FIS: PI060339; 06/1354; 02/0905; 01/0089/01–02; PI12/01293, PS09/01, PS09/01897/01370; G03/136;); and Asociación Española Contra el Cáncer (GCB120981SAN), Spain. J.F.S.M, J.J.L., L.R., M.V.M, and J.B. designed and wrote the manuscript. All authors reviewed and approved the final version of the manuscript

Conflict of Interest

J.J.L. and L.R. have received honoraria from Janssen and Celgene. J.B. and M.V.M. have received honoraria for lectures and advisory boards from Janssen, Celgene, and Millenium. J.F.S.M. has received honoraria for lectures and advisory boards from Janssen, Millennium and Celgene, Novartis, and Amgen.

References

1. Blokhin N, Larionov L, Perevodchikova N, Chebotareva L, Merkulova N. Clinical experiences with sarcolysin in neoplastic diseases. *Ann N Y Acad Sci* 1958;68:1128–32.

2. Alexanian R, Bergsagel DE, Migliore PJ, Vaughn WK, Howe CD. Melphalan therapy for plasma cell myeloma. *Blood* 1968;31:1–10.

3. Group MTC. Combination Chemotherapy *versus* melphalan plus prednisone as treatment for multiple myeloma: An overwiev of 6.633 patients from 27 randomized studies. *J Clin Oncol* 1998; 16:3832–42.

4. Larkin M. Low-dose thalidomide seems to be effective in multiple myeloma. *Lancet* 1999;354:925.

5. Twombly R. First proteasome inhibitor approved for multiple myeloma. *J Natl Cancer Inst* 2003;95:845.

6. Gore ME, Selby PJ, Viner C, *et al.* Intensive treatment of multiple myeloma and criteria for complete remission. *Lancet* 1989;2:879–82.

7. Alexanian R, Dimopoulos M. The treatment of multiple myeloma. *N Engl J Med* 1994;330:484–9.

8. Myeloma Trialists' Collaborative Group. Interferon as therapy for multiple myeloma: an individual patient data overview of 24 randomized trials and 4012 patients. *Br J Haematol* 2001;113:1020–34.

9. Siegel DS, Desikan KR, Mehta J, *et al.* Age is not a prognostic variable with autotransplants for multiple myeloma. *Blood* 1999;93:51–4.

10. Attal M, Harousseau JL, Stoppa AM, *et al.* A prospective, randomized trial of autologous bone marrow transplantation and chemotherapy in multiple myeloma. Intergroupe Francais du Myelome. *N Engl J Med* 1996;335:91–7.

11. Barlogie B, Kyle RA, Anderson KC, *et al.* Standard chemotherapy compared with high-dose chemoradiotherapy for multiple myeloma: final results of phase III US Intergroup Trial S9321. *J Clin Oncol* 2006;24:929–36.

12. Blade J, Rosinol L, Sureda A, *et al.* High-dose therapy intensification

compared with continued standard chemotherapy in multiple myeloma patients responding to the initial chemotherapy: long-term results from a prospective randomized trial from the Spanish cooperative group PETHEMA. *Blood* 2005;106:3755–9.

13. Child JA, Morgan GJ, Davies FE, *et al.* High-dose chemotherapy with hematopoietic stem-cell rescue for multiple myeloma. *N Engl J Med* 2003;348:1875–83.

14. Fermand JP, Katsahian S, Divine M, *et al.* High-dose therapy and autologous blood stem-cell transplantation compared with conventional treatment in myeloma patients aged 55 to 65 years: long-term results of a randomized control trial from the Group Myelome-Autogreffe. *J Clin Oncol* 2005;23:9227–33.

15. Fermand JP, Ravaud P, Chevret S, *et al.* High-dose therapy and autologous peripheral blood stem cell transplantation in multiple myeloma: up-front or rescue treatment? Results of a multicenter sequential randomized clinical trial. *Blood* 1998;92:3131–6.

16. Palumbo A, Bringhen S, Petrucci MT, *et al.* Intermediate-dose melphalan improves survival of myeloma patients aged 50 to 70: results of a randomized controlled trial. *Blood* 2004;104:3052–7.

17. Segeren CM, Sonneveld P, van der Holt B, *et al.* Overall and event-free survival are not improved by the use of myeloablative therapy following intensified chemotherapy in previously untreated patients with multiple myeloma: a prospective randomized phase 3 study. *Blood* 2003;101:2144–51.

18. Palumbo A, Triolo S, Argentino C, *et al.* Dose-intensive melphalan with stem cell support (MEL100) is superior to standard treatment in elderly myeloma patients. *Blood* 1999;94:1248–53.

19. Koreth J, Cutler CS, Djulbegovic B, *et al.* High-dose therapy with single autologous transplantation *versus* chemotherapy for newly diagnosed multiple myeloma: A systematic review and meta-analysis of randomized controlled trials. *Biol Blood Marrow Transplant* 2007;13:183–96.

20. Ludwig H, Bolejack V, Crowley J, *et al.* Survival and years of life lost in different age cohorts of patients with multiple myeloma. *J Clin Oncol* 2010;28:1599–605.

21. Turesson I, Velez R, Kristinsson SY, Landgren O. Patterns of improved survival in patients with multiple myeloma in the twenty-first century: a population-based study. *J Clin Oncol* 2010;28:830–4.

22. Lokhorst HM, van der Holt B, Zweegman S, *et al.* A randomized phase 3 study on the effect of thalidomide combined with adriamycin, dexamethasone, and high-dose melphalan, followed by thalidomide maintenance in patients with multiple myeloma. *Blood* 2010;115:1113–20.

23. Morgan GJ, Davies FE, Gregory WM, *et al.* Long-term follow-up of MRC Myeloma IX trial: Survival outcomes with bisphosphonate and thalidomide treatment. *Clin Cancer Res* 2013;19:6030–8.

24. Zervas K, Mihou D, Katodritou E, *et al.* VAD-doxil *versus* VAD-doxil plus thalidomide as initial treatment for multiple myeloma: results of a multicenter randomized trial of the Greek Myeloma Study Group. *Ann Oncol* 2007;18:1369–75.

25. Cavo M, Tacchetti P, Patriarca F, *et al.* Bortezomib with thalidomide plus dexamethasone compared with thalidomide plus dexamethasone as induction therapy before, and consolidation therapy after, double autologous stem-cell transplantation in newly diagnosed multiple myeloma: a randomised phase 3 study. *Lancet* 2010;376:2075–85.

26. Rosinol L, Oriol A, Teruel AI, *et al.* Superiority of bortezomib, thalidomide, and dexamethasone (VTD) as induction pretransplantation therapy in multiple myeloma: a randomized phase 3 PETHEMA/GEM study. *Blood* 2012;120:1589–96.

27. Moreau P, Hulin C, Macro M, *et al.* VTD is superior to VCD prior to intensive therapy in multiple myeloma: results of the prospective IFM2013-04 trial. *Blood* 2016;127:2569–74.

28. Rajkumar SV, Jacobus S, Callander NS, *et al.* Lenalidomide plus high-dose dexamethasone *versus* lenalidomide plus low-dose dexamethasone as initial therapy for newly diagnosed multiple myeloma: an open-label randomised controlled trial. *Lancet Oncol* 2010;11:29–37.

29. Zonder JA, Crowley J, Hussein MA, *et al.* Lenalidomide and high-dose dexamethasone compared with

dexamethasone as initial therapy for multiple myeloma: a randomized Southwest Oncology Group trial (S0232). *Blood* 2010;116:5838–41.

30. Sonneveld P, Goldschmidt H, Rosinol L, *et al.* Bortezomib-based *versus* nonbortezomib-based induction treatment before autologous stem-cell transplantation in patients with previously untreated multiple myeloma: a meta-analysis of phase III randomized, controlled trials. *J Clin Oncol* 2013;31:3279–87.

31. Popat R, Oakervee HE, Hallam S, *et al.* Bortezomib, doxorubicin and dexamethasone (PAD) front-line treatment of multiple myeloma: updated results after long-term follow-up. *Br J Haematol* 2008;141:512–6.

32. Cavo M, Pantani L, Petrucci MT, *et al.* Bortezomib-thalidomide-dexamethasone is superior to thalidomide-dexamethasone as consolidation therapy after autologous hematopoietic stem cell transplantation in patients with newly diagnosed multiple myeloma. *Blood* 2013;120:9–19.

33. Jakubowiak AJ, Dytfeld D, Griffith KA, *et al.* A phase 1/2 study of carfilzomib in combination with lenalidomide and low-dose dexamethasone as a frontline treatment for multiple myeloma. *Blood* 2012;120:1801–9.

34. Sonneveld P, Asselberg-Hacker E, Zweegman S, *et al.* Dose escalation Phase 2 trial of Carfilzomib combined with thalidomide and low-dose dexamethason In newly diagnosed, transplant eligible patients with multiple myeloma. A trial of the European Myeloma Network. *Blood* 2013;122:688.

35. Kumar S, Flinn I, Richardson PG, *et al.* Randomized, multicenter, phase 2 study (EVOLUTION) of combinations of bortezomib, dexamethasone, cyclophosphamide, and lenalidomide in previously untreated multiple myeloma. *Blood* 2012;119:4375–82.

36. Reeder CB, Libby EN, Costa LJ, *et al.* A phase I/II trial of cyclophosphamide, carfilzomib, thalidomide and dexamethasone (CYCLONE) in patients with newly diagnosed multiple myeloma: final results of MTD expansion cohort. *Blood* 2013;122:3179.

37. Bhutani D, Zonder J, Valent J, *et al.* Evaluating the effects of lenalidomide induction therapy on peripheral stem

cells collection in patients undergoing autologous stem cell transplant for multiple myeloma. *Support Care Cancer* 2013;21:2437–42.

38. Cavo M, Pantani L, Pezzi A. Bortezomib-thalidomide-dexamethasone (VTD) is superior to bortezomib-cyclophosphamide-dexamethasone (VCD) as induction therapy prior to autologous stem cell transplantation in multiple myeloma. *Leukemia* 2015;29(12):2429 31.

39. Cavo M, Salwender H, Rosiñol L, *et al*. Double vs single autologous stem cell transplantation after bortezomib-based induction regimens for multiple myeloma: an integrated analysis of patient-level data from phase European III studies. *Blood* 2013;122:767.

40. Harousseau JL, Attal M, Avet-Loiseau H, *et al*. Bortezomib plus dexamethasone is superior to vincristine plus doxorubicin plus dexamethasone as induction treatment prior to autologous stem-cell transplantation in newly diagnosed multiple myeloma: results of the IFM 2005-01 phase III trial. *J Clin Oncol* 2010;28:4621–9.

41. Moreau P, Facon T, Attal M, *et al*. Comparison of 200 mg/m^2 melphalan and 8 Gy total body irradiation plus 140 mg/m^2 melphalan as conditioning regimens for peripheral blood stem cell transplantation in patients with newly diagnosed multiple myeloma: final analysis of the Intergroupe Francophone du Myelome 9502 randomized trial. *Blood* 2002;99:731–5.

42. Lahuerta JJ, Mateos MV, Martinez-Lopez J, *et al*. Busulfan 12 mg/kg plus melphalan 140 mg/m^2 *versus* melphalan 200 mg/m^2 as conditioning regimens for autologous transplantation in newly diagnosed multiple myeloma patients included in the PETHEMA/GEM2000 study. *Haematologica* 2010;95:1913–20.

43. Lonial S, Kaufman J, Tighiouart M, *et al*. A phase I/II trial combining high-dose melphalan and autologous transplant with bortezomib for multiple myeloma: a dose- and schedule-finding study. *Clin Cancer Res* 2010;16:5079–86.

44. Roussel M, Moreau P, Huynh A, *et al*. Bortezomib and high-dose melphalan as conditioning regimen before autologous stem cell transplantation in

patients with de novo multiple myeloma: a phase 2 study of the Intergroupe Francophone du Myelome (IFM). *Blood* 2010;115:32–7.

45. Lazarus HM, Phillips GL, Herzig RH, Hurd DD, Wolff SN, Herzig GP. High-dose melphalan and the development of hematopoietic stem-cell transplantation: 25 years later. *J Clin Oncol* 2008;26:2240–3.

46. Bayraktar UD, Bashir Q, Qazilbash M, Champlin RE, Ciurea SO. Fifty years of melphalan use in hematopoietic stem cell transplantation. *Biol Blood Marrow Transplant* 2013;19:344–56.

47. Shaw PJ, C.E. N, Lazarus HM. Not too little, not too much – just right! (Better ways to give high dose melphalan). *Bone Marrow Transplant* (in press).

48. Barlogie B, Attal M, Crowley J, *et al*. Long-term follow-up of autotransplantation trials for multiple myeloma: update of protocols conducted by the intergroupe francophone du myelome, southwest oncology group, and university of arkansas for medical sciences. *J Clin Oncol* 2010;28:1209–14.

49. Ladetto M, Pagliano G, Ferrero S, *et al*. Major tumor shrinking and persistent molecular remissions after consolidation with bortezomib, thalidomide, and dexamethasone in patients with autografted myeloma. *J Clin Oncol* 2010;28:2077–84.

50. Berenson JR, Crowley JJ, Grogan TM, *et al*. Maintenance therapy with alternate-day prednisone improves survival in multiple myeloma patients. *Blood* 2002;99:3163–8.

51. Attal M, Harousseau JL, Leyvraz S, *et al*. Maintenance therapy with thalidomide improves survival in patients with multiple myeloma. *Blood* 2006;108:3289–94.

52. Barlogie B, Pineda-Roman M, van Rhee F, *et al*. Thalidomide arm of Total Therapy 2 improves complete remission duration and survival in myeloma patients with metaphase cytogenetic abnormalities. *Blood* 2008;112:3115–21.

53. Maiolino A, Hungria VT, Garnica M, *et al*. Thalidomide plus dexamethasone as a maintenance therapy after autologous hematopoietic stem cell transplantation improves progression-free survival in multiple myeloma. *Am J Hematol* 2012;87:948–52.

54. Spencer A, Prince HM, Roberts AW, *et al*. Consolidation therapy with low-dose thalidomide and prednisolone prolongs the survival of multiple myeloma patients undergoing a single autologous stem-cell transplantation procedure. *J Clin Oncol* 2009;27:1788–93.

55. Stewart AK, Trudel S, Bahlis NJ, *et al*. A randomized phase 3 trial of thalidomide and prednisone as maintenance therapy after ASCT in patients with MM with a quality-of-life assessment: the National Cancer Institute of Canada Clinicals Trials Group Myeloma 10 Trial. *Blood* 2013;121:1517–23.

56. Kalff A, Kennedy N, Smiley A, *et al*. Thalidomide consolidation post autologous stem cell transplant (ASCT) for multiple myeloma (MM) is cost-effective with durable survival benefit at 5 years post randomisation: final analysis of the ALLG MM6 Study. *Blood* 2013;122:537.

57. Lokhorst H, Holt Bvd, Zweegman S, *et al*. Thalidomide combined with high dose melphalan improves event free and overall survival in patients with newly diagnosed multiple myeloma: extended follow-up of the HOVON-50 Trial. *Blood* 2013;122:3332.

58. Hahn-Ast C, von Lilienfeld-Toal M, van Heteren P, Mückter S, Brossart P, Glasmacher A. Improved progression-free and overall survival with thalidomide maintenance therapy after autologous stem cell transplantation in multiple myeloma: a metaanalyis of five randomized trials. *Haematologica* 2011;96:368.

59. Hicks LK, Haynes AE, Reece DE, *et al*. A meta-analysis and systematic review of thalidomide for patients with previously untreated multiple myeloma. *Cancer Treat Rev* 2008;34:442–52.

60. Kagoya Y, Nannya Y, Kurokawa M. Thalidomide maintenance therapy for patients with multiple myeloma: meta-analysis. *Leuk Res* 2012;36:1016–21.

61. Ludwig H, Durie BG, McCarthy P, *et al*. IMWG consensus on maintenance therapy in multiple myeloma. *Blood* 2012;119:3003–15.

62. Nooka AK, Behera M, Boise LH, Watson M, Kaufman JL, Lonial S. Thalidomide as maintenance therapy in multiple myeloma (MM) improves progression free survival (PFS) and

overall survival (OS): a meta-analysis. *ASH Annual Meeting Abstracts* 2011;118:1855.

63. Attal M, Lauwers-Cances V, Marit G, *et al.* Lenalidomide maintenance after stem-cell transplantation for multiple myeloma. *N Engl J Med* 2012;366:1782–91.

64. McCarthy PL, Owzar K, Hofmeister CC, *et al.* Lenalidomide after stem-cell transplantation for multiple myeloma. *N Engl J Med* 2012;366:1770–81.

65. Palumbo A, Cavallo F, Gay F, *et al.* Autologous transplantation and maintenance therapy in multiple myeloma. *N Engl J Med* 2014;371:895–905.

66. Palumbo A, Bringhen S, Kumar SK, *et al.* Second primary malignancies with lenalidomide therapy for newly diagnosed myeloma: a meta-analysis of individual patient data. *Lancet Oncol* 2014;15:333–42.

67. Sonneveld P, Schmidt-Wolf IG, van der Holt B, *et al.* Bortezomib induction and maintenance treatment in patients with newly diagnosed multiple myeloma: results of the randomized phase III HOVON-65/ GMMG-HD4 trial. *J Clin Oncol* 2012;30:2946–55.

68. Sonneveld P, Scheid C, van der Holt B, *et al.* Bortezomib induction and maintenance treatment improves survival in patients with newly diagnosed multiple myeloma:extended follow-up of the HOVON-65/GMMG-HD4 Trial. *Blood* 2013;122:404.

69. Rosinol L, Oriol A, Teruel AI, *et al.* Maintenance therapy after stem-cell transplantation for multiple myeloma with bortezomib/thalidomide *versus* thalidomide vs. alfa2b-interferon: final results of a phase III Pethema/GEM randomized trial. *ASH Annual Meeting Abstracts* 2012;120:334.

70. Barlogie B, Jagannath S, Desikan KR, *et al.* Total therapy with tandem transplants for newly diagnosed multiple myeloma. *Blood* 1999;93:55–65.

71. Naumann-Winter F, Greb A, Borchmann P, Bohlius J, Engert A, Schnell R. First-line tandem high-dose chemotherapy and autologous stem cell transplantation *versus* single high-dose chemotherapy and autologous stem cell transplantation in multiple myeloma, a systematic review of controlled studies. *Cochrane Database Syst Rev* 2012;10: CD004626.

72. Attal M, Harousseau J-L, Facon T, *et al.* Single *versus* double autologous stem-cell transplantation for multiple myeloma. *N Engl J Med* 2003;349:2495–502.

73. Cavo M, Tosi P, Zamagni E, *et al.* Prospective, randomized study of single compared with double autologous stem-cell transplantation for multiple myeloma: Bologna 96 clinical study. *J Clin Oncol* 2007;25:2434–41.

74. Einsele H, Liebisch P, Bargou R, Meisner C, Metzner B, Wandt H. Single high-dose chemoradiotherapy *versus* tandem high-dose melphalan followed by autologous stem cell transplantation: preliminary analysis [Xth International Myeloma Foundation Workshop, Sydney]. *Haematologica* 2005;90:131.

75. Fermand JP. High does therapy supported with autologous blood stem cell transplantation in multiple myeloma: long term follow-up of the prospective studies of the MAG group [Xth International Myeloma Workshop, Sydney 2005]. *Haematologica* 2005;90:40.

76. Goldschmidt H. Single vs. double high-dose therapy in multiple myeloma: second analysis of the GMMG-HD2 trial [International Myeloma Workshop, Syndey 2005]. *Haematologica* 2005;90:38.

77. Kumar A, Kharfan-Dabaja MA, Glasmacher A, Djulbegovic B. Tandem *versus* single autologous hematopoietic cell transplantation for the treatment of multiple myeloma: a systematic review and meta-analysis. *J Natl Cancer Inst* 2009;101:100–6.

78. Giralt S, Vesole DH, Somlo G, *et al.* Re: Tandem vs single autologous hematopoietic cell transplantation for the treatment of multiple myeloma: a systematic review and meta-analysis. *J Natl Cancer Inst* 2009;101:964; author reply 6–7.

79. Mehta J. Re: Tandem vs single autologous hematopoietic cell transplantation for the treatment of multiple myeloma: a systematic review and meta-analysis. *J Natl Cancer Inst* 2009;101:1430–1; author reply 1–3.

80. Tricot G, Kern SE, Barlogie B. Re: Tandem vs single autologous hematopoietic cell transplantation for the treatment of multiple myeloma: a systematic review and meta-analysis. *J Natl Cancer Inst* 2009;101:964–6; author reply 6–7.

81. Sonneveld P, van der Holt B, Segeren CM, *et al.* Intermediate-dose melphalan compared with myeloablative treatment in multiple myeloma: long-term follow-up of the Dutch Cooperative Group HOVON 24 trial. *Haematologica* 2007;92:928–35.

82. Abdelkefi A, Ladeb S, Torjman L, *et al.* Single autologous stem cell transplantation followed by maintenance therapy with thalidomide is superior to double autologous transplantation in multiple myeloma: results of a multicenter randomized clinical trial. *Blood* 2008;111(4):1805–10.

83. Bruno B, Rotta M, Patriarca F, *et al.* A comparison of allografting with autografting for newly diagnosed myeloma. *N Engl J Med* 2007;356:1110–20.

84. Gahrton G, Iacobelli S, Bjorkstrand B, *et al.* Autologous/reduced-intensity allogeneic stem cell transplantation vs autologous transplantation in multiple myeloma: long-term results of the EBMT-NMAM2000 study. *Blood* 2013;121:5055–63.

85. Garban F, Attal M, Michallet M, *et al.* Prospective comparison of autologous stem cell transplantation followed by dose-reduced allograft (IFM99-03 trial) with tandem autologous stem cell transplantation (IFM99-04 trial) in high-risk de novo multiple myeloma. *Blood* 2006;107:3474–80.

86. Krishnan A, Pasquini MC, Logan B, *et al.* Autologous haemopoietic stem-cell transplantation followed by allogeneic or autologous haemopoietic stem-cell transplantation in patients with multiple myeloma (BMT CTN 0102): a phase 3 biological assignment trial. *Lancet Oncol* 2011;12:1195–203.

87. Lokhorst HM, van der Holt B, Cornelissen JJ, *et al.* Donor *versus* no-donor comparison of newly diagnosed myeloma patients included in the HOVON-50 multiple myeloma study. *Blood* 2012;119:6219–25.

88. Rosinol L, Perez-Simon JA, Sureda A, *et al.* A prospective PETHEMA study of tandem autologous transplantation *versus* autograft followed by reduced-intensity conditioning allogeneic transplantation in newly diagnosed multiple myeloma. *Blood* 2008;112:3591–3.

89. Costa L, Armeson K, Hill E. Tandem autologous transplantation *versus* autologous plus reduced-intensity conditioning allogeneic transplantation in the management of newly diagnosed multiple myeloma: meta-analysis of all prospective trials with biological randomisation. *Bone Marrow Transplant* 2013;47:S45.

90. Kharfan-Dabaja M, M. H, Reljic T, Bensinger W, Djulbegovic B, Kumar A. Comparative efficacy of tandem autologous-autologous *versus* tandem autologous-reduced intensity allogeneic haematopoietic cell transplantation in multiple myeloma: results of a systematic review and meta-analysis. *Bone Marrow Transplant* 2013;47:S44.

91. Institute for Quality and Efficiency in Health Care: Executive Summaries. Stem cell transplantation for multiple myeloma: Executive summary of final report: N05-03C, Version 1.0. 2005–2011 Sep19. Epub Date 2014/05/01.

92. Lokhorst H, van deHolt B, Cornelissen J, *et al*. No improvement of overall survival after extended follow-up of donor versus no donor analysis of newly diagnosed myeloma patients included in the HOVON 50/54 Study. *Blood* 2013;122(21):2132–2.

93. Crawley C, Iacobelli S, Bjorkstrand B, Apperley JF, Niederwieser D, Gahrton G. Reduced-intensity conditioning for myeloma: lower nonrelapse mortality but higher relapse rates compared with myeloablative conditioning. *Blood* 2007;109:3588–94.

94. Qazilbash MH, Saliba R, De Lima M, *et al*. Second autologous or allogeneic transplantation after the failure of first autograft in patients with multiple myeloma. *Cancer* 2006;106:1084–9.

95. Nishihori T, Alsina M. Advances in the autologous and allogeneic transplantation strategies for multiple myeloma. *Cancer Control* 2011;18:258–67.

96. Rajkumar SV, Gahrton G, Bergsagel PL. Approach to the treatment of multiple myeloma: a clash of philosophies. *Blood* 2011;118:3205–11.

97. Russell SJ, Rajkumar SV. Multiple myeloma and the road to personalised medicine. *Lancet Oncol* 2011;12:617–9.

98. Siegel DSd, Jacobus S, Rajkumar SV, *et al*. Outcome with lenalidomide plus dexamethasone followed by early autologous stem cell transplantation in the ECOG E4A03 Randomized Clinical Trial. *ASH Annual Meeting Abstracts* 2010;116:38.

99. Cavallo F, Spencer A, Gay F, *et al*. Early autologous stem cell transplantation improves survival in newly diagnosed multiple myeloma patients. *Haematologica* 2014;99:520.

100. Palumbo A, Gay F, Spencer A, *et al*. A Phase III study of ASCT vs cyclophosphamide-lenalidomide-dexamethasone and lenalidomide-prednisone maintenance vs lenalidomide alone in newly diagnosed myeloma patients. *Blood* 2013;122:763.

Maintenance Therapy in Plasma Cell Myeloma after Autologous Transplant

Sarah A. Holstein and Philip L. McCarthy

Introduction

Immunomodulatory drugs (IMiDs) and proteasome inhibitors (PIs) have markedly improved the outcomes of plasma cell myeloma (multiple myeloma, MM) patients. For those patients eligible for high-dose therapy, induction therapy consisting of IMiD and/or PI-based therapy, followed by consolidation with autologous hematopoietic cell transplant (HCT) remains a standard of care. As nearly all patients will eventually relapse following HCT, there has been significant interest in the use of post-transplant maintenance therapy as a strategy to delay recurrence and improve survival. Early studies focused on the use of interferon or thalidomide maintenance therapy, but the side effect profiles of these agents, coupled with a lack of clear overall survival (OS) benefit, have limited their routine use. We present and discuss recent studies which have focused on lenalidomide- or bortezomib-based post-HCT maintenance strategies.

Lenalidomide Maintenance after Autologous Transplant: Does It Improve Overall Survival?

The first study to incorporate lenalidomide post-HCT was a phase II study in which patients received induction therapy with bortezomib, doxorubicin, and dexamethasone followed by tandem transplant with melphalan ($100\,mg/m^2$)[1]. Patients then received consolidation therapy with four cycles of lenalidomide ($25\,mg/day$ on days 1–21) plus prednisone ($50\,mg$ every other day) followed by maintenance lenalidomide ($10\,mg/day$ on days 1–21) until relapse. This study demonstrated the feasibility of lenalidomide consolidation/maintenance with the most frequent grade 3–4 adverse events being neutropenia (16%), thrombocytopenia (6%), and pneumonia (4%). Upgrading of responses was seen in 16% of patients following the lenalidomide/prednisone consolidation and an additional 4% of patients during maintenance lenalidomide. Since then three randomized trials involving lenalidomide maintenance after autologous HCT have been reported and are summarized in Table 47.1.

CALGB 100104

In the United States, the CALGB 100104 trial was the first pivotal phase 3 trial to evaluate the role of lenalidomide maintenance post-HCT (Table 47.1). This study included 460 patients who were randomized to receive lenalidomide *versus* placebo following HCT[2]. Treatment was initiated at day 100 at a dose level of $10\,mg/day$ and was escalated to 15 mg/day after 3 months or decreased to $5\,mg/day$ daily or from days 1 to 21 of each month as tolerated. Notably, the primary endpoint of time to progression (TTP) was met early on (46 months *versus* 27 months, HR=0.48, $P<0.001$) and thus the study was unblinded. Following unblinding, the majority of nonprogressing patients still on the placebo arm (86 of 128) crossed over and received lenalidomide. Not only did this study demonstrate a significant improvement in TTP, it also yielded a substantial improvement in OS: at 34 months the OS was 85% in the lenalidomide arm compared with 77% in the placebo arm ($P=0.03$). An updated analysis with a 65-month median follow-up for OS continues to show significant improvements in both TTP (53 *versus* 27 months, HR=0.54, $P<0.001$) and OS (median OS not reached for lenalidomide *versus* 76 months for placebo; $P=0.001$[3].

IFM 2005-02

The most directly comparable European trial was the IFM 2005-02 trial which included 614 patients (Table 47.1). In this trial, all patients following HCT received two cycles of consolidation therapy with lenalidomide ($25\,mg/day$ for days 1–21) prior to starting maintenance therapy (lenalidomide *versus* placebo)[4]. As with the CALGB 100104 study, the initial dose of lenalidomide maintenance was $10\,mg/day$ and was then escalated to $15\,mg/day$ after 3 months. This study was also unblinded early after the primary endpoint of PFS was met (median PFS of 41 months *versus* 23 months, HR 0.5, $P<0.001$). Crossover to lenalidomide was not permitted. Maintenance therapy was discontinued at a median time of 2 years (range 1–3 years) following randomization due to a concern regarding second primary malignancies (SPMs). In contrast to the CALGB study, there was no improvement in OS on the lenalidomide arm; the 3-year OS in the lenalidomide was 80% *versus* 84% in the placebo arm (HR 1.25, $P=0.29$). Longer follow-up of this trial has been reported and at 60 months after randomization the PFS benefit is maintained for the lenalidomide arm (42% *versus* 18%, $P<0.0001$) but the 5-year OS rates are equivalent (68% *versus* 67%)[5]. An analysis of the

Table 47.1 Randomized trials involving lenalidomide maintenance therapy after autologous HCT

Study	n	Induction therapy	Dosing schedule	Duration of maintenance	TTP or PFS (maintenance *versus* no)	OS (maintenance *versus* no)
McCarthy *et al.*[2] Holstein *et al.*[3]	460	<2 regimens; 94% received a regimen containing Thal, Len, and/or Bor	10 mg continuous, increase up to 15 mg	Until progression	Median TTP: 53 *versus* 27 months ($P<0.001$) 3-year TTP: 66% (95% CI 59–73) *versus* 39% (95% CI 33–48) ($P<0.001$)	Median follow-up 65 months: Not reached *versus* 76 months ($P=0.001$) 3-year OS: 88% (95% CO 84–93) *versus* 80% (95% CI 74–86) ($P=0.03$)
Attal *et al.* [4,5]	614	46% received vincristine, doxorubicin, Dex and 46% received Bor and Dex 21% received tandem transplant 25% received induction reinforcement with DCEP	All patients received 2 cycles of consolidation (25 mg/day, 21 out of 28 days) Maintenance: 10 mg continuous, increase up to 15 mg	Stopped due to concerns regarding second primary malignancies at a median time of 2 years (range 1–3 years)	Median PFS: 41 *versus* 23 months ($P<0.001$) 4-year PFS: 43% *versus* 22% ($P<0.001$)	Median follow-up 45 months: 74% *versus* 76% ($P=0.7$) 4-year OS: 73% *versus* 75% ($P=0.7$) 5-year OS: 68% *versus* 67 (HR=1)
Palumbo *et al.*[6]	402	4 cycles Len/Dex followed by either tandem transplant (MEL200) or melphalan/Len/prednisone (MPR)	10 mg (3 weeks on, 1 week off)	Until progression	Median PFS: 42 *versus* 22 months ($P<0.001$)	34-year OS[a]: 88% *versus* 79% ($P=0.14$)

[a] Combining MEL200 and MPR groups.
Abbreviations: Thal (thalidomide), Len (lenalidomide), Dex (dexamethasone), Bor (bortezomib), DCEP (dexamethasone, cyclophosphamide, etoposide, cisplatin).

median second PFS (defined as time from progression in first-line to the second progression or death) was inferior in the lenalidomide arm (10 months) compared with the placebo arm (18 months, $P<0.0001$). In addition, the OS after progression on the lenalidomide arm was inferior to the placebo arm. It will be interesting to examine the salvage regimens used after progression on both arms.

GIMEMA RV-209

Although not directly comparable to the American and French studies, the Italian tandem autologous HCT and maintenance study (GIMEMA RV-209) has provided further evidence for the benefit of lenalidomide post-HCT (Table 47.1)[6]. This study design incorporated two randomizations. Following induction therapy with four cycles of lenalidomide/dexamethasone, patients were randomized to consolidation with either tandem HCT (melphalan 200 mg/m^2) *versus* six cycles of oral melphalan/lenalidomide/prednisone (MPR). Subsequently patients on both arms were randomized to either lenalidomide maintenance (10 mg/day days 1–21) or no maintenance therapy. An analysis which combined the MPR and HCT arms revealed that patients who received lenalidomide maintenance

had a significantly improved median PFS (42 months) compared with those who received no maintenance (22 months, $P<0.001$). Furthermore, the 3-year OS was 88% for the lenalidomide arm and 79% for the observation arm ($P=0.14$). It was noted that lenalidomide maintenance improved the CR rate in both arms.

Meta-analysis of the CALGB 100104, IFM 2005-02 and GIMEMA RV-209 Trials

Recently a meta-analysis of the CALGB 100104, IFM 2005-02 and GIMEMA RV-209 studies was performed in order to assess the impact of lenalidomide on OS[7]. In total, this included 1209 patients (605 received lenalidomide and 604 received placebo or control). Median OS for lenalidomide was not reached while the median for the placebo/control group was 86 months (HR=0.74, 95% CI 0.62-0.89, log-rank $P=0.001$). The median OS at 5, 6, and 7 years was longer with lenalidomide compared to placebo/control (71% *versus* 66%, 65% *versus* 58%, 62% *versus* 50%). Notably, patients who achieved less than a partial response (PR) benefited from lenalidomide (HR=0.86, 95% CI 0.65-1.15) as did patients who achieved a very good PR (VGPR) or CR (HR=0.70, 95% CI 0.54–0.90).

Adverse Events Associated with Lenalidomide Maintenance after Autologous HCT: Is It Worth the Try?

The primary adverse events associated with lenalidomide maintenance have been hematologic in nature. In the IFM 2005–02 study, 74% of patients on the lenalidomide arm and 43% on the placebo arm had grade 3 or 4 events, of which 58% and 22%, respectively, were hematologic[4]. In this study a quarter of the patients (27%) in the lenalidomide group discontinued therapy due to adverse events as compared with 15% of patients receiving placebo. Fairly similar adverse event rates were reported for the CALGB 100104 study: 69% of patients on the lenalidomide arm and 30% on the placebo arm developed grade 3/4 adverse events, of which 48% and 17%, respectively, were hematologic[2]. Lower rates of discontinuation of therapy due to adverse events were reported in this study: in the lenalidomide arm, 10% of patients stopped therapy, compared with 1% in the placebo arm, and 6% of patients who crossed over to lenalidomide maintenance. The lower discontinuation rates observed in the American study may be in part related to the use of less myelosuppressive induction regimens as compared with those used in the French study.

Differences Among the Three Randomized Lenalidomide Maintenance Trials

There has been intense debate regarding why the American and French studies demonstrated similar PFS benefit but different OS outcomes[8]. Factors which need to be considered include induction regimen differences, the presence or absence of consolidation therapy, and duration of maintenance therapy (Table 47.1). With respect to induction therapy, patients enrolled in the French trial did not receive an IMiD as part of their induction therapy while 74% of patients in the CALGB received either thalidomide- or lenalidomide-containing regimens. In addition, in the French trial, 25% of patients received high-dose alkylator therapy (DCEP; dexamethasone, cyclophosphamide, etoposide, cisplatin) and 21% of patients underwent tandem autologous HCT. Subgroup analysis of the American study revealed that the hazard ratio for OS favored the lenalidomide arm for subgroups that either had received lenalidomide induction or had not received thalidomide induction, but did not reach statistical significance for patients who either had thalidomide induction or did not have lenalidomide induction [2]. However, all of these subgroups achieved PFS benefit from lenalidomide maintenance. These results suggest that the nature of the induction regimen, specifically whether a patient received lenalidomide *versus* thalidomide, has an impact on OS which may in part be due to the induction regimen but is also likely to be due to disease responsiveness to subsequent lines of

therapy after relapse post-maintenance therapy. The American study did not report stratified outcomes based on whether bortezomib was used pre-HCT. Approximately 15% of patients received both lenalidomide and bortezomib as part of their induction regimen. Currently, as many patients receive both lenalidomide and bortezomib with dexamethsone (the classic RVD regimen) as induction therapy in the United States, it may be assumed that these patients also have an OS benefit with lenalidomide maintenance based on the subset analysis.

As noted above, all patients in the French trial received two cycles of standard dosing lenalidomide as consolidation prior to being randomized to lenalidomide *versus* placebo. We do not know how this impacted on the effect of maintenance on both arms. Further, this consolidation was given between days 60 and 100 post-HCT and thus may have affected the recovering marrow following HCT.

Finally, another important key difference among the two trials was that in the French study lenalidomide was discontinued after a median of 2 years of therapy (range 1–3 years) while in the American study lenalidomide was continued until progression. As equivalent second primary malignancy (SPM) rates (discussed below) were noted in both studies, this indicates that there is not an increased risk for continuing lenalidomide beyond 2 years and also suggests that the OS benefit observed in the American study is in part due to the extended use of lenalidomide.

Progression-Free Survival 2

Of interest, the European Medicine Agency defines PFS2 as the time from initial randomization to time of object disease progression (PD) after next-line of therapy or death from any cause. It has been proposed as a surrogate for OS, particularly for trials evaluating maintenance therapy (EMA guideline, http://www.ema.europa.eu/docs/en_GB/document_library/Scientific_guideline/2011/12/WC500119966.pdf). The definition of PFS2 in the IFM 05-02 update was slightly different as it was the sum of the PFS1 and PFS2. It remains to be determined if PFS2 will be used as a surrogate for OS. Also, it will be important to determine the PFS2 for the CALGB 100104 study. It is expected that the PFS2 for the lenalidomide arm will be prolonged when compared to placebo.

Lenalidomide Maintenance Therapy after Autologous HCT and SPMs

Following the initial reports of the American and French studies, there was significant concern that a signal was arising that revealed an increased rate of SPMs in patients receiving lenalidomide maintenance. McCarthy *et al.*[9] reported a SPM incidence of 2.6% in the lenalidomide arm *versus* 1.7% in the placebo arm while Attal *et al.*[10] reported rates of 2.6% and 0.04%, respectively. After further follow-up, the CALGB study reported that 14 (6.1%) hematologic malignancies and 11

(4.8%) solid tumors developed in patients receiving lenalido-mide as compared with 3 (1%) and 7 (3.1%), respectively, in the placebo arm[23]. Although the cumulative incidence risk of SPM was greater in the lenalidomide arm as compared with the placebo arm ($P<0.005$), the cumulative incidence risk of progression and death was higher in the placebo arm ($P< 0.001$)[3]. The IFM study subsequently reported a total of 20 (6.6%) hematologic malignancies and 24 (7.8%) solid tumors in 35 patients in the lenalidomide arm and 6 (1.9%) hemato-logic malignancies and 22 (7.2%) solid tumors in 20 patients in the placebo arm[5]. No significant differences in the incidence of nonmelanoma skin cancers were reported in either study.

Subsequently there have been several reports which have tried to determine whether the observed increase in SPMs can be attributed solely to lenalidomide or whether there are other factors, which contribute to this risk. Multiple studies have demonstrated that monoclonal gammopathy of undetermined significance and MM, even in the absence of therapy, are associated with an increased risk of hematologic malignan-cies[11–13]. Krishnan *et al.* conducted a retrospective cohort study to assess the risk of SPM after autologous HCT[14]. They found that the overall cumulative incidence was 5.3% at 5 years and 11.2% at 10 years (excluding nonmelanoma skin cancers). There was a trend, which was not statistically signifi-cant (odds ratio 3.5, $P=0.15$) towards increased risk of SPM with thalidomide.

Duration of Lenalidomide Therapy and SPM Risk

The Arkansas group analyzed outcomes from Total Therapy (TT) 2 (no lenalidomide) and TT3 (lenalidomide-containing) trials and found no difference in the SPM incidence[15]. Dur-ation of lenalidomide therapy does not appear to be an import-ant factor. An analysis of patients who received long-term lenalidomide therapy with the BiRd regimen (clarithromycin, lenalidomide, dexamethasone) demonstrated that the develop-ment of SPMs was not associated with age, HCT, or number of cycles of lenalidomide[16]. Furthermore, the incidence of SPM in this cohort was not statistically different than expected based on SEER data (2.85 *versus* 2.1 per 100 person-yrs). A retro-spective study of patients treated with lenalidomide/dexa-methasone for a minimum of 2 years (median duration of 3 years) showed an annual incidence rate of SPM of 1.96%[17].

SPMs with Lenalidomide and Alkylator Therapy

Evidence is emerging that the combination of lenalidomide and alkylator therapy contributes more to the risk of SPMs, particularly hematologic SPMs, than does lenalidomide alone. A pooled analysis of 2459 newly diagnosed MM patients from nine European Myeloma network trials showed that the cumu-lative incidence of SPM at 3 years was 2.0% for patients who had received lenalidomide and alkylator therapy as compared with 1.1% for those who did not receive lenalidomide[18]. The

cumulative incidence of death from MM was lower in the group which received lenalidomide (13.8% *versus* 26.1%), demonstrating a benefit–risk ratio that favors lenalidomide. A meta-analysis of 3254 newly diagnosed patients treated on seven randomized, controlled phase 3 trials revealed that the cumulative 5-year incidence of all SPMs at 5 years was 6.9% in patients who received lenalidomide *versus* 4.8% in those who did not ($P=0.037$)[19]. Notably, there was an increased risk in hematologic malignancies (3.1% *versus* 1.4%, $P=0.029$) and not solid tumors. Furthermore, exposure to lenalidomide and lower dose oral melphalan was associated with an increased risk of hematologic SPMs, but not lenalidomide and higher dose intravenous melphalan. In contrast, exposure to lenalidomide and cyclophosphamide or lenalidomide and dexamethasone was not associated with increased SPM risk. As with other studies, the cumulative incidences of death due to MM or treatment-related events were higher than those due to SPMs.

Practice Points

In aggregate these studies show a small but measurable increased risk of SPMs, particularly hematologic SPMs, with lenalidomide. However, it is also quite clear that lenalidomide is associated with a decreased risk of progression and death from MM. Thus we would advise that patients be counseled about this risk of SPMs and that they should also be counseled regarding the body of literature which demonstrates the PFS, as well as the meta-analysis which demonstrates the OS bene-fits of lenalidomide in the post-HCT setting. Patients should undergo routine age-appropriate cancer screening and there should be a low threshold for further evaluation, including bone marrow biopsy, if unexpected cytopenias occur.

Bortezomib Maintenance Therapy after Autologous HCT

There have been no randomized trials which directly compare single-agent bortezomib to placebo post-transplant. The study that is most commonly cited as providing rationale for borte-zomib maintenance is the HOVON-65/GMMG-HD4 trial, which included 827 newly diagnosed patients[20]. Patients were randomized to induction therapy consisting of either VAD (vincristine, doxorubicin, dexamethasone) or PAD (bor-tezomib, doxorubicin, dexamethasone) followed by single or tandem HCT. Maintenance therapy consisted of thalidomide for patients on the VAD arm and bortezomib (every other week for 2 years) on the PAD arm. The nature of the study design introduces some difficulties when trying to directly compare the maintenance regimens. However, several notable conclusions were reached. First, maintenance bortezomib was better tolerated than thalidomide. Second, bortezomib main-tenance significantly improved the nCR + CR rates. Third, when PFS was calculated from time of transplant, there was a statistically significant benefit to bortezomib. Fourth, the OS for the PAD arm was superior when adjusted for International Scoring System (ISS) (HR=0.80, 95% CI 0.65–1.00, P=0.047). Fifth, the PFS and OS benefit was statistically improved for the PAD arm primarily for patients in renal failure. Based on this study, many providers use bortezomib every other week schedule post-HCT. Given the lack of a placebo-controlled study, it is difficult to counsel patients about the expected PFS or OS benefit of bortezomib maintenance and the development or worsening of existing peripheral neuropathy limits the prolonged use of bortezomib.

A placebo-controlled bortezomib consolidation study was conducted by the Nordic Myeloma Study Group[21]. In this study, 370 patients were randomized to receive bortezomib consolidation (days 1, 4, 8, 11 out of a 3- week cycle for two cycles then once weekly days 1, 8, 15 in a 4-week cycle for four cycles) *versus* no consolidation after autologous HCT. The PFS favored the bortezomib arm (27 months *versus* 20 months, P=0.05) but no difference in OS was observed. Straka *et al.* have reported the outcomes of two randomized studies which evaluated bortezomib consolidation *versus* observation post-HCT. Although consolidation improved response rates (> VGPR rates for bortezomib improved from 55% to 62% *versus* 59% to 48% in the observation group) and median PFS (33.6 months for bortezomib *versus* 27.8 months for observation (P=0.0058), there was not a difference in median OS (not reached for either arm, P =0.75)[22].

Bortezomib Plus Thalidomide Maintenance Therapy After Autologous HCT

Several trials have evaluated bortezomib in combination with thalidomide post-transplant. The Spanish Myeloma Group reported their results from a trial in which newly diagnosed MM patients received different induction regimens. After a single autologous HCT, patients were randomized to single-agent thalidomide, bortezomib plus thalidomide, or single-agent interferon[23]. While the PFS was better in the thalidomide-bortezomib arm, there were no differences among the arms for OS and the bortezomib-containing arm did not overcome the poor prognosis associated with high-risk cytogenetics. Cavo *et al.* evaluated thalidomide/dexamethasone (TD) with or without bortezomib (VTD) as induction therapy followed by tandem transplant followed by two additional cycles of TD/VTD[24]. Although higher response rates were achieved in the bortezomib-containing arm, this arm was associated with a higher incidence of adverse events, including peripheral neuropathy. There was an improved PFS with VTD induction and consolidation without OS benefit. Finally, Arkansas's TT3 regimen incorporated bortezomib into both the induction phase (VDT-PACE) and maintenance phase (VTD)[25]. Results of this phase-2 study demonstrated that bortezomib could be safely combined with multiagent chemotherapy, effecting nCR status and 2-year survival rates in more than 80% of patients.

Bortezomib and SPMs

There has not been a signal for an increased SPM risk associated with bortezomib. The VISTA trial, which compared bortezomib/melphalan/prednisone (VMP) to melphalan/prednisone (MP) in transplant-ineligible patients, had equivalent numbers of hematologic malignancies and solid tumors in both arms[26]. SPM rates from other bortezomib trials have not been reported.

Adverse Risk Cytogenetics and Implications for Maintenance Therapy

Patients with adverse risk cytogenetic features such as del17p, monosomy 13 (not by FISH), t(4;14), and t(14;16) represent a difficult population to manage as they have inferior outcomes despite treatment with novel agents and HCT. Whether maintenance strategies exist that provide substantial benefit to this patient population has yet to be proven. The CALGB lenalidomide maintenance trial did not report outcomes based on cytogenetics. The IFM 2005-02 study did report the baseline cytogenetic features of the patients and showed that the hazard ratio for progression or death favored the lenalidomide arm for patients with 13q deletion, without 13q deletion, and without (t4;14) or 17p deletion, but did not reach significance for patients with either t(4;14) or 17p deletion[10]. Avet-Loiseau *et al.*, in their published ASH abstract, reported that for patients with t(4:14) the PFS was 27 months in the lenalidomide arm *versus* 15 months in the placebo arm and for patients with del(17p) the PFS was 29 months *versus* 14 months for lenalidomide and placebo, respectively[27]. However, in an oral presentation discussing high-risk MM patients, including this abstract, the PFS for patients with t(4:14) in the placebo arm was reported to be 24 months, suggesting that there is not a significant benefit of lenalidomide maintenance for patients with t(4:14) (International Myeloma Workshop, June 2014, J. San Miguel, personal communication).

Bortezomib has previously been shown to partially overcome the adverse prognosis associated with t(4;14) and chromosome 13 deletion[24,28,29]. The HOVON trial did demonstrate that patients who had del17 abnormalities had improved OS rates in the bortezomib-containing arm compared with the thalidomide arm. However, patients with other high-risk cytogenetic abnormalities did not obtain a benefit from bortezomib when compared to thalidomide[20,30,31].

RVD Maintenance Program for Subjects with High-Risk Cytogenetics

Should Multi-Agent Maintenance Therapy (Or Extended Consolidation Therapy) Be Used for High-Risk Patients?

Nooka *et al.* treated patients with high-risk disease (deletion p53, deletion 1p, t(4;14), t(14;16), or plasma cell leukemia)

Table 47.2 Techniques used to determine MRD in plasma cell myeloma

Technique	Methodology	Sensitivity	Applicability rate	Limitations
Multiparametric flow cytometry (MFC)	Flow cytometric detection using fluorescently labeled antibodies which differentiates between normal and malignant plasma cells	10^{-4}–10^{-5}[40]	>97%[36,41]	Different panels of antibodies used by different groups Operator-dependent
Allele-specific oligonucleotide PCR (ASO-PCR)	Preparation of patient-specific primers from the rearranged region of the immunoglobulin (Ig) heavy chain genes; extraction of RNA from myeloma cells; reverse transcription	10^{-5}[41]	<70%[43–45]	Expense Difficulties with primer design, failure to amplify or sequencing
High-throughput sequencing (HTS)	Consensus primer sets used to amplify and sequence all rearranged Ig gene segments in myeloma cells	10^{-6}[46]	91%[46]	Some discordancy with MFC and ASO-PCR[47]

with up to 3 years of lenalidomide/bortezomib/dexamethasone (RVD) followed by single-agent lenalidomide[32]. This study demonstrated the feasibility of such an approach and the 3-year OS rate was noted to be 93%. Arkansas's 2006–66 study, which followed TT3, also included 3 years of post-transplant RVD[33]. In comparison with TT3, which had 3 years of VTD post-transplant therapy, RVD post-transplant therapy did not improve the outcome of patients with high-risk disease based on gene expression profiling.

Practice Points

In conclusion, at this point there is insufficient evidence to support the sole choice of a maintenance agent based on cytogenetics or gene expression profiling; however, early data favor more aggressive maintenance programs in certain high-risk cytogenetic populations. Further analyses of already completed trials (e.g., CALGB 100104) as well as additional clinical trials are needed to better define what approach should be used for patients with adverse cytogenetic features.

Minimal Residual Disease

Multiple studies have demonstrated that achieving a CR after HCT correlates with prolonged survival[34]. The definition of CR continues to evolve as the ability to detect smaller and smaller numbers of residual malignant plasma cells, also referred to as minimal residual disease (MRD), improves. Multiparametric flow cytometry (MFC), allele-specific oligonucleotide PCR (ASO-PCR), and high-throughput sequencing (HTS) are techniques which are currently under investigation (Table 47.2). These methodologies differ in their sensitivity and applicability and further studies are needed to determine which approach will become the gold standard. All of these techniques are limited by their ability to detect only disease that is present in the bone marrow, thus patients may be MRD-negative in the marrow but have residual extramedullary disease (see Chapter 46). The International Myeloma Working Group has recently released guidelines regarding MRD

assessment and has incorporated MRD status into the response criteria[50].

The results of studies which have assessed MRD in the post-HCT setting are summarized in Table 47.3. In aggregate, these studies show significantly superior outcomes for patients who achieve MRD negativity. Paiva et al. assessed MRD by MFC at day 100 post-HCT in 295 newly diagnosed patients treated on the GEM2000 protocol and found that both PFS and OS were prolonged in patients who were MRD-negative [35]. Rawstron et al. also examined MRD status in patients post-HCT (MRC Myeloma IX trial) via MFC and determined that MRD positivity at day 100 post-HCT was associated with inferior PFS and OS[36]. This study also demonstrated that the use of thalidomide maintenance was associated with a significant improvement in PFS in the MRD-positive patients but not in the MRD-negative patients. Furthermore, MRD status was reassessed after 7 months. At that time, 28% of MRD-positive patients on thalidomide maintenance had converted to MRD-negative as compared with 3% of patients who did not receive thalidomide. While it is tempting to speculate that the use of any maintenance therapy could be restricted to only patients who do not achieve MRD-negative status post-HCT, further studies are needed. In particular, prospective trials involving randomization of MRD-negative patients to maintenance therapy versus monitoring are ongoing and planned to further explore this hypothesis. As MM is currently an incurable disease, until curative agents are available, patients who come off maintenance therapy will need to be closely monitored.

Progression on Maintenance Therapy

While disease relapse post-transplant can manifest in different ways, it is not uncommon for the first signs to be subtle changes in the free light chain ratio or re-emergence of a monoclonal protein on immunofixation electrophoresis (i.e., biochemical progression). In the absence of active disease per CRAB (hypercalcemia, renal insufficiency, anemia, bone

Table 47.3. Summary of studies measuring MRD status at day +100 post-HCT

Study	n	MRD technique	Outcome (MRD-positive *versus* MRD-negative)
Paiva et al.[51]	295	MFC	Median PFS: 37 *versus* 71 months (*P*<0.001) Median OS: 89 months *versus* not reached (*P*=0.002)
Paiva et al.[48] (GEM2000 and GEM2005 studies)	241	MFC	TTP: 58% *versus* 86% at 3 years (*P*<0.001) OS: 80% *versus* 90% at 3 years (*P*=0.001)
Rawstron et al.[36] (MRC Myeloma IX study)	397	MFC	Median PFS: 15.5 *versus* 28.6 months (*P*<0.001) Median OS: 59.0 *versus* 80.6 months (*P*=0.0183)
Putkonen et al.[49]	37 (included 7 patients s/p allogeneic SCT)	ASO-PCR	Median PFS: 19 *versus* 70 months (*P*=0.003)
Sarasquete et al.[44]	32	MFC and ASO-PCR	Median PFS: 10 *versus* 27 months (*P*=0.05) *via* MFC and 15 *versus* 34 months (*P*=0.04) *via* ASO-PCR

disease) criteria, it is uncertain whether the optimal strategy should be to continue the maintenance therapy and monitor for further signs of progression, to escalate the dose of maintenance therapy, to add dexamethasone, or to switch to a completely different regimen. There are several ongoing trials which are attempting to answer these questions. One trial takes patients with biochemical progression on lenalidomide maintenance and intervenes by increasing the dose of lenalidomide and adding dexamethasone (NCT01463670). Another trial takes a similar patient population and adds thalidomide to the maintenance lenalidomide (NCT01927718).

Quality of Life on Maintenance Therapy

The impact that post-HCT maintenance therapy has on quality of life has not been vigorously investigated. There have been relatively few randomized trials that have included formal health-related quality of life (HRQoL) assessments as either the primary or secondary endpoints [37]. HRQoL assessment was reported with the National Cancer Institute of Canada Clinical Trials Group Myeloma 10 Trial which randomized patients to thalidomide-prednisone maintenance therapy *versus* observation following autologous HCT[38]. Given thalidomide's side effect profile, it is not surprising that the HRQoL assessment revealed that patients receiving thalidomide and prednisone had worse HRQoL scores for cognitive function and for symptoms of dyspnea, constipation, thirst, leg swelling, numbness, dry mouth, and balance problems. While lenalidomide is generally much better tolerated than thalidomide, neither the CALGB 100104[2] nor IFM 05-02[4] studies included HRQoL assessment as an endpoint. Given that many patients remain on lenalidomide for several years post-transplant, it is important to address the effects that this prolonged therapy has on quality of life.

The Mayo group have published the results of a study in which more than 700 MM patients were surveyed about their attitudes regarding maintenance therapy including side effects that they were most worried about, whether they would choose maintenance therapy if it caused mild *versus* moderate toxicity, whether the cost of maintenance therapy is a factor in decision-making, and whether maintenance therapy that improved OS but not PFS would be considered beneficial [39]. Their results demonstrate that patients are worried about common side effects such as neuropathy, blood clots, and cytopenias. In addition, patients would choose maintenance therapy if there was only a PFS benefit, but were less likely to do so if toxicities were moderate (*versus* mild) or as the cost per month of treatment increased.

Financial Cost Considerations for Maintenance Therapy Programs

The cost of treatment is a factor which should not be ignored. In the United States, lenalidomide and bortezomib are both expensive. Lenalidomide maintenance requires monthly blood count checks and answering a questionnaire. Bortezomib requires blood count checks as well as patient travel and drug administration. While it is assumed that subcutaneous administration of bortezomib would be equivalent to intravenous (as used in the HOVON65 GMMG4 study), this has not been studied in the maintenance setting. The extent to which insurance covers these medication costs is variable, and for many patients, out-of-pocket expenses represent a significant, and sometimes insurmountable, financial burden. If the results of ongoing and planned maintenance studies are successful, this financial burden may be further increased as these studies are investigating strategies which include multiple novel agents (e.g., lenalidomide plus ixazomib, lenalidomide plus vorinostat, bortezomib plus vorinostat, lenalidomide plus monoclonal antibodies).

More Controversies and Future Directions

In the setting of a malignancy where (currently) the intent of therapy is not curative, it is important that both patient and physician weigh the relative benefits *versus* risks of maintenance therapy. It is clear that lenalidomide maintenance prolongs PFS and based on the most recent meta-analysis improves OS. What the true impact of prolonged lenalidomide therapy is on patient quality of life has not been fully determined. There is an increase in hematologic SPMs associated with lenalidomide and patients should be counseled of this risk. However, all of the available data show that the magnitude of benefit from lenalidomide for improving PFS and OS exceeds the risk of SPMs. In this context, lenalidomide represents the current standard of care for the majority of patients in the post-HCT setting. There are fewer definitive data on bortezomib maintenance that would support the routine use of this agent. However, most patients will eventually relapse despite lenalidomide or bortezomib maintenance and patients with adverse cytogenetic features continue to have inferior outcomes. It is clear that the future of maintenance therapy will move beyond single-agent lenalidomide or bortezomib. We anticipate that not only will novel agents be incorporated into the post-transplant setting (e.g., monoclonal antibodies), but that a more individualized approach to maintenance therapy selection will become possible based on factors such as cytogenetics, genome expression profiling, and MRD detection.

References

1. Palumbo A, Gay F, Falco P *et al.* Bortezomib as induction before autologous transplantation, followed by lenalidomide as consolidation-maintenance in untreated multiple myeloma patients. *J Clin Oncol* 28(5), 800–807 (2010).

2. McCarthy PL, Owzar K, Hofmeister CC *et al.* Lenalidomide after stem-cell transplantation for multiple myeloma. *N Engl J Med* 366(19), 1770–1781 (2012).

3. Holstein SA, Owzar K, Richardson PG, *et al.* Updated analysis of CALGB/ECOG/BMT CTN 100104: lenalidomide (Len) vs. placebo (PBO) maintenance therapy after single autologous stem cell transplant (ASCT) for multiple myeloma. *J Clin Oncol.* 2015;33(suppl) abstract 8523.

4. Attal M, Lauwers-Cances V, Marit G *et al.* Lenalidomide maintenance after stem-cell transplantation for multiple myeloma. *N Engl J Med* 366(19), 1782–1791 (2012).

5. Attal M, Lauwers-Cances V, Marit G *et al.* Lenalidomide maintenance after stem-cell transplantation for multiple myeloma: follow-up analysis of the IFM 2005–02 Trial. *Blood* 122(21), 406 (2013).

6. Palumbo A, Cavallo F, Caravita T *et al.* Autologous transplantation and maintenance therapy in multiple myeloma. *N Engl J Med* 371(10), 895–905 (2014).

7. Attal M, Palumbo A, Holstein SA, *et al.* Lenalidomide (LEN) maintenance (MNTC) after high-dose melphalan and autologous stem cell transplant (ASCT)

in multiple myeloma (MM): a meta-analysis (MA) of overall survival (OS). *J Clin Oncol* 34(suppl), abstract 8001 (2016).

8. McCarthy PL, Einsele H, Attal M, Giralt S. The emerging role of consolidation and maintenance therapy for transplant-eligible multiple myeloma patients. *Expert Rev Hematol* 7(1), 55–66 (2014).

9. McCarthy PL, Owzar K, Anderson KC *et al.* Phase III intergroup study of lenalidomide *versus* placebo maintenance therapy following single autologous hematopoietic stem cell transplantation (AHSCT) for multiple myeloma: CALGB 100104. *ASH Annual Meeting Abstracts* 116(21), 37 (2010).

10. Attal M, Lauwers VC, Marit G *et al.* Maintenance treatment with lenalidomide after transplantation for myeloma: final analysis of the IFM 2005–02. *ASH Annual Meeting Abstracts* 116(21), 310 (2010).

11. Tzeng HE, Lin CL, Tsai CH *et al.* Time trend of multiple myeloma and associated secondary primary malignancies in Asian patients: a Taiwan population-based study. *PLoS One* 8(7), e68041 (2013).

12. Razavi P, Rand KA, Cozen W, Chanan-Khan A, Usmani S, Ailawadhi S. Patterns of second primary malignancy risk in multiple myeloma patients before and after the introduction of novel therapeutics. *Blood Cancer J* 3, e121 (2013).

13. Mailankody S, Pfeiffer RM, Kristinsson SY *et al.* Risk of acute myeloid leukemia and myelodysplastic syndromes after multiple myeloma and its precursor

disease (MGUS). *Blood* 118(15), 4086–4092 (2011).

14. Krishnan AY, Mei M, Sun CL *et al.* Second primary malignancies after autologous hematopoietic cell transplantation for multiple myeloma. *Biol Blood Marrow Transplant* 19(2), 260–265 (2013).

15. Usmani SZ, Sexton R, Hoering A *et al.* Second malignancies in total therapy 2 and 3 for newly diagnosed multiple myeloma: influence of thalidomide and lenalidomide during maintenance. *Blood* 120(8), 1597–1600 (2012).

16. Rossi A, Mark T, Jayabalan D *et al.* BiRd (clarithromycin, lenalidomide, dexamethasone): an update on long-term lenalidomide therapy in previously untreated patients with multiple myeloma. *Blood* 121(11), 1982–1985 (2013).

17. Fouquet G, Tardy S, Demarquette H *et al.* Efficacy and safety profile of long-term exposure to lenalidomide in patients with recurrent multiple myeloma. *Cancer* 119(20), 3680–3686 (2013).

18. Palumbo A, Larocca A, Zweegman S *et al.* Second primary malignancies in newly diagnosed multiple myeloma patients treated with lenalidomide: analysis of pooled data in 2459 patients. *ASH Annual Meeting Abstracts* 118(21), 996 (2011).

19. Palumbo A, Bringhen S, Kumar SK *et al.* Second primary malignancies with lenalidomide therapy for newly diagnosed myeloma: a meta-analysis of individual patient data. *Lancet Oncol* 15(3), 333–342 (2014).

20. Sonneveld P, Schmidt-Wolf IG, Van Der Holt B *et al.* Bortezomib induction and maintenance treatment in patients

with newly diagnosed multiple myeloma: results of the randomized phase III HOVON-65/ GMMG-HD4 trial. *J Clin Oncol* 30(24), 2946–2955 (2012).

21. Mellqvist U-H, Gimsing P, Hjertner O *et al.* Bortezomib consolidation after autologous stem cell transplantation in multiple myeloma: a Nordic Myeloma Study Group randomized phase 3 trial. *Blood* 121(23), 4647–4654 (2013).

22. Straka C, Vogel M, Muller J, *et al.* Results from two phase III studies of bortezomib (BTZ) consolidation vs observation (OBS) post-transplant in patients (pts) with newly diagnosed multiple myeloma (NDMM). *J Clin Oncol* 33(suppl), abstract 8511 (2015).

23. Rosinol L, Oriol A, Teruel AI *et al.* Superiority of bortezomib, thalidomide, and dexamethasone (VTD) as induction pretransplantation therapy in multiple myeloma: a randomized phase 3 PETHEMA/GEM study. *Blood* 120(8), 1589–1596 (2012).

24. Cavo M, Tacchetti P, Patriarca F *et al.* Bortezomib with thalidomide plus dexamethasone compared with thalidomide plus dexamethasone as induction therapy before, and consolidation therapy after, double autologous stem-cell transplantation in newly diagnosed multiple myeloma: a randomised phase 3 study. *Lancet* 376(9758), 2075–2085 (2010).

25. Barlogie B, Anaissie E, Van Rhee F *et al.* Incorporating bortezomib into upfront treatment for multiple myeloma: early results of total therapy 3. *Br J Haematol* 138(2), 176–185 (2007).

26. San Miguel JF, Schlag R, Khuageva NK *et al.* Persistent overall survival benefit and no increased risk of second malignancies with bortezomib-melphalan-prednisone *versus* melphalan-prednisone in patients with previously untreated multiple myeloma. *J Clin Oncol* 31(4), 448–455 (2013).

27. Avet-Loiseau H, Caillot D, Marit G *et al.* Long-term maintenance with lenalidomide improves progression free survival in myeloma patients with high-risk cytogenetics: an IFM study. *ASH Annual Meeting Abstracts* 116(21), 1944 (2010).

28. Avet-Loiseau H, Leleu X, Roussel M *et al.* Bortezomib plus dexamethasone induction improves outcome of patients with t(4;14) myeloma but not outcome

of patients with del(17p). *J Clin Oncol* 28(30), 4630–4634 (2010).

29. Jagannath S, Richardson PG, Sonneveld P *et al.* Bortezomib appears to overcome the poor prognosis conferred by chromosome 13 deletion in phase 2 and 3 trials. *Leukemia* 21(1), 151–157 (2007).

30. Scheid C, Sonneveld P, Schmidt-Wolf IG *et al.* Bortezomib before and after autologous stem cell transplantation overcomes the negative prognostic impact of renal impairment in newly diagnosed multiple myeloma: a subgroup analysis from the HOVON-65/GMMG-HD4 trial. *Haematologica* 99(1), 148–154 (2014).

31. Neben K, Lokhorst HM, Jauch A *et al.* Administration of bortezomib before and after autologous stem cell transplantation improves outcome in multiple myeloma patients with deletion 17p. *Blood* 119(4), 940–948 (2012).

32. Nooka AK, Kaufman JL, Muppidi S *et al.* Consolidation and maintenance therapy with lenalidomide, bortezomib and dexamethasone (RVD) in high-risk myeloma patients. *Leukemia* 28(3), 690–693 (2014).

33. Nair B, Van Rhee F, Shaughnessy JD, Jr. *et al.* Superior results of Total Therapy 3 (2003-33) in gene expression profiling-defined low-risk multiple myeloma confirmed in subsequent trial 2006-66 with VRD maintenance. *Blood* 115(21), 4168–4173 (2010).

34. Van De Velde HJ, Liu X, Chen G, Cakana A, Deraedt W, Bayssas M. Complete response correlates with long-term survival and progression-free survival in high-dose therapy in multiple myeloma. *Haematologica* 92(10), 1399–1406 (2007).

35. Paiva B, Vidriales MB, Cervero J *et al.* Multiparameter flow cytometric remission is the most relevant prognostic factor for multiple myeloma patients who undergo autologous stem cell transplantation. *Blood* 112(10), 4017–4023 (2008).

36. Rawstron AC, Child JA, De Tute RM *et al.* Minimal residual disease assessed by multiparameter flow cytometry in multiple myeloma: impact on outcome in the Medical Research Council Myeloma IX Study. *J Clin Oncol* 31(20), 2540–2547 (2013).

37. Kvam AK, Fayers P, Hjermstad M, Gulbrandsen N, Wisloff F. Health-

related quality of life assessment in randomised controlled trials in multiple myeloma: a critical review of methodology and impact on treatment recommendations. *Eur J Haematol* 83(4), 279–289 (2009).

38. Stewart AK, Trudel S, Bahlis NJ *et al.* A randomized phase 3 trial of thalidomide and prednisone as maintenance therapy after ASCT in patients with MM with a quality-of-life assessment: the National Cancer Institute of Canada Clinicals Trials Group Myeloma 10 Trial. *Blood* 121(9), 1517–1523 (2013).

39. Burnette BL, Dispenzieri A, Kumar S *et al.* Treatment trade-offs in myeloma: A survey of consecutive patients about contemporary maintenance strategies. *Cancer* 119(24), 4308–4315 (2013).

40. Rawstron AC, Davies FE, Dasgupta R *et al.* Flow cytometric disease monitoring in multiple myeloma: the relationship between normal and neoplastic plasma cells predicts outcome after transplantation. *Blood* 100(9), 3095–3100 (2002).

41. Paiva B, Martinez-Lopez J, Vidriales MB *et al.* Comparison of immunofixation, serum free light chain, and immunophenotyping for response evaluation and prognostication in multiple myeloma. *J Clin Oncol* 29(12), 1627–1633 (2011).

42. Van Der Velden VH, Cazzaniga G, Schrauder A *et al.* Analysis of minimal residual disease by Ig/TCR gene rearrangements: guidelines for interpretation of real-time quantitative PCR data. *Leukemia* 21(4), 604–611 (2007).

43. Puig N, Sarasquete ME, Balanzategui A *et al.* Critical evaluation of ASO RQ-PCR for minimal residual disease evaluation in multiple myeloma. A comparative analysis with flow cytometry. *Leukemia* 28(2), 391–397 (2014).

44. Sarasquete ME, Garcia-Sanz R, Gonzalez D *et al.* Minimal residual disease monitoring in multiple myeloma: a comparison between allelic-specific oligonucleotide real-time quantitative polymerase chain reaction and flow cytometry. *Haematologica* 90(10), 1365–1372 (2005).

45. Puig N, Sarasquete ME, Alcoceba M *et al.* The use of CD138 positively selected marrow samples increases the applicability of minimal residual disease

assessment by PCR in patients with multiple myeloma. *Ann Hematol* 92(1), 97–100 (2013).

46. Faham M, Zheng J, Moorhead M *et al.* Deep-sequencing approach for minimal residual disease detection in acute lymphoblastic leukemia. *Blood* 120(26), 5173–5180 (2012).

47. Martinez-Lopez J, Lahuerta JJ, Pepin F *et al.* Prognostic value of deep sequencing method for minimal residual disease detection in multiple myeloma. *Blood* 123(20), 3073–3079 (2014).

48. Paiva B, Gutierrez NC, Rosinol L *et al.* High-risk cytogenetics and persistent minimal residual disease by multiparameter flow cytometry predict unsustained complete response after autologous stem cell transplantation in multiple myeloma. *Blood* 119(3), 687–691 (2012).

49. Putkonen M, Kairisto V, Juvonen V *et al.* Depth of response assessed by quantitative ASO-PCR predicts the outcome after stem cell transplantation in multiple myeloma. *Eur J Haematol* 85(5), 416–423 (2010).

50. Kumar S, Paiva B, Anderson KC, *et al.* International Myeloma Working Group consensus criteria for response and minimal residual disease assessment in multiple myeloma. *Lancet Oncol* 17(8), e328–e346 (2016).

51. Paiva B, Vidriales MB, Cervero J, *et al.* Multiparametric flow cytometric remission is the most relevant prognostic factor for multiple myeloma patients who undergo autologous stem cell transplantation. *Blood* 112(10), 4017–23 (2008).

48

Allogeneic Hematopoietic Cell Transplants for Plasma Cell Myeloma

Thomas Giever and Parameswaran Hari

Introduction

Allogeneic hematopoietic cell transplant (allo-HCT) has had a poorly defined and controversial role in the treatment of plasma cell myeloma (PCM). While PCM has become the most common indication for autologous hematopoietic cell transplantation (auto-HCT) in North America[1], most patients invariably relapse after an auto-HCT even in the era of modern induction regimens, post-auto-HCT maintenance, and salvage therapies (see Chapters 46 and 47). Although an infrequently utilized option in PCM, interest has remained high in pursuing allo-HCT[2] given the use of a myeloma-free donor cell graft and the possibility of a donor-driven, immune-mediated graft-versus-myeloma (GvM) effect[3–5]. Based on reporting to the Center for International Blood and Marrow Transplant Research (CIBMTR), fewer than 300 patients underwent an allo-HCT for PCM between 2011 and 2013. Here we discuss the current evidence, clinical settings, and emerging clinical trials in the allo-HCT setting for PCM.

Early History of Allo-HCT in Plasma Cell Myeloma

Allo-HCT with traditional myeloablative conditioning regimens was first utilized for PCM in the late 1980s and early 1990s but was found to have an unacceptably high treatment-related mortality (TRM) of 40–60%[4]. The US Intergroup S9321 notably had its allo-HCT arm terminated after an early TRM of 53% was observed[6]. However, survivors of allo-HCT in the study demonstrated a plateau in survival at 22% with no late relapses indicating that allo-HCT responses are long sustained. The combination of high TRM in this study and the emergence of novel agents for PCM (such as lenalidomide and bortezomib) led to declining interest in allo-HCT.

Subsequent development of nonmyeloablative and reduced intensity conditioning (NST/RIC) approaches offered the prospect of reducing TRM for allo-HCT[7,8] and there was an increase in patients receiving allo-HCT in the 2000s[9]. Several phase 2 studies utilized an initial auto-HCT followed (usually after 3–6 months) by allo-HCT using NST/RIC. The rationale was to uncouple myeloablation and disease control achieved by the auto-HCT from the GvM benefits of the allo-HCT. Early

results suggested that for newly diagnosed patients, this tandem auto-HCT-allo-HCT approach resulted in excellent outcomes at 24 months, with TRM ranging from 11–26% for related donor grafts and unrelated donor grafts respectively [7,10,11]. Long-term follow-up of tandem auto-HCT-allo-HCT from the Seattle group indicated a post-allo-HCT complete response (CR) rate of 60% and TRM of 18% at 5 years [12]. The median time to progression was 5 years with the 5-year overall survival (OS) and event-free survival (EFS) at 64% and 36%. The GITMO (Gruppo Italiano Trapianti di Midollo) experience in 100 newly diagnosed patients who received tandem auto-HCT-allo-HCT was similar and although CR rates increased to 53% after allo-HCT, median EFS was only 37 months[13]. The lack of an apparent cure with ongoing late relapses was disappointing in both studies however.

A CIBMTR analysis demonstrated a switch to NST/RIC-based regimens for allo-HCT in PCM with concomitant reduction in the use of traditional myeloablative conditioning in the years 2001–2005 compared to the preceding time frame [14]. These advances expanded the eligibility for allo-HCT to older PCM patients and increased the number of allo-HCTs performed after auto-HCT in a tandem auto-HCT-allo-HCT fashion. However the decline in TRM was negated by an increase in relapse risk with longer follow-up[14].

Upfront Allo-HCT in Plasma Cell Myeloma

Several randomized trials summarized in Table 48.1 have evaluated sequenced auto-HCT-allo-HCT approach *versus* tandem auto-HCT in the upfront setting after initial induction therapy. In 2007 Bruno *et al.* described the outcomes of 245 patients, less than 65 years old, genetically assigned (on sibling donor availability) to allo-HCT *versus* a second tandem auto-HCT after an initial auto-HCT[15]. Eighty patients with an HLA-identical sibling underwent allo-HCT with 2 Gy total body irradiation (TBI)-based conditioning while 82 patients without an HLA-identical sibling were assigned to receive a second auto-HCT. In a donor-*versus*-no-donor analysis, at a median follow-up of 45 months, OS and EFS were significantly superior in patients with sibling donors (80 *versus* 54 months and 35 *versus* 29 months, respectively). The auto-HCT-allo-HCT and tandem auto-HCT approaches resulted in CR rates of 55% *versus* 26% and TRM rates of 10% and 2%, respectively.

Table 48.1 Randomized comparisons of auto- versus allo-transplantation

Author	n total/ n allo	Trial setting	Conditioning regimen	cGvHD allo-HCT	TRM	OS	PFS	Conclusion
Bruno et al. [15,16]	245/58	Postinduction biologic assignment based on sibling match donor	Mel auto-HCT followed by TBI 2 Gy versus Mel doses 100–200 mg/m^2	32%	10%	Median 80 versus 54 months (P=0.01)	Median 35 versus 29 months (P= 0.02)	Clear benefit for allo-HCT in intention-to-treat donor-versus-no-donor analysis
IFM 9903-04 [32]	284/65	Parallel prospective studies limited to high-risk disease	Mel 200 auto-HCT followed by Flu Bu + ATG allo-HCT versus Mel 200 auto-HCT	42%	11%	Median 34 versus 48 months (P=0.07)	Median 19 versus 22 months (P=0.58)	30% did not complete allo-HCT. No benefit to allo-HCT in this study
Rosinol et al.[83]	110/25	Limited to patients not in CR after a first auto-HCT	Flu Mel allo-HCT versus auto-HCT	66%	16%	Median NR versus 58 months (P=0.9)	Median 20 versus 26 months (P= 0.4)	Higher CR rate after allo-HCT but no survival benefit
Knop et al.[46]	199/126	Limited to patients with 13q- by FISH, unrelated donor grafts in 60%	Mel 200 auto-HCT followed by Flu Mel versus Mel 200 auto-HCT	N/R	12%	Median NR @ 49 months	Median 34.5 versus 22 months (P= 0.005)	Largest trial in high-risk patients and with unrelated donors. Del17p subgroup with OS benefit
EBMT-NMAM [18]	357/108	Postinduction biologic assignment based on sibling match donor	Mel 200 auto-HCT followed by Flu-TBI 2 Gy versus Mel 200 auto-HCT	54%	13%	8-year OS 49% versus 39% (P=0.03)	8-year PFS 22% versus 12% (P= 0.02)	Allo-HCT with lower risk of relapse and improved PFS. Benefit for higher risk del 13 subset
BMT CTN 0102 [17]	710/226	Postinduction biologic assignment based on matched sibling donor	Mel 200 auto-HCT followed by TBI 2 Gy allo-HCT versus Mel 200 auto-HCT	54%	11%	3-year OS 77% versus 80%	3-year PFS 43% versus 46%	No benefit to allo-HCT in this study
HOVON 54[84]	Not strictly a randomized study – donor versus no-donor analysis of HOVON 50		Mel 200 auto-HCT followed by TBI 2 Gy allo-HCT	64%	16%	6-year OS 55% in both groups	6-year PFS 28% (donor group) versus 22% (no-donor group)	No benefit to having a related donor but allo-HCT was by center preference. Relapse lower for those with donors

Mel – melphalan, Flu –fludarabine, Bu – busulfan, Gy – gray, TBI – total body irradiation, ATG – antithymocyte globulin, N/R – not reported.

Updated results after 7 years follow-up showed median OS was not reached (P=0.02) and PFS was 39 months (P=0.02) in the 58 patients who received an allo-HCT whereas median OS was 5.3 years and EFS 33 months in the 46 who received tandem auto-HCT[16]. Of those obtaining a CR after allo-HCT, 53% were in a sustained CR compared with 19% for those in CR following tandem auto-HCT.

The Blood and Marrow Transplant Clinical Trials Network (BMT CTN) 0102 multicenter trial in the United States performed a larger study along similar lines comparing tandem auto-HCT with auto-HCT-allo-HCT based upon matched sibling donor availability[17]. The two arms were similar for the primary endpoint of 3-year PFS with 46% in the tandem auto-

HCT group versus 43% in the auto-HCT-allo-HCT group. Higher risk patients (defined by a high beta-2-microglobulin and chromosome 13 abnormalities) also did not benefit from the auto-HCT-allo-HCT approach in terms of 3-year PFS. Incidence of grade 3–4 graft-versus-host disease (GvHD) was high with 26% acute and 47% chronic GvHD at 1 year after allo-HCT.

Another European study (NMAM 2000) conducted by the European Group for Blood and Marrow Transplantation (EBMT) with an extended 8-year follow-up demonstrated sustained improved PFS and OS for the auto-HCT-allo-HCT approach versus tandem auto-HCT[18,19]. At 96 months, PFS and OS were 22% and 49% favoring auto-HCT-allo-HCT *versus* 12% (*P*=0.027) and 36% (*P*= 0.030) for tandem auto-HCT. Relapse was lower in the allo-HCT cohort (60% *versus* 82%, *P*=0.0002) although TRM was higher. In high-risk patients with deletion 13 chromosome abnormality, PFS (21% *versus* 5%, *P*=0.26) and OS (47% *versus* 31%, *P*=0.154) favored the allo-HCT cohort. Interestingly, patients who relapsed or progressed following allo-HCT had a significantly higher OS than the patients who relapsed after tandem auto-HCT. The GvM effect is thought to have played a major role in this phenomenon.

Meta-analyses of allo-HCT *versus* auto-HCT studies have confirmed that while CR rates are higher for allo-HCT, a consistent survival benefit cannot be demonstrated[20]. The discordant results of the randomized trials of allo-HCT in upfront therapy of PCM are illustrated in Table 48.1. The trials vary in conditioning regimens, patient selection, PCM risk profile, and the use of agents such as ATG (antithymocyte globulin) which may reduce the potential for GvM effect[21]. Variable follow-up duration may also contribute to the disparity.

In the absence of a clear cut survival advantage across studies and with recent improvements in induction and maintenance therapy, some experts have suggested abandoning allo-HCTs in PCM[22]. However, PCM remains incurable with induction followed by auto-HCT and while two randomized studies have shown a survival benefit for allo-HCT, no study has suggested an inferior outcome with allo-HCT. Also notable is that the completed allo-HCT studies were in patients who had not received highly effective modern induction regimens.

Evidence for a GvM Effect

While not specific to PCM, the key indicators of the existence of a clinically beneficial graft-*versus*-malignancy are the induction of sustained antineoplastic effect by infused allogeneic donor lymphocytes, the association of GvHD with disease responses and lower relapse rates in recipients of unmanipulated (T-cell replete) allografts compared with those receiving T-cell depleted grafts or syngeneic grafts [23–25]. In the setting of PCM idiotype-specific CD4 T-cell response could be transferred from an immunized donor marrow to patients in early studies[26]. The success of donor lymphocyte infusions (DLI) in patients with residual or progressive PCM after allo-HCT is corroborative evidence [27,28]. Although the durability of responses after DLI is modest, the occurrence of GvHD after DLI appears to be the most powerful predictor of a response[29,30]. The prospective BMT CTN 0102 study and a retrospective CIBMTR study also found that the occurrence of chronic GvHD after allo-HCT correlated with freedom from progressive PCM [17,31]. Additionally, *in-vitro* or *in-vivo* T-cell depletion has been associated with higher relapse rates and a need for subsequent DLI after allo-HCT[32,33].

Risk Assessment and Allo-HCT in High-Risk Plasma Cell Myeloma

Multiple biologic factors that influence risk and prognosis in myeloma also inform and influence the choice of therapy in order to provide a risk-adapted algorithm to patients[34,35]. Most experts recommend testing for biologic risk at diagnosis which differentiates patients into high, intermediate, and standard-risk groups[36]. Even with modern therapy, high-risk patients have a median OS of approximately 3 years while intermediate and standard-risk patients have an OS of 5 and 10 years respectively. According to the Mayo Stratification of Myeloma And Risk-adapted Therapy (mSMART) guidelines, in the absence of concurrent trisomies, patients with t(4;14) are considered intermediate risk while 17p deletion, t(14;16), and t(14;20) are considered high risk[36]. In those with t(4:14) intermediate-risk disease, bortezomib-based induction therapy followed by bortezomib-based maintenance may overcome the higher risk[37]. Prospective data from the Dutch-Belgian Hemato-Oncology Cooperative Group (HOVON) and the German Multicenter Myeloma Group (GMMG) study HOVON-65–GMMG-HD4 indicated that a bortezomib-based induction followed by a single or tandem auto-HCT and consolidation/maintenance therapy produced durable remissions even in high-risk subsets[38].

Patients with high-risk PCM have a shorter PFS compared to those with standard-risk myeloma[39,40]. High-risk PCM patients also may acquire new clonal abnormalities and present with rapidly progressing relapses or secondary plasma cell leukemia[41,42]. The benefits of novel agent therapy have not accrued to this subgroup of patients. In the absence of an effective established standard of care, these patients should be enrolled in clinical trials whenever possible. In the EBMT NMAM 2000 study, at a median follow-up of 96 months, 21% of patients with the higher risk deletion 13 abnormality receiving tandem auto-HCT-allo-HCT were progression free compared to 5% in the tandem auto-HCT group[18]. A survival benefit was noted with auto-HCT-allo-HCT in spite of the higher TRM associated with the regimen. Thus the higher initial risk of mortality and morbidity from allo-HCT might be acceptable in subgroups whose expected benefit from standard regimens is limited.

Recent attempts have been made to combine novel PCM drugs and immunomodulatory strategies with tandem auto-HCT-allo-HCT in higher risk patients. Michallet *et al.*[43] utilized vincristine/doxorubicin/high-dose dexamethasone (VAD) or bortezomib/dexamethasone (VD) as induction therapy followed by auto-HCT with melphalan conditioning, and those with better than a partial response were offered an RIC allo-HCT. Those not in CR at day 90 were given four cycles of bortezomib; subsequently if a CR was not attained they would be given DLIs. In 12 patients, this combination resulted in the median OS not being reached and a median PFS of 49 months. Acute and chronic GvHD was limited with four patients (three grade II and one grade I) and four patients (three limited and one extensive) respectively. Three deaths were reported, all due to disease progression.

A designation of "ultra-high-risk PCM" is used to characterize patients who have a predicted median survival of 24 months or less based upon initial risk stratification[44]. This group includes patients presenting with International Stage (ISS) stage III disease in addition to specific genetic abnormalities such as deletion 17p, immunoglobulin heavy chain gene translocations t(4;14) or t(14;16), and chromosome 1q21 amplification (>3 copies)[34,44]. A subgroup analysis of the HOVON-65-GMMG-HD4 study identified a high-risk population comprising approximately 18% of patients, characterized by the presence of del(17p13)/t(4;14)/1q21 (>3 copies) and an ISS score of II or III, with median PFS of only 18.7 months[34].

A review of allo-HCT in high-risk patients showed similar remission rate, PFS, OS, and relapse rate when those with del (17p)/t(4;14) were compared with the non-del(17p)/t(4;14) patients and identified achievement of mCR as the major factor for outcome[45]. In a prospective randomized study restricted to MM patients with del 13q by FISH, Knop et al. [46] have recently reported the results of a prospective randomized allo-HCT trial for patients with genetically defined high-risk (del 13q) PCM. Patients with newly diagnosed PCM carrying del 13q abnormality were randomized to either tandem auto-HCT- allo-HCT from an HLA-matched related or unrelated donors (with fludarabine/melphalan conditioning) or tandem auto-HCT. At 49 months of follow-up, PFS was superior for the allo-HCTed group and in the highest risk subgroup with del 17p and del 13 q abnormality, OS was superior for the allo-HCTation.

In summary, the outcomes for high-risk PCM remain poor despite the best available standard therapies and promising initial data suggest that allo-HCT should ideally be explored in this subset. In this subgroup of patients the adverse risk–benefit ratio for allo-HCT over standard therapies is balanced by the lack of efficacy of standard approaches.

Allo-HCT for Plasma Cell Myeloma at Relapse

Allogeneic transplantation for curative intent as an adjunct or an alternative to an auto-HCT has the best long-term outcomes and highest curative potential when utilized as part of a planned upfront strategy. However, given the higher risk of TRM and chronic GvHD, many patients may choose to defer allo-HCT completely or to a later line of therapy after relapse at which time the benefits are lower. Patients relapsing early after modern induction following auto-HCT (<18 months from transplant) represent another group with an expected survival of <12 months from relapse. Although there has been interest in considering allo-HCT in this subgroup[47], no randomized prospective data exist comparing allo-HCT with other alternatives in this group.

In the setting of multiply relapsed PCM, a CIBMTR analysis[48] and several single-center studies[49–51] have suggested that allo-HCT does not offer significant advantages in survival or offer a prospect of cure. In the CIBMTR study, 152 patients who had received a NST/RIC allo-HCT after relapse following a prior auto-HCT (50% relapsed within 24 months) were studied. Despite an acceptable TRM of 13% in the first year, the 3-year PFS and OS were 6% and 20% respectively[48]. A retrospective analysis from MD Anderson Cancer Center reported a 5-year PFS of 15% after allo-HCT in a cohort of patients with mostly (81%) relapsed patients[50]. Multivariate analysis showed allo-HCT to be most beneficial when used for consolidation in an initial remission.

Allo-HCT in Plasma Cell Leukemia

Plasma cell leukemia (PCL) is an aggressive plasma cell disorder which presents either *de novo* as primary PCL or as a leukemic transformation of end-stage PCM[52]. Primary PCL is an aggressive neoplasm and patients generally present at a younger age, with worse performance status at diagnosis, and have a high incidence of extramedullary involvement with extensive bone marrow disease[53]. Patients with t(4;14), del 1p21, and *MYC* gene rearrangements have been shown to have worse outcomes[35,40].

The Intergroupe Francophone du Myelome (IFM) showed that novel agents improved PCL survival from 8 months to 15 months[54]. The EBMT reported the comparative outcomes of 272 patients with primary PCL and of 20844 PCM patients who received an auto-HCT between 1980 and 2006[55]. Patients with PCL were more likely to achieve a CR but were additionally more likely to suffer TRM and OS was inferior to the PCM patients due to nonsustained responses. A CIBMTR study of 97 primary PCL patients who underwent an upfront auto-HCT (within 18 months of diagnosis) reported a 3-year PFS and OS of 34% and 64% respectively [56]. In the same analysis, 50 patients received allo-HCT for PCL (16 with NST/RIC regimens). At 3 years, the PFS was 18% and OS was 56% in the NST/RIC cohort with a significant relapse rate of 39%.

Conversely, while specific treatment data were not available, a review utilizing the Surveillance Epidemiology and End Results (SEER) program of 445 PCL patients noted the median OS improved between the cohorts of 1996–2000 and 2006–2009 from 5 months and 12 months respectively[57]. The review did not demonstrate an improvement between the cohorts of 1996–2000 and 2001–2005 when auto-HCT became a more viable treatment option. The authors suggest that although novel therapies were available starting in 2001, they were not approved for the frontline setting until 2006 and the increased use of more effective medical treatment is responsible for the OS improvement seen in the later cohort[57]. Additionally, a review focusing on HCT in PCL recommended evaluation for HCT consolidation only in eligible patients who initially respond to induction systemic therapy given the poor prognosis for frontline nonresponders [58].

Maintenance Therapy after Allo-HCT

Lenalidomide is a potent antimyeloma agent that also up-regulates NK cells and NK T-cells, and has been shown to improve time to disease progression and OS when used as ongoing maintenance therapy after auto-HCT[59]. Lenalidomide maintenance after allo-HCT is attractive since the GvM effect could be augmented by lenalidomide induced stimulation of the alloreactive lymphocytes and NK cells. In a phase 1/2 study, within the first week of lenalidomide treatment, peripheral CD4 and CD8 T-cells increased with improved NK cell-derived antimyeloma activity and was followed by a delayed increase in the regulatory T-cells[60]. Lenalidomide promotes T-cell proliferation augmenting response to a myeloma-specific tumor vaccine[61,62]. Objective responses to salvage treatment with lenalidomide were noted in 83% of patients (including 29% CR) relapsing after an allo-HCT. On lenalidomide therapy, 31% developed or exacerbated an acute GvHD episode which was significantly associated with an improved antimyeloma response; however at least one death was attributed to GvHD[63]. These studies suggested that in the post-allo-HCT setting, lenalidomide may induce disease response and also GvHD.

In daily practice, the feasibility of lenalidomide maintenance after allo-HCT has been questioned. The HOVON 76 trial assessed maintenance lenalidomide starting 1 to 6 months after allo-HCT for newly diagnosed PCM[64]. Unfortunately, 53% developed GvHD with 37% acute GvHD (at a median of 18 days on lenalidomide) and 17% chronic GvHD leading to premature discontinuation of therapy in 43% of the patients. A recent US phase 2 study reported the use of lenalidomide maintenance starting at a median of 96 days post-transplant in 30 high-risk patients after allo-HCT[65]. The cumulative incidence of PCM progression from start of maintenance was 37% with a low TRM of 11%. Acute GvHD was noted in 37% while PFS and OS at 18 months from initiation of lenalidomide was 63% and 78% respectively, suggesting benefit and manageable GvHD risk in this high-risk subgroup.

The intrinsic antimyeloma activity of proteasome inhibitors (PI) and their ability to suppress GvHD[66,67] without mitigating the GvM effect makes bortezomib an ideal option for post-allo-HCT maintenance. Kroger et al. investigated the use of bortezomib for at least two cycles and a median of 8 months following a RIC allo-HCT[68]. In patients with measurable disease, CR was seen in 30%, PR in 50%, and a minor response was seen in 20% of patients. There was no major increase in GvHD. More studies are needed to more definitively define the role of bortezomib and other PIs as planned maintenance post-allo-HCT. In this regard, the BMT CTN is planning to initiate a national US allo-HCT study (BMT CTN 1301) for high-risk PCM patients either in the upfront setting or after an early relapse following auto-HCT. This trial incorporates a proteasome inhibitor (bortezomib) in the conditioning regimen and also the second-generation oral proteasome inhibitor (ixazomib) in planned post-allo-HCT maintenance.

Measuring Responses after Transplant: Going Beyond the Complete Response

Deeper levels of remission in PCM correlate with superior PFS but there is no defined level of remission that equates to a cure. For those in an immunofixation-defined CR after transplantation, outcomes may be further predicted by evaluating for a complete molecular remission[69,70]. In a study of patients in CR following allo-HCT, those who were polymerase chain reaction negative for plasma cell clone-specific markers were relapse-free at 5 years[71]. In another study comparing auto-HCT recipients and allo-HCT recipients, allo-HCT patients were more likely to be in molecular CR (mCR) which in turn predicted for lower relapse rates[69]. These results support the concept that mCR is associated with longer relapse-free survival and reduced relapse rates[45].

Similar or even greater depths of remission including minimal residual disease (MRD) can be assessed by the newer technique of deep sequencing or by monitoring for the presence of aberrant plasma cells in remission bone marrows using multiparametric flow cytometry (MFC) at serial time points [72,73]. Patients with no detectable malignant plasma cells at both 3 and 6 months post-auto-HCT by MFC were noted to have a 5-year OS of 100% in early studies[72]. A study evaluating the prognostic value of MRD by deep sequencing after induction therapy showed those who were MRD-negative had an increased median time to progression compared with MRD-positive patients (80 months versus 31 months) and an increased OS (median not reached versus 81 months)[73]. Concordance between deep sequencing and MFC can be high at 83%[73]. Newer MRD techniques validated in the auto-HCT [74] setting need to be validated in the allo-HCT setting too. The lack of a validated residual disease negative state that equates to cure and the current nonavailability of such testing outside of academic centers are drawbacks.

Treatment for Relapsed Plasma Cell Myeloma after Allo-HCT

Treatment options for relapsed PCM after allo-HCT include donor lymphocyte infusion (DLI) alone or in combination with salvage chemotherapy. Novel agents and combinations involving novel agents have been used successfully[63,75]. A higher risk of GvHD has been reported in those treated with lenalidomide but no special precautions other than close monitoring are required.

DLIs are able to induce a clinically meaningful GvM effect in some relapsed patients after allo-HCT[37]. However, DLI treatment is also associated with a risk of inducing severe GvHD[76]. A series of 54 patients receiving DLI reported overall responses and CR rates of 52% and 17% with acute and chronic GvHD in 57% and 47% respectively[77]. Disease control from DLI was superior for those in remissions and in those who developed GvHD. An alternative strategy is the use of prophylactic DLI at defined time points (usually 6 months)

Table 48.2 Controversies and practical guidelines for allogeneic hematopoietic cell transplant patient selection

A. Patient factors:
1. Age:
Approximately 15% of patients with MM are <55 years old. Allo-HCT is an option in these patients.
2. Performance status (PS) and comorbidity:
Allo-HCT is feasible with low TRM in those with good PS and low comorbidity scores.
Younger patients with MM (<55 years) with good PS and low comorbidity scores are considered allo-HCT eligible at our center.

B. Disease factors:
1. Newly diagnosed MM:
We attempt karyotypic, plasma cell enriched FISH based and Gene Expression Profiling (GEP) based (Arkansas model) risk stratification in allo-HCT eligible patients at diagnosis. If any of the following are discovered, we proceed to donor search:
- Ultra-high-risk MM: defined by ISS stage 3 or a high plasma cell proliferation index AND the presence of any or a combination of the following specific genetic changes: del 17p, chromosome 1q gains, t(14:20), t(14:16), OR a high-risk gene expression profile.
- Primary plasma cell leukemia.
- Primary refractory MM: patients who are refractory to or progressing on combination therapy involving both full doses of lenalidomide and a proteasome inhibitor (bortezomib/carfilzomib) after 4 cycles.
2. Relapsed MM:
Early relapse after auto-HCT: defined as those relapsing with clinical disease (NOT biochemical progression) within 18 months after induction and auto-HCT. These patients are candidates if they achieve a VGPR or better disease status with salvage therapy.
We advise allo-HCT consultation to patients fulfilling the above criteria since current therapies and auto-HCT are associated with short survival in these subgroups.

C. Donor evaluation:
1. Ideal donor: Matched sibling or an unrelated donor matched at all A,B,C,DR loci using high-resolution typing:
If an ideal donor has been identified, allo-HCT is offered either on a clinical trial protocol or as standard of care for patients defined above AFTER risks and benefits have been reviewed.
2. Alternative donor/unavailable ideal donor:
We offer allo-HCT using a haploidentical or other mismatched donor only on a clinical trial protocol and only for those without an ideal donor.

D. Conditioning therapy:
For those who have not had an auto-HCT or more than 1 year from an auto-HCT, we offer myeloablative or reduced intensity conditioning regimens. Nonmyeloablative conditioning regimens are not used.

E. Post-allo-HCT therapy:
At day 100, patients with no GvHD and adequate performance status, we initiate maintenance therapy either on a clinical trial or as standard of care with lenalidomide or bortezomib with intent to continue such therapy for 3 years.

or in graded incremental T-cell doses for improving donor-derived T-cell immunity and to convert those with partial donor T-cell chimerism to full donor hematopoiesis[78]. The future of DLI is an area of increasing research and includes the use of donor-derived T-cells directed at PCM-associated antigens such as WT1 or those in the cancer testis antigen family [79,80].

The Future of Allo-HCT for Plasma Cell Myeloma

Current strategies in allo-HCT-based therapy for PCM are restricted to high-risk patients and aim to achieve deeper molecular and MRD-negative remissions prior to allograft infusion. Additional topics of interest include evaluating novel combination therapies during the pre- and post-allograft phase aimed at sustaining CR. It is generally accepted that for patients with high-risk PCM, achieving and maintaining deep remissions offer the best prospect of long-term survival[81,82]. Regarding the allo-HCT itself, designing more effective conditioning regimens beyond NST/RIC is probably necessary to

improve PCM specific outcomes. Additional cellular therapy approaches such as chimeric antigen receptor T-cells directed at myeloma-specific targets are also in development.

Controversies and Practice Points

Allo-HCT could be offered either on a clinical trial (ideally) or as standard of care to patients with well-defined high- or ultra-high-risk features (Table 48.2) if they are otherwise eligible for an allo-HCT. In relapsed PCM, it is our institutional practice to offer allo-HCT to patients who remain therapy sensitive and are in early relapse or to patients after they achieve a deep remission such as VGPR or CR. We discourage allo-HCT in multiply relapsed patients or in those with uncontrolled PCM. In young persons with PCL, given the extremely high risk of relapse after an auto-HCT, the option of allo-HCT should be explored and its risks and benefits should be discussed. It is our practice to consider DLI after salvage therapy to augment donor-derived anti-PCM immunity in patients who relapse after allo-HCT (see Chapter 25).

References

1. Pasquini MC Wang Z. Current use and outcome of hematopoietic stem cell transplantation: CIBMTR Summary Slides, 2012. Available at: http://www.cibmtr.org. (Accessed March 30, 2013).

2. Bensinger WI, Buckner CD, Anasetti C, *et al.* Allogeneic marrow transplantation for multiple myeloma: an analysis of risk factors on outcome. *Blood* 1996;88:2787–93.

3. Gahrton G, Tura S, Flesch M, *et al.* Allogeneic bone marrow transplantation in 24 patients with multiple myeloma reported to the EBMT registry. *Hematol Oncol* 1988;6:181–6.

4. Gahrton G, Tura S, Ljungman P, *et al.* Allogeneic bone marrow transplantation in multiple myeloma. European Group for Bone Marrow Transplantation. *N Engl J Med* 1991;325:1267–73.

5. Gahrton G, Tura S, Ljungman P, *et al.* Prognostic factors in allogeneic bone marrow transplantation for multiple myeloma. *J Clin Oncol* 1995;13:1312–22.

6. Barlogie B, Kyle RA, Anderson KC, *et al.* Standard chemotherapy compared with high-dose chemoradiotherapy for multiple myeloma: final results of phase III US Intergroup Trial S9321. *J Clin Oncol* 2006;24:929–36.

7. Kroger N, Schwerdtfeger R, Kiehl M, *et al.* Autologous stem cell transplantation followed by a dose-reduced allograft induces high complete remission rate in multiple myeloma. *Blood* 2002;100:755–60.

8. Giralt S, Estey E, Albitar M, *et al.* Engraftment of allogeneic hematopoietic progenitor cells with purine analog-containing chemotherapy: harnessing graft-*versus*-leukemia without myeloablative therapy. *Blood* 1997;89:4531–6.

9. Bacigalupo A, Ballen K, Rizzo D, *et al.* Defining the intensity of conditioning regimens: working definitions. *Biol Blood Marrow Transplant* 2009;15:1628–33.

10. Maloney DG, Molina AJ, Sahebi F, *et al.* Allografting with nonmyeloablative conditioning following cytoreductive autografts for the treatment of patients with multiple myeloma. *Blood* 2003;102:3447–54.

11. Kroger N, Sayer HG, Schwerdtfeger R, *et al.* Unrelated stem cell transplantation in multiple myeloma after a reduced-intensity conditioning with pretransplantation antithymocyte globulin is highly effective with low transplantation-related mortality. *Blood* 2002;100:3919–24.

12. Rotta M, Storer BE, Sahebi F, *et al.* Long-term outcome of patients with multiple myeloma after autologous hematopoietic cell transplantation and nonmyeloablative allografting. *Blood* 2009;113:3383–91.

13. Bruno B, Rotta M, Patriarca F, *et al.* Nonmyeloablative allografting for newly diagnosed multiple myeloma: the experience of the Gruppo Italiano Trapianti di Midollo. *Blood* 2009;113:3375–82.

14. Kumar S, Zhang MJ, Li P, *et al.* Trends in allogeneic stem cell transplantation for multiple myeloma: a CIBMTR analysis. *Blood* 2011;118:1979–88.

15. Bruno B, Rotta M, Patriarca F, *et al.* A comparison of allografting with autografting for newly diagnosed myeloma. *N Engl J Med* 2007;356:1110–20.

16. Giaccone L, Storer B, Patriarca F, *et al.* Long-term follow-up of a comparison of nonmyeloablative allografting with autografting for newly diagnosed myeloma. *Blood* 2011;117:6721–7.

17. Krishnan A, Pasquini MC, Logan B, *et al.* Autologous haemopoietic stem-cell transplantation followed by allogeneic or autologous haemopoietic stem-cell transplantation in patients with multiple myeloma (BMT CTN 0102): a phase 3 biological assignment trial. *Lancet Oncol* 2011;12:1195–203.

18. Gahrton G, Iacobelli S, Bjorkstrand B, *et al.* Autologous/reduced-intensity allogeneic stem cell transplantation *versus* autologous transplantation in multiple myeloma: long-term results of the EBMT-NMAM2000 study. *Blood* 2013;121:5055–63.

19. Bjorkstrand B, Iacobelli S, Hegenbart U, *et al.* Tandem autologous/reduced-intensity conditioning allogeneic stem-cell transplantation *versus* autologous transplantation in myeloma: long-term follow-up. *J Clin Oncol* 2011;29:3016–22.

20. Armeson KE, Hill EG, Costa LJ. Tandem autologous vs autologous plus reduced intensity allogeneic transplantation in the upfront management of multiple myeloma: meta-analysis of trials with biological assignment. *Bone Marrow Transplant* 2013;48:562–7.

21. Moreau P, Garban F, Attal M, *et al.* Long-term follow-up results of IFM99-03 and IFM99-04 trials comparing nonmyeloablative allo-HCTation with autologous transplantation in high-risk de novo multiple myeloma. *Blood* 2008;112:3914–5.

22. Stewart AK. Reduced-intensity allogeneic transplantation for myeloma: reality bites. *Blood* 2009;113:3135–6.

23. Weiden PL, Sullivan KM, Flournoy N, Storb R, Thomas ED. Antileukemic effect of chronic graft-*versus*-host disease: contribution to improved survival after allogeneic marrow transplantation. *N Engl J Med* 1981;304:1529–33.

24. Sullivan KM, Fefer A, Witherspoon R, *et al.* Graft-*versus*-leukemia in man: relationship of acute and chronic graft-*versus*-host disease to relapse of acute leukemia following allogeneic bone marrow transplantation. *Prog Clin Biol Res* 1987;244:391–9.

25. Horowitz MM, Gale RP, Sondel PM, *et al.* Graft-*versus*-leukemia reactions after bone marrow transplantation. *Blood* 1990;75:555–62.

26. Kwak LW, Taub DD, Duffey PL, *et al.* Transfer of myeloma idiotype-specific immunity from an actively immunised marrow donor. *Lancet* 1995;345:1016–20.

27. Salama M, Nevill T, Marcellus D, *et al.* Donor leukocyte infusions for multiple myeloma. *Bone Marrow Transplant* 2000;26:1179–84.

28. Verdonck LF, Lokhorst HM, Dekker AW, Nieuwenhuis HK, Petersen EJ. Graft-*versus*-myeloma effect in two cases. *Lancet* 1996;347:800–1.

29. Lokhorst HM, Schattenberg A, Cornelissen JJ, *et al.* Donor lymphocyte infusions for relapsed multiple myeloma after allogeneic stem-cell transplantation: predictive factors for response and long-term outcome. *J Clin Oncol* 2000;18:3031–7.

30. van de Donk NW, Kroger N, Hegenbart U, *et al.* Prognostic factors for donor lymphocyte infusions following non-myeloablative allogeneic stem cell transplantation in multiple myeloma.

Bone Marrow Transplant
2006;37:1135–41.

31. Ringden O, Shrestha S, da Silva GT, *et al.* Effect of acute and chronic GVHD on relapse and survival after reduced-intensity conditioning allogeneic transplantation for myeloma. *Bone Marrow Transplant* 2012;47:831–7.

32. Garban F, Attal M, Michallet M, *et al.* Prospective comparison of autologous stem cell transplantation followed by dose-reduced allograft (IFM99-03 trial) with tandem autologous stem cell transplantation (IFM99-04 trial) in high-risk de novo multiple myeloma. *Blood* 2006;107:3474–80.

33. Alyea E, Weller E, Schlossman R, *et al.* T-cell–depleted allogeneic bone marrow transplantation followed by donor lymphocyte infusion in patients with multiple myeloma: induction of graft-*versus*-myeloma effect. *Blood* 2001;98:934–9.

34. Neben K, Lokhorst HM, Jauch A, *et al.* Administration of bortezomib before and after autologous stem cell transplantation improves outcome in multiple myeloma patients with deletion 17p. *Blood* 2012;119:940–8.

35. Avet-Loiseau H, Daviet A, Brigaudeau C, *et al.* Cytogenetic, interphase, and multicolor fluorescence in situ hybridization analyses in primary plasma cell leukemia: a study of 40 patients at diagnosis, on behalf of the Intergroupe Francophone du Myelome and the Groupe Francais de Cytogenetique Hematologique. *Blood* 2001;97:822–5.

36. Mikhael JR, Dingli D, Roy V, *et al.* Management of newly diagnosed symptomatic multiple myeloma: updated Mayo Stratification of Myeloma and Risk-Adapted Therapy (mSMART) Consensus Guidelines 2013. *Mayo Clin Proc* 2013;88:360–76.

37. Mateos M, Oriol A, Martínez-López J, *et al.* Bortezomib, melphalan, and prednisone *versus* bortezomib, thalidomide, and prednisone as induction therapy followed by maintenance treatment with bortezomib and thalidomide *versus* bortezomib and prednisone in elderly patients with untreated multiple myeloma: a randomised trial. *The Lancet Oncology* 2010;11:934–41.

38. Sonneveld P, Schmidt-Wolf IG, van der Holt B, *et al.* Bortezomib induction and maintenance treatment in patients with

newly diagnosed multiple myeloma: results of the randomized phase III HOVON-65/ GMMG-HD4 trial. *J Clin Oncol* 2012;30:2946–55.

39. Chang H, Qi X, Yeung J, Reece D, Xu W, Patterson B. Genetic aberrations including chromosome 1 abnormalities and clinical features of plasma cell leukemia. *Leuk Res* 2009;33:259–62.

40. Tiedemann RE, Gonzalez-Paz N, Kyle RA, *et al.* Genetic aberrations and survival in plasma cell leukemia. *Leukemia* 2008;22:1044–52.

41. Bahlis NJ. Darwinian evolution and tiding clones in multiple myeloma. *Blood* 2012;120:927–8.

42. Egan JB, Shi CX, Tembe W, *et al.* Whole-genome sequencing of multiple myeloma from diagnosis to plasma cell leukemia reveals genomic initiating events, evolution, and clonal tides. *Blood* 2012;120:1060–6.

43. Michallet M, Sobh M, El-Cheikh J, *et al.* Evolving strategies with immunomodulating drugs and tandem autologous/allogeneic hematopoietic stem cell transplantation in first line high risk multiple myeloma patients. *Exp Hematol* 2013;41:1008–15.

44. Avet-Loiseau H. Ultra high-risk myeloma. *Hematology Am Soc Hematol Educ Program* 2010;2010:489–93.

45. Kroger N, Badbaran A, Zabelina T, *et al.* Impact of high-risk cytogenetics and achievement of molecular remission on long-term freedom from disease after autologous-allogeneic tandem transplantation in patients with multiple myeloma. *Biol Blood Marrow Transplant* 2013;19:398–404.

46. Knop S, Liebisch P, Hebart H, *et al.* Autologous followed by allogeneic *versus* tandem-autologous stem cell transplant in newly diagnosed FISH-del13q myeloma. *ASH Annual Meeting Abstracts* 2014; 124:43.

47. Kroger N, Shimoni A, Schilling G, *et al.* Unrelated stem cell transplantation after reduced intensity conditioning for patients with multiple myeloma relapsing after autologous transplantation. *Br J Haematol* 2010;148:323–31.

48. Freytes CO, Vesole DH, Zhong X, *et al.* Second transplants in relapsed multiple myeloma (MM): autologous (AUTO-HCT) *versus* non-myeloablative/reduced intensity (NST/RIC) allogeneic

transplantation (AlloHCT). *ASH Annual Meeting Abstracts* 2011;118:824.

49. Mehta J, Tricot G, Jagannath S, *et al.* Salvage autologous or allogeneic transplantation for multiple myeloma refractory to or relapsing after a first-line autograft? *Bone Marrow Transplant* 1998;21:887–92.

50. Bashir Q, Khan H, Orlowski RZ, *et al.* Predictors of prolonged survival after allogeneic hematopoietic stem cell transplantation for multiple myeloma. *Am J Hematol* 2012;87:272–6.

51. Lee CK, Barlogie B, Zangari M, *et al.* Transplantation as salvage therapy for high-risk patients with myeloma in relapse. *Bone Marrow Transplant* 2002;30:873–8.

52. Jimenez-Zepeda VH, Dominguez VJ. Plasma cell leukemia: a rare condition. *Ann Hematol* 2006;85:263–7.

53. Garcia-Sanz R, Orfao A, Gonzalez M, *et al.* Primary plasma cell leukemia: clinical, immunophenotypic, DNA ploidy, and cytogenetic characteristics. *Blood* 1999;93:1032–7.

54. Chaoui D, Leleu X, Roussel M, Royer B, Rubio MT, Ducastelle S, *et al.* Has the prognostic of primary plasma cell leukemia improved with new drugs? *ASH Annual Meeting Abstracts* 2009;114:3869.

55. Drake MB, Iacobelli S, van Biezen A, *et al.* Primary plasma cell leukemia and autologous stem cell transplantation. *Haematologica* 2010;95:804–9.

56. Mahindra A, Kalaycio ME, Vela-Ojeda J, *et al.* Hematopoietic cell transplantation for primary plasma cell leukemia: results from the Center for International Blood and Marrow Transplant Research. *Leukemia* 2012;26:1091–7.

57. Gonsalves WI, Rajkumar SV, Go RS, *et al.* Trends in survival of patients with primary plasma cell leukemia: a population-based analysis. *Blood* 2014;124:907–12.

58. Nishihori T, Abu Kar SM, Baz R, *et al.* Therapeutic advances in the treatment of primary plasma cell leukemia: a focus on hematopoietic cell transplantation. *Biol Blood Marrow Transplant* 2013;19:1144–51.

59. McCarthy PL, Owzar K, Hofmeister CC, *et al.* Lenalidomide after stem-cell transplantation for multiple myeloma. *N Engl J Med* 2012;366:1770–81.

60. Wolschke C, Stubig T, Hegenbart U, *et al.* Postallograft lenalidomide induces strong NK cell-mediated antimyeloma activity and risk for T cell-mediated GvHD: Results from a phase I/II dose-finding study. *Exp Hematol* 2013;41:134–142 e3.

61. Luptakova K, Rosenblatt J, Glotzbecker B, *et al.* Lenalidomide enhances anti-myeloma cellular immunity. *Cancer Immunol Immunother* 2013;62:39–49.

62. Rosenblatt J, Vasir B, Uhl L, *et al.* Vaccination with dendritic cell/tumor fusion cells results in cellular and humoral antitumor immune responses in patients with multiple myeloma. *Blood* 2011;117:393–402.

63. Coman T, Bachy E, Michallet M, *et al.* Lenalidomide as salvage treatment for multiple myeloma relapsing after allogeneic hematopoietic stem cell transplantation: a report from the SFGM-TC. *Haematologica* 2013;98:776–83.

64. Kneppers E, van der Holt B, Kersten MJ, *et al.* Lenalidomide maintenance after nonmyeloablative allogeneic stem cell transplantation in multiple myeloma is not feasible: results of the HOVON 76 Trial. *Blood* 2011;118:2413–9.

65. Alsina M, Becker P, Zhong X, *et al.* Lenalidomide maintenance for high-risk multiple myeloma after allogeneic hematopoietic cell transplantation. *Biol Blood Marrow Transplant* 2014;20:1183–9.

66. Vodanovic-Jankovic S, Hari P, Jacobs P, Komorowski R, Drobyski WR. NF-kappaB as a target for the prevention of graft-*versus*-host disease: comparative efficacy of bortezomib and PS-1145. *Blood* 2006;107:827–34.

67. Koreth J, Stevenson KE, Kim HT, *et al.* Bortezomib-based graft-*versus*-host disease prophylaxis in HLA-mismatched unrelated donor transplantation. *J Clin Oncol* 2012;30:3202–8.

68. Kroger N, Zabelina T, Ayuk F, *et al.* Bortezomib after dose-reduced allogeneic stem cell transplantation for multiple myeloma to enhance or maintain remission status. *Exp Hematol* 2006;34:770–5.

69. Martinelli G, Terragna C, Zamagni E, *et al.* Molecular remission after allogeneic or autologous transplantation of hematopoietic stem cells for multiple myeloma. *J Clin Oncol* 2000;18:2273–81.

70. Cavo M, Terragna C, Martinelli G, *et al.* Molecular monitoring of minimal residual disease in patients in long-term complete remission after allogeneic stem cell transplantation for multiple myeloma. *Blood* 2000;96:355–7.

71. Corradini P, Cavo M, Lokhorst H, *et al.* Molecular remission after myeloablative allogeneic stem cell transplantation predicts a better relapse-free survival in patients with multiple myeloma. *Blood* 2003;102:1927–9.

72. Rawstron AC, Davies FE, DasGupta R, *et al.* Flow cytometric disease monitoring in multiple myeloma: the relationship between normal and neoplastic plasma cells predicts outcome after transplantation. *Blood* 2002;100:3095–100.

73. Martinez-Lopez J, Lahuerta JJ, Pepin F, *et al.* Prognostic value of deep sequencing method for minimal residual disease detection in multiple myeloma. *Blood* 2014;123:2073–9.

74. Paiva B, Martinez-Lopez J, Vidriales MB, *et al.* Comparison of immunofixation, serum free light chain, and immunophenotyping for response evaluation and prognostication in multiple myeloma. *J Clin Oncol* 2011;29:1627–33.

75. El-Cheikh J, Crocchiolo R, Boher JM, *et al.* Comparable outcomes between unrelated and related donors after reduced-intensity conditioning allogeneic hematopoietic stem cell transplantation in patients with high-risk multiple myeloma. *Eur J Haematol* 2012;88:497–503.

76. Kroger N, Kruger W, Renges H, *et al.* Donor lymphocyte infusion enhances remission status in patients with persistent disease after allografting for multiple myeloma. *Br J Haematol* 2001;112:421–3.

77. Lokhorst HM, Wu K, Verdonck LF, *et al.* The occurrence of graft-*versus*-host disease is the major predictive factor for response to donor lymphocyte infusions in multiple myeloma. *Blood* 2004;103:4362–4.

78. Bellucci R, Alyea EP, Weller E, *et al.* Immunologic effects of prophylactic donor lymphocyte infusion after allogeneic marrow transplantation for multiple myeloma. *Blood* 2002;99:4610–7.

79. de Carvalho F, Alves VL, Braga WM, Xavier CV,Jr, Colleoni GW. MAGE-C1/CT7 and MAGE-C2/CT10 are frequently expressed in multiple myeloma and can be explored in combined immunotherapy for this malignancy. *Cancer Immunol Immunother* 2013;62:191–5.

80. Tyler EM, Jungbluth AA, O'Reilly RJ, Koehne G. WT1-specific T-cell responses in high-risk multiple myeloma patients undergoing allogeneic T cell-depleted hematopoietic stem cell transplantation and donor lymphocyte infusions. *Blood* 2013;121:308–17.

81. Haessler J, Shaughnessy JD Jr, Zhan F, *et al.* Benefit of complete response in multiple myeloma limited to high-risk subgroup identified by gene expression profiling. *Clin Cancer Res* 2007;13:7073–9.

82. Hoering A, Crowley J, Shaughnessy JD Jr, *et al.* Complete remission in multiple myeloma examined as time-dependent variable in terms of both onset and duration in Total Therapy protocols. *Blood* 2009;114:1299–305.

83. Rosinol L, Perez-Simon JA, Sureda A, *et al.* A prospective PETHEMA study of tandem autologous transplantation *versus* autograft followed by reduced-intensity conditioning allogeneic transplantation in newly diagnosed multiple myeloma. *Blood* 2008;112:3591–3.

84. Lokhorst HM, van der Holt B, Cornelissen JJ, *et al.* Donor *versus* no-donor comparison of newly diagnosed myeloma patients included in the HOVON-50 multiple myeloma study. *Blood* 2012;119:6219,25; quiz 6399.

Hematopoietic Cell Transplantation for Immunoglobulin Light Chain (AL) Amyloidosis

Taimur Sher and Morie A. Gertz

Introduction

Immunoglobulin light chain amyloidosis (AL), the most common form of systemic amyloidosis, is a plasma cell dyscrasia characterized by extracellular deposition of amyloidogenic light chain fragments that result in progressive organ dysfunction. AL is a fatal disease with a median survival of 12–17 months[1]. Death results from rapid clinical deterioration due to the involvement of heart, kidneys, liver, and the gastrointestinal tract. Treatment of AL involves the use of multiagent therapy aiming at eradicating the underlying transformed plasma cells, the source of amyloidogenic light chains, and providing organ-directed supportive care. Antiplasma cell therapy in AL has evolved along the lines of multiple myeloma (MM). In this review we focus on the evolution of the role of auto-HCT in AL, the unique challenges it poses in the management of persons with AL, and its evolving role in the era of new treatment modalities.

Autologous Hematopoietic Cell Transplantation

A Historical Perspective and Barriers to Auto-HCT in AL

Oral melphalan in combination with steroids such as dexamethasone (MelDex) demonstrated significant activity in AL in early clinical investigations. The MelDex combination delivered high hematologic CRs that exceeded CR rates observed in MM and resulted in improvement in survival [2]. Therapeutic benefit from MelDex and other steroid combinations required prolonged treatment over the course of 12–18 months. This long-term use has been associated with a high incidence of therapy-related myeloid neoplasms (up to 20%) and other metabolic and cardiovascular toxicities[3]. The success of auto-HCT in MM in the 1980s established high-dose melphalan as the standard of care (see Chapter 46). This medical advancement inspired the exploration of auto-HCT in AL; however, organ dysfunction and rapid clinical deterioration in these patients presented a formidable barrier and it was not until the mid-1990s that the first experience with this modality was reported in AL[4]. The role and practice of auto-HCT in AL has significantly evolved over the last two decades

with significant improvement in safety primarily as a result of better patient selection.

How Important Is Patient and Center Selection for Auto-HCT in AL?

Comenzo et al. reported their experience with auto-HCT in a select group of 25 AL patients with a median age of 48 (range 29–60) years. At a median follow-up of 2 years 68% of the patients were alive with an early transplant-related mortality (TRM) of 20%[5]. The hematologic complete response, by criteria predating the immunoglobulin light chain assay, was achieved in 60% of patients. To explore this further, several groups over the course of 5–6 years reported their experience. Using a melphalan dose of between 100 and 200 mg/m^2 these series demonstrated that high-dose melphalan was associated with higher hematologic response rates, including CRs in up to 40% of patients and organ responses in up to 45%[6,7]. Consequently it was established that auto-HCT was effective in targeting the neoplastic plasma cells in AL; however, the main lesson from these studies was the unacceptably high TRM of 10–43% at 3 months[7]. The primary cause of this mortality was sudden cardiac death, gastrointestinal hemorrhage, hypotension, and sepsis with multiorgan failure. Another major challenge witnessed was the lack of sensitive prognostic and predictive biologic markers to assist patient selection for auto-HCT.

These experiences led the IFM (Intergroupe Francophone du Myélome) to conduct one of the most important studies in AL therapeutics, which to date remains the only randomized study comparing auto-HCT to the standard of care oral MelDex regimen (total of 100 patients). Compared to MelDex there was no difference in the hematologic and organ response rates between the auto-HCT and MelDex arms (66% versus 68% and 39% versus 45%, respectively). Intriguingly, patients in the MelDex arm survived much longer than auto-HCT patients (56.9 months versus 22.2 months)[8]. The TRM of auto-HCT was 24%. A closer look at these data revealed several findings: 26% of patients randomized to undergo auto-HCT were dropped due to early mortality; 12% of patients with advanced cardiac disease underwent auto-HCT, which might have been excluded from the auto-HCT arm elsewhere; and the dose basis for melphalan was not clear but the majority of

Table 49.1 Guidelines for patient selection for autologous hematopoietic cell transplant

Absolute contraindications
(evolving conditions and might improve with therapy)

Clinical congestive heart failure

Total bilirubin >3.0 mg/dL

Left ventricular ejection fraction <30%

Troponin T >0.06 ng/mL[a]

Relative contraindications
(evolving conditions and might improve with therapy except age)

Serum creatinine >2.0 mg/dL

Interventricular septal thickness >1.5 cm

Age >60 years

More than two visceral organs involvement

[a] While troponin T >0.06 ng/mL is not an absolute contraindication, due to day 100 all-cause mortality of 28%, it is strongly recommended to consider alternative therapies in such patients.

Table 49.2 Risk-adapted approach for patient selection and chemotherapy dosing for autologous hematopoietic cell transplant in AL

Good risk

One or two organs involved

No cardiac involvement

Creatinine clearance ≥51 mL/min

Any age

Intermediate risk

Younger than 61 years old

One or two organs involved

Asymptomatic or compensated cardiac involvement

Creatinine clearance <51 mL/min

Poor risk

Three organs involved

Advanced cardiac involvement

Melphalan dosing for autologous hematopoietic cell transplant based on risk group and age:

	Good risk			Intermediate risk		Poor risk
Age	≤60	61–70	≥71	≤60	61–70	Any age
Melphalan dose (mg/m²)	200	140	100	140	100	Avoid SCT

Modified from ref [10].

patients received ≥140 mg/m². Additionally, as has been demonstrated in a study from the Center of International Blood and Marrow Transplantation Registry (CIBMTR), it is possible that the inclusion of multiple centers might have contributed to the high rate of mortality and complications due to the inexperience of the transplant team treating AL.

In our opinion, the IFM and CIBMTR studies highlight the importance of patient and center selection to offset the adverse outcomes associated with auto-HCT in persons with AL.

Major Strides To Improve Safety of Auto-HCT in AL: What Else Is Important to Predict Outcomes?

During the mid to late 2000s, significant progress was made in addressing the critical issues of high mortality and morbidity of auto-HCT in AL. Experience from centers with large volumes of AL patients identified several patient, disease, and treatment-related factors that could predict high TRM and morbidity. Prominent among these predictive factors were advanced age, presence of syncope, suboptimal left ventricular ejection fraction, thickened interventricular septum, and advanced kidney disease (Table 49.1)[9]. In the 587 AL patients who have undergone auto-HCT at the Mayo Clinic since the start of program, the number of involved organs proved to be a very important prognostic marker, with a median survival of 45 months, 104 months, and not reached for patients with more than two, two, or one involved organ, respectively (Figure 49.1).

This experience led to the proposal of a risk-adapted approach for the use of auto-HCT that advises not only about the decision to choose for or against auto-HCT but also provide guidelines about the melphalan dosing in various risk

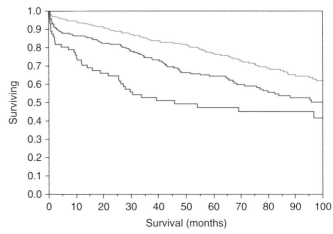

Figure 49.1. Overall survival in 587 AL patients treated with auto-HCT at the Mayo Clinic according to the number of involved organs: red = ≥2; blue = 2; green = 1. *P*<0.0001.

groups (Table 49.2) [10]. Although this approach has not been evaluated prospectively in randomized fashion it has been adapted both in the United States and Europe and has contributed to the improved safety of auto-HCT. In a large series of 422 AL patients treated with auto-HCT at Mayo Clinic, we noted a 40% reduction in TRM in patients treated after

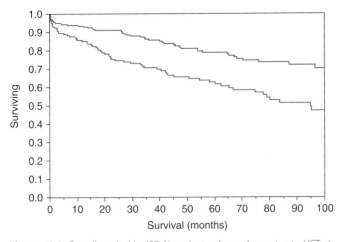

Figure 49.2 Overall survival in 437 AL patients who underwent auto-HCT at the Mayo Clinic depending upon the difference between the involved and uninvolved free light chain in serum. Red = dFLC ≤18mg/dL; blue = dFLC >18mg/dL; P<0.0001.

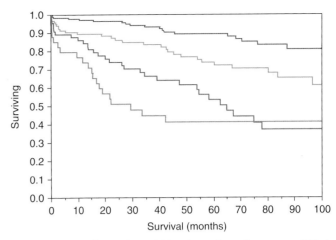

Figure 49.3 Overall survival in 410 AL patients who underwent auto-HCT at the Mayo Clinic based on the revised Mayo prognostic score. Patients are assigned a score of 1 for each of dFLC (difference between involved and uninvolved free light chain) ≥18mg/dL, cTnT ≥0.025ng/mL, and NT-ProBNP ≥1800pg/mL, creating scores of 0 (no risk factor present; represented by red line), 1 (one risk factor present; represented by green line), 2 (two risk factors present; represented by blue line), or 3 (all risk factors present; represented by brown line), respectively. P<0.0001.

January 2006 compared to those treated before January 2006 (day 100 mortality of 7% *versus* 12%). Corresponding 2-year overall survival increased from 78% to 82 [11]. Similarly, in a large series of 522 patients who underwent auto-HCT at Boston University Medical Center, the investigators reported successive improvement in day 100 mortality in the second decade of their experience versus the first (4% *versus* 17%) for an overall TRM of 12% for the group[12].

One of the major advancements in the management of AL was the development of the three-tiered Mayo staging system (MSS), devised in 2004 by measuring serum levels of readily available biomarkers of myocardial stress and injury, i.e., cardiac troponin T (cTNT) and N-terminal of the pro-hormone of beta natriuretic peptide (NT-ProBNP)[13]. This staging system, for the first time, provided a reproducible and quantifiable framework that could prognosticate the outcomes of AL patients both in the auto-HCT and nontransplant setting. In 434 AL patients who underwent auto-HCT at the Mayo Clinic between 1996 and 2010 the MSS emerged as one of the most important determinants of outcome with a median survival not reached at the time of data cut-off for stages 1 and 2 and 58 months for stage 3 disease[14]. In addition to being prognostic, MSS proved very valuable in comparing patients across different studies and became an influential tool in selecting patients not only for auto-HCT but also as an important inclusion and exclusion criteria in the next generation of clinical trials. The introduction of serum-free light chain assay (SFLA), providing quantitative measurements of circulating free light chains, is another advance that has proven indispensable in defining the hematologic response to treatment. Several studies have confirmed hematologic response as the most important determinant of overall outcome and subsequent organ response[15]. In the Mayo Clinic series, the median survival of patients with no response, partial hematologic response, or complete hematologic response to auto-HCT

was 32 months, 107 months, and not reached, respectively [14]. Investigators at Boston University reported an impressive 53% survival at 10 years in patients achieving hematologic CR after auto-HCT[16]. In addition to serving as the defining factor for hematologic response, SFLA has also emerged as a prognostic indicator [17]. As a marker of the amyloidogenic light chain burden the difference between involved and uninvolved (dFLC), free light chain at baseline was able to separate 437 AL patients who underwent auto-HCT at the Mayo Clinic into two prognostic groups with median survival of 95 *versus* 162 months for dFLC >18mg/dL and ≤8mg/dL, respectively (Figure 49.2). Most recently, dFLC has been combined with cTNT and NT-ProBNP to generate a *modified* MSS that can reliably separate AL patients undergoing auto-HCT into four groups (Figure 49.3) with distinct prognosis [18].

Caution with Hematopoietic Cell Mobilization: Why?

Supportive care forms the cornerstone of auto-HCT in AL. Without aggressive supportive care, improvements in TRM could not be achieved. Major morbidities arising during the process of auto-HCT and their management are listed in Table 49.3. Patients with AL experience unique toxicities of fluid retention and noncardiogenic pulmonary edema during the course of hematopoietic stem and progenitor cell mobilization that can lead to mortality of 2–3% prior to high-dose therapy[19,20]. Some patients cannot proceed beyond mobilization due to exacerbation of congestive heart failure or onset of cardiac dysrhythmias. Management includes close monitoring of weight during growth factor administration, salt restriction, judicious use of diuretics (excessive use and hypotension should be avoided), use of lower dose and split

Table 49.3 Complications during various stages of AL therapy and suggested management strategies

Stage/process	Complication	Comments and management
Hematopoietic cell mobilization/collection	Fluid retention	Seen in up to 50% of patients. Adversely affects 1-year survival. Likely results from proinflammatory effect of mobilization cytokines. More pronounced with severe albuminuria and patients with cardiac involvement but can also happen without significant cardiac involvement. Management includes optimal use of diuretics and split dosing schedule of G-CSF (twice a day *versus* once daily)
	Mortality	Approximately 2% during the mobilization phase. Primarily results from fluid retention and exacerbation of heart failure. Careful patient selection, close monitoring of weight gain, and aggressive management of fluid retention are expected to reduce early mortality
Regimen-related toxicity	Fluid retention	Very common especially in patients with severe nephrotic syndrome. Careful monitoring of fluid balance is critical. Overzealous diuresis should be avoided due to risk of hypotension. Albumin infusion should be used if edema progresses despite diuretics or serum albumin is less than 2g/dL. Avoid use of G-CSF to enhance engraftment as it can result in significant exacerbation of volume overload
	Hypotension	Common complication and usually results from intravascular volume depletion from severe nephrosis, autonomic neuropathy, impaired adrenergic responses, or as a result of medications. May be an early sign of sepsis so prompt cultures should be taken and antibiotics instituted as clinically appropriate. Avoid overly aggressive diuresis. It is preferable to tolerate some degree of edema in order to avoid hypotension. Use of albumin infusions is helpful in hypotension from severe hypoalbuminemia and in cases of refractory edema. Medication list should be carefully reviewed and adjusted. Adequate fall precautions should be in place due to increased risk of syncope and potential for head injury especially with severe thrombocytopenia. In refractory cases judicious use of α-adrenergic stimulants such as midodrine should be used
	Gastrointestinal (GI) bleeding	Unique toxicity of auto-HCT for AL. Seen in up to 17% of patients. Associated with high mortality. Likely results from amyloid angiopathy and mucosal injury from chemotherapy. Hepatic involvement with AL and Factor X deficiency may exacerbate bleeding. Patients should undergo pretransplant stool occult blood test. Heme positive cases should undergo endoscopic evaluation. If bleeding occurs platelets should be kept above 50000/μL. With risk-adapted melphalan dosage incidence of clinically significant GI bleeding decreases
	Nausea, vomiting, and mucositis	Fairly common and is multifactorial with higher incidence with 200mg/m^2 dose of melphalan. Hypotension and intravascular volume depletion are common precipitants. May exacerbate GI bleeding. Use of opioids for mucositis may exacerbate nausea and hypotension
	Sepsis and multiorgan failure	Second most common cause of the death after cardiac causes. Critical to recognize that fever may be absent with severe sepsis. Prompt recognition and early institution of broad-spectrum antimicrobials is the key to survival
	Cardiac arrhythmias and sudden cardiac death	Cardiac arrhythmias are frequent even in patients with minimal cardiac involvement. High-grade arrhythmias such as sustained ventricular tachycardia and undetected torsades can be fatal. Hypotension, fluid and electrolyte imbalance, and use of high-risk medications are common precipitating factors. Careful patient selection, continuous telemetry monitoring, and prompt correction of electrolyte abnormalities are imperative. In asymptomatic low-risk arrhythmias, antiarrhythmic agents with negative inotropic effects should be avoided
	Rare but important complications	Patients may develop renal failure requiring renal replacement therapy, which may be challenging due to hypotension and cardiac dysrhythmias Visceral rupture especially splenic and hepatic rupture has been reported. This usually requires surgical intervention and is associated with high mortality and morbidity. The authors have seen a few patients survive this dreaded complication as long as no advanced cardiac involvement was present
Post-auto-HCT recovery period	Fluid retention and infectious complications	Fluid retention and edema may continue to be a challenge in the post-transplant course. Some degree of edema is acceptable to avoid overzealous diuresis and hypotension Opportunistic infections such as herpes zoster and pneumocystis can develop during this period and patients should be placed on prophylaxis

schedule of G-CSF, and avoiding chemotherapy as part of the mobilization regimen.

What About Gastrointestinal Hemorrhage?

Gastrointestinal hemorrhage is another rather unique complication of AL and can be seen in up to 15–20% of cases [21,22]. This may be from a primary coagulation defect such as acquired factor X deficiency or from a complex interplay of amyloid angiopathy and chemotherapy-induced mucosal damage[22,23]. Occasionally this bleeding may be fatal. In the case of active bleeding, platelets should be kept above 50 000 and hemoglobin at 9 g/dL.

Multidisciplinary Planning to Improve Outcomes in AL

Cardiovascular complications may include worsening of congestive heart failure, cardiac dysrhythmias, hypotension, and sudden cardiac death[24]. It is important to anticipate and proactively manage these complications. The use of a risk-adapted approach is expected to result in improved outcomes over time as the majority of these complications depend upon the melphalan dose. We would like to emphasize here that the delivery of appropriate organ-directed supportive care during auto-HCT for AL requires a multidisciplinary approach with close coordination between the hematologist, nephrologist, cardiologist, and blood bank experts and as such we recommend that this procedure should be conducted at centers experienced in dealing with challenges unique to persons with AL.

Where Are the Data to Support Auto-HCT in AL?

The overall experience of the first 5 years of auto-HCT in AL seriously questioned the clinical benefit of this modality. Results of the IFM study in particular questioned the legitimacy of auto-HCT. However, remarkable improvement in mortality and morbidity in the last decade has established the clinical benefit of auto-HCT in AL and shifted the debate from legitimacy of auto-HCT to whom to transplant? The critics of auto-HCT in AL consider the patient selection process for auto-HCT as a selection bias and use this argument to question the clinical benefit of transplant in AL. While the only way to conclusively demonstrate the true benefit is to conduct a randomized controlled trial comparing standard therapy with auto-HCT, clinical experience from over 1000 patients treated at two large centers has demonstrated that most AL patients who survive beyond 10 years had undergone auto-HCT. Furthermore, a case–control study carried out by our group at the Mayo Clinic noted a significant difference in OS in 63 AL patients who underwent auto-HCT in comparison to 63 age-, sex-, and AL-specific-variable-matched patients who underwent conventional therapy (2-year survival 81% versus 55%; 4-year survival 71% versus 41%, respectively) [25]. Table 49.4 lists some of the pros and cons of auto-HCT in AL.

Table 49.4 Critical review of pros and cons of autologous hematopoietic cell transplant in AL

Autologous hematopoietic cell transplantation *versus* no transplant	
Pros and cons	**Comments**
Improved hematologic and organ response	Response rates are higher with increasing melphalan dose 200 > 140 > 100. So is the toxicity
Improved survival outcomes	Yet to be proven in randomized controlled studies. Emerging experience favors transplant in eligible patients
Higher mortality and morbidity	With improved patient selection TRM has decreased from 40% to 7% in experienced centers. The treatment-related mortality from standard therapy is less than 2%. With risk-adapted approach, cardiovascular, GI, and renal mortality and morbidity is expected to decline
Auto-HCT is not for all patients	Patient selection process is critical and leaves 3 in 4 AL patients ineligible for transplant. This can be considered as a selection bias but retrospective evidence has noted potential survival benefit

Current Challenges, Controversies, and Future Directions

Can We Improve Cardiac-Related Mortality in AL?

In our opinion, the feasibility and safety of auto-HCT is established for AL; nevertheless, two important issues remain outstanding: the majority of patients with AL are not candidates for auto-HCT; and a significant number of patients undergoing auto-HCT do not achieve hematologic CR – a prerequisite for long-term survival.

Currently, approximately three out of every four AL patients seen at the Mayo Clinic do not qualify for auto-HCT due to one or more contraindications. This is primarily from advanced cardiac involvement, which remains the principal cause of a persistent 40% 1-year mortality in AL[26]. This is by far the most significant and outstanding challenge in the management of AL, as early mortality from a cardiac standpoint has not changed over the course of the last 4 decades. Theoretically, there are two possible ways to deal with this problem – diagnose AL early and achieve effective disease control with sequential cardiac transplantation.

The most cost-effective way to pursue the aim of early diagnosis is to create awareness among the internists and cardiologists to consider AL in the differential diagnosis of any patient who is presenting with signs and symptoms of heart disease with a negative evaluation for coronary or valvular disease. The second option of solid organ transplantation, while appealing, is associated with several technical, ethical, and medical issues and cannot be practiced routinely [27,28]. Nonetheless, we consider sequential cardiac transplantation and auto-HCT in young patients who present with disease limited to the heart and who do not have concurrent MM.

In some patients who are not candidates for auto-HCT but are not too sick an "induction type" approach with the use of oral melphalan and prednisone for a few months has been explored, but this did not result in clinical improvement. The recent introduction of proteasome inhibitors and immunomodulatory drugs (IMiDs) for the treatment of MM and their impressive activity in relapsed and newly diagnosed AL have renewed the hopes for "myeloma-like induction therapy" in AL patients who are borderline candidates for auto-HCT. The efficacy of this approach remains to be evaluated in a prospective and randomized trial. A retrospective analysis of CyBorD (cyclophosphamide, dexamethasone, and bortezomib) in 17 patients with AL[29] has been reported. Three of these patients initially were considered not suitable as candidates but subsequently had improvement in disease status and physical condition and underwent auto-HCT. Hematologic response rate in this series of patients was over 90%.

Auto-HCT in Persons with Less Than CR with Frontline Therapy?

A significant number of AL patients who undergo auto-HCT fail to achieve hematologic CR, the most important predictor of long-term survival. Some investigators have pursued the tandem transplant approach akin to MM but no consistent improvement has been reported. In a pilot study, investigators at Boston University gave four doses of bortezomib at $1\,mg/m^2$ on days -6, -2, $+1$, and $+4$ together with 140 to $200\,mg/m^2$ of melphalan to nine patients. Eight out nine patients responded and six (67%) achieved hematologic CR[30]. This approach warrants further evaluation. Another group explored post-transplant consolidation in a phase 2 study of 40 newly diagnosed AL patients who were treated with risk-adapted auto-

HCT followed by consolidation with bortezomib and dexamethasone beginning at day 100 in those who did not achieve hematologic CR. The day 100 TRM was 10% with 27% of patients achieving hematologic CR at 3 months. At 1 year the CR rate was 60% with the use of consolidation bortezomib and dexamethasone[31].

What About Relapse After Auto-HCT in AL?

AL patients who achieve hematologic CR with auto-HCT have prolonged responses but the risk of relapse is much higher in patients with partial remission or less prior to auto-HCT. The optimal treatment of patients who relapse after auto-HCT is not known. Both lenalidomide and bortezomib in various combinations have demonstrated very high response rates in patients with relapsed AL. Recent analysis of 146 patients who experienced disease relapse after auto-HCT at Mayo Clinic demonstrated a median OS of 51 months after hematologic relapse; the majority of these patients received IMiDs and/or proteasome inhibitors indicating significant activity of these agents[32].

Conclusion

In summary, recent years have seen an unprecedented improvement in the care of AL patients. Auto-HCT for AL is a highly specialized intervention and tremendous progress has been made to improve its safety. At the Mayo Clinic 149 out of 601 (25%) auto-HCTs for AL have been completed entirely on an outpatient basis. With careful patient selection and the use of aggressive supportive care the TRM mortality has dropped from 20–43% recorded 15 years ago to less than 7% in experienced centers. In parallel with the improved safety of auto-HCT, tremendous progress has been made in the therapeutic arena of antineoplastic therapy for plasma cell disorders. Together these advances will help to address some outstanding challenges. The greatest challenge in the management of AL remains an unacceptably high early (1 year) disease-related mortality. Advances in proteomics and regenerative medicine have high hopes attached to them as they may help to turnaround the notorious legacy associated with AL.

References

1. Kyle RA, Gertz MA. Primary systemic amyloidosis: clinical and laboratory features in 474 cases. *Semin Hematol*, 32(1), 45–59 (1995).

2. Palladini G, Perfetti V, Obici L *et al*. Association of melphalan and high-dose dexamethasone is effective and well tolerated in patients with AL (primary) amyloidosis who are ineligible for stem cell transplantation. *Blood*, 103(8), 2936–2938 (2004).

3. Gertz MA, Kyle RA. Acute leukemia and cytogenetic abnormalities

complicating melphalan treatment of primary systemic amyloidosis. *Archiv Intern Med*, 150(3), 629–633 (1990).

4. Comenzo RL, Vosburgh E, Simms RW *et al*. Dose-intensive melphalan with blood stem cell support for the treatment of AL amyloidosis: one-year follow-up in five patients. *Blood*, 88(7), 2801–2806 (1996).

5. Comenzo RL, Vosburgh E, Falk RH *et al*. Dose-intensive melphalan with blood stem-cell support for the treatment of AL (amyloid light-chain) amyloidosis: survival and responses in

25 patients. *Blood*, 91(10), 3662–3670 (1998).

6. Gertz MA, Lacy MQ, Dispenzieri A *et al*. Stem cell transplantation for the management of primary systemic amyloidosis. *Am J Med*, 113(7), 549–555 (2002).

7. Moreau P, Leblond V, Bourquelot P *et al*. Prognostic factors for survival and response after high-dose therapy and autologous stem cell transplantation in systemic AL amyloidosis: a report on 21 patients. *Br J Haematol*, 101(4), 766–769 (1998).

8. Jaccard A, Moreau P, Leblond V *et al.* High-dose melphalan *versus* melphalan plus dexamethasone for AL amyloidosis. *New Engl J Med*, 357(11), 1083–1093 (2007).

9. Migrino RQ, Mareedu RK, Eastwood D, Bowers M, Harmann L, Hari P. Left ventricular ejection time on echocardiography predicts long-term mortality in light chain amyloidosis. *J Am Soc Echocardiogr*, 22(12), 1396–1402 (2009).

10. Comenzo RL, Gertz MA. Autologous stem cell transplantation for primary systemic amyloidosis. *Blood*, 99(12), 4276–4282 (2002).

11. Gertz MA, Lacy MQ, Dispenzieri A *et al.* Trends in day 100 and 2-year survival after auto-SCT for AL amyloidosis: outcomes before and after 2006. *Bone Marrow Transplant*, 46(7), 970–975 (2011).

12. Tsai SB, Seldin DC, Quillen K *et al.* High-dose melphalan and stem cell transplantation for patients with AL amyloidosis: trends in treatment-related mortality over the past 17 years at a single referral center. *Blood*, 120(22), 4445–4446 (2012).

13. Dispenzieri A, Gertz MA, Kyle RA *et al.* Serum cardiac troponins and N-terminal pro-brain natriuretic peptide: a staging system for primary systemic amyloidosis. *J Clin Oncol*, 22(18), 3751–3757 (2004).

14. Gertz MA, Lacy MQ, Dispenzieri A *et al.* Autologous stem cell transplant for immunoglobulin light chain amyloidosis: a status report. *Leuk Lymphoma*, 51(12), 2181–2187 (2010).

15. Gertz MA, Lacy MQ, Dispenzieri A *et al.* Effect of hematologic response on outcome of patients undergoing transplantation for primary amyloidosis: importance of achieving a complete response. *Haematologica*, 92(10), 1415–1418 (2007).

16. Girnius S, Seldin DC, Skinner M *et al.* Short and long-term outcome of treatment with high-dose melphalan and stem cell transplantation for multiple myeloma-associated AL amyloidosis. *Ann Hematol*, 89(6), 579–584 (2010).

17. Dispenzieri A, Lacy MQ, Katzmann JA *et al.* Absolute values of immunoglobulin free light chains are prognostic in patients with primary systemic amyloidosis undergoing peripheral blood stem cell transplantation. *Blood*, 107(8), 3378–3383 (2006).

18. Kumar S, Dispenzieri A, Lacy MQ *et al.* Revised prognostic staging system for light chain amyloidosis incorporating cardiac biomarkers and serum free light chain measurements. *J Clin Oncol*, 30(9), 989–995 (2012).

19. Johnston PB, Lacy MQ, Dispenzieri A, *et al.* Toxicities associated with stem cell mobilization utilizing cyclophosphamide and grown factor *versus* G-CSF alone in primary systemic amyloidosis [abstract]. *Blood*, 96, 182a (2000).

20. Leung N, Leung TR, Cha SS, Dispenzieri A, Lacy MQ, Gertz MA. Excessive fluid accumulation during stem cell mobilization: a novel prognostic factor of first-year survival after stem cell transplantation in AL amyloidosis patients. *Blood*, 106(10), 3353–3357 (2005).

21. Kumar S, Dispenzieri A, Lacy MQ, Litzow MR, Gertz MA. High incidence of gastrointestinal tract bleeding after autologous stem cell transplant for primary systemic amyloidosis. *Bone Marrow Transplant*, 28(4), 381–385 (2001).

22. Hoshino Y, Hatake K, Muroi K *et al.* Bleeding tendency caused by the deposit of amyloid substance in the perivascular region. *Intern Med*, 32(11), 879–881 (1993).

23. Choufani EB, Sanchorawala V, Ernst T *et al.* Acquired factor X deficiency in patients with amyloid light-chain amyloidosis: incidence, bleeding manifestations, and response to high-dose chemotherapy. *Blood*, 97(6), 1885–1887 (2001).

24. Falk RH, Rubinow A, Cohen AS. Cardiac arrhythmias in systemic amyloidosis: correlation with echocardiographic abnormalities. *J Am College Cardiol*, 3(1), 107–113 (1984).

25. Dispenzieri A, Kyle RA, Lacy MQ *et al.* Superior survival in primary systemic amyloidosis patients undergoing peripheral blood stem cell transplantation: a case-control study. *Blood*, 103(10), 3960–3963 (2004).

26. Kumar S, Gertz M, Lacy M *et al.* Recent improvements in survival in light chain amyloidosis and the importance of an early mortality risk score. *Blood*, 19, 116–121 (2010).

27. Dubrey SW, Burke MM, Hawkins PN, Banner NR. Cardiac transplantation for amyloid heart disease: the United Kingdom experience. *J Heart Lung Transplant*, 23(10), 1142–1153 (2004).

28. Gillmore JD, Goodman HJ, Lachmann HJ *et al.* Sequential heart and autologous stem cell transplantation for systemic AL amyloidosis. *Blood*, 107(3), 1227–1229 (2006).

29. Mikhael JR, Schuster SR, Jimenez-Zepeda VH *et al.* Cyclophosphamide-bortezomib-dexamethasone (CyBorD) produces rapid and complete hematologic response in patients with AL amyloidosis. *Blood*, 119(19), 4391–4394 (2012).

30. Sanchorawala V, Quillen K, Sloan JM, Andrea NT, Seldin DC. Bortezomib and high-dose melphalan conditioning for stem cell transplantation for AL amyloidosis: a pilot study. *Haematologica*, 96(12), 1890–1892 (2011).

31. Landau H, Hassoun H, Bello C *et al.* Consolidation with bortezomib and dexamethasone following risk-adapted melphalan and stem cell transplant in systemic AL amyloidosis. *Amyloid*, 18 Suppl 1, 130–131 (2011).

32. Warsame R, Bang SM, Kumar SK *et al.* Outcomes and treatments of patients with immunoglobulin light chain amyloidosis who progress or relapse postautologous stem cell transplant. *Eur J Haematol*, 92(6), 485–490 (2014).

Chapter

50

Autotransplants for Germ Cell Tumor: How Best To Do It

Craig Nichols, Christian Kollmannsberger, and Lawrence Einhorn

Overview

Almost exactly 40 years ago, the first patient with disseminated germ cell tumor entered a cisplatin combination chemotherapy trial and ushered in an era of unprecedented favorable outcomes for patients with this uncommon solid tumor[1]. Prior to the introduction of cisplatin, fewer than 10% of patients with disseminated disease were cured and in patients with regional disease, some cures were obtained through radical surgeries or extensive high-dose radiation. Today, more than 95% of the 8300 patients diagnosed with testicular cancer annually in the United States can anticipate cure. The incredibly effective chemotherapy safety net has allowed the majority of patients presenting with early stage to be cured without further therapeutic interventions beyond orchiectomy and reserves other active treatments for the small percentage of patients recurring after removal of the primary source. For those presenting with regional or disseminated disease, brief systemic chemotherapy almost always renders these patients cured. In only the patients with dire presentations is there a significant chance to fail to be cured with application of modern chemotherapy with or without adjunctive postchemotherapy surgery.

In the modern context, the need for effective salvage therapy beyond initial cisplatin combination primary chemotherapy is unusual. However, over the last 25 years, ongoing investigations have refined the effectiveness and tolerability of salvage systemic therapies and overall management strategies. Incorporating multidisciplinary management by experienced teams renders roughly half of patients who fail to be cured with primary systemic chemotherapy to long-term disease-free status. Currently, while not often required, high-dose chemotherapy followed by hematopoietic cell rescue represents the most effective salvage management strategy for relapsed testicular cancer in all of Oncology.

Historical Perspective on High-Dose Therapy Followed by Hematopoietic Cell Rescue

The modern era of testing high-dose chemotherapy strategies in germ cell tumors began in the late 1980s with studies conducted at Indiana University and subsequently validated in the multi-institutional setting in the Eastern Cooperative

Oncology Group (ECOG). The initial phase 1/2 trial at Indiana University and the subsequent phase II ECOG trial used a basic high-dose carboplatin and etoposide backbone and demonstrated that high-dose chemotherapy was tolerable in the setting of recurrent or refractory disseminated germ cell tumor and that a significant portion of patients despite extensive prior treatment were cured [2,3]. About 15% of patients with high-dose chemotherapy as third-line therapy appeared to be cured. However, an equal proportion of patients suffered fatal consequences of treatment.

Subsequently other groups in the United States and in Europe formally began to investigate high-dose salvage approaches. Similar lessons were learned and some original hypotheses validated. It appeared as if there were certain subsets of patients who consistently failed high-dose treatment (highly cisplatin refractory and mediastinal primary nonseminoma) and results seemed to improve both in terms of treatment-related deaths and therapeutic outcomes when high-dose therapy was moved forward in the succession of treatments after primary standard dose therapy. As well, growing general experience with management of patients receiving high-dose chemotherapy and growing familiarity with multidisciplinary management improved the therapeutic index for high-dose chemotherapy in germ cell tumors.

Development in Technical Aspects of High-Dose Chemotherapy in Germ Cell Tumors

The initial studies of high-dose chemotherapy in germ cell tumors began in earnest in the late 1980s. At this time, hematopoietic cell source was primarily from bone marrow, growth factor support was inconsistent, and experience in patient selection and supportive care was in its infancy. Not surprisingly, particularly at centers where there was not a long tradition of autologous transplantation, toxicity encountered was stout and therapy-related death was not infrequent. As experience grew and technology improved, the ease and safety of high-dose chemotherapy improved. In modern series, the incidence of therapy-related deaths is 2–3% with the standard doublet of high-dose carboplatin and etoposide.

There have been a number of attempts to increase the therapeutic effect of high-dose chemotherapy by increasing doses of the primary chemotherapy constituents, adding third or fourth drugs to the standard two-drug backbone, or adding more cycles of high-dose chemotherapy (usually from two to three cycles). In general, dose increases, additional drugs, and additional cycles of treatment did not consistently result in improved therapeutic outcomes. A large randomized trial comparing conventional salvage chemotherapy plus a single cycle of high-dose chemotherapy with three drugs (cyclophosphamide, etoposide and carboplatin) to conventional salvage therapy for one cycle followed by three high-dose cycles with two drugs (carboplatin and etoposide) was performed in a relatively favorable prognosis group of recurrent germ cell tumor patients [4]. No statistically significant differences in response, progression-free survival (PFS), or overall survival (OS) were detected. Overall, however, both arms were disappointing with low OS compared to large single-institution series.

Practice Points

Outside the context of a clinical trial, the best studied approach appears to be conventional dose salvage chemotherapy for one to two cycles (TIP, VIP, or VeIP) followed by two cycles of high-dose carboplatin and etoposide supported with peripheral blood autologous transplant. The best studied doses and schedule are carboplatin $700 \, mg/m^2$ and etoposide $750 \, mg/m^2$ daily for 3 consecutive days ($-5, -4, -3$) prior to hematopoietic progenitor cell infusion at a minimum of 1 million CD34+ cells per kilogram of body weight with each cycle of chemotherapy[5]. The second cycle is given in short order immediately upon recovery from the first cycle. Such chemotherapy and the requisite intense supportive care only should be delivered in centers with significant experience with hematopoietic cell collection and support of patients undergoing high-dose chemotherapy. As well, centers best suited to undertake such complex patients should have significant experience in applying multimodal approaches to management of germ cell tumors; especially incorporating aggressive surgery in the postchemotherapy setting.

Factors Predicting Outcomes with High-Dose Chemotherapy and Autologous Transplant in Subjects with Recurrent Germ Cell Tumors

As accumulated experience grew and large-scale collaborations formed, the field was able to mount some studies to define predictive parameters for successful outcome using high-dose chemotherapy followed by autologous transplant for patients with recurrent germ cell tumors

Premier among these was the collective effort by the International Prognostic Factor Study Group to develop a predictive classification for relapsed patients which included individual data from almost 2000 relapsed patients collected at high volume centers around the world (Table 50.1)[6]. This effort was similar to the development of the original

Table 50.1 International prognostic group classification

Factors		Points
Primary site	Gonadal	0
	Retroperitoneal	1
	Mediastinal	3
Response to first-line therapy	CR/PR−	0
	PR+/ SD	1
	PD	2
PFS interval after first-line therapy	>3 months	0
	≤3 months	1
Serum HCG level	≤1000IU/L	0
	>1000IU/L	1
Serum AFP level	Normal	0
	≤1000IU/L	1
	>1000IU/L	2
Liver, bone, brain metastases	Absent	0
	Present	1

1. Add up points for preliminary score (0–10)
2. Regroup into category score: (0): 0; (1–2): 1; (3–4): 2; (5 or more):
3. Add histology points as below to category score to determine final risk category

Histology	Seminoma	−1
	Nonseminoma	0

Stratification	Points	2-year progression-free survival/3-year overall survival
Very low risk	-1	75.1%/77%
Low risk	0	51%/65.6%
Intermediate risk	1	40.1%/58.3%
High risk	2	25.9%/27.1%
Very high risk	3	5.6%/6.1%

International Germ Cell Classification Consensus (IGCCC) which successfully developed a predictive model for untreated germ cell tumor patients.

Based on seven significant factors on multivariate analysis in (histology-seminoma *versus* nonseminoma, primary tumor site (mediastinal *versus* retroperitoneal *versus* gonadal), response to first-line chemotherapy (CR *versus* PR *versus* other), progression-free interval following first-line chemotherapy, AFP and HCG levels at diagnosis of relapse, and the presence of nonpulmonary visceral metastases the model is able to differentiate five distinct risk groups ranging from very low to very high (Table 50.1). Owing to the large, international, and multicenter patient population included, this model is widely applicable and is now considered the new standard predictive model for relapsed patients. Largely confirmatory single-institution efforts were also reported.

In practical terms and like the IGCCC, predictive models separate the population of patients with recurrent germ cell tumors into three fairly distinct groups each with different clinical implications [5,6]. The first is a very low-risk group in which application of high-dose chemotherapy approaches would be expected to result in long-term disease control for 70–80% of the population. This includes patients with recurrent seminoma as well as testicular nonseminoma patients with early presentations of recurrent disease and, in whom, a favorable response and duration of response with initial cisplatin-based systemic therapy has been seen. The second group is an intermediate-risk group who have roughly a 50% chance of favorable long-term outcome with high-dose chemotherapy. This is the largest subset of recurrent patients and includes those who have retroperitoneal primaries and can include those with significant degrees of cisplatin-resistance. Finally there is a poor-risk group in whom even application of high-dose chemotherapy and maximum multidisciplinary management rarely is curative with an overall long-term survival in the 5–10% range. This group contains biologically distinct subsets that include mediastinal primary nonseminoma, those with nongerm cell malignant elements, late relapsing germ cell tumors, and the rare patients who have primary absolute resistance to standard dose cisplatin-based chemotherapy. In the good-risk group, the question becomes whether similar good results might be achieved with conventional dose salvage therapies reserving high-dose chemotherapy as a third-line option. For the poor-risk group, the primary clinical question is whether even high-dose chemotherapy is futile and such patients should be considered for highly investigational, molecular approaches, serial standard single-agent therapy, or early palliative care. A number of high-volume germ cell tumor institutions exclude such patients from clinical management with high-dose chemotherapy[5]. The larger intermediate-risk group of recurrent germ cell tumors mirrors the untreated poor-risk group of the IGCCC with an approximately 50% chance of successful outcome – a group in which patients are willing to accept more toxic therapy in order to achieve better results and a group for which toxicity reduction is not the primary endpoint. The rarity of each of these subsets makes defining best approaches by conventional randomized clinical trials very difficult.

Several retrospective and prospective phase 2 studies have established salvage high-dose chemotherapy as a standard option for patients with initial relapse of disease, and in particular for those with unfavorable prognostic criteria. Two randomized trials have been published. The only randomized trial to date of patients with favorable prognostic features comparing salvage high-dose chemotherapy programs with salvage conventional dose programs showed no benefit for the high-dose treatment[7]. This trial has been criticized because only one cycle of high-dose chemotherapy was used, patients with platinum-refractory disease were excluded, and patients in the conventional dose arm were able to receive high-dose chemotherapy as third-line treatment. An additional randomized trial comparing single-dose with sequential high-dose chemotherapy cycles demonstrated improved tolerability for the sequential chemotherapy group[8]. No conclusions regarding superior efficacy could be drawn from this trial as specific patient subgroups made the interpretation of this trial difficult. Significant differences in drug dosing between the high-dose portions of each arm, as well as the fact that one contained three drugs and the other only two, are the main critical points of this trial.

Data Favoring Autologous Transplant in Germ Cell Tumors

Several large important retrospective data sets have been published in recent years.

Einhorn and colleagues published the largest retrospective, institutional series to date including 184 patients treated at Indiana University with tandem autologous transplants using carboplatin and etoposide since 1996[5]. One hundred and 70 patients received two consecutive courses of high-dose carboplatin and etoposide and 110 of the 184 patients underwent 1–2 cycles of conventional dose salvage chemotherapy with vinblastine, cisplatin, and ifosfamide prior to salvage high-dose chemotherapy and autologous transplant. All patients underwent aggressive resection of residual masses after chemotherapy whenever technically feasible. Very high cure rates were reported in both prognostically favorable and unfavorable patients including cisplatin refractory patients. Of note, it is important to remember that patients with mediastinal nonseminoma as well as patients experiencing late relapse were not included in this large retrospective trial.

The second large retrospective analysis was performed by the International Prognostic Factor Group and included 1594 patients with initial relapse of germ cell tumor treated with either conventional dose salvage chemotherapy or salvage high-dose programs[9]. This trial did include mediastinal nonseminoma patients and late relapsing patients as well as those with extreme cisplatin refractory disease. Patient characteristics at relapse were relatively balanced with the conventional salvage group being slightly younger with slightly higher favorable initial response to treatment and lower median HCG elevation. The high-dose chemotherapy group had a somewhat higher incidence of visceral metastases. In this very large multi-institutional multinational effort, a significant advantage in favor of high-dose chemotherapy was seen across all subgroups according to the International Prognostic Classification even after adjustment for all known prognostic factors (Hazard ratio for death ranging from 0.18 to 0.47 favoring high-dose chemotherapy followed by autologous transplant across the five distinct subgroups). While not a randomized trial, the directionality of the data is compelling, strongly suggesting benefit in OS in all prognostic subsets.

Based on these studies, several conclusions can be drawn. First, sequential high-dose chemotherapy with two to three consecutive high-dose cycles of two drugs (carboplatin/etoposide) appears to be more effective and in particular significantly safer (mortality in experienced centers 2–4%) than a single high-dose chemotherapy cycle including three chemotherapy agents (mortality up to 10%) and should therefore be the preferred high-dose approach. Outcomes after high-dose chemotherapy in the third or later line setting are substantially worse than for the use of high-dose chemotherapy as second-line treatment[8,10]. There should be little or no debate on the use of high-dose chemotherapy for a patient with poor prognosis features but a benefit of high-dose chemotherapy appears to emerge even in patients with favorable predictive criteria at initial relapse. These findings can serve as the rationale to treat all germ cell tumor patients who have relapsed with high-dose programs until we can identify those good-risk patients who have equivalent cure rates with conventional dose salvage therapy. Sequential high-dose chemotherapy with one or two conventional chemotherapy cycles followed by two high-dose cycles of carboplatin and etoposide with hematopoietic cell support represents the best studied standard as management of initial recurrence of germ cell tumors.

Multidisciplinary approaches remain an important part of any salvage strategy and residual lesions should be completely resected, whenever possible. The rate of residual active germ cell tumor and the frequency of residual teratoma appear significantly higher after salvage therapy as compared to first line therapy. Desperation surgery can even offer long-term survival in selected patients. Salvage surgery is particularly effective if recurrent disease is localized to the retroperitoneum[10–12].

Limitations to Autologous Transplant in Germ Cell Tumors

The management of patients with primary mediastinal non-seminoma or with late relapse, defined as recurrence of disease 2 years or longer after cisplatin-based therapy, remains controversial. These patients exhibit an extremely poor prognosis. Some studies have suggested responses to high-dose chemotherapy but the results for these patients with either salvage standard or high-dose chemotherapy followed by aggressive resection of all residual masses remain disappointing.

Because of the complexity of relapsed disease and the difficult therapeutic situation, as well as the necessity of close multidisciplinary cooperation between medical oncologists, urologists, radiologists, pathologists, and radiation oncologists, all patients who have relapsed should be referred to high-volume specialized centers.

Poor-risk Germ Cell Tumors and Autologous Transplant

There have not been significant changes in the therapeutic recommendations for management of poor-risk germ cell tumors for more than two decades despite a number of attempts to investigate new and more intense strategies by adding more active agents, increasing dose intensity, increasing dose density, and incorporating early high-dose chemotherapy with hematopoietic cell support. For all intents and purposes, the standard remains four cycles of bleomycin, etoposide, and cisplatin (BEP) with multimodal considerations for selective postchemotherapy surgery and early initiation of salvage therapy for those who are identified as having persistent or recurrent malignant germ cell elements. While the therapeutic recommendations have not changed for some time, outcomes seem to be improving for reasons that are not entirely clear. Through favorable stage migration, very precise application of standard treatments and appropriate consideration of aggressive postchemotherapy surgery, approximately 70% of patients classically defined as IGCCC poor-risk disease will be cured and, for IGCCC intermediate-risk patients, approximately 85–90% will be cured[13,14]. These modern results stand in significant contrast to the original IGCCC predictions of 50% for poor-risk patients and 75% for intermediate-risk patients.

There have been a number of clinical investigations looking at early introduction of high-dose chemotherapy with hematopoietic cell rescue. Several phase 2 studies investigating initial high-dose chemotherapy and hematopoietic cell support reported promising 2-year survival rates of 70–80% indicating that a 10–20% survival advantage might be achievable with first-line high-dose chemotherapy and hematopoietic cell rescue compared with standard BEP therapy [15–17]. Droz and colleagues were among the first to use this approach for patients with an unfavorable risk profile. In the trial conducted in the late 1980s, 28 poor-risk patients received two cycles of double-dose vinblastine-BEP (v-BEP) and one cycle of high-dose chemotherapy with double-dose cisplatin, etoposide, and cyclophosphamide followed by autologous transplant. Complete remission rates of (61%) and 12 (42%) were alive disease-free at a median follow-up of 66 months. A small randomized trial followed in which high-dose chemotherapy was incorporated as part of the first-line chemotherapy, applying high-dose chemotherapy as consolidation after three cycles at standard doses. In that study, 114 patients received either four cycles of v-BEP or three cycles at standard doses followed by one cycle of high-dose cisplatin, etoposide, and cyclophosphamide [16]. The study failed to show a survival advantage for the high-dose chemotherapy arm. However, the results of this trial are difficult to interpret as the four-drug regimen used for the control arm is not considered standard treatment, particularly as the dose intensity in the experimental arm was very low. Results were confounded by the finding that 30% of the patients randomized to the experimental arm did not complete therapy because of toxicity or early death.

Motzer et al. showed that first-line high-dose chemotherapy was well tolerated, and also found a survival advantage after this approach compared with a historical control group treated with vinblastine, actinomycin-D, cyclophosphamide, cisplatin, and bleomycin[17]. In this phase 2 trial, patients with a slow clearance of elevated serum marker levels, as shown by a prolonged half-life (>7 days for AFP and >3 days for HCG) indicating resistance to standard cisplatin-based therapy, were included. Patients received first-line high-dose chemotherapy with a combination of carboplatin and etoposide and autologous transplant after two cycles of vinblastine, actinomycin-D, bleomycin, cyclophosphamide, and cisplatin. Twenty-two patients were treated with this regimen; the complete response and the "no evident disease" (NED) rates were 54% and 48%, respectively.

In a subsequent trial by the same investigators, poor-prognosis patients with an insufficient decline in tumor markers after two cycles of standard dose VIP therapy received two cycles of high-dose carboplatin and etoposide and cyclophosphamide (CEC), followed by autologous transplant.

In all, 30 patients were entered into the trial and treated with an initial two cycles of VIP. Fourteen patients with delayed tumor marker decline after the first two cycles were switched to subsequent tandem autologous transplants, while the 16 with a normal decline in tumor markers completed four VIP cycles. Only nine of the patients in the transplant group received two cycles of CEC, as the other five developed progressive disease after the first cycle. Of the nine receiving tandem high-dose chemotherapy, seven had a complete remission. In all, 17 patients (57%) had a complete remission and 15 (50%) were alive and with NED at a median follow-up of 30 months. When compared with the previous experience in poor-risk patients with GCT, i.e., conventional dose cisplatin-containing therapy at Memorial Sloan-Kettering Cancer Center (MSKCC), these studies suggested that poor-risk patients selected for a high likelihood of failure by predicted marker half-life and treated with a program that includes high-dose chemotherapy might have both improved median overall and event-free survival rates.

The German Testicular Cancer Study Group (GTCSG) investigated a sequential high-dose chemotherapy strategy consisting of one standard VIP cycle followed by three consecutive high-dose cycles of carboplatin and etoposide and ifosfamide within a phase 1/2 study [18]. The results were very promising, with long-term cure rates of 75% among poor-prognosis patients. When patients from this study were compared within a matched pair analysis including patients from randomized trials using conventional dose chemotherapy, an 11% improvement in the 2-year OS rate was suggested, and a multivariate analysis showed the use of first-line high-dose chemotherapy to be an independent favorable factor for improved survival.

Based on the results from the MSKCC and the GTCSG two randomized studies were initiated. The European Organization for the Research and Treatment of Cancer (EORTC) study randomized patients to either four cycles of standard VIP or one standard VIP cycle followed by three consecutive high-dose VIP cycles. The study was closed in 2008 but no results have yet been reported.

A parallel intergroup effort in the United States allocated 219 patients with intermediate- or poor-prognosis characteristics to either four cycles of standard BEP or two cycles of standard BEP followed by two cycles of high-dose carboplatin, etoposide, plus cyclophosphamide [19]. There was no difference in the whole group of patients for the 1-year durable CR rates, being 48% and 52% in the standard BEP and experimental high-dose chemotherapy group, respectively. Patients with an unsatisfactory tumor marker decline during days 7–49 appeared to have a significantly worse outcome than those with a timely decrease in marker levels. Within an unplanned subgroup analysis of the 67 patients with an unsatisfactory decline in marker levels, high-dose chemotherapy seemed to improve the outcome for this group, with a 1-year durable CR rate of 61% for those on high-dose chemotherapy *versus* 34% for those receiving BEP alone ($P<0.03$). The toxicity in the high-dose chemotherapy arm was significantly higher than with BEP regimen.

Four cycles of BEP therefore remain the standard of care for IGCCC poor-prognosis patients, with four cycles of VIP being an accepted alternative, in particular in those with pre-existing lung problems or extensive lung disease, and the expectancy of extensive surgery for residual lesions.

Practice Points and Future Directions

Over the 25 years of investigation of high-dose chemotherapy with hematopoietic cell support, significant lessons have been learned that have brought forward a treatment strategy that is much safer and more thoughtfully integrated into the therapeutic timeline. In terms of technical refinements, the best studied and standard approach is using tandem cycles of high-dose etoposide and carboplatin with peripheral blood hematopoietic cell support delivered in a center with sufficient experience and facilities to safely deliver such potentially toxic treatments. Adding additional high-dose chemotherapeutic agents or using either one or three or more cycles remains experimental.

In terms of incorporating high-dose chemotherapy in the treatment timeline for germ cell tumors, there is currently no proven role for use of high-dose chemotherapy as part of initial management of poor-risk germ cell tumors. Even in subsets in whom outcomes are unfavorable (primary mediastinal nonseminoma or patients with worse than predicted marker decline), there remains no proven role for early initiation of high-dose chemotherapy.

There is consensus that the best studied and standard indication for high-dose chemotherapy with stem cell support for patients with germ cell tumors is in the setting of recurrent disease after primary management. Predictive factors have been generally defined and agreed upon. Classification systems suggest a surprisingly good-risk group of recurrent patients for whom a sizable majority are cured (recurrent seminoma, recurrence after CR to primary therapy and low volume recurrent disease, high-dose chemotherapy as second-line treatment). In contrast, there is a very unfavorable group of patients with single or a combination of predictive factors for whom even application of high-dose chemotherapy is highly likely to be futile with cure rates well under 10% (mediastinal primary nonseminoma, late relapsing patients, non germ cell elements, high-dose chemotherapy as third-line therapy, progressive disease on prior cisplatin therapy). The largest group of patients exist between these favorable and unfavorable categories and have a roughly 50% chance of being cured with high-dose chemotherapy as second-line therapy.

It is unlikely that there will be meaningful modifications to the doses and schedule of the high-dose chemotherapy backbone because of the few patients available for study and the relatively good outcomes produced with a standard high-dose

treatment program. That said, there is a study being launched that will investigate the best timing of high-dose chemotherapy in patients with recurrent germ cell tumors. The TIGER trial is an international effort to compare in a randomized fashion standard salvage therapy in patients with initial recurrence of germ cell tumors with standard dose paclitaxel, ifosfamide, and cisplatin with TICE with standard dose cycles of paclitaxel and ifosfamide (TI) followed by three high-dose cycles of carboplatin and etoposide (CE). The power calculations suggest the need for a large number of patients and investigators from the United States, Europe, and Australia are coming together to enroll patients. A number of countries and large institutions remain concerned about the potential value and impact of the study and have opted not to participate.

References

1. Einhorn LH. Treatment of testicular cancer: a new and improved model. *JClin Oncol* 8:1777–1781, 1990

2. Nichols CR, Tricot G, Williams SD *et al*. Dose-intensive chemotherapy in refractory germ cell cancer. A phase I/II trial of high-dose carboplatin and etoposide with autologous bone marrow transplantation. *J Clin Oncol* 7:932–939, 1989

3. Nichols CR, Anderson J, Lazarus HM, *et al*. High dose carboplatin and etoposide with autologous bone marrow transplantation in refractory germ cell cancer: an Eastern Cooperative Oncology Group Protocol. *J Clin Oncol* 10:558–563, 1992

4. Lorch A, Kollmannsberger C, Hartmann JT, *et al*. Single *versus* sequential high-dose chemotherapy in patients with relapsed or refractory germ cell tumors: a prospective randomized multicenter trial of the German Testicular Cancer Study Group. *J Clin Oncol* 25:2778–84, 2007

5. Einhorn LH, Williams SD, Chamness A, *et al*. High-dose chemotherapy and stem-cell rescue for metastatic germ-cell tumors. *N Engl J Med* 357:340–8, 2007

6. Lorch A, Beyer J, Bascoul-Mollevi C, *et al*. Prognostic factors in patients with metastatic germ cell tumors who experienced treatment failure with cisplatin-based first-line chemotherapy. *J Clin Oncol* 28:4906–11, 2010

7. Pico JL, Rosti G, Kramar A, *et al*. A randomised trial of high-dose chemotherapy in the salvage treatment of patients failing first-line platinum chemotherapy for advanced germ cell tumours. *Ann Oncol* 16:1152–9, 2005

8. Lorch A, Kleinhans A, Kramar A, *et al*. Sequential *versus* single high-dose chemotherapy in patients with relapsed or refractory germ cell tumors: long-term results of a prospective randomized trial. *J Clin Oncol* 30:800–5, 2012

9. Lorch A, Bascoul-Mollevi C, Kramar A, *et al*. Conventional-dose *versus* high-dose chemotherapy as first salvage treatment in male patients with metastatic germ cell tumors: evidence from a large international database. *J Clin Oncol* 29:2178–84, 2011

10. Albers P, Ganz A, Hannig E, *et al*. Salvage surgery of chemorefractory germ cell tumors with elevated tumor markers. *J Urol* 164:381–4, 2000

11. Coogan CL, Foster RS, Rowland RG, *et al*. Postchemotherapy retroperitoneal lymph node dissection is effective therapy in selected patients with elevated tumor markers after primary chemotherapy alone. *Urology* 50:957–62, 1997

12. Beck SD, Foster RS, Bihrle R, *et al*. Pathologic findings and therapeutic outcome of desperation post-chemotherapy retroperitoneal lymph node dissection in advanced germ cell cancer. *Urol Oncol* 23:423–30, 2005

13. Olofsson SE, Tandstad T, Jerkeman M, *et al*. Population-based study of treatment guided by tumor marker decline in patients with metastatic nonseminomatous germ cell tumor: a report from the Swedish-Norwegian Testicular Cancer Group *J Clin Oncol* 29:2032–9, 2011

14. Adra N, Albany C, Sonnenburg D, Tong Y, Hanna NH, Einhorn LH. A retrospective analysis of patients with poor-risk germ cell tumor (PRGCT) treated at Indiana University from

2000 to 2010. *J Clin Oncol* 31:Suppl; abstr 4557, 2013

15. Chevreau C, Droz JP, Pico JL *et al*. Early intensified chemotherapy with autologous bone marrow transplantation in first line treatment of poor risk non- seminomatous germ cell tumours. Preliminary results of a French randomized trial. *Eur Urol* 23:213–7, 1993

16. Droz JP, Kramar A, Biron P *et al*. Failure of high-dose cyclophosphamide and etoposide combined with double-dose cisplatin and bone marrow support in patients with high-Volume metastatic nonseminomatous germ-cell tumours: mature results of a randomised trial. *Eur Urol* 51:739–46, 2007

17. Motzer RJ, Mazumdar M, Gulati SC *et al*. Phase II trial of high-dose carboplatin and etoposide with autologous bone marrow transplantation in first-line therapy for patients with poor-risk germ cell tumors. *J Natl Cancer Inst* 85:1828–35, 1993

18. Bokemeyer C, Kollmannsberger C, Meisner C *et al*. First-line high-dose chemotherapy compared to standard-dose PEB/VIP chemotherapy in patients with advanced germ cell tumors. A multivariate and matched pair analysis. *J Clin Oncol*; 17:3450–6, 1999

19. Motzer RJ, Nichols CJ, Margolin KA *et al*. Phase III randomized trial of conventional-dose chemotherapy with or without high-dose chemotherapy and autologous hematopoietic stem-cell rescue as first-line treatment for patients with poor-prognosis metastatic germ cell tumors. *J Clin Oncol* 25:247–56, 2007

Chapter

51

Autotransplants for Neuroblastoma

Kimberly A. Kasow and Gregory A. Hale

Introduction

Neuroblastoma is the most common extracranial solid tumor of childhood, comprising approximately 10% of pediatric cancers and arising from the developing sympathetic nervous system. The majority of children have metastatic disease at diagnosis and require aggressive multidisciplinary therapy consisting of induction chemotherapy, surgery, consolidation therapy with autologous hematopoietic cell transplantation (HCT), radiation therapy, and immunotherapy [1]. In a large randomized clinical trial conducted by the Children's Cancer Group (CCG), autologous HCT for patients with high-risk disease has been proven to result in improved event-free survival (EFS) compared to standard chemotherapy, with these observations being confirmed on long-term follow-up of this cohort [2,3]. Despite this aggressive therapy, the most common cause of treatment failure remains disease recurrence. Even when post-transplant anti-GD2 antibody immunotherapy is incorporated, the 3-year disease-free survival (DFS) rate is 65% at best [4]. Other options that have been explored to improve outcomes in this high-risk cohort include allogeneic transplantation, graft manipulation to reduce tumor cell content and enhance immunogenicity, cellular therapies, and nontransplant modalities to reduce the tumor burden within the patient at the time of HCT.

Role of Autologous Hematopoietic Cell Transplantation

Historical Perspective

High-risk neuroblastoma (Table 51.1) is one of the few pediatric malignancies in which autologous HCT has been clearly proven in randomized clinical trials to be superior to non-transplant therapies. From 1991 to 1996, the Children's Cancer Group (CCG) conducted a clinical trial involving 539 patients, with participants randomly assigned to two different treatments [2,3]. The first randomization point occurred following the second cycle of induction chemotherapy. At this point in therapy, 379 patients with high-risk neuroblastoma were randomized to receive either myeloablative conditioning with melphalan, etoposide, carboplatin, and TBI followed by infusion of a purged autologous marrow graft or three additional

Table 51.1 High-risk neuroblastoma patients who are candidates for autologous HCT

INSS Stage 4 are eligible with the following:

a. MYCN amplification (>4-fold increase in MYCN signals as compared to reference signals) and age ≥365 days regardless of additional biologic features

b. Age >18 months (>547 days) regardless of biologic features

c. Age 12–18 months (365–547 days) with any one of the following 3 unfavorable biologic features: MYCN amplification, unfavorable pathology, and/or DNA index = 1 or any biologic feature that is indeterminant/unsatisfactory/unknown

OR

Patients with newly diagnosed neuroblastoma with INSS Stage 3 are eligible with the following:

a. MYCN amplification (>4-fold increase in MYCN signals as compared to reference signals) and age ≥365 days, regardless of additional biologic features

b. Age >18 months (>547 days) with unfavorable pathology, regardless of MYCN status

c. Patients with newly diagnosed INSS Stage 2a/2b with MYCN amplification (>4-fold increase in MYCN signals as compared to reference signals) and age ≥365 days, regardless of additional biologic features

OR

Patients ≥365 days initially diagnosed with: INSS Stage 1, 2, 4S who progressed to a Stage 4 without interval chemotherapy

cycles of conventional chemotherapy without HCT. Following completion of the first randomization therapy, 258 participants were randomized a second time to receive either 13-cis-retinoic acid or not, resulting in a total of four treatment groups. The initial analysis of this trial reported an improved 3-year event-free survival (EFS) for those patients receiving autologous HCT compared to those receiving intensive chemotherapy (34% versus 22%, P=0.034) [2]. Patients randomized to receive 13-cis-retinoic acid had improved outcomes compared to those who did not receive this medication (3-year EFS of 46% versus 29%, P=0.027). A follow-up analysis confirmed these initial findings with a 5-year EFS of 30% for the HCT group compared with 19% for the conventional chemotherapy

(A)

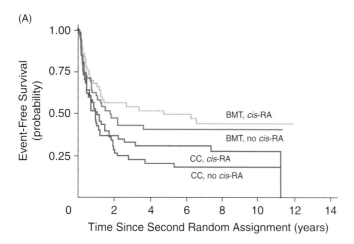

(B)

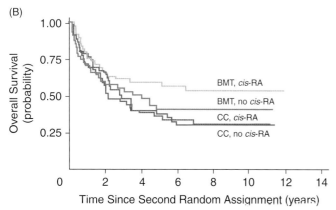

Figure 51.1 Event-free survival for patients with high-risk neuroblastoma who participated in both the first and second randomization assignment Reprinted from reference [3] with permission. Copyright 2009 American Society of Clinical Oncology. All rights reserved.

group (P=0.04) [3]. The survival benefit was also confirmed for the 13-*cis*-retinoic acid recipients (Figure 51.1) [3]. Patients randomized to receive both autologous BMT and 13-*cis*-retinoic acid had the best outcomes while those randomized to not receive either intervention had the lowest EFS. This trial experienced significant dropout during its course: enrolling 539 patients with only 379 undergoing first randomization for transplantation *versus* 3 additional cycles of chemotherapy and only 258 undergoing randomization to receive *cis*-retinoic acid. The treatment regimen in this trial differs from the current treatment in several ways. First, bone marrow was used as the graft cell source rather than peripheral blood hematopoietic cells (HCs). Second, radiotherapy occurred between courses cycle 4 and 5 prior to transplantation; currently radiation is administered after transplantation. Third, the conditioning regimen was melphalan, etoposide, and carboplatin with TBI. Fourth, the marrow graft was purged in an attempt to remove tumor cells. An analysis by The Cochrane Collaboration included the CCG trial along with two European randomized clinical trials of autologous HCT for this disease, totaling 739 patients [5–7]. They found a statistically significant difference in EFS in favor of "myeloablative" therapy over

low-dose maintenance chemotherapy or no further treatment (HR 0.78, P=0.00006) [5]. While the CCG study utilized a TBI-based conditioning regimen with purged marrow grafts, the other studies used non-TBI-containing regimens and peripheral blood HC grafts. Despite these differences, the 5-year EFS was 30% in the CCG study compared with 38% for each of the other two trials. Given this current knowledge, autologous hematopoietic cell transplantation (HCT) remains a necessary component of neuroblastoma therapy for patients with high-risk disease.

Tandem or Sequential Autologous HCT: Does It Matter?

Tandem transplantation has been successfully used with favorable outcomes in this population through an increase in treatment intensity [8,9]. A pilot study of tandem high-dose chemotherapy with HC rescue was conducted by the Children's Oncology Group (COG) with an initial transplant using thiotepa and cyclophosphamide followed by a second transplant using melphalan, carboplatin, and etoposide [10]. Each course of high-dose chemotherapy was followed by an infusion of autologous peripheral blood HCs. Initially all grafts were processed by CD34 positive selection; however this graft processing was discontinued during the study due to an observed increase in viral infections. Of 41 patients treated on this trial, 8 did not receive either transplant procedure and 7 underwent a single procedure. However, 79% of those receiving a first transplant underwent the second transplant procedure. The median time from first to second transplant was 52 days. Two of 41 died of nonrelapse causes (4.9%). Three-year EFS was 44.8%, demonstrating feasibility and leading to a COG randomized trial between a tandem and single transplant procedure, which has been completed but not yet analyzed.

Practice Points

While a single course of "myeloablative" therapy remains the standard of care for patients with high-risk neuroblastoma, tandem autologous HCT remains a viable option for patients while we await the results of the COG randomized clinical trial [11].

Transplant Conditioning Regimen: Is There a Standard?

Historically a conditioning regimen of melphalan, carboplatin, and etoposide has been the most commonly used regimen for autologous HCT in neuroblastoma[12]. However, platinum toxicity has been a significant problem for patients treated with this regimen. TBI has been removed from most autologous transplant conditioning regimens. This is not due to TBI's inferiority in survival rates compared to chemotherapy-based regimens, but rather to its long-term complications. In preference, local radiation therapy is delivered to the primary tumor bed and MIBG-avid sites of disease evident on pretransplant imaging [13,14]. Thiotepa-based regimens, such as topotecan, thiotepa, and carboplatin, have been used to treat other patients as well, in an attempt to control CNS disease [15]. Using this regimen, one study demonstrated that 10 out of 11 neuroblastoma patients were alive in remission at 6 to 32 months after HCT. This regimen is attractive because most patients have had extensive exposure to topoisomerase II inhibitors pretransplantation. Topotecan has the advantages of not being affected by the most common mechanisms of drug resistance, being synergistic with most alkylating agents, and having excellent CNS penetration [15]. Busulfan and melphalan regimens have been used over the past two decades with promising results published in small series [16–18]. More recently, in a retrospective analysis using registry data, European investigators concluded that patients receiving busulfan and melphalan had improved outcomes and EFS compared to other regimens [19]. Multivariate analysis, which included 3974 autograft recipients transplanted from 1978 to 2006, showed improved overall survival for patients less than 2 years of age, with less disease at the time of HCT in those who received peripheral blood HCs, those who received autologous HCT, and those who received the busulfan/melphalan conditioning regimen. In first remission, those who received the busulfan/melphalan conditioning regiman had an overall survival of 48% compared with 35% for those receiving other regimens ($P < 0.001$). In this same retrospective analysis, no patient who underwent second autologous HCT survived.

Transplant Conditioning Regimen: What About 131-I-MIBG?

More recently 131-I-MIBG has been added to conditioning regimens in an attempt to gain disease-specific antitumor effect, without enhancing organ toxicity [20–22]. MIBG, a norepinephrine analog, is selectively taken up by neuroblastoma cells in 90% of patients. As a single agent, MIBG administered alone to patients with relapsed or refractory neuroblastoma demonstrated a response rate of 37% [23]. An early trial employed 131-I-MIBG 2 weeks prior to melphalan, carboplatin, and etoposide and autologous HCT with a response rate of 27% and a 3-year EFS of 31% [24]. In a more recent trial, eight patients received MIBG followed by autologous HCT followed again by busulfan and melphalan with autologous HCT 6 weeks later with no graft failure and one patient death from sinusoidal obstructive syndrome [22]. Five of the eight patients had a response to MIBG alone. Three patients attained a CR, two a PR, and one a minor response with one nonevaluable patient.

Practice Point

The present standard of care is to administer a chemotherapy-based conditioning regimen most commonly consisting of melphalan, etoposide, and carboplatin or busulfan and melphalan.

Purging of Autologous Hematopoietic Graft: Methodologies

Most series of autologous HCT demonstrate that disease recurrence is the most commonly observed reason for treatment failure, suggesting that residual tumor within the patient and/or contaminated HCs may contribute to disease recurrence [2,3,25]. In an elegant study of neomycin resistance gene marking grafts in patients undergoing autologous HCT for neuroblastoma, Brenner et al. demonstrated the presence of the marker gene in tumors at the time of relapse after transplant in both marrow and extramedullary sites [25]. Since the marrow grafts were collected in morphologic remission, this observation suggested that relapse occurred at least in part due to occult tumor being reinfused with the hematopoietic cell graft. There are two basic methodologies for cell processing to "remove tumor cells" from hematopoietic grafts: positive selection and negative selection (see Chapter 30). In positive selection, the HCs are targeted using an antigen expressed preferentially on hematopoietic progenitor cells such as CD34+ or CD133+ [26,27]. CD34+ selection was used in the recent European clinical trial [6]. The CD34+ antigen is the most common antigen used in positive selection and is thought to be expressed on hematopoietic stem cells and hematopoietic progenitor cells of all lineages. Using the Isolex 300i device or the CliniMACS device, highly purified HC ("stem and progenitor') products can be obtained. CD34 antigen is reported to be expressed on neuroblastoma cells leading to concerns that tumor cells may be copurified with the progenitors; therefore, alternate antigens expressed on HC such as CD133 have been studied. In negative selection the tumor cells are destroyed through the use of tumor-specific antigens.

Purging of Autologous Hematopoietic Graft: The Data and the Unanswered Questions?

In a subsequent trial investigators reported a retrospective study of 24 patients with high-risk neuroblastoma who received CD34+-selected peripheral blood HC grafts; 4 patients whose graft contained more than 2000 tumor cells were all alive at 5 years compared to 20 patients whose grafts contained no tumor cells and who had a 5-year DFS of 33% ($P = 0.04$) [28]. These physicians concluded that residual tumor cells in the hematopoietic graft may have a protective effect, suggesting that residual disease persisting in the patient after transplantation may primarily contribute to relapse rather than reinfused occult malignant cells within the graft.

In a randomized trial of purged *versus* unpurged peripheral blood HC grafts, COG demonstrated that there was no difference in outcome between the two groups [29]. Preliminary analysis demonstrated the 2-year EFS for recipients of unpurged products was 51% compared with 47% for those receiving purged products ($P = 0.47$). Recent COG trials have proven that tumor cannot be identified in peripheral blood

HCs of neuroblastoma patients who underwent apheresis even when marrow had persistent disease [30].

The COG study described that immunomagnetic purging of peripheral blood HCs for autologous HCT for neuroblastoma did not impact outcome. Interestingly, this study also demonstrated that patients who still have tumor cells in the hematopoietic graft did significantly worse after myeloablative therapy than did those patients whose grafts had no tumor cells detected. One question raised is whether other purging techniques that result in a greater degree of tumor cell depletion may result in higher survival rates? Immunomagnetic purging used in the COG study may not have been sensitive enough to eradicate the entire tumor content. The COG study did not answer the question as to whether patients with no detectable tumor after purging have improved outcomes compared with those with detectable tumor after purging. Finally purging may be more important in peripheral blood HC grafts since the tumor content of these grafts is lower than that of marrow grafts, which were the main source of HCs in earlier trials of graft purging in neuroblastoma.

Practice Points

Currently there is no proven efficacy to the purging of patients undergoing autologous HCT for neuroblastoma. Future studies will likely study alternate methodologies of cell processing as a means of purifying the hematopoietic graft from tumor cells, such as CD34+ or CD133+ positive selection.

Minimal "Measurable" Residual Disease

Minimal residual disease (MRD) is increasingly used (or talked about) in patients with hematologic malignancies in order to identify high-risk patients and to assess response to therapy (see Chapters 23 and 24). Similarly, MRD is currently being investigated in neuroblastoma as MRD assessment of the HC product from bone marrow aspirates or blood may be useful in assessing tumor contamination or response to therapy. Currently, though, no standard interpretation of MRD in this disease exists in correlation with clinical outcomes. While neuroblastoma cells express well-defined antigens, with diganglioside (GD2) being the best described, a standard way to study MRD in this disease has not been developed [31]. MRD assessment of the HC product or bone marrow aspirates may be useful in assessing tumor contamination or response to therapy. Investigators have examined tumor markers including gene expression profiling in addition to analyzing GD2 expression, and both blood and marrow have been studied. In COG trials, hematopoietic grafts have been purged of neuroblastoma cells by immunomagnetic methodologies using the following five monoclonal antibodies directed against neuroblastoma cell surface markers: 459, HSAN 1.2, BA-1, HNK-1, and 126–4 [29]. In this same study, after purging grafts were tested by using assays quantifying *CHGA*, *DCX*, *DDC*, *PHOX2B*, and *TH* mRNA expression. In a study of quantitative reverse transcriptase PCR analysis of GD2 expression, the detection of

MRD by this method correlated with radiographic disease scores. Interestingly of 120 patients studied, 62 had evidence of GD2 expression: 11 in both marrow and blood, 38 in marrow only, and 13 in blood only, with the highest transcript numbers detected in those patients with transcripts in both blood and marrow [29]. Patients in whom the marker was detected in either the marrow or blood had higher risks of disease progression and death compared with those with negative markers. Gene profiling of markers is an active area of investigation. Eight genes have been identified as being abundantly expressed in stage 4 neuroblastoma and are thought to be worth evaluating: *CCND1*, *CRMP1*, *DDC*, *GABRB3*, *ISL1*, *KIF1A*, *PHOX2B*, and *TACC2* [32]. MRD assessment will be increasingly studied in the future with the goals of quantifying response to therapy and assessing tumor contamination of stem cell products.

Practice Points

Currently there is no demonstrated role for the monitoring of MRD in neuroblastoma patients *in-vivo* during therapy. Future efforts should focus on identifying novel antigens or gene markers or combinations of these.

Role of Allogeneic Hematopoietic Cell Transplant

Allogeneic HCT has been used successfully in neuroblastoma, but primarily in case reports and small series. Allogeneic HCT avoids the possibility of infusing tumor cells with the marrow product, obviating any concerns for purging, but at the expense of complications of allogeneic HCT such as graft failure, graft-*versus*-host disease (GvHD), and infections resulting from protracted immune incompetence. Patients potentially treatable by allogeneic HCT include those with inadequate numbers of autologous hematopoietic progenitor cells collected, unable to have tumor-free grafts obtained, or with progressive disease making them ineligible for autologous HCT. Historically, allogeneic HCT for neuroblastoma patients has been characterized by unacceptably high rates of regimen-related mortality and disease recurrence [19,33]. The largest series of allogeneic HCT to date is published by the Center for International Blood and Marrow Transplant Research (CIBMTR) and demonstrates inferior disease-free survival (DFS) for those who underwent allogeneic HCT after an autologous HCT [34]. No relationship between GvHD and survival after allogeneic HCT was observed. Randomized trials between allogeneic and autologous HCT for this disease have not been possible due to the rarity of neuroblastoma and the small number of patients. Recent improvements in supportive care and HLA typing, along with the advent of reduced intensity conditioning regimens, have resulted in physicians re-exploring the use of allogeneic HCT for neuroblastoma [35–39]. The addition of MIBG therapy to allogeneic transplant conditioning regimens is being explored with case reports of transient or sustained response in refractory patients [40–42].

One clinical trial treated five high-risk neuroblastoma patients (four recurrent after autologous HCT and one induction failure) with 131-I-MIBG followed by melphalan, fludarabine, and thiotepa followed by HLA haplotype mismatch HCT with mesenchymal cells (see Chapter 68) [41]. Two children remain in remission. Given the low toxicity, investigators have proposed further trials to evaluate immune-mediated therapy. Additionally, investigators have suggested that allogeneic HCT may be considered for patients without autologous products to treat the pancytopenia occurring after therapeutic MIBG.

The published literature largely consists of case reports and small series, with many suggesting that a graft-versus-malignancy effect may be operational in neuroblastoma, but investigators are unable to quantify the survival advantage, if any, that is seen with this modality [35–38,43]. Certainly, there is indirect evidence that neuroblastoma may respond to a graft-versus-tumor (GvT) effect after allogeneic HCT. It is noteworthy that even patients with chemotherapy-resistant disease were curable in some series, suggesting that in some cases an immunologic GvT effect may be operational, although there has been no relationship to visible acute or chronic GvHD [35–38,43]. It is possible that another immunologic mechanism distinct from GvHD may be mediating the antitumor effects [44–46]. Most studies support the observation that chemotherapy-resistant disease is a marker for poor outcome, but should be viewed as a prognostic factor and not an absolute contraindication to allogeneic HCT. It is postulated that T-cell alloreactivity or natural killer cell mediated cell destruction may be operational. Reduced intensity conditioning regimens are increasingly becoming employed as a way to reduce transplant-related mortality. In one publication, 46 pediatric patients underwent allogeneic HCT from HLA-matched related and unrelated volunteer donors following a conditioning regimen of busulfan, fludarabine, and antithymocyte globulin [39]. The 3-year EFS for the seven neuroblastoma patients in this study was 28.6%, with patients with measurable disease at allogeneic HCT having inferior outcomes. Two of the neuroblastoma patients improved from very good partial remission to complete remission after transplantation; one of four patients with progressive disease at the time of HCT had stable disease at 47 months and another of these four patients had a 3-month-long partial remission after a DLI prior to disease progression. No transplant-related toxicity was noted in this subgroup of neuroblastoma patients, but it was only 6.9% for the entire cohort.

The largest series of allogeneic transplantation was published by the CIBMTR [34]. In this retrospective trial of 143 neuroblastoma patients undergoing allogeneic transplantation from 1990 to 2007, 46 had not undergone prior autologous HCT and 97 had undergone prior autologous HCT. For recipients who had not received a prior autologous HCT, 59% were in remission at 1-year post-allogeneic HCT, compared to 29% at 5 years post-allogeneic HCT. For patients who had undergone a prior autologous HCT, 50% were in remission at 1-year post-allo-HCT, with 7% in remission at 5 years post-allogeneic HCT. However, when examining patients who underwent allogeneic HCT with no prior autologous HCT, the DFS rates compare favorably given the degree of HLA mismatch between donors and recipients, the percentage of recipients with poor performance scores, and the extensive prior therapy of this patient population. Theoretical reasons for the improved outcomes for this group without a prior autologous HCT could be that there was more immunocompetence allowing more antitumor effect, there was less prior therapy (since many who relapsed after autologous HCT received salvage chemotherapy and may have received more therapy to obtain tumor-free stem cells prior to the autograft), and earlier performance of allogeneic HCT prevented the development of tumor resistance. However, only 39% of patients who underwent prior autologous HCT had chemosensitive disease while only 23% of patients who had not received a prior autologous HCT had chemosensitive disease, suggesting that an immunologic intervention such as allogeneic HCT may have been more beneficial than the additional chemotherapy patients receive in autologous HCT. Alternatively there are reports of HLA haplotype mismatch HCT with and without GvHD in patients with neuroblastoma, suggesting a possible therapeutic effect of T or natural killer (NK) lymphocyte populations [37,43].

Immunotherapies: Challenges Moving Forward

Antibody Therapy Following HCT

Disease recurrence following autologous HCT is a significant cause of treatment failure. Therefore, once remission has been achieved, the primary barrier to successful outcomes is the eradication of residual chemotherapy-resistant tumor cells that reside within the patient. Administration of antibody therapy is one venue to eradicate these malignant cells, particularly at the completion of therapy in the setting of minimal residual disease. Several antibodies directed against the diganglioside antigens (GD2) have been studied in neuroblastoma patients, with the anti-GD2 antibody ch14.18 being the most commonly studied after autologous HCT. Ch14.18 is a monoclonal chimeric (human murine) antibody with activity against neuroblastoma. When the antibody is administered in combination with interleukin-2 (IL-2) or granulocyte-macrophage colony-stimulating factor (GM-CSF), antitumor effects are enhanced by increasing the numbers of neutrophils, macrophages, and natural killer cells, leading to increased antibody-dependent cell-mediated cytotoxicity [47,48]. Recently, the COG conducted a randomized clinical trial of 226 high-risk neuroblastoma patients undergoing autologous HCT, assigning them randomly to receive post-transplantation standard therapy (six cycles of 13-cis-retinoic acid) or immunotherapy with six cycles of 13-cis-retinoic acid and five concomitant cycles of ch14.18 in combination with alternating GM-CSF and IL-2 [4]. At a median follow-up of 2.1 years, immunotherapy had improved EFS compared to standard therapy (66% *versus* 46%, $P=0.01$). OS survival was 86% for the immunotherapy group compared to 46% for the standard therapy group ($P=0.02$). Of note, patients in the immunotherapy group experienced pain (52%), capillary leak syndrome (23%), and hypersensitivity reactions (25%). This randomized trial confirmed earlier pilot studies of ch14.18 in combination with GM-CSF alone or in combination with IL-2 [49,50]. Efforts to develop new antibodies to novel neuroblastoma antigens or alternate formulation of an anti-GD2 antibody, such as a humanized version, are underway to decrease toxicity or to enhance antitumor efficacy.

Cellular Therapy

The possibility of cellular therapeutic antitumor effect in neuroblastoma is supported by the use of immunomodulatory therapies to treat this disorder using dendritic cells, NK cells, and anti-GD2 antibodies [44,45,51,52]. The use of novel agents such as immunomodulatory agents and radioactive treatments may further increase survival. Following autologous HCT, patients with neuroblastoma who did not express the corresponding KIR ligand demonstrated improved survival after HCT (Figure 51.2) [52]. An initial prospective trial at St. Jude studied 16 patients with lymphomas or solid tumors undergoing high-dose chemotherapy with busulfan and melphalan followed by infusion of an autologous graft of CD133+-selected hematopoietic peripheral blood hematopoietic cells. [53]. Eight of the 16 patients experienced disease progression after HCT, including 5 of the 6 patients (83%) with no inhibitory KIR-HLA mismatch and 3 of the 6 patients (50%)

with 1 mismatched pair; none of the 4 (0%) patients with 2 mismatched pairs experienced disease progression. Multivariate analyses for DFS showed that inhibitory KIR-HLA mismatch was the only significant prognostic variable ($P=0.01$), being even more prominent than disease stage. A subsequent retrospective study of 169 patients undergoing autologous HCT for stage IV neuroblastoma found that patients lacking an HLA ligand had a 46% lower risk of death and a 34% lower risk of disease progression at 3 years compared to patients who possessed all ligand for the inhibitory KIR [54]. Survival was strongly correlated with the missing KIR ligand, more than with MYCN gene amplification. These latter two analyses, taken together, suggest that an autoreactive mechanism mediated via natural killer cells may eliminate residual neuroblastoma (see Chapter 62).

Lymphodepletion Prior to Autologous Transplants

Recent publications have highlighted observations that in the setting of lymphodepletion, selective expansion of certain lymphocyte populations occurs more rapidly in an environment with no competition [55–59]. CD34+ positive selection is currently the most commonly used method of T-cell-depleting hematopoietic grafts, while theoretically serving as a means of purging grafts of tumor cells. This CD34+ selection results in a highly purified product for HCs and has been associated with increased risk of infection and post-transplantation lymphoproliferative disease [10]. In addition, other studies have shown increased varicella reactivation in patients who received CD34+ selected hematopoietic grafts [27], affecting up to 21% of patients (see Chapters 29 and 30).

Other investigators have shown that infusion of autologous T-cells early after transplant improves long-term immune recovery in neuroblastoma patients [60]. Nineteen patients were enrolled in a pilot trial to receive autologous expanded T-lymphocytes on day 2, 12, or 90 after the second infusion of HCs (as part of a tandem autologous HCT) and 23 were enrolled in a subsequent randomized trial to received expanded T-lymphocytes on day 2 (early) or day 90 (late) after the second HCT. On days 12 and 60 after the second HCT, influenza vaccine and pneumococcal vaccine were administered; no IVIG was given. Patients who received the infusion on day 2 had better T-cell count recovery and T-cell proliferation than those who received T-lymphocytes on day 90. While antitumor effects were not described in this publication, it certainly raises the possibility of administration of certain lymphocyte populations such as antigen-specific T-cells or NK cells to eradicate residual neuroblastoma after autologous HCT, particularly in combination with antibody therapy.

Practice Points

Currently there is no advantage to EFS and due to reported delayed immune reconstitution for processed grafts as described above, unprocessed and unmodified hematopoietic grafts are the standard graft source for autologous HCT for neuroblastoma.

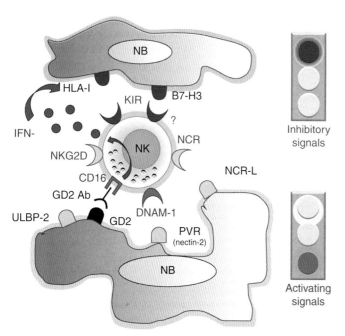

Figure 51.2 Inhibitory and activating interactions between human NK cells and neuroblasts
Reprinted with permission from reference [52].

Controversies

Despite a standardized treatment approach to high-risk neuroblastoma, several controversies still exist regarding optimal treatment. First, while TBI has been omitted from the conditioning regimen, the precise chemotherapeutic agents to be used in the conditioning regimen vary. Second, a recently completed randomized clinical trial comparing single *versus* tandem autologous HCT has been completed with analyses pending. The results will be instrumental in the design of future clinical trials. Third, MIBG seems to be promising in the treatment of certain patients with relapsed disease; however, how MIBG will be incorporated into frontline therapy has not been decided. Certainly tandem autologous HCT with MIBG conditioning as one conditioning regimen could be a consideration. Fourth, peripheral blood hematopoietic cells are currently the most common graft source; the role of purging appears to be unnecessary as studied in an early COG study. However with improved purging methodologies, purging may theoretically become beneficial. Contrariwise, small amounts of tumor contamination may evoke an immunologic antineuroblastoma effect during immune recovery throughout the lymphopenic period after autologous HCT.

Fifth, immunotherapy with a chimeric anti-GD2 antibody following autologous HCT has resulted in the greatest improvements in outcomes for high-risk neuroblastoma. Building on the immunotherapeutic principles, the roles of humanized anti-GD2 antibodies, other antineuroblastoma antibodies, natural killer cell infusions, and/or the use of ALK inhibitors, while promising, remain to be elucidated. Finally, allogeneic HCT does not currently seem to have a role in frontline therapy.

Future Directions

Currently autologous HCT remains a cornerstone in the treatment of high-risk neuroblastoma in combination with induction chemotherapy, surgical resection, radiation therapy, and post-transplant immunomodulatory therapies. Allogeneic HCT and other cellular therapies, particularly NK-cells, are promising and may be considered in specific circumstances within clinical trials. Overall outcomes remain less than optimal, with future trials focusing on the use of allogeneic cellular therapies in neuroblastoma, the exploration of the lymphopenic environment to enhance immunologic recovery, and the development of novel interventions to further reduce disease recurrence.

References

1. Pizzo PA, Poplack DG. *Principles and Practice of Pediatric Oncology*, 4th edn. Philadelphia: Lippincott Williams & Wilkins; 2002.

2. Matthay KK, Villablanca JG, Seeger RC *et al.* Treatment of high-risk neuroblastoma with intensive chemotherapy, radiotherapy, autologous bone marrow transplantation, and 13-cis-retinoic acid. *N Engl J Med* 1999; 341; 1165–1173.

3. Matthay KK, Reynolds CP, Seeger RC *et al.* Long-term results for children with high-risk neuroblastoma treated on a randomized trial of myeloablative therapy followed by 13-cis-retinoic acid: a Children's Oncology Group study. *J Clin Oncol* 2009; 27: 1007–1013.

4. Yu AL, Gilman AL, Ozkaynak O *et al.* Anti-GD2 antibody with GM-CSF, interleukin-2, and isotretinoin for neuroblastoma. *N Engl J Med* 2010; 363: 1324–1334.

5. Yalcin B, Kremer LC, Caron HN, van Dalen EC. High-dose chemotherapy and autologous haematopoietic stem cell rescue for children with high-risk neuroblastoma. *Cochrane Database Syst Rev* 2013; 8: 1–41.

6. Berthold F, Boos J, Burcahc S *et al.* Myeloablative megatherapy with autologous stem-cell rescue *versus* oral maintenance chemotherapy as consolidation treatment in patients with high-risk neuroblastoma. A randomized controlled trial. *Lancet Oncol* 2005; 6: 649–658.

7. Pritchard J, Cotterill SJ, Germond SM *et al.* High dose melphalan in the treatment of advanced neuroblastoma: results of a randomized trial (ENSG-1) by the European Neuroblastoma Study Group. *Cancer* 2005; 44: 348–357.

8. Cheung NV, Heller G. Chemotherapy dose intensity correlates strongly with the response, median survival, and median progression-free survival in metastatic neuroblastoma. *J Clin Oncol* 1991; 9: 1050–1058.

9. Kletzel M, Katzenstein HM, Hauk PR *et al.* Treatment of high-risk neuroblastoma with triple-tandem high-dose therapy and stem cell rescue: results of the Chicago pilot II study. *J Clin Oncol* 2002: 20: 2284–2292.

10. Seif AE, Naranjo A, Baker DL *et al.* A pilot study of tandem high-dose chemotherapy with stem cell rescue as consolidation for high-risk neuroblastoma: Children's Oncology Group study ANBL00P1. *Bone Marrow Transplant.* 2013; 48: 947–952.

11. Grupp SA, Dvorak CC, Nieder ML *et al.* COG Stem Cell Transplant Scientific Committee. Children's Oncology Group's 2013 blueprint for research: Stem cell transplantation. *Pediatr Blood Cancer.* 2013; 60: 1044–1047.

12. Gadner H, Emminger W, Ladenstein R, Peters C. High-dose melphalan, etoposide, and carboplatin (MEC) +/- fractionated total body irradiation for treatment of advanced solid tumors. *Pediatr Hematol Oncol.* 1992; 9: v-viii.

13. Flandin I, Hartmann O, Michon J *et al.* Impact of TBI on late effects in children treated by megatherapy for stage IV neuroblastoma. A study for the French Society of Pediatric Oncology. *In J Radiat Oncol Biol Phys* 2006: 64; 1424–1431.

14. Hobbie WL, Moshang T, Carlson CA *et al.* Late effects in survivors of tandem peripheral blood stem cell transplant for high-risk neuroblastoma. *Pediatr Blood Cancer* 2008; 51: 679–683.

15. Kushner BH, Cheung NKV, Kramer K, Dunkel IJ, Calleja E, Boulad F. Topotecan combined with myeloablative doses of thiotepa and carboplatin for neuroblastoma, brain tumors, and other poor-risk solid tumors in children and young adults. *Bone Marrow Transplant* 2001; 28: 551–556.

16. DE Ioris MA, Contoli B, Jenkner A *et al*. Comparison of two different conditioning regimens before autologous transplantation for children with high-risk neuroblastoma. *Anticancer Res* 2012; 32: 5427–5434.

17. Molina B, Alonso L, Gonzalez-Vicent M *et al*. High-dose busulfan and melphalan as conditioning regimen for autologous peripheral blood progenitor cell transplantation in high-risk neuroblastama patients. *Pediatr Hematol Oncol* 2011; 28: 115–123.

18. Boland I, Vassal G, J Morizet J, *et al*. Busulphan is active against neuroblastoma and medulloblastoma xenografts in athymic mice at clinically achievable plasma drug concentrations. *Br J Cancer* 1999; 79: 787–792.

19. Ladenstein R, Potschger U, Hartman O *et al*. 28 years of high-dose therapy and SCT for neuroblastoma in Europe: lessons from more than 4000 procedures. *Bone Marrow Transplant* 2008; 41(Suppl 2): S118–127.

20. Hamidieh AA, Beiki D, Paragomi P, *et al*. The potential role of pretransplant MIBG diagnosic scintigraphy in targeted administration of I-MIBG accompanied by ASCT for high-risk and relapsed neuroblastoma: A pilot study. *Pediatr Transplant* 2014; 18: 510–517.

21. Atas E, Kesik V, Kismet E, Kosseoglu V. 131I-Metaiodobenzylguanidine conditioning regimen in children with neuroblastoma undergoing stem cell transplantation. *Pediatr Transplant* 2013; 17: 407–408.

22. French S, Dubois SG, Horn B *et al*. I-MIBG followed by consolidation with busulfan, melphalan and autologous stem cell transplantation for refractory neuroblastoma. *Pediatr Blood Cancer*. 2013; 60: 879–884.

23. Matthay KK, DeSantes K, Hasagawa B *et al*. Phase 1 dose escalation of I131-metaiodobenzylguanidine with autologous bone marrow support in refractory neuroblastoma. *J Clin Oncol* 1998; 16: 229–236.

24. Matthay KK, Tan JC, Villablanca JG *et al*. Phase 1 dose escalation of iodine-131-metaiodobenzylguanidine with myeloablative chemotherapy and autologous stem cell transplantation in refractory neuroblastoma: a New Approaches to Neuroblastoma therapy Consortium Study. *J Clin Oncol* 2006; 24: 500–506.

25. Rill DR, Santana VM, Roberts WM *et al*. Direct demonstration that autologous bone marrow transplantation for solid tumors can return a multiplicity of tumorigenic cells. *Blood* 1994; 84: 380–383.

26. Donovan J, Temel J, Zuckerman A *et al*. CD34 selection as a stem cell purging strategy for neuroblastoma: preclinical and clinical studies. *Med Pediatr Oncol* 2000; 35: 677–682.

27. Marabelle A, Merlin E, Halle P *et al*. CD34+ immunoselection of autologous grafts for the treatment of high-risk neuroblastoma. *Pediatr Blood Cancer* 2011; 56: 134–142.

28. Handgretinger R, Leung W, Ihm K *et al*. Tumour cell contamination of autologous stem cell grafts in high-risk neuroblastoma: the good news? *Br J Cancer* 2003; 88: 1874–1877.

29. Kreissman SG, Seeger RC, Matthay KM *et al*. Purged *versus* non-purged peripheral blood stem-cell transplantation for high-risk neuroblastoma (COG A3973): a randomized phase 3 trial. *Lancet Oncol* 2013; 14: 999–1008.

30. Park JE, Scott JR, Stewart JF *et al*. Pilot induction regimen incorporating pharmacokinetically guided topotecan for newly diagnosed high-risk neuroblastoma: a Children's Oncology Group study. *J Clin Oncol* 2011; 29: 4351–4357.

31. Beiske K, Burchill SA, Cheung IY *et al*. Consensus criteria for sensitive detection of minimal neuroblastoma cells in bone marrow, blood and stem cell preparations by immunocytology and QRT-PCR: recommendations by the International Neuroblastoma Risk Group Task Force. *Br J Cancer* 2009; 100: 1627–1637.

32. Cheung IY, Feng Y, Gerald W, Cheung NV. Exploiting gene expression profiling to novel minimal residual disease markers of neuroblastoma. *Clin Cancer Res* 2008; 14: 7020–7027.

33. Ladenstein R, Lasset C, Hartmann O *et al*. Comparison of auto *versus* allografting as consolidation of primary treatments in advanced neuroblastoma over one year of age at diagnosis: Report from the European Group for Bone Marrow Transplantation. *Bone Marrow Transplant* 1994; 14: 37–46.

34. Hale GA, Arora M, Ahn KW *et al*. Allogeneic hematopoietic cell transplantation for neuroblastoma: the CIBMTR experience. *Bone Marrow Transplant* 2013; 48: 1056–1064.

35. Jubert C, Wall DA, Grimley M *et al*. Engraftment of unrelated cord blood after reduced-intensity conditioning regimen in children with refractory neuroblastoma: a feasibility trial. *Bone Marrow Transplant* 2011; 46: 232–237.

36. Geyer MB, Jacobson JS, Freedman J *et al*. A comparison of immune reconstitution and graft-*versus*-host disease following myeloablative conditioning (MAC) vs. reduced toxicity conditioning (RTC) and umbilical cord blood transplantation (UCBT) in paediatric recipients. *Br J Haematol* 2011; 155: 218–234.

37. Pession A, Masetti R, Di Leo C *et al*. HLA-mismatched hematopoietic stem cell transplantation for pediatric solid tumors. *Pediatr Rep* 2011; 3(Suppl 2): e12.

38. Sung KW, Park JE, Cheuh HW *et al*. Reduced-intensity allogeneic stem cell transplantation for children with neuroblastoma who failed tandem autologous stem cell transplantation. *Pediatr Blood Cancer* 2011; 57: 680–685.

39. Paillard C, Rochette E, Lutz P *et al*. Reduced-intensity conditioning followed by allogeneic transplantation in pediatric malignancies: a report from the Société Française des Cancers de l'Enfant and the Société Française de Greffe de Moelle et de Thérapie Cellulaire. *Bone Marrow Transplant* 2013; 48: 1401–1408.

40. Sato Y, Kurosawa H, Fukushima K *et al*. I-131-Metaiodobenzylguanidine therapy with allogeneic cord blood stem cell transplantation for recurrent neuroblastoma. *Ital J Pediatr* 2012; 15: 1–3.

41. Toporski J, Garkavij M, Tennvall J *et al*. High dose iodine-131-metaiodobenzylguadine with haploidentical stem cell transplantation and posttransplant immunotherapt in children with relapsed/refractory neuroblastoma. *Biol Blood Marrow Transplant* 2009; 12: 1077–1085.

42. Takahashi H, Manabe A, Aoyama C *et al*. Iodine 131-metaiodobenzylguanidine therapy with reduced-intensity allogeneic stem cell transplantation in recurrent neuroblastoma. *Pediatr Blood Cancer* 2008; 50: 676–678.

43. Inoue M, Nakano T, Yoneda A *et al.* Graft-*versus*-tumor effect in a patient with advanced neuroblastoma who received HLA haplo-identical bone marrow transplantation. *Bone Marrow Transplant* 2003; 32: 103–106.

44. Ash S, Stein J, Ashenasv N, Yaniv I. Immunomodulation with dendritic cells and donor lymphocyte infusion converge to induce graft vs neuroblastoma reactions without GVHD after allogeneic bone marrow transplantation. *Br J Cancer* 2010; 103: 1597–1605.

45. Ash S, Gigi V, Askenasy N *et al.* Graft *versus* neuroblastoma reaction is efficiently elicited by allogeneic bone marrow transplantation through cytolytic activity in the absence of GVHD. *Cancer Immunol Immunother* 2009; 58 : 2073–2084.

46. Venstrom JM, Zheng J, Noor N *et al.* KIR and HLA genotypes are associated with disease progression and survival following autologous hematopoietic stem cell transplantation for high-risk neuroblastoma. *Clin Cancer Res* 2009; 15: 7330–7334.

47. Barker E, Mueller BM, Handgretinger R, Herter M, Yu AL, Reisfeld A. Effect of a chimeric anti-ganglioside GDS2 antibody on cell-mediated lysis of human neuroblastoma cells. *Cancer Res* 1991; 51: 144–149.

48. Hank JA, Robinson RR, Surfus J *et al.* Augmentation of antibody dependent cell mediated cytotoxicity following in vivo therapy with recombinant interleukin 2. *Cancer Res* 1990; 50: 5234–5239.

49. Gilman AL, Ozkaynak MF, Matthay KK *et al.* Phase 1 study of ch14.18 with granulocyte-macrophage colony-stimulating factor and interleukin-2 in children with neuroblastoma after autologous bone marrow transplantation or stem-cell rescue: a report from the Children's Oncology Group. *J Clin Oncol* 2009; 27: 85–91.

50. Ozkaynak MF, Sondel PM, Krailo MD *et al.* Phase 1 study of chimeric human/murine anti-ganglioside G9D2) monoclonal antibody (ch14.18) with granulocyte-macrophage colony-stimulating factor in children with neuroblastoma immediately after hematopoietic stem-cell transplantation: a Children's Cancer Group Study. *J Clin Oncol* 2000; 18: 4077–4085.

51. Delgado DC, Hank JA, Kolesar J *et al.* Genotypes of NK cell KIR receptros, their ligands, and Fc gamma recdiptors in the response of neuroblastoma patients to Hu14.18-IL2 immunotherapy. *Cancer Res* 2010; 70: 9554–9561.

52. Bottino C, Dondero A, Bellora F *et al.* Natural killer cells and neuroblastoma: tumor recognition, escape mechanisms, and possible novel immunotherapeutic approaches. *Front Immunol* 2014; 5: 1–11.

53. Leung W, Handgretinger R, Iyengar R, Turner V, M S Holladay MS, Hale GA Inhibitory KIR-HLA receptor–ligand mismatch in autologous haematopoietic stem cell transplantation for solid tumour and lymphoma. *Br J Cancer* 2007; 97: 539–542.

54. Venstrom JM, Zheng J, Noor N *et al.* KIR and HLA genotypes are associated with disease progression and survival following autologous hematopoietic stem cell transplantation for high-risk neuroblastoma. *Clin Cancer Res* 2009; 15: 7330–7334.

55. Jing W, Gershan JA, Johnson BD. Depletion of CD4 T cells enhances immunotherapy for neuroblastoma after syngeneic HSCT but compromises development of anti-tumor immune memory. *Blood* 2009; 113: 4449–4457.

56. Cui Y, Zhang H, Meadors J, Poon R, Guimond M, Mackall CL. Harnessing the physiology of lymphopenia to support adoptive immunotherapy in lymphoreplete hosts. *Blood* 2009; 114: 3831–3840.

57. Miller JS, Weisdorf DJ, Burns LJ *et al.* Lymphodepletion followed by donor lymphocyte infusion (DLI) causes significantly more acute graft-*versus*-host disease than DLI alone. *Blood* 2007; 110: 2761–2763.

58. Baba J, Watanabe S, Saida Y *et al.* Depletion of radio-resistant regulatory T cells enhances antitumor immunity during recovery from lymphopenia. *Blood* 2012; 120: 2417–2427.

59. Louis CU, Straathof K, Bollard CM *et al.* Enhancing the in vivo expansion of adoptively transferred EBV-specific CTL with lymphodepleting CD45 monoclonal antibodies in NPC patients. *Blood* 2009; 113: 2442–2450.

60. Grupp SA, Prak EL, Boyer J *et al.* Adoptive transfer of autologous T cells improves T-cell repertoire diversity and long-term B-cell function in pediatric patients with neuroblastoma. *Clin Cancer Res.* 2012; 18: 6732–6741.

Chapter

52

Hematopoietic Cell Transplants for Bone Marrow Failure Disorders

Régis Peffault de Latour, Judith C.W. Marsh, and Jakob R. Passweg

Introduction

Bone marrow failure syndromes (BMF) include acquired diseases, such as severe aplastic anemia (SAA), which is generally considered an autoimmune disease, and congenital BMF disorders. Acquired SAA is the more common disease and also needs to be differentiated from hypoplastic myelodysplastic syndrome (MDS) and paroxysmal nocturnal hemoglobinuria (PNH). The congenital diseases are disorders that include those due to (i) failure of DNA repair such as Fanconi anemia, (ii) more rarely, the ribosomopathies such as Diamond Black-fan anemia, and (iii) disorders of telomere maintenance, i.e., dyskeratosis congenita. In contrast to acquired SAA, for constitutional SAA: (i) standard doses of chemotherapy and/or irradiation should be absolutely avoided in Fanconi anemia, due to the underlying defect in DNA repair; and (ii) matched siblings who may also have BMF should also be avoided. Allo-HCT will not correct the underlying disease but will address the bone marrow failure. The indication and assessment of patients for transplantation, and the subsequent allo-HCT, should be performed with access to specialized centers that have the latest molecular tests and the clinical expertise to ensure that appropriate conditioning regimens are used to mitigate increased susceptibilities to toxicities and secondary cancer.

Figure 52.1 shows the absolute numbers of allo-HCT for marrow failure as reported to the European Group for Blood and Marrow Transplantation (EBMT) and also shows the continued increase of allo-HCT for these indications from 2004 to 2011 in Europe.

Allogeneic Hematopoietic Cell Transplant for Acquired Aplastic Anemia

SAA is defined as pancytopenia with marrow hypocellularity. The incidence of acquired aplastic anemia in the western world is around 2 per million persons per year, but is higher in East Asia. There are two incidence peaks, one in childhood and adolescence and the second in patients aged >60 years. Patients with SAA frequently present with anemia, neutropenic infection, or bleeding. A watch and wait strategy is often used initially if there is milder pancytopenia, but, conversely, a long interval from diagnosis to allo-HCT is associated with

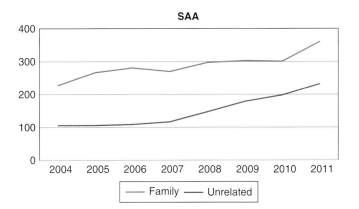

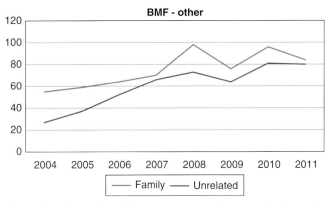

Figure 52.1 Frequencies of allogeneic transplants for severe aplastic anemia (SAA) and other marrow failure syndromes (BMF – other) most of which are Fanconi anemia. It is evident that the number of transplants for marrow failure done within the EBMT network continues to increase for acquired as well as for congenital marrow failure and from sibling as well as from unrelated donors. Data from the Activity Survey of the European Group of Blood and Marrow Transplantation.

higher mortality risks[1]. Prior to treatment the patient should ideally be stable clinically with control of bleeding and infections. Once the diagnosis is confirmed, and the disease severity is assessed, family HLA typing is done and treatment initiated.

Initial Therapy in Acquired Aplastic Anemia: What Is the Best Strategy?

The choice of first-line treatment will depend on the age of the patient, the availability of an HLA-identical sibling donor, and disease severity[2] (Figure 52.2). Family HLA typing is

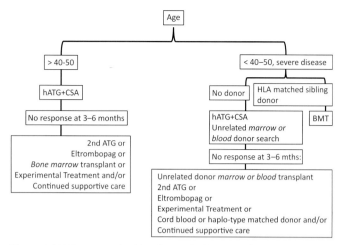

Figure 52.2 Treatment algorithm for acquired severe aplastic anemia.

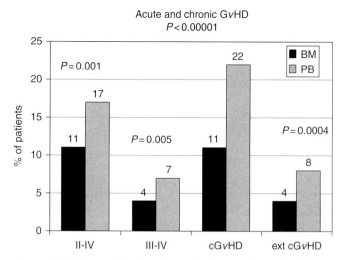

Figure 52.3 Differences in rates and severity of acute and chronic GvHD by graft source comparing bone marrow versus peripheral blood in HLA-matched sibling donor transplantation reported to the EBMT. Rates and severity of acute and chronic GvHD is higher in recipients of peripheral blood transplants (PB) as compared to marrow transplants (BM). Reproduced from reference [1].

therefore required at first diagnosis of pancytopenia, even if the diagnosis of SAA awaits confirmation. The standard first-line treatment for a newly diagnosed patient with SAA is allogeneic bone marrow transplant (BMT) from an HLA-identical sibling donor or immunosuppression using a combination of horse antithymocyte globulin (ATG) and cyclosporine A (ATG+CSA). In an observational study comparing the two strategies[2], survival was better with BMT as a first-line treatment in young patients with very low neutrophil counts, and better with immunosuppression in older patients with higher neutrophil counts. Owing to the rarity of SAA, no randomized clinical trials of first-line sibling BMT or immunosuppressive therapy (IST) have been performed.

Allogeneic BMT from an HLA-identical sibling donor is recommended as first-line treatment for severe or very severe SAA (VSAA) (VSAA is defined as neutrophil count $<0.2 \times 10^9/L$) and if the patient is younger than 50 years of age.

Donor Source

HLA-Matched Sibling: Best Case Scenario

Results of BMT for SAA from an HLA-identical sibling donor have improved steadily over the years with a 75–80% chance of long-term cure in more recent cohorts, and exceeding 90% for children. Unresolved issues are graft failure rates of 4–14% including late graft failure, and graft-*versus*-host disease (GvHD). Severe acute GvHD (grade III–IV) appears to occur less commonly now, but without a corresponding improvement in survival. The incidence of chronic GvHD remains around 30–40%.

In cohorts of patients reported more recently to the EBMT, outcome in the age categories of 20–30, 30–40, and 40–50 years are similar. The option to treat a patient initially with IST and transplanting those who fail to respond to IST is attractive; however, the outcomes of patients undergoing transplant after failing IST are worse than undergoing transplant as first-line treatment[3]. In one study, the hazard ratio for mortality was 1.7 in patients receiving a transplant as part

of a second-line treatment compared to patients receiving upfront transplant[3]. More recent data may show lower risks. Optimal transplant strategies for HLA-identical sibling BMT are well described. It is recommended to use bone marrow hematopoietic cells, rather than G-CSF mobilized peripheral blood hematopoietic cells for ATG-based conditioning regimens. In retrospective studies, earlier engraftment occurred with peripheral blood but peripheral blood hematopoietic cells resulted in more chronic GvHD and poorer survival, compared with bone marrow[1,4]. Figure 52.3 shows acute and chronic GvHD in recipients of peripheral blood and marrow transplants from sibling donors as reported to the EBMT[1]. In this study, acute and chronic GvHD, and in particular severe forms of the disease, were more frequent with peripheral blood as a hematopoietic cell source.

Donor Gender and T-Cell Depletion: How Do They Influence Outcomes of Allo-HCT?

The effect of donor–recipient gender-mismatch has been analyzed and shows better survival in patients with donors from the same sex. Male patients with female donors had an increased risk of acute GvHD compared to male into male transplants; female patients with male donors had an increased risk of graft failure[5]. The preparative regimens and GvHD prevention regimens described below refer mainly to patients with acquired SAA. In young patients with SAA the standard conditioning used is cyclophosphamide 50 mg/kg×4 days + ATG (varying doses and schedules have been published) (see Chapters 12 and 29). This preparative regimen is not "myeloablative" but highly immunosuppressive to help prevent graft failure and GvHD. The advantage of adding ATG to cyclophosphamide is not fully established. A small randomized trial

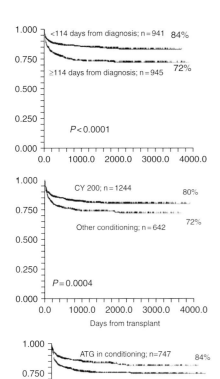

Figure 52.4 Survival of patients receiving HLA-matched sibling donor transplantation for aplastic anemia by disease duration prior to transplant, and use of conditioning regimens with cyclophosphamide and antithymocyte globulin. Higher long-term survival is seen for patients receiving an early transplant and when cyclophosphamide is given at a dose of 4×50mg/kg (=200mg/kg) and with incorporation of ATG. Reproduced from reference [1].

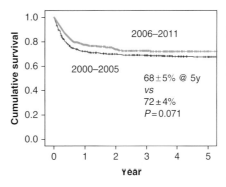

Figure 52.5 Survival after allogeneic transplantation from HLA-matched unrelated donors in 2000–2005 compared to transplants in 2006–2011. Long-term survival is much improved over the 30–40% survival rates reported in the early 1990s. Survival probabilities continue to improve in the 2000s but the differences are small.

did not show a significant difference adding in ATG, but two retrospective studies show improved survival if ATG was used[1,6] (Figure 52.4). The recommended post-transplant GvHD prophylaxis regimen is cyclosporine A (CSA) maintained for a minimum of 12 months with slow tapering and a short course of methotrexate (Mtx). The superiority of the combined treatment has been confirmed in a randomized trial comparing CSA+Mtx to Mtx alone.

Allo-HCT in Older Adults

Because of unsatisfactory results with older patients transplanted from sibling donor transplant, and considering that many of these patients received a transplant not as first-line but as second-line treatment, with a long interval from diagnosis to transplant and a high transfusion load, several studies have tried to modify the preparative regimen by adding fludarabine and by reducing the cyclophosphamide dose. Some interesting data have been published[7] showing higher survival of fludarabine-containing regimens, but data are still limited. Another approach warranting further exploration is to use alemtuzumab instead of ATG, as the risk of chronic GvHD is lower and Mtx is not required post-transplant[8].

Nonsibling Donors for Allo-HCT

Unrelated HLA-Matched Volunteer Donor: What Are the Issues to Optimize Outcomes?

The outcome of unrelated donor transplants for patients with SAA has improved in the last decade[9,10] from about 30–40% survival at 5 years to approximately 70–80%. Improved selection of better HLA-matched donors has most likely played a major role. Since the progress of high-resolution typing with greater availability of HLA-A, B, C, DRB1, DQB1 matched donors, the number of unrelated donor transplants for marrow failure has increased (Figure 52.1). Outcomes after unrelated donor transplant for AA continue to improve as shown by the results from the EBMT database (Figure 52.5) with 72% 5-year survival in patients transplanted between 2006 and 2011. Slightly higher survival rates are reported in phase 2 studies: 73–80%[11,12]. However, smaller phase 2 studies may show better results from centers with a special expertise but may also reflect a selection bias by entering only patients qualifying through specific inclusion and exclusion criteria. More recent data from EBMT report overall survival rates after unrelated donor transplantation that are similar to matched sibling donor transplantation, albeit with increased risk of acute and chronic GvHD[6].

The appropriate time to start an unrelated donor search is an important issue. For patients who may be candidates for unrelated donor transplant, the donor search should start at the time of diagnosis, as response to IST usually occurs after around 3–4 months, during which time an appropriate donor may be identified. Pediatric groups, in particular, currently discuss upfront unrelated donor transplant, provided a fully matched donor is readily available[13]. With the increasing size of the donor pool and the increasing proportion of unrelated donor type at high-resolution level donor search duration may be shortened.

As for sibling transplants, using ATG-based conditioning regimens, outcomes are improved if marrow is used rather than peripheral blood[14]. Bone marrow failure patients derive little, if any, benefit from the higher T-cell dose found in peripheral blood with the associated higher risks of chronic GvHD. Optimal conditioning regimens in unrelated donor transplant are not known. Increasingly, regimens incorporating fludarabine, ATG or the monoclonal antibody alemtuzumab, and small doses of total body irradiation (e.g., 2 Gy of TBI) are being used[11,15–17] in combination with variable doses of cyclophosphamide. Of interest is a study that examined a dose de-escalation of cyclophosphamide[16] in combination with fludarabine, ATG, and low-dose TBI. There was excessive toxicity with cyclophosphamide doses of ≥ 150 mg/kg and graft failure with doses of <50 mg/kg. Similar regimens are used successfully in patients with congenital marrow failure[18].

Cord Blood Transplant

Umbilical cord blood has been used in a limited number of patients with SAA who lack a suitably matched marrow donor [19]. Cord blood transplant (CBT) has increased the availability of HCT in the absence of a suitable matched adult donor. Outcome is excellent if an identical sibling cord is available (unpublished data from the EBMT database), but this is a rare situation, limited to the affected child whose mother is pregnant. Outcomes are less successful in unrelated cord blood transplants. Data from the EBMT SAA working party database indicate long-term survival of only 35% for unselected patients undergoing CBT. Results from smaller phase 2 studies are more variable[19,20]. Transplant of two partially HLA-matched cord blood units thus enables salvage treatment of high-risk patients. In a series of 71 patients[20], with a median age of 13 years, the cumulative incidence of neutrophil recovery at day 60 was only 51±6%, with a shorter time to engraftment using higher nucleated cell counts ($>3.9\times10^7$/kg). The incidence of acute GvHD was 20±5% and of chronic GvHD was 18±5%. Three-year overall survival was 38±6%. Therefore, CBT results are currently not equivalent to sibling or unrelated marrow allo-transplant and further studies are needed.

Haplotype Matched Transplant

In parallel to CBT, HLA haplotype matched hematopoietic cell transplant has undergone major modifications and progress. The main advantages of HLA haplotype-matched hematopoietic cell transplantation is the ready availability of a one-haplotype-matched donor for almost all patients, and the lower cost of the transplant. The most commonly used transplant technology is using T-cell depleted grafts with a high dose of CD34 + cells[21]. More recently, unmanipulated haplotype-matched bone marrow transplant with post-transplant cyclophosphamide (50 mg/kg×2 on days +3 and +4) as GvHD prophylaxis has been reported[22], although few patients with aplastic anemia have been treated. Problems with this approach include primary graft failure (see Chapter 9), GvHD, and poor immune reconstitution[23]. Haplotype-matched transplants have been used only on an individual basis in subjects with aplastic anemia and no large studies have been performed. In a series of 19 Chinese patients receiving a combination of

G-CSF-primed marrow and G-CSF-mobilized peripheral blood hematopoietic cells from haplotype-matched family donors, using a conditioning regimen with busulfan, cyclophosphamide and ATG, all patients engrafted and overall survival was 64% with 56% reported as having chronic GvHD[24]. More recently, a single center series of eight patients using reduced intensity conditioning with post-transplant high-dose cyclophosphamide, showed engraftment failure in two patients with donor-directed HLA antibodies, but engraftment in six without antibodies, and only one case of skin grade II acute GvHD and no chronic GvHD[25]. As for CBT, all patients must be screened for donor-directed HLA antibodies, and their presence precludes the use of that donor.

Paroxysmal Nocturnal Hemoglobinuria

Paroxysmal nocturnal hemoglobinuria (PNH) is a disease with highly variable clinical manifestations. The symptoms may resemble aplastic anemia but it is more commonly associated with classical hemolytic or thromboembolic disease. In a recent comparative study[26] of transplanted patients from the EBMT registry matched to patients without transplantation from a cohort of the French Hematological Society, the 5-year survival of transplanted patients was 68% ± 3 (54% ± 7 in patients with thromboembolic presentation, 69% ± 5 in

Table 52.1 Controversies in bone marrow failure syndromes and allo-HCT

Controversy	Comments by authors
Upfront HLA-matched unrelated donor allograft	May be appropriate in children and adolescents: observational studies as prospective studies unlikely
Appropriate use of CBT	Prospective studies in refractory SAA, e.g., APCORD by the French BMT society
Appropriate use of HLA haplotype-matched transplant	Observational studies as prospective studies unlikely
Conditioning regimens in older adults	Appropriate intensity, observational studies as prospective studies unlikely
Immunosuppressive therapy (IST) for treatment of subjects with moderate AA	hATG+CSA *versus* CSA alone *versus* observation: influence of transfusion dependence, observational studies; increasing awareness of constitutional AA in moderate AA
IST strategies in the older adults	hATG+CSA *versus* CSA alone
Incorporating thrombopoietin analogs into treatment strategies	Prospective studies underway or planned incorporating thrombopoietin analogs into IST treatment or using them upfront

patients with an aplastic anemia presentation and 86% ± 6 in patients with hemolytic presentation). Patients with a thromboembolic presentation did not benefit from transplantation, whereas for patients presenting with aplastic anemia, a matched pair analysis could not be performed. The outcome of this latter subgroup of patients is, however, similar to other patients with marrow failure reported to the registries. Of note, most of the patients in the transplant cohort, as well among the control cohort, were treated prior to the availability of complement inhibitors.

Controversies in Bone Marrow Failure Syndromes and Allo-HCT

Table 52.1 cites current controversies discussed in allogeneic HCT for marrow failure.

References

1. Bacigalupo A, Socié G, Schrezenmeier H, et al. Bone marrow versus peripheral blood as the stem cell source for sibling transplants in acquired aplastic anemia: survival advantage for bone marrow in all age groups. Haematologica. 2012;97(8):1142–8.

2. Bacigalupo A, Brand R, Oneto R, et al. Treatment of acquired severe aplastic anemia: bone marrow transplantation compared with immunosuppressive therapy–The European Group for Blood and Marrow Transplantation experience. Semin Hematol. 2000;37(1):69–80.

3. Ades L, Mary JY, Robin M, et al. Long-term outcome after bone marrow transplantation for severe aplastic anemia. Blood. 2004;103(7):2490–7.

4. Schrezenmeier H, Passweg JR, Marsh JC, et al. Worse outcome and more chronic GVHD with peripheral blood progenitor cells than bone marrow in HLA-matched sibling donor transplants for young patients with severe acquired aplastic anemia. Blood. 2007;110(4):1397–400.

5. Stern, M, Passweg, J, Locasciulli, A, et al. Influence of donor/recipient sex matching on outcome of allogeneic hematopoietic stem cell transplantation. Transplantation. 2006;82(2):218–26.

6. Bacigalupo A, Socie A, Hamladji RM, et al. Current outcome of HLA identical sibling versus unrelated donor transplants in severe aplastic anemia. Haematologica. 2015;100:696–702.

7. Maury S, Bacigalupo A, Anderlini P, et al. Improved outcome of patients older than 30 years receiving HLA-identical sibling hematopoietic stem cell transplantation for severe acquired aplastic anemia using fludarabine-based conditioning: a comparison with conventional conditioning regimen. Haematologica. 2009;94(9):1312–5.

8. Locatelli F, Bruno B, Zecca M, et al. Cyclosporin A and short-term methotrexate versus cyclosporin A as graft versus host disease prophylaxis in patients with severe aplastic anemia given allogeneic bone marrow transplantation from an HLA-identical sibling: results of a GITMO/EBMT randomized trial. Blood. 2000;96(5):1690–7.

9. Maury S, Balere-Appert ML, Chir Z, et al. French Society of Bone Marrow Transplantation and Cellular Therapy (SFGM-TC). Unrelated stem cell transplantation for severe acquired aplastic anemia: improved outcome in the era of high-resolution HLA matching between donor and recipient. Haematologica. 2007;92:589–96.

10. Viollier R, Socié G, Tichelli A, et al. Recent improvement in outcome of unrelated donor transplantation for aplastic anemia. Bone Marrow Transplant. 2008;41(1):45–50.

11. Bacigalupo A, Marsh JC. Unrelated donor search and unrelated donor transplantation in the adult aplastic anaemia patient aged 18–40 years without an HLA-identical sibling and failing immunosuppression. Bone Marrow Transplant. 2013;48(2):198–200.

12. Marsh JC, Gupta V, Lim Z, et al. Alemtuzumab with fludarabine and cyclophosphamide reduces chronic graft versus host disease after allogeneic stem cell transplantation for acquired aplastic anemia Blood. 2011;118(8):2351–7

13. Samarasinghe S, Steward C, Hiwarkar P, et al. Excellent outcome of matched unrelated donor transplantation in paediatric aplastic anaemia following failure with immunosuppressive therapy: a United Kingdom multicentre retrospective experience. Br J Haematol. 2012;157(3):339–46.

14. Eapen M, Rademacher JL, Antin JH, et al. Effect of stem cell source on outcomes after unrelated donor transplantation in severe aplastic anemia. Blood 2011;118:2618–21.

15. Deeg HJ, Amylon ID, Harris RE, et al. Marrow transplants from unrelated donors for patients with aplastic anemia: minimum effective dose of total body irradiation. Biol Blood Marrow Transplant. 2001;7:208–15.

16. Tolar J, Deeg HJ, Arai S, Horwitz M, et al. Fludarabine-based conditioning for marrow transplantation from unrelated donors in severe aplastic anemia: early results of a cyclophosphamide dose deescalation study show life-threatening adverse events at predefined cyclophosphamide dose levels. Biol Blood Marrow Transplant. 2012;18(7):1007–11.

17. Kojima S, Matsuyama T, Kato S, et al. Outcome of 154 patients with severe aplastic anemia who received transplants from unrelated donors: the Japan Marrow Donor Program. Blood. 2002;100:799–803.

18. Shimada A, Takahashi Y, Muramatsu H, et al. Excellent outcome of allogeneic bone marrow transplantation for Fanconi anemia using fludarabine-based reduced-intensity conditioning regimen. Int J Hematol. 2012;95(6):675–9.

19. Peffault de Latour R, Rocha V, Socié G. Cord blood transplantation in aplastic anemia. Bone Marrow Transplant. 2013;48(2):201–2.

20. Peffault de Latour R, Purtill D, Ruggeri, et al. Influence of nucleated cell dose on overall survival of unrelated cord blood transplantation for patients with severe acquired aplastic anemia: a study by Eurocord and the Aplastic Anemia Working Party of the European Group for Blood and Marrow Transplantation. Biol Blood Marrow Transplant. 2010;1:78–85.

21. Reisner Y, Hagin D, Martelli MF. Haploidentical hematopoietic

transplantation: current status and future perspectives. *Blood.* 2011;118(23):6006–17.

22. Luznik L, O'Donnell PV, Fuchs EJ. Post-transplantation cyclophosphamide for tolerance induction in HLA-haploidentical bone marrow transplantation. *Semin Oncol.* 2012;39(6):683–93.

23. Ciceri F , Lupo-Stanghellini MT, Korthof ET, on behalf of the SAA-WP EBMT. Haploidentical transplantation in patients with acquired aplastic anemia. *Bone Marrow Transplant.* 2012;48:183.

24. Clay J, Kulasekarara AG, Potter V, *et al.* Non-myeloablative peripheral blood haploidentical stem cell transplantation for refractory severe aplastic anemia. *Biol Blood Marrow Transplant.* 2014;20(11):1711–6.

25. Xu LP, Liu KY, Liu DH, *et al.* A novel protocol for haploidentical hematopoietic SCT without in vitro T-cell depletion in the treatment of severe acquired aplastic anemia. *Bone Marrow Transplant.* 2012;47(12):1507–12.

26. Peffault de Latour R, Schrezenmeier H, Bacigalupo A, *et al.* Allogeneic stem cell transplantation in paroxysmal nocturnal hemoglobinuria. *Haematologica.* 2012;97(11):1666–73.

Chapter 53

Hematopoietic Cell Transplants for Fanconi Anemia

Carlo Dufour and Maurizio Miano

Introduction

Fanconi Anemia (FA) is a rare autosomal recessive disease characterized by a defect on genes of the FA/BRCA pathway critical for the DNA repair, which results in physical abnormalities, cancer predisposition, and progressive bone marrow failure (BMF). Clinical phenotype can be very heterogeneous ranging from mild to very severe forms.

BMF usually occurs at a median of 7 years of age and is present in about 90% of patients by the age of 40 years. Improvement of hematopoiesis has been described and sometimes shown to be due to spontaneous genetic reversion also known as mosaicism. Haematological abnormalities also include a predisposition to develop clonal evolution to myelodysplasia (MDS) and/or acute leukemia[1], that mostly occurs during adolescence or young adulthood. In older ages, a higher incidence of solid cancer is reported.

Malformations may range from subtle ones like small facial dysmorphysms, skin café au lait spots and short stature to more evident and severe ones that involve upper limb, particularly thumb and radius deformities, kidney, heart, genitourinary tract, and skeleton. Noteworthy, the proportion of patients with minor or no somatic malformations may account to up 20% pointing to the fact that the lack of a striking malformation picture cannot exclude diagnosis of FA. The correct diagnosis of FA is crucial for treatment and follow-up.

In patients who lack typical physical stigmata of FA, BMF may be misdiagnosed as that of Acquired Aplastic Anemia (AA), would not be responsive to the immunosuppressive therapy, and also would not tolerate the conditioning regimen for AA. So far the golden standard for diagnosis of FA is the chromosomal fragility test (DEB or MMC) that needs to be carried out in all patients with marrow failure with and without malformations.

Hematopoietic Cell Transplantation
Conditioning Regimens: Concerns and Progress

Haematopoietic cell transplantation (HCT) represents the only proven treatment to restore normal hematopoiesis in patients with FA, although it cannot cure other clinical abnormalities and cancer predisposition. Over the last 2 decades tremendous improvements on HCT outcome have occurred due to the

better approaches to overcome disease-related toxicity in turn depending on the tissue fragility. In fact, FA patients are characterized by a high sensitivity to DNA alkylating agents and to irradiation which has been used for many years within the preparative regimens. For this reason, the first transplants resulted in a dismal outcome due to the severe, unexpected toxicities following the use of classical myeloablative conditioning regimen including total body irradiation (TBI) and high dose of Cyclophosphamide (Cy) as used in severe aplastic anemia (SAA)[2,3]. Results ameliorated over time thanks to the attenuation of preparative regimens that overcame excessive toxicities. These lighter regimens consisted of single doses of thoraco-abdominal irradiation (500 cGy) and low doses of Cy (20 mg/kg)[4]. Since 2000, the aim to reduce toxicity and the risk of late malignancies by eliminating irradiation has been pursued by the introduction of fludarabine (Flu)-based reduced intensity conditioning (RIC) that has resulted in a further improvement of the outcome of HCT.

Graft *versus* host disease (GvHD) represents another cause of morbidity and mortality after HCT and a generator of increased risk for late, post-transplant malignancies. FA patients are considered to be at a higher risk to develop GvHD due to their underlying DNA repair impairment and the higher tendency to cell apoptosis.

The results from the largest published study on about 800 FA transplanted patients in the period between 1972 to 2009 show an OS of 71% and 49% at 15 and 20 years, respectively[5]. However, a significant improvement of OS occurred in transplants performed after 2000, particularly in the HLA-matched unrelated donor (MUD) setting whose outcomes have significantly improved (3-year OS of 77% with Flu-based conditioning regimens) compared with the older studies (Figure 53.1).

What Is the "Ideal" Time for Allo-HCT in FA?

It has been shown that patients undergoing HCT before the onset of transfusion dependency and androgen treatments have a better outcome and so do those with no evidence of clonal evolution or leukemia[6]. Transplant should be performed prior to heavy transfusion load (studies indicate not to overcome the threshold of 20 red cells/platelets transfusion) to avoid immunization that may compromise engraftment.

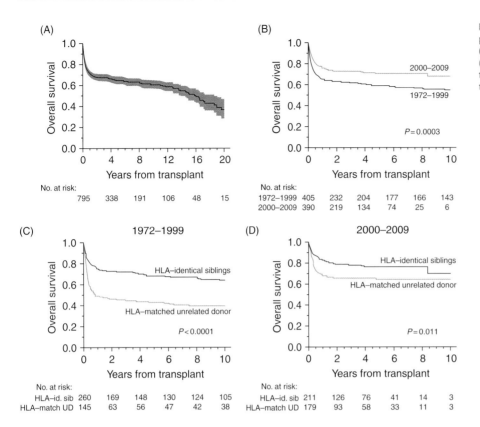

Figure 53.1 Survival of 795 FA transplanted patients in the period between 1972 and 2009 (71% and 49% at 15 and 20 years, respectively). (A) Overall survival. (B) Survival by year of transplant. (C–D) Survival by year and type of transplant. From reference [5].

Patients who had received a large number of transfusions should be evaluated for iron overload and appropriate chelating treatment should be established before HCT. Patients receiving androgen therapy should interrupt treatment at least one month before transplant and accurately be controlled for the presence of liver adenomas, which can represent a heavy complication after transplant[7].

Studies showed that patients transplanted prior to the age of 10 years have a better survival rate[8] and lower risk of late malignancies[5]. However, these studies did not compare patients who underwent HCT with those who did not. Interestingly, in a recent analysis which considered as time zero the moment in which the patient reaches hematological criteria currently recommended for transplant, the long-term survival rate was superior for nontransplanted patients (5-year cumulative risk of mortality of 11%) over transplanted ones (5-year cumulative mortality risk of 64% in HLA-MUD and of 33% in MFD HCTs) ($P=0.0029$)[9]. These differences are in part explained by the duration of the follow-up since earlier deaths occurred more in transplanted patients whereas later deaths occurred in nontransplanted ones. However, it is of note that FA patients eligible for HCT may become long-term survivors. This might be due to the improvement of supportive care for marrow failure and possibly to the occurrence of mosaicism.

For these reasons, age should be not considered "per se" as a stringent indication to the HCT unless associated to other criterion, thus pointing to the need of a single patient-based decision.

Practice Points

The search of a HLA-matched sibling or of an alternative donor should be performed at the moment of diagnosis in order to have him available when haematological criteria for transplant are reached. Patients should be followed up with regular blood counts and annual bone marrow evaluations in order to intercept the time at which persistent, moderate to severe pancytopenia, preferably still without cytogenetic abnormalities, develops. It has to be underlined that in a minority of cases pancytopenia can improve spontaneously returning to normal levels or may temporarily worsen due to infections. Timing should also be anticipated in case of signs of clonal evolution or postponed to enable treatments aimed to improve organ damage or severe infections. Patients carrying high-risk mutations for clonal evolution like those of FANCD2 should also be considered for an earlier transplant [10].

What Is the Best Donor and Graft Source for Transplant in FA?

The best results have been obtained following a HLA-matched sibling donor (MSD) transplant. However, FA patients, as affected from a genetic disease, have a lower chance of getting an available HLA-MSD since siblings themselves are at risk of having the same disorder. The development of other strategies for patients lacking a HLA-MSD has clearly improved results in the past 15 years. The possibility of finding a HLA-matched unrelated donor (MUD) has progressively increased due to the growing number of donors in the worldwide registries. Also, the improvements of the HLA typing contributed to amelioration of donor selection and consequently to the outcome. The same typing improvements apply to cord blood (CB) that represents an important source of cells in patients lacking a HLA matched donor. Recent advances in the management of haploidentical transplants are also giving promising results and may open the possibility to almost all patients of finding a donor in the future.

Bone marrow cells are considered the best graft source in the setting of FA patients whereas the use of peripheral blood hematopoietic cells (PBHC) has been proven to be associated with a higher incidence of GvHD[5] and for this reason should not be encouraged.

HLA-Matched Sibling Donor Transplant

Transplant from a HLA-MSD still represents the best choice for patients with FA. Hystorical data indicate survival rates above 80%[11]. These figures have been confirmed by the recent, largest retrospective study conducted by the SAAWP of the European Blood and Marrow Transplant (EBMT)[5] that shows an OS of about 82% (with Flu-based conditioning regimens). The use of irradiation in the MDS HCT setting has now been substantially abandoned, and most centers use Cy alone[10] or in association with Flu. This was based on the evidence that, as compared to irradiation containing regimens, nonirradiation ones did not show differences in OS (78% versus 81% respectively; p=ns), neutrophil recovery (94% versus 89%, respectively; p=ns), and GvHD (23% versus 21%, respectively; p=ns)[8]. In particular, in the largest single-center study, 43 patients who received Cy alone at the dose of 15mg/kg × 4 days showed an OS of 93%[12]. In a further evaluation of a total of 67 patients (including 9 who received HLA-related nonsibling donor HCT) this regimen showed a better OS (93% versus 73%) and short-term TRM (6% versus 9%) in patients aged <10 years versus the older ones (BONFIM CM, personal communication).

A conditioning regimen with lower doses of Cy (20–40mg/kg,) plus Flu (150–175mg/kg) with or without anti-thymocyte globulin (ATG) has also been adopted resulting in an OS of 80–100%, although follow-up was short[6,13,14].

Busulfan has also been used as an alternative option to irradiation in order to reduce toxicity following MSD transplant[15]. In the largest reported experience dose was 6mg/kg associated with low-dose Cy (40mg/kg). Sustained engraftment was 93% and toxicity consisted of mucositis >grade II (94%), CSA neuro-toxicity and cytomegalovirus (CMV) disease (11%), veno-occlusive disease (5%), and bronchiolitis obliterans (5%)[16].

HLA-Matched Unrelated Donor Transplant

HLA-MUD HCT represents the most accessible option for patients with FA lacking a HLA-MSD. However, before the last decade, the outcome of patients undergoing HCT was very poor compared to those transplanted from a HLA-MSD. The use of Flu in the conditioning regimen dramatically improved the outcome of these transplants. A large Center for International Blood and Marrow Transplant (CIBMTR) study comparing the outcome of 98 patients undergoing Flu-based regimens versus other non-Flu regimens showed far better results in terms of neutrophil engraftment (89% versus 69%; $P=0.02$) and OS (52% versus 13%; $P=0.001$) for the first population[17]. Further improvement has been obtained thanks to the attempt to reduce/avoid irradiation. A descalation TBI dose study showed 300cGy [18] as the lowest possible when used within a Flu/Cy-based conditioning regimen in the HLA-MUD HCT setting. Attempts to eliminate irradiation by increasing the dose of Cy have also been successfully performed. In a study of 49 patients conditioned with Flu 125mg/m^2, Cy 60mg/kg, and ATG 4mg/kg, OS was 81% for those who received 8/8 HLA-matched stem cells. In this respect the EBMT study[5] showed that radiation-free regimens provided a better (70%), although not significantly OS versus radiation containing regimens (67%). The same study shows in HLA-MUD HCTs a far better OS after Flu-based conditioning (77%) over Flu-free (57%; $P=0.008$) regimens. The association of "ex vivo" T-cell depletion to Flu-containing regimen also produced a significant better survival rate (78% versus 58%; $P=0.013$).

Although in some smaller studies with shorter follow-up [19,20] GvHD rate was lower, this complication still represents the most burning issue in the HLA-MUD HCT setting with an overall incidence in the EBMT study of 36% for acute and 12% for chronic GvHD. These figures are still higher than those seen in the MSD HCTs, particularly for acute GvHD (36% versus 19%)[5]. GvHD not only acts as a detrimental factor on the short-term quality of life of the survivors, but also works as one of the major determinants for the occurrence of late malignancies, as shown by its association with an over 4-fold increased risk of late tumors[5]. Overall, despite the remarkable improvements achieved during the last years, the outcome of HLA-MUD HCT, although very satisfactory, still has to be considered slightly inferior to that of HLA-MSD.

Cord Blood Transplant

The use of CB has been associated with a lower incidence of GvHD[21] and for this reason it may be considered as an attractive option in the setting of patients with a nonmalignant disease that do not benefit from GvL effect. However, the increased risk of graft failure due to the low number of cells is a limitation for adult patients. In a Eurocord Registry study of FA patients transplanted worldwide mostly from unrelated CD, Flu-based conditioning regimens provided a better neutrophil recovery (72% versus 42%; $P=0.02$) and OS (50% versus 25%; $P=0.01$) over conditioning without Flu. Therefore, also in the CB setting, Flu was found to be associated with a better outcome. A cell dose of >6×10^7

nuclear cells/kg at cryopreservation and $>5 \times 10^7$ NC/kg upon thawing correlated with a faster neutrophil recovery (70% *versus* 50%; $P=0.01$) and a longer survival rate (49% *versus* 31%; $P=0.04$)[22].

Halo-type matched Transplant

The first experiences of haploidentical transplants in FA have been published since 2000 and included patients who received a T-cell depleted (TCD) transplant after a Flu-based conditioning regimen[20,23–25]. Further experiences showed seven patients receiving haplo-grafts out of a larger series of FA with an estimated OS rate of 69%[26].

In the largest reported series, 12 patients received TCD peripheral stem cells following a Flu 30 mg/m^2 (4 days), Cy 300 mg/m^2 (4 days), and ATG 10 mg/kg (4 days) as a conditioning regimen. Haematopoietic recovery was obtained in all patients but two who needed an additional successful HCT from the other parent. This regimen was well tolerated with a rather low GvHD incidence (17%), an OS of 83%, but with an EFS of 67%.

TCD has been used in three FA patients who achieved complete donor chimerism following the administration of CD3+ negatively selected cells associated with Rituximab-based *in vivo* B-cell depletion[27]. A further approach of *in vivo* selective depletion of activated T cells has also been used in three patients by administering low doses of Cy on day +3. In these cases engraftment was obtained but was complicated by severe aGvDH and infections[28].

Clonal Evolution and Transplant

The risk of clonal evolution for patients affected with FA is very high, especially during and after adolescence[29]. The diagnosis of MDS in FA patients can be particularly challenging. In fact, although signs of MDS in FA patients are often related to chromosomal abnormalities, mostly 1q, 3q, 5q, or monosomy 7, it may also happen that marrow morphological signs of dysplasia do not necessarily correlate with a real clonal evolution. Amongst chromosomal abnormalities, aberrations of chromosome 3 and 7 seem to be more related to an increased risk of clonal evolution[30,31]. At variance from what has been reported in the past, the clones once established do not tend to disappear[32].

It appears difficult to define an approach for patients requiring transplant once transformation has already occurred. This is because the need for a more aggressive treatment has to be balanced with the increased risk of toxicity. The use of dose-adjusted Busulfan as part of the conditioning regimen, under investigation in an ongoing study, may contribute to this aim.

So far, different approaches have been proposed in the rare series of FA patients treated with overt MDS/AML. A report from the Cincinnati Group suggested that a Mini FLAG (fludarabine 30 mg/m^2, cytarabine 300 mg/m^2 days −2 to 4) pre-HCT was well tolerated[33]. A similar approach has been used by the St Louis Group that applied full conventional FLAG followed by allo-HCT with RIC regimen and TBI 200 cGy to six transformed FA patients who are all alive and with no clonal disease after a median follow-up of 30 months[34]. The Minneapolis Group encourages going directly to a TCD HCT, with a regimen including TBI 300 cGy with thymic shielding Cy 40 mg, Flu 140, ATG 150 mg/kg, TCD, cyclosporine with no previous cytoreduction[10,35]. The largest retrospective study on 113 transplanted patients with clonal transformation, some of whom received pre-HCT cytoreduction, showed survival probabilities of 64% and 55% at 1 and 5 years post-transplant, respectively. A better outcome was shown in patients with cytogenetic abnormalities (67%) *versus* those with MDS/AML (AML, 43%). Age <14 years was associated with better outcome (69% *versus* 39%) for patients with both MDS and AML.

On the whole, based on current evidence, the best approach looks to be performing the transplant before the onset of clonal evolution. To allow this, a strict monitoring of haematological parameters including bone marrow studies with cytogenetics is highly recommended in all FA patients but in a more strict fashion in those close to or in open marrow failure phase.

Risk of Late Malignancies and Transplant

Patients with FA have an estimated risk of malignancies between 48- to 500-fold higher than the normal population. Apart from MDS and leukemia, representing the clonal

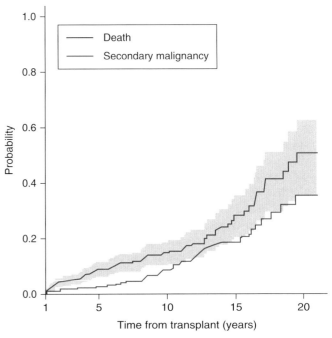

Figure 53.2. Cumulative incidence of deaths (blue) and secondary malignancies (red) in 1 year-survivor. From reference [5].

evolution consequent to bone marrow failure, patients are subject to a high incidence of solid tumors, in particular head and neck or anogenital squamous cell carcinomas (SCC).

The influence of HCT on secondary tumors, in an already "per se" high-risk population, has been evaluated in many studies. Patients undergoing HCT have a higher and earlier incidence of cancer compared with nontransplanted ones[36]. Approximately 40% of patients develop tumors 15 to 20 years after transplant. Head and neck SCC may occur earlier, about 8 years after HCT, and seems to be correlated to the TAI+Cy conditioning regimen and to the occurrence of GvHD[37].

In the recent EBMT study, age at transplant, prior cGvHD, use of PBHC, and the presence of clonal evolution at the time of transplant were shown to be associated with an increased risk of secondary malignancies. In the same study the curve of late malignancies over long-term follow-up paralleled that of deaths, pointing to these late events as one of the major determinants for death in the FA transplanted population (Figure 53.2).

Practice Point

Based on available evidence it is clear that future approaches should aim to reduce factors that increase the risk of malignancies such as irradiation in preparative regimen and GvHD. In this respect the well-established use of Flu might further show its beneficial effect and individualized dose of busulfan may prove to be a useful tool.

References

1. Kutler DI, Singh B, Satagopan J, et al. Auerbach AD A 20-year perspective on the International Fanconi Anemia Registry (IFAR). *Blood.* 2003;101(4):1249–56.

2. Berger R, Bernheim A, Gluckman E, Gisselbrecht C. In vitro effect of cyclophosphamide metabolites on chromosomes of Fanconi. anaemia patients. *Br J Haematol.* 1980;45, 565–8.

3. Gluckman E, Berger R, Dutreix J. Bone marrow transplantation for Fanconi anemia. *Sem Hematol.* 1984;21, 20–6.

4. Socié G, Devergie A, Girinski T, et al. Transplantation for Fanconi's anaemia: long-term follow-up of fifty patients transplanted from a sibling donor after low-dose cyclophosphamide and thoraco-abdominal irradiation for conditioning. *Br J Haematol.* 1998;103(1):249–55.

5. Peffault de Latour R, Porcher R, Dalle JH, et al; FA Committee of the Severe Aplastic Anemia Working Party; Pediatric Working Party of the European Group for Blood and Marrow Transplantation. Allogeneic hematopoietic stem cell transplantation in Fanconi anemia: the European Group for Blood and Marrow Transplantation experience. *Blood.* 2013;122(26):4279–86. doi:10.1182/blood-2013-01-479733. Epub 2013 Oct 21.

6. Ayas M, Saber W, Davies SM, et al. Allogeneic hematopoietic cell transplantation for fanconi anemia in patients with pretransplantation cytogenetic abnormalities, myelodysplastic syndrome, or acute leukemia. *J Clin Oncol.* 2013;31(13):1669–76. doi: 10.1200/JCO.2012.45.9719. Epub 2013 Apr 1.

7. Kumar AR, Wagner JE, Auerbach AD, et al. Fatal hemorrhage from androgen-related hepatic adenoma after hematopoietic cell transplantation. *J Pediatr Hematol/Oncol.* 2004;26:16–18.

8. Pasquini R, Carreras J, Pasquini MC, et al. HLA-matched sibling hematopoietic stem cell transplantation for fanconi anemia: comparison of irradiation and non irradiation containing conditioning regimens. *Biol Blood Marrow Transplant.* 2008;14(10):1141–7.

9. Svahn J, Onofrillo D, Cappelli E, et al. Long-term hematologic follow-up in Fanconi anemia and impact on survival in 97 patients in a national data base. The 26th Fanconi Anemia Research Fund Scientific Symposium, 18–21 Sept, 2014. Abstract, pp. 117–118.

10. MacMillan ML, Wagner JE. Haematopoietic cell transplantation for Fanconi anaemia – when and how? *Br J Haematol.* 2010;149(1):14–21. Review.

11. Dufour C, Rondelli R, Locatelli F, et al. Stem cell transplantation from HLA-matched related donor for Fanconi's anaemia: a retrospective review of the multicentric Italian experience on behalf of AIEOP-GITMO. *Br J Haematol.* 2001;112:796–805.

12. Bonfim CM, de Medeiros CR, Bitencourt MA, et al. HLA-matched related donor hematopoietic cell transplantation in 43 patients with Fanconi anemia conditioned with 60 mg/kg of cyclophosphamide. *Biol Blood Marrow Transplant.* 2007;13, 1455–60.

13. Locatelli F, Zecca M, Pession A, et al.; Italian Pediatric Group. The outcome of children with Fanconi anemia given hematopoietic stem cell transplantation and the influence of fludarabine in the conditioning regimen: a report from the Italian pediatric group. *Haematologica.* 2007;92(10):1381–8.

14. Tan PL, Wagner JE, Auerbach AD, Defor TE, Slungaard A, MacMillan ML. Successful engraftment without radiation after fludarabine-based regimen in Fanconi anemia patients undergoing genotypically identical donor hematopoietic cell transplantation. *Pediatr Blood Cancer.* 2006;46:630–6.

15. Ertem M, Ileri T, Azik F, Uysal Z, Gozdasoglu S. Related donor hematopoietic stem cell transplantation for Fanconi anemia without radiation: a single center experience in Turkey. *Pediatr Transplant.* 2009;13(1):88–95. doi: 10.1111/j.1399–3046.2008.00952.x. Epub 2008 Apr 22.

16. Torjemane L, Ladeb S, Ben Othman T, Abdelkefi A, Lakhal A, Ben Abdeladhim, A. Bone marrow transplantation from matched related donors for patients with Fanconi anemia using low dose busulfan and cyclophosphamide as conditioning. *Pediatr Blood Cancer.* 2006;46:496–500.

17. Wagner JE, Eapen M, MacMillan ML, et al. Unrelated donor bone marrow transplantation for the treatment of Fanconi anemia. *Blood.* 2007;109:2256–62.

18. MacMillan ML, Blazar Br, DeFor Te, Ma L, Tolar J, Zierhut H, Wagner E.

Alternate donor HCT for Fanconi Anemia (FA): results of a total body irradiation (TBI) dose de-escalation study. *Biol Blood Marrow Transplant.* 2009;15:2–4.

19. MacMillan ML, Hughes MR, Agarwal S, Daley GQ. Cellular therapy for Fanconi anemia: the past, present, and future. *Biol Blood Marrow Transplant.* 2011;17(1 Suppl):S109–14. doi: 10.1016/j.bbmt.2010.11.027. Review.

20. Chaudhury S, Auerbach AD, Kernan NA, *et al.* Fludarabine-based cytoreductive regimen and T-cell-depleted grafts from alternative donors for the treatment of high-risk patients with Fanconi anaemia. *Br J Haematol.* 2008;140(6):644–55. doi: 10.1111/j.1365–2141.2007.06975. Review.

21. Gluckman E, Rocha V, Boyer-Chammard A, *et al*; Eurocord Transplant Group and the European Blood and Marrow Transplantation Group. Outcome of cord-blood transplantation from related and unrelated donors. *N Engl J Med.* 1997;337(6):373–381.

22. Gluckman E, Rocha V, Ionescu I, Alternate donor HCT for Fanconi Anemia (FA): results of a total body irradiation (TBI) dose de-escalation study; Eurocord-Netcord and EBMT. Results of unrelated cord blood transplant in fanconi anemia patients: risk factor analysis for engraftment and survival. *Biol Blood Marrow Transplant.* 2007;13(9):1073–82. Epub 2007 Jul 20.

23. Motwani J, Lawson SE, Darbyshire PJ. Successful HSCT using nonradiotherapy-based conditioning regimens and alternative donors in patients with Fanconi anaemia – experience in a single UK centre. *Bone Marrow Transplant.* 2005;36:405–10. doi:10.1038/sj.bmt.1705071.

24. Yabe H, Inoue H, Matsumoto M, *et al.* Unmanipulated HLA-haploidentical bone marrow transplantation for the treatment of fatal, nonmalignant diseases in children and adolescents. *Int J Hematology.* 2004, 80(1):78–82.

25. Rihani R, Lataifeh I, Halalsheh H, *et al.* Haploidentical stem cell transplantation as a salvage therapy for cord blood engraftment failure in a patient with Fanconi anemia. *Pediatr Blood Cancer.* 2010;55:580–2. doi: 10.1002/pbc.22584.

26. Locatelli F, Zecca M, Pession A, *et al.* The outcome of children with Fanconi anemia given hematopoietic stem cell transplantation and the influence of fludarabine in the conditioning regimen: a report from the Italian Pediatric Group. *Haematologica.* 2007;92:1381–8. doi:10.3324/haematol.11436.

27. Dufort G, Pisano S, Incoronato A, *et al.* Feasibility and outcome of haploidentical SCT in pediatric high-risk hematologic malignancies and Fanconi anemia in Uruguay. *Bone Marrow Transplant.* 2012;47:663–8. doi:10.1038/bmt.2011.148; published online 18 July 2011.

28. Thakar MS, Bonfim C, Sandmaier BM, *et al.* Cyclophosphamide-based in vivo T-cell depletion for HLA-haploidentical transplantation in Fanconi anemia. *Pediatr Hematol Oncol.* 2012;29(6):568–78. doi: 10.3109/08880018.2012.708708. Epub 2012 Jul 27.

29. Butturini A, Gale RP, Verlander PC, *et al.* Hematologic abnormalities in Fanconi anemia: An International Fanconi Anemia Registry study. *Blood.* 1994;84:1650–5.

30. Tonnies H, Huber S, Kuhl JS, *et al.* Clonal chromosomal aberrations in bone marrow cells of Fanconi anemia patients: Gains of the chromosomal segment 3q26q29 as an adverse risk factor. *Blood.* 2003;101:3872–4.

31. Mehta PA, Harris RE, Davies SM, *et al.* Numerical chromosomal changes and risk of developmentof myelodysplastic syndrome: acute myeloid leukemia in patients with Fanconi anemia. *Cancer Genet Cytogenet.* 2010;203:180–6.

32. Cioc AM, Wagner JE, MacMillan ML, DeFor T, Hirsch B. Diagnosis of myelodysplastic syndrome among a cohort of 119 patients with fanconi anemia: morphologic and cytogenetic characteristics. *Am J Clin Pathol.* 2010;133(1):92–100.

33. Mehta PA, Ileri T, Harris RE, *et al* . Chemotherapy for myeloid malignancy in children with Fanconi anemia. *Pediatr Blood Cancer*, 48 (2007), pp. 668–672.

34. Talbot A, Peffault de Latour R, Buchbinder N, *et al.* Sequential treatment with chemotherapy and reduced-intensity conditioning for allogeneic hematopoietic stem cell transplantation in Fanconi anemia patients with acute myeloid leukemia or myelodysplastic syndrome. *Blood: ASH Annual Meeting Abstracts.* 2012;120: 2363.

35. Mitchell R, Wagner JE, Hirsch B, DeFor TE, Zierhut H, MacMillan ML. Haematopoietic cell transplantation for acute leukaemia and advanced myelodysplastic syndrome in Fanconi anaemia. *Br J Haematol.* 2014;164(3):384–95. doi: 10.1111/bjh.12634. Epub 2013 Oct 30.

36. Rosenberg PS, Socié G, Alter BP, Gluckman E. Risk of head and neck squamous cell cancer and death in patients with Fanconi anemia who did and did not receive transplants. *Blood.* 2005;105(1):67–73. Epub 2004 Aug 26.

37. Curtis RE, Metayer C, Rizzo JD, *et al.* Impact of chronic GVHD therapy on the development of squamous-cell cancers after hematopoietic stem-cell transplantation: an international case-control study. *Blood.* 2005;105(10):3802–11. Epub 2005 Feb 1.

Chapter 54

Allogeneic Hematopoietic Cell Transplants for Thalassemia

Javid Gaziev and Guido Lucarelli

Introduction

Thalassemias are the most common inherited single-gene disorders in the world with the highest prevalence in areas where malaria was endemic. Currently, it poses a major public health concern not only in countries where thalassemia is endemic but also in countries where the disease was not common due to migration. The β-thalassemia is caused by more than 200 point mutations in the β-globin gene with either absent or reduced beta chain production, which leads to the development of hemolytic anemia[1]. The most severe form of disease is characterized by the complete absence of β-globin production and results from the inheritance of two β^0 thalassemia alleles, homozygous or compound heterozygous states. These combinations usually result in β-thalassemia major and the patients present within 6 months of life with severe anemia, and if not treated with blood transfusions, die within a few years. The current conventional treatment of β-thalassemia major consists of lifelong regular blood transfusions combined with iron chelation therapy. Advances in transfusion practices and chelation therapy have improved the life expectancy in β-thalassemia major. However, patients continue to develop debilitating chronic disease and treatment-related complications, particularly in adulthood, that lead to morbidity and premature mortality[2,3]. Allogeneic hematopoietic cell transplant (allo-HCT) for patients with thalassemia is a curative therapeutic option that enables patients to resume their normal lives[4–6]. It should be acknowledged that the acute toxicities of allo-HCT are challenged by the observation that in high-income countries where patients with thalassemia are well served by medical treatment they could have a better survival rate. However, these same patients with increasing age currently experience poor outcome on conventional treatment, even in well-resourced countries with universal access to good medical treatment[2,3].

Allogeneic Hematopoietic Cell Transplant for β-Thalassemia Major

Historical Perspective

The first two bone marrow transplantations for β-thalassemia major from HLA-matched sibling donors were simultaneously performed in December 1981, in Seattle, USA and in Pesaro, Italy. The patient transplanted in Seattle was a 14-month-old untransfused child who had successful engraftment and was cured from thalassemia. Restricting transplants to untransfused patients was impracticable and the Pesaro team performed the transplant in a 16-year-old patient who had received 150 RBC transfusions. This patient rejected the allograft and was the first of an extensive series of transplants for thalassemia performed at a single center.

Pretransplant Conditioning Regimen: Does One Size Fits All?

Patients with thalassemia have some disease and treatment-related characteristics that must be considered before transplantation. The disease is characterized by extreme marrow hyperplasia with aggressive extension of a rapidly proliferating erythroid lineage into intra- and extramedullary areas not usually occupied by marrow. This results in major bone remodeling together with marked hepatomegaly and splenomegaly. It might be hypothesized that this large mass of rapidly proliferating hematopoietic tissue would be more difficult to eradicate than normal hematopoietic tissue. Another consideration is that thalassemia patients are exposed to chronic blood transfusions which increase the likelihood of immunization to minor histocompatibility antigens leading to increased risk of rejection. Therefore, pretransplant preparation of these patients must be sufficiently myeloablative and immunosuppressive to overcome these barriers and ensure sustained engraftment. Total body irradiation (TBI) can satisfy both these objectives; however, there are many reasons, such as the known growth-retarding effects of TBI in young children and the increased risk of secondary malignancies, to avoid its use especially in very young patients with potential for a long life span. There is a considerable body of experience with the use of busulfan (Bu) in ablating marrow in patients undergoing allo-HCT for the treatment of nonmalignant conditions. Cyclophosphamide (Cy) is an agent that is well established as providing immunosuppression adequate for allogeneic hematopoietic engraftment of patients with aplastic anemia. Experimental data and clinical experience in the use of chemotherapy-only transplant regimens for the treatment of malignant diseases[7,8] have been pivotal in developing regimens appropriate for the treatment of thalassemia for transplantation using a combination of Bu and Cy, which can eradicate the thalassemia and facilitate sustained allogeneic hematopoietic engraftment. High-dose Bu combined with Cy is the preferred preparatory regimen for patients with thalassemia and is a valid alternative to regimens that include total body irradiation. Busulfan pharmacokinetic (PK) variability following oral administration is well documented in both adult and especially in pediatric patients. Therefore therapeutic drug monitoring of Bu with targeted area under the concentration-*versus*-time (AUC) curve is recommended because of the relationship between systemic exposure to the drug and both toxicity and success of treatment[9,10]. The recently developed intravenous formulation of Bu showed good tolerability, less toxicity profile, and high inter-and intrapatient pharmacokinetics consistency, allowing for predictable systemic exposure without PK monitoring[11]. Our experience with intravenous Bu in thalassemia for the first time showed that the first-dose Bu clearance is significantly higher than subsequent daily doses, which remains unchanged during the following days [12]. The differences in Bu clearance after the first dose and subsequent daily doses allowed us to adapt a new dose adjustment strategy targeting the lower end of the AUC range (900–1350 µmol/min), which successfully avoided unnecessary dose increases during subsequent days.

In an attempt to reduce transplant-related toxicity, reduced toxicity/intensity conditioning regimens have been developed. Treosulfan/fludarabine/thiotepa-based conditioning has been used in patients with thalassemia with discordant results [13–15]. In a recent study sequential use of pretransplant immunosuppression with 1–2 cycles of fludarabine (Flu) and dexamethasone followed by reduced toxicity conditioning with fludarabine, busulfan, and antithymoglobulin (ATG) in 18 patients with high risk resulted in OS and thalassemia-free survival (TFS) of 89%[16]. All patients received hydroxyurea for at least 3 months before starting preparation.

A Risk Class-Based Approach to Allo-HCT in β-Thalassemia Major

Analysis of transplant outcomes in a group of 167 β-thalassemia major patients aged less than 17 years who were treated with the same conditioning regimen revealed three negative prognostic factors such as hepatomegaly >2cm, portal fibrosis, and irregular chelation history for survival[17,18]. Class 1 patients have none of these risk factors, class 2 patients have one or two risk factors, and class 3 patients have all three risk factors (Table 54.1). Chelation history was defined as regular when desferoxamine therapy was initiated no later than 18 months after the first transfusion and administered subcutaneously for 8–10 hours continuously for at least 5 days each week and any deviation from this regimen was considered as irregular. Definition of risk classes allowed us to adopt treatment protocols tailored to the patient clinical conditions associated with quality of previous conventional treatment.

Table 54.1 Risk factors and risk classes

	Risk factors		
	Hepatomegaly >2 cm	Liver fibrosis	Chelation history[a]
Class 1	No	No	Regular
Class 2	No/Yes	No/Yes	Regular/irregular
Class 3	Yes	Yes	Irregular

[a] Chelation history was defined as regular when desferoxamine therapy was initiated no later than 18 months after the first transfusion and administered subcutaneously for 8–10 h continuously for at least 5 days each week and any deviation from this regimen was considered as irregular.

The prognostic significance of this risk class classification was confirmed by transplant centers outside Pesaro.

Early Experience (1982–2002)
Class 1 and Class 2 Risk Groups

Class 1 and class 2 young patients (<17 years of age) were treated with Bu 14mg/kg and Cy 200mg/kg as conditioning regimen, and they received graft-*versus*-host disease (GvHD) prophylaxis with cyclosporine (CsA) and low-dose methylprednisolone. The probability of thalassemia-free survival (TFS) in class 1 (n=124) and class 2 (n=297) patients treated between 1985 and 1992 was 91% and 84%, respectively[19].

Class 3 Group

Before the risk class adopted approach, class 3 younger patients (age <17 years) treated with Bu 14mg/kg and Cy 200mg/kg had a low probability of TFS (53%) and a higher probability of treatment-related mortality (TRM) (39%) mainly due to drug-related toxicity[20]. In an attempt to reduce high TRM the dose of Cy was reduced to 160–120mg/kg in the conditioning regimen for class 3 patients. Although OS was improved from 53% to 79% TFS was not changed due to increased rejection probability from 7% to 30%. This experience clearly showed the important role of Cy in promoting hematopoietic engraftment. A new approach aimed at decreasing the higher rejection rate through reducing erythroid expansion and increasing immunosuppression over time to avoid an unacceptable peritransplant drug toxicity in class 3 patients was then undertaken (April 1997). This novel approach included an intensified pretransplant preparation with 3mg/kg of azathioprine and 30mg/kg hydroxyurea daily from day −45 from the allo-HCT, Flu at the dose of 20mg/m² from day −17 through day −13, followed by conditioning regimen with Bu 14mg/kg and Cy 160mg/kg. GvHD prophylaxis consisted of CSA, low-dose methylprednisolone, and a modified "short course" of methotrexate (Protocol 26). Preliminary results were very encouraging with improved TFS from 58% to 85%, and reduced rejection probability from 30% to 8% as compared with previous preparative regimens

[21]. However, updated results from 38 class 3 patients treated with this new approach showed the probabilities of OS, TFS, rejection, and TRM of 94%, 80%, 14%, and 7%, respectively indicating that rejection, although decreased, still remains high in these patients[22].

Allo-HCT in Young Adult with β-Thalassemia Major: Outcomes

Adult patients (age >17 years old) have more advanced disease and treatment-related organ damage mainly due to prolonged exposure to iron overload and/or hepatitis C. Consequently, most adult patients belong to class 3 of risk. One hundred and seven adult patients with median age of 20 years (range 17–35 years) were given transplants from HLA-identical siblings[23]. There were 18 class 2 patients treated with Bu 14 mg/kg and Cy 200 mg/kg, and 89 class 3 patients treated with Bu 14–16 mg/kg and Cy 120–160 mg/kg as preparatory regimen. TFS in adults was not optimal (62%) due to unacceptably high TRM (37%). Interestingly despite a reduced dose of Cy the probability of rejection in adults was low (4%), suggesting that donor–host tolerance might be induced even among extensively transfused patients. This was an unexpected observation indicating that adult patients could benefit from less-intensive conditioning regimens with reduced transplant-related toxicity. Therefore, we subsequently reduced the dose of Cy to 90 mg/kg total dose in the conditioning regimen for adults and decided to apply the preconditioning phase preparation of the Protocol 26 to them. A recent analysis of 15 "high-risk" for transplantation adult patients treated with this regimen showed probabilities of OS, TFS, rejection, and TRM of 65%, 65%, 7%, and 28%, respectively[24].

Current Experience (2004–2015)

In 2004 some members of the Pesaro team including the authors of this chapter moved to Rome to establish a new transplant program at the International Center for Transplantation in Thalassemia and Sickle Cell Anemia of the Mediterranean Institute of Hematology. The patient population treated in Rome was different from that treated in Pesaro: patients were ethnically very heterogeneous, and the vast majority were immunized to minor histocompatibility antigens due to their repeated red blood cell transfusions mainly without the use of leukodepletion filters, which is known to be a factor contributing to graft rejection. Taking these into consideration, we have modified treatment protocols for transplantation. Between June 2004 and June 2015 29 class 1 patients with median age of 3 years (range 2–5 years), and 37 class 2 patients with median age of 6 years (range 2–16 years) were treated at our Institute. The OS, TFS, rejection, and TRM for class 1 and class 2 patients were 93% (95% CI 74–98%), 90% (95% CI 73–97%), 3% (95% CI 0–16%), 7% (95% CI 0–8%) and 94% (95% CI 80–98%), 89% (95% CI 74–95%), 5% (95% CI 74–95%), 6% (95% CI 0–7%), respectively (Figure 54.1 and

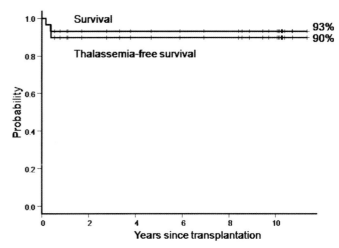

Figure 54.1 Overall survival and thalassemia-free survival in 29 class 1 patients treated with BuCy ± thiotepa.

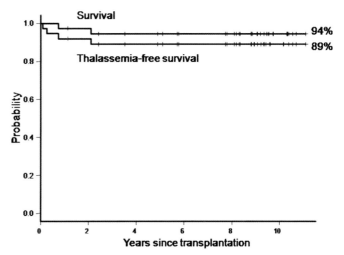

Figure 54.2 Overall survival and thalassemia-free survival in 37 class 2 patients treated with BuCy ± thiotepa.

54.2). Among 26 class 3 risk group patients with median age of 12 years (range 5–16 years) and treated with Protocol 26 between June 2004 and February 2007, the probability of OS, TFS, rejection, and TRM was 85% (95% CI 44–94%), 73% (95% CI 51–86%), 15%(95% CI 5–32%), and 15% (95% CI 0–28%), respectively (Figure 54.3)[25]. Therefore, in February 2007 we modified this treatment protocol increasing the dose of fludarabine from 20 mg/m^2 to 30 mg/m^2 during the preconditioning phase and added thiotepa 10 mg/kg/day to the conditioning regimen to further decrease rejection in these patients. Since then we have been using modified Protocol 26 for class 3 patients aged <18 years old. Between February 2007 and June 2015, we treated 42 class 3 patients with median age of 9.8 years (range 5.9–16.6 years) with this protocol. The 5-year probabilities of thalassemia-free survival were 93% with modified protocol and 73% with original protocol (P=0.032). The respective probabilities of overall survival were 93% and 85% (P=0.37). Modified treatment protocol effectively and

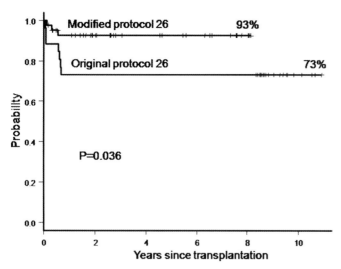

Figure 54.3 Thalassemia-free survival in class 3 patients treated with original Protocol 26 or modified Protocol 26.

safely prevented graft rejection and significantly improved thalassemia-free survival of class 3 patients. Importantly, the treatment intensification was not associated with increased nonhematological toxicity, even though these patients suffer from pre-existing organ damage due to iron overload and/or hepatitis. This treatment protocol makes allogeneic BMT accessible to all class 3 younger patients with results equal to class 1 or class 2 patients with thalassemia [25].

Updates on Global Experience of Allo-HCT for β-Thalassemia Major

Currently bone marrow transplant programs for thalassemia have been established in several countries worldwide. Transplant outcomes in class 1 and class 2 patients are excellent and are similar to those obtained in Pesaro[26–36]. However, results of transplantation in class 3 patients are not optimal due to high rejection rates and/or TRM especially in patients treated with standard BuCy±ATG conditioning regimens (Table 54.2).

Alternative Donors and Limitations
Allo-HCT from Alternative Related Donors

Allogeneic HCT is often limited by a lack of suitable donors. Approximately 70% of patients lack a suitable sibling donor. For these patients, alternative related or unrelated donors can be found, but many countries lack appropriate registries and the high cost of a search can make it practically impossible to find an unrelated donor. Thus, patients without a matched sibling donor could benefit from a related HLA-phenotypically matched or one-antigen mismatched donor. Historically, the use of related alternative donors (either phenotypically identical or one-antigen mismatched donors) has been associated with high engraftment failure, severe

GvHD, and low disease-free survival in cases of hematologic malignancies or aplastic anemia[37]. In 2000, our group published a study examining alternative related unmanipulated bone marrow transplantation for thalassemia, and we reported high rates of graft failure and GvHD, and low disease-free survival rates[38]. The results of this study clearly showed that the conditioning regimens used were not adequately myeloablative and immunosuppressive to ensure a high sustained engraftment rate, prevent severe GvHD, and promote a high thalassemia-free survival probability. Therefore, we adopted a new intensified treatment protocol for alternative donor transplantation in thalassemia. This protocol was initially designed for second transplants[39] but the very encouraging results led us to also apply it in patients receiving transplants from donors who are not HLA-matched siblings. Sixteen thalassemia patients with median age of 9.6 years (range, 1.4–24 years) who received BMT from phenotypically HLA-identical (n=11) or one-antigen mismatched relatives (n=5) were treated according to this new protocol[40]. All patients had sustained engraftment. One patient died due to chronic GvHD-related causes. The probability of OS, TFS, and TRM was 94% (95% CI 63–99%), 94% (95% CI 63–99%), and 6% (95% CI 1–26%), respectively. Importantly, the use of phenotypically matched or 1-antigen mismatched related donors resulted in outcomes similar to the use of matched sibling donor grafts providing that patients are treated with this treatment protocol. These data support the use of related HLA-phenotypically matched or one-antigen mismatched donors as an acceptable alternative to matched unrelated donors in patients with thalassemia.

HLA Haplotype Mismatch Family Donors

An HLA-haplotype mismatch transplant program for thalassemia was started in 2002 when the authors of this chapter were working in Pesaro. Patients who lacked either HLA-matched family or unrelated donor were eligible for this study. Between 2002 and 2008 22 patients with thalassemia major (median age of 7 years; range 3–14 years) were given grafts from their mothers (n=20) or brothers (n=2). Patients received preconditioning preparation with 3 mg/kg of azathioprine and 60 mg/kg hydroxyurea daily from day –59 from the transplant, and Flu 30 mg/m² from day –17 through day –13. Conditioning regimen consisted of Bu14Thiotepa10Cy200 and ATG. All patients received cyclosporine for GvHD prophylaxis for the first 2 months after transplantation. Eight patients received T-cell depleted peripheral blood grafts (CD34+ immunoselection) and CD3+/CD19+-depleted bone marrow, and 14 patients received CD34+ selected peripheral blood and bone marrow hematopoietic cells using the CliniMACS system. Median infused cell doses were CD34+ 15.2×10⁶/kg, CD3+ 1.8×10⁵/kg, and CD19+ 0.27×10⁶/kg in the first eight patients and CD34+14.2×10⁶/kg, CD3+ 2×10⁵/kg, and CD19+ 0.19×10⁶/kg in the last 14 patients. Overall,

Table 54.2 Recent transplant outcomes reported after HLA-matched sibling allografts for thalassemia

	Patients	Risk class (patients)	Conditioning	Stem cells source	OS, %	TFS, %	Rejection,%	TRM,%	Comments
Lawson et al.[26]	55	1 (17) 2 (27) 3 (11)	BuCy±Campath or ALG ±Fludarabine	BM	94.5	81.8	13.2	5.4	Decreased rejection with Campath, ALG, or Fludarabine
DiBartolomeo et al.[27]	115	No class categorization	Bu16Cy200	BM	89.2	85.7	6.7	8.7	Long-term results
Ghavamzadeh et al.[28]	183	1 (88) 2 (95)	Bu16Cy200	BM (96), PB (87)	BM: 89 PB: 83	BM: 76 PB: 76	BM: 9 PB: 18	BM: 9 PB: 14	High chronic GvHD rate with PB graft
Irfan et al.[29]	56	1 (20) 2 (20) 3 (16)	Bu14Cy200 ±ALG Protocol 26	BM (29), PB (27)	BM: 73 PB: 65	BM: 67 PB: 55	Class 2: 10 Class 3: 25	31	Low OS and TFS rates High rejection rate
Chiesa et al.[30]	53	1 (2) 2 (26) 3 (25)	i.v. BuCy200±TT Class 3 i.v. BuCy160 ±ATG	BM	Class 1–2: 96 Class 3: 96	Class 1–2: 91 Class 3: 66	Class 3: 34	4	High graft rejection rate in class 3 patients
Gaziev et al.[12]	68	1 (6) 2 (23) 3 (39)	i.v. BuCy200±TT Class 3 i.v. BuCy160±TT	BM	91	87	5.8	3	Targeted Bu was associated with low TRM and high TFS
Iravani et al.[31]	52	3	Bu16Cy160	BM (32) PB (20)	BM: 81 PB: 80	BM: 65 PB: 65	BM: 22 PB: 15	BM: 19 PB: 14	High chronic GvHD rate with PB graft
Sabloff et al.[32]	179	2 (75) 3 (64)	BuCy in 77 BuCyATG in 102	BM	Class 2: 91 Class 3: 64	Class 2: 88 Class 3: 62	Class 2: 6 Class 3: 12	Class 2: 6 Class 3: 6	High TRM in patients >7 years & hepatomegaly
Yesilipek et al.[33]	245	1 (41) 2 (130) 3 (63)	BuCy ± TG BuCyTT Protocol 26	BM (88), PB (137), CB (20)	82.9 89.1 76.1	80.5 67.8 62.2	17%	9.75 7.69 6.35	High chronic GvHD rate with PBHC High rejection rate
Goussetis et al.[34]	75	1 (16) 2 (38) 3 (17)	BuCyATG BuCyFluATG	BM±CB (73), PB (2)	100 97 94	94 97 88	5.8 0 5.8	4	ATG use improved transplant outcomes
Galambrun et al.[35]	108	All classes	BuCy200 BuFlu ±TT±ATG	BM (96), PB/CB (11)	86.8	69.4	23.4	12	ATG use significantly improved TFS
Hussein et al.[36]	44	1 (7) 2 (24) 3 (13)	Bu16cy200ATG Bu8FluTLIATG	BM	97.8	86.4	11.4	2.3	High rejection rate (23%) in class 3 with reduced intensity
Mathews et al.[15]	50	3	Treo-TT-Flu	BM (13), PB (37)	BM: 63,6 PB: 87.4	BM: 57.3 PB: 78.8	8	12	Improved transplant outcomes
Choudhary et al.[14]	28	2 (7) 3 (21)	Treo-TT-Flu	BM, PB± CB	78.5	71.4	7	21.4	High TRM. Three fatal SOS

Abbreviations: ALG = antilymphocyte globulin; ATG = antithymocyte globulin; BM = bone marrow; PB = peripheral blood; Treo = treosulfan, TT = thiotepa; Flu = fludarabine; TLI = total lymphoid irradiation; Protocol 26 = Bu14Cy160 preceded by azathioprine, hydroxyurea, and fludarabine; SOS = sinusoidal obstructive syndrome .

six patients had rejected their grafts, two patients died from EBV-related cerebral lymphoma or CMV-related pneumonia, and 14 patients are alive and cured from thalassemia. The probability of OS, TFS, rejection, and TRM was 90%, 61%, 29%, and 14%, respectively[41]. Although a pediatric patient population, immune reconstitution, especially CD4+ cell recovery, was delayed in these patients. These data showed the feasibility of haploidentical stem cell transplantation for patients with thalassemia and, therefore, should be considered for those younger patients who lack either a suitable related or unrelated donor.

Cord Blood Transplants from Related or Unrelated Donors

A recent study from the Eurocord cooperative group reported the outcomes of related cord blood transplantation on 33 patients with class 1 or class 2 thalassemia, and 11 with sickle cell disease[42]. As conditioning regimen most patients received BuCy or BuFlu and ATG. Thiotepa was added to BuCy or BuFlu in 17 patients. The incidence of rejection was high (21%), although no patient died from transplant-related complications. Few patients have experienced either acute (11%) or chronic (6%) GvHD, which is encouraging. The 2-year event-free survival was 79%, which is not excellent considering that patients were in a low/intermediate-risk group. An increased risk of graft failure after cord blood transplantation compared with patients given bone marrow transplants has already been reported. One log fewer cell dose in cord blood grafts, which is a well-known disadvantage, probably has a negative influence on sustained engraftment in recipients with nonmalignant diseases. Recently the outcome of transplants in 13 children with hemoglobinopathies after the co-infusion of cord blood and bone marrow from sibling donors has been reported[43]. Patients who received a co-transplant had low incidence of grade ≥2 acute (0% *versus* 26.3%) and chronic (0% *versus* 21%) GvHD compared to patients given BMT. The 5-year probability of EFS was 100% in the co-transplant group, 90% after BMT, and 86% after cord blood transplantation. Although interesting, these data should be interpreted with caution given the very small sample size.

Encouraging results of sibling cord blood transplantation for children with nonmalignant diseases including thalassemia and accumulating experience of successful application of unrelated HLA-mismatched cord blood in hematologic malignancies have allowed unrelated cord blood transplantation to be applied in patients with thalassemia. Recently, the outcome of unrelated cord blood transplantation for 45 patients with nonmalignant diseases with median age of 4.5 years (range 0.1–16.2 years) has been reported[44]. Cord blood units were 4/6 or higher HLA-matched on antigen level for HLA-A and -B, and allele-level for HLA-DRB1. There were 32 transfusion-dependent thalassemia patients with 21 class 1 and 9 class 2 characteristics. Conditioning regimen of these patients consisted of BuCy. Five patients (16%) had graft failure and all five

had sustained engraftment following second transplantation. Although there was a high incidence of grade II–IV and grade III–IV acute GvHD (76% and 42%, respectively), only one patient experienced extensive chronic GvHD. However, in a recent Eurocord/CIBMTR/New York Blood Center study researchers evaluated the outcome of 51 patients with thalassemia (n=35, median age 4 years) and sickle cell disease (n=16, median age 6 years) treated with unrelated cord blood[45]. Seven patients received 6/6 matched (HLA-A, -B antigen, and DRB1 allele levels), 18 patients 5/6 matched, 25 patients 4/6 matched, and 1 patient 3/6 matched cord blood grafts following myeloablative (n=39) or reduced intensity (n=12) conditioning regimens. Most patients were also given ATG or alemtuzumab before allo-HCT. Overall and disease-free survival for patients with thalassemia and sickle cell disease were 50% and 21%, and 94% and 62%, respectively. A reduced intensity conditioning regimen (Flu 150 mg/m^2, melphalan 140 mg/m^2, and alemtuzumab 60 mg for patients weighing >30 kg and 0.9 mg/kg for those weighing <30 kg) has been utilized in six patients with hemoglobinopathies (four patients with sickle cell disease and two patients with thalassemia) who received allele- or antigen-mismatched unrelated cord blood transplantation. Patients were also given third-party mesenchymal stromal cells in an attempt to promote engraftment[46]. This study was prematurely closed due to the lack of improved engraftment and unacceptably high transplant related mortality. Better transplant outcomes have been observed following a novel reduced intensity conditioning regimen which included hydroxyurea, distal alemtuzumab, fludarabine, melphalan, and thiotepa in 22 patients with non-malignant diseases (including four patients with thalassemia major) who received unrelated cord blood transplantation[47]. Most cord blood units were HLA-mismatched with median infused total nucleated cell dose of 7.9×10^7/kg. One-year overall and event-free survival were 77.3% and 68.2%, respectively. This study showed the importance of pretransplant cytoreduction and increased myeloablative potential of conditioning regimen by adding thiotepa in promoting engraftment in this setting.

Allo-HCT from Unrelated Donors

Results of allo-HCT from unrelated donors for the treatment of hematologic diseases have improved steadily, mainly due to the introduction of high-resolution molecular techniques for histocompatibility testing and improvements in the management of post-transplant complications. In a recent study the outcome of BMT from HLA-matched unrelated donors prospectively selected using high-resolution molecular typing for HLA class I and class II loci for 68 patients with thalassemia major who received BuCy or Bu-Flu and/or thiotepa as conditioning regimen has been reported[48]. The OS, TFS, rejection, and TRM for the entire cohort of patients was 79.3%, 65.8%, 14.4%, and 20.7% respectively. The incidence of acute grade II–IV or grade III–IV GvHD was 40% and 17%, respectively.

Ten out of 56 evaluable patients (18%) developed chronic GvHD. Class 1 and class 2 patients had much better overall and disease-free survival (96.7% and 80%, respectively) than class 3 patients (65.5% and 54.5%, respectively). Similar results have been reported from China. Fifty-two patients with thalassemia major were treated with unrelated PB grafts following intravenous Bu, Cy, Flu, and thiotepa[49]. Three-year OS and TFS were 92.3% and 90.4%, respectively. Adult patients treated with unrelated BMT had high TRM (30%), and inferior TFS (70%)[50]. Provided that selection of the donor is based on stringent criteria of HLA compatibility and that individuals have limited organ damage from iron overload, the results of unrelated BMT are comparable to those obtained when the donor is an HLA-matched sibling. The main limitation of the experience with unrelated BMT for thalassemia is that, using stringent criteria of HLA-matching, only about one-third of thalassemia patients who started the search found a suitable donor in a median time of 3–4 months. Using less-stringent criteria of HLA-matching for donor selection with one or two allelic disparity could increase the donor pool, but the results of such transplants remain to be determined.

Mixed Chimerism Following Allo-HCT: What Does This Imply in Thalassemia Transplants?

Up to one-third of patients with thalassemia have mixed hematopoietic chimerism (MC) at 2 months and approximately 10% of these patients will become persistent chimeras at 2 years after transplantation[19]. Patients with persistent MC are transfusion independent, suggesting that low levels of engrafted donor cells are able to cure disease phenotype. The level of residual host hematopoietic cells (RHCs) determined at 2 months after transplant was predictive for graft rejection with nearly all patients experiencing graft rejection when RHCs exceeded 25%, and only 13% of patients showing rejection when RHCs were less than 10%. The risk of rejection for patients who had RHCs between 10% and 25% was 41% [51]. These data indicate that unlike hematologic malignancies where residual host cells are predictive of relapse, patients with thalassemia could have lifelong stable MC without rejection following allo-HCT. These observations could be useful for developing gene therapy in patients with thalassemia.

Focus on Transplant-Related Complications

Graft Failure or Rejection

Unlike hematologic malignancies, patients with thalassemia have a substantial incidence of graft rejection after most myeloablative preparatory regimens, and this seems to be related to the stage of disease at the time of transplant. In fact, the probability of graft rejection is low in class 1 patients (3%), whereas the rates are in the ranges of 12% to 34% in the class 3 risk group[15,29,32,36]. Patients with engraftment failure and without functioning marrow have a bleak prospect because an early second transplant with a second course of

conditioning is usually not a reasonable option. Patients who reject their grafts (and have a return of host hematopoiesis) do not have an urgent need for second transplants, and such interventions can be delayed until the toxic effects of the conditioning regimen for the first transplants have been ameliorated. At least a year should be allowed to elapse between the first and second transplant. Our historical experience with second transplants showed a low thalassemia-free survival rate and high rejection probability. In 2003 we devised a new treatment protocol for 2nd allo-HCT aimed at reducing a high graft rejection rate and increasing DFS. Sixteen patients with a median age of 9 years (range 4–20 years) underwent 2nd transplant following allograft rejection using either bone marrow or peripheral blood graft[39]. All but two patients received allografts from the same donor. The sustained engraftment rate was high (94%) with only one patient having graft failure. The probability of OS, TFS, graft failure, and TRM were 79%, 79%, 6%, and 16%, respectively. This treatment protocol for 2nd allo-HCT in patients with thalassemia recurrence from the same donor is highly effective in terms of sustained engraftment and DFS.

Graft-*versus*-Host Disease

Graft-*versus*-host disease is one of the principal causes of morbidity and mortality after allo-HCT. In a recent prospective study we have evaluated GvHD in children who underwent BMT for thalassemia. All patients were given CSA, methylprednisolone, and a modified short course of Mtx (Cy or Mtx on day +1, and Mtx on days +3 and +6) as GvHD prophylaxis. The incidence of grade II–IV and III–IV acute GvHD was 35% and 9%, respectively. In multivariate analysis, high CD3+ (HR 4.6; 95% CI 1.4–14.7; $P=0.010$) and CD34+ (HR 4.3; 95% CI 1.4–12.7; $P=0.011$) cell doses in the graft were associated with grade II–IV aGvHD. Cumulative incidence of extensive chronic GvHD was 10%[52]. The incidence of chronic GvHD was significantly higher (20–48%) in patients given peripheral blood compared with bone marrow (18–19%) grafts[28,31,33]. These data indicate that the use of grafts from peripheral blood should be avoided in patients with thalassemia.

Ex-thalassemic after Successful Allo-HCT: What Still Needs to Be Monitored?

Thalassemia patients after successful BMT we called "ex-thalassemic". Most ex-thalassemics still carry the clinical sequelae of iron overload including cardiac, hepatic, and endocrine dysfunction. Therefore management of these complications in ex-thalassemics is an important issue. Iron stores in patients with class 2 and class 3 risk groups remain elevated even 7 years after allo-HCT[53]. Natural history of liver fibrosis following BMT for thalassemia showed that ion overload and hepatitis C virus infection are independent risk factors for liver fibrosis progression[54]. Therefore, the toxic effect of iron overload contributing to progression of already-present organ damage should be avoided as soon as possible using post-transplant iron depletion. Either regular phlebotomy or chelation therapy can successfully remove excess iron from the body by normalizing the iron pool.

Growth failure and endocrine dysfunction are common and well-known complications occurring in thalassemia patients treated by conventional treatment. We have shown that children receiving transplant before 8 years of age showed a normal growth rate, while older children, class 3 risk group patients, and patients who developed chronic GvHD had impaired growth. Gonadal damage is a common side effect of BuCy conditioning. Nevertheless some patients can restore their fertility after transplant, which is supported by our observations of 10 successful pregnancies and six spontaneous paternities in ex-thalassemics (unpublished data) which indicate that patients exposed to BuCy regimen are not inevitably infertile.

Another important issue in ex-thalassemics is lifelong monitoring for post-transplant malignancies, although their incidence in this patient population is low (0.8%). In our ex-thalassemics we have observed three early and one late non-Hodgkin lymphomas, and five solid tumors.

Controversies and Expert Point Of View

1. What is the Role of Allo-HCT in the Era of Current Conventional Therapy?

Advances in blood transfusion and iron chelation therapy have substantially improved the life expectancy of patients with thalassemia in high-income countries. However, in low- and middle-income countries, many children with beta-thalassemia die each year due to the lack of adequate blood transfusion facilities and chelation therapy. Furthermore, the aging of this population leads to increasing development of new chronic complications such as heart disease, lung disease, and endocrine disorders, leading to additional morbidity and premature mortality. Hematopoietic cell transplantation is the only well-established curative treatment for thalassemia and shows excellent long-term results. Current results of allo-HCT demonstrate that up to 90% of the patients with class 1 or class 2 risk group could be cured if transplant is performed at a younger age. Results of allo-HCT in patients with class 3 risk group treated with a modified treatment protocol are similar to class 1 or class 2 risk groups.

2. What is the Optimal Conditioning Regimen for Transplantation in Patients with Thalassemia?

Class 1 and class 2 risk group treated with standard conditioning regimen including BuCy have a high thalassemia-free survival rate. Allo-HCT for class 3 risk group is challenging due to high rates of graft rejection and transplant-related mortality. Our current modified treatment protocol for this high-risk group is highly effective in terms of rejection and thalassemia-free survival with results equal to intermediate/low-risk groups (class 1 or class 2). Nonmyeloablative but profoundly immunosuppressive conditioning regimens have been used in the treatment of transfusion-dependent hemoglobinopathies to offset toxicities. Although well tolerated, nearly all patients rejected their grafts. Reduced toxicity conditioning regimen consisting of treosulfan, fludarabine, and thiotepa for thalassemia produced mixed results. Although rates of graft rejection were similar (7% to 9%), thalassemia-free survival in these studies varied between 71% and 84%. Therefore, the use of such conditioning regimens should be reserved for selected patients who have advanced organ system dysfunction.

3. What are the Data with Alternate Graft Source in Thalassemia?

As the incidence of chronic GvHD is particularly high with the use of peripheral blood, bone marrow is the graft of choice for patients with thalassemia.

4. What Is the Role of Alternative Source of Allo-HCT in Thalassemia?

A substantial proportion of patients without a matched sibling donor could benefit from a matched unrelated bone marrow donor transplantation. Outcomes after unrelated BMT for thalassemia in class 1 or class 2 risk groups are comparable to those observed after sibling marrow transplantation. Our data support the use of related HLA-phenotypically matched or one-antigen mismatched donors as an acceptable alternative to matched unrelated donors in patients with thalassemia. The use of mismatched unrelated cord blood grafts in thalassemia should be avoided due to a high failure rate. Encouraging results have been obtained using T-cell-depleted HLA-haplotype mismatch transplant in thalassemia.

5. What Is the Role of Allo-HCT for Adult Patients with Thalassemia?

Adult patients have more advanced disease and treatment-related organ damage mainly due to prolonged exposure to iron overload. Allo-HCT controls iron overload-related organ damage. Therefore we recommend allo-HCT in adults who have a matched sibling donor using our current conditioning regimen.

6. Should Thalassemia Patients Be Given a Second Allograft from the Same Donor?

Our current treatment protocol for second transplantation is highly effective in terms of sustained engraftment and thalassemia-free survival. We recommend offering second transplants from the same donor to all patients who reject their first grafts with autologous recovery.

7. Does Allo-HCT Address the Clinical Sequelae of Iron Overload?

Most ex-thalassemics still carry the clinical sequelae of iron overload including cardiac, hepatic, and endocrine dysfunction. We recommend removal of iron overload by phlebotomy or chelators to avoid the progression of iron overload-related tissue damage and therefore to restore organ system function following transplantation.

Future Directions

Future research should focus on decreasing the transplantation-related morbidity and mortality and on further increasing thalassemia-free survival. This will include designing effective, reduced toxicity conditioning regimens (see Chapter 27), discovering targeted therapies to prevent and treat GvHD, *in-vitro* expansion and modification of allograft, and using embryonic stem cells to eliminate the need for HLA typing and toxic conditioning regimens (see Chapters 13 and 68). Use of gene therapy with targeting of autologous or allogeneic stem cells (see Chapter 67) may also hold promise for the correction of genetic diseases such as thalassemia and sickle cell anemia.

References

1. D.J. Weatheral, J.B. Clegg. *The Thalassemia Syndromes.* 4th ed. Oxford: Blackwell Science. 2001.

2. B. Modell, M. Khan, M. Darlison. Survival in beta-thalassemia major in the UK: data from the UK Thalassemia Register. *Lancet* 2000; 355: 2051–2.

3. M.J. Cunningham, E.A. Macklin, E.J. Neueld, *et al.* Thalassemia Clinical Research Network. Complications of beta–thalassemia major in North America. *Blood* 2002; 99: 36–43.

4. E.D. Thomas, C.D. Buckner, J.E. Sanders, *et al.* Marrow transplantation for thalassaemia. *Lancet* 1982; ii: 227–5.

5. G. Lucarelli, M. Galimberti, C. Delfini, *et al.* Marrow transplantation for thalassemia following busulfan and cyclophosphamide. *Lancet* 1985, 1(8442): 1355–1357.

6. G. Lucarelli, M. Galimberti, P. Polchi, *et al.* Marrow transplantation in patients with advanced thalassemia. *N Engl J Med* 1987; 316: 1050–5.

7. P.J. Tutschka, G.J. Elfenbein, L.L. Sensenbrenner, *et al.* Preparative regimens for marrow transplantation in acute leukemia and aplastic anemia. Baltimore experience. *Am J Ped Hematol Oncol* 1980; 2: 363–70.

8. G.W. Santos, P.J. Tutschka, R. Brookmeyer, *et al.* Marrow transplantation for acute nonlymphocytic leukemia after treatment with busulfan and cyclophosphamide. *N Engl J Med* 1983; 309: 1347–53.

9. A.M. Bolinger, A.B. Zangwill, J.T. Slattery, *et al.* Target dose adjustment of busulfan in pediatric patients undergoing bone marrow transplantation. *Bone Marrow Transplant* 2001; 28: 1013–18.

10. M. Chandy, P. Balasubramanian, S.V. Ramachandran, *et al.* Randomized trial of two different conditioning regimens for bone marrow transplantation in thalassemia-the role of busulfan pharmacokinetics in determining outcome. *Bone Marrow Transplant* 2005; 36: 839–45.

11. B.S. Andersson, A. Kashyap, V. Gian, *et al.* Conditioning therapy with intravenous busulfan and cyclophosphamide (IV BuCy2) for hematologic malignancies prior to allogeneic stem cell transplantation: a phase II study. *Biol Blood Marrow Transplant* 2002; 8: 145–54.

12. J. Gaziev, L. Nguyen, C. Puozzo, *et al.* Novel pharmacokinetic behavior of intravenous busulfan in children with thalassemia undergoing hematopoietic stem cell transplantation: a prospective evaluation of pharmacokinetic and pharmacodynamic profile with therapeutic drug monitoring. *Blood* 2010; 115(22): 4597–604.

13. M.E. Bernardo, E. Piras, A. Vacca, *et al.* Allogeneic hematopoietic stem cell transplantation in thalassemia major: results of a reduced-toxicity conditioning regimen based on the use of threosulfan. *Blood* 2014; 120: 473–6.

14. D. Choudhary, S.K. Sharma, N. Gupta, *et al.* Treosulfan-thiotepa-fludarabinee based conditioning regimen for allogeneic aransplantation in patients with thalassemia major: a single-Center experience from North India. *Biol Blood Marrow Transplant* 2013; 9: 492–503.

15. V. Mathews, V. George, A. Viswabandya, *et al.* Improved clinical outcomes of high risk b thalassemia major patients undergoing a HLA-matched related allogeneic stem cell transplant with a treosulfan based conditioning regimen and peripheral blood stem cell grafts. *PlosOne* 2013; 8: 1–8.

16. U. Anurathapan, S. Pakakasama, P. Rujkijyanont, *et al.* Pretransplant immunosuppression followed by reduced-toxicity conditioning and stem cell transplantation in high-risk thalassemia: a safe approach to disease control. *Biol Blood Marrow Transplant* 2013; 19: 1254–70.

17. G. Lucarelli, M. Galimberti, P. Polchi, *et al.* Bone marrow transplantation in patients with thalassemia. *N Engl J Med* 1990; 322: 417–21.

18. G. Lucarelli, M. Galimberti, P. Polchi, *et al.* Bone marrow transplantation in thalassemia. *Hematol Oncol Clin North Am* 1991; 5(3): 549–56.

19. G. Lucarelli, M. Andreani, E. Angelucci. The cure of thalassemia by bone marrow transplantation. *Blood Reviews* 2002; 16: 81–5.

20. G. Lucarelli, R. Clift, M. Galimberti, *et al.* Marrow transplantation for patients with thalassemia: results in Class 3 patients. *Blood* 1996; 87: 2082–88.

21. P. Sodani, J. Gaziev, P. Polchi, *et al.* New approach for bone marrow transplantation in patients with class 3 thalassemia aged younger than 17 years. *Blood* 2004; 104: 1201–3.

22. J. Gaziev, G. Lucarelli. Stem cell transplantation for thalassemia. *RBM Online* 2005;10:111–15.

23. G. Lucarelli, R.A. Clift, M. Galimberti, *et al.* Bone marrow transplantation in adult thalassemic patients. *Blood* 1999; 93: 1164–7.

24. J. Gaziev, P. Sodani, P. Polchi, *et al.* Bone marrow transplantation in adults with thalassemia. Treatment and long-term follow-up. *Ann NY Acad Sci* 2005; 1054: 196–205.

25. J. Gaziev, A. Isgrò, P. Sodani, *et al.* Optimal outcomes in young class 3 patients with thalassemia undergoing HLA-identical sibling bone marrow transplantation. *Transplantation* 2016; 100(4): 925–32.

26. S.E. Lawson, I.A. Roberts, P. Amrolia, I. Dokal, R. Szydlo, P.J. Darbyshire. Bone marrow transplantation for beta-thalassaemia major: the UK experience in two paediatric centres. *Br J Haematol* 2003; 120(2): 289–95.

27. P. Di Bartolomeo, S. Santarone, E. Di Bartolomeo, *et al.* Long-term results of survival in patients with thalassemia major treated with bone marrow transplantation. *Am J Hematol* 2008; 83(7): 528–30.

28. A. Ghavamzadeh, A. Iravani, A. Ashouri, *et al.* Peripheral blood *versus* bone marrow as a source of hematopoietic stem cells for allogeneic transplantation in children with class I and II beta thalassemia major. *Biol Blood Marrow Transplant* 2008; 14(3): 301–8.

29. M. Irfan, K. Hashmi, S. Adil, *et al.* Beta-thalassaemia major: bone marrow *versus* peripheral blood stem cell transplantation. *J Pak Med Assoc* 2008; 58(3): 107–10.

30. R. Chiesa, B. Cappelli, R. Crocchiolo, *et al.* Unpredictability of intravenous busulfan pharmacokinetics in children undergoing hematopoietic stem cell transplantation for advanced beta thalassemia: limited toxicity with a dose-adjustment policy. *Biol Blood Marrow Transplant* 2010;16(5):622–8.

31. M. Iravani, E. Tavakoli, M.H. Babaie, A. Ashouri, F. Khatami, A. Ghavamzadeh. Comparison of peripheral blood stem cell transplant with bone marrow transplant in class 3 thalassemic patients. *Exp Clin Transplant* 2010; 8(1): 66–73

32. M. Sabloff, M. Chandy, Z. Wang, *et al.* HLA-matched sibling bone marrow transplantation for beta-thalassemia major. *Blood* 2011; 117(5): 1745–50.

33. M.A. Yesilipek, M. Ertem, M. Cetin, *et al.* HLA-matched family hematopoetic stem cell transplantation in children with beta thalassemia major: the experience of the Turkish Pediatric Bone Marrow Transplantation Group. *Pediatr Transplant* 2012; 16(8): 846–51.

34. E. Goussetis, I. Peristeri, V. Kitra, *et al.* HLA-matched sibling stem cell transplantation in children with ß-thalassemia with anti-thymocyte globulina s part of the preparative regimen: the Greek experience. *Bone Marrow Transplant* 2012; 47: 1061–6.

35. C. Galambrun, C. Pondarre, Y. Bertrand, *et al.* French multicenter 22-year experience in stem cell transplantation for beta-thalassemia major: lessons and future directions. *Biol Blood Marrow Transplant* 2013; 19(1): 62–8.

36. A.A. Hussein, A. Al-Zaben, L. Ghatasheh, *et al.* Risk adopted allogeneic hematopoietic stem cell transplantation using a reduced intensity regimen for children with thalassemia major. *Pediatr Blood Cancer* 2013; 60(8): 1345–9.

37. P.J. Shaw, F. Kan, K.W. Ahn, *et al.* Outcomes of pediatric bone marrow transplantation for leukemia and myelodysplasia using matched sibling, mismatched related, or matched unrelated donors. *Blood* 2010; 116(11):4007–15.

38. D. Gaziev, M. Galimberti, G. Lucarelli, *et al.* Bone marrow transplantation from alternative donors for thalassemia: HLA-phenotypically identical relative and HLA-nonidentical sibling or parent transplants. *Bone Marrow Transplant* 2000; 25(8): 815–21.

39. J. Gaziev, P. Sodani, G. Lucarelli, *et al.* Second hematopoietic SCT in patients with thalassemia recurrence following rejection of the first graft. *Bone Marrow Transplant* 2008; 42(6): 397–404.

40. J. Gaziev, M. Marziali, A. Isgrò, *et al.* Bone marrow transplantation for thalassemia from alternative related donors: improved outcomes with a new approach. *Blood* 2013; 122(15): 2751–6.

41. P. Sodani, A. Isgro, J. Gaziev, *et al.* Purified T-depleted, CD34+ peripheral blood and bone marrow cell transplantation from haploidentical mother to child with Thalassemia. *Blood* 2010; 115: 1296–302.

42. F. Locatelli, V. Rocha, W. Reed, *et al.* Related unbilical cord blood transplantation in patients with thalassemia and sickle cell disease. *Blood* 2003; 101: 2137–43.

43. S. Soni, F. Boulad, M.D. Cowan, *et al.* Combined umbilical cord blood and bone marrow from HLA-identical sibling donors for hematopoietic stem cell transplantation in children with hemoglobinopathies. *Pediatr Blood Cancer* 2014; 61(9): 1690–4.

44. T-H. Jaing, I-J. Hung, C.H. Yang, *et al.* Unrelated cord blood transplantation for thalassemia: a single institution experience of 35 patients. *Bone Marrow Transplant* 2012; 47: 33–39.

45. A. Ruggeri, M. Eapen, A. Scaravadou *et al.* Umblical cord blood transplantation for children with thalassemia and sickle cell disease. The Eurocord Registry, the Center for Iternational Blood and Marrow Transplant Research, and the New York Blood Center. *Biol Blood Marrow Transplant* 2011; 17(9): 1375–82.

46. S. Kharbanda, A.R. Smith, S.K. Hutchinson, *et al.* Unrelated donor allogeneic hematopoietic stem cell transplantation for patients with hemoglobinopathies using a reduced-intensity conditioning regimen and third-party mesenchymal stromal cells. *Biol Blood Marrow Transplant* 2014; 20: 577–92.

47. S.H. Parikh, A. Mendizabal, C.L. Benjamin, *et al.* A novel reduced-intensity conditioning regimen for unrelated umbilical cord blood transplantation in children with non-malignant diseases. *Biol Blood Marrow Transplant* 2014; 20: 326–36.

48. G. La Nasa, C. Giardini, F. Argiolu, *et al.* Unrelated donor bone marrow transplantation for thalassemia: the effect of extended haplotypes. *Blood* 2002; 99(12): 4350–6.

49. Li. Chunfu, Wu. Xuedong, Feng. Xiaoping, *et al.* A novel conditioning regimen improves outcomes in ß-thalassemia major patients using unrelated donor peripheral blood stem cell transplantation. *Blood* 2012; 120: 3875–81.

50. G. La Nasa, G. Caocci, F. Argiolu, *et al.* Unrelated donor stem cell transplantation in adult patients with thalassemia. *Bone Marrow Transplant* 2005; 36: 971–5.

51. M. Andreani, M. Testi, M. Battarra, *et al.* Realtionship between mixed chimerism and rejection after bone marrow transplantation in thalassemia. *Blood Transfus* 2008; 6: 143–9.

52. J. Gaziev, A. Isgro, M. Marziali, *et al.* High CD3+ and CD34+ cell doses in the graft increase the incidence of acute GVHD in children receiving BMT for thalassemia. *Bone Marrow Transplant* 2012; 47: 107–14.

53. G. Lucarelli, E. Angelucci, C. Giardini, *et al.* Fate of iron stores in thalassemia after bone marrow transplantation. *Lancet* 1993; 342: 1388–91.

54. E. Angelucci, P. Muretto, A. Nicolucci, *et al.* Effects of iron overload and hepatitis C virus positivity in determining progression of liver fibrosis in thalassemia following bone marrow transplantation. *Blood* 2002; 100: 17–21.

Chapter

55

Allogeneic Hematopoietic Cell Transplants for Sickle Cell Disease

R. Patrick Weitzel, Courtney D. Fitzhugh, and John F. Tisdale

Introduction

Sickle cell disease (SCD) is an autosomal recessive disorder caused by a single nucleotide mutation in the β -globin gene of hemoglobin and is characterized by chronic hemolysis and sickle-shaped red blood cells and its consequences. It was the first identified and is one of the most prevalent and severe monogenetic disorders, affecting more than 100 000 individuals in the United States and several million around the world, primarily populations in regions of Africa, the Caribbean, Middle East, and India[1]. The substitution of the amino acid valine for glutamate at the sixth position of the β-globin peptide sequence promotes the formation of the hemoglobin S (HbS) protein tetramer, consisting of two pairs of α-globin chains and two pairs of abnormal β-globin chains. Sickle hemoglobin (HbS) polymerizes in deoxygenated states, inducing alteration of the normal biconcave erythrocyte shape to a crescent shape, and producing abnormally high cellular rigidity. Repeated episodes of sickling result in structural damage to the cell membrane and impairment of the cell's elasticity. These changes enhance adherence to the vascular endothelium, cause obstruction of blood flow, and promote hemolysis, thereby resulting in the many acute and chronic complications of sickle cell disease. These include, but are not limited to, pain crises, increased risk of infection from splenic dysfunction, and renal failure. Progressive destruction of the microvasculature can also result in end-stage organ failure and amplify painful episodes.

Allogeneic hematopoietic cell transplant (allo-HCT) is the only established curative treatment for SCD patients. Supportive treatments for SCD exist and include hydroxyurea and transfusion therapy, though these have limitations that warrant further exploration of alternative treatments[2]. For many years, hydroxyurea has been shown to reduce the frequency and severity of SCD complications including vaso-occlusive crises and acute chest syndrome. Hydroxyurea's benefit has been shown to largely be due to fetal hemoglobin (HbF) reactivation. Unfortunately, these supportive therapies are neither curative nor have they been shown to reverse established end-organ damage. In patients receiving frequent transfusion, iron overload requires chelation therapy in order to remove extra iron from the body, or alloimmunization may be caused, which will limit the ability to administer subsequent transfusions as well as produce severe inflammatory consequences.

Defining or predicting a patient's disease severity poses a problem for hematologists treating patients with SCD. As tolerance for conditioning therapies including radiation and/ or chemotherapy may be poor in patients with higher disease severity and hematologists are not able to predict beforehand who will have the most severe phenotype, risk *versus* benefit for allo-HCT becomes a difficult calculation. In addition, allo-HCT is associated with an inherent risk of graft rejection and graft-*versus*-host disease (GvHD).

Indications for Allo-HCT

The indications for allo-HCT in children and adults with SCD are constantly evolving. Some of the limitations to predicting disease severity include the high phenotypic variability of the disease. Often physicians are left weighing the risks of transplant with the perceived benefit as it relates to the specific patient's disease course and the potential complications of their disease over time. Waiting to intervene once major disease complications arise and clearly establish SCD severity limits its therapeutic application because the patient is less likely to tolerate the conditioning regimen and much end-organ damage may be irreversible at that time.

The most common indications for transplant include frequent vaso-occlusive crises, priapism, acute chest syndrome, symptomatic silent infarction, and osteonecrosis of multiple joints[3]. Persons with SCD who require long-term management with transfusion for prevention of primary cerebrovascular attack (CVA) but have difficulty finding compatible units to continue transfusion therapy and are at risk for recurrent stroke, are often directed to transplant.

Transcranial Doppler (TCD) examination has proven effective in predicting the risk of CVA in these patients. The detection of abnormal TCD in persons with SCD allows interventions which have been shown to reduce the risk of the subsequent CVA; however, red cell transfusion carry its own risk[4,5]. Unfortunately, to date there are no reliable predictors of which patients will have persistently abnormal TCDs, or will develop a second CVA or alloimmunization. Therefore, early administration with allo-HCT is becoming a preferred intervention.

Recent studies have regrettably shown that hydroxyurea does not always reduce the severity of SCD. Despite improved

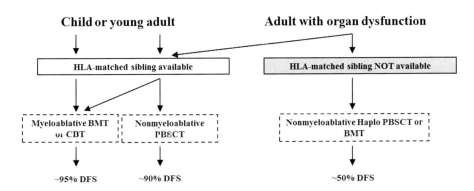

Figure 55.1 Algorithm for selecting transplantation options for individuals with SCD.

supportive care, the average patient with SCD only lives around 40 years, which is not significantly improved from the median age of death reported more than one decade ago [6,7]. Although the prediction of who will have the most severe disease is not certain among pediatric patients, considerable certainty exists in adult patients.

Donor for Allo-HCT: Matched Sibling?

Matched sibling allo-HCT with myeloablative conditioning (MAC) regimen is the preferred strategy (Figure 55.1). The first successful transplant for SCD was in 1984 in an 8-year-old female patient being treated for acute myelogenous leukemia (AML)[8]. The transplant was successful in ameliorating her AML, and reduction of HbS was further observed to match the levels in the sickle-trait donor after transplant. Subsequent reports from Belgium[9] and France[10] reported extremely favorable overall and disease-free survival rates near or above 90% in 42 and 14 patients, respectively.

The first American multicenter study reported[11] 22 young patients with severe comorbidities and recurrent clinical events who received grafts from HLA-MSD and MAC regimen with cyclophosphamide (Cy) busulfan (Bu) plus *in-vivo* lymphocyte depletion using antithymocyte globulin or the specific CD52-targeting antibody Campath™. GvHD prophylaxis was approached with cyclosporine, methotrexate, and/or prednisone. Sixteen of the 20 surviving patients achieved stable donor engraftment, with another patient displaying mixed chimerism. Seizures were noted in some patients although most resolved with treatment; these neurologic complications were noted as the cause of death for two patients. Rejection was observed in four patients, reflecting an event-free survival rate of 73% (events defined as death, graft rejection, or SCD recurrence), a very promising result in a particularly high-risk patient cohort.

In 2000, 50 pediatric patients were reported at a longer follow-up (median 39 months)[12] in another multicenter study. All but three patients survived and of those, 38 exhibited complete donor chimerism and four stable mixed chimerism. Graft rejection and/or SCD recurrence was observed in about

10% of patients. Of note were the lack of comorbidities and improvement of end-organ damage observed among the patients with longer follow-up of at least two years; incidents of acute chest syndrome and CVA were completely eliminated in the patients exhibiting full engraftment. Similar results were obtained in Europe[13], and the large majority of these patients remain alive today without any SCD-related symptoms.

The largest group reported a retrospective analysis of 87 patients transplanted between 1989 and 2002[14]. Cerebral vasculopathy was the primary comorbid indication for transplant. Overall and event-free survival was similar to previous multicenter studies, at 93% and 86%, respectively (95% CI). A major finding of this study was the profound reduction in 5-year graft rejection after the addition of antithymocyte globulin to the pretransplant conditioning regimen around 1992. The EFS approached 95% in patients transplanted after 2000. Moderate to high-grade (II–IV) acute GvHD was present in 20% of patients and correlated with older patient age, noncord blood graft source, and higher degree of HLA disparity. Importantly, further evidence of accumulating cerebral complications such as stroke or ischemic lesions was not observed post-transplant in patients with successful engraftment. Evaluation of transplanted SCD patients over a similar time range [15] for additional markers of end-organ damage revealed stable or improved pulmonary function, improved MRI, and improved kidney score.

Does Age at Allo-HCT Matter in SCD?

The majority of transplantation for SCD has been carried out in pediatric patients. Indeed, lower patient age appears to predict improved engraftment outcomes and may allow for the prevention of any SCD-related end-organ damage if performed early enough. However, no accurate predictors of future SCD severity in children have been identified. Whether to transplant the pediatric SCD patient before the onset of severe complications is a source of controversy due to the severity of pretransplant conditioning regimens and potential effects on future gonadal function. However, data suggest that whenever a matched sibling donor is available, HCT is indeed safe and effective enough to become the standard intervention for the pediatric or young adult SCD patient. SCD patients have received donor grafts from normal homozygous HbA or sickle cell trait (HbAS) siblings. In one retrospective evaluation, early transplantation (before the patient had received a maximum of three blood transfusions) was shown to have benefits of higher overall survival (100% *versus* 88%, 95% CI) and reduced adverse events including relapse[13]. We recommend that for patients with homozygous SCD and an HLA-matched sibling donor but without severe complications, discussion should take place between the patient, parents, and transplant physician regarding benefits and risks, so that an informed decision may be made regarding this highly effective therapy in this setting.

What Is the Role of Allo-HCT in Adults with SCD?

A dearth of therapeutic options has been noted for the adult SCD patient who has become refractory to hydroxyurea therapy and transfusion through alloimmunization. Studies were therefore initiated with the goal of filling this void and applying allo-HCT to these sicker patients. These trials have included substantially fewer patients and have shown comparatively less success, although a much wider variety of conditioning and treatment approaches have been attempted. The majority of these studies have included a low-intensity TBI and chemotherapeutic approach to achieve nonmycloablative conditioning pretransplant, in contrast to earlier pediatric studies. These patients have included a cohort of young adults (all <28 years) reported to show a disease-free survival of 93% at a median follow-up of 3.4 years[16]. Acute GvHD was not severe and manageable with prednisone and ongoing immunosuppression was unnecessary. In our practice, we transplant adult patients with SCD who frequently have multiple comorbidities including recurrent painful crises, kidney and liver damage, stroke, and elevated pulmonary pressures as determined by transthoracic echocardiogram. We recently reported our results in the HLA-matched sibling setting using a nonmyeloablative approach with alemtuzumab, 300 cGy TBI, and sirolimus for GvHD prophylaxis[17]. Twenty-six of 30 patients (87%) reported patients are free of SCD without evidence of GvHD, therefore approaching the success rate seen in the pediatric setting.

What Should Be the Intensity of Conditioning Regimen for Allo-HCT in SCD?

Nonmyeloablative conditioning (NMA) regimens have been investigated with considerable interest; however, incidence of graft rejection and GvHD has been more frequent in these studies. Early experiences required ongoing immunosuppression to maintain engraftment[18,19]; however, recent reports have showed promising success in initiating long-term bidirectional tolerance to avoid rejection caused by alloimmune

response. As discussed above, our report included 30 adults across a wider age range (17–65 years) and a NMA regimen [17]. The large majority of the 87% of patients with positive transplant outcomes initially showed a chimeric pattern of engraftment which remained stable, approximately half of which no longer required sirolimus to maintain after one year post-transplant. This chimerism is very often compartmentalized, with the same patients exhibiting sufficient or even complete donor myeloid engraftment and much lower or even no stable lymphoid engraftment. Importantly, significantly reduced narcotic dosing and hospital visits were measured among this patient group. Neither acute nor chronic GvHD were observed, even after withdrawal of immunosuppression in the weaned patients.

Most notably, however, was the observation that as little as ~15% donor myeloid chimerism in the chimeric patient still reduces serum HbS levels to a point sufficient to reverse the SCD phenotype. This has indicated to transplanting physicians that reduced intensity conditioning (RIC) regimens combined with immune modulation may be an equally effective yet much less toxic approach than MAC regimen, particularly in the older patient affected by SCD complications and organ damage likely to be exacerbated by chemotherapy. Unlike allo-HCT for malignant disease, a graft-*versus*-SCD effect is not necessary for therapeutic benefit in SCD and other hemaglobinopathies. Additionally, patients receiving these conditioning regimens have fathered and mothered children naturally, indicating these reduced intensity approaches may be useful in preserving younger patients' fertility in contrast to conventional MAC regimen, which has been shown to be extremely deleterious to patients' fertility. However, comparatively fewer long-term follow-up results are available, and it remains to be seen whether immunosuppression and its withdrawal post-transplant truly lack long-term risks in these patients. Therefore, long-term follow-up studies of patients undergoing MAC and non-MAC regimens which are being performed at our institution and others are crucial to assess both the positive and negative impacts of transplant.

Allo-HCT Barriers in Subjects with SCD

While the results of HLA MSD transplant have been promising, many barriers exist. First, HLA typing is not explored in a significant proportion of patients. Among almost 5000 pediatric patients with SCD, 6.5% met eligibility criteria for allo-HCT[20]. Yet, HLA typing was performed on only 41% of eligible (or 2.6% of total) patients. Patients did not undergo HLA typing because of physician refusal (4%), parental refusal (9.5%), insufficient psychosocial or financial support (10.5%), and absence of any potential sibling donor (24%). More recently, a study reported that parents of children with SCD are more likely to participate in research studies if they believe that their child's SCD is moderate to severe and if they believe that more research in SCD is needed[21]. However, the major limitation to allo-HCT for patients with SCD is lack of HLA-matched sibling donors. We reported that of 287 patients screened at the National Institutes of Health by HLA typing, 102 (36%) were found to have an HLA-matched sibling[19]. This percentage is likely exaggerated because many patients evaluated were already known to have an HLA-matched sibling by virtue of their inclusion in other NIH trials. In contrast, in the previous study, only 14% of eligible patients had an HLA-matched sibling[20]. Hence, an alternative donor source is necessary to expand the donor pool so that most patients with severe SCD can have access to this potentially curative procedure.

Alternative Graft Sources
Umbilical Cord Blood as Source of Graft in SCD

Cord blood transplantation (CBT) has increasingly been employed for patients with malignant and nonmalignant hematologic diseases. For patients with SCD, related CBT, performed in general using 6/6 HLA-matched cords, displays results comparative to the success seen with HLA-matched sibling *bone marrow* or *peripheral* mobilized hematopoietic cells. In a recent report where 160 patients with SCD received HLA-identical *related* CBT or BMT[22], 30 underwent *related* CBT. Disease-free survival (DFS) 6 years post-HCT was 92% after BMT and 90% post-CBT (*P*=NS). No patients who underwent CBT experienced grade IV acute GvHD and none developed chronic extensive GvHD as compared to 2% and 5% (95% CI), respectively, in patients who received BMT.

In contrast, *unrelated* CBT, where the cords are mostly 4/6 and 5/6 HLA-matched, has been less successful. The largest study to date reported 16 patients with SCD[23]. Though the OS was 94%, DFS was unacceptably low at 50%. Further, the rate of grade 2–4 acute GvHD in the patients with SCD as well as in the 35 patients with β-thalassemia major was 22%, with 3% developing chronic GvHD. Another study was stopped early because five of eight transplanted patients rejected their grafts, two experienced grade II acute GvHD, and one developed chronic extensive GvHD[24]. Therefore, additional research in areas such as *ex-vivo* expansion, immune modulation with pharmacologic and cell-based approaches, and optimal allelic HLA-matching is needed to improve outcome for patients with SCD who undergo unrelated CBT. Given the results reported to date, we recommend that patients undergo unrelated CBT only in the setting of a clinical trial designed specifically to address the current limitations of CBT.

Matched Unrelated Donor as a Graft Source for SCD

In order to explore other alternative donor options, Krishnamurti *et al.* sought to determine the probability for patients with SCD to find a potential matched unrelated donor (MUD)[25]. Therefore, the National Marrow Donor Program (NMDP) database was evaluated to discover patients with SCD for whom a donor search was commenced. They found that 34% of patients had 1–2 potential donors who were 6/6 HLA-matched. In contrast, we performed a donor search via the NMDP and Bone Marrow Donors Worldwide for 10 adults with disease severe enough to be eligible for PB HCT on our protocols but who lacked an HLA-matched sibling donor. We discovered that only one patient had more than a 1% chance of having a 6/6 HLA-matched donor per the Haplogic algorithm[26]. Nevertheless, due to insufficient donor availability and scarcity of trials, data are scarce regarding MUD transplants for patients with SCD. Two trials are currently ongoing: one for pediatric patients with SCD, the Sickle Cell Unrelated Transplant (SCURT) trial (NCT00745420), and another for young adults with SCD, the Sickle Cell Transplantation to Prevent Disease Exacerbation (STRIDE) trial (NCT01565616). The results of these studies will be necessary to begin to explore MUD transplant outcomes for patients with SCD, with the goal of expanding of the donor pool and making many more patients eligible for transplant over the coming decades.

Haplotype Matched Transplant for Patients with SCD

Many benefits exist for this alternative donor option including a large donor pool since children, parents, and half-matched siblings can potentially be donors (as compared to HLA-matched siblings and MUD), the possibility for multiple donor collections and larger cell doses (unlike CBT donors), and comparatively fast time to donor collection (as compared to MUD). Because of the greater immunologic barrier to engraftment, however, HLA haplotype mismatch HCT has been associated with a higher risk for GvHD, graft rejection, and transplant-related mortality. Two small studies have been published. The first involved 14 children and young adults who received nonmyeloablative conditioning[27]. Seven (50%) of the patients were free from SCD, and one additional patient with mixed erythroid chimerism was free from painful crises and transfusions but was anemic. None of the reported patients experienced GvHD, and 75% of engrafted patients were weaned off of immunosuppressive therapy. The second study included eight pediatric patients who received more intensive conditioning[28]. The DFS was 38%. Further, two of the patients experienced grade II–IV GvHD and two patients developed chronic extensive GvHD; both these patients died from chronic GvHD. Therefore, studies which optimize conditioning, immunosuppression, and donor-recipient matching are necessary to achieve better results in haplotype-matched transplant for adult and pediatric patients with SCD. Though the success rates with haplotype transplants are lower than desirable, the availability of a donor for virtually all patients makes this option highly desirable for further development. Additionally, regimens that are nonablative allowing autologous recovery if unsuccessful should add to the safety of this approach as has been documented thus far. At present, given that the success rate for haplotype-matched transplant is not significantly better as related to unrelated CBT, the type of alternative donor transplant recommended should be based on institutional experience and done in the context of a clinical trial.

Gene Therapy for Patients with SCD

For those lacking a matched allogeneic HSC donor, genetic strategies targeting autologous hematopoietic CD34+ cells remain logical alternatives. The permanent integration of potentially therapeutic genes into primary autologous HSCs has been rigorously pursued, and steady progress in the field has resulted in proof-of-concept through clinical successes in the immunodeficiencies[29–37]. The globin disorders, though long held as a therapeutic target, have proven much more difficult because of the necessity of regulated, lineage-specific, high-level globin expression. Incorporation of elements of the human β-globin locus-control region (LCR), which functions as a tissue-specific enhancer, led to the evolution of a new generation of globin retroviral vectors incorporating four or five hypersensitive LCR elements, yet these vectors were unstable and proved unreliable for directing high-level human β-globin expression. The incorporation of these elements became feasible with the development of lentiviral vector systems, allowing for the first time sustained, high-level, regulated human β-globin expression sufficient to revert the phenotype in a murine model of β-thalassemia[38]. These results were confirmed and extended in both thalassemia and SCD models[39–45], and clinical trials testing lentiviral vectors in patients SCD have now been initiated. Finally, the landmark development of human iPS cells by Takahashi and Yamanaka [46] through the introduction of specific reprogramming factors allows the creation of embryonic-like stem cells circumventing the ethical issues surrounding embryonic stem cells. Furthermore, advances in genome editing with methods including zinc finger nucleases, TALENs, and CRISPR/Cas9 [47] have the potential to transform our approach to the hemoglobinopathies.

Controversies in SCD HCT

While there have been remarkable advances in the application of curative allo-HCT in SCD such that children with an HLA-matched sibling have a 95% chance of being free of SCD with this approach, there are a number of controversies that limit application. Despite significant effort, predictors of disease severity that reliably identify patients at long-term risk for serious complications and earlier mortality remain lacking. This lack results in a difficulty in identifying patients for whom potentially risky strategies employing HCT can be justified, especially in the research setting where in contrast

to the MAC regimen HCT setting in children, results are either less mature or not yet proven. This is especially true for both the HLA haplotype mismatched HCT setting and the autologous HCT gene therapy/editing setting. While these approaches are highly promising, their place in the management of SCD remains to be determined. As such, it remains controversial as to which patients are appropriate to consider for such interventions, and efforts to minimize toxicity while improving efficacy represent one way to circumvent the current controversy. Additionally, the majority of current and future envisioned regimens render patients sterile, and sterility preservation is a significant factor that prevents many families from moving to HCT during childhood. Interestingly, our own experience suggests that gonadal function, similar to other organ function, is limited in adult patients with SCD. Attempts to further characterize gonadal function along with efforts to preserve existing fertility are thus justified. Allo-HCT approaches are also high-cost interventions. Given that SCD disproportionally affects individuals at the lower end of the socioeconomic spectrum, the high cost presents an additional barrier which must be overcome. It deserves note that SCD itself also entails high-costs, especially among adults with accumulated end-organ damage[48], and allo-HCT represents a cost-effective strategy [49], especially when viewed in the long-term[50]. Minimizing the risk for morbidity (including GvHD and sterility) and mortality while aiming to achieve the already highly efficacious results of MAC allo-HCT in children should address the major controversies limiting application of curative approaches in SCD.

Conclusions and Recommendations

Over the past 20 years, allogeneic HCT has become a more readily available opportunity for patients with SCD. Particularly when an HLA-matched sibling has been available as a donor, studies to date show that BMT and PB HCT have a high success rate and low rates of GvHD and transplant-related mortality not only in pediatric patients, but also in adults with severe disease. The success rate is similar for patients who undergo related CBT. *Unrelated* CBT and HLA haplotype mismatch transplant outcomes are suboptimal, and institutional expertise and available research protocols should help determine which option to explore (Figure 55.1). Matched unrelated donor and gene therapy trials are ongoing, and recommendations regarding both can be made when results are available. Therefore, while overall allo-HCT results have improved substantially in the HLA-matched sibling setting, more work is required to improve results in patients without an HLA-matched sibling donor option. Allo-HCT, particularly if donor pools can be expanded and more transplants can eventually be performed in African clinics, has the potential to make the first significant global impact in SCD incidence and severity in decades.

References

1. Piel, F.B., *et al.*, Global burden of sickle cell anaemia in children under five, 2010–2050: modelling based on demographics, excess mortality, and interventions. *PLoS Med*, 2013. 10(7): p. e1001484.

2. Charache, S., *et al.*, Effect of hydroxyurea on the frequency of painful crises in sickle cell anemia. *N Engl J Med*, 1995. 332(20). p. 1317–1322.

3. Fitzhugh, C.D., *et al.*, Hematopoietic stem cell transplantation for patients with sickle cell disease: progress and future directions. *Hematol Oncol Clin North Am*, 2014. 28(6): p. 1171–85.

4. Adams, R.J., *et al.*, Prevention of a first stroke by transfusions in children with sickle cell anemia and abnormal results on transcranial Doppler ultrasonography [see comments]. *N Engl J Med*, 1998. 339(1): p. 5–11.

5. Kwiatkowski, J.L., *et al.*, Effect of transfusion therapy on transcranial doppler ultrasonography velocities in children with sickle cell disease. *Pediatr Blood Cancer*. 56(5): p. 777–782.

6. Fitzhugh, C.D., *et al.*, Cardiopulmonary complications leading to premature deaths in adult patients with sickle cell disease. *Am J Hematol*, 2010. 85(1): p. 36–40.

7. Platt, O.S., *et al.*, Mortality in sickle cell disease. Life expectancy and risk factors for early death [see comments]. *N Engl J Med*, 1994. 330(23): p. 1639–44.

8. Johnson, F.L., *et al.*, Bone-marrow transplantation in a patient with sickle-cell anemia. *N Engl J Med*, 1984. 311(12): p. 780–3.

9. Vermylen, C. and G. Cornu, Bone marrow transplantation for sickle cell disease. The European experience. *Am J Pediatr Hematol Oncol*, 1994. 16(1): p. 18–21.

10. Bernaudin, F., *et al.*, Bone marrow transplantation (BMT) in 14 children with severe sickle cell disease (SCD): the French experience. GEGMO. *Bone Marrow Transplant*, 1993. 12(Suppl 1): p. 118–21.

11. Walters, M.C., *et al.*, Bone marrow transplantation for sickle cell disease. *N Engl J Med*, 1996. 335(6): p. 369–76.

12. Walters, M.C., *et al.*, Impact of bone marrow transplantation for symptomatic sickle cell disease: an interim report. Multicenter investigation of bone marrow transplantation for sickle cell disease. *Blood*, 2000. 95(6): p. 1918–24.

13. Vermylen, C. and G. Cornu, Hematopoietic stem cell transplantation for sickle cell anemia. *Curr Opin Hematol*, 1997. 4(6): p. 377–80.

14. Bernaudin, F., *et al.*, Long-term results of related myeloablative stem-cell transplantation to cure sickle cell disease. *Blood*, 2007. 110(7): p. 2749–56.

15. Walters, M.C., *et al.*, Pulmonary, gonadal, and central nervous system status after bone marrow transplantation for sickle cell disease. *Biol Blood Marrow Transplant*, 2010. 16(2): p. 263–72.

16. Kuentz, M., Peripheral blood stem cell allograft from HLA-unrelated donors. *Hematol Cell Ther*, 1996. 38(5): p. 453–4.

17. Hsieh, M.M., *et al.*, Nonmyeloablative HLA-matched sibling allogeneic hematopoietic stem cell transplantation for severe sickle cell phenotype. *JAMA*, 2014. 312(1): p. 48–56.

18. Iannone, R., *et al.*, Results of minimally toxic nonmyeloablative transplantation in patients with sickle cell anemia and beta-thalassemia. *Biol Blood Marrow Transplant*, 2003. 9(8): p. 519–28.

19. Horan, J.T., *et al.*, Hematopoietic stem cell transplantation for multiply transfused patients with sickle cell disease and thalassemia after low-dose total body irradiation, fludarabine, and rabbit anti-thymocyte globulin. *Bone Marrow Transplant*, 2005. 35(2): p. 171–7.

20. Walters, M.C., *et al.*, Barriers to bone marrow transplantation for sickle cell anemia. *Biol Blood Marrow Transplant*, 1996. 2(2): p. 100–4.

21. Liem, R.I., *et al.*, Parental attitudes toward research participation in pediatric sickle cell disease. *Pediatr Blood Cancer*, 2010. 55(1): p. 129–33.

22. Locatelli, F., *et al.*, Outcome of patients with hemoglobinopathies given either cord blood or bone marrow transplantation from an HLA-identical sibling. *Blood*, 2013. 122(6): p. 1072–8.

23. Ruggeri, A., *et al.*, Umbilical cord blood transplantation for children with thalassemia and sickle cell disease. *Biol Blood Marrow Transplant*, 2011. 17(9): p. 1375–82.

24. Kamani, N.R., *et al.*, Unrelated donor cord blood transplantation for children with severe sickle cell disease: results of one cohort from the phase II study from the Blood and Marrow Transplant Clinical Trials Network (BMT CTN). *Biol Blood Marrow Transplant*, 2012. 18(8): p. 1265–72.

25. Krishnamurti, L., *et al.*, Availability of unrelated donors for hematopoietic stem cell transplantation for hemoglobinopathies. *Bone Marrow Transplant*, 2003. 31(7): p. 547–50.

26. Hsieh, M., J. Wilder, C. Fitzhugh, B. Link, J.F. Tisdale. Results of Alternative Donor Search in Adult Patients with Severe Sickle Cell Disease (SCD) Eligible for Hematopoietic Stem Cell Transplantation (HSCT). The American Society of Hematology Annual Meeting. 2007.

27. Bolanos-Meade, J., *et al.*, HLA-haploidentical bone marrow transplantation with posttransplant cyclophosphamide expands the donor pool for patients with sickle cell disease. *Blood*, 2012. 120(22): p. 4285–91.

28. Dallas, M.H., *et al.*, Long-term outcome and evaluation of organ function in pediatric patients undergoing haploidentical and matched related hematopoietic cell transplantation for sickle cell disease. *Biol Blood Marrow Transplant*, 2013. 19(5): p. 820–30.

29. Cavazzana-Calvo, M., *et al.*, Gene therapy of human severe combined immunodeficiency (SCID)-X1 disease [see comments]. *Science*, 2000. 288(5466): p. 669–72.

30. Aiuti, A., *et al.*, Immune reconstitution in ADA-SCID after PBL gene therapy and discontinuation of enzyme replacement. *Nat Med*, 2002. 8(5): p. 423–5.

31. Aiuti, A., *et al.*, Correction of ADA-SCID by stem cell gene therapy combined with nonmyeloablative conditioning. *Science*, 2002. 296(5577): p. 2410–3.

32. Ott, M.G., *et al.*, Correction of X-linked chronic granulomatous disease by gene therapy, augmented by insertional activation of MDS1-EVI1, PRDM16 or SETBP1. *Nat Med*, 2006. 12(4): p. 401–9.

33. Aiuti, A., *et al.*, Multilineage hematopoietic reconstitution without clonal selection in ADA-SCID patients

treated with stem cell gene therapy. *J Clin Invest*, 2007. 117(8): p. 2233–40.

34. Aiuti, A., *et al.*, Gene therapy for immunodeficiency due to adenosine deaminase deficiency. *N Engl J Med*, 2009. 360(5): p. 447–58.

35. Gaspar, H.B., *et al.*, Hematopoietic stem cell gene therapy for adenosine deaminase-deficient severe combined immunodeficiency leads to long-term immunological recovery and metabolic correction. *Sci Transl Med*, 2011. 3(97): p. 97ra80.

36. Hacein-Bey-Abina, S., *et al.*, Efficacy of gene therapy for X-linked severe combined immunodeficiency. *New Engl J Med*, 2010. 363(4): p. 355–64.

37. Hacein-Bey-Abina, S., *et al.*, A modified gamma-retrovirus vector for X-linked severe combined immunodeficiency. *New Engl J Med*, 2014. 371(15): p. 1407–17.

38. May, C., *et al.*, Therapeutic haemoglobin synthesis in beta-thalassaemic mice expressing lentivirus-encoded human beta-globin. *Nature*, 2000. 406(6791): p. 82–6.

39. Persons, D.A., *et al.*, Successful treatment of murine beta-thalassemia using in vivo selection of genetically modified, drug-resistant hematopoietic stem cells. *Blood*, 2003. 102(2): p. 506–13.

40. Persons, D.A., *et al.*, The degree of phenotypic correction of murine beta-thalassemia intermedia following lentiviral-mediated transfer of a human gamma-globin gene is influenced by chromosomal position effects and vector copy number. *Blood*, 2003. 101(6): p. 2175–83.

41. Pawliuk, R., *et al.*, Correction of sickle cell disease in transgenic mouse models by gene therapy. *Science*, 2001. 294(5550): p. 2368–71.

42. Imren, S., *et al.*, Permanent and panerythroid correction of murine beta thalassemia by multiple lentiviral integration in hematopoietic stem cells. *Proc Natl Acad Sci U S A*, 2002. 99(22): p. 14380–5.

43. Moreau-Gaudry, F., *et al.*, High-level erythroid-specific gene expression in primary human and murine hematopoietic cells with self-inactivating lentiviral vectors. *Blood*, 2001. 98(9): p. 2664–72.

44. Perumbeti, A., *et al.*, A novel human gamma-globin gene vector for genetic correction of sickle cell anemia in a humanized sickle mouse model: critical determinants for successful correction. *Blood*, 2009. 114(6): p. 1174–85.

45. Arumugam, P.I., *et al.*, Improved human beta-globin expression from self-inactivating lentiviral vectors carrying the chicken hypersensitive site-4 (cHS4) insulator element. *Mol Ther*, 2007. 15(10): p. 1863–71.

46. Takahashi, K. and S. Yamanaka, Induction of pluripotent stem cells from mouse embryonic and adult fibroblast cultures by defined factors. *Cell*, 2006. 126(4): p. 663–76.

47. Gaj, T., C.A. Gersbach, and C.F. Barbas, 3rd, ZFN, TALEN, and CRISPR/Cas-based methods for genome engineering. *Trends Biotechnol*, 2013. 31(7): p. 397–405.

48. Ballas, S.K., The cost of health care for patients with sickle cell disease. *Am J Hematol*, 2009. 84(6): p. 320–2.

49. Arnold, S.D., *et al.*, Allogeneic hematopoietic cell transplantation for children with sickle cell disease is beneficial and cost-effective: a single-center analysis. *Biol Blood Marrow Transplant*, 2015. 21(7): p. 1258–65.

50. Saenz, C. and J.F. Tisdale, Assessing costs, benefits, and risks in chronic disease: taking the long view. *Biol Blood Marrow Transplant*, 2015. 21(7): p. 1149–50.

56

Chapter

Autologous Hematopoietic Cell Transplants for Autoimmune Diseases: Therapeutic Rationale and Limitations

Marcelo C. Pasquini and Robert Peter Gale

Introduction

Autoimmune diseases are caused by imbalanced immune regulation. One approach to treating these diseases is to reset the immune system by destroying or severely altering the abnormal immune system with high doses of immune suppressive drugs and/or radiation, infusing autologous or allogeneic blood or bone marrow cells, and encouraging normal immune reconstitution from cells in the graft, residual cells in the subject, or both[1]. This process can be likened to rebooting a computer, the first advice one receives from information technology experts when something is akimbo or a program is not working correctly. There are, of course, several fundamental issues with this approach such as whether a blood or bone marrow cell infusion is needed, why, in autotransplants infusing abnormal cells should correct the immune abnormality, and others. In this chapter we review fundamental aspects of hematopoietic cell transplants focusing mostly on autotransplants for autoimmune diseases. The chapter which follows reviews results of this intervention in persons with specific autoimmune diseases.

Rationale

The rationale for hematopoietic cell transplants in autoimmune diseases is to give immune suppressive drugs to alter or eradicate the immune abnormality(ies) underlying the disease. Hematopoietic cell transplants build on this strategy by allowing for high-dose immune suppression by subsequently infusing autologous or allogeneic blood or bone marrow cells [1,2]. Severity of the autoimmune abnormality as evidenced by the clinical features, disease evolution, and response to therapy influences the type and intensity of immune suppression given. Although autoimmune diseases are common, there is a wide spectrum of clinical features, severities, chronicity, and health impacts. For example, the natural history of diseases such as vitiligo or psoriasis is very different from systemic sclerosis or multiple sclerosis. Even within systemic sclerosis and multiple sclerosis there is a wide spectrum of disease severity with some persons having rapid physical and end-organ deterioration whereas others have a more chronic and less symptomatic disease. Early identification of persons likely to have a more severe disease course is important in selecting therapy(ies).

The hypothesis is that an imbalance in immune cells, say between autoreactive *versus* regulatory or suppressor cells, will be normalized when the immune system recovers after transplantation. Considerable data from animal models of autoimmune diseases support this notion. However, these are selected models and there is substantial publication bias; negative reports or models where this approach fails are rarely published. Also, there is considerable controversy regarding how accurately these models reflect autoimmune disease in humans. For example, many of these experiments are done in young, healthy animals without comorbidities and before there is irreversible end-organ damage. However, due to the weight of evidence from these data it is reasonable to consider appropriately conducted clinical trials of this approach in humans. Also, some data from uncontrolled studies in humans support this approach. For example, in persons with multiple sclerosis receiving high-dose therapy and an autotransplant there is a substantial decrease in autoreactive lymphocytes post-transplant and re-establishment of a normal T-cell regulatory phenotype [2–4]. These data are encouraging but are an invalidated surrogate for clinical benefit. Moreover, they reflect an association from which one should not assume causality. As we will discuss, use of surrogate endpoints for clinical benefit in uncontrolled studies of autotransplants is a widespread and fundamental problem in interpreting outcomes.

Autotransplants for autoimmune diseases differ in rationale and strategic objectives from autotransplants for neoplastic diseases. In neoplastic diseases the goal is to use high doses of drugs and/or radiation to eradicate the neoplastic clone followed by a transplant to reverse bone marrow damage. Although there may be anticancer effects associated with engraftment, the main objective is not to reset the immune system. In contrast, in autotransplants for autoimmune diseases the main role of pretransplant therapy is altering or destroying what is believed to be an abnormal immune system, not eradication of a neoplasm. This distinction explains, at least in part, why less intensive pretransplant regimens (termed nonmyeloablative) are increasingly used. Specifics of these regimens and comparison of outcomes with conventional pretransplant regimens are discussed in Chapter 27.

Technique

Grafts used for autotransplants for autoimmune diseases are typically from mobilized blood cells rather than bone marrow cells. Blood cell mobilization approaches in autoimmune diseases are discussed in Chapters 10 and 57. The potential therapy impact of hematopoietic cell transplants in autoimmune diseases relies on several steps including: (1) blood cell mobilization; (2) collection; (3) the conditioning regimen; and (4) potential modification(s) of the graft. Common mobilization strategies include giving hematopoietic growth factor such as granulocyte colony-stimulating factor (G-CSF) with or without high doses of drugs such as cyclophosphamide. Sometime later, the range typically being a month to several years later, the subject receives a pretransplant conditioning regimen follow by one or more infusions of autologous blood cells. Pretransplant regimens range from very intensive, such as high doses of drugs like cyclophosphamide and whole body radiation with doses up to 12 Gy, to less intensive regimens such as fludarabine and cyclophosphamide. Sometimes the graft is manipulated by selecting CD34-positive cells and/or by depleting T-cells. Some persons receive high doses of antithymocyte globulin (ATG) before or after infusing the graft.

The complex procedures of giving G-CSF and/or cyclophosphamide to facilitate collecting autologous blood cells and use of diverse pretransplant conditioning regimens make critical interpretation of clinical trials outcomes difficult. For example, G-CSF and cyclophosphamide have independent immune-modulating effects. As such, one possible explanation of clinical outcomes could be this intervention alone. The next complexity comes from the apheresis. There are no studies using apheresis alone to treat autoimmune disease. Removing large numbers of blood mononuclear cells including B- and T-cells could affect clinical outcomes independent of drugs given for blood cell mobilization and for pretransplant conditioning. A third complexity is drugs and/or radiation given pretransplant. Finally, there is frequent use of ATG pre- and/or post-transplant which can affect the recipient, the graft, or both. These interventions are highly immune suppressive and may alter the course of autoimmune disease independent of the subject receiving an infusion of autologous blood cells. For example, there are no convincing data in persons with autoimmune diseases that bone marrow or immune cells detected post-transplant are derived from cells in the graft. This issue raises questions whether the blood cell infusion should be termed a graft and whether the entire procedure should be termed an autotransplant. Undoubtedly subjects receiving less-intensive pretransplant regimens would recover without a blood cell infusion and no convincing evidence that the post-transplant immune system is derived from cells in the graft. Nevertheless, we will stick with these terms in our subsequent discussion. Importantly, the bottom line is when we consider post-transplant outcomes we are uncertain which component of this complex, multistep procedure, if any, operates.

In allotransplants for autoimmune diseases the objective is complete replacement of the recipient abnormal immune system. This approach has been successful in children with primary immune deficiency disorders some of which are associated with autoimmunity. Allotransplants are less commonly done in young adults with typical autoimmune disorders such as juvenile rheumatoid arthritis because of concerns about transplant-related mortality and long-term complications. Although the concept of replacing the recipient immune system is simple, however, the dynamics of graft-*versus*-host disease, itself associated with autoimmune features, and residual autoimmunity are complex.

Transplant Activity

The first transplants for autoimmune diseases were in the mid-1990s[5–10] and they are now done at more than 250 transplant centers worldwide[5–13]. Allogeneic transplants for autoimmune diseases are relatively uncommon but the rate is increasing; more than 200 are reported to the Center for International Blood and Marrow Research (CIBMTR) and European Blood and Marrow Transplant (EBMT) Group (Figures 56.1 and 56.2) (see Chapter 2). The most common autoimmune diseases treated by autotransplants are multiple sclerosis, systemic sclerosis, systemic lupus erythematosus, and Crohn's disease[14,15]. Other diseases sometimes treated by this approach include diabetes mellitus type 1, juvenile rheumatoid arthritis, autoimmune cytopenias, vasculitis, and others.

Subject Selection and Timing

The question of who should receive an autotransplant for an autoimmune disease and when is complex but critical to evaluating outcomes. The first autotransplants were done in persons with advanced disease failing many prior therapies. However, this strategy is problematic. Most autoimmune diseases begin with an inflammatory phase follow by a phase in which irreversible end-organ damage dominates the clinical picture. Because there are many drugs for autoimmune diseases that have proved effective, it is appropriate to use these before considering an autotransplant. However, waiting until a subject fails many therapies and has advanced disease poses several problems. The most important is irreversible end-organ damage which may have already occurred. A second consequence of this strategy is subjects typically acquire comorbidities some of which are a direct consequence of the disease whereas others are an accumulation of adverse effects of prior therapies. The net result is to substantially decrease the potential benefit of an autotransplant, increase morbidity and possibly mortality, select for subjects least likely to improve, and decrease the pool of potential autotransplant recipients. Transplant physicians are well acquainted with these issues which operate in many or most other transplant settings.

The alternative is to use autotransplants in persons with less advanced disease. However, this approach is also problematic. For example, some subjects will miss the chance to receive

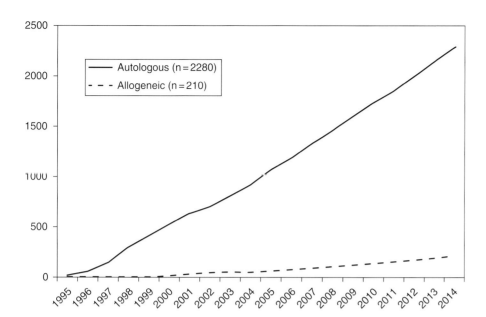

Figure 56.1. Cumulative numbers of auto- and allotransplants for autoimmune diseases reported to the Center for International Blood and Marrow Transplant and European Blood and Marrow Transplant Group.

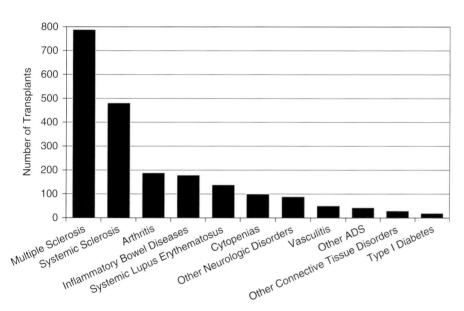

Figure 56.2. Autoimmune diseases treated by autotransplants 1996–2013 reported to the Center for International Blood and Marrow Transplant and European Blood and Marrow Transplant Group. ADs, autoimmune diseases.

drugs proved effective if an autotransplant is done early. But the most important problems are the variable nature of these diseases and our inability to accurately identify subjects with a sufficiently poor short-term prognosis in whom an autotransplant is appropriate. Because of this an early autotransplant strategy mandates doing randomized trials, ideally double-blind and placebo-controlled. These are difficult to do for many reasons. This conundrum of early *versus* late transplants is nothing new to transplant experts or clinical trialists. There is no easy solution.

Limitations

Expertise

Autotransplants for autoimmune diseases require collaboration with specialists from diverse areas not usually part of the transplant team such as rheumatology, neurology, and dermatology. Transplant center expertise is also important. With few exceptions most transplant centers do fewer than one autotransplant for an autoimmune disease per year. This low transplant center activity is associated with higher morbidity and mortality. Other issues differing between typical auto- and allotransplants include variables used for subject selection, pretransplant evaluation, and types of supportive care.

Funding

Health insurance coverage for transplants for autoimmune diseases is heterogeneous and requests are often denied. This lack of coverage, public and private, especially in the United States, results in low activity limiting implementation of clinical trials. This partly explains the fewer transplants in the United States for autoimmune diseases compared with Europe and Latin America. In Brazil, for example, autoimmune diseases such as multiple sclerosis and systemic sclerosis are funded by the federal government.

Considerations

– Autotransplants for autoimmune diseases are a form of intense immune suppression.
– Appropriate subject selection and timing are critical.
– Which elements of the complex, confounded autotransplant scheme are important for favorable outcomes is unknown.
– Randomized, placebo-controlled, double-blind trials are needed to determine efficacy.
– A multidisciplinary team is needed for successful implementation.

Future Directions

There is considerable progress in using autotransplants to treat autoimmune diseases despite the complexities we

discuss. Several randomized trials are in progress or completed and some report favorable results (discussed in Chapter 57). Transplants are increasingly done before there is irreversible end-organ damage. If benefits are convincingly proved in controlled trials it will be important to determine which elements of this complex intervention are effective. For example, is infusion of hematopoietic cells necessary in persons receiving less-intensive pretransplant conditioning regimens? We also need to know to what extent subject selection rather than the transplant procedure determines outcomes. The field of autotransplants for autoimmune diseases is still young and developing. Rigorously designed clinical trials in earlier stage diseases are now needed.

Acknowledgments

Professors D. Farge and M. Badoglio from the EBMT Autoimmune Diseases Working Party kindly provided unpublished data on autotransplant activity.

References

1. Muraro PA, Abrahamsson SV. Resetting autoimmunity in the nervous system: The role of hematopoietic stem cell transplantation. *Curr Opin Investig Drugs*. 2010;11(11):1265–75.

2. Muraro PA, Douek DC, Packer A, Chung K, Guenaga FJ, Cassiani-Ingoni R, et al. Thymic output generates a new and diverse TCR repertoire after autologous stem cell transplantation in multiple sclerosis patients. *J Exp Med*. 2005;201(5):805–16.

3. Arruda LCM, Lorenzi JCC, Sousa APA, Zanette DL, Palma PVB, Panepucci RA, et al. Autologous hematopoietic SCT normalizes miR-16, -155 and -142–3p expression in multiple sclerosis patients. *Bone Marrow Transplant*. 2015;50(3):380–9.

4. Muraro PA, Robins H, Malhotra S, Howell M, Phippard D, Desmarais C, et al. T cell repertoire following autologous stem cell transplantation for multiple sclerosis. *J Clin Invest*. 2014;124(3):1168–72.

5. Euler HH, Marmont AM, Bacigalupo A, Fastenrath S, Dreger P, Hoffknecht M, et al. Early recurrence or persistence of autoimmune diseases after unmanipulated autologous stem cell transplantation. *Blood*. 1996;88(9):3621–5.

6. Burt RK. BMT for severe autoimmune diseases: an idea whose time has come. *Oncology (Williston Park)*. 1997;11(7):1001–14; 17, discussion 18–24.

7. Cooley HM, Snowden JA, Grigg AP, Wicks IP. Outcome of rheumatoid arthritis and psoriasis following autologous stem cell transplantation for hematologic malignancy. *Arthritis Rheum*. 1997;40(9):1712–5.

8. Fassas A, Anagnostopoulos A, Kazis A, Kapinas K, Sakellari I, Kimiskidis V, et al. Peripheral blood stem cell transplantation in the treatment of progressive multiple sclerosis: first results of a pilot study. *Bone Marrow Transplant*. 1997;20(8):631–8.

9. Marmont AM, van Lint MT, Gualandi F, Bacigalupo A. Autologous marrow stem cell transplantation for severe systemic lupus erythematosus of long duration. *Lupus*. 1997;6(6):545–8.

10. Brodsky RA, Petri M, Smith BD, Seifter EJ, Spivak JL, Styler M, et al. Immunoablative high-dose cyclophosphamide without stem-cell rescue for refractory, severe autoimmune disease. *Ann Intern Med*. 1998;129(12):1031–5.

11. Binks M, Passweg JR, Furst D, McSweeney P, Sullivan K, Besenthal C, et al. Phase I/II trial of autologous stem cell transplantation in systemic sclerosis: procedure related mortality and impact on skin disease. *Ann Rheum Dis*. 2001;60(6):577–84.

12. Burt RK, Traynor AE, Cohen B, Karlin KH, Davis FA, Stefoski D, et al. T cell-depleted autologous hematopoietic stem cell transplantation for multiple sclerosis: report on the first three patients. *Bone Marrow Transplant*. 1998;21(6):537–41.

13. McSweeney PA, Nash RA, Sullivan KM, Storek J, Crofford LJ, Dansey R, et al. High-dose immunosuppressive therapy for severe systemic sclerosis: initial outcomes. *Blood*. 2002;100(5):1602–10.

14. Farge D, Labopin M, Tyndall A, Fassas A, Mancardi GL, Van Laar J, et al. Autologous hematopoietic stem cell transplantation (HSCT) for autoimmune diseases: an observational study on 12 years of experience from the European Group for Blood and Marrow Transplantation (EBMT) Working Party on Autoimmune Diseases. *Haematologica*. 2009;95(2):284–92.

15. Pasquini MC, Voltarelli J, Atkins HL, Hamerschlak N, Zhong X, Ahn KW, et al. Transplantation for autoimmune diseases in north and South america: a report of the center for international blood and marrow transplant research. *Biol Blood Marrow Transplant*. 2012;18(10):1471–8.

Chapter

57

Autologous Hematopoietic Cell Transplants for Autoimmune Diseases: Specific Diseases and Controversies

L.C.M. Arruda, M.C. Oliveira, K.C.R. Malmegrim, E. Gluckman, and D. Farge

Introduction

Autologous hematopoietic cell transplantation (auto-HCT) has been intensely investigated as a new therapeutic approach for autoimmune diseases (ADs). Almost 20 years after the first transplant, concise data show that auto-HCT can induce long-term disease stabilization and this new therapeutic approach has been increasingly accepted in several ADs for its combination of safety and efficacy[1–5]. More than 2000 AD patients worldwide (European Blood and Marrow Transplant (EBMT), Center for International Blood and Marrow Research (CIBMTR), Asian registry) have already undergone hematopoietic cell transplantation, mainly autologous, for treatment of AD[3–12], including multiple sclerosis (MS)[13–28], systemic sclerosis (SSc)[29–34], Crohn's disease (CD)[35–39], systemic lupus erythematosus (SLE)[40–44], and type 1 diabetes (T1D)[45–47], among others[3,5,7,8,48].

Preclinical studies[49–55], early case reports[56,57], and phase 1 and 2 clinical studies[5,13,19,20,31–33,35,36,40,45,46,58–60] have determined key points for effective auto-HCT and evidenced the heterogeneity of AD. More recently, randomized phase 2 and 3 clinical trials have demonstrated the superior therapeutic efficacy of auto-HCT *versus* conventional therapies in rapidly progressive SSc [31,34], severe MS[26], and in CD refractory to prior therapy. With time, knowledge on clinical management and on immunologic mechanisms associated with auto-HCT for ADs has evolved into a very pronounced *learning curve*, leading to significant improvements in transplant-related safety and in disease-free survival. In fact, there is a noticeable center effect among the hundreds of auto-HCT already reported, in which centers that are more experienced, with larger patient series, report better outcomes[4,5]. This underscores the importance of having educational events and of creating a network of teaching professionals with both experts in ADs and in hematopoietic cell transplant (HCT) aiming to expand AD transplant activity, yet preserving quality of healthcare[3,61,62]. There is currently little interest of the pharmaceutical companies to participate in such investigations; however transplant interest for ADs has remained concentrated in academic centers[63] (see Chapter 56).

Patient selection has improved in most ADs, and there is a current tendency to include patients at earlier stages of disease, while organ function is still preserved and reversal of lesions still possible. However, inclusions for auto-HCT have been limited by a growing competition from newly released pharmaceutic medications, especially new biologics. Therefore, large randomized trials aiming to compare auto-HCT to the best available conventional therapies have been jeopardized by low patient accrual. Our chapter will complement Chapter 56 and will include an in-depth discussion of indications and current trends as well as controversies surrounding auto-HCT in ADs.

Indications for Auto-HCT in Autoimmune Diseases: Disease Type and Timing of Auto-HCT?

Connective Tissue Diseases

Systemic Sclerosis (SSc) is currently one of the main ADs enrolled for auto-HCT[5,10,12]. In this heterogeneous AD, microvascular lesions, autoantibody formation, and low-grade inflammations are associated with different degrees of skin and internal organ fibrosis, mostly affecting cardiopulmonary, renal, and gastrointestinal functions. This rare disease (prevalence 50–300 per million persons) leads to progressive disability, and severe or rapidly progressive cases are associated with high mortality rates up to 30% at 5 years after diagnosis[64,65]. Indications for auto-HCT have changed since transplant activity first began as patient selection has been proven to directly affect transplant outcomes[5,30,66]. Nowadays transplantation is indicated for patients earlier in the disease course. Research groups have been concerned about the cardiac function of SSc patients[30,66], which may not be detected by conventional methods[62,67] (cardiac echography alone), becoming clinically overt during transplant procedure, under the stress of fluid overload, cyclophosphamide administration, and possible infections[66]. Furthermore, such SSc patients present worse outcomes on long-term follow-up, with shorter disease progression-free survival (PFS)[30]. In fact, the recently published phase 3 randomized, double-blind ASTIS study showed that, although over a 10-year follow-up auto-HCT promoted higher PFS and overall survival (OS) than patients treated with 12 monthly intravenous cyclophosphamide pulses, transplant-related mortality (TRM) reached 10%[34]. These results are partially due to enrolling patients over a very long period of time and to have included patients at times when patient selection was not considered so relevant. As pointed out by Burt *et al.*[67], most of the deaths among patients enrolled for auto-HCT in ASTIS were related to cardiopulmonary dysfunction. To avoid future inclusion of patients with excessive cardiac involvement, a more complete series of evaluations is suggested[30] including cardiac magnetic resonance (MRI) with gadolinium enhancement, right heart catheterization with fluid overload, and 24-hour cardiac rhythm registration (Holter), besides the conventionally used echocardiography and electrocardiography. Updated recommendations are currently under discussion by the Autoimmune Disease Working Party (ADWP) of the EBMT and should be incorporated in the EBMT guidelines for auto-HCT in SSc. There are still no specific criteria to determine cut-off values for these recently instated heart evaluations and they are mainly guided but subjective analyses. Ongoing studies should shortly define more specific parameters.

A second approach aiming to improve auto-HCT outcomes for SSc is to enroll patients with shorter prior disease duration. Current patient inclusion directions determine maximum non-Raynaud's disease duration of 4 years, aiming to select patients in more reversible stages of disease[3]. The recommendation was initially adopted by the randomized phase 3 ASTIS trial. However, after 3 years of patient inclusion in the ASTIS trial, this limit was decreased. Overall, 82% (128 out of 156 subjects) of ASTIS recruited patients had up to 2 years of first non-Raynaud's phenomenon disease duration. However, no difference in patients' outcomes was detected between groups[34].

Systemic Lupus Erythematosus (SLE) patients, although more prevalent in the population (40–50/100000 habitants), are much less frequently enrolled for auto-HCT than SSc. SLE is a heterogeneous chronic AD predominantly affecting females (>85%) where response rates to standard first therapy with the classical NIH regimen or the Eurolupus regimen vary according to extent of visceral involvement, ethnic origin, and socioeconomic profile[68–70]. Even with modern treatments, around 5–15% of patients with SLE evolve towards end-stage disease, and 10–15% die within 10 years[71]. In severe SLE patients, refractory to conventional immunosuppressive therapies, auto-HCT has been shown to achieve sustained clinical remissions in around half of patients with qualitative immunologic changes not seen with other forms of therapy[40–43,72,73]. In this high-risk population, TRM has been significant in multicenter[42,44] (as opposed to single center[40,41]) settings, and highlights the need for careful patient selection and recognition of the intrinsic immune suppression and other risks associated with advanced SLE. Despite the declining TRM over the years[5,12], there is current competition with biologic drugs, especially rituximab, belimumab, and more recently epratuzumab. Patients are frequently referred for auto-HCT with significant delay, when the window of opportunity has already been exceeded due to installation of end-stage organ disease and other irreversible damage.

Arthritis

Rheumatoid Arthritis (RA) was the most frequently transplanted AD in the mid-1990s[74–79]. However, in spite of the low transplant-related toxicity for this disease and high short-term remission rates, most patients reactivate their disease within 6 months to 2 years after auto-HCT[5,74,75,79]. Today, there is little controversy regarding the exceptional indication of auto-HCT for RA patients. Indeed, the high number of available biologic drugs to treat RA deems conventional treatment more effective than auto-HCT. An exception is **juvenile rheumatoid arthritis (JIA),** especially the systemic forms, which have been successfully treated by auto-HCT, with long-term remission of articular and systemic manifestations [80–82].

Neurologic diseases

Multiple Sclerosis (MS) is the most frequent chronic inflammatory demyelinating disease, and also the AD most frequently enrolled for auto-HCT in the last 18 years[5,10]. This is probably due to the high prevalence of MS (1/700 adults), but also because until recent years, very limited therapeutic alternatives were available for these patients. MS may be categorized into relapsing-remitting (RR-MS), primary (PP-MS) or secondary progressive (SP-MS) forms, and a rapidly evolving malignant (or Marburg) form. Various immunomodulators, such as glatiramer-acetate, β-interferon, and fingolimod are used as first-line treatments and second-line treatments include mitoxantrone and various types of monoclonal antibodies (natalizumab). In the beginning of the transplant activity, patients with progressive and relapsing-remitting forms of MS were enrolled for auto-HCT, irrespective of inflammation on MRI or on clinical evaluations. This scenario has changed. Today, auto-HCT is formally indicated for those patients with RR-MS forms or for those with progressive disease having inflammatory lesions on MRI[3,14]. The trend began when researchers noticed significantly better long-term outcomes in patients with lower Expanded Disability Status Scale (EDSS) scores than in those with higher scores [18,59].

Over the years, studies have repeatedly shown that better outcomes after auto-HCT are achieved by RR-MS patients [14,18] than by those with progressive forms of MS who tend to present worse PFS[13,16,22,59,83,84]. Patients with higher levels of accumulated disability present higher mortality and worse neurologic outcomes than those less neurologically disabled[16,19,84]. Patients at a younger age (<40 years old) also tend to perform better after auto-HCT, irrespective of prior disease duration[19,83]. Additionally, the presence of inflammatory lesions on MRI evaluations also correlated with better transplant outcomes[14]. Therefore, current auto-HCT studies tend to preferentially enroll RR-MS patients with

MRI-detected inflammation[14,85]. A study exclusively enrolling RR-MS patients reported PFS of 100% in the 3-year follow-up[13]. A recent update described 145 RR-MS patients evaluated in longer follow-up, with improvement of disability and quality of life scores, besides decreasing of lesion volume on MRI[24]. Similar results were also shown by an interim analysis of an American multicenter study enrolling 25 inflammatory, RR-MS patients, of whom 24 underwent auto-HCT with BEAM plus ATG regimen[25]. Besides a non-EDSS survival curve above 90% in 3 years of follow-up, fall in EDSS scores also showed neurologic improvement after auto-HCT. These studies are important to demonstrate how disability can be reversed when patients are enrolled for transplant early in their disease course, while lesions are still inflammatory. For the progressive forms of MS, however, the presence of inflammation on MRI may become conditional for auto-HCT indication.

Despite successful clinical results, patient recruitment has been localized in a few academic centers worldwide and over time few prospective auto-HCT studies in MS are available. A good example is the ASTIMS study, recently published on behalf of the ADWP of the EBMT as the first phase 2 randomized study on MS patients to be disclosed[26]. Twenty-one MS patients with inflammatory lesions on MRI were randomized into 12 treated with auto-HCT and 9 receiving conventional treatment with mitoxantrone. During 4 years of follow-up, auto-HCT patients had no gadolinium-enhancing lesions and 79% less new lesions besides stabilization of disability (EDSS) compared to the mitoxantrone-treated group (rate ratio = 0.21, P=0.00016). Annual relapse rates were lower in the auto-HCT-treated patients and, at end of follow-up, disease progression was similar between groups. Although this is an important study, ASTIMS faced important problems. First, patient recruitment has been low, due to the competition with new disease-modifying drugs. Second, although very recently published, ASTIMS is already outdated, since mitoxantrone has been replaced by other more effective second-line medications, such as natalizumab and fingolimod, among others. Still, auto-HCT for MS has the appeal of being a single-time treatment, and possibly with lower side effects over time and less overall cost. Moreover, auto-HCT has a higher impact on the quality of life of MS patients, achieving results more pronounced than in those treated with conventional drugs[20,24,26,86].

Other rare autoimmune neurologic disorders, including **neuromyelitis optica (NMO) or Devick disease** (prevalence 1.5/10000) and **chronic idiopathic demyelinating polyneuropathy (CIDP)** (prevalence 2–7.7/100000), have been reported in small series of cases[87–89]. These diseases are less frequently enrolled for transplantation and the absence of guidelines has rendered them susceptible to neurologist referral. Therefore, the main point of debate is whether disease evaluation is optimal in these patients who are most frequently referred for auto-HCT at end-stage disease, when all previous available options have failed. Unfortunately, it may be too late for auto-HCT, due to chronic lesions and irreversible damage. Awareness of the neurologists about successful use of auto-HCT in a few patients and of its potential indication for treatment as a 'clinical option' at an earlier stage of neurologic diseases is warranted to progress in the field[3].

Inflammatory Bowel Disease

Crohn's Disease (CD)s is a chronic inflammatory bowel disease (IBD) with prevalence around 0.1%, affecting both adults and children. Despite immunosuppressive therapies (corticosteroids, thiopurines, methotrexate) and biologics (mainly anti-TNF monoclonal antibodies), some patients fail all available therapies. Surgery in this disease may lead to short bowel syndrome or to a definitive stoma and is not an attractive option. In the subset of CD patients in whom the disease runs an aggressive course with potentially reduced life expectancy[90], auto-HCT has been investigated for the past 15 years[37]. It has been suggested that auto-HCT is superior to best available medical care at 1 year[38], and that at longer follow-up, very few patients benefit from transplantation. However, auto-HCT is considered as third-line treatment, after failing disease-modifying drugs and biologic agents. In our opinion, it is important to identify "high-risk "subjects early in the disease course (who are deemed to fail other therapeutic options) for auto-HCT to reduce morbidity and mortality[90].

Refractory Celiac Disease patients (at high risk of enteropathy-associated T-cell lymphoma) potentially respond, but experience of auto-HCT has been relatively recent and the ADWP recommendation is that patients should only be treated on an IRB/REC (institutional review board/research ethics committee) approved prospective clinical trial[3].

Type 1 Diabetes

Small numbers of type 1 diabetes mellitus (DM1) patients with acute early onset of diseases have been transplanted in South American, European, and Asian centers[45–47,91–93]. The rationale for such an approach is to halt immune-mediated pancreatic β-cell destruction, therefore preserving residual insulin production. Patients were enrolled within 3 months after diagnosis, while still bearing an estimated 20–30% of the original β-cell mass[94]. Ongoing investigations suggest that a key element in DM1 patient recruitment for auto-HCT is time from diagnosis, since it is essential that immune "resetting" (auto-HCT) interventions precede complete destruction of the insulin-producing cells. Initial studies included DM1 patients with up to 6 weeks from diagnosis, with successful rates of 84% of insulin independence after the procedure[45,46]. Recent analyses of 65 patients treated in Chinese and Polish transplant centers, under a similar protocol, evidenced that patients transplanted later after DM1 diagnosis had lower remission rates than those treated earlier after disease onset[47]. Although no cut-off value for the time from diagnosis to transplant was established, six months after diagnosis may be too late for patient enrollment. In addition, suboptimal outcomes with auto-HCT were observed in subjects with a history of keto-acidosis[47,91,92]. To date, indications for auto-HCT in DM1 are short disease duration from diagnosis (less than 6 weeks) and without a history of ketoacidosis.

Controversies in Transplant Procedure: Still Unresolved Questions?

Peripheral Blood Hematopoietic Cells Mobilization: 2 g/m² versus 4 g/m² Intravenous Cyclophosphamide

Few cases of auto-HCT for ADs have been performed using hematopoietic cells from BM, but most of the subjects undergo mobilization via peripheral blood leukapheresis. Association of 2 to 4 g/m² intravenous cyclophosphamide (Cy) to granulocyte colony-stimulating factor (G-CSF) enables the harvesting of higher numbers of peripheral PB hematopoietic cells (PBHC) and decreases the risk of G-CSF-induced AD flair. The higher 4 mg/m²) dose of cyclophosphamide contributes to strengthen the immunoablative potential of the subsequently administered transplant conditioning regimen. There are no specific recommendations concerning Cy doses at mobilization regimen, nor have comparative studies been conducted. Some centers, mostly in North or South America, mobilize with 2 g/m², while others, mostly in Europe, use higher dosages, usually 4 g/m². A retrospective EBMT and Northwestern University (Chicago, Il, USA) study described 174 peripheral blood mobilizations with either G-CSF alone or combined with 2 or 4 g/m² intravenous Cy[95]. Patient mobilization with Cy-containing regimens yielded collection of higher CD34+ counts than G-CSF-only regimens, with a small, but nonsignificant advantage for the 4 g/m²-containing combinations. On the other hand, Cy-including mobilization regimens were more frequently followed by adverse complications, especially infections. A more recent report on DM1 patients described safe and effective mobilization of CD34+ cells after 2 g/m² plus G-CSF-stimulation[96]. In summary, there is no consensus about the ideal PBHC mobilization scheme, which probably must be evaluated case by case and according to the baseline autoimmune disease.

Ex-vivo Graft Selection: Yes or No?

In 2002, Moore et al. reported that CD34+ selection of the graft did not influence safety or outcomes of auto-HCT for RA [74]. However, in the context of RA, a disease highly refractory to auto-HCT, the results from graft selection in this setting may have lost their importance. Since then, a consensus has not yet been achieved, and divergent opinions persist, mainly regarding the risk of disease reactivation in nonmanipulated grafts versus high costs, cell loss, and excessive immunosuppression in cell-selected grafts. Importantly, high rates of viral infections have been frequently reported in auto-HCT with CD34+-selected grafts, mostly herpes zoster, herpes simplex, and Epstein–Barr virus, especially in those associated with in-vivo lymphodepletion[42,97–100].

In 2006, a single North American center reported the outcomes of 50 SLE patients treated with auto-HCT[40]. All had CD34+ selected grafts and were conditioned with Cy+ antithymocyte globulin (ATG). The 5-year OS was 84%, the relapse incidence increased over time, leading to a PFS of 50% at 5 years[40]. Considering that after CD34+ enrichment with the Isolex (Baxter, Chicago, IL, USA) "stem cell separation device," T-cell clones are undetectable in the selected graft [97], we may assume that the relapses originated from residual circulating T-cells that survived the conditioning regimen, rather than from the graft. On the other hand, in an EBMT study where only 10 out of 28 SLE patients had received CD34 +-enriched grafts, the disease-free survival decreased progressively over time, reaching 29% at 5 years post-auto-HCT[42]. In this study, however, only 39% of auto-HCT procedures used Cy+ATG as conditioning regimens and the cell selection devices were different. Although heterogeneity in the data does not allow proper comparisons, rough conclusions indicate that CD34+ selection may decrease SLE reactivations after auto-HCT[42].

Conversely, the EBMT ADWP has recently completed a multicenter nonrandomized retrospective study to compare CD34+ selected versus nonselected auto-HCT for 138 systemic sclerosis subjects[100]. Preliminary data did not show differences in overall- and progression-free survivals, or relapse incidence after auto-HCT, between SSc patients with and without ex-vivo CD34+ selection of PBHC. Conflicting information was provided by a Japanese study presented at the 2014 European League Against Rheumatism (EULAR) conference, reporting higher efficacy, albeit with higher incidence of viral infections, in a group of 11 SSc patients transplanted with CD34+-selected versus 8 nonselected grafts[99].

Collectively, these data do not allow for conclusions, mostly due to the heterogeneity in studies. The results are under the influence of numerous parameters, such as multiple conditioning regimens, different types of disease, and incidence of infections, among others. While well-designed randomized prospective studies are still warranted to settle this issue, it is possible that graft CD34 selection is more important in some diseases than in others.

Conditioning Regimens: What Is Best?

From the practical standpoint, the key to an ideal conditioning regimen is the balance between safety and efficacy. In experimental models, higher intensity conditioning regimens are associated with better clinical outcomes[51–55]. In humans, the same relationship is also observed; however, intensity of the regimen is directly associated with higher transplant-related mortality (TRM) especially with use of total body irradiation (TBI) in AD patients[4,5]. In Europe, early EBMT-EULAR guidelines favored nonmyeloablative conditioning regimen and restricted the use of TBI in subjects undergoing allogeneic transplantation for simultaneous AD and hematologic malignancy[2]. Currently, there is a divergence between the experts who support the more "myeloablative" from those who are using less ablative (albeit more immunosuppressive) regimens for auto-HCT in AD[58,63,101,102]. Conditioning regimens were initially based on the experience of hematologists with autologous and allogeneic transplantation for malignant diseases. In consequence, the first myeloablative approaches led to unexpectedly high rates of transplant-related toxicity with unacceptable TRM for AD patients[59,103,104]. TBI was associated with 100-day mortality of 21% (16% TRM in subjects with systemic sclerosis[103] and with possible impairment of neuronal recovery in severely disabled MS subjects)[59]. In a Brazilian study, more myeloablative combinations of BEAM (carmustine, etoposide, cytarabine, and melphalan) plus horse ATG were also associated with TRM of 7.5% in MS patients, subsequently reduced to zero after transition to Cy + rabbit ATG[21]. Importantly, other factors such as the center experience[5] to deal with ADs and specific tissue sensitivity to the conditioning agent (radiation for brain tissue and lung or kidney in systemic sclerosis)[16] may have contributed to the poor results.

Conditioning regimens are essential to decrease autoreactivity and enable the installation of a new and tolerant immune system, thus enabling immunologic balance. Effective immunoablation is proportional to the intensity of the conditioning regimen and myeloablative schemes are usually associated with higher rates of eradication of autoimmunity. Nevertheless, the intensity of the conditioning regimen is also associated with higher transplant-related toxicity and TRM, especially in patients with severe tissue injuries and previous organ dysfunctions. A prospective EBMT study evaluated 900 subjects with ADs treated under multiple regimens[5]. Although no association between regimen intensity and toxicity was identified, higher transplant mortality rates were observed in visceral-involving diseases, such as in systemic sclerosis and SLE, than in others[5]. The TRM and morbidity depend on the intensity of the conditioning regimen, the expertise of personnel at the transplant center, and general medical condition and functional status of the subject with AD[63].

Auto-HCT Efficacy: Why Does It Vary According to AD Type, Patient Selection, and Center Activity?

In systemic sclerosis subjects, baseline organ dysfunction determines auto-HCT outcomes and may also be influenced by the conditioning regimen. On the European side, it is the consensus that TBI-based combinations should be avoided due to lung toxicity, and most of the transplant centers use cyclophosphamide plus ATG combinations, with or without graft manipulation[2,3]. In the early days of auto-HCT, a North American multicenter study reported high incidence of TRM and toxicity associated with TBI in SSc patients[103]. Acquisition of experience in patient management and installation of lung shielding decreased the incidence of adverse events, as reported in later publications[101].

However, a sensitive debate remains as to whether TBI is safe in these already injured patients[102]. A still ongoing North American multicenter study (SCOT) compares myeloablative TBI-containing regimens with the nontransplant strategy of 12 intravenous monthly boluses of Cy for severe SSc subjects using the same inclusion criteria as the ASTIS trial, and should disclose important information about safety of the procedure (NCT00114530 at www.clinicaltrials.gov).

Another issue to be discussed in SSc is whether high doses of Cy are safe[105]. Scleroderma (i.e. systemic sclerosis) is known to affect heart function leading to arrhythmia, myocardial dysfunctions due to fibrosis, or restrictive pericarditis, frequently subclinical and not detected by conventional echocardiography, but that can become overt during transplant procedure[30,62,66]. In an early phase I-II feasibility French multicenter study, one out of 12 enrolled systemic sclerosis patients had cardiac involvement and received a melphalan based transplant regimen[33]. However, this patient developed fever followed by pneumonia while neutropenic (day +3 after cell infusion) and died four weeks later. Therefore, an ongoing trial aims to evaluate whether high doses of Cy are safe in well selected and nonheart dysfunctional SSc patients or if regimens with fludarabine associated with lower doses of Cy are safer and effective (NCT01445821 at www.clinicaltrials.gov). Recently, a pilot study evaluated the outcomes of six heart-affected systemic sclerosis subjects transplanted under a thiotepa plus reduced-Cy conditioning regimen[106]. Transplant-related toxicity was low, but two patients progressed, with one death, in median follow-up of 19 months. Interestingly, all patients received as implantable cardioverter defibrillator before transplant and in three out of the six patients, abnormal cardiac "discharges" were registered on follow-up, indicating that their cardiac function remained impaired after auto-HCT. A larger prospective trial is currently recruiting patients (www.clinicaltrials.gov; NCT01895244, last accessed in March 2015).

In MS patients treated by auto-HCT, PFS still ranges from 29 to 65%, irrespective of the transplant protocol used [19,22,84,107]. In 2012, an Italian group reported 74 MS patients transplanted under the intermediately myeloablative BEAM + ATG regimen, with low TRM (2.7%), although not negligible[83]. This study showed 66% of PFS over a five-year follow-up, and outcomes of the RR-MS patients were better than those of the secondary progressive MS patients. The same group published a second study evaluating auto-HCT with low-intensity lymphoablative regimen with cyclophosphamide 120mg/kg (Cy120) plus rabbit ATG followed by unmanipulated autologous graft, in 7 RR-MS patients[108]. Although effective, the conditioning treatment was not ablative enough to completely abrogate disease activity, and only two (28%) remained neurologically stable with a follow-up of at least 36 months after auto-HCT. Despite the absence of deaths, high transplant-related toxicity led the authors to conclude that use of less ablative (Cy120 + ATG) regimens do not offer advantages compared to the intermediate-intensity regimens

(BEAM + ATG)[108]. On the other hand, Burt *et al.* favor the use cyclophosphamide 200mg/kg added to serotherapy (ATG, ALG or alemtuzumab), aiming to achieve higher lymphocyte depletion with fewer toxic effects[13]. In Burt study, PFS was 100% after a mean follow-up of 36 months, although 23% of the MS patients experienced relapses after auto-HCT. Such outstanding results may be due to the enrollment of patients in earlier stages of MS highly inflammatory and with low EDSS scores.

In neuromyelitis optica (NMO), the EBMT ADWP recently published a retrospective study of 16 NMO patients treated with auto-HCT[87]. Although TRM was zero and immediate outcomes were successful, most patients relapsed over time and five years after auto-HCT, PFS and relapse-free survival had declined to 48 and 10%, respectively. Similar results are also described by other isolated case reports or case series[23,88]. Higher post-auto-HCT relapse rates in NMO than in MS patients have also been previously underlined [23]. The reasons for such high incidence of disease reactivation after auto-HCT are still unknown. A more recent report of 3 NMO patients, refractory to auto-HCT but successfully treated with subsequent allogeneic HCT leads to conceive that either the conditioning regimen in auto-HCT was insufficiently immunoablative or the "graft-*versus* autoimmunity" effect after allogeneic HCT was determinant for long-term disease control[109]. Another debated approach is to associate rituximab to the conditioning regimen, since NMO is an antibody-mediated disorder. Indeed, recently a case report described resolution of aquaporin-4 antibodies and clinical remission after auto-HCT using a combination of Cy, ATG, and rituximab as conditioning regimen[110]. An ongoing trial estimating to enroll and transplant 10 patients with a rituximab-containing cyclophosphamide plus ATG autologous conditioning regimen should contribute to clarify this question (www.clinicaltrials.org; NCT00787722, last accessed in April 2015).

In SLE, a still debated question is whether the cyclophosphamide and ATG (Cy+ATG) regimen is able to induce prolonged disease remission[40]. Cyclophosphamide is used as conventional treatment for lupus, with high rates of remission [68–70]. Most of the transplant-enrolled SLE patients have previously failed IV or oral cyclophosphamide[44,70]. On the one hand, it feels logical to use high doses of this same drug to achieve disease remission, due to its already tested and usually effective therapeutic mechanism. On the other, perhaps a substitution of cyclophosphamide for another drug with different mechanism of action might be more effective in these Cy-resistant patients. In addition, associating ATG, a T-lymphocyte-depleting drug, may not target the most precise immune components in SLE pathogenesis. Since more intense regimens may further increase transplant-related toxicity, it sounds reasonable to add drugs with disease-specific targets. Therefore, some modifications of the widely used Cy+ATG conditioning for SLE patients are suggested, such as the association of rituximab, alemtuzumab, and other B-lymphocyte depleting schemes[40].

In DM1, although some patients remain insulin-free after several years from auto-HCT, disease reactivation after auto-HCT is still a major concern. In 2007, a Brazilian group reported their initial experience on auto-HCT for DM1 subjects. Twenty-one out of 25 DM1 subjects became insulin-free after transplantation[45,46], but most patients resumed insulin on median follow-up of 67 months, and currently only three patients remain completely and continuously insulin-free (personal communication). In parallel, C-peptide levels, a marker for β-cell function, increased after auto-HCT, remaining above initial values for at least 48 months, and not different from baseline until 60 months. These results indicate that auto-HCT is able to at least temporarily discontinue autoimmune destruction of pancreatic β-cells, and that this effect correlates with clinical outcomes[45,46]. Longer follow-up of the patients will determine if the immunologic intervention mediated by auto-HCT changes the incidence and severity of chronic complications of DM1 in these patients.

In CD, auto-HCT has shown great short-term efficacy in patients with severe and refractory forms, who remain at high-risk for auto-HCT procedure, but CD tends to reactivate over time. In 2010, a center reported their long-term experience with 24 CD patients treated with auto-HCT[36]. Conditioning regimen included Cy 200mg/kg plus rabbit ATG, followed by CD34+ autologous grafts. TRM was zero and there was dramatic improvement of the disease activity indexes shortly after auto-HCT, but relapse-free survival progressively declined to 19% at 5 years after auto-HCT[36]. Similar results were reported by other small studies, with or without graft selection[39,111–113]. A German group reported low remission rates and high incidence of relapses in 12 CD patients transplanted with high-dose cyclophosphamide and CD34+ selected cells, but without any serotherapy[114]. The ongoing EBMT Autologous Stem Cell Transplantation International Crohn's Disease (ASTIC) randomized study compared immediate auto-HCT with best medical care followed by transplantation delayed by 1 year (NCT00297193). The preliminary results in 23 auto-HCT patients and 22 controls showed that auto-HCT did not increase the likelihood of sustained disease remission (a composite primary endpoint that required clinical remission (CDAI ≤150) without corticosteroids or immunosuppressive/biologic drugs for at least the last 3 months with no endoscopic/radiologic evidence of active (erosive) disease anywhere in the GI tract) at 1 year. Only two auto-HCT patients achieved all criteria for sustained disease remission *versus* one control, and one HCT patient died during auto-HCT. A suggested but not proven observation described by most studies is that disease refractoriness decreases after auto-HCT and AD patients tend to respond to drugs that were ineffective before transplant [112,114]. Further evaluations with larger numbers of patients are still required and the ASTIC trial will hopefully contribute to answer the question regarding response to conventional treatment after transplant (NCT00297193).

Strategies to prevent disease reactivation are currently being discussed, including more aggressive conditioning and addition of maintenance therapies, but so far nothing has been proposed.

Outcome Measurements: Can AD Specialists and Hematologists Use the Same Endpoint?

It is a challenge for the AD specialist to detect severe disease subpopulations of patients, predict their poor life expectancy, and indicate auto-HCT. Nevertheless, natural outcomes of AD patients treated under standard care are now well established both in North American and in European prospective large cohorts of AD patients. These figures must be considered when deciding whether auto-HCT should be considered for a AD patient who is refractory to first- or second-line standard therapy according to each AD subtype. In SSc, mortality rates vary widely among different subpopulations of patients with mild to severe disease and predictors of mortality have only recently been identified in Europe with the large prospective European Scleroderma Trials and Research group (EUSTAR) cohort analyses[64,65,105,115–117]. Because SSc is a rare disease, many SSc patients are still diagnosed at a late disease stage at which heart, lung, or kidney fibrosis has already progressed to irreversible visceral damage, which will be a contraindication for auto-HCT. In SSc, mortality rates in patients followed by tertiary centers range from 11.4 to 28.7%[64,65,115]. However, when SSc patients are stratified according to disease severity, mortality rates increase to approximately 30% in patients with more risk factors[65]. In SLE, large North American (NIH), European (Eurolupus), and Chinese cohorts identified subsets of patients with early organ/tissue damage, especially renal and cardiovascular damage, who may reach mortality rates of up to 25% in 10 years[118]. Even for MS, the belief that it is a disease mostly associated with high disability and low quality of life, rather than with poor survival, has become outdated. A study that compared approximately 30000 MS patients to a non-MS cohort using an insurance database showed that survival in MS patients was significantly shortened to a mean of 6 years[119]. In IBD, a meta-analysis including data from 35 publications identified mortality rates of ulcerative colitis and Crohn's disease patients as being 19% and 38% above the general population, respectively[90]. Although some of these reports are outdated due to further improvements in mortality rates, these data show that there is severe AD-related morbidity and that auto-HCT may have a role to play in the treatment of subpopulations of patients with a poor prognosis.

It has been debated whether the tools used to measure patient outcomes are adequate and whether they truly reflect auto-HCT effectiveness and efficacy. Although definitions such as overall survival and non relapse mortality (NMR) at day 100 are very precise and homogeneous among auto-HCT for AD studies, other frequently used endpoints are subject to different interpretation and variability. Such definitions were adopted from the hematologic field, and are somewhat unfamiliar to AD specialists. In the recently published ASTIS

trial for SSc, the primary study endpoint was event-free survival, which involved death from any cause or end-stage organ failure due to impairment of heart, lung, or kidney function [34]. For example, in the ASTIS study, PFS, defined as patients without worsening of skin or visceral function above baseline, was not evaluated, impairing proper comparisons with other similar studies[67]. In MS, PFS may be considered as the amount of time during which the MS patient is either free from disease activity, or from persistent worsening in disability [83,120]. In addition, some studies may define progression as any increase of EDSS, while others will consider that the patient has not progressed until EDSS worsens above baseline levels. More than only a matter of semantics, these variations impose very different interpretations in reported results and may misleadingly determine whether auto-HCT is suitable to treat patients or not. To choose the best endpoints to evaluate transplant outcomes, and that they become homogeneous among studies, is therefore fundamental for the field to advance.

Furthermore, parameters used to measure disease activity are also excessively variable among studies and translate as a lack of consensus among AD specialists in establishing the best markers of activity. In SSc, skin involvement, pulmonary measures, gastrointestinal malabsorption, proteinuria, need for post-auto-HCT treatment, or even autoantibody titers may be used to calculate outcomes. In MS, disease activity may be measured through disability scores (EDSS), clinical relapses, or multiple types of MRI findings. Neurologists debate whether EDSS or the more complex composite scale should be used in the follow-up of transplanted patients. An MS patient, for instance, may present with gadolinium-enhancing lesions on MRI, but no clinical increase in EDSS. Similarly, in DM1, endpoints may range from insulin independency to C-peptide levels. In addition, relapse and progression may be biologically and clinically distinct and a DM1 patient may present increasing C-peptide levels, and yet require high doses of insulin injections. Therefore, clear definitions of relapse and progression must be identified for each autoimmune disease, if possible combining the expertise of both transplant professional and AD specialist.

Post-transplant Complications: How to Decrease the Risk?

Early Events and Complications

Profound immunodepletion is a fundamental step and an expected consequence of auto-HCT. However, it is frequently followed by infections, which may jeopardize patient outcomes and account for most of the transplant-related mortality rates. These infective risks and other risks can be minimized with prophylactic, preemptive, and adequate supportive care strategies. Facilities for treating patients with AD with auto-HCT should be broadly similar to those available for allogeneic HCT practice[3]. During the neutropenic phase of auto-HCT, bacterial and, less frequently, fungal infections prevail. Later, when neutrophil engraftment is already settled, but lymphocyte ontogeny is still ongoing, viral infections are mostly detected. Herpes, cytomegalovirus, and Epstein–Barr virus reactivations have been described, especially in graft-selected transplants[42,98,121]. Deaths due to viral infections have been reported and are a concern to investigators. Adequate pretransplant testing should include screening for CMV, HSV, VZV, EBV, HIV, HTLV1 and HTLV2, hepatitis viruses, and toxoplasmosis in all patients. During hospitalization for the HCT procedure: (a) CMV antibody-positive patients receiving ATG or other serotherapy, or receiving manipulated autografts, are recommended to undergo CMV PCR or antigenemia screening for the first 100 days post-transplant; and (b) EBV antibody-positive patients receiving ATG or other serotherapy, or manipulated autografts are recommended to undergo EBV PCR screening for the first 100 days with active surveillance for post-transplant lymphoproliferative disease (PTLD) according to local practice. All patients should be accommodated in isolation facilities, with appropriate clean air facilities in accordance with the Joint Accreditation Committee-ISCT & EBMT (JACIE) accreditation standards during bone marrow aplasia/severe neutropenia and receive adequate bacterial, fungal, and viral prophylaxis according to local practice in the expert transplant center[3].

However, when adding these potential complications, one must take into account the fact that conventional therapy also leads to a higher incidence of infections. Natalizumab, an immunomodulating drug extensively used in MS treatment, may contribute to JC-virus reactivation and progressive multifocal leukoencephalopathy (PML), the risk increasing with longer duration of the immunosuppressive therapy and viral status of the patient[122]. Similarly, fingolimod may facilitate herpes zoster infections, among other neurologic manifestations, while anti-TNF increases the risk for tuberculosis. In addition, current knowledge and improvements in patient care have ameliorated infection rates after auto-HCT and not so many late complications are observed nowadays. Moreover, lymphodepletion is limited to the initial years after auto-HCT, beyond which infection rate decreases significantly.

Late but Important Complications and Considerations
Impact on Fertility
Loss of fertility has been a matter of concern in auto-HCT, especially in the face of the current tendency to enroll patients in earlier stages of disease and, therefore, at younger ages. On the other hand, pregnancy in AD patients, such as SSC and SLE, poses a high risk both for the mother and the baby, and can favor a flare-up of AD post-delivery. In AD patients treated by auto-HCT, Cy-based regimens are associated with higher post-transplant fertility rates, but other combined agents, including irradiation, may decrease this probability [123,124]. Moreover, as a general rule, younger female patients

tend to preserve fertility at higher rates than older women [123]. The EBMT ADWP has reported a survey on post-auto-HCT pregnancies[125]. Twenty-two out of 324 female patients became pregnant at some time point after auto-HCT, 15 of which (68%) had healthy live births. The study does not enable calculation of fertility rates, since the proportion of women that desired to become pregnant after auto-HCT remains unknown. Nevertheless, it demonstrates that pregnancies are possible after auto-HCT.

In men, fertility after auto-HCT may be evaluated by post-transplant sperm analyses. A small study evaluating fertility in DM1 male subjects showed that the number and motility of spermatozoids decreased significantly after auto-HCT using cyclophosphamide plus ATG regimen[126]. Two years after transplantation, sperm motility and morphology tended to achieve pretransplantation levels. Interestingly, all type 1 diabetes patients already had abnormal sperm motility and morphology before auto-HCT, which worsened further (but transiently) after the procedure. Whether auto-HCT might contribute to normalize sperm function on long-term follow-up is still unknown.

In summary, infertility after auto-HCT for ADs is probably less concerning nowadays than when data were based on transplants for malignant and hematologic indications. Nevertheless, it has not yet been established whether pregnancy increases the risk of baseline disease relapse.

Secondary Malignancies
As patient follow-up increases after auto-HCT, chronic complications such as secondary malignancies emerge as a concern. In 2012, the EBMT reported five patients who developed malignancies among 900 who had been treated with auto-HCT for autoimmune disease indications[127]. However, since most autoimmune disease patients have already been heavily treated with several immunosuppressive regimens, and since the autoimmune disease itself may predispose to development of malignancies, it is difficult to define the exact influence of auto-HCT in this scenario.

Secondary Autoimmune Diseases
Modifications due to the induced immunologic resetting after auto-HCT, in the context of a persisting genetic background, may trigger secondary ADs. A review of the literature evidenced development of ADs after auto-HCT for both hematologic and autoimmune indications[128]. In a different review of AUTO-HCTs for AD as primary indication, the incidence of secondary AD varied from 3.9% to 9.8%, mostly organ-limited[129]. Among those, the largest case series from the ADWP EBMT reported a 9.8% cumulative incidence in the 5-year follow-up among 347 patients who developed at least one secondary AD within 22 (0.6–49) months after auto-HCT [130]. In this study, lupus erythematosus as primary AD and antithymocyte globulin use plus CD34+ graft selection were the main risk factors for secondary AD by multivariate analysis. Moreover, in a type 1 diabetes series of 25 patients,

five patients developed thyroid disorders and one presented with mild SLE after auto-HCT (Malmegrim *et al.*, unpublished data). However, it must be considered that thyroid disorders are naturally more frequent in DM1 subjects and therefore it is difficult to estimate the role of auto-HCT in this incidence. Lymphodepleting agents added to the conditioning regimen have been shown as predisposing factors. In a study including 155 patients, alemtuzumab and ATG were associated with a 16% and 1.9% incidence of secondary autoimmune manifestations, respectively[131].

Mechanistic Studies: How to Assess the Predictors of Response to Auto-HCT?

The rationale for auto-HCT involves nonspecific abrogation of autoreactivity, mainly T- and B-lymphocytes, followed by reconstitution of a more tolerant immune system, in the ideal context that environmental triggering factors will no longer be present and/or effective[132–134]. Indeed, mechanistic studies in different ADs have shown renewal of the immune repertoire and reinstatement of immunoregulatory mechanisms as events associated with successful clinical outcomes[135–139] (Figure 57.1). These mechanisms are synergistic and their relative contribution may depend on the conditioning regimen and on the underlying disease[132–136,140,141].

Immunologic evaluations have followed clinical studies since the early years of auto-HCT for autoimmune diseases, with great progress. Despite increasing rates of success associated with auto-HCT, it is still necessary to improve outcomes, especially progression-free survival. Therefore, it is essential to fully understand the immunologic mechanisms involved with the procedure, as a means to establish more specific and effective strategies of therapeutic intervention.

In 2005, Farge *et al.* reported the first analyses of immunologic mechanisms involved with clinical remission after auto-HCT for SSc[138]. The study was able to show that shortly after auto-HCT, B-cell levels were inversely associated with clinical response to the procedure. Later, other studies also demonstrated reduction of autoreactivity following auto-HCT. In SLE patients, significant inhibition of autoreactive T-cell response against self-peptides was detected, and transplant-induced remission was associated with negativation of pathogenic anti-double-stranded DNA (dsDNA) antibodies [139,142]. In addition, depletion of IL-17 producing mucosal-associated invariant T-cells was described in post-mortem brain tissue from MS patients, for up to 2 years after auto-HCT[143]. These findings were supported by an observation of lower Th17 blood levels in MS patients that responded to transplantation[144]. In CD subjects, toll-like receptor 4 (TLR4)-expressing cell frequencies, as well as tumor necrosis factor-alpha (TNF-α) and interleukin (IL)-10 levels, significantly decreased after auto-HCT[36]. Persistent inversion of the Th2/Th1 ratio was described in SSc patients, up to 3 years post-transplantation[145], and in type 1 diabetes, decreased levels of serum autoantibodies, IL-1, IL-17, and TNF-α were

detected after transplantation[146]. Recently, incomplete immunologic ablation with persistence of islet-specific auto-reactive T-cells was demonstrated after auto-HCT (Malmegrim *et al.*, unpublished data). The frequency of these cells inversely correlated with C-peptide levels and insulin independence.

Besides the decrease in autoreactivity, studies have also demonstrated the emergence of a new immune repertoire after auto-HCT. Alexander *et al.* detected the reconstitution of naïve B-cells within 1 year after transplantation in responsive SLE patients[139]. Additionally, regeneration of thymic-derived FoxP3+ regulatory T-cells and diverse TCR repertoire due to increased thymic-derived naïve T-cell output were also observed in this study. Furthermore, in another study, responsive SSc patients unexpectedly presented lower signal joint T-cell receptor excision circles (sjTREC levels), used for quantification of thymic output[147]. The authors suggested that profound suppression of thymic function might be associated with clinical response. In MS patients, regeneration of a new and diverse TCR ("T-cell receptor") repertoire was described in MS patients at 2 years post-auto-HCT[136]. The authors proposed that *de novo* regeneration of the T-cell compartment, rather than the persisting lymphopenia that followed transplantation, was associated with suppression of the inflammatory activity. A more recent study confirmed these results, showing higher TCR repertoire diversity in MS patients that responded to transplantation than in those that failed to respond[135].

Finally, studies have reported improvement of regulatory mechanisms and of immunologic tolerance after auto-HCT. A pilot study demonstrated effective restoration of regulatory T-cells (Tregs) and of their suppressive function after auto-HCT for SSc patients, possibly contributing to clinical remission[137]. Transient expansion of Tregs was also detected in MS patients at 6 months post-transplantation[143]. Concurrently, frequency of both conventional CD4+CD25highFoxp3 + and unusual TGF-β-producing-CD8+FoxP3+ Tregs was found to be increased in SLE patients who underwent auto-HCT[142]. In CD, clinical remission after transplant correlated with expansion of CD4+CD25bright regulatory T-cells [36]. Similar results were detected in seven patients with refractory CD who were treated with auto-HCT without graft manipulation[111]. Fully responsive patients presented higher Treg counts and lower IFN-gamma and IL-12 levels. In one patient who relapsed after transplant, regulatory T-cell counts decreased while IL-12 and TLR2 expression increased. In type 1 diabetes, up-regulation of fas and fasL pro-apoptotic genes were detected post-auto-HCT, possibly contributing to re-establishment of immunologic tolerance[148]. Finally, in a recent study, expressions of microRNAs and of their target immunoregulatory genes were normalized shortly after auto-HCT for MS, as a possible mechanism to improve tolerance [149].

Collectively, these results demonstrate that auto-HCT favorably modifies the immune balance of autoimmune

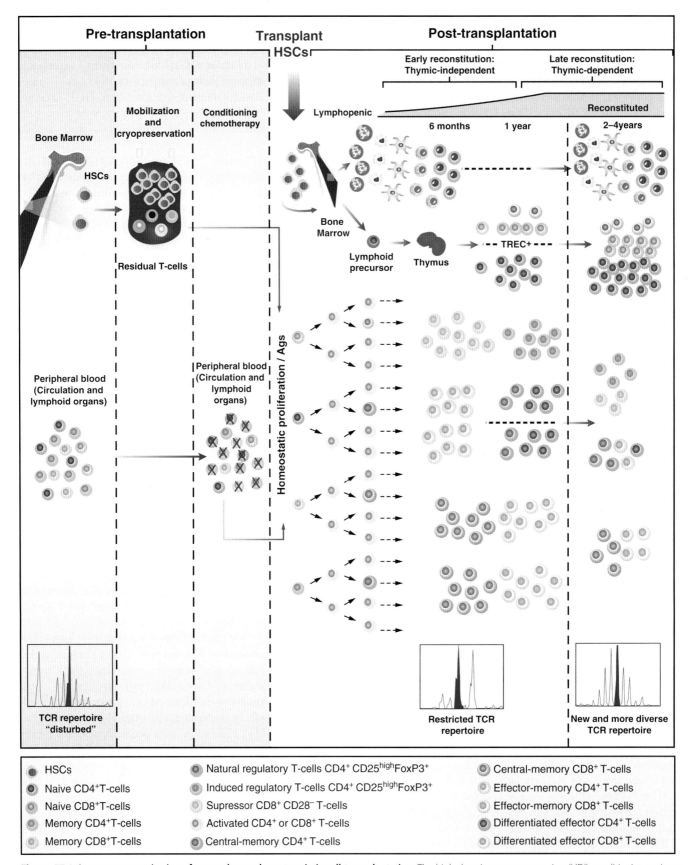

Figure 57.1 Immune reconstitution after autologous hematopoietic cell transplantation. The high-dose immunosuppression (HDI) conditioning regimen promotes intense ablation of the myeloid and lymphoid systems. Infused hematopoietic stem cells (HSCs) migrate to the bone marrow (BM), repopulating the empty space and stimulating the generation of new lymphoid and myeloid precursors. Shortly after auto-HCT, neutrophils, monocytes, eosinophils, dendritic cells, NK cells, and B-cells are rapidly reconstituted in the BM. Lymphoid precursors migrate to the thymus, where they undergo positive and negative selection, generating new naïve T-cells, at this time tolerant to patient auto-antigens. The post-HDI lymphopenic environment triggers homeostatic proliferation and promotes expansion of mature residual T-cells that were not deleted by HDI or that were reinfused with the graft. In these initial periods after transplantation (up to 1–2 years), the early reconstitution is thymic-independent and mainly due to oligoclonal expansion of CD8+ memory T-cells and of CD8+CD28-suppressive T-cells. The CD4/CD8 ratio remains inverted for long-periods. Induced regulatory T-cells (Tregs) are generated by acquisition of FoxP3 expression by conventional CD4+CD25 T-cells. Thymic output of newly generated naïve T-cells begins approximately 1 to 2 years post-transplantation (depending on patient age) and increases with time, determining long-term diversification and renovation of the T-cell repertoire. Along with thymic reactivation, new natural CD4+CD25hiFoxP3+ Tregs are generated, contributing to self-tolerance. Over time, homeostatic proliferation declines, the peripheral blood compartment being replaced by self-tolerant T- and B-cells.

disease patients towards a more tolerant and self-protective profile. Several mechanisms have been identified in this process, such as depletion of autoreactive cells, thymic rebound, epigenetic changes, activation of suppressive pathways, among others (Figure 57.1). Several questions remain, such as how to predict which subsets of patients are at higher risk of relapse, which of the post-transplant mechanisms are more important to warrant prolonged remission, and even what is the duration of these immunologic transplant-induced effects. For the future, taking into account the fact that some of the therapeutic mechanisms of auto-HCT may be disease-specific, investigations should be continued in search of potential biomarkers of response and of strategies to improve efficacy.

Conclusions and Future Directions

In conclusion, auto-HCT should be considered as part of the therapeutic strategies for ADs. While toxicity and relapse rates after auto-HCT are still not negligible, indications stand as second- or third-line therapy in severe AD patients who may lose the chance of recovery when referred too late for auto-HCT. Nevertheless, further understanding of the mechanistic events associated with the auto-HCT process is important to improve clinical outcomes. Time and experience have contributed to establish clinical and biobanking guidelines[3,61] and to improve auto-HCT protocols. Some of these modifications have already afforded lower transplant-related toxicity and better clinical outcomes, and in the future, auto-HCT or other procedures derived from it may become standard approaches for severe autoimmune disorders.

Other cell-based strategies for treatment of ADs have been attempted as a less toxic alternative to auto-HCT. In this setting, mesenchymal cells play a central position, having been investigated in multiple disorders[150–152]. However, available studies provide very heterogeneous and sometimes discordant results, and have poor reproducibility. The effectiveness of such cells is still controversial and not well determined; however safety and low immunogenicity stand as the main advantages. For the future, further investigations and possible minor manipulations, enhancing and extending cell effectiveness through time, may show some benefit in AD treatment. Additionally, other interventions, such as injections of *ex-vivo*-expanded regulatory cells, may be proven effective.

Acknowledgments

We thank Manuela Badoglio, ADWP EBMT study coordinator, for providing the latest activity figures and all members from the ADWP EBMT for their collaboration. We also thank Dr. Marcelo Pasquini and colleagues from the CIBMTR for updating us on stem cell transplant activity for autoimmune disease in the CIBMTR registry.

References

1. Marmont AM. Stem cell transplantation for severe autoimmune diseases: progress and problems. *Haematologica* 1998; 83(8): 733–743.

2. Tyndall A, Gratwohl A. Blood and marrow stem cell transplants in autoimmune disease. A consensus report written on behalf of the European League Against Rheumatism (EULAR) and the European Group for Blood and Marrow Transplantation (EBMT). *Br J Rheumatol* 1997; 36(3): 390–392.

3. Snowden JA, Saccardi R, Allez M, Ardizzone S, Arnold R, Cervera R *et al.* Haematopoietic SCT in severe autoimmune diseases: updated guidelines of the European Group for Blood and Marrow Transplantation. *Bone Marrow Transplant* 2012; 47(6): 770–790. doi: 10.1038/bmt.2011.185

4. Gratwohl A, Passweg J, Bocelli-Tyndall C, Fassas A, van Laar JM, Farge D *et al.* Autologous hematopoietic stem cell transplantation for autoimmune diseases. *Bone Marrow Transplant* 2005; 35(9): 869–879. doi: 10.1038/sj.bmt.1704892

5. Farge D, Labopin M, Tyndall A, Fassas A, Mancardi GL, Van Laar J *et al.* Autologous hematopoietic stem cell transplantation for autoimmune diseases: an observational study on 12 years' experience from the European Group for Blood and Marrow Transplantation Working Party on Autoimmune Diseases. *Haematologica* 2010; 95(2): 284–292. doi: 10.3324/haematol.2009.013458

6. Sun L. Stem cell transplantation: progress in Asia. *Lupus* 2010; 19(12): 1468–1473. doi: 10.1177/0961203310370051

7. Passweg JR, Baldomero H, Peters C, Gaspar HB, Cesaro S, Dreger P *et al.* Hematopoietic SCT in Europe: data and trends in 2012 with special consideration of pediatric transplantation. *Bone Marrow Transplant* 2014; 49(6): 744–750. doi: 10.1038/bmt.2014.55

8. Gratwohl A, Baldomero H, Gratwohl M, Aljurf M, Bouzas LF, Horowitz M *et al.* Quantitative and qualitative differences in use and trends of hematopoietic stem cell transplantation: a Global Observational Study. *Haematologica* 2013; 98(8): 1282–1290. doi: 10.3324/haematol.2012.076349

9. Snowden JA, Pearce RM, Lee J, Kirkland K, Gilleece M, Veys P *et al.* Haematopoietic stem cell transplantation (HSCT) in severe autoimmune diseases: analysis of UK outcomes from the British Society of Blood and Marrow Transplantation (BSBMT) data registry 1997–2009. *Br J Haematol* 2012; 157(6): 742–746. doi: 10.1111/j.1365-2141.2012.09122.x

10. Pasquini MC, Voltarelli J, Atkins HL, Hamerschlak N, Zhong X, Ahn KW *et al.* Transplantation for autoimmune diseases in north and South America: a report of the Center for International Blood and Marrow Transplant Research. *Biol Blood Marrow Transplant* 2012; 18(10): 1471–1478. doi: 10.1016/j.bbmt.2012.06.003

11. Sullivan KM, Muraro P, Tyndall A. Hematopoietic cell transplantation for autoimmune disease: updates from Europe and the United States. *Biol Blood Marrow Transplant* 2010; 16(1 Suppl): S48–56. doi: 10.1016/j.bbmt.2009.10.034

12. Sureda A, Bader P, Cesaro S, Dreger P, Duarte RF, Dufour C *et al.* Indications for allo- and auto-SCT for haematological diseases, solid tumours and immune disorders: current practice

in Europe, 2015. *Bone Marrow Transplant* 2015; 50(8):1037–1056. doi: 10.1038/bmt.2015.6

13. Burt RK, Loh Y, Cohen B, Stefoski D, Stefosky D, Balabanov R et al. Autologous non-myeloablative haemopoietic stem cell transplantation in relapsing-remitting multiple sclerosis: a phase I/II study. *Lancet Neurol* 2009; 8(3): 244–253. doi: 10.1016/S1474-4422(09)70017-1

14. Burt RK, Balabanov R, Voltarelli J, Barreira A, Burman J. Autologous hematopoietic stem cell transplantation for multiple sclerosis – if confused or hesitant, remember: 'treat with standard immune suppressive drugs and if no inflammation, no response'. *Mult Scler* 2012; 18(6): 772–775. doi: 10.1177/1352458512442993

15. Reston JT, Uhl S, Treadwell JR, Nash RA, Schoelles K. Autologous hematopoietic cell transplantation for multiple sclerosis: a systematic review. *Mult Scler* 2011; 17(2): 204–213. doi: 10.1177/1352458510383609

16. Burt RK, Kozak T. Hematopoietic stem cell transplantation for multiple sclerosis: finding equipoise. *Bone Marrow Transplant* 2003; 32 (Suppl 1): S45–48. doi: 10.1038/sj.bmt.1703942

17. Nash RA, Bowen JD, McSweeney PA, Pavletic SZ, Maravilla KR, Park MS et al. High-dose immunosuppressive therapy and autologous peripheral blood stem cell transplantation for severe multiple sclerosis. *Blood* 2003; 102(7): 2364–2372. doi: 10.1182/blood-2002-12-3908

18. Burt RK, Cohen B, Rose J, Petersen F, Oyama Y, Stefoski D et al. Hematopoietic stem cell transplantation for multiple sclerosis. *Arch Neurol* 2005; 62(6): 860–864. doi: 10.1001/archneur.62.6.860

19. Saccardi R, Kozak T, Bocelli-Tyndall C, Fassas A, Kazis A, Havrdova E et al. Autologous stem cell transplantation for progressive multiple sclerosis: update of the European Group for Blood and Marrow Transplantation autoimmune diseases working party database. *Mult Scler* 2006; 12(6): 814–823.

20. Saccardi R, Mancardi GL, Solari A, Bosi A, Bruzzi P, Di Bartolomeo P et al. Autologous HSCT for severe progressive multiple sclerosis in a multicenter trial: impact on disease activity and quality of life. *Blood* 2005; 105(6): 2601–2607. doi: 10.1182/blood-2004-08-3205

21. Hamerschlak N, Rodrigues M, Moraes DA, Oliveira MC, Stracieri AB, Pieroni F et al. Brazilian experience with two conditioning regimens in patients with multiple sclerosis: BEAM/horse ATG and CY/rabbit ATG. *Bone Marrow Transplant* 2010; 45(2): 239–248. doi: 10.1038/bmt.2009.127

22. Krasulová E, Trneny M, Kozák T, Vacková B, Pohlreich D, Kemlink D et al. High-dose immunoablation with autologous haematopoietic stem cell transplantation in aggressive multiple sclerosis: a single centre 10-year experience. *Mult Scler* 2010; 16(6): 685–693. doi: 10.1177/1352458510364538

23. Xu J, Ji BX, Su L, Dong HQ, Sun WL, Wan SG et al. Clinical outcome of autologous peripheral blood stem cell transplantation in opticospinal and conventional forms of secondary progressive multiple sclerosis in a Chinese population. *Ann Hematol* 2011; 90(3): 343–348. doi: 10.1007/s00277-010-1071-5

24. Burt RK, Balabanov R, Han X, Sharrack B, Morgan A, Quigley K et al. Association of nonmyeloablative hematopoietic stem cell transplantation with neurological disability in patients with relapsing-remitting multiple sclerosis. *JAMA* 2015; 313(3): 275–284. doi: 10.1001/jama.2014.17986

25. Nash RA, Hutton GJ, Racke MK, Popat U, Devine SM, Griffith LM et al. High-dose immunosuppressive therapy and autologous hematopoietic cell transplantation for relapsing-remitting multiple sclerosis (HALT-MS): a 3-year interim report. *JAMA Neurol* 2015; 72(2): 159–169. doi: 10.1001/jamaneurol.2014.3780

26. Mancardi GL, Sormani MP, Gualandi F, Saiz A, Carreras E, Merelli E et al. Autologous hematopoietic stem cell transplantation in multiple sclerosis: a phase II trial. *Neurology* 2015; 84(10): 981–988. doi: 10.1212/WNL.0000000000001329

27. Burman J, Iacobaeus E, Svenningsson A, Lycke J, Gunnarsson M, Nilsson P et al. Autologous haematopoietic stem cell transplantation for aggressive multiple sclerosis: the Swedish experience. *J Neurol Neurosurg Psychiatry* 2014; 85(10):1116–1121. doi: 10.1136/jnnp-2013-307207

28. Carreras E, Saiz A, Marín P, Martínez C, Rovira M, Villamor N et al. CD34+ selected autologous peripheral blood stem cell transplantation for multiple sclerosis: report of toxicity and treatment results at one year of follow-up in 15 patients. *Haematologica* 2003; 88(3): 306–314.

29. van Laar JM, Farge D, Tyndall A. Stem cell transplantation: a treatment option for severe systemic sclerosis? *Ann Rheum Dis* 2008; 67 (**Suppl** 3): iii35–38. doi: 10.1136/ard.2008.098384

30. Burt RK, Oliveira MC, Shah SJ, Moraes DA, Simoes B, Gheorghiade M et al. Cardiac involvement and treatment-related mortality after non-myeloablative haemopoietic stem-cell transplantation with unselected autologous peripheral blood for patients with systemic sclerosis: a retrospective analysis. *Lancet* 2013; 381(9872): 1116–1124. doi: 10.1016/S0140-6736(12)62114-X

31. Burt RK, Shah SJ, Dill K, Grant T, Gheorghiade M, Schroeder J et al. Autologous non-myeloablative haemopoietic stem-cell transplantation compared with pulse cyclophosphamide once per month for systemic sclerosis (ASSIST): an open-label, randomised phase 2 trial. *Lancet* 2011; 378(9790): 498–506. doi: 10.1016/S0140-6736(11)60982-3

32. Binks M, Passweg JR, Furst D, McSweeney P, Sullivan K, Besenthal C et al. Phase I/II trial of autologous stem cell transplantation in systemic sclerosis: procedure related mortality and impact on skin disease. *Ann Rheum Dis* 2001; 60(6): 577–584.

33. Farge D, Marolleau JP, Zohar S, Marjanovic Z, Cabane J, Mounier N et al. Autologous bone marrow transplantation in the treatment of refractory systemic sclerosis: early results from a French multicentre phase I-II study. *Br J Haematol* 2002; 119(3): 726–739.

34. van Laar JM, Farge D, Sont JK, Naraghi K, Marjanovic Z, Larghero J et al. Autologous hematopoietic stem cell transplantation vs intravenous pulse cyclophosphamide in diffuse cutaneous systemic sclerosis: a randomized clinical trial. *JAMA* 2014; 311(24): 2490–2498. doi: 10.1001/jama.2014.6368

35. Oyama Y, Craig RM, Traynor AE, Quigley K, Statkute L, Halverson A et al. Autologous hematopoietic stem cell transplantation in patients with refractory Crohn's disease. *Gastroenterology* 2005; 128(3): 552–563.

36. Burt RK, Craig RM, Milanetti F, Quigley K, Gozdziak P, Bucha J et al. Autologous nonmyeloablative hematopoietic stem cell transplantation in patients with severe anti-TNF refractory Crohn disease: long-term follow-up. *Blood* 2010; 116(26): 6123–6132. doi: 10.1182/blood-2010-06-292391

37. Craig RM, Traynor A, Oyama Y, Burt RK. Hematopoietic stem cell transplantation for severe Crohn's disease. *Bone Marrow Transplant* 2003; 32 (Suppl 1): S57–59. doi: 10.1038/sj.bmt.1703945

38. Nash RA, McDonald GB. Crohn disease: remissions but no cure. *Blood* 2010; 116(26): 5790–5791. doi: 10.1182/blood-2010-09-309252

39. Hommes DW, Duijvestein M, Zelinkova Z, Stokkers PC, Ley MH, Stoker J et al. Long-term follow-up of autologous hematopoietic stem cell transplantation for severe refractory Crohn's disease. *J Crohns Colitis* 2011; 5(6): 543–549. doi: 10.1016/j.crohns.2011.05.004

40. Burt RK, Traynor A, Statkute L, Barr WG, Rosa R, Schroeder J et al. Nonmyeloablative hematopoietic stem cell transplantation for systemic lupus erythematosus. *JAMA* 2006; 295(5): 527–535. doi: 10.1001/jama.295.5.527

41. Traynor AE, Schroeder J, Rosa RM, Cheng D, Stefka J, Mujais S et al. Treatment of severe systemic lupus erythematosus with high-dose chemotherapy and haemopoietic stem-cell transplantation: a phase I study. *Lancet* 2000; 356(9231): 701–707. doi: 10.1016/S0140-6736(00)02627-1

42. Alchi B, Jayne D, Labopin M, Demin A, Sergeevicheva V, Alexander T et al. Autologous haematopoietic stem cell transplantation for systemic lupus erythematosus: data from the European Group for Blood and Marrow Transplantation registry. *Lupus* 2013; 22(3): 245–253. doi: 10.1177/0961203312470729

43. Marmont du Haut Champ AM. Hematopoietic stem cell transplantation for systemic lupus erythematosus. *Clin Dev Immunol* 2012; 2012: 380391. doi: 10.1155/2012/380391

44. Illei GG, Cervera R, Burt RK, Doria A, Hiepe F, Jayne D et al. Current state and future directions of autologous hematopoietic stem cell transplantation in systemic lupus erythematosus. *Ann Rheum Dis* 2011; 70(12): 2071–2074. doi: 10.1136/ard.2010.148049

45. Couri CE, Oliveira MC, Stracieri AB, Moraes DA, Pieroni F, Barros GM et al. C-peptide levels and insulin independence following autologous nonmyeloablative hematopoietic stem cell transplantation in newly diagnosed type 1 diabetes mellitus. *JAMA* 2009; 301(15): 1573–1579. doi: 10.1001/jama.2009.470

46. Voltarelli JC, Couri CE, Stracieri AB, Oliveira MC, Moraes DA, Pieroni F et al. Autologous nonmyeloablative hematopoietic stem cell transplantation in newly diagnosed type 1 diabetes mellitus. *JAMA* 2007; 297(14): 1568–1576. doi: 10.1001/jama.297.14.1568

47. D'Addio F, Valderrama Vasquez A, Ben Nasr M, Franek E, Zhu D, Li L et al. Autologous nonmyeloablative hematopoietic stem cell transplantation in new-onset type 1 diabetes: a multicenter analysis. *Diabetes* 2014. doi: 10.2337/db14-0295

48. Burt RK, Loh Y, Pearce W, Beohar N, Barr WG, Craig R et al. Clinical applications of blood-derived and marrow-derived stem cells for nonmalignant diseases. *JAMA* 2008; 299(8): 925–936. doi: 10.1001/jama.299.8.925

49. Ikehara S. Bone marrow transplantation for autoimmune diseases. *Acta Haematol* 1998; 99(3): 116–132. doi: 40826

50. Ikehara S, Good RA, Nakamura T, Sekita K, Inoue S, Oo MM et al. Rationale for bone marrow transplantation in the treatment of autoimmune diseases. *Proc Natl Acad Sci U S A* 1985; 82(8): 2483–2487.

51. van Bekkum DW. Stem cell transplantation for autoimmune disorders. Preclinical experiments. *Best Pract Res Clin Haematol* 2004; 17(2): 201–222. doi: 10.1016/j.beha.2004.04.003

52. van Bekkum DW. Stem cell transplantation in experimental models of autoimmune disease. *J Clin Immunol* 2000; 20(1): 10–16.

53. Van Bekkum DW. Experimental basis for the treatment of autoimmune diseases with autologous hematopoietic stem cell transplantation. *Bone Marrow Transplant* 2003; 32 (Suppl 1): S37–39. doi: 10.1038/sj.bmt.1703941

54. van Bekkum DW. Experimental basis of hematopoietic stem cell transplantation for treatment of autoimmune diseases. *J Leukoc Biol* 2002; 72(4): 609–620.

55. van Bekkum DW. Autologous stem cell transplantation for treatment of autoimmune diseases. *Stem Cells* 1999; 17(3): 172–178. doi: 10.1002/stem.170172

56. Nelson JL, Torrez R, Louie FM, Choe OS, Storb R, Sullivan KM. Pre-existing autoimmune disease in patients with long-term survival after allogeneic bone marrow transplantation. *J Rheumatol Suppl* 1997; 48: 23–29.

57. Marmont AM. Stem cell transplantation for autoimmune disorders. Coincidental autoimmune disease in patients transplanted for conventional indications. *Best Pract Res Clin Haematol* 2004; 17(2): 223–232. doi: 10.1016/j.beha.2004.04.004

58. Burt RK, Traynor AE, Pope R, Schroeder J, Cohen B, Karlin KH et al. Treatment of autoimmune disease by intense immunosuppressive conditioning and autologous hematopoietic stem cell transplantation. *Blood* 1998; 92(10): 3505–3514.

59. Burt RK, Cohen BA, Russell E, Spero K, Joshi A, Oyama Y et al. Hematopoietic stem cell transplantation for progressive multiple sclerosis: failure of a total body irradiation-based conditioning regimen to prevent disease progression in patients with high disability scores. *Blood* 2003; 102(7): 2373–2378. doi: 10.1182/blood-2003-03-0877

60. Tyndall A, Saccardi R. Haematopoietic stem cell transplantation in the treatment of severe autoimmune disease: results from phase I/II studies, prospective randomized trials and future directions. *Clin Exp Immunol* 2005; 141(1): 1–9. doi: 10.1111/j.1365-2249.2005.02806.x

61. Alexander T, Bondanza A, Muraro PA, Greco R, Saccardi R, Daikeler T et al. SCT for severe autoimmune diseases: consensus guidelines of the European Society for Blood and Marrow Transplantation for immune monitoring and biobanking. *Bone*

Marrow Transplant 2015; 50(2):173–80. doi: 10.1038/bmt.2014.251

62. Saccardi R, Tyndall A, Coghlan G, Denton C, Edan G, Emdin M *et al.* Consensus statement concerning cardiotoxicity occurring during haematopoietic stem cell transplantation in the treatment of autoimmune diseases, with special reference to systemic sclerosis and multiple sclerosis. *Bone Marrow Transplant* 2004; 34(10): 877–881. doi: 10.1038/sj.bmt.1704656

63. Illei GG. Hematopoietic stem cell transplantation in autoimmune diseases: is the glass half full or half empty? *Arthritis Rheum* 2006; 54(12): 3730–3734. doi: 10.1002/art.22257

64. Domsic RT, Medsger TA. Connective tissue diseases: Predicting death in SSc: planning and cooperation are needed. *Nat Rev Rheumatol* 2011; 7(11): 628–630. doi: 10.1038/nrrheum.2011.152

65. Fransen J, Popa-Diaconu D, Hesselstrand R, Carreira P, Valentini G, Beretta L *et al.* Clinical prediction of 5-year survival in systemic sclerosis: validation of a simple prognostic model in EUSTAR centres. *Ann Rheum Dis* 2011; 70(10): 1788–1792. doi: 10.1136/ard.2010.144360

66. Burt RK, Shah SJ, Gheorghiade M, Ruderman E, Schroeder J. Hematopoietic stem cell transplantation for systemic sclerosis: if you are confused, remember: "it is a matter of the heart". *J Rheumatol* 2012; 39(2): 206–209. doi: 10.3899/jrheum.111302

67. Burt RK, Oliveira MC, Shah SJ. Cardiac assessment before stem cell transplantation for systemic sclerosis. *JAMA* 2014; 312(17): 1803. doi: 10.1001/jama.2014.12566

68. Houssiau FA, Vasconcelos C, D'Cruz D, Sebastiani GD, Garrido Ed Ede E, Danieli MG *et al.* Immunosuppressive therapy in lupus nephritis: the Euro-Lupus Nephritis Trial, a randomized trial of low-dose *versus* high-dose intravenous cyclophosphamide. *Arthritis Rheum* 2002; 46(8): 2121–2131. doi: 10.1002/art.10461

69. Contreras G, Pardo V, Leclercq B, Lenz O, Tozman E, O'Nan P *et al.* Sequential therapies for proliferative lupus nephritis. *N Engl J Med* 2004; 350(10): 971–980. doi: 10.1056/NEJMoa031855

70. Illei GG, Austin HA, Crane M, Collins L, Gourley MF, Yarboro CH *et al.* Combination therapy with pulse cyclophosphamide plus pulse methylprednisolone improves long-term renal outcome without adding toxicity in patients with lupus nephritis. *Ann Intern Med* 2001; 135(4): 248–257.

71. Doria A, Iaccarino L, Ghirardello A, Zampieri S, Arienti S, Sarzi-Puttini P *et al.* Long-term prognosis and causes of death in systemic lupus erythematosus. *Am J Med* 2006; 119(8): 700–706. doi: 10.1016/j.amjmed.2005.11.034

72. Jayne D, Tyndall A. Autologous stem cell transplantation for systemic lupus erythematosus. *Lupus* 2004; 13(5): 359–365.

73. Traynor AE, Barr WG, Rosa RM, Rodriguez J, Oyama Y, Baker S *et al.* Hematopoietic stem cell transplantation for severe and refractory lupus. Analysis after five years and fifteen patients. *Arthritis Rheum* 2002; 46(11): 2917–2923. doi: 10.1002/art.10594

74. Moore J, Brooks P, Milliken S, Biggs J, Ma D, Handel M *et al.* A pilot randomized trial comparing CD34-selected *versus* unmanipulated hemopoietic stem cell transplantation for severe, refractory rheumatoid arthritis. *Arthritis Rheum* 2002; 46(9): 2301–2309. doi: 10.1002/art.10495

75. Snowden JA, Passweg J, Moore JJ, Milliken S, Cannell P, Van Laar J *et al.* Autologous hemopoietic stem cell transplantation in severe rheumatoid arthritis: a report from the EBMT and ABMTR. *J Rheumatol* 2004; 31(3): 482–488.

76. Snowden JA, Kapoor S, Wilson AG. Stem cell transplantation in rheumatoid arthritis. *Autoimmunity* 2008; 41(8): 625–631. doi: 10.1080/08916930802198550

77. Verburg RJ, Sont JK, van Laar JM. Reduction of joint damage in severe rheumatoid arthritis by high-dose chemotherapy and autologous stem cell transplantation. *Arthritis Rheum* 2005; 52(2): 421–424. doi: 10.1002/art.20859

78. Teng YK, Verburg RJ, Sont JK, van den Hout WB, Breedveld FC, van Laar JM. Long-term followup of health status in patients with severe rheumatoid arthritis after high-dose chemotherapy followed by autologous hematopoietic stem cell transplantation. *Arthritis*

Rheum 2005; 52(8): 2272–2276. doi: 10.1002/art.21219

79. Moore J, Ma D, Will R, Cannell P, Handel M, Milliken S. A phase II study of Rituximab in rheumatoid arthritis patients with recurrent disease following haematopoietic stem cell transplantation. *Bone Marrow Transplant* 2004; 34(3): 241–247. doi: 10.1038/sj.bmt.1704570

80. Roord ST, de Jager W, Boon L, Wulffraat N, Martens A, Prakken B *et al.* Autologous bone marrow transplantation in autoimmune arthritis restores immune homeostasis through CD4+CD25+Foxp3+ regulatory T cells. *Blood* 2008; 111(10): 5233–5241. doi: 10.1182/blood-2007-12-128488

81. Wulffraat NM, de Kleer IM, Prakken B. Refractory juvenile idiopathic arthritis: using autologous stem cell transplantation as a treatment strategy. *Expert Rev Mol Med* 2006; 8(26): 1–11. doi: 10.1017/S1462399406000135

82. Wu Q, Pesenacker AM, Stansfield A, King D, Barge D, Foster HE *et al.* Immunological characteristics and T-cell receptor clonal diversity in children with systemic juvenile idiopathic arthritis undergoing T-cell-depleted autologous stem cell transplantation. *Immunology* 2014; 142(2): 227–236. doi: 10.1111/imm.12245

83. Mancardi GL, Sormani MP, Di Gioia M, Vuolo L, Gualandi F, Amato MP *et al.* Autologous haematopoietic stem cell transplantation with an intermediate intensity conditioning regimen in multiple sclerosis: the Italian multi-centre experience. *Mult Scler* 2012; 18(6): 835–842. doi: 10.1177/1352458511429320

84. Bowen JD, Kraft GH, Wundes A, Guan Q, Maravilla KR, Gooley TA *et al.* Autologous hematopoietic cell transplantation following high-dose immunosuppressive therapy for advanced multiple sclerosis: long-term results. *Bone Marrow Transplant* 2012; 47(7): 946–951. doi: 10.1038/bmt.2011.208

85. Saccardi R, Freedman MS, Sormani MP, Atkins H, Farge D, Griffith LM *et al.* A prospective, randomized, controlled trial of autologous haematopoietic stem cell transplantation for aggressive multiple sclerosis: a position paper. *Mult Scler*

2012; 18(6): 825–834. doi: 10.1177/1352458512438454

86. Phillips JT, Giovannoni G, Lublin FD, O'Connor PW, Polman CH, Willoughby E *et al.* Sustained improvement in Expanded Disability Status Scale as a new efficacy measure of neurological change in multiple sclerosis: treatment effects with natalizumab in patients with relapsing multiple sclerosis. *Mult Scler* 2011; 17(8): 970–979. doi: 10.1177/1352458511399611

87. Greco R, Bondanza A, Oliveira MC, Badoglio M, Burman J, Piehl F *et al.* Autologous hematopoietic stem cell transplantation in neuromyelitis optica: a registry study of the EBMT Autoimmune Diseases Working Party. *Mult Scler* 2015; 21(2): 189–197. doi: 10.1177/1352458514541978

88. Matiello M, Pittock SJ, Porrata L, Weinshenker BG. Failure of autologous hematopoietic stem cell transplantation to prevent relapse of neuromyelitis optica. *Arch Neurol* 2011; 68(7): 953–955. doi: 10.1001/archneurol.2011.38

89. Peng F, Qiu W, Li J, Hu X, Huang R, Lin D *et al.* A preliminary result of treatment of neuromyelitis optica with autologous peripheral hematopoietic stem cell transplantation. *Neurologist* 2010; 16(6): 375–378. doi: 10.1097/NRL.0b013e3181b126e3

90. Bewtra M, Kaiser LM, TenHave T, Lewis JD. Crohn's disease and ulcerative colitis are associated with elevated standardized mortality ratios: a meta-analysis. *Inflamm Bowel Dis* 2013; 19(3): 599–613. doi: 10.1097/MIB.0b013e31827f27ae

91. Gu Y, Gong C, Peng X, Wei L, Su C, Qin M *et al.* Autologous hematopoietic stem cell transplantation and conventional insulin therapy in the treatment of children with newly diagnosed type 1 diabetes: long term follow-up. *Chin Med J (Engl)* 2014; 127(14): 2618–2622.

92. Gu W, Hu J, Wang W, Li L, Tang W, Sun S *et al.* Diabetic ketoacidosis at diagnosis influences complete remission after treatment with hematopoietic stem cell transplantation in adolescents with type 1 diabetes. *Diabetes Care* 2012; 35(7): 1413–1419. doi: 10.2337/dc11-2161

93. Snarski E, Milczarczyk A, Torosian T, Paluszewska M, Urbanowska E, Król M *et al.* Independence of exogenous insulin following immunoablation and stem cell reconstitution in newly diagnosed diabetes type I. *Bone Marrow Transplant* 2011; 46(4): 562–566. doi: 10.1038/bmt.2010.147

94. Notkins AL, Lernmark A. Autoimmune type 1 diabetes: resolved and unresolved issues. *J Clin Invest* 2001; 108(9): 1247–1252. doi: 10.1172/JCI14257

95. Burt RK, Fassas A, Snowden J, van Laar JM, Kozak T, Wulffraat NM *et al.* Collection of hematopoietic stem cells from patients with autoimmune diseases. *Bone Marrow Transplant* 2001; 28(1): 1–12. doi: 10.1038/sj.bmt.1703081

96. De Santis GC, de Pina Almeida Prado B, de Lima Prata K, Brunetta DM, Orellana MD, Palma PV *et al.* Mobilization and harvesting of PBPC in newly diagnosed type 1 diabetes mellitus. *Bone Marrow Transplant* 2012; 47(7): 993–994. doi: 10.1038/bmt.2011.188

97. Dubinsky AN, Burt RK, Martin R, Muraro PA. T-cell clones persisting in the circulation after autologous hematopoietic SCT are undetectable in the peripheral CD34+ selected graft. *Bone Marrow Transplant* 2010; 45(2): 325–331. doi: 10.1038/bmt.2009.139

98. Nash RA, Dansey R, Storek J, Georges GE, Bowen JD, Holmberg LA *et al.* Epstein–Barr virus-associated posttransplantation lymphoproliferative disorder after high-dose immunosuppressive therapy and autologous CD34-selected hematopoietic stem cell transplantation for severe autoimmune diseases. *Biol Blood Marrow Transplant* 2003; 9(9): 583–591.

99. Tsukamoto H, Ayano M, Miyamoto T, Niiro H, Arinobu Y, Akahoshi M *et al.* Comparison of CD34-selected and unmanipulated autologous hematopoietic stem cell transplantation for systemic sclerosis: four-year follow-up results. *EULAR Conference* 2014; 73 (Suppl 2): 96–97.

100. Oliveira M, Labopin M, Henes J, Moore J, Del Papa N, Stanciu S *et al.* Does ex vivo CD34+ cell selection change the outcome of systemic sclerosis patients treated with autologous hematopoietic stem cell transplantation (AHSCT), an ADWP EBMT Study? *ASH Conference* 2014; 124(21).

101. Nash RA, McSweeney PA, Crofford LJ, Abidi M, Chen CS, Godwin JD *et al.* High-dose immunosuppressive therapy and autologous hematopoietic cell transplantation for severe systemic sclerosis: long-term follow-up of the US multicenter pilot study. *Blood* 2007; 110(4): 1388–1396. doi: 10.1182/blood-2007-02-072389

102. Burt RK, Marmont A, Oyama Y, Slavin S, Arnold R, Hiepe F *et al.* Randomized controlled trials of autologous hematopoietic stem cell transplantation for autoimmune diseases: the evolution from myeloablative to lymphoablative transplant regimens. *Arthritis Rheum* 2006; 54(12): 3750–3760. doi: 10.1002/art.22256

103. McSweeney PA, Nash RA, Sullivan KM, Storek J, Crofford LJ, Dansey R *et al.* High-dose immunosuppressive therapy for severe systemic sclerosis: initial outcomes. *Blood* 2002; 100(5): 1602–1610.

104. Openshaw H, Lund BT, Kashyap A, Atkinson R, Sniecinski I, Weiner LP *et al.* Peripheral blood stem cell transplantation in multiple sclerosis with busulfan and cyclophosphamide conditioning: report of toxicity and immunological monitoring. *Biol Blood Marrow Transplant* 2000; 6(5A): 563–575.

105. Nannini C, West CP, Erwin PJ, Matteson EL. Effects of cyclophosphamide on pulmonary function in patients with scleroderma and interstitial lung disease: a systematic review and meta-analysis of randomized controlled trials and observational prospective cohort studies. *Arthritis Res Ther* 2008; 10(5): R124. doi: 10.1186/ar2534

106. Henes JC, Koetter I, Horger M, Schmalzing M, Mueller K, Eick C *et al.* Autologous stem cell transplantation with thiotepa-based conditioning in patients with systemic sclerosis and cardiac manifestations. *Rheumatology (Oxford)* 2014; 53(5): 919–922. doi: 10.1093/rheumatology/ket464

107. Chen B, Zhou M, Ouyang J, Zhou R, Xu J, Zhang Q *et al.* Long-term efficacy of autologous haematopoietic stem cell transplantation in multiple sclerosis at a single institution in China. *Neurol Sci* 2012; 33(4): 881–886. doi: 10.1007/s10072-011-0859-y

108. Curro' D, Vuolo L, Gualandi F, Bacigalupo A, Roccatagliata L, Capello

E *et al.* Low intensity lympho-ablative regimen followed by autologous hematopoietic stem cell transplantation in severe forms of multiple sclerosis: A MRI-based clinical study. *Mult Scler* 2015; 21(11):1423–1430. doi: 10.1177/1352458514564484

109. Greco R, Bondanza A, Vago L, Moiola L, Rossi P, Furlan R *et al.* Allogeneic hematopoietic stem cell transplantation for neuromyelitis optica. *Ann Neurol* 2014; 75(3): 447–453. doi: 10.1002/ana.24079

110. Aouad P, Li J, Arthur C, Burt R, Fernando S, Parratt J. Resolution of aquaporin-4 antibodies in a woman with neuromyelitis optica treated with human autologous stem cell transplant. *J Clin Neurosci* 2015; 22(7): 1215–1217. doi: 10.1016/j.jocn.2015.02.007

111. Clerici M, Cassinotti A, Onida F, Trabattoni D, Annaloro C, Della Volpe A *et al.* Immunomodulatory effects of unselected haematopoietic stem cells autotransplantation in refractory Crohn's disease. *Dig Liver Dis* 2011; 43(12): 946–952. doi: 10.1016/j.dld.2011.07.021

112. Kriván G, Szabó D, Kállay K, Benyó G, Kassa C, Sinkó J *et al.* [Successful autologous haematopoietic stem cell transplantation in severe, therapy-resistant childhood Crohn's disease. Report on the first case in Hungary]. *Orv Hetil* 2014; 155(20): 789–792. doi: 10.1556/OH.2014.29892

113. Kountouras J, Sakellari I, Tsarouchas G, Tsiaousi E, Michael S, Zavos C *et al.* Autologous haematopoietic stem cell transplantation in a patient with refractory Crohn's disease. *J Crohns Colitis* 2011; 5(3): 275–276. doi: 10.1016/j.crohns.2011.03.004

114. Hasselblatt P, Drognitz K, Potthoff K, Bertz H, Kruis W, Schmidt C *et al.* Remission of refractory Crohn's disease by high-dose cyclophosphamide and autologous peripheral blood stem cell transplantation. *Aliment Pharmacol Ther* 2012; 36(8): 725–735. doi: 10.1111/apt.12032

115. Bryan C, Knight C, Black CM, Silman AJ. Prediction of five-year survival following presentation with scleroderma: development of a simple model using three disease factors at first visit. *Arthritis Rheum* 1999; 42(12): 2660–2665. doi: 10.1002/1529-0131 (199912)42:12<2660::AID-ANR23>3.0.CO;2-N

116. Hussein H, Lee P, Chau C, Johnson SR. The effect of male sex on survival in systemic sclerosis. *J Rheumatol* 2014; 41(11): 2193–2200. doi: 10.3899/jrheum.140006

117. Sampaio-Barros PD, Bortoluzzo AB, Marangoni RG, Rocha LF, Del Rio AP, Samara AM *et al.* Survival, causes of death, and prognostic factors in systemic sclerosis: analysis of 947 Brazilian patients. *J Rheumatol* 2012; 39(10): 1971–1978. doi: 10.3899/jrheum.111582

118. Rahman P, Gladman DD, Urowitz MB, Hallett D, Tam LS. Early damage as measured by the SLICC/ACR damage index is a predictor of mortality in systemic lupus erythematosus. *Lupus* 2001; 10(2): 93–96.

119. Kaufman DW, Reshef S, Golub HL, Peucker M, Corwin MJ, Goodin DS *et al.* Survival in commercially insured multiple sclerosis patients and comparator subjects in the U.S. *Mult Scler Relat Disord* 2014; 3(3): 364–371. doi: 10.1016/j.msard.2013.12.003

120. Mancardi G, Saccardi R. Autologous haematopoietic stem-cell transplantation in multiple sclerosis. *Lancet Neurol* 2008; 7(7): 626–636. doi: 10.1016/S1474-4422(08)70138-8

121. Kohno K, Nagafuji K, Tsukamoto H, Horiuchi T, Takase K, Aoki K *et al.* Infectious complications in patients receiving autologous CD34-selected hematopoietic stem cell transplantation for severe autoimmune diseases. *Transpl Infect Dis* 2009; 11(4): 318–323. doi: 10.1111/j.1399-3062.2009.00401.x

122. Bloomgren G, Richman S, Hotermans C, Subramanyam M, Goelz S, Natarajan A *et al.* Risk of natalizumab-associated progressive multifocal leukoencephalopathy. *N Engl J Med* 2012; 366(20): 1870–1880. doi: 10.1056/NEJMoa1107829

123. Pfitzer C, Orawa H, Balcerek M, Langer T, Dirksen U, Keslova P *et al.* Dynamics of fertility impairment and recovery after allogeneic haematopoietic stem cell transplantation in childhood and adolescence: results from a longitudinal study. *J Cancer Res Clin Oncol* 2015; 141(1): 135–142. doi: 10.1007/s00432-014-1781-5

124. Nabhan SK, Bitencourt MA, Duval M, Abecasis M, Dufour C, Boudjedir K *et al.* Fertility recovery and pregnancy after allogeneic hematopoietic stem cell transplantation in Fanconi anemia

patients. *Haematologica* 2010; 95(10): 1783–1787. doi: 10.3324/haematol.2010.023929

125. Snarski E, Snowden JA, Oliveira MC, Simoes B, Badoglio M, Carlson K *et al.* Onset and outcome of pregnancy after autologous haematopoietic SCT (AHSCT) for autoimmune diseases: a retrospective study of the EBMT autoimmune diseases working party (ADWP). *Bone Marrow Transplant* 2015; 50(2): 216–220. doi: 10.1038/bmt.2014.248

126. Leal AM, Oliveira MC, Couri CE, Moraes DA, Stracieri AB, Pieroni F *et al.* Testicular function in patients with type 1 diabetes treated with high-dose CY and autologous hematopoietic SCT. *Bone Marrow Transplant* 2012; 47(3): 467–468. doi: 10.1038/bmt.2011.113

127. Daikeler T, Tichelli A, Passweg J. Complications of autologous hematopoietic stem cell transplantation for patients with autoimmune diseases. *Pediatr Res* 2012; 71(4 Pt 2): 439–444. doi: 10.1038/pr.2011.57

128. Bohgaki T, Atsumi T, Koike T. Autoimmune disease after autologous hematopoietic stem cell transplantation. *Autoimmun Rev* 2008; 7(3): 198–203. doi: 10.1016/j.autrev.2007.11.005

129. Holbro A, Abinun M, Daikeler T. Management of autoimmune diseases after haematopoietic stem cell transplantation. *Br J Haematol* 2012; 157(3): 281–290. doi: 10.1111/j.1365-2141.2012.09070.x

130. Daikeler T, Labopin M, Di Gioia M, Abinun M, Alexander T, Miniati I *et al.* Secondary autoimmune diseases occurring after HSCT for an autoimmune disease: a retrospective study of the EBMT Autoimmune Disease Working Party. *Blood* 2011; 118(6): 1693–1698. doi: 10.1182/blood-2011-02-336156

131. Loh Y, Oyama Y, Statkute L, Quigley K, Yaung K, Gonda E *et al.* Development of a secondary autoimmune disorder after hematopoietic stem cell transplantation for autoimmune diseases: role of conditioning regimen used. *Blood* 2007; 109(6): 2643–2548. doi: 10.1182/blood-2006-07-035766

132. Muraro PA, Douek DC. Renewing the T cell repertoire to arrest autoimmune aggression. *Trends Immunol* 2006; 27(2): 61–67. doi: 10.1016/j.it.2005.12.003

133. Abrahamsson S, Muraro PA. Immune re-education following autologous hematopoietic stem cell transplantation. *Autoimmunity* 2008; 41(8): 577–584. doi: 10.1080/08916930802197081

134. Hügle T, Daikeler T. Stem cell transplantation for autoimmune diseases. *Haematologica* 2010; 95(2): 185–188. doi: 10.3324/haematol.2009.017038

135. Muraro PA, Robins H, Malhotra S, Howell M, Phippard D, Desmarais C et al. T cell repertoire following autologous stem cell transplantation for multiple sclerosis. *J Clin Invest* 2014; 124(3): 1168–1172. doi: 10.1172/JCI71691

136. Muraro PA, Douek DC, Packer A, Chung K, Guenaga FJ, Cassiani-Ingoni R et al. Thymic output generates a new and diverse TCR repertoire after autologous stem cell transplantation in multiple sclerosis patients. *J Exp Med* 2005; 201(5): 805–816. doi: 10.1084/jem.20041679

137. Baraut J, Grigore EI, Jean-Louis F, Khelifa SH, Durand C, Verrecchia F et al. Peripheral blood regulatory T cells in patients with diffuse systemic sclerosis (SSc) before and after autologous hematopoietic SCT: a pilot study. *Bone Marrow Transplant* 2014; 49(3): 349–354. doi: 10.1038/bmt.2013.202

138. Farge D, Henegar C, Carmagnat M, Daneshpouy M, Marjanovic Z, Rabian C et al. Analysis of immune reconstitution after autologous bone marrow transplantation in systemic sclerosis. *Arthritis Rheum* 2005; 52(5): 1555–1563. doi: 10.1002/art.21036

139. Alexander T, Thiel A, Rosen O, Massenkeil G, Sattler A, Kohler S et al. Depletion of autoreactive immunologic memory followed by autologous hematopoietic stem cell transplantation in patients with refractory SLE induces long-term remission through de novo generation of a juvenile and tolerant immune system. *Blood* 2009; 113(1): 214–223. doi: 10.1182/blood-2008-07-168286

140. Li HW, Sykes M. Emerging concepts in haematopoietic cell transplantation. *Nat Rev Immunol* 2012; 12(6): 403–416. doi: 10.1038/nri3226

141. Sykes M, Nikolic B. Treatment of severe autoimmune disease by stem-cell transplantation. *Nature* 2005; 435(7042): 620–627. doi: 10.1038/nature03728

142. Zhang L, Bertucci AM, Ramsey-Goldman R, Burt RK, Datta SK. Regulatory T cell (Treg) subsets return in patients with refractory lupus following stem cell transplantation, and TGF-beta-producing CD8+ Treg cells are associated with immunological remission of lupus. *J Immunol* 2009; 183(10): 6346–6358. doi: 10.4049/jimmunol.0901773

143. Abrahamsson SV, Angelini DF, Dubinsky AN, Morel E, Oh U, Jones JL et al. Non-myeloablative autologous haematopoietic stem cell transplantation expands regulatory cells and depletes IL-17 producing mucosal-associated invariant T cells in multiple sclerosis. *Brain* 2013; 136(Pt 9): 2888–2903. doi: 10.1093/brain/awt182

144. Darlington PJ, Touil T, Doucet JS, Gaucher D, Zeidan J, Gauchat D et al. Diminished Th17 (not Th1) responses underlie multiple sclerosis disease abrogation after hematopoietic stem cell transplantation. *Ann Neurol* 2013; 73(3): 341–354. doi: 10.1002/ana.23784

145. Tsukamoto H, Nagafuji K, Horiuchi T, Mitoma H, Niiro H, Arinobu Y et al. Analysis of immune reconstitution after autologous CD34+ stem/progenitor cell transplantation for systemic sclerosis: predominant reconstitution of Th1 CD4+ T cells. *Rheumatology (Oxford)* 2011; 50(5): 944–952. doi: 10.1093/rheumatology/keq414

146. Li L, Shen S, Ouyang J, Hu Y, Hu L, Cui W et al. Autologous hematopoietic stem cell transplantation modulates immunocompetent cells and improves β-cell function in Chinese patients with new onset of type 1 diabetes. *J Clin Endocrinol Metab* 2012; 97(5): 1729–1736. doi: 10.1210/jc.2011–2188

147. Bohgaki T, Atsumi T, Bohgaki M, Furusaki A, Kondo M, Sato-Matsumura KC et al. Immunological reconstitution after autologous hematopoietic stem cell transplantation in patients with systemic sclerosis: relationship between clinical benefits and intensity of immunosuppression. *J Rheumatol* 2009; 36(6): 1240–1248. doi: 10.3899/jrheum.081025

148. de Oliveira GL, Malmegrim KC, Ferreira AF, Tognon R, Kashima S, Couri CE et al. Up-regulation of fas and fasL pro-apoptotic genes expression in type 1 diabetes patients after autologous haematopoietic stem cell transplantation. *Clin Exp Immunol* 2012; 168(3): 291–302. doi: 10.1111/j.1365–2249.2012.04583.x

149. Arruda LC, Lorenzi JC, Sousa AP, Zanette DL, Palma PV, Panepucci RA et al. Autologous hematopoietic SCT normalizes miR-16, -155 and -142–3p expression in multiple sclerosis patients. *Bone Marrow Transplant* 2014;50:380–389

150. Connick P, Kolappan M, Crawley C, Webber DJ, Patani R, Michell AW et al. Autologous mesenchymal stem cells for the treatment of secondary progressive multiple sclerosis: an open-label phase 2a proof-of-concept study. *Lancet Neurol* 2012; 11(2): 150–156. doi: 10.1016/S1474-4422(11)70305-2

151. Gu F, Wang D, Zhang H, Feng X, Gilkeson GS, Shi S et al. Allogeneic mesenchymal stem cell transplantation for lupus nephritis patients refractory to conventional therapy. *Clin Rheumatol* 2014; 33(11): 1611–1619. doi: 10.1007/s10067-014-2754-4

152. Carlsson PO, Schwarcz E, Korsgren O, Le Blanc K. Preserved β-cell function in type 1 diabetes by mesenchymal stromal cells. *Diabetes* 2015; 64(2): 587–592. doi: 10.2337/db14-0656

551

Chapter

58

Hematopoietic Cell Transplants for Human Immunodeficiency Virus-Related Lymphomas

Amrita Krishnan

Introduction

It has long been recognized that chronically immunosuppressed individuals are at increased risk of malignancy. In the case of HIV-infected individuals, the potential causes for AIDS-related lymphoma (ARL) include chronic antigenic stimulation, decrease in T-cell immunity, an abnormal cytokine milieu, and infection by oncogenic viruses[1]. There is a high rate of association with Epstein–Barr virus (EBV) with *in situ* hybridization studies demonstrating viral DNA present in 50% or more ARL samples[2]. Human herpes virus-8 (HHV8) also plays a pathogenic role in the development of some subtypes of ARL, including primary effusion lymphoma (PEL)[3]. Based upon the discovery of a 60- to 100-fold increased risk of non-Hodgkin lymphoma (NHL) in HIV-infected patients, the diagnostic criteria for AIDS defining illnesses were expanded to include NHL[4]. Following the widespread use of combination antiretroviral therapy (cART), the risk of ARL has fallen by 50%[5]. In addition the subtypes of ARL also have changed significantly with a marked decline in primary CNS lymphoma (PCNSL) but a continued increase in subtypes associated with preserved immunity such as Hodgkin lymphoma (HL)[6].

Treatment and Prognosis of HIV-Associated Non-Hodgkin Lymphomas: Are We Making Progress?

In the era of cART, there has been a shift towards use of standard-intensity regimens for patients with ARL and HL which has resulted in significant improvements in patient outcomes. Gopal *et al.* evaluated a cohort of patients with ARL who were diagnosed between 1996 and 2010. They reported 5-year OS rates of 61.6% for HL, 50.0% for Burkitt lymphoma (BL), 44.1% for diffuse large cell lymphoma (DLBCL), and 22.8% for PCNSL[7]. Survival rates for HIV-infected patients with appropriately controlled HIV and NHL now approach those of non-HIV-infected patients[8]. The most active frontline regimen for HIV-associated DLBCL is infusional dose-adjusted EPOCH-R (etoposide, prednisone, vincristine, cyclophosphamide, doxorubicin, rituximab)[9]. In a trial reported in 2003, 39 patients with ARL (diffuse large cell and Burkitt lymphoma) were treated with dose-adjusted EPOCH-R for six cycles[10]. At a median follow-up of 53

months, OS and PFS rates were 60% and 73%, respectively. Recent efforts have been focused on shortening the number of cycles of chemoimmunotherapy while maintaining high remission rates. The potential efficacy of this approach was seen in a small trial of 33 patients with AIDS-related DLCBL who received a short course of EPOCH with double-dose rituximab (EPOCH-RR)[11]. Patients were treated with three to six cycles of therapy based upon their response on interim FDG PET imaging. Patients received a median of three cycles. Thirty patients (91%) achieved a CR. At a median follow-up of 5 years, OS and PFS were 68% and 84%, respectively. Burkitt lymphoma (BL) remains a challenge in both the HIV-negative and positive patient. Intensive regimens with rituximab used in the HIV-negative patients are also being used in HIV-related Burkitts. These include the hyperCVAD regimen (cyclophosphamide, vincristine, doxorubicin, dexamethasone alternating with high-dose methotrexate/cytarabine), CODOX-M/IVAC[12,13]. These intensive approaches produce 1-year PFS rates of up to 74.1%, but they remain associated with significant toxicity [12]. A potentially less toxic approach for BL is also EPOCH-RR, which appears to be both effective and well tolerated in HIV-infected patients with BL. Dunleavy *et al.* published their experience using EPOCH-RR in 11 patients with HIV BL[10]. There were no treatment-related deaths and at a median follow-up of 73 months, OS was 100% with a PFS of 90%.

Mobilization of Hematopoietic Progenitor Cells (HPC) from HIV-Infected Subjects

The ability for HIV patients to mobilize hematopoietic cells has important implications not only for high-dose chemotherapy trials but also for gene therapy trials which often require a larger number of hematopoietic cells for transduction. Re *et al.* reviewed the outcomes for 155 HIV-infected patients with HL and NHLs[14]. Eighty-six percent of the patients had chemotherapy mobilization while 14% underwent mobilization with G-CSF alone. A total of 113 patients achieved collection goals while 42 failed to mobilize adequately. In a multivariate analysis, predictors of poor mobilization were refractory lymphoma ($P=0.03$) and a CD4+ count less than 237/mm^3 ($P=0.009$). Plerixafor is now being used for poor mobilizers in a similar fashion to the HIV-negative lymphoma patients[15]. In fact in our gene therapy trials, we use "pre-planned" plerixafor rather than "on-demand" plerixafor.

Autologous Transplantation for AIDS-Related Lymphomas

Autologous hematopoietic cell transplant in HIV-positive patients was initially attempted prior to the era of cART, and while the post-transplant course was complicated by multiple opportunistic infections, it demonstrated the feasibility of hematopoietic cell mobilization and successful engraftment in the bone marrow milieu of active viral replication. The first success using autologous transplantation in the setting of HIV infection came in the post-cART era in patients who had lymphoma, and controlled HIV viral load at the time of treatment[16]. However, relapse rates were high, likely reflecting the advanced refractory nature of the lymphoma at the time of transplant. The City of Hope transplant experience with advanced lymphoma and HIV focused on chemosensitive lymphoma patients, i.e., criteria similar to HIV-negative lymphoma patients[17]. In an initial series of 20 NHL and HL patients on cART with viral loads less than 10000 gc/mL by RT PCR, the safety feasibility and efficacy of the procedure was demonstrated. With the exception of one patient who had

delayed engraftment until day 23, timing of engraftment of hematopoietic cells was similar to that seen in HIV-negative patients. At the time of the initial report, the PFS was 85% and OS 81%, with a low TRM and no deaths from opportunistic infection. This experience was updated and evaluated as a case–control analysis of patients with HIV-1-related lymphoma compared to HIV-negative patients with the same lymphoma histologies[18]. The nonrelapse mortality was similar between groups and 2-year DFS and OS were similar at 75% (Figure 58.1)[18].

These results, i.e., similar outcome post-transplant regardless of HIV status, were confirmed in another retrospective case–control study comparing 53 HIV-infected lymphoma patients with negative controls adjusted for histology, IPI, and disease status at transplant. The OS was 61% in the HIV group *versus* 70% in the HIV-negative cohort, respectively[19]. In addition, an European Blood and Marrow Transplant (EBMT) retrospective multicenter experience with 68 high-risk patients with HIV and lymphoma in first CR at 20 institutions reported a PFS of 56% after autologous HCT, which was similar to the US studies[20]. Table 58.1[21] summarizes the largest series of autologous HCT trials for HIV lymphoma. Most recently the US intergroup BMT CTN (blood and marrow clinical trials network) confirmed the high PFS and low transplant related mortality of this autologous transplant approach[22].

Influence of Autologous HCT on HIV Replication: Increase, Decrease, or No Effect?

An area of study that remains is the effect of the apheresis and conditioning regimen on the HIV-1 reservoir. Cillo *et al.* performed a retrospective analysis of pre-and post-transplant plasma specimens on HIV lymphoma patients who received high-dose chemotherapy[23]. The patients had no detectable HIV levels in the blood by conventional assays. Single-copy-sensitive assays for HIV RNA and DNA as a surrogate measure of the HIV-1 reservoir were performed. Nine of the 10 patients were found to have detectable HIV-1 DNA. The transplant recipients were likely "re-infected" with endogenous virus under cover of cART, possibly from the apheresis product or from the endogenous reservoir. The conclusion was that the

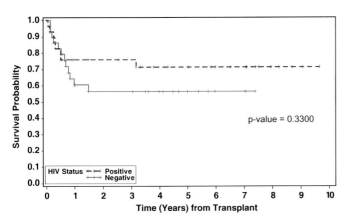

Figure 58.1 Probability of disease-free survival by HIV status. Reproduced with permission from reference[18].

Table 58.1 Autologous transplant trials for HIV lymphomas

References	Patient number	Conditioning regimens	PFS (%)	Time to follow-up
Gabarre *et al.* 2004[46]	14	BEAM/Cy TBI/ other	29	49 months
Krishnan *et al.* 2005[17]	29	Cy/VP16/TBI	76	24 months
Spitzer *et al.* 2008[25]	20	Bu/Cy	50	23 weeks
Re *et al.* 2009[20]	27	BEAM	76	24 months
Balsalobre *et al.* 2009[47]	68	Not reported	56	32 months
Diez-Martin *et al.* 2009[19]	53	BEAM	61	30 months

Adapted from Forman S, Negrin R, Appelbaum F, Antin J, eds. *Thomas' Hematopoietic Cell Transplantation*, 5th ed. Hoboken, NJ, Wiley-Blackwell, 2014.

high-dose "myeloablative" chemotherapy, followed by cART, did not have a substantive effect on the HIV-1 reservoir, thus suggesting that dose-intense cytoreductive therapy by itself was not sufficient to eliminate HIV-1 infection.

Immunologic Recovery after Transplant

A number of the studies detailed above demonstrate that patients may have spikes in HIV viral load post-HCT [16,24,25]. This may in part be due to the difficulty of consistently administering cART during the peritransplant period. In our original series 11 of 20 patients could not take antiretrovirals during the transplant due to nausea or mucositis. Despite this, T-cell reconstitution post-transplant is comparable to that of noninfected patients if patients are able to resume antiretrovirals early post-transplant. CD8+ cells may recover numerically 2 months post-HCT; CD4+ T-cells frequently fail to reach normal levels, even by 12 months and recovery of naïve CD4+ T-cells may be quite delayed. Even among HIV-negative patients there is evidence of qualitative abnormalities of T-cell reconstitution that may persist up to 1 year post-transplant[26] (see Chapter 22). An important component of immunologic reconstitution following autologous HCT is thymic maturation of T-cells, during which excision of circular fragments of DNA occur, which can serve as markers of the rate of T-cell development. These are termed T-cell excision circles, or TRECS, and they may serve as markers of T-cell recovery following immunosuppressive or myeloablative therapy[27].

Simonelli and colleagues prospectively assessed immunologic recovery post-transplant in both HIV-infected and noninfected patients[28]. Both groups were similar in regards to histologic subtypes, number of prior regimens, and disease status at transplant. There was no difference in pre-HCT CD4+ T-cell counts or TREC levels counts between the groups. The groups only differed in that HIV-infected patients had a higher CD8+ cell count prior to transplant ($P=0.004$) and therefore had a lower CD4+/CD8+ ratio ($P<0.001$). There was a nadir in CD4+ T-cell counts following HCT, which took approximately 24 months to recover, when the HIV-infected and noninfected groups reached 58% and 47% of their pretransplant values, respectively. TREC recovery was comparable between the two groups with both groups achieving higher than baseline levels by 12 months. Other series have shown similar patterns of T-cell recovery post-transplant in HIV-infected patients[29,30].

Allogeneic Transplantation in Subjects with HIV: The "Ideal" Donor and Recipient

Solid organ transplantation paved the way for allogeneic hematopoietic cell transplant in the HIV-infected patients. It demonstrated that continued immunosuppression was possible in the already immunodeficient host. The so-called "Berlin patient" subsequently showed the potential of the -allogeneic hematopoietic approach when a HIV-positive

leukemia patient received hematopoietic cells from a donor who was homozygous for a constitutional deletion of the CCR5 receptor. This rendered the patient functionally cured of his HIV infection[31]. Now with over 6 years of follow-up the patient remains with no detectable virus off cART[32].

A summary of the allogeneic experience in patients with HIV and malignancy including 14 case reports and small trials of allogeneic HCT were reviewed by Hütter and Zaia who reported an OS of approximately 50%[33]. Gupta et al. in a review of the Center for International Blood and Marrow Transplant Research (CIBMTR) data reported that four of the nine patients transplanted in the cART era remained alive at a median follow-up of 59 months[34]. Not surprisingly the survival of patients transplanted prior to the use of antiretrovirals was dismal.

The "Berlin case" (discussed above) put the spotlight on hematopoietic cell transplantation. However, the reproducibility of this experience is highly limited. The gene mutation referred to as the CCR5 Δ32 allele is found in up to 16% of people of northern European descent and is encountered far less frequently in individuals of Asian and African descent[35]. Approximately 1% of the Caucasian population is homozygous for this gene. In the case of the Berlin patient, he was fortunate to have multiple HLA-matched donor choices and an ethnic background with a higher incidence of the mutation, leading to the identification of a donor with this mutation.

Could similar results be achieved with a heterozygous CCR5 delta 32 donor? This would potentially increase the donor pool. Investigators in Boston treated two patients with HIV infection for relapsed HL and DLBCL, respectively. Both patients underwent allogeneic transplant on cART and received grafts from CCR5 wild-type donors. Patients were evaluated for persistence of HIV using PCR quantification of HIV DNA and two long terminal repeat (LTR) circles. While HIV was detected in peripheral blood mononuclear cells prior to transplant and up to 3 months post-HCT, subsequent follow-up to 3.5 years post-transplant did not demonstrate evidence of detectable HIV. This loss of detectable HIV-1 correlated with full donor chimerism, development of graft-versus-host disease, and decreases in HIV-specific antibody levels. The investigators raised the question as to whether the transplant procedure may have led to a sustained reduction in the HIV-1 reservoir. However, both patients demonstrated detectable HIV at 12 and 32 weeks, respectively, following cessation of cART[36].

A formal intergroup trial is being conducted by the Blood and Marrow Clinical Trials Network (BMT CTN), NCT01410344. This trial will study allogeneic transplantation under a variety of conditioning regimens in HIV-positive patients. Important endpoints beyond toxicity will include microbial translocation, and impact of conditioning on viral reservoirs. However, even if this approach shows long-term control of the virus and depletion of the viral reservoir, the transplant-related mortality and risks of graft-versus-host disease limit the widespread applicability of this approach.

Another potential approach to identifying donor sources with natural HIV resistance utilizes umbilical cord blood cells. Studies conducted initially at the City of Hope by Zaia and Rossi demonstrated that cord blood units could be identified that are either heterozygous or homozygous for the CCR5 deletion[37]. To date, no successful transplant has shown that this would lead to cure of HIV infection, similar to the "Berlin patient", but a pediatric patient with relapsed ALL was transplanted at the University of Minnesota with cord blood identified to be CCR5 double mutant; due to complications, the patient did not survive long enough to determine the impact of the donor graft on the HIV infection[38].

Gene Therapy: Rationale and Clinical Trials

Alternately genetic modification of autologous hematopoietic cells circumvents the issues of identifying suitable donors, avoids the risks of graft-*versus*-host disease, and given the far lower morbidity of autologous transplantation allows a more viable approach to hematopoietic cell therapy for HIV-1.

A large phase 2 trial of genetically modified autologous hematopoietic cells, infused cells without conditioning therapy, but follow-up demonstrated only minimal detection of gene-marked cells in peripheral blood as well as lack of significant effect on HIV-1 levels[39]. The study did utilize analytical treatment interruption (ATI) of cART to more accurately assess the effects of the genetically modified cells on the HIV infection. There were no long-term deleterious effects of the ATI in regards to infection or hematologic parameters and thus this approach set the platform for future trials as a way to demonstrate efficacy of the modified hematopoietic cells.

At City of Hope, we tested a myeloablative conditioning regimen as we felt this would be the best milieu to allow maximal engraftment of genetically modified autologous hematopoietic cells. However, the challenge was also to identify suitable patients for whom myeloablation could be justified. The lymphoma population was a justifiable group given the poor long-term survival of patients with relapsed HIV lymphoma. Our pilot trial treated four relapsed HIV-1 positive NHL patients with hematopoietic cells transduced with a lentivirus encoding three anti-HIV-1 RNAs, namely TAR, siRNA to tat/rev, and a ribozyme targeting CCR5[40]. High-dose CBV (cyclophosphamide, BCNU, VP16) chemotherapy was used for conditioning, the modified cells were infused, and 24 hours later unmodified cells were infused. There were no serious adverse events associated with the infusion of genetically modified cells, but, similar to the Mitsuyasu study, levels of gene marking were low at 0.35%[41,42]. This was surmised to be due in part to competition with the much higher levels of unmodified hematopoietic cells that were infused.

The success of gene therapy is likely contingent upon high levels of only genetically modified hematopoietic cells being infused or post-transplant *in-vivo* selection of the protected cells. Ultimately, the "proof is in the pudding", i.e., the test of this method will be in the true target population, those with

HIV and no malignancy. Initial trials are being done using nonmyeloablative conditioning with infusion of maximal doses of only genetically modified cells in patients in remission from HIV-1-related NHL. The rationale for this is that these patients have already been exposed to chemotherapy risks and hence the addition of nonmyeloablative conditioning beyond their NHL chemotherapy would not significantly increase the risk already incurred from chemotherapy. Infusion of only genetically modified hematopoietic cells could be justified in the nonmyeloablative setting since early or late graft failure in this setting would not have the same devastating consequences as following ablative chemotherapy. A pilot trial using busulfan at nonmyeloablative doses in first remission of HIV-1-positive NHL patients is open at City of Hope (NCT01961063; www.clinicaltrials.gov).

The choice of busulfan was solely to facilitate engraftment as it is not considered an antilymphoma therapy. Its efficacy has been demonstrated in previous clinical trials in human genetic diseases, especially in the pediatric populations using solely gene-modified hematopoietic cells. In this regard, in adenosine deaminase-deficient children, busulfan was first used at 2 mg/kg intravenously for 2 days followed by infusion of CD34+ transduced bone marrow cells[43]. Subsequently, AUC-based dosing by Candotti *et al.* demonstrating doses ranging from 65 to 90 mg/m^2 (equivalent to ~4 mg/kg) achieved an AUC in the range of 4000–4800 mU*min and was associated with engraftment[44]. Toxicity was mild with transient neutropenia, mild thrombocytopenia, and transient elevated liver enzymes. The final step for the HIV-1 trials is to use this AUC targeted busulfan-based conditioning in HIV-1 infected patients without malignancy. Such a trial is planned at City of Hope and will use this nonmyeloablative conditioning followed by infusion of a CCR5-negative product edited by a zinc finger nuclease.

The zinc finger nuclease construct has already been successfully tested with reinfusion of autologous T-lymphocytes [45]. Limitations of cell number have been one of the challenges of using CD34+ selected cells and thus T-lymphocytes are attractive targets for gene therapy and they can be expanded to large numbers *in-vitro*. Targeting mature T-lymphocytes for gene therapy has the added advantage that the effect of the therapeutic gene can be rapidly monitored for effects on cell survival, viral load, and other parameters. Zinc finger nucleases combine the DNA recognition specificity of zinc finger proteins with the strong enzymatic activity of the cleavage domain of the restriction enzyme FokI. The T-cell trial included 12 patients who had chronic aviremic HIV-1 infection and had infusion of the CCR5-negative ZFN-edited T-cell product without any conditioning[45]. Patients in cohort 1 (n=6) underwent a 12-week analytic treatment interruption (ATI) of cART beginning 4 weeks after the T-cell infusion. HIV-1 viral load was undetectable at the start of ATI and became detectable in four of the six patients at 2–4 weeks after cessation of cART. There was a decline of CD4+ counts during ATI, however the decline in CCR5-modified cells (1.81 cells/day) was significantly less than the unmodified cells (7.25 cells/day). There was one serious adverse event associated with the cell infusion which was attributed to a transfusion reaction. This trial sets the platform for ZFN-editing of cells as a feasible and well-tolerated approach that may lead to in-vivo resistance to HIV-1 of these CCR5 edited cells. The planned trial of ZFN-1-modified hematopoietic cells in conjunction with nonmyeloablative busulfan conditioning in selected HIV-1-positive immune nonresponders may be the ultimate proof-of-principle of this concept.

References

1. E. C. Breen, Hussain S. K., Magpantay L., *et al.* B-cell stimulatory cytokines and markers of immune activation are elevated several years prior to the diagnosis of systemic AIDS-associated non-Hodgkin B-cell lymphoma. *Cancer Epidemiol Biomarkers Prev* 2011; 20: 1303–14.

2. D. Shibata, Weiss L. M., Hernandez A. M., Nathwani B. N., Bernstein L., Levine A. M. Epstein–Barr virus-associated non-Hodgkin's lymphoma in patients infected with the human immunodeficiency virus. *Blood* 1993; 81: 2102–9.

3. S. H. Swerdlow, International Agency for Research on Cancer, World Health Organization. *WHO Classification of Tumours of Haematopoietic and Lymphoid Tissues*, 4th ed. Lyon, France, International Agency for Research on Cancer, 2008.

4. Centers for Disease Control. Revision of the CDC surveillance case definition for acquired immunodeficiency syndrome. Council of State and Territorial Epidemiologists; AIDS Program, Center for Infectious Diseases. *MMWR Morb Mortal Wkly Rep* 1987; 36: 1S–15S.

5. R. F. Little, Dunleavy K. Update on the treatment of HIV-associated hematologic malignancies. *Hematology Am Soc Hematol Educ Program* 2013; 2013: 382–8.

6. N. Martis, Mounier N. Hodgkin lymphoma in patients with HIV infection: a review. *Curr Hematol Malig Rep* 2012; 7: 228–34.

7. S. Gopal, Patel M. R., Yanik E. L., *et al.* Temporal trends in presentation and survival for HIV-associated lymphoma in the antiretroviral therapy era. *J Natl Cancer Inst* 2013; 105: 1221–9.

8. K. Dunleavy, Wilson W. H. Implications of the shifting pathobiology of AIDS-related lymphoma. *J Natl Cancer Inst* 2013; 105: 1170–1.

9. K. Dunleavy, Wilson W. H. How I treat HIV-associated lymphoma. *Blood* 2012; 119: 3245–55.

10. K. Dunleavy, Pittaluga S., Shovlin M., *et al.* Low-intensity therapy in adults with Burkitt's lymphoma. *N Engl J Med* 2013; 369: 1915–25.

11. K. Dunleavy, Little R. F., Pittaluga S., *et al.* The role of tumor histogenesis, FDG-PET, and short-course EPOCH with dose-dense rituximab (SC-EPOCH-RR) in HIV-associated diffuse large B-cell lymphoma. *Blood* 2010; 115: 3017–24.

12. B. Xicoy, Ribera J. M., Muller M., *et al.* Dose-intensive chemotherapy including rituximab is highly effective but toxic in human immunodeficiency virus-infected patients with Burkitt lymphoma/leukemia: parallel study of 81 patients. *Leuk Lymphoma* 2014; 55(10): 2341–8.

13. A. Noy, Kaplan L., Lee J. Y. A modified dose intensive R-CODOX-M/IVAC for HIV-associated Burkitt and atypical Burkitt lymphoma(BL) demonstrates high cure rates and low toxicity: prospective multicenter phase II trial of the AIDS Malignancy Consortium (AMC 048). *Blood* 2013; 122: 2.

14. A. Re, Cattaneo C., Skert C., *et al.* Stem cell mobilization in HIV seropositive patients with lymphoma. *Haematologica* 2013; 98: 1762–8.

15. I. Attolico, Pavone V., Ostuni A., *et al.* Plerixafor added to chemotherapy plus G-CSF is safe and allows adequate PBSC collection in predicted poor mobilizer patients with multiple myeloma or lymphoma. *Biol Blood Marrow Transplant* 2012; 18: 241–9.

16. J. Gabarre, Azar N., Autran B., Katlama C., Leblond V. High-dose therapy and autologous haematopoietic stem-cell transplantation for HIV-1-associated lymphoma. *Lancet* 2000; 355: 1071–2.

17. A. Krishnan, Molina A., Zaia J., *et al.* Durable remissions with autologous stem cell transplantation for high-risk HIV-associated lymphomas. *Blood* 2005; 105: 874–8.

18. A. Krishnan, Palmer J. M., Zaia J. A., Tsai N. C., Alvarnas J., Forman S. J. HIV status does not affect the outcome of autologous stem cell transplantation (ASCT) for non-Hodgkin lymphoma (NHL). *Biol Blood Marrow Transplant* 2010; 16: 1302–8.

19. J. L. Diez-Martin, Balsalobre P., Re A., *et al.* Comparable survival between HIV + and HIV– non-Hodgkin and Hodgkin lymphoma patients undergoing autologous peripheral blood stem cell transplantation. *Blood* 2009; 113: 6011–4.

20. A. Re, Michieli M., Casari S., *et al.* High-dose therapy and autologous peripheral blood stem cell transplantation as salvage treatment for AIDS-related lymphoma: long-term results of the Italian Cooperative Group on AIDS and Tumors (GICAT) study with analysis of prognostic factors. *Blood* 2009; 114: 1306–13.

21. J. Zaia, Krishnan A., Rossi J. Hematopoietic cell transplantation for patients with human immunodeficiency virus infection. In: *Thomas' Hematopoietic Cell Transplantation.* Hoboken, NJ, Wiley-Blackwell, 2008: p. 1001.

22. J.C. Alvarnas, Le Rademacher J., Wang, Y., *et al.* Autologous hematopoietic cell transplantation for HIV-related lymphoma. *Blood* 2016; 128:1050–8.

23. A. R. Cillo, Krishnan A., Mitsuyasu R. T., *et al.* Plasma viremia and cellular HIV-1 DNA persist despite autologous hematopoietic stem cell transplantation for HIV-related lymphoma. *J Acquir Immune Defic Syndr* 2013; 63: 438–41.

24. D. Serrano, Carrion R., Balsalobre P., *et al.* HIV-associated lymphoma successfully treated with peripheral blood stem cell transplantation. *Exp Hematol* 2005; 33: 487–94.

25. T. R. Spitzer, Ambinder R. F., Lee J. Y., *et al.* Dose-reduced busulfan, cyclophosphamide, and autologous stem cell transplantation for human immunodeficiency virus-associated lymphoma: AIDS Malignancy Consortium study 020. *Biol Blood Marrow Transplant* 2008; 14: 59–66.

26. P. A. Te Boekhorst, Lamers C. H., Schipperus M. R., *et al.* T-lymphocyte reconstitution following rigorously

T-cell-depleted *versus* unmodified autologous stem cell transplants. *Bone Marrow Transplant* 2006; 37: 763–72.

27. C. Pratesi, Simonelli C., Zanussi S., *et al.* Recent thymic emigrants in lymphoma patients with and without human immunodeficiency virus infection candidates for autologous peripheral stem cell transplantation. *Clin Exp Immunol* 2008; 151: 101–9.

28. C. Simonelli, Zanussi S., Pratesi C., *et al.* Immune recovery after autologous stem cell transplantation is not different for HIV-infected *versus* HIV-uninfected patients with relapsed or refractory lymphoma. *Clin Infect Dis* 2010; 50: 1672–9.

29. T. Benicchi, Ghidini C., Re A., *et al.* T-cell immune reconstitution after hematopoietic stem cell transplantation for HIV-associated lymphoma. *Transplantation* 2005; 80: 673–82.

30. S. Resino, Perez A., Seoane E., *et al.* Short communication: Immune reconstitution after autologous peripheral blood stem cell transplantation in HIV-infected patients: might be better than expected? *AIDS Res Hum Retroviruses* 2007; 23: 543–8.

31. G. Hutter, Nowak D., Mossner M., *et al.* Long-term control of HIV by CCR5 Delta32/Delta32 stem-cell transplantation. *N Engl J Med* 2009; 360: 692–8.

32. K. Allers, Hutter G., Hofmann J., *et al.* Evidence for the cure of HIV infection by CCR5Delta32/Delta32 stem cell transplantation. *Blood* 2011; 117: 2791–9.

33. G. Hutter, Zaia J. A. Allogeneic haematopoietic stem cell transplantation in patients with human immunodeficiency virus: the experiences of more than 25 years. *Clin Exp Immunol* 2011; 163: 284–95.

34. V. Gupta, Tomblyn M., Pedersen T. L., *et al.* Allogeneic hematopoietic cell transplantation in human immunodeficiency virus-positive patients with hematologic disorders: a report from the center for international blood and marrow transplant research. *Biol Blood Marrow Transplant* 2009; 15: 864–71.

35. J. Novembre, Galvani A. P., Slatkin M. The geographic spread of the CCR5 Delta32 HIV-resistance allele. *PLoS Biol* 2005; 3: e339.

36. R. Sanchez, Wills S., Young S. HIV returns in two patients after bone marrow transplant. CNN. December 9, 2013; Sect. Health. http://www.cnn.com/2013/12/07/health/hiv-patients/ (accessed July 29, 2014).

37. L. D. Petz, Redei I., Bryson Y., *et al.* Hematopoietic cell transplantation with cord blood for cure of HIV infections. *Biol Blood Marrow Transplant* 2013; 19: 393–7.

38. G. Gonzalez, Park S., Chen D., Armitage S., Shpall E., Behringer R. Identification and frequency of CCR5Delta32/Delta32 HIV-resistant cord blood units from Houston area hospitals. *HIV Med* 2011; 12: 481–6.

39. R. T. Mitsuyasu, Merigan T. C., Carr A., *et al.* Phase 2 gene therapy trial of an anti-HIV ribozyme in autologous CD34+ cells. *Nat Med* 2009; 15: 285–92.

40. D. L. DiGiusto, Krishnan A., Li L., *et al.* RNA-based gene therapy for HIV with lentiviral vector-modified CD34(+) cells in patients undergoing transplantation for AIDS-related lymphoma. *Sci Transl Med* 2010; 2: 36ra43.

41. D. L. DiGiusto, Stan R., Krishnan A., Li H., Rossi J. J., Zaia J. A. Development of hematopoietic stem cell based gene therapy for HIV-1 infection: considerations for proof of concept studies and translation to standard medical practice. *Viruses* 2013; 5: 2898–919.

42. A. Y. Krishnan, Zaia J. A., Rossi J. J., *et al.* Autologous stem cell transplantation (ASCT) for AIDS-related lymphomas (ARL) and the potential role of HIV-resistant stem cells. *Blood* 2006; 108: Abstract 491a.

43. A. Aiuti, Slavin S., Aker M., *et al.* Correction of ADA-SCID by stem cell gene therapy combined with nonmyeloablative conditioning. *Science* 2002; 296: 2410–3.

44. F. Candotti, Shaw K. L., Muul L., *et al.* Gene therapy for adenosine deaminase-deficient severe combined immune deficiency: clinical comparison of retroviral vectors and treatment plans. *Blood* 2012; 120: 3635–46.

45. P. Tebas, Stein D., Tang W. W., *et al.* Gene editing of CCR5 in autologous CD4 T cells of persons infected with HIV. *N Engl J Med* 2014; 370: 901–10.

46. J. Gabarre, Marcelin A. G., Azar N., *et al.* High-dose therapy plus autologous hematopoietic stem cell transplantation for human immunodeficiency virus (HIV)-related lymphoma: results and impact on HIV disease. *Haematologica* 2004; 89: 1100–8.

47. P. Balsalobre, Diez-Martin J. L., Re A., *et al.* Autologous stem-cell transplantation in patients with HIV-related lymphoma. *J Clin Oncol* 2009; 27: 2192–8.

Chapter

59

Human Leukocyte Antigen-Haplotype Mismatch Transplants: Overcoming Major Genetic Barriers

Andrea Bacigalupo and Franco Aversa

Graft Manipulation in HLA-haplotype Mismatched Transplant

For many years, relevant obstacles to a wide use of human leukocyte antigen (HLA)-haplotype mismatch family donors have been represented by graft-*versus*-host disease (GvHD) and graft rejection, mediated by donor and host alloreactive T-cell responses, respectively. In particular, in this context of great immune genetic disparity between patient and donor, although mature donor T-cells present in the graft facilitate T-cell reconstitution, they are responsible for the occurrence of GvHD, which impairs a patient's immune reconstitution. Strategies to prevent GvHD after HLA-haplotype mismatch transplant based on either pharmacologic immunosuppression or T cell depletion (TCD) of the graft have been developed over time. In particular, a milestone in the history of haplotype mismatch transplant was the demonstration that an efficient TCD of the graft is able to prevent both acute and chronic GvHD even when using a related donor differing at the three major HLA loci. The other major breakthrough in the field of HLA-haplotype mismatch transplant was the use of "megadoses" of G-CSF-mobilized peripheral blood donor hematopoietic progenitor cells (HPCs). Indeed, the infusion of huge numbers of hematopoietic progenitors has been shown in the experimental model to be able to overcome the barrier of HLA incompatibility in the donor/recipient pair and to elude the residual (after the conditioning regimen) antidonor cytotoxic T-lymphocyte activity from the recipient side.

The first successful haplotype mismatch transplants were carried out in the early 1980s in severe combined immunodeficiency (SCID) patients, in whom host *versus* graft (HvG) reactivity is minimal, allowing the study of GvH prevention[1]. TCD initially combined soybean agglutinin (SBA) and E-rosetting with sheep red blood cells, and was able to prevent GvHD in the absence of any additional post-transplant GvHD prophylaxis[1]. This approach has been successfully implemented over the years in hundreds of SCID patients with a very long follow-up, demonstrating an impressive cure rate, especially in patients receiving the transplant within the first year after birth[2]. In contrast, the first series of leukemia patients who subsequently received TCD HLA-haplotype mismatch transplants, exhibited a high rate of graft rejection[3].

In immune-competent hosts (as opposed to SCID patients), resistance to engraftment is mediated by recipient antidonor cytotoxic T-lymphocyte precursors (CTLp) which survive the standard conditioning regimens. With TCD grafts, the balance between competing host and donor T-cells shifts in favor of the host, resulting in unopposed HvG reaction[3]. The breakthrough came with the clinical use of a graft containing a "megadose" of TCD HPCs, a principle that Reisner and co-workers successfully pioneered in animal models[4,5]. *In-vitro* studies showed that cells within the human CD34+ cell population exhibit "veto" activity favoring engraftment, i.e., "CD34+ cells" from the donor exhert a veto effect by specifically neutralizing host CTLp responsible for graft failure[6]. Furthermore, early myeloid CD33+ cells, which rapidly expand after engraftment, are also endowed with marked "veto" activity, which is not found in late myeloid cells expressing CD14 or CD11b[7].

The "Megadose" of CD34+ Cells with TCD: Data with MAC Regimens

After a "myeloablative" conditioning (MAC) regimen (sTBI, thiotepa, ATG, and, after 1995, fludarabine instead of the original cyclophosphamide), the infusion of ≥ 10 million CD34+ cells/kg with a very low T-cell content ($\leq 1 \times 10^4$ CD3$^+$ cells/kg) ensured primary engraftment in 95% of patients with acute leukemia in the original experience of Perugia[8,9]. With the fludarabine-based conditioning regimen and the positive selection of the CD34+ cells, both rejection and GvHD were prevented even in the absence of any further post-transplant immunosuppression[9,10]. Despite the absence of GvHD in these high-risk leukemia patients, the leukemia relapse rate was 18% in acute myeloid leukemia (AML) and 30% in acute lymphoid leukemia (ALL) patients who were transplanted in any complete remission (CR)[11]. The high-dose MAC regimen may have compensated for the lack of T-cell mediated graft-*versus*-leukemia (GvL) effect and, in the absence of post-transplant immunosuppression, the few T-cells in the graft may have exerted a subclinical GvL/GvHD effect. Furthermore, in AML, donor-*versus*-recipient NK alloreactivity[12–14] prevented relapse. In an updated analysis of 154 patients with AML, transplantation from NK-alloreactive donors was associated with a significantly lower relapse rate (7% *versus* 36%) (*P=0.02*) and better survival (59% *versus* 33%, *P=0.05*) [11]. Therefore, given this evidence, donor-*versus*-recipient NK alloreactivity should be exploited when selecting the optimal graft from among the mismatched family members. Apart from the NK alloreactivity, 43% of AML and 30% of ALL patients who were in any CR at transplant survive event-free with a maximum follow-up of 20 years. Although patients with chemoresistant relapse at the time of transplant had poor outcomes, disease-free survival (DFS) for AML was 18%. Finally, all long-term survivors enjoy an excellent quality of life with no chronic GvHD[11]. An European Blood and Marrow Transplant (EBMT) retrospective study reported similar results with 48% DFS in AML patients in first CR[15].

Natural Killer Cells and Killer Cell Immunoglobulin-Like Receptors

Human NK cell function is regulated by a balance between activating and inhibitory receptors[14,16,17] (see Chapter 63). Clonally distributed inhibitory receptors termed "killer cell immunoglobulin-like receptors" (KIRs) recognize human leukocyte antigen (HLA) class I allele groups ("KIR ligands"): HLA-C alleles with a Lys80 residue ("Group 2" alleles), HLA-C with an Asn80 residue ("Group 1" alleles), and HLA-B alleles sharing the Bw4 specificity. All KIR genes are randomly expressed and KIR distribution varies on NK cells. Only NK cells which express inhibitory KIRs for "self HLA ligands" become "licensed/educated"[16,18]. When educated NK cells with a single inhibitory KIR confront allogeneic targets, that do not express an HLA ligand for that KIR, the NK cells sense the missing expression of their inhibitory ligand and mediate alloreactions ("missing self" recognition). Combined evidence from *in-vitro* studies, murine models, and clinical trials indicated the ability of NK cells to mediate donor-*versus*-recipient alloreactivity rested on "missing self recognition"[12,13,18]. In HLA-haplotype mismatch transplants, engrafted progenitor cells give rise to an NK cell repertoire of donor origin which included alloreactive clones, capable of killing the recipient's cryopreserved leukemic cells[12–14,19]. Thus, these donor-derived NK cells are "licensed and educated" by donor HLA antigens, within the bone marrow microenvironment. This process shapes their repertoire to be both donor-tolerant and recipient alloreactive. They are, therefore, enabled to recognize, and react to, missing self on recipient targets[12–14,18]. The same educational process can be observed in HLA-mismatched unrelated donor transplants[20].

Post-Transplant Imunologic Reconstitution

One major problem, at least in adults, which appears to be common to all TCD transplants, is the slow recovery of the antimicrobial and antiviral responses (see Chapter 30). Because of the minimal number of residual T-lymphocytes in the graft, and because of *in-vivo* ATG-linked T-cell depletion (TCD), post-transplant immunologic reconstitution is delayed, exposing haplo-transplant recipients to life-threatening opportunistic infections for several months[3,8–11]. In a study of 255 patients, the overall transplant-related nonrelapse mortality (TRM) was 36% for 145 patients in CR at transplant and 58% for 110 patients transplanted in relapse[10,11]. To reduce TRM, several groups are focusing on rebuilding post-transplant immunity, in order to improve clinical outcomes and to separate GvHD from favorable donor immune responses[11]. Adoptive immune therapies have been explored with pathogen-specific T-lymphocytes or broad repertoire T-cells that were depleted of alloreactive T-cells or engineered with a suicide gene.

Perruccio *et al.* generated T-cell clones specific for *Aspergillus* or CMV antigens, screened them for cross-reactivity against recipient alloantigens, and infused the nonalloreactive clones soon after HCT[21]. CMV reactivation and *Aspergillus* galactomannan antigenemia disappeared over time, while the frequencies of anti-*Aspergillus*- and anti-CMV-specific T-cell clones increased. Pathogen-specific T-cells persisted over time, did not cause GvHD, and were associated with control of *Aspergillus* and CMV antigenemia and infectious mortality (see Chapter 64). In another study, CMV-specific T-cells were generated by *ex-vivo* stimulation with CMV pp65 and infused to control refractory CMV viremia or disease after HLA-MVD or HLA-haplotype mismatch transplant[22]. Similar approaches were used to prevent or control adenovirus or Epstein–Barr virus infections[23–25]. Photodepletion of donor-*versus*-recipient alloreactive T-lymphocytes in a mixed lymphocyte reaction using dibromorhodamine (TH9402) efficiently eliminates alloreactivity[26–28]. In a phase 1 clinical trial, grade II acute GvHD developed in 4 of 19 patients and extensive chronic GvHD in 5 patients. Immunologic reconstitution was dose-dependent as infection and TRM rates improved with the highest T-cell doses[28]. Although effective, such approaches are time consuming and labor intensive and thus not broadly applicable.

For adoptive transfer of T-cells with a wide T-cell receptor repertoire, polyclonal donor T-cells were engineered to express suicide genes, e.g., the herpes simplex thymidine kinase (HSV-TK) gene, to guarantee lysis of engineered T-cells in case they triggered GvHD[29]. Most of the patients who received TK-engineered T-cell add-back after HLA-haplotype mismatch transplant obtained a rapid and broad immune reconstitution, protective against pathogens, and apparently benefited from a low rate of infection-related mortality[30]. Although TK-engineered T-cell engraftment appeared necessary and sufficient to promote a robust T-cell recovery, the immune reconstitution was progressively enriched by T-lymphocytes negative for transgene expression and retroviral integration[29–31]. Vago *et al.* reported that donor-derived transgene-negative T-cells, observed in TK007, were enriched for recent thymic emigrants, denoting their *de novo* generation in the host thymus[32]. These data indicate that immune reconstitution after TK-cell infusion is supported by a thymic-dependent pathway and results in the maturation and differentiation of donor hematopoietic precursors in the recipient thymus. The low incidence of GvHD observed in the absence of any pharmacologic immunosuppressive treatment suggests that the high numbers of T-cells circulating in these patients had achieved central tolerance in the patient thymus, with negative selection of host-reactive cells. This was also confirmed by the fact that the activation of the suicide gene machinery, sufficient to control GvHD, did not affect immune reconstitution (see Chapter 22).

From Positive Selection to Negative Depletion: Why?

More recently, negative selection of peripheral blood progenitor cells has been used instead of CD34+ cell immunoselection with the aim of reducing TRM. In contrast to CD34+ selection, in negative selection other immune components, such as NK cells, dendritic cells and monocytes, are not lost during the separation procedure and may be used to generate antileukemic, antiviral or graft-facilitating effects. Infusing CD3+/CD19 + depleted HLA-haplotype mismatch transplant in children with acute leukemia after a conditioning that included fludarabine, thiotepa, melphalan, and OKT-3 or ATG, primary engraftment was achieved in 88% of patients, acute GvHD grade II and III–IV occurred in 20% and 7%, and chronic GvHD in 21%. The TRM was 8% at 1 year and 20% at 5 years[33,34]. The EFS at 3 years was: 25% (whole group), 46% (any CR, first HCT) *versus* 8% (active disease) and 20% (no first HCT, any disease status). A concern with this approach of negative selection is the higher incidence of GvHD in comparison with the CD34+ selection. In addition, using CD3+/CD19+ depletion techniques, gamma/delta T-cell receptors (TcRγδ) on T-cells are also eliminated, despite not being involved in classic GvHD. Subsequently, in an innovative approach, the Handgretinger's group depleted the leukapheresis product of only TcR alpha/beta + (αβ+) cells, thus retaining large numbers of effector cells such as TcRγδ+ T-cells and NK cells[35–37]. TcRγδ+ T-cells combine conventional adaptive features with direct, rapid responses against sterile stresses and a variety of pathogens[38]. Furthermore TcRγδ+ T-cells appear to exert antileukemic activity since they directly recognized stress-induced self antigens expressed by malignant cells. They are not expected to initiate GvHD since they do not recognize specific processed peptide antigens as presented on major histocompability complex (MHC) molecules. To remove TcRαβ+ T-cells a biotinylated anti-TcR αβ antibody was employed, followed by an antibiotin antibody conjugated to magnetic microbeads. CD19+ B-lymphocytes were also immuno-depleted to prevent post-transplant EBV-associated lymphoproliferative disorders (see Chapter 20) [36,37]. Recovery of CD34+ cells (74%) was similar to CD34 + enrichment procedures. In Tubingen, children with advanced acute leukemia were transplanted with TcRαβ+/CD19+ depleted grafts following chemotherapy-based conditioning[37]. Locatelli *et al.* in Rome employed the same

method for graft processing and a TBI-based conditioning regimen[39]. In both cohorts no post-transplant GvHD prophylaxis was given, although anti-T antibodies (OKT3 or ATG) in the conditioning regimen exerted additional *in-vivo* TCD of the inoculum. Very rapid full donor-type engraftment occurred in all patients. Few had acute grade I and II GvHD and no patient developed chronic GvHD, confirming that TcRγδ+ T-cells do not cause GvHD. Immune reconstitution was rapid in these children. A longer follow-up and more patients are required to assess the post-transplant relapse rate. This novel graft manipulation strategy has also been tested in 23 children with nonmalignant disorders undergoing HLA-haplotype mismatch transplant[40]. With no post-transplantation pharmacologic prophylaxis for GvHD, three patients experienced skin-only grade I to II acute GvHD. No cases of visceral acute or chronic GvHD was observed. The 2-year probability of DFS is 91.1%[40].

Negative Selection in Adults

To determine whether the post-transplant immunologic reconstitution can be improved even in adult patients, this approach has been recently tested in 16 patients with high-risk acute leukemia (12 AML, 4 ALL)[41,42]. Median age was 45 years (range 19–65), nine were in CR and seven in chemoresistant relapse. Conditioning consisted of ATG (Thymoglobulin, Sanofi Genzyen, France) (1.5mg/kg from day −13 to day −10), treosulfan (12g/m^2 from day −9 to −7), fludarabine (30mg/m^2 from day −6 to −2), and thiotepa (5mg/kg on days −5 and −4). No immune suppression was given after transplantation as GvHD prophylaxis; no G-CSF was administered post-transplantation. All but one patient, who required a second graft from the same donor to boost hematopoietic reconstitution, achieved a full donor sustained engraftment. Tending to confirm the working hypothesis, there was a rapid, sustained increase in peripheral blood T-cell subpopulations. CD4+ and CD8+ cell counts reached a median of 200/μL on days 45 (range 19–98) and 38 (range 13–69), respectively. Naïve and memory T-cell subsets increased significantly over the first year after transplantation. B-cell reconstitution was rapid and sustained and immunoglobulin serum levels normalized within 3 months. Two patients had skin grade I/II acute GvHD, one grade III–IV. No patient has so far developed moderate to severe chronic GvHD. The CMV reactivation occurred in only two cases; both were successfully treated with ganciclovir. No patient had EBV-related PTLD and no invasive fungal disease occurred. Relapse was the main cause of failure (6/7) for patients transplanted with active disease. On the other hand, of the nine patients who were in any CR at transplant, one died from acute GvHD, one from leukemia relapse, and seven survived disease-free at a median follow-up of 7 months (range 5–18).

Regulatory T-Cells (Tregs)

In the search for an alternative strategy to improve immune recovery without the risk of GvHD, attention focused on thymic-derived CD4+CD25+ FoxP3+ regulatory T-cells (Tregs) that play a physiologic role in maintaining immunologic self-tolerance and immune homeostasis[43–46]. Adoptive immunotherapy with a high number of broad repertoire T-cells, co-infused with freshly isolated CD4+CD25+ FOXP3+ Tregs, has been recently exploited in a cohort of high-risk leukemia patients[47]. Only 6/43 evaluable patients developed grade II–IV acute GvHD. No patient had chronic GvHD. The pattern of post-transplant immune reconstitution was markedly different from standard TCD HLA-haplotype mismatch transplant. Co-infused conventional T-lymphocytes (Tcons) developed a wide T-cell repertoire, high frequencies of pathogen-specific CD4+ and CD8+ T-cell precursors were detected as early as 2 months post-transplant, and the incidence of CMV disease decreased markedly. Vaccination against pandemic influenza with MF59-H1N1 California resulted in strong antiviral protection, showing that patients had become immunologically competent 3–4 months after transplant. In patients transplanted from NK-alloreactive donors, adoptive transfer of Tregs did not impair NK cell post-transplant regeneration/maturation. It was faster than in standard TCD HLA-haplotype mismatch transplant, with enhanced donor *versus* recipient alloreactive NK cell repertoires against KIR-ligand mismatched targets[48–50]. The infusion of Tcons under the Treg protective umbrella, in the absence of post-transplant pharmacologic immunosuppression, guaranteed almost total control of AML and ALL relapse. The leukemia relapse rate was 0.05 at a median follow-up of 46 months. The probability of DFS was 0.56 at a median follow-up of 46 months[50]. These results demonstrate that the immunosuppressive potential of Tregs can be used to suppress GvHD without loss of the benefits of GvL activity. Humanized murine models provided insights into the mechanisms underlying separation of GvL from GvHD, suggesting the GvL effect is due to largely unopposed Tcon alloantigen recognition in the bone marrow.

After reports that adoptive immunotherapy with Tregs controls the alloreactivity of conventional T-lymphocytes in animal models, tomorrow's world of HLA-haplotype transplantation will focus on newly "designed" grafts[50]. An interesting step forward from grafts with a high Tcon content under the protective Treg umbrella are grafts that also contain NK cells, TCRγδ+ T-cells, and other accessory cells. NK cells would be expected to provide an antileukemic effect immediately after administration and afford better protection against infections. TCRγδ+ T-cells would improve resistance to pathogens in the critical early post-transplant phase and hopefully contribute to GvL effect. Switching graft processing techniques from CD34+ enrichment to TCRαβ+/CD19+ depletion, followed by the addition of naturally occurring Tregs and Tcons, is a way to achieve fast immune reconstitution and a powerful GvL effect with a low incidence of GvHD and no need for post-transplant pharmacologic prophylaxis.

Unmanipulated HLA-Haplotype Mismatch Transplant

Early Trials with Unmanipulated Grafts: Data and Challenges

HLA-mismatched family donors have been used for over four decades. The problems were, as expected, graft-*versus*-host disease (GvHD) and graft rejection, and both have been shown to correlate with the degree of HLA disparity[51–53]. In an attempt to reduce the risk of GvHD, the combination of cyclosporine and methotrexate (CyA+MTX) was used in the early 1980s[54]; a small number of patients did survive, although the procedure remained extremely toxic and associated with high mortality. The results were so poor that the number of family mismatched allogeneic transplants performed in Europe remained stable until around 2005[55].

The Chinese Experience with Unmanipulated Grafts: A Ray of Hope for HLA-Haplotype Mismatch Transplant

In 2006 the Chinese group led by Dao-Pei Lu compared the outcome of 158 leukemia patients grafted from HLA-identical siblings with 135 leukemia patients grafted from HLA-haplotype mismatch family members, after a myeloablative conditioning regimen[56]. The results were astonishing – the OS and DFS were identical for both groups. The conditioning regimen was a modified busulfan cyclophosphamide (BuCy) for both groups, and all patients received CyA, MTX, and mycophenolate (MMF); the HLA-mismatch group received in addition ATG[56]. The graft source was a combination of G-CSF (G) mobilized bone marrow (G-BM) and G-mobilized PB. The cohort in HLA-haplotype mismatch group had a higher risk of acute GvHD ($P=0.02$) and of TRM ($P=0.05$), but OS was comparable ($P=0.6$). This is the first report on a relatively large number of family mismatched grafts with outcome comparable to sibling HLA-matched grafts, and this led to the emergence of other programs.

G-CSF Mobilized Marrow and Basiliximab and Myeloablative Conditioning Regimens

Another group of Chinese investigators developed a program incorporating unmanipulated G-BM mobilized. They incorporated intensive GvHD prophylaxis, ATG, CyA, MTX, and MMF with basiliximab, an anti-CD25 antibody[57]. The same GvHD prophylaxis has been recently reported by an Italian consortium[58]: acute GvHD grade II–IV and III–IV was respectively 24% and 5%, which is extremely low in a family HLA-haplotype mismatch, T-cell replete, transplant. The TRM was not negligible, being 30% for "standard" and 45% for "high-risk" patients[58]. Overall 3-year survival was 54% for standard and 33% for high-risk patients. Infections were no different from what is reported for unrelated donor grafts: 47%

bacterial, 70% CMV, and 16% invasive fungal infections[58]. Di Bartolomeo *et al.* used for most patients a conditioning regimen combining thiotepa, intravenous busulfan, and fludarabine (TBF), originally described by Sanz and coworkers for cord blood (CB) transplants[59].

G-CSF Mobilized PB and Sirolimus and MAC Regimens

A Milan group has reported HLA haplotype mismatch transplants using unmanipulated PB cells, with GvHD prophylaxis consisting of ATG and sirolimus[60]: in the initial 113 patients, acute GvHD II–IV was reported to be 40% and GvHD III–IV 20%, with an overall TRM of 30% and actuarial 3-year survival of 45% for early and 20% for advanced leukemias. Therefore the attempt of eliminating a calcineurin inhibitor, and substituting with sirolimus, was successful only in a proportion of patients.

Post-Transplant Cyclophosphamide with Marrow Graft in the Setting of Nonmyeloablative Conditioning

The Johns Hopkins group is to be commended for bringing to the clinic a protocol originally described by them 40 years ago in rats[61]. The hypothesis is simple: after infusion of an unmanipulated HLA-haplotype mismatch graft (day 0), alloreactive T-cells will proliferate, in the absence of a calcineurin inhibitor, and on day +3 most will be in the S-phase of the cell cycle; patients then receive a large dose of Cy (50 mg/kg) on days +3 and +4, killing these alloreactive T-cells. This phenomenon of "post-transplant purging" would spare T-cells not undergoing active proliferation, which may include donor's antigen-specific T-cells, and hopefully some T-cells exerting a GvL effect. In 2008 the Johns Hopkins group, in collaboration with the Fred Hutchinson Cancer Research Center, reported the first series of patients to receive unmanipulated marrow following a nonmyeloablative conditioning (NMA) regimen of low-dose Cy, fludarabine, and TBI 2 Gy. Cy was then given at the dose of 50 mg/kg on days +3 and +4 with tacrolimus and MMF initiation on day +5[62]. Engraftment was achieved in 87% of patients at a median interval from transplant of day +16 for neutrophils and day +24 for platelets; acute GvHD grades II–IV and III–IV were respectively 34% and 6% and chronic GvHD was 4% with two doses of Cy (days +3 and +4) (patient cohort at Johns Hopkins) and 25% with one dose of Cy (day +3) (patient cohort at Fred Hutchinson Cancer Research Center). The TRM was less than 20%, though relapse was significant at over 60%. The OS was in the 40% range for lymphoid and in the 20% range for myeloid malignancies. This study proved that post-transplant Cy (PT-Cy) was feasible, prevented GvHD, and allowed engraftment, though relapse was high. Whether the latter observation was due to the PT-Cy killing GvL T-cells, or to the NMA regimen remained to be

determined. The experience at Johns Hopkins has been recently updated[63] on 372 patients: all patients received the uniform conditioning regimen originally described[62], with bone marrow as a graft source and PT-Cy, tracrolimus, and mycophenolate for GvHD prophylaxis. The 6-month nonrelapse mortality remains very low (8%) and the 4-year probability of relapse and survival was 46% and 50%, respectively. After stratifying patients for disease risk index (DRI) survival was 71%, 48%, and 35% for patients with low, intermediate, and high DRI[63].

PT-Cy with Marrow Grafts in the Setting of Myeloablative Conditioning: Are the Outcomes Better?

The problem with NMA regimens is a significant risk of relapse, especially for patients with acute leukemia, and most of all if not in remission. A recent study using PT-Cy and myeloablative conditioning (MAC) regimens has shown a low incidence of graft failure (<5%), a low incidence of GvHD (18%), and relapse as expected with a conventional CyA+MTX GvHD prophylaxis[64]. The OS of leukemia patients in remission was close to 70%. An update on 225 patients, allografted from haploidentical family members, in the San Martino Unit in Genoa (unpublished data), can be seen in Figure 59.1. The diagnosis of these patients was acute leukemia (n=116, 51%), refractory anemia with excess blasts (RAEB) (n=54, 24%), myelofibrosis (n=20, 9%), and other diagnoses (n=35, 16%). The median age of the entire group was 52 years (range 17–74). The actuarial 3-year survival of first remission patients (CR1) is 77%, for CR2 it is 50%, and for patients with active disease at the time of transplant it is 38%.

PT-Cy Using G-Mobilized Peripheral Blood Grafts

Some centers have elected to use unmanipulated PB, instead of unmanipulated marrow and PT-Cy. Results depend on the intensity of the conditioning regimen: with an NMA regimen, rates of GvHD and mortality remain low[65]; however, with a MAC regimen, acute GvHD grade III–IV has been reported to be as high as 22%[66].

The Two-Step Approach of PT-Cy

One group has devised a so-called two-step approach[67]: patients receive a conventional dose of total body irradiation (12 Gy) over 4 days, then a high dose of haploidentical donor lymphocytes (2×10^8/kg), followed after 72 hours by Cy 50 mg/kg^2, followed by tacrolimus + mycophenolate on day 1. Finally, on day zero, patients receive CD34 selected cells, from G-mobilized peripheral blood[67]. Results, although in patients in hematologic remission, were very good with a 2-year nonrelapse mortality of 3.6% and a disease-free-survival of 74%[67].

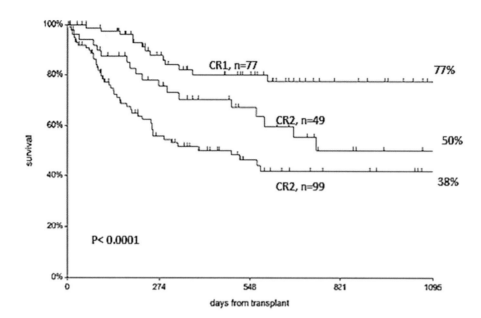

Figure 59 1 Actuarial survival of 225 patients grafted with a haplo-mismatched family donor with post-transplant Cy + CyA + MMF for GvHD prophylaxis (unpublished data).

Controversies Surrounding Unmanipulated HLA-Haplotype Mismatch Transplants

Controversy #1: What Is the Best Platform?

There are basically two platforms for unmanipulated haploidentical stem cell transplants: one based on PT-Cy with a calcineurin inhibitor and MMF, and a second based on ATG with CyA, MTX, MMF, and often a second antibody. Several variations of these two platforms exist, with different conditioning regimens, different graft sources, and different combinations of agents for GvHD prophylaxis. All these platforms seem to achieve a high rate of engraftment, but severe acute GvHD can vary from as low as 3% to as high as 30%. Consequently TRM is also quite different in different programs. Some centers are trying already to combine the two basic platforms (PT-Cy and ATG) and early results seem very promising. A registry-based study from EBMT (unpublished) would suggest a lower TRM and better survival for PT-CY-based haplo transplants, compared to the ATG-based platforms. For the time being, as in every early medical procedure, the only recommendation is to enroll patients in prospective clinical trials, and time will possibly show differences in survival.

Controversy #2: Should We Use Marrow or PB?

Donation of stem cells is hazardous, as shown by five deaths in 51024 donations in Europe[68]; of these five deaths, four were in 23254 PB donors (172 deaths per 10000 donations) and one in 2770 BM donors (0.36 deaths in 10000 donations); severe adverse events were significantly more frequent with PB (10.76/10000) as compared to marrow (4.32/10000)[68]. So PB donation is no safer than marrow donation, despite what is generally thought. Of course harvesting both, as in programs of G-BM + G-PB, exposes the donor to a double hazard, and may not be recommended from a safety point of view. When

used alone, HLA-haplotype mismatched unmanipulated G-CSF mobilized PB causes significantly more GvHD if combined with a MAC regimen as compared to unmanipulated BM[64,66]. The rates of engraftment, transplant-related mortality, and relapse are the same. So, in the short term, there may be no advantage in using PB, for the donor and the patient, and only time will tell us whether differences in chronic GvHD will become evident when using PB instead of BM as a graft source.

In keeping with a significant difference between BM and PB, it has now been shown that PT-Cy can be used as the sole GvHD prophylaxis (without a calcineurin inhibitor and mycophenolate) when patients receive a sibling or unrelated BM graft[69]. This is not the case for PB grafts[70] with a very high rate of lethal acute GvHD.

Controversy #3: What Is the Optimal Dose of PT-Cy?

The dose of cyclophosphamide must be significant: whether 100 mg/kg is necessary or optimal remains to be determined. Some trials already exist with doses different from 50 mg/kg × 2: we would expect GvHD risk to rise when reducing the dose of PT-Cy, as confirmed by the original Luznik paper, in which patients receiving Cy 50 mg/kg , had more chronic GvHD compared to patients receiving Cy 100 mg/kg[62]. For the time being it would seem reasonable to stick to the original dose of 50 mg/kg × 2.

Controversy #4: What Is the Optimal Timing of PT-Cy?

Most reports are based on the original day +3, day +4 regimen, with a calcineurin inhibitor starting on day +5[62]. However, one group has used PT-Cy on days +3 and +5[64], together with CyA and MMF starting on day 0: patients have shown excellent engraftment and very low incidence of acute and chronic GvHD, and standard relapse rates, suggesting the platform is suitable also for modifications[64].

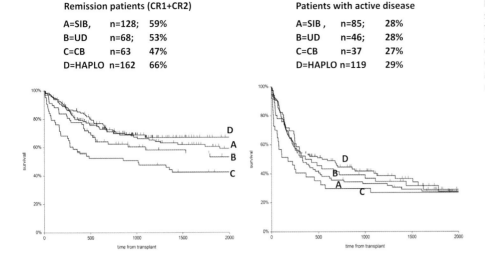

Remission patients (CR1+CR2)

A=SIB,   n=128; 59%
B=UD   n=68;   53%
C=CB   n=63   47%
D=HAPLO n=162   66%

Patients with active disease

A=SIB , n=85;   28%
B=UD   n=46;   28%
C=CB   n=37   27%
D=HAPLO n=119   29%

Figure 59.2 Actuarial survival of 708 patients stratified according to disease status at the time of transplant: on the left remission patients: A = siblings (SIB), B = unrelated (UD); 3 = cord blood (CB), D = HLA haplotype mismatched family donors (HAPLO) grafted between 2007 and 2015 in San Martino, Genoa, Italy (unpublished) data. On the right patients with active disease at transplant.

Controversy #5: Should We Use PT-Cy Also for Matched Siblings and Unrelated Donor Transplants

If PT-Cy is so effective in controlling acute, and especially chronic GvHD, in patients receiving HLA-haplotype grafts, why not expand its use to include HLA MSD/MUD transplants. This has already been tested in single-center studies [69] as well as in a multicenter study[71]. The use of PB from sibling or unrelated donors and PT-Cy alone resulted in high rates of grade III–IV acute GvHD[70,72]. The authors of the OCTET-Cy study[72] concluded that PT-Cy should not be used alone as GvHD prophylaxis after MAC-based regimen in PB HLA MSD and MUD and favored the addition of mToR inhibitor for future studies. Whether the GvHD prophylaxis used for haplo-grafts (PT-Cy, MMF and a CNI) is suitable for UD grafts needs to be tested prospectively.

Controversy #6: How Do Unmanipulated HLA-Haplotype Mismatch Grafts Compare with Other Donor Transplants?

The original Lu *et al.* paper[56] showed comparable outcomes of unmanipulated HLA-haplotype mismatch, using ATG-based GvHD prophylaxis *versus* sibling grafts

A report from the Atlanta group confirmed this report years later, using a PT-Cy-based GvHD prophylaxis, comparing 53 HLA-haplotype mismatch transplants with 117 sibling and 101 unrelated donor transplants[73]: TRM was respectively 7%, 13% ,16%; acute GvHD grades III–IV occurred in 8%, 11%, and 11%; and extensive chronic GvHD in 38%, 54%, and 54%, respectively. The OS and DFS did not differ[73]. It should be noted that 35/53 of the HLA-haplotype mismatch transplant patients in this report received an NMA regimen, and this may explain the low rate of GvHD. A similar report on 459 patients has been recently reported[74]: in a multivariate Cox analysis disease phase was the strongest predictor of survival; on the other hand, transplants from family mismatched HLA-haplotype mismatch donors, matched unrelated donors, and HLA-identical siblings had comparable outcome. An unpublished update on 708 patients grafted from siblings, unrelated,

or family haplo-mismatched donors in the San Martino Unit in Genoa is shown in Figure 59.2. For remission patients HAPLO grafts are not inferior to SIB o UD grafts, and if anything, perhaps better; for patients with active disease the actuarial 7-year survival is identical with all 4 donor types.

A confirmatory study has recently been completed by the Center for International Blood and Marrow Transplant Research (CIBMTR)[75]: unrelated 10/10 matched grafts for AML in remission (n=1982) were matched with family haploidentical grafts, using PT-Cy, a calcineurin inhibitor, and mycophenolate as GvHD prophylaxis (n=192). Survival and disease-free survival were superimposable[75]. These initial reports suggest that HLA-identical siblings, matched unrelated individuals, and family HLA-haplotype mismatch members are alternative options to perform a transplant when indicated. HLA-mismatched unrelated donors and cord blood transplants have perhaps a somewhat inferior outcome, due to a combination of more GvHD (in the mismatched unrelated setting) and more infections (cord blood transplants)[76].

Conclusions

After a pioneering decade led by the Perugia group, HLA-haplotype mismatch family transplants are rapidly increasing in numbers, possibly because of the expansion of programs using unmanipulated stem cell grafts, with encouraging results in several centers. This is particularly true in Italy, as shown by the EBMT survey[55], with a rapid increase of HLA-haplotype mismatch grafts in the last years, to over $35/10^6$ inhabitants, compared to $15/10^6$ in Germany. and less than $10/10^6$ inhabitants in France[55]. Data from the Italian transplant registry, presented in 2014 (unpublished data), have shown an increase of HLA-haplotype mismatch transplants from 151 in 2008 to 415 in 2013: almost a 3-fold increase in 6 years. How T-cell-depleted HLA-haplotype mismatch grafts compare with unmanipulated grafts is currently being investigated: there has not been a head-to-head comparison, but early matched paired or restrospective studies show comparable results. The current trend would suggest the use of selective T-cell depletion on one side, and post-transplant Cy on the other. For the latter BM is used in many centers, although several centers are now exploring the use of unmanipulated mobilized PB, although the risk of GvHD is always increased when increasing the number of mature T-cells infused, especially in the MAC regimen setting. HLA-haplotype mismatch transplants remain an alternative donor procedure and should be regarded as such:

complications, including blood stream infections, invasive fungal disease, viral infections, GvHD, and toxicity may occur with significant frequency and expose the patients to the risk of transplant-related mortality. For this reason HLA-haplotype mismatch grafts, whether T-cell-depleted or unmanipulated, should be performed in centers with expertise in unrelated donor or cord blood transplants, and should follow clinical protocols.

References

1. Reisner Y, Kapoor N, Kirkpatrick D, *et al.* Transplantation for severe combined immunodeficiency with HLA-A,B,D,DR incompatible parental marrow cells fractionated by soybean agglutinin and sheep red blood cells. *Blood.* 1983;61(2):341–8.

2. Friedrich W, Hönig M. HLA-haploidentical donor transplantation in severe combined immunodeficiency. *Immunol Allergy Clin North Am.* 2010;30(1):31–44.

3. Martelli MF, Aversa F, Bachar-Lustig E, *et al.* Transplants across human leukocyte antigen barriers. *Semin Hematol.* 2002;39(1):48–56.

4. Bachar-Lusting E, Rachamim N, Li HW, *et al.* Megadose of T cell-depleted bone marrow overcomes MHC barriers in sublethally irradiated mice. *Nat Med* 1995;1:1268–73.

5. Rachamin N, Gan J, Segall H, Krauthgamer R, *et al.* Tolerance induction by "megadose" hematopoietic transplants: donor-type human CD34 stem cells induce potent specific reduction of host anti-donor cytotoxic T lymphocyte precursors in mixed lymphocyte culture. *Transplantation.* 1998;65:1386–93.

6. Gur H, Krauthgamer R, Berrebi A, *et al.* Tolerance induction by megadose hematopoietic progenitor cells: expansion of veto cells by short-term culture of purified human CD34(+) cells. *Blood.* 2002;99:4174–81.

7. Gur H, Krauthgamer R, Bachar-Lustig E, *et al.* Immune regulatory activity of CD34+ progenitor cells: evidence for a deletion-based mechanism mediated by TNF-alpha. *Blood.* 2005;105(6):2585–93.

8. Aversa F, Tabilio A, Terenzi A, *et al.* Successful engraftment of T-cell-depleted haploidentical "three-loci" incompatible transplants in leukemia patients by addition of recombinant human granulocyte colony-stimulating factor-mobilized peripheral blood progenitor cells to bone marrow inoculum. *Blood.* 1994;84:3948–55.

9. Aversa F, Tabilio A, Velardi A, *et al.* Treatment of high risk acute leukemia with T-cell-depleted stem cells from related donors with one fully mismatched HLA haplotype. *N Engl J Med.* 1998;339:1186–93.

10. Aversa F, Terenzi A, Tabilio A, *et al.* Full haplotype-mismatched hematopoietic stem-cell transplantation: a phase II study in patients with acute leukemia at high risk of relapse. *J Clin Oncol.* 2005;23(15):3447–54.

11. Aversa F, Martelli MF, Velardi A. Haploidentical hematopoietic stem cell transplantation with a megadose T-cell-depleted graft: harnessing natural and adaptive immunity. *Semin Oncol.* 2012;39(6):643–52.

12. Ruggeri L, Capanni M, Urbani E, *et al.* Effectiveness of donor natural killer cell alloreactivity in mismatched hematopoietic transplants. *Science.* 2002;295:2097–2100.

13. Ruggeri L, Aversa F, Martelli MF, Velardi A. Allogeneic hematopoietic transplantation and natural killer cell recognition of missing self. *Immunol Rev.* 2006;214:202–18.

14. Velardi A, Ruggeri L, Mancusi A, Aversa F, Christiansen FT. Natural killer cell allorecognition of missing self in allogeneic hematopoietic transplantation: a tool for immunotherapy of leukemia. *Curr Opin Immunol.* 2009;21(5):525–30.

15. Ciceri F, Labopin M, Aversa F, *et al.* Acute Leukemia Working Party (ALWP) of European Blood and Marrow Transplant (EBMT) Group. A survey of fully haploidentical hematopoietic stem cell transplantation in adults with high-risk acute leukemia: a risk factor analysis of outcomes for patients in remission at transplantation. *Blood.* 2008;112(9):3574–81.

16. Moretta L, Moretta A. Killer immunoglobulin-like receptors. *Curr Opin Immunol.* 2004;16:626–33.

17. Moretta L, Locatelli F, Pende D, Marcenaro E, Mingari MC, Moretta A. Killer Ig-like receptor-mediated control of natural killer cell alloreactivity in haploidentical hematopoietic stem cell transplantation. *Blood.* 2011;117(3):764–71.

18. Yawata M, Yawata N, Draghi M, Little AM, Parteniou F, Parham P. Roles for HLA and KIR polymorphisms in natural killer cell repertoire selection and modulation of effector function. *J Exp Med.* 2006;203:633–45.

19. Leung W, Iyengar R, Turner V, *et al.* Determinants of antileukemia effects of allogeneic NK cells. *J Immunol.* 2004;172:644–50.

20. Haas P, Loiseau P, Tamouza R, *et al.* NK-cell education is shaped by donor HLA genotype after unrelated allogeneic hematopoietic stem cell transplantation. *Blood.* 2011;117(3):1021–9.

21. Perruccio K, Tosti A, Burchielli E, *et al.* Transferring functional immune responses to pathogens after haploidentical hematopoietic transplantation. *Blood.* 2005;106(13):4397–406.

22. Feuchtinger T, Opherk K, Bethge WA, Topp MS, Schuster FR, Weissinger EM *et al.* Adoptive transfer of pp65-specific T cells for the treatment of chemorefractory cytomegalovirus disease or reactivation after haploidentical and matched unrelated stem cell transplantation. *Blood.* 2010;116(20):4360–7.

23. Leen AM, Christin A, Myers GD, *et al.* Cytotoxic T lymphocyte therapy with donor T cells prevents and treats adenovirus and Epstein–Barr virus infections after haploidentical and matched unrelated stem cell

transplantation. *Blood*. 2009;114(19):4283–92.

24. Comoli P, Schilham MW, Basso S, *et al.* T-cell lines specific for peptides of adenovirus hexon protein and devoid of alloreactivity against recipient cells can be obtained from HLA-haploidentical donors. *J Immunother*. 2008;31(6):529–36.

25. Comoli P, Basso S, Zecca M, *et al.* Preemptive Therapy of EBV-related lymphoproliferative disease after pediatric haploidentical stem cell transplantation. *Am J Transplant*. 2007;7(6):1648–55.

26. Perruccio K, Topini F, Tosti A, *et al.* Photodynamic purging of alloreactive T cells for adoptive immunotherapy after haploidentical stem cell transplantation. *Blood Cells Mol Dis*. 2008; 40(1):76–83.

27. Mielke S, Nunes R, Rezvani K, *et al.* A clinical-scale selective allodepletion approach for the treatment of HLA-mismatched and matched donor-recipient pairs using expanded T lymphocytes as antigen-presenting cells and a TH9402-based photodepletion technique. *Blood*. 2008;111(8):4392–402.

28. Roy DC, Guerin M, Boumedine RS, *et al.* Reduction in incidence of severe infections by transplantation of high doses of haploidentical T cells selectively depleted of alloreactive units. *ASH Annual Meeting Abstracts*. 2011;118(21):3020.

29. Marktel S, Magnani Z, Ciceri F, *et al.* Immunologic potential of donor lymphocytes expressing a suicide gene for early immune reconstitution after hematopoietic T-cell-depleted stem cell transplantation. *Blood*. 2003;101(4):1290–8.

30. Ciceri F, Bonini C, Gallo-Stampino C, Bordignon C. Modulation of GvHD by suicide-gene transduced donor T lymphocytes: clinical applications in mismatched transplantation. *Cytotherapy*. 2005;7(2):144–9.

31. Ciceri F, Bonini C, Stanghellini MTL, *et al.* Infusion of suicide-gene-engineered donor lymphocytes after family haploidentical haemopoietic stem-cell transplantation for leukaemia (the TK007 trial): a non-randomised phase I-II study. *Lancet Oncol* 2009; 10(5):489–500.

32. Vago L, Oliveira G, Bondanza A. T-cell suicide gene therapy prompts thymic

renewal in adults after hematopoietic stem cell transplantation. *Blood*. 2012;120(9):1820–30.

33. Bader P, Soerensen J, Jarisch A, *et al.* Rapid immune recovery and low TRM in haploidentical stem cell transplantation in children and adolescence using CD3/CD19 depleted stem cells. *Best Pract Res Clin Haematol*. 2011;24(3):331–7.

34. Bethge WA, Haegele M, Faul C, *et al.* Haploidentical allogeneic hematopoietic cell transplantation in adults using CD3/CD19 depletion and reduced intensity conditioning: an update. *Blood Cells Mol Dis*. 2008;40(1):13–9.

35. Chaleff S, Otto M, Barfield RC, *et al.* A large-scale method for the selective depletion of alphabeta T lymphocytes from PBSC for allogeneic transplantation. *Cytotherapy*. 2007;9(8):746–54.

36. Handgretinger R. New approaches to graft engineering for haploidentical bone marrow transplantation. *Semin Oncol*. 2012;39(6):664–73.

37. Handgretinger R, Lang P, Feuchtinger TF, *et al.* Transplantation of TcR {alpha}{beta}/CD19 depleted stem cells from haploidentical donors: robust engraftment and rapid immune reconstitution in children with high risk leukemia. *ASH Annual Meeting Abstracts*. 2011;118:1005.

38. Carding SR, Egan PJ. Gammadelta T cells: functional plasticity and heterogeneity. *Nat Rev Immunol*. 2002;2(5):336–45.

39. Locatelli F, Bauquet A, Palumbo G, Moretta F, Bertaina A. Negative depletion of α/β+ T cells and of CD19+ B lymphocytes: a novel frontier to optimize the effect of innate immunity in HLA-mismatched hematopoietic stem cell transplantation. *Immunol Lett* 2013;155(1–2):21–3.

40. Bertaina A, Merli P, Rutella S, *et al.* HLA-haploidentical stem cell transplantation after removal of αβ+ T and B cells in children with nonmalignant disorders *Blood*. 2014;124(5):822–6.

41. Prezioso L, Bonomini S, Lambertini C, *et al.* Haploidentical stem cell transplantation after negative depletion of T cells expressing the αβ chain of the T-cell receptor (TCR) for adults with hematological malignancies. *Blood* 2013;122:4609 (Abstract).

42. Aversa F. *Ex vivo* TCRα/β/CD19 T and B cell depletion in HSCT for treatment of adult patients with hematological disease. Milteni Symposium on Cellular therapy: Facts, developments, future visions, EBMT meeting, Milan 2014 (Abstract).

43. Hoffmann P, Ermann J, Edinger M, Fathman CG, Strober S. Donor-type CD4+CD25+ regulatory T cells suppress lethal acute graft-*versus*-host disease after allogeneic bone marrow transplantation. *J Exp Med*. 2002;196(3):389–99.

44. Nguyen VH, Shashidhar S, Chang DS, *et al.* The impact of regulatory T cells on T-cell immunity following hematopoietic cell transplantation. *Blood*. 2008;111(2):945–53.

45. Edinger M, Hoffmann P, Ermann J, *et al.* CD4+CD25+ regulatory T cells preserve graft-*versus*-tumor activity while inhibiting graft-*versus*-host disease after bone marrow transplantation. *Nat Med*. 2003;9(9):1144–50.

46. Di Ianni M, Del Papa B, Cecchini D, *et al.* Immunomagnetic isolation of CD4+CD25+FoxP3+ natural T regulatory lymphocytes for clinical applications. *Clin Exp Immunol*. 2009;156:246–53.

47. Di Ianni M, Falzetti F, Carotti A, *et al.* Tregs prevent GVHD and promote immune reconstitution in HLA-haploidentical transplantation. *Blood*. 2011;117(14):3921–8.

48. Trenado A, Charlotte F, Fisson S, *et al.* Recipient-type specific CD4+CD25+ regulatory T cells favor immune reconstitution and control graft-*versus*-host disease while maintaining graft-*versus*-leukemia. *J Clin Invest*. 2003;112(11):1688–96.

49. Martelli MF, Di Ianni M, Ruggeri L, *et al.* A Donor natural killer cell allorecognition of missing self in haploidentical hematopoietic transplantation for acute myeloid leukemia: challenging its predictive value. *Blood*. 2007;110(1):433–40.

50. Martelli MF, Di Ianni M, Ruggeri L, *et al.* "Designed" grafts for HLA-haploidentical stem cell transplantation. *Blood* 2014;123(7):967–73.

51. Anasetti C, Beatty PG, Storb R, *et al.* Effect of HLA incompatibility on graft-*versus*-host disease, relapse, and survival after marrow transplantation for

patients with leukemia or lymphoma. *Hum Immunol.* 1990;29(2):79–91. PubMed PMID: 2249952.

52. Anasetti C, Amos D, Beatty PG, *et al.* Effect of HLA compatibility on engraftment of bone marrow transplants in patients with leukemia or lymphoma. *N Engl J Med.* 1989;320(4):197–204. PubMed PMID: 2643045.

53. Beatty PG, Clift RA,. Mickelson EM, *et al.* Marrow transplantation from related donors other than HLA-identical siblings. *N Engl J Med.* 1985;313(13):765–771.

54. Powles RL, Morgenstern GR, Kay HE, *et al.* Mismatched family donors for bone-marrow transplantation as treatment for acute leukaemia. *Lancet.* 1983;1(8325):612–615.

55. Passweg. JR, Baldomero H, Gratwohl A, *et al.* and for the European Group for Blood and Marrow Transplantation (EBMT). The EBMT activity survey: 1990–2010. *Bone Marrow Transplant.* 2012;47:906–23.

56. Lu D-P, Dong L, Wu T, *et al.* Conditioning including antithymocyte globulin followed by unmanipulated HLA-mismatched/haploidentical blood and marrow transplantation can achieve comparable outcomes with HLA-identical sibling transplantation. *Blood.* 2006;107(8):3065–73.

57. Ji S-Q, Chen H-R, Yan H-M, *et al.* Anti-CD25 monoclonal antibody (basiliximab) for prevention of graft-*versus*-host disease after haploidentical bone marrow transplantation for hematological malignancies. *Bone Marrow Transplant.* 2005;36(4):349–54.

58. Di Bartolomeo P, Santarone S, De Angelis G, *et al.* Unmanipulated bone marrow transplantation from haploidentical related donors for patients with high risk hematologic malignancies. *Blood* 2010;116:Abstract 2350.

59. Sanz J, Boluda JCH, Martín C, *et al.* Single-unit umbilical cord blood transplantation from unrelated donors in patients with hematological malignancy using busulfan, thiotepa, fludarabine and ATG as myeloablative conditioning regimen. *Bone Marrow Transplantation.* 2012;47(10):1287–93.

60. Noviello M, Forcina A, Lupo-Stanghellini MT, *et al.* Early reconstitution of T-cell immunity to CMV after HLA-haploidentical hematopoietic stem cell transplantation is a strong surrogate biomarker for lower non-relapse mortality rates. *ASH Annual Meeting Abstracts* 2012;120:4191

61. Santos GW, Owens AH. Production of graft-*versus*-host disease in the rat and its treatment with cytotoxic agents. *Nature.* 1966;210(5032):139–40.

62. Luznik L, O'Donnell PV, Symons HJ, *et al.* HLA-haploidentical bone marrow ransplantation for hematologic malignancies using nonmyeloablative conditioning and high-dose, posttransplantation cyclophosphamide. *Biol Blood Marrow Transplant.* 2008;14(6):641–50.

63. McCurdy SR, Kanakry JA, Showel MM, *et al.* Risk-stratified outcomes of nonmyeloablative HLA-haploidentical BMT with high-dose posttransplantation cyclophosphamide. *Blood.* 2015;125(19):3024–31.

64. Raiola AM, Dominietto A, Ghiso A, *et al.* Unmanipulated haploidentical bone marrow transplant and posttransplantation cyclophosphamide for hematologic malignancies after myeloablative conditioning. *Biol Blood Marrow Transplant.* 2013;19;117–22.

65. Castagna L, Crocchiolo R, Furst S, *et al.* Bone marrow compared with peripheral blood stem cells for haploidentical transplantation with a nonmyeloablative conditioning regimen and post-transplantation cyclophosphamide. *Biol Blood Marrow Transplant.* 2014;20:724–9.

66. Solomon S, Sizemore C, Zhang Z, *et al.* TBI-based myeloablative haploidentical stem cell transplantation is a safe and effective alternative to unrelated donor transplantation in patients without matched sibling donors. *Blood.* 2014;124:426(Abstract).

67. Grosso D, Gaballa S, Alpdogan O, *et al.* A two-step approach to myeloablative haploidentical transplantation: low nonrelapse mortality and high survival confirmed in patients with earlier stage disease. *Biol Blood Marrrow Transplant.* 2015;21(4):646–52.

68. Halter J, Kodera Y, Urbano-Ispizua A, *et al.* for the European Group for Blood and Marrow Transplantation (EBMT) Activity Survey Office. Severe events in donors after allogeneic hematopoietic stem cell donation. *Haematologica.* 2009;94:94–101.

69. Kanakry CG, Tsai HL, Bolan͂os-Meade J, *et al.* Single-agent GVHD prophylaxis with posttransplantation cyclophosphamide after myeloablative, HLA-matched BMT for AML, ALL, and MDS. *Blood.* 2014;124:3817–27.

70. Bradstock KF, Bilmon I, Kwan J, *et al.* Single-agent high-dose cyclophosphamide for graft-*versus*-host disease prophylaxis in human leukocyte antigen matched reduced-intensity peripheral blood stem cell transplantation results in an unacceptably high rate of severe acute graft-*versus*-host disease. *Biol Blood Marrow Transplant.* 2015;21:934–53.

71. Kanakry CG, O'Donnell PV, Furlong T, *et al.* Multi-institutional study of post-transplantation cyclophosphamide as single-agent graft-*versus*-host disease prophylaxis after allogeneic bone marrow transplantation using myeloablative busulfan and fludarabine conditioning. *J Clin Oncol.* 2014;32(31):3497–505.

72. Holtick U, Chemnitz JM, Shimabukuro-Vornhagen A, *et al.* OCTET-CY: a phase II study to investigate the efficacy of post-transplant cyclophosphamide as sole graft-*versus*-host prophylaxis after allogeneic peripheral blood stem cell transplantation. *Eur J Haematol.* 2016;96(1):27–35.

73. Bashey A, Zhang X, Sizemore CA., *et al.* T-cell–replete HLA-haploidentical hematopoietic transplantation for hematologic malignancies using post-transplantation cyclophosphamide results in outcomes equivalent to those of contemporaneous HLA-matched related and unrelated donor transplantation. *J Clin Oncol.* 2013;31:1310–16.

74. Raiola AM, Dominietto A, di Grazia C, *et al.* Unmanipulated haploidentical transplants compared with other alternative donors and matched sibling grafts. *Biol Blood Marrow Transplant.* 2014;20:1573–9.

75. Ciurea SO, Zhang MJ, Bacigalupo AA, *et al.* Haploidentical transplant with post-transplant cyclophosphamide versus matched unrelated donor transplant for acute myeloid leukemia. *Blood.* 2015;126(8):1033–40.

76. Kekre N, Antin J. Hemopoietic stem cell transplant sources in the 21st century: choosing the ideal donor when a perfect match does not exist. *Blood.* 2014;124:334–9.

60

Cord Blood Cell Transplants: Donor Selection, Volume, and Controversies

Karen K. Ballen

Cord Blood: The Need

Since the first umbilical cord blood transplantation (UCBT) in France in 1988, the field of UCB banking and transplantation has continued to grow exponentially. An estimated 600 000 UCB units have been donated worldwide for public use, and over 30 000 UCBTs have been performed. The chance of each patient's sibling being a complete human leukocyte antigen (HLA)-matched donor is 25%; given the small size of most families in developed countries, only 30% of patients who require an allograft will have an HLA-matched sibling donor. Despite intense efforts to increase the diversity of the National Marrow Donor Program and affiliated registries, many patients, particularly patients of diverse racial/ethnic backgrounds, will not be able to identify a suitably matched unrelated volunteer donor. UCBT, therefore, is an important option, especially for patients from racial/ethnic minorities.

History of Umbilical Cord Blood Transplantation

The history of UCBT illustrates the important collaboration between basic science, industry, and clinical medicine, as well as the strength of international collaboration. Initial work by Broxmeyer and colleagues established that UCB hematopoietic progenitor cells had proliferative capacity, and could engraft in a murine model[1]. The Biocyte Corporation was then founded to help fund this research. Dr. Eliane Gluckman performed the first UCBT, treating a child with Fanconi anemia, in Paris in 1988[2]. The first transplants were done with unwashed cells. Fanconi anemia was chosen, as work by Arleen Auerbach in New York had previously described accurate prenatal diagnosis, so an unaffected sibling could serve as the UCB donor[3]. The first UCB was a success, and the growth of UCB banking followed.

Umbilical Cord Blood Banking

The realization that a single UCB unit could successfully engraft a human patient, that UCB could safely be collected after delivery, and that UCB could be cryopreserved for many years opened the field of UCB banking. In Europe, UCB banks were initially established in Milan, Dusseldorf, London, and Paris. Dr. Pablo Rubinstein established one of the largest unrelated UCB banks at the New York Blood Center, and

published procedures for processing and thawing UCB units [4]. There are currently over 100 UCB banks, collecting units for public use in North America, South America, Australia, Europe, Asia, and the Middle East. In the United States, federal regulations established guidelines for HPC, Cord Blood manufacturing, and testing to ensure the safety, purity, potency, and identity of the product. UCB must either be licensed by the Food and Drug Administration (FDA) or considered investigational, and used as an Investigational New Drug (IND). The FDA provides specific regulatory requirements for process verification and validation in 21 CFR section 1271. Accrediting organizations for cord blood banks, including the AABB and the Foundation for Accreditation of Cellular Therapy (FACT), provide a series of guidelines and requirements to ensure safety.

Pediatric Umbilical Cord Blood Transplants

Kurtzberg and colleagues reported the first unrelated UCBT in 25 children with a variety of malignant and nonmalignant diseases[5]. The 100-day overall survival (OS) was 64% in this group of high-risk children. Wagner et al. showed the influence of CD34+ dose on outcome[6]. No randomized studies have been done in children comparing graft sources, but several retrospective studies have shown comparable or superior survival in children receiving UCBT compared to other graft sources. The Eurocord group compared outcomes of matched unrelated BMT (HLA 6 out of 6) either unmanipulated or T-depleted to mismatched UCBT[7]. Engraftment was delayed after UCBT. Graft-*versus*-host disease (GvHD) was similar between UCBT and T-cell depleted BMT and decreased compared to the T-replete patients; relapse and leukemia-free survival (LFS) were similar. The Center for International Blood and Marrow Transplant Research (CIBMTR) compared outcomes of pediatric patients with acute leukemia receiving unrelated mismatched UCBT (n = 503) to children receiving a MUD-HCT (n = 282)[8]. The best results were seen in children receiving fully matched UCBT. LFS was similar between BM and one or two HLA-mismatched UCBTs. Results for children and adults treated with UCBT have improved over time, as illustrated in Figure 60.1.

The results have been particularly good for children with inherited metabolic disorders (IMDs) undergoing UCBT. Prasad and colleagues treated 159 children (median age 1.5 years) with single, myeloablative UCBT for IMDs, most commonly

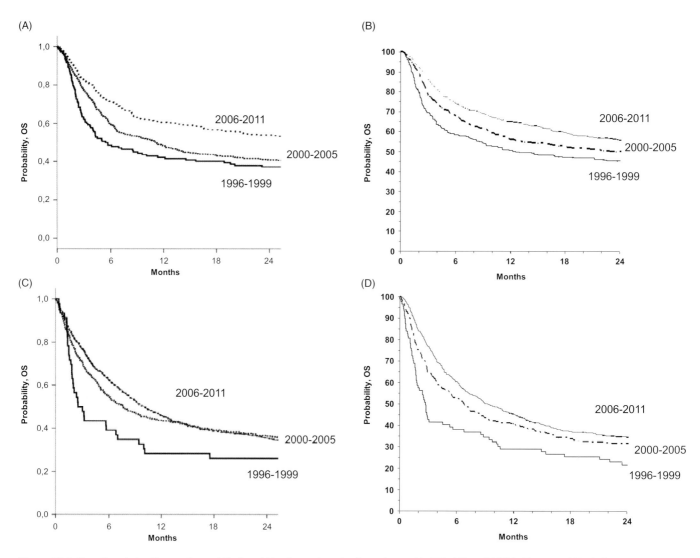

Figure 60.1 Overall survival at 2 years after umbilical cord blood transplantation for patients with AML, ALL, and MDS in Europe and North America.
(**A**) Children (≤16 years) from Europe: UCBT period 1996–1999 (n=142), OS: 37±4%; 2000–2005 (n=441), OS: 41±2%; 2006–2011 (n=749), OS: 54 ±2%.
(**B**) Children (≤16 years) from North America: UCBT period 1996–1999 (n=276), OS: 45±6%; 2000–2005 (n=843), OS: 50±3%; 2006–2011 (n=993), OS: 56±6%.
(**C**) Adults from Europe: UCBT period 1996–1999 (n=46), OS: 26±6; 2000–2005 (n=339), OS: 37±3%; 2006–2011 (n=1595), OS: 36±2%. (**D**) Adults from North America:
UCBT period 1996–1999 (n=87), OS: 22±8%; 2000–2005 (n=359), OS: 31±4%; 2006–2011 (n=1210), OS: 34±3%. Reproduced from Ballen KK, Gluckman E, Broxmeyer
HE. Umbilical cord blood transplantation: the first 25 years and beyond. Blood 2013; 122 (4): 491–8, reprinted with permission.

Hurler syndrome, Krabbe A disease, and Sanfilippo syndrome [9]. Overall survival at 5 years was 58% and 76% for those patients with a good performance status. Patients transplanted earlier in their disease course did better.

Preliminary analysis of a randomized study comparing double UCBT to single UCBT showed similar survival and engraftment, suggesting that in pediatric UCBT, there is no need for a double UCBT, assuming an adequate cell dose for the single UCBT (BMT CTN 0501, Clinicaltrials.gov NCT00412360)[10].

Controversy: Is There a Role for Double UCBT in Pediatric Patients?

Comment: The preliminary results of the randomized CTN trial cited above showed no advantage in engraftment, relapse,

or survival to double UCBT. Therefore, if there is a single UCBT with adequate cell dose (>2.5×10⁷ NC/kg), given the added cost of a second UCBT, a single UCBT should be performed. Double UCBT in children should be limited to those older or larger children for whom a single UCB unit does not have an adequate cell dose.

Adult Umbilical Cord Blood Transplants
High-Dose Myeloablative Single-Unit UCBT

After promising results in children, several investigators extended these principles to adults. The initial results in single UCBT using a myeloablative conditioning regimen in adults were poor, with a very high 100-day transplant-related mortality of 40%[11]. Results improved with changes in patient selection, supportive care including growth factors, and the use of UCBT with higher cell doses (Figure 60.1). The Japanese groups have had outstanding results with a disease-free-survival (DFS) of 63% for patients with AML and 70% for patients with myelodysplastic syndromes; these excellent outcomes may be related to patient size, genetic homogeneity in an island nation, or practice patterns, such as longer hospitalizations and no antithymocyte globulin use[12]. A prospective, multicenter study confirmed a DFS of 42% in adults with high-risk malignancies, using a conditioning regimen of cyclophosphamide, cytarabine, and total body radiation[13]. Sanz et al. have reported encouraging results in early stage hematologic malignancies with DFS of 46%[14].

Improving Adult UCBT Outcomes

Double Cord Blood Transplantation and Reduced Intensity Conditioning

Early studies in adult UCBT showed that cell dose was critical for engraftment and survival, which naturally lead to studies on double UCBT[11]. Double UCBT has been implemented more widely in the United States than in Europe, likely due to the higher weight of the US population[15]. Non myeloablative or reduced intensity conditioning (RIC), the "mini" transplant, was introduced in the 1990s to reduce transplant-related mortality and allow older patients to proceed safely to transplant.

The Minnesota group used a RIC regimen of fludarabine, cyclophosphamide, and low-dose total body radiation, with double UCBT, and published a 38% long-term disease-free survival[16]. These results were confirmed in several other studies[17]. Decreased GvHD was seen with the use of sirolimus as part of the GvHD prophylaxis regimen[18]. Multiple investigators have attempted to predict the dominant unit on the basis of cell dose, HLA type, viable CD34+ count, CD3+, and order of infusion[19].

The advantage of single versus double UCBT in adults is controversial. The second cord UCB unit is expensive, and may increase the risk of GvHD. Verneris et al. reported a decreased relapse rate for adults receiving double versus single UCBT[20]. No randomized studies have compared single versus double UCBT in adults. Data from France showed improved survival with double UCBT versus single UCBT (62% versus 47%). The relapse rate was less with double UCBT (21% versus 42%)[21]. Therefore, for adults, the question of single versus double UCBT requires further investigation.

Controversy: Is There an Advantage for Double versus Single UCBT in Adults?

Comment: There are no randomized data to answer this question. The Eurocord data above suggest an advantage to double UCBT with acute leukemia patients in CR 1 but the study is small and no advantage was seen for CR 2 patients. In the

Mother	A 3, A2	B 1, B8	DRB1*03:01, DRB1*15:02
CB unit	A 3, A4	B 1, B44	DRB1*03:01, DRB1*11:01
Patient	A 3, A2	B 10, B44	DRB1*03:01, DRB1*11:01

Figure 60.2 Noninherited maternal allele in UCBT Matching cord blood unit is HLA mismatched but NIMA matched to the patient.

absence of clear data, either double UCBT or single UCBT with adequate cell dose ($>3.0 \times 10^7$ NC/kg) are acceptable, depending on institutional preference.

Selection of the Best Umbilical Cord Blood Unit

HLA Typing

Advances in UCB unit selection have contributed to the improvement in survival after UCBT. Selection of the optimal UCB unit is complex and involves other factors besides cell dose and HLA type. The interaction between cell dose and HLA match was best demonstrated in an analysis of 1061 recipients of single UCBT after myeloablative conditioning regimen; the lowest TRM was seen in recipients of 6/6 HLA-A,-B antigen, -DRB1 allele-matched units, regardless of cell dose[22]. A higher cell dose overcame the degree of HLA mismatch so that an UCB unit that was a 4/6 HLA-match to the recipient required a TNC $>5.0 \times 10^7$/kg to achieve a similar TRM as 5/6 units with a TNC $>2.5 \times 10^7$/kg.

The presence of preformed HLA antibodies against the UCB units has been shown to be a negative prognostic factor for engraftment and survival for both single and double UCBT [23][24]. Maternal HLA typing on the UCB units is not available for many UCB units, but when available, matching of the UCB unit to the noninherited maternal allele (NIMA) of the patient may be important. The mother gets exposed to fetal antigens during pregnancy, and the fetus gets exposed to maternal cells and develops immunity and T-regulatory cells against the NIMA, as illustrated in Figure 60.2. In 2009, van Rood and colleagues published a series of 1121 patients undergoing single-unit, myeloablative UCBT. Patients who received HLA-mismatched but NIMA-matched grafts had equivalent survival to patients receiving 6/6 HLA-matched grafts[25]. In a study of 118 patients, Rocha et al. showed improved survival (5-year OS of 55% versus 38%) in favor of NIMA matched versus NIMA mismatched grafts[26]. Thus, when maternal typing is available, there may be an advantage to selection of a UCB unit matched at the NIMA.

Traditionally, UCB units had been matched to the patient at the intermediate level for HLA-A and HLA-B and at the allele level for HLA-DR. However, recent data suggest that matching at HLA-C, at least for myeloablative, single-unit UCBT, may be helpful[27]. The impact of matching at HLA-C in double UCBT or RIC UCBT is not clear[28]. Allele-level typing at class I may also affect UCBT outcomes, and this would entail a shift in clinical practice for some centers[29]. In addition, there are conflicting studies on the importance of matching for killer

Table 60.1 Suggested cord blood selection strategy

HLA antibody
- Perform HLA antibody screen
- Repeat HLA antibody screen just prior to ordering UCB units
- Do not select UCB units against which patients have preformed antibodies

HLA typing
- 6/6 match is optimal, regardless of cell dose
- Avoid double UCB units completely matching each other, unless a 6/6 match with the patient
- Double mismatches at any given locus should be avoided
- Perform high-resolution typing for class I and class II
- Match UCB unit to patient at the allele level (high resolution) whenever possible
- HLA-C matching may be beneficial, for single-unit, myeloablative UCBT. Importance for double RIC UCBT unclear
- DQ typing not used in search strategy
- Confirm UCB identity just prior to transplant on an attached segment

Viability
- Select UCB units with viability >90%

Cell dose
- Total TNC must be at least 3.5×10^7 NC/kg
- Each unit must be at least 1.5×10^7 NC/kg
- Higher cell dose triumphs over HLA match when TNC is $\leq 2.0 \times 10^7$ NC/kg for each single CBU
- Closer HLA match triumphs over cell dose when TNC is $>2.0 \times 10^7$ NC/kg for each single CBU unless there is a >50% higher cell dose in the less well-matched cord blood unit

Reproduced from reference[61].

immunoglobulin (KIR) ligand[30,31,32]. A sample strategy for selecting UCB units is displayed in Table 60.1.

Additional Factors Affecting Umbilical Cord Blood Unit Choice

A higher CD34+ dose has been associated with improved engraftment in both children and adults receiving UCBT. Because of laboratory variability in the CD34+ count, using the CD34+ count as a selection criterion for UCB unit selection may be problematic. Recently, a higher viable CD34+ cell dose has been shown to correlate with the dominant unit and the speed of engraftment[33].

Controversy: How to Select the Optimal Umbilical Cord Blood Unit

Comment: There are many more factors to consider besides HLA typing and cell dose. A 6/6 matched unit, if available, should be selected regardless of cell dose. Matching at HLA-C and at the allele level has been shown to be associated with improved survival in a retrospective study. It is unclear

which allele is the most important to have matched. If maternal typing is available, a NIMA matched unit should be selected. No units should be selected to which there are preformed HLA antibodies.

Comparison of Graft Sources: What is the Optimal Graft Source for Adults without a Matched Sibling Donor?

Unfortunately, there are no completed randomized prospective studies to determine the optimal graft source for adults. Multiple retrospective studies have indicated comparable survival between either single or double UCBT and other graft sources for both myeloablative and reduced intensity conditioning. The CIBMTR studied 165 single UCBT adult patients, 888 MUD PBHC patients, and 472 MUD BM patients[34]. TRM was higher for the UCBT patients, but since acute and chronic GvHD were lower, DFS was comparable among UCBT, fully matched MUD, and mismatched MUD patients. DFS was comparable among UCBT, fully matched MUD, and mismatched MUD patients. This study indicated that the disease status of the patient, rather than the graft source, was the most important predictor of survival. Similar findings have been seen with double UCBT. Brunstein and colleagues showed comparable survival among patients (myeloablative preparative regimen) receiving double UCBT, matched related donor, and matched or mismatched MUD-HCT[35].

In the reduced intensity setting, several retrospective studies have shown comparable survival among double UCBT recipients and recipients of other graft sources. Chen *et al.* described comparable survival among patients treated with a reduced intensity fludarabine-based preparative regimen and receiving either double UCBT or MUD-HCT[36]. A multicenter study also showed comparable survival between MUD and double UCBT recipients receiving a RIC[37]. A recent study by Milano and colleagues showed that for AML patients with minimal residual disease, the relapse rate was lower with UCBT compared to MUD or mismatched MUD[38]. Table 60.2 outlines some of the studies comparing UCBT with other graft sources.

Results with HLA-haplotype mismatch transplant continue to improve, with a major advance being the use of post-transplant cyclophosphamide to induce immunologic tolerance. The US Clinical Trials Network (CTN) sponsored two parallel phase 2 trials using RIC regimen for patients with hematologic malignancy, one using a haploidentical donor as graft source and the other double UCBT[39]. Each study enrolled 50 patients. The transplant-related mortality was lower in the haploidentical patients (7% *versus* 24%) but the relapse rate was higher with the haploidentical approach (45% *versus* 31%). Therefore, the 1-year DFS was comparable at 48% for haploidentical patients and 46% for the double UCBT recipients. The CTN is currently accruing patients to a randomized study of haploidentical *versus* double UCBT using the same RIC regimen. This is an important study for the transplant community to complete.

Table 60.2 Comparison of survival after transplantation of single or double-unit UCBT with other graft sources

Series	No. of patients	Conditioning	Graft source	Follow-up (years)	Median age (years)	Survival (PFS or DFS) (%)	Comment
Brunstein[35] Leukemia	128	Myeloablative	dUCB	5	25	51	UCB similar to MRD, MUD
	204		MRD		40	33	
	152		MUD		31	48	
	52		MMUD		31	38	
Ponce[63] Heme malignancy	75	Myeloablative	dUCBT	2	37	55	UCB similar to MUD
	108		MRD		47	66	
	184		MUD		40	55	
Brunstein[39] Leukemia and lymphoma	50	RIC	dUCB	1	58	46	Now a randomized CTN study
	50		haplo BM		48	48	
Chen[36] Hematologic malignancy	64	RIC	dUCB	3	53	30	UCB similar to MUD
	221		MUD		58	40	
Marks[64] Acute lymphoid leukemia	116	Myeloablative	sUCB	3	25	44	Less extensive chronic GvHD with UCBT
	546		MUD		32	44	
	140		MMUD		33	43	

Abbreviations: sUCB: single umbilical cord blood; dUCB: double umbilical cord blood; MMUD: mismatched unrelated donor; MUD: matched unrelated donor; RIC: reduced intensity conditioning; haplo: haploidentical; PFS: progression-free survival; MRD: matched related donor; DFS: disease-free survival.

Controversy: What Is the Best Alternative Graft Source for Adults?

Comment: There are no randomized data to support the choice of mismatched unrelated donor, haploidentical donor, or single or double UCBT. Multiple retrospective studies have indicated similar survival; some studies have demonstrated an increased transplant-related mortality but a decreased relapse rate for UCBT. This important question is best answered in a prospective, randomized study. All eligible patients are encouraged to enroll in the US CTN double UCBT *versus* HLA-haplotype mismatch transplant study.

Improving Cord Blood Transplant Outcomes

Several strategies are under investigation to improve engraftment and reduce the risk of infection. The Spanish groups pioneered the concept of combining a haploidentical donor with a single UCBT; the rationale is that the haploidentical donor provides initial early engraftment and that the UCB provides durable engraftment when the haploidentical donor is rejected[40]. Using a similar concept with a reduced intensity approach of fludarabine, melphalan, and thymoglobulin, Liu *et al.* demonstrated rapid neutrophil engraftment at 11 days and a low incidence of acute GvHD of 25%[41]. The Spanish group has extended this concept by using mismatched unrelated donors in combination with UCBT. Finally, Ponce *et al.* have used double UCBT plus a haploidentical graft; days to engraftment and length of stay were improved with this approach[42].

A novel strategy is injecting the UCB cell directly into the bone marrow in an attempt to bypass the homing process needed after the usual IV cell infusion[43]. A Eurocord study confirmed an improvement in engraftment with decreased GvHD, although this advantage was not seen in an American study[44].

Cord Blood Expansion and Homing Techniques

Cord blood expansion is a possible strategy to circumvent the issue of low cell dose. The Notch gene family codes for transmembrane proteins that inhibit differentiation and affect hematopoietic progenitor cell engraftment. Using the notch ligand Delta 1, Delaney *et al.* showed an expansion of short-term repopulating cells and an improvement in the time of neutrophil engraftment to 16 days in 10 patients receiving myeloablative conditioning and one expanded and one unmanipulated unit[45]. Mesenchymal progenitor cell expansion has been attempted by the MD Anderson group with success; there was a 30-fold expansion in CD34+ count, and median time to engraftment of 15 days, which compared favorably to a historical control group with a 24-day median engraftment [46]. The expanded unit provided early engraftment while the unmanipulated unit provided long-term engraftment in most of the patients. A randomized clinical trial of unmanipulated double UCBT *versus* one mesenchyal stem cell expanded unit and one unmanipulated unit is ongoing at several centers (ClinicalTrials.gov NCT01854567).

Another approach is to use a nicotinamide-based system in combination with cytokines to *ex-vivo* expand CD 133+ UCB

Table 60.3 Novel strategies for improving engraftment

Agent	Mechanism	Investigator	n	Days to ANC >500	Current trial
FT-VI	Fucosylation	Popat[51]	7	14	NCT01471067
PGE2	Homing	Cutler[50]	12	17	NCT01527838
Sitagliptin	DPP-IV inhibition	Farag[52]	24	21	NCT01720264
Notch	Inhibit differentiation	Delaney[45]	10	16	NCT01690520
Mesenchymal stem cells	Improve stroma	De Lima[46]	31	15	NCT01854567
Nicotinamide	Inhibit enzymes that require NAD+	Horwitz[47]	11	13	NCT01816230
Stem Ex	Copper chelation	Montesinos[48]	101	21	NCT01484470

Abbreviations: FT: fucosyltransferase; PGE2: prostaglandin E2; DPP: dipeptidyl peptidase; NAD+: nicotinamide adenine dinucleotide.

cells[47]. Intracellular copper concentration regulates the differentiation of hematopoietic progenitor cells. Therefore, one approach has been to use a copper chelator to reduce intracellular copper concentration. Using the copper chelator system Stem Ex, investigators compared 101 patients receiving single-unit expanded cells with historical controls. Neutrophil and platelet engraftment and 100-day survival were improved in the patients receiving the expanded UCB unit[48]. A concern is the specialized expertise cord blood expansion would require and the cost of the *ex-vivo* expansion.

Another approach is to increase the homing of the UCBT to the bone marrow and hematopoietic microenvironment. The Boston group has investigated the use of prostaglandin (PG) E2 incubation of the UCB unit to upregulate CXCR4 expression[49]. One of two UCB units was treated with PGE2 in a reduced intensity double UCBT[50]. Engraftment was improved by 4 days compared to historical controls and the PGE2 treated UCB provided long-term hematopoiesis in 10 of 12 patients. A large randomized phase 2 study (one PGE2 treated UCB and one unmanipulated UCB *versus* two unmanipulated UCB) is ongoing in double UCBT with either a myeloablative or reduced intensity conditioning regimen (ClinicalTrials.govNCT01627314). Selectins are needed to initiate homing of hematopoietic stem cells, and selectins are modified for this purpose via a fucosylation process. Therefore, fucosylation of UCB cells is an investigational method to improve homing and engraftment. A multicenter double UCB trial (ClinicalTrials.govNTC1471067) is underway, with the smaller unit being treated. Preliminary results in the first seven patients indicate a time to neutrophil engraftment of 14 days [51]. The SDF-1a:CXCR4 axis plays a pivotal role in stem cell homing and is controlled by the enzyme CD26/dipeptidylpeptidase 4(DPP-IV). Sitagliptin is an oral DPP-IV inhibitor approved by the US Food and Drug Administration (FDA) for the treatment of type II diabetes mellitus. The Indianopolis group reported the results of 24 patients undergoing single UCBT with myeloablative conditioning followed by sitagliptin 600 mg orally daily, given on day –1 to +2[52]. The dose was well tolerated but there was no sustained inhibition of DPP-IV. An every 8-hour dosing schedule resulted in capillary leak

syndrome; therefore, a new clinical trial is ongoing with a dose of 600 mg every 12 hours (ClinicalTrials.gov: NCT0170264). Future trials may seek to combine homing approaches, such as *ex-vivo* priming with PGE2 combined with DPP-IV inhibition. These novel approaches are outlined in Table 60.3[53].

Controversy: What is the Role of *Ex-vivo* Expansion in Adult UCBT?

Comment: There are no randomized data to support the use of *ex-vivo* expansion. Small phase 1 and 2 studies have shown an improvement in engraftment with a variety of approaches. While engraftment is an easier endpoint to measure, it may be less important clinically than survival or immune reconstitution. *Ex-vivo* expansion remains experimental at present.

Reducing Infections and Enhancing Adaptive Immunity

Opportunistic infection remains a major cause of morbidity and mortality after UCBT. Late viral infections, occurring after the first 100 days, can be fatal[54].

T-cell reconstitution is delayed after UCBT, which helps to contribute to the increased risk of infections, particularly viral infections, in the first several months after UCBT. UCB components may be used to enhance immunomodulation. Active T-cells expanded from naïve UCB T-cell populations can recognize cytomegalovirus, adenovirus, and Epstein–Barr virus. These T-cells have been used to treat refractory viral infections after transplant[55]. *Ex-vivo* expanded UCB T-regulatory cells have been infused post-UCBT and have been shown to decrease acute GvHD[56].

Increasing Access to Transplant

A purported goal of UCB banking has been to provide units for patients who cannot find matched unrelated donors in the registry. Since it is particularly difficult for non-white patients to find matched unrelated donors, UCBT is a particularly attractive option for patients of diverse racial and ethnic

Table 60.4 Regenerative medicine

Approach	Disease	Investigators	n	Results	Current trial
Fresh auto-UCB	Hypoxic brain injury at birth	Cotten et al.[61]	23	Improved function at 1 year	NCT01072370
Auto-UCB	Cerebral palsy	Sun et al.[65]	184	Parental reports of improved function	NCT01072370
BM-MSC	Acute MI	Jeevanantham et al.[66]	Meta-analysis	Improved LV function	NCT01569178
Frozen auto-UCB	Diabetes mellitus	Haller et al.[67]	24	No decrease in insulin needs	

Abbreviations: UCB: umbilical cord blood; auto: autologous; BM-MSC: bone marrow-mesenchymal stem cell; MI: myocardial infarction; LV: left ventricle.

background. However, a registry study reported worse outcomes for black patients compared to white patients receiving UCBT. In addition, black patients were more likely to receive UCB units that were smaller and less well matched[57]. Black patients were also more likely to have a longer hospital length of stay, particularly after myeloablative conditioning regimens. [58] For black patients, they may be more likely to find an HLA-matched unit from a black donor, but the UCB contains fewer numbers of cells. Thus, the UCB inventory would need to be a lot larger to provide adequate UCB units for a diverse group of patients.

Regenerative Medicine

UCB cells, compared to adult bone marrow, are less mature, have longer telomeres, and greater proliferative potential. Adaptation of this therapy may be important in the treatment of cardiac, neurologic, and vascular disease. Mesenchymal stem cells can be isolated from the umbilical cord, and have been used to treat peripheral vascular disease and Buerger's disease[59].

Cerebral vascular accident (CVA) is the third leading cause of death among adults, and a major cause of disability. Reducing the extension of stroke is a major focus of regenerative medicine techniques. Administration of UCB cells has produced functional recovery and vascular remodeling after stroke [60].

Trials are underway using UCB to treat children with cerebral palsy, traumatic brain injury, autism, and hypoxic ischemic encephalopathy (NCT01072370, NCT 01700166, NCT 01988584, NCT 01251003, and NCT 01638819). In a study at Duke with infants who had suffered hypoxic brain injury at birth, those infants who received fresh autologous UCB collected at birth and hypothermia had improved functional status at 1 year, compared to infants treated with hypothermia without the UCB infusion (74% versus 41%, $P=0.05$) [61]. Some of these approaches are outlined in Table 60.4.

If UCBT proves successful as regenerative medicine therapy, the numbers of UCBT may rise sharply as a treatment for common diseases of children and adults; in addition, there may be momentum to bank UCB privately, and thereby limit public access.

Conclusions and Controversies

The results of UCBT have improved since 1988, but several challenges and controversies still exist. In cord blood banking, while increased diversity is a goal of UCB banking, black patients are more likely to receive smaller, less well-matched units. Additional efforts are needed to increase the collection of larger units from non-white donors. In pediatric UCBT, recent data have shown no advantage to double versus single UCBT, assuming an adequate cell dose is collected. UCBT is an accepted transplant modality for children, but in adults, cost and the risk of infection have limited use of UCBT. The recent interest in post-transplant cyclophosphamide for haploidentical HCT has decreased the use of UCBT in some situations. A critical question is which is better: haploidentical or UCBT? This question can only be answered in a randomized trial and participation in the randomized CTN trial comparing double UCBT to haploidentical HCT is strongly encouraged.

There have been multiple attempts at UCB expansion, but no trials have demonstrated a survival advantage. These techniques are expensive, and may be difficult to do outside of large centers. In addition, while engraftment is the endpoint of many of these trials, it is poor immune recovery that contributes to the late infections in UCBT patients, and this endpoint is much harder to measure. Future trials will need to explore immune recovery and survival as the endpoints of interest. Regenerative medicine is a fertile area of investigation for the use of UCB outside of oncology. If the use of UCB to repair injured brain or myocardial tissue proves effective, the use of UCB is likely to increase dramatically. As we begin the second quarter century of UCBT, we hope to answer some of these important controversies.

References

1. HE Broxmeyer, GW Gordon, G Hangoc G, et al. Human umbilial cord blood as a potential source of transplantable hematopoietic stem/progenitor cells. Proc Natl Acad Sci USA 1989;86.10: 3828–32.

2. E Gluckman, HE Broxmeyer, AD Auerbach, et al. Hematopoietic reconstitution in a patient with Fanconi anemia by means of umbilical-cord blood from an HLA-identical sibling. N Eng J Med 1989;321.17: 1174–78.

3. AD Auerbach, O Liu, R Ghosh, *et al.* Prenatal identification of potential donors for umbilical cord blood transplantation for Fanconi anemia. *Transfusion* 1990;30.8: 682–7.

4. P Rubinstein, L Dobrila, RE Rosenfield, *et al.* Processing and cryopreservation of placental/umbilical cord blood for unrelated bone marrow reconstitution. *Proc Natl Acad Sci USA* 1995;92: 10119–22.

5. J Kurtzberg, M Laughlin, ML Graham, *et al.* Placental blood as a source of hematopoietic stem cells for transplantation into unrelated recipients. *New Engl J Med* 1996;335.3: 157–66.

6. JE Wagner, JN Barker, TE Defor, *et al.* Transplantation of unrelated donor umbilical cord blood in 102 patients with malignant and nonmalignant diseases. *Blood* 2002;100: 1611–8.

7. V Rocha, J Cornish, E Sievers. Comparison of outcomes of unrelated bone marrow and umbilical cord blood transplants in children with acute leukemia. *Blood* 2010;97.10: 2962–71.

8. M Eapen, P Rubinstein, MJ Zhang, *et al.* Outcomes of transplantation of unrelated donor umbilical cord blood and bone marrow in children with acute leukemia: a comparison study . *Lancet* 2007;369.9577: 1947–54.

9. VK Prasad, A Mendizabal, SH Parikh, *et al.* Unrelated donor umbilical cord blood transplantation for inherited metabolic disorders in 159 pediatric patients from a single center: influence of cellular composisiton of the graft on transplantation outcomes. *Blood* 2008;112.7: 2979–89.

10. JE Wagner, M Eapen, SL Carter, *et al.* No survival advantage after double vs single cord blood transplantation in children with hematologic malignancy. *Blood* 2012;120.21: 359a.

11. MJ Laughlin, J Barker, B Bambach, *et al.* Hematopoietic engraftment and survival in adult recipients of umbilical-cord blood from unrelated donors. *N Engl J Med* 2001;344.24: 1815–22.

12. J Ooi, S Takahashi, A Tomonari, *et al.* Unrelated cord blood transplantation after myeloablative conditioning in adults with acute myelogeneous leukemia. *Biol Blood Marrow Transplant* 2008;14.12: 1341–47.

13. T Mori, S Tanaka, N Tsukada, *et al.* Prospective multicenter study of single-unit cord blood transplantation with myeloablative conditioning for adult patients with high-risk malignancies. *Biol Blood Marrow Transplant* 2013;19: 486–91.

14. J Sanz, JC Boluda, C Martin, *et al.* Single-unit umbilical cord blood transplantation from unrelated donors in patients with hematologic malignancy using busulfan, thiotepa, fludarabine, and ATG as myeloablative conditioning regimen. *Bone Marrow Transplant* 2012;47.10: 1287–93.

15. KK Ballen, E Gluckman, H Broxmeyer. Umbilical cord blood transplantation: The first 25 years and beyond. *Blood* 2013;122.4: 491–8.

16. JN Barker, DJ Weisdorf, TE DeFor, *et al.* Rapid and complete donor chimerism in adult recipients of unrelated donor umbilical cord blood transplantation after reduced intensity conditioning. *Blood* 2003;102.5: 1915–19.

17. KK Ballen, TR Spitzer, BY Yeap, *et al.* Double unrelated reduced-intensity umbilical cord blood transplantation in adults. *Biol Blood Marrow Transplant* 2007;13.1: 82–89.

18. C Cutler, K Stevenson, HT Kim, *et al.* Double umbilical cord blood transplantation with reduced intensity conditioning and sirolimus based GVHD prophylaxis. *Bone Marrow Transplant* 2011;46.5: 273–77.

19. P Ramirez, JE Wagner, TE DeFor, *et al.* Factors predicting single-unit predominance after double umbilical cord blood transplantation. *Bone Marrow Transplant* 2012;47.6: 799–803.

20. MR Verneris, CG Brunstein, J Barker, *et al.* Relapse risk after umbilical cord blood transplantation: enhanced graft-*versus*-leukemia effect in recipients of 2 units. *Blood* 2009;114.9: 4293–9.

21. M Labopin, M Ruggeri, NC Gorin, *et al.* Cost-effectiveness and clinical outcomes of double vs single cord blood transplants in adults with acute leukemia in France. *Leukemia* 2014;99.3: 535–40.

22. JN Barker, A Scaradavou, CE Stevens, *et al.* Combined effect of total nucleated cell dose and HLA match on transplantation outcome in 1061 cord blood recipients with hematologic malignancies. *Blood* 2010;115.9: 1843–49.

23. M Takanashi, YAtsuta, K Fujiwara, *et al.* The impact of anti-HLA antibodies on unrelated cord blood transplantations. *Blood* 2010;116.15: 2839–46.

24. C Cutler C, HT Kim, L Sun, *et al.* Donor-specific anti-HLA antibodies predict outcome in double umbilical cord blood transplantation. *Blood* 2011;118.25: 6691–97.

25. JJ van Rood, CE Stevens, J Smits, *et al.* Reexposure of cord blood to noninherited maternal HLA antigens improves transplant outcomes in hematological malignancies. *Proc Natl Acad Sci USA* 2009;106.47: 19952–7.

26. V Rocha, S Spellman, MJ Zhang, *et al.* Effect of HLA-matching recipients to donor noninherited maternal antigens on outcomes after mismatched umbilical cord blood transplantation for hematologic malignancy. *Biol Blood Marrow Transplant* 2012;18.12: 1890–96.

27. M Eapen, JP Klein, GF Sanz, *et al.* Effect of donor-recipient matching at HLA A, B, C and DRB1 on outcomes after umbilical cord blood transplantation for leukemia and myelodysplastic syndrome: a retrospective analysis. *Lancet Oncol* 2011,12.13: 1214–21.

28. A Garfall, H Kim, C Cutler, *et al.* Allele level matching at HLA-C or DRB1 is associated with improved survival after reduced intensity cord blood transplantation. *Blood* 2012;120.21: 2010a (Abstract).

29. M Eapen, JP,Klein, A Ruggeri, *et al.* Impact of allele-level HLA matching on outcomes after myeloablative single unit umbilical cord blood transplantation for hematologic malignancy. *Blood* 2014;123.1: 133–40.

30. A Garfall, HT Kim,L Sun, *et al.* KIR-ligand incompatibility is not associated with relapse reduction after double umbilical cord blood transplantation. *Bone Marrow Transplant* 2013 ;48.7: 1000–2.

31. CG Brunstein, JE Wagner, DJ Weisdorf, *et al.* Negative effect of KIR alloreactivity in recipients of umbilical cord blood transplants depends on transplantation conditioning intensity. *Blood* 2009;113.22: 5628–34.

32. R Willemze, CA Rogrigues, M Labopin, *et al.* KIR-ligand incompatibility in the graft-*versus*-host direction improves outcomes after umbilical cord transplantation for acute leukemia. *Leukemia* 2009;23.3: 492–500.

33. KM Smith. Analysis of 402 cord blood units to assess factors influencing infused viable CD 34+ cell dose: the critical determinant of engraftment. *Blood* 2013;122.21: 296–300.

34. M Eapen, V Rocha, G Sanz, *et al.* Effect of graft source on unrelated donor hematopoietic stem-cell transplantation in adults with acute leukemia: a retrospective analysis. *Lancet Oncol* 2010;11.7: 653–60.

35. CG Brunstein, JA Gutman, DJ Weisdorf, *et al.* Allogeneic hematopoietic cell transplantation for hematologic malignancy: relative risks and benefits of double umbilical cord blood. *Blood* 2010;116.22: 4693–9.

36. YB Chen, J Aldridge, HT Kim, *et al.* Reduced-intensity conditioning stem cell transplantation: comparison of double umbilical cord blood and unrelated donor grafts. *Biology Blood Marrow Transplant* 2012;8: 805–12.

37. CG Brunstein, M Eapen, KW Ah, *et al.* Reduced-intensity conditioning transplantation in acute leukemia: the effect of source of unrelated donor stem cells on outcomes. *Blood* 2012;119.23: 5591–98.

38. F Milano, T Gooley, B Wood, *et al.* Cord-blood transplantation in patients with minimal residual disease. New Engl J Med 2016;375(10): 444-53.

39. CG Brunstein, EJ Fuchs EJ, SJ Carter, *et al.* Alternative donor transplantation after reduced intensity conditioning: results of parallel phase 2 trials using partially HLA-mismatched related bone marrow or unrelated double umbilical cord blood grafts. *Blood* 2011 ;118.2: 282–88.

40. G Bautista, JR Cabreza, C Regidor, *et al.* Cord blood transplants supported by co-infusion of mobilized hematopoietic stem cells from a third-party donor. *Bone Marrow Transplant* 2009;43.5: 365–73.

41. H Liu, ES Rich, L Godley, *et al.* Reduced-intensity conditioning with combined haploidentical and cord blood transplantation results in rapid engraftment, low GVHD, and durable remissions. *Blood* 2011;118.24: 6438–45.

42. DM Ponce, PB Dahi, S Devlin, *et al.* Double-unit cord blood transplantation combined with haplo-identical CD34+ selected PBSC results in 100% CB engraftment and enhanced myeloid recovery. *Blood* 2013;122:298.

43. F Frassoni, F Gualandi, M Podesta, *et al.* Direct intrabone transplant of unrelated cord-blood cells in acute leukemia: a phase I/II study. *Lancet Oncol* 2008;9.9: 831–39.

44. C Brunstein, JN Barker, DJ Weisdorf, *et al.* Intra-BM injection to enhance engraftment after myeloablative umbilical cord blood transplantation with two partially HLA-matched units. *Bone Marrow Transplant* 2009;43.12: 935–40.

45. C Delaney, S Heimfeld, C Brashem-Stein, *et al.* Notch-mediated expansion of human cord blood progenitor cells capable of rapid myeloid reconstitution. *Nature Med* 2010;16.2: 232–36.

46. M de Lima, I McNiece, SN Robinson, *et al.* Cord-blood engraftment with ex vivo mesenchymal-cell coculture. *N Engl J Med* 2012;367.24: 2305–15.

47. ME Horwitz, NJ Chao. DA Rizzieri, *et al.* Umbilical cord blood expansion with nicotinamide provides long-term mulitlineage engraftment. *J Clin Invest* 2014;124.7: 3121–8.

48. P Montesinos P, T Peled, E Landau, *et al.* Stem-Ex (copper chelation based) ex vivo expanded cord blood umbilical cord blood stem cell transplantation (UCBT) accelerates engraftment and improves 100 day survival in myeloablated patients compared to a registry cohort undergoing double-unit UCBT: results of a multicenter study of 101 patients with hematologic malignancies. *Blood* 2013;122: 295 (Abstract).

49. W Goessling, RS Allen, X Guan, *et al.* Prostaglandin E2 enhances human cord blood stem cell xenotransplants and shows long-term safety in preclinical nonhuman primate transplant models. *Stem Cell* 2011;8.4: 445–58.

50. C Cutler, P Multani, D Robbins, *et al.* Prostaglandin-modulated umbilical cord blood hematopoietic stem cell transplantation. *Blood* 2013;122: 3074–81.

51. UR Popat, B Oran B, CM Hosing, *et al.* Ex vivo fucosylation of cord blood accelerates neutrophil and platelet engraftment. *Blood* 2013;122: 691–95.

52. SS Farag, S Srivastava, S Messina-Graham, *et al.* In-vivo DPP-4 inhibition to enhance engraftment of single-unit cord blood transplants in adults with hematologic malignancies. *Stem Cell Dev* 2013;22: 1007–15.

53. M Norkin, HM Lazarus, JR Wingard. Umbilical cord blood graft enhancement strategies: has the time come to move these into the clinic? *Bone Marrow Transplant* 2013;48.7: 884–9.

54. C Sauter, M Abboud, X Jia, *et al.* Serious infection risk and immune recovery after double-unit cord blood transplantation without antithymocyte globulin. *Biol Blood Marrow Transplant* 2011;17.10: 1–12.

55. P Hanley P, CR Cruz, B Savoldo, *et al.* Functionally active virus-specific T cells that target CMV, adenovirus, and EBV can be expanded from naive T-cell populations in cord blood and will target a range of viral epitopes. *Blood* 2009;114.9: 1958–67.

56. CG Brunstein, J Miller, Q Cao, *et al.* Infusion of ex vivo expanded T regulatory cells in adults transplanted with umbilical cord blood: safety profile and detection kinetics. *Blood* 2011;117.3: 1061–70.

57. KK Ballen, JP Klein, TL Pedersen, *et al.* Relationship of race/ethnicity and survival after single umbilical cord blood transplantation for adults and children with leukemia and myelodysplastic syndromes. *Biol Blood Marrow Transplant* 2012;18.6: 903–12.

58. KK Ballen, S Joffe, R Brazauskas, *et al.* Hospital length of stay in the first 100 days after allogeneic hematopoietic cell transplantation for acute leukemia in remission: comparison among alternative graft sources. *Biol Blood Marrow Transplant* 2014;20.11:1819–27.

59. T Deuse, M Stubbendorff. Immunogenicity and immunomodulatory properties of umbilical cord lining mesenchymal stem cells. *Cell Transplant* 2011;20.5: 655–67.

60. X Cui, M Choppe, A Zacharek, *et al.* Combination treatment of stroke with subtherapeutic doses of Simvastatin and human umbilical cord blood cells enhances vascular remodeling and improves functional outcomes. *Neuroscience* 2012;227: 223–31.

61. CM Cotten, AP Murtha, RN Goldberg, *et al.* Feasibility of autologous cord blood cells for infants wtih hypoxic-ischemic encephalopathy. *J Pediatr* 2014;164: 973–9.

62. JN Barker, C Byam, A Scaradavou. How I treat: the selection and acquisition of

unrelated cord blood grafts. *Blood* 2011;117.8: 2332–9.

63. DM Ponce, J Zheng, AM Gonzales, *et al.* Reduced late mortality risk contributes to similar survival after double-unit cord blood transplantation compared with related and unrelated donor hematopoietic stem cell transplantation. *Biol Blood Marrow Transplant* 2011;17.9: 1316–26.

64. DI Marks, KA Woo, X Zhong, *et al.* Unrelated umbilical cord blood transplantation for adult acute lymphoid leukemia in first or second complete remission. *Hematologica.* 2014;99.2: 322–8.

65. J Sun, J Allison, C McLaughlin, *et al.* Differences in quality between privately and publicly banked umbilical cord blood units: a pilot study of autologous cord blood infusion in children with acquired neurologic disorders. *Transfusion* 2010;50.9: 1980–7.

66. V Jeevanantham, M Butler, A Saad, *et al.* Adult bone marrow cell therapy improves survival and induces long-term improvement in cardiac parameters: a systematic review and meta-analysis. *Circulation* 2012;126.5: 551–68.

67. MJ Haller, CH Wasserfall, MA Hulme, *et al.* Autologous umbilical cord blood infusion followed by oral docosahexaenoic acid and vitamin D supplementation for C-peptide preservation in children with Type 1 diabetes. *Biol Blood Marrow Transplant* 2013;19.7: 1126–9.

Chapter

61

Selecting Human Leukocyte Antigen Haplotype Mismatch *versus* Cord Blood Graft

Asad Bashey

Introduction

An human leukocyte antigen (HLA) match sibling donor (MSD) has been considered the optimal donor for allogeneic hematopoietic cell transplant (HCT) because historically outcomes have been superior with this donor source. However, with the size of the average family in most industrialized nations, MSD are available for only 30% of the patients for allo-HCT (see Chapters 7 and 8). An 8 of 8 (*A, B, C,* and *DRB1* HLA loci) HLA match unrelated donor (MUD) has been considered a suitable alternative in patients who lack an MSD for allo-HCT[1,2]. However, rates of acute and chronic GvHD may be higher following MUD allogeneic HCT (allo-HCT). The probability of obtaining a fully HLA match unrelated MUD is highly dependent upon the patient's ethnicity. Such a donor may be available for more than 70% of white patients of European origin but can be found for less than 20% for some groups of Americans of African origin[3]. For most other ethnicities the frequency is intermediate between these two percentages. Finding an unrelated HLA MUD can be particularly challenging for patients of mixed ethnicity. Furthermore, the acquisition of a hematopoietic cell (HC) product from an unrelated HLA MUD can take several months on average in North America making this an unsuitable option for patients with aggressive malignancies who are in precarious remission. In practice, HLA MSD and HLA MUD donors can be accessed in a timely fashion in only about 60% of patients.

For the patients without timely access to a HLA- MSD or -MUD, options were historically very limited. Most patients would succumb to their malignancy before an allo-HCT could be performed. Recently two alternative donor strategies, namely cord blood (CB) and HLA haplotype mismatch donors, have emerged as suitable graft source for patients who are unable to obtain HC from HLA-MSD or -MUD. Emerging data suggest that for suitably selected patients, results from transplants performed using CB and HLA haplotype mismatch may not be inferior to those performed using HLA MUD[4–9]. No randomized comparisons between allografts using CB unit(s) and HLA haplotype mismatch have been reported. The Blood and Marrow Transplant Clinical Trials Network (BMT CTN) is currently conducting such a randomized comparison using nonmyeloablative conditioning (NMA) for both donor sources (BMT CTN trial 1101).

In the meantime, patients who have access to both unrelated CB - and HLA haplotype- graft sources must choose based on data from studies that have already been completed.

HLA Haplotype Mismatch Transplant or Cord Blood Transplant: How Best to Select

In comparing outcomes between CBT and HLA haplotype mismatch transplant it is important to recognize the different technical approaches that have been developed for using each of these graft sources and to understand the advantages and limitations of these differing technical approaches.

HLA haplotype Mismatch Transplant

HLA haplotype mismatch transplant performed using T-cell-replete (unmanipulated) grafts that used similar GvHD prophylaxis to that used for T-replete HLA-MSD or –MUD HCT (e.g., cyclosporine and methotrexate) resulted in severe T-cell-mediated alloreactivity with high rates of severe GvHD and nonrelapse mortality (NRM)[10,11]. Attempts to reduce this using *ex-vivo* T-cell depletion resulted in high rates of graft rejection and increased the risk of post-transplant relapse and infections[12]. This remained a considerable obstacle until successful strategies were developed to ameliorate these problems.

Correct Method to Suppress Donor's Alloreactive T-Cells: Is Post-Transplant Cyclophosphamide the Correct Answer?

Approaches to control alloreactivity have coalesced into three major categories:

1. *Ex-vivo* T-cell depletion. This strategy was first characterized by the use of *ex-vivo* T-cell depletion and was primarily developed by investigators in Perugia. They used a large dose of G-CSF mobilized peripheral blood HCs ("mega dose," median CD34+ cells 13.8×10^6/kg) that was subjected to *ex-vivo* T-cell depletion resulting in a residual dose of $\leq 3 \times 10^4$ CD3+ cells/kg[13]. This product was combined with a preparative regimen consisting of thiotepa, total body radiation (TBI), fludarabine, and antithymocyte globulin (ATG). No additional immunosuppression was used post-transplant. Primary engraftment occurred in 91% of patients. GvHD occurred

in a small minority of patients. However, NRM was high at the rates of 37% and 44% in patients who were in remission and not in remission at the time of transplant, respectively. Infection was the primary cause of nonrelapse death.

A newer iteration of this approach recently published by the Perugia group uses a CD34+ cell-selected graft followed by infusion of controlled numbers of regulatory (Treg) and conventional (Tcon) T-cells on day −4 and day 0, respectively[14]. Using this approach rates of acute and chronic GvHD were similarly low to those seen using their original approach although rates of relapse were lower (5% *versus* 21%). However, again the rate of NRM continues to be relatively high (40%) and deaths once again are primarily due to infection (see Chapter 59).

2. *In-vivo* T-cell depletion using anti-T-cell antibodies. The group at Peking University has treated the most patients using this approach. Over the last 9 years the group has transplanted 756 patients with leukemia from HLA haplotype mismatch donors using a graft that comprises G-CSF stimulated bone marrow-HC and PB-HC without *ex-vivo* T-depletion[15]. A myeloablative preparative regimen with multiple alkylators and intense pre- and post-transplant immunosuppression using ATG, cyclosporine, mycophenolate, and methotrexate was used. Patients received a median CD34+ and CD3+ cell dose of 2.21×10^6/kg and 1.53×10^8/kg, respectively. This approach was associated with high rates of neutrophil and platelet engraftment (99% and 92%, respectively). Three-year cumulative incidence of NRM was 18%. Maximum cumulative incidences of acute (grade II–IV) and chronic GvHD were 43% and 53%, respectively. Three-year leukemia-free survival (LFS) rates of 68% and 49% were seen in "standard-risk" and "high-risk" patients, respectively. Rizzieri *et al.* have used a reduced intensity (RIC) regimen with high doses of PB-HC and *in-vivo* T-depletion using alemtuzumab to achieve a 94% engraftment rate[16]. Cumulative rates of NRM and severe acute GvHD were 10.8% and 8%, respectively. However the 1-year survival rate was only 31%. In a later modification of this approach the dose of alemtuzumab was reduced and cyclophosphamide was replaced with either busulfan or melphalan in order to reduce the rate of infections and relapse seen in the prior study[17]. However, in a comparison of transplants from various donor sources using this regimen, survival was significantly inferior in patients transplanted from HLA haplotype mismatch donor *versus* MSD grafts.

3. pt-Cy without *ex-vivo* or *in-vivo* nonselective T-depletion. Work pioneered in Baltimore has demonstrated that high-dose cyclophosphamide administered on day +3 and +4 (pt-Cy) combined with tacrolimus and mycophenolate administered post-transplant can effectively control alloreactivity following HLA haplotype mismatch transplant[18,19]. Unlike the nonselective strategies of T-cell depletion, this approach appears to selectively target highly activated and proliferative alloreactive T-cells in the early post-transplant period while "sparing" effector memory T-cells, which are important for anti-infection immunity and Treg cells[20,21]. Consistent with this observation, rates of opportunistic infections appear to be no higher than those seen following conventional HLA match allo-HCT. Although randomized comparisons have not yet been completed, a nonrandomized comparison of contemporaneous patients transplanted at a single center demonstrated that rates of acute and chronic GvHD, NRM, relapse, and disease-free and overall survival were not inferior in patients undergoing HLA haplotype mismatch transplant plus pt-Cy when compared to patients who underwent conventional HLA match donor transplants (MSD and MUD)[4]. It has also been demonstrated that the degree of HLA mismatch on the nonshared (mismatch) haplotype does not appear to affect outcomes following HLA haplotype mismatch transplant plus pt-Cy[22]. While the original approach to HLA haplotype mismatch transplant with pt-Cy developed in Baltimore utilized a *bone marrow* graft with NMA conditioning, they can also be safely performed using PB HCs and "myeloablative" conditioning (MAC) regimens[23–26].

There are no randomized comparisons between the approaches using nonselective *in-vivo* or *ex-vivo* T-depletion. However, Ciurea *et al.*[27] have demonstrated in a single-center retrospective comparison that HLA haplotype mismatch transplant plus pt-Cy produced lower rates of infection, NRM, and chronic GvHD and superior rates of OS and progression-free survival (PFS) compared to an approach using *ex-vivo* and *in-vivo* nonselective T-depletion. The simplicity and efficacy of pt-Cy in the setting of HLA haplotype mismatch transplant has made it perhaps the most easily disseminated method in comparison to the other approaches. Furthermore, it appears to be the most economically viable. It is therefore likely that pt-Cy will be significantly more popular than other approaches (as described above) in the setting of HLA haplotype mismatch transplant in the foreseeable future. Furthermore, the BMT CTN has chosen this approach as the one to assess in multicenter trials and to directly compare to dCBT.

Cord Blood Transplant

CBT was first performed just over 25 years ago and since then in excess of 30 000 of these transplants have been performed worldwide. It is clear that a greater HLA mismatch is tolerable for unrelated donor CBT than for HLA mismatch *bone marrow* or PB HC grafts, particularly if the available cord blood cell dose is adequate ($\geq3\times10^7$ total nucleated cells/kg). In the pediatric setting CBT is an established donor source and there appears to be no benefit to using tow or double units of cord blood for transplant when a single CB unit is available with adequate cell dose[28]. In retrospective comparisons, unrelated CBT was associated with slower engraftment, less

GvHD, and similar leukemia-free survival and OS to HLA MUD transplants[7,8,29] (see Chapter 60).

When adult recipients of a single CB unit with a cell dose $\geq 2.5 \times 10^7$ TNC/kg were compared to recipients of HLA MUD transplants, CBT was associated with a higher NRM and lower chronic GvHD than 8/8 HLA MUD transplants; however, the LFS was not different[30]. However, single CB units often fail to provide an adequate cell dose for adult patients and for such patients the use of two or double CB units is the only viable strategy in the absence of a commercialized method of CBU expansion (see Chapter 66). In a retrospective comparison to single CBT, dCBT was associated with better outcomes in adult patients treated in CR1 but not in CR2[31]. Also in a retrospective comparison from two transplant centers, where a "myeloablative" TBI-based regimen was used in both groups, dCBT was associated with slower engraftment and higher NRM than HLA MUD transplant. However, relapse risk was lower after dCBT than HLA MUD and LFS was not different[6]. The role of ATG during conditioning for CBT remains uncertain. In a comparison performed in pediatric recipients of CBT, ATG was associated with higher rates of post-transplant infections and lower rates of acute but not chronic GvHD than CBT performed without ATG[32]. Many investigators eschew the use of ATG for CBT given the already slow rate of immune reconstitution following such transplants, particularly in adults. Older adult patients are also unable to tolerate the MAC regimen used in many pediatric protocols of CBT. Thus RIC and NMA conditioning regimens have been developed to enable such patients to access CBT (Minnesota and DFCI studies). Among these regimens, the TCF (low-dose TBI, cyclophosphamide, fludarabine without ATG) regimen developed by investigators in Minnesota remains among the most widely reported and employed [33]. Indeed, in a comparison performed with HLA MUD transplants, dCBT using the TCF regimen had similar NRM and overall mortality to 8 of 8 HLA MUD whereas the outcomes for dCBT performed using other regimens were inferior[5]. Thus in the absence of randomized comparisons, the TCF regimen appears to represent the current standard of care for dCBT. Furthermore, the similarity of the TCF regimen in dCBT to the regimen most commonly used for T-replete HLA haplotype mismatch transplant (with pt-Cy) represents the most appropriate comparative method between the two allograft strategies. Indeed these two regimens have been formally used by the BMT CTN to compare dCBT to HLA haplotype mismatch transplant in parallel phase 2 studies[34] and the ongoing randomized phase 3 trial (BMT CTN 1101).

Comparison of Cord Blood Transplant with HLA Haplotype Mismatch Transplant: Is This a Fair Comparison?

Graft Composition and Immunologic Recovery
Graft composition differs significantly between CB grafts and marrow or PB derived from conventional donors. Compared to grafts from living volunteer donors, CB grafts contain very few antigen-specific memory T-cells and a greater proportion of naïve T-cells[35]. Thus, whereas thymic-independent peripheral expansion of donor-derived memory T-cells is the primary mechanism of early immune reconstitution following conventional donor transplantation, it is greatly deficient following CBT[36,37]. However, thymic-dependent late immune reconstitution beyond 6 months may be equivalent following CBT compared to conventional donor transplants, particularly in pediatric patients. In older adult patients, the slow immune reconstitution following CBT may be further exacerbated because of thymic atrophy[38,39]. In contrast, unmanipulated marrow or PB-derived grafts from volunteer related donors as used for HLA haplotype mismatch transplant with pt-Cy are rich in effector memory cells targeting common infectious pathogens, which may provide effective immunity against those pathogens in the early transplant period. Since these cells are not alloreactive, are likely quiescent in the first few days following HLA haplotype mismatch transplant, and proliferate more slowly in response to lymphopenia they are relatively spared by the lethal effect of pt-Cy, which is effective in eliminating the alloreactive cells that would otherwise produce unacceptable rates of GvHD or graft rejection in this setting[21].CB grafts are also relatively deficient in Treg cells, whereas these cells are present in the graft used for HLA haplotype mismatch transplant with pt-Cy and are relatively spared the lethality of pt-Cy because of their high expression of aldehyde dehydrogenase[20]. Consistent with these differences in graft composition several investigators have found significantly delayed recovery in cellular immunity following CBT when compared to that seen following conventional donor (MSD and MUD) transplants[36,40], whereas recovery of cellular immunity following HLA haplotype mismatch transplant with pt-Cy is rapid and not substantially different from that seen following T-replete transplants from conventional donors [9,41]. Consistent with these differences in graft composition and immune recovery, some investigators have demonstrated a higher incidence of mortality from infections in the first 6 months following CBT when compared to transplants from HLA MUD[9,37], although no clear increase in deaths from infections has been reported following HLA haplotype mismatch transplant with pt-Cy than with HLA MUD transplants [9]. These infections are a major component of the higher NRM often observed in recipients of CBT in comparison to recipients of conventional HLA match donor (sibling and unrelated) transplants.

Comparisons of Post-Transplant Outcomes between Cord Blood Transplant and HLA Haplotype Mismatch Transplant
CBT and HLA haplotype mismatch transplant are the often both available as options for patients who lack a conventional donor, and both approaches have demonstrated acceptable

outcomes for such patients. However, as yet there have been no prospective randomized comparisons between haploidentical donor transplant (HIDT) and CBT. The BMT CTN is currently conducting such a randomized comparison but until its results are available we must rely on available nonrandomized and mostly retrospective comparisons (summarized in Table 61.1). In the only prospective comparison hitherto reported, the BMT CTN conducted two parallel prospective studies (0603 and 0604)of HLA haplotype mismatch transplant with pt-Cy and dCBT, respectively[34]. The eligibility criteria were identical and the trials used a common study design and were simultaneously conducted. The most widely reported approaches to nonmyeloablative conditioning with T-replete HLA haplotype mismatch transplant with pt-Cy and dCBT, namely the regimen developed by the Baltimore group and the TCF regimen developed by the Minnesota group respectively, were used in these studies. The regimens were remarkably similar to each other and neither employed *in-vivo* T-depletion with ATG. The results of these studies showed that neutrophil recovery to ANC 500/µL occurred at a median of 16 and 15 days for HLA haplotype mismatch transplant with pt-Cy and dCBT, respectively. However, median time to platelet recovery to 50000/mL was shorter after HLA haplotype mismatch transplant with pt-Cy than dCBT at 26 and 43 days, respectively. Acute GvHD grade III–IV occurred in 0% *versus* 21%, respectively. One-year estimated probabilities were as follows for HLA haplotype mismatch transplant with pt-Cy *versus* dCBT: NRM 7% *versus* 24%; relapse 45% *versus* 31%; chronic GvHD 13% *versus* 25%; PFS 48% *versus* 46%, and survival 62% *versus* 54%. These data suggest that these two approaches are both valid and effective alternatives in patients who do not have timely access to a conventional donor. The differences observed between HLA haplotype mismatch transplant with pt-Cy and dCBT are intriguing. However, the studies were not designed to directly compare HLA haplotype mismatch transplant with pt-CY and dCBT. Also, given the small size of the studies and their nonrandomized design the effect of imbalances in patient selection can be substantial and must be treated with caution. These trials represent a foundation for the ongoing randomized trial rather than a conclusive comparison of these graft sources.

Other direct comparisons of HLA haplotype mismatch transplant with pt-Cy and CBT have relied on retrospective analysis. El-Cheikh *et al.*[42] compared 69 patients who underwent HIDT-pt-Cy to 81 patients who underwent UCBT at their centers. Patient characteristics were similar except there was a significantly greater proportion of patients with acute leukemias in the CBT group and with Hodgkin lymphoma (HL) in the HLA haplotype mismatch transplant with pt-Cy group. The nonmyeloablative regimen used for both groups consisted of cyclophosphamide, fludarabine, and 2Gy TBI. Post-transplant GvHD prophylaxis was also the same in both groups and consisted of cyclosporine A and MMF. However, the HLA haplotype mismatch transplant patients received the standard dose of pt-Cy (50mg/kg/day on days 3 and 4).

Supportive care measures, including management of CMV infections, were similar. Follow-up was longer in the CBT patients (59 months *versus* 18 months). Non-engraftment rates were similar (11% *versus* 12%) as was time to neutrophil recovery (22 *versus* 20 days) but platelet recovery was delayed in the CBT (41 *versus* 29 days). More RBC and platelet transfusions were used for the CBT patients. Rates of NRM were not different but acute and chronic GvHD was greater in the CBT patients and both overall survival (45% *versus* 69%) and PFS (36% *versus* 65%) were superior following HLA haplotype mismatch transplant with pt-Cy. The differences in rates of GvHD, survival, and PFS need to be treated with caution given the differences in patient characteristics between the two groups. Raiola *et al.*[9] recently reported on a retrospective comparison of 105 CBT to 92 HLA haplotype mismatch transplants with pt-Cy. The CBT were infused directly into the marrow cavity and all the HLA haplotype mismatch transplants with pt-Cy were performed using marrow grafts. Unlike the study by El-Cheikh *et al.*, the majority of patients for both the CBT and HLA haplotype mismatch transplant with pt-Cy groups in the study by Raiola *et al.* received myeloablative conditioning. HLA haplotype mismatch transplants with pt-Cy were performed using cyclosporine A and MMF (starting day 0 and day +1 respectively for GvHD prophylaxis with the standard dose of pt-Cy (50mg/kg on days 3 and 4)). The CBT patients received cyclosporine A, MMF, and ATG. HLA haplotype mismatch transplant with pt-Cy patients were somewhat older, had more advanced disease, and fewer had acute leukemias and more had lymphoid malignancies than the CBT patients. Neutrophil and platelet recovery was significantly slower following CBT compared to HLA haplotype mismatch transplant with pt-Cy. CD4 counts were comparable in MSD and HLA haplotype mismatch transplant with pt-Cy after 50 days but were lower in CBT than MSD until 180 days. All groups had comparable CD4+ counts after 1 year. While total rates of reported viral, fungal, and bacterial infections were not clearly different between HLA haplotype mismatch transplant with pt-Cy and CBT, lethal infections occurred in 17% of CBT *versus* 11% of HLA haplotype mismatch transplant with pt-Cy. Rates of acute and chronic GvHD and discontinuation of immunosuppressive therapy were not significantly different between CBT and HLA haplotype mismatch transplant with pt-CY although it is important to appreciate that CBT received ATG as part of their conditioning whereas HLA haplotype mismatch transplant with pt-Cy did not. Cumulative incidence of TRM was not statistically different when comparing all patients. However, patients in CR1 had a TRM of 37% in CBT and 17% in HLA haplotype mismatch transplant with pt-Cy (*P*=0.06). Relapse rates were not different. Actuarial 4-year survival was 34% *versus* 52% for UCBT and HIDT-pt-Cy respectively (*P*=NS). For patients in CR1 and CR2, the rates were 33% and 57%, respectively (*P*=0.09). Similarly, for CR1 and CR2 patients, disease-free survival was 38% for CBT *versus* 60% for HLA haplotype mismatch transplant with pt-Cy (*P*= 0.10). In a multivariate analysis, the use of CBT *versus* HLA-

Table 61.1 Studies comparing cord blood transplantation to haplotype mismatch donor transplantation

	Brunstein et al.[34]	El-Cheikh et al.[42]		Raiola et al.[9]		González-Vicent et al.[43]		Mo et al.[44]		
Trial design	Parallel prospective trials#	Retrospective comparison		Retrospective comparison		Retrospective comparison		Retrospective match analysis		
	CBT	HHMT	CBT	HHMT	CBT	HHMT	CBT	HHMT	CBT	HHMT
n	50	50	81	69	105	92	38	29	37	111
Median age	58	48	47	44	40	4	6	9	9	15
Gender M/F	NA	NA	46/35	39/30	NA	NA	18/20	21/8	23/14	78/33
Diagnoses										
AML	29	22	37	3	70	39	24	18	18	54
ALL	6	6	14	1			14	11	9	27
MDS/MPD	0	0	8	2	23	14	0	0	9	27
NHL/HL	14	19	16	54 *	10	25	0	0	1	3
Others	1	3	6	9	2	4	0	0	0	0
Preparative regimen	(RIC)TCF	(RIC)JHU	(RIC) JHU	RIC (JHU)	(MAC) TBF or TBI based (RIC) FluCyTBI	(MAC)TBF or TBI based (RIC) FluCyTBI	(MAC) BuCy or FluBuCy or FluBuThio	(RIC) FluBuThio	(MAC) AraC Bu Cy Simustine ATG	(MAC) AraC Bu Cy Simustine ATG
GvHD prophylaxis	CSA, MMF	pt-Cy tacrolimus MMF	CSA MMF	pt-Cy CSA MMF	ATG CSA MMF	pt-Cy CSA MMF	CSA ATG methylpred	CSA Mtx or CSA methylpr	CSA MMF methylpred	CSA MMF Mtx
Median follow-up (months)	12	12	59	18	12.5	19	57	16	40	36
Engraftment										
ANC >0.5K median days	15	16	22	20	23	18	20	* 13	18 *	13
Platelets >20K median days	38	24	41	29	NA	NA	56	11 *	33	16 *
Acute GvHD										
II–IV (% CI)	40	32	52	29 *	19	14	44	19	42	49

Table 61.1 (cont.)

Trial design	Brunstein et al.[34] Parallel prospective trials#	El-Cheikh et al.[42] Retrospective comparison		Raiola et al.[9] Retrospective comparison		González-Vicent et al.[43] Retrospective comparison		Mo et al.[44] Retrospective match analysis		
	CBT	HHMT	CBT	HHMT	CBT	HHMT	CBT	HHMT	CBT	HHMT
III–IV (%CI)	21	0	NA	NA	1	4	NA	NA	11	16
Chronic GvHD (% CI)	25	13	12	* 6	23	˜5	NA	NA	20.5	* 60.5
NRM/TRM (%CI)	24 @ 1 yr	7 @ 1 yr	23 @ 1 yr	17 @1 yr	35 @ 2.7 yrs	˜8 @ 2.7 yrs	47	* 25		
Relapse (%CI)	31 @ 1 yr	45 @ 1 yr	NA	NA	30	35	25	48	11	18
DFS/PFS (KM %)	46 @ 1 yr	48 @ 1 yr	36@ 2 yrs	* 65 @ 2 yrs	33 @ 4 yrs	43 @ y rs	32	* 44	54 @ 1 yr	68@ 1 yr
OS (KM %)	54 @ 1 yr	62 @ 1 yr	45 @ 2 yrs	69 @ 2 yrs	34 @ 4 yrs	52 @ 4 yrs	NA	NA	57@ 1 yr	73 @ 1 yr *

* = difference between CBT and HHMT is statistically significant
# - parallel trials not intended for direct comparison therefore no statistical significance provided
RIC= reduced intensity or nonmyeloablative conditioning; MAC = myeloablative conditioning regimen;
TCF= TBI 200cGy d-1, cyclophosphamide 50mg/m^2 d -6, fludarabine 40mg/m^2/d d-6 to -2
JHU = TBI 200cGy d -1, cyclophosphamide 14.5mg/kg/d -6 & -5, fludarabine 30mg/m^2/d d-6 to -2 (or very similar regimen)
TBF = thiotepa, busulfan, fludarabine
AraC= cytarabine, Bu= busulfan, Cy = cyclophosphamide, CSA = cyclosporine A, MMF = mycophenolate mofetil, Mtx = methotrexate
CI = cumulative incidence, KM = Kaplan-Meier, OS = overall survival, DFS = disease-free survival, PFS = progression-free survival
HHMT=HLA haplotype mismatch transplant

MSD but not HLA haplotype mismatch transplant with pt-Cy *versus* HLA-MSD was a negative predictor for survival (HR 1.4, $P=0.03$ and HR 0.95, $P=NS$, respectively).

The studies described above allow a direct comparison of CBT to HLA haplotype mismatch transplant with pt-Cy but they are each subject to flaws that limit the conclusions that can be drawn. The studies reported in the paper by Brunstein *et al.*[34] were prospective and had identical eligibility criteria and study plans with similar nonmyeloablative conditioning regimens. However, they were relatively small parallel phase 2 studies subject to selection bias and not designed to directly compare the outcomes of CBT and HLA haplotype mismatch transplant with pt-Cy. The study by El-Cheikl *et al.*[42] was also small, retrospective, and subject to significant differences in patient characteristics between the CBT and HLA haplotype mismatch transplant with pt-Cy groups. However, the conditioning regimens were similar. Although larger, the study by Raiola *et al.*[9] was also retrospective and was compromised by the use of different conditioning and GvHD prophylaxis regimens between the CBT and HLA haplotype mismatch transplant with pt-Cy groups, in particular the use of ATG for CBT. Nevertheless, these reports suggest that HLA haplotype mismatch transplant with pt-Cy does not produce inferior outcomes to UCBT and chronic GvHD appears to be lower following HLA haplotype mismatch transplant with pt-Cy when ATG is not used with CBT.

Two additional reported studies have compared HLA haplotype mismatch transplant performed using methods other than pt-Cy with CBT in pediatric patients. A study by González-Vicent *et al.*[43] compared 29 patients who received an HLA haplotype mismatch transplant using *ex-vivo* T-cell depletion by either CD34+ cell selection or CD3+/CD19+ cell depletion using the *Milltenyi device* with 39 unmanipulated CBT. The study was compromised by its small size, differences in patient characteristics, regimen intensity, and GvHD prophylaxis between the HLA haplotype mismatch transplant and CBT groups. They found that NRM and acute GvHD rates were lower and leukemia-free survival was higher following HLA haplotype mismatch transplant than CBT. Mo *et al.*[44] compared 33 single CBTs to 337 HLA haplotype mismatch transplants. Both groups of patients were treated using the Peking University approach consisting of intense conditioning regimen and rabbit ATG and unmanipulated grafts. CBT received methylprednisone instead of methotrexate for GvHD prophylaxis. The strengths of this study include the relatively similar conditioning regimen between HLA haplotype mismatch transplant and CBT and matching of each CBT patient with three HLA haplotype mismatch transplant patients for baseline characteristics. The results showed that the HLA haplotype mismatch transplant patients had more rapid engraftment, higher rates of acute GvHD, lower rates of NRM, and better 1-year survival.

Other Considerations

In deciding whether CBT or HLA haplotype mismatch transplant is the option chosen for patients who lack a conventional donor, comparative outcomes – both those summarized in the above section and forthcoming comparisons from randomized studies – will be primary determinants, However, other evident differences between these graft sources may also be considered (Table 61.2).

Table 61.2 Relative advantages and disadvantages of cord blood transplant *versus* HLA haplotype mismatch transplant post-transplant cyclophosphamide

	CBT	HHMT-pt-Cy
Donor availability	Greater availability for ethnic minorities than HLA MUD but limited for large/obese recipients	Almost universal donor availability with more than two donors available for average recipient
Availability in developing nations	Poor due to lack of CB banks and expense	Readily available and relatively inexpensive
Graft acquisition expense	High – greater graft acquisition cost than HLA MUD if dCBT used	Costs significantly lower – limited to collection of graft by marrow harvest or leukapheresis
Time from search initiation to transplant	More rapid progression from search initiation to transplant than HLA MUD	Most rapid progress from search initiation to transplant – most control over access to donor
DLI for relapse of malignancy	Not available – major limitation in relapsing patients	Readily available – safety & efficacy now demonstrated using low doses of T-cells or post-DLI immunosuppression
Use in donors sensitized to HLA antigens	Rapid immune reconstitution from memory T-cells in graft. Similar risk of early infections to conventional donor transplants	Rapid immune reconstitution from memory T-cells in graft. Similar risk of early infections to conventional donor transplants
Immune reconstitution	Slow immune reconstitution particularly in adults. Lack of memory T-cells and thymic atrophy in adults. Use of ATG exacerbates this problem	Rapid immune reconstitution from memory T-cells in graft. Similar risk of early infections to conventional donor transplant

Availability of DLI

Donor lymphocyte infusion (DLI) is an important therapeutic option for patients who experience relapse of malignancy following transplants from HLA- MSD and - MUD
(see Chapter 25). DLI may be used alone particularly in
highly immunogenic, slow-growing malignancies and in disease that is detected using molecular techniques prior to
frank clinical relapse. It may also be used in combination
with chemotherapy and other antineoplastic agents in other
malignancies. CBT typically involves administration of the
entire cryopreserved product at the time of transplantation
and DLI is therefore typically not available, potentially
limiting therapeutic options at the time of relapse following
this type of transplant. In contrast, additional lymphocytes
are usually relatively easily acquired from a living related
HLA-haploidentical donor. Experience using DLI to treat
relapse is more limited following HLA haplotype mismatch
transplant than following conventional donor transplants.
Initially there were concerns that the administration of
DLI from HLA-haploidentical donors without additional
pt-Cy or other forms of controlling alloreactivity would
result in severe and potentially fatal GvHD. However, both
the Baltimore group and the group at Peking University
have demonstrated the safety and efficacy of HLA haplotype
mismatch donor-derived DLI using different approaches (see
Chapter 59).

Huang *et al.* reported on the use of G-CSF primed DLI in
patients who had relapsed following HLA haplotype mismatch
transplant for leukemias[45]. Twenty patients were treated of
which eight achieved a CR. Acute GvHD grade III–IV
occurred in six patients. The two-year probability of
leukemia-free survival was 40%. In a later analysis of
124 patients treated with such DLI for relapse, preemption of
relapse, or prophylaxis, the authors determined that prophylactic immunosuppression with cyclosporine or methotrexate
for up to 6 weeks post-DLI was associated with a significantly
reduced rate of severe acute GvHD[46]. Zeidan *et al.* reported
on 40 patients who received DLI after relapse of malignancy
following HLA haplotype mismatch transplant with pt-Cy[47].
In contrast to the studies from Beijing, the DLI were not G-
CSF primed and no post-DLI immunosuppression was used.
Initial CD3+ cell dose was 1×10^5/kg with the most commonly
administered dose being 1×10^6/kg. No post-DLI immunosuppression was used. Acute GvHD grades II–IV and III–IV
developed in 10 and 6 patients, respectively. Twelve patients
(30%) achieved a CR. These data suggest that the use of DLI to
treat or prevent relapse following HLA haplotype mismatch
transplant can be safe and effective. The use of appropriate
precautions such as low doses of T-cells or post-DLI immunosuppression may be necessary given the greater potential for
alloreactivity in this setting than seen following DLI from
conventional donors.

As additional donor-derived lymphocytes are usually not
available to treat relapse of malignancy after CBT (see

Chapter 66), this represents a tangible and significant
advantage on the use of HLA haplotype mismatch transplant over CBT.

Cost

As financial pressures on healthcare resources increase the
relative costs of alternative donor sources will come under
greater scrutiny. CB has to be obtained from cord blood banks
at significant acquisition costs estimated at US$40000 or
greater per unit. These costs are amplified in dCBT, which is
the dominant form of CBT in adults. Technologies designed to
expand the number of hematopoietic cells in each CBU are
currently being investigated. If successful, they may potentially
lower the costs of CBT by allowing the use of single rather than
double CB for adult transplantation. However, it is also possible that they may increase the costs of CBT depending upon
the rate at which these technologies are priced at commercialization. Acquisition cost for an HLA haplotype mismatch
donor graft is considerably lower than for CBT and is equivalent to that for HLA MSD. Furthermore, the use of HLA
haplotype mismatch transplant with pt-Cy avoids the expense
of graft engineering associated with *ex-vivo* T-depletion and/or
ATG associated with other methods of HLA haplotype mismatch transplant. Thus the advantage here currently lies with
HLA haplotype mismatch transplant with pt-Cy. If HLA haplotype mismatch transplant with pt-Cy is indeed associated
with a lower incidence of early infections than CBT then that
may also be associated with a cost advantage.

The relative costs of HLA haplotype mismatch transplant
with pt-Cy and dCBT will be formally compared as part of the
objectives of BMT CTN clinical trial 1101[48]. Consenting
patients will provide health insurance information to allow
calculation of direct medical costs from reimbursement
records, and will provide out-of-pocket costs, time costs, and
health-related quality of life measures through an online
survey. The results of this analysis will establish the relative
cost-effectiveness of the two alternative donor sources as an
important adjunct to the clinical outcomes measured.

Availability of CB Units

Since the original CBT performed in 1988, unrelated cord
blood banks have been established in almost all developed
nations. More than 600000 CB units are now available for
transplantation in such banks. However, there remains a
lack of such facilities in many developing nations. Ethnic
disparities between these nations and the developed nations
where CB units are acquired and stored, as well as the
significant cost of acquiring these units for transplantation,
has been a major barrier to the development of CBT in these
nations. In contrast, the local availability of the donor, the
much lower acquisition cost, and the lack of need for sophisticated technology make HLA haplotype mismatch transplant with pt-Cy in particular a more feasible strategy for
developing nations.

Summary

Significant progress has recently been made in developing alternative donor sources for patients who need hematopoietic cell transplantation but do not have timely access to a conventional donor. Both CB and HLA haplotype mismatch donors have now become established graft sources for alternative donor transplantation in such patients. This has been a particularly important development for patients from ethnic minority and mixed race backgrounds in Western nations and has significantly expanded access to hematopoietic cell transplantation for these groups. Patients with aggressive malignancies who may suffer relapse of their disease during the time required to acquire a HLA MUD graft have also benefited from these developments.

In patients for whom both suitable CB and HLA haplotype mismatch donors are available, which is the preferred strategy? Data presented here suggest that while there may be equipoise in the most important outcomes, i.e., overall and disease-free survival, until the results of large randomized comparisons become available, it appears that in adult patients, HLA haplotype mismatch transplant particularly using T-replete graft and pt-Cy is associated with less chronic GvHD and a more robust early immune reconstitution perhaps resulting in a lower rate of early infections and NRM than CBT. Whether these advantages to HLA haplotype mismatch transplant with pt-Cy will be countered by a higher rate of relapse in these patients will be answered by the results of current randomized trials. In the largest retrospective comparisons between HLA haplotype mismatch transplant with pt-Cy and other types of allografts including CB (HLA-MSD, -MUD, and CB transplants), the HLA haplotype mismatch transplant with pt-Cy does not appear to be associated with a higher relapse rate[4,9]. Costs and practicality appear to favor HLA haplotype mismatch transplant with pt-Cy (and not necessarily other types/methods of HLA haplotype mismatch transplant) when compared to CBT. More comprehensive analyses of these issues will be forthcoming from randomized studies. So far there is greater worldwide experience and more long-term outcome data with CBT than HLA haplotype mismatch transplant although that may change in the future. Center experience may contribute to NRM and treatment success and thus may be an important determinant of the preferred option in individual locations. The experience hitherto reported with CBT and HLA haplotype mismatch transplant has largely been concentrated within centers that specialize in and thus disproportionately use one of these graft sources over the other. Thus only in randomized comparisons will the bias associated with center experience be relatively diminished. These are exciting times in the field of alternative donor transplantation. Both CBT and HLA haplotype mismatch transplant appear to have taken us closer to the goal of universal donor availability.

References

1. Lee SJ, Klein J, Haagenson M, Baxter-Lowe LA, Confer DL, Eapen M, *et al.* High-resolution donor-recipient HLA matching contributes to the success of unrelated donor marrow transplantation. *Blood* 2007;110(13):4576–83.

2. Woolfrey A, Klein JP, Haagenson M, Spellman S, Petersdorf E, Oudshoorn M, *et al.* HLA-C antigen mismatch is associated with worse outcome in unrelated donor peripheral blood stem cell transplantation. *Biol Blood Marrow Transplant* 2011;17(6):885–92.

3. Gragert L, Eapen M, Williams E, Freeman J, Spellman S, Baitty R, *et al.* HLA match likelihoods for hematopoietic stem-cell grafts in the U.S. registry. *N Engl J Med* 2014;371(4):339–48.

4. Bashey A, Zhang X, Sizemore CA, Manion K, Brown S, Holland HK, *et al.* T-cell-replete HLA-haploidentical hematopoietic transplantation for hematologic malignancies using post-transplantation cyclophosphamide results in outcomes equivalent to those of contemporaneous HLA-match related and unrelated donor transplantation. *J Clin Oncol* 2013;31(10):1310–6.

5. Brunstein CG, Eapen M, Ahn KW, Appelbaum FR, Ballen KK, Champlin RE, *et al.* Reduced-intensity conditioning transplantation in acute leukemia: the effect of source of unrelated donor stem cells on outcomes. *Blood* 2012;119(23):5591–8.

6. Brunstein CG, Gutman JA, Weisdorf DJ, Woolfrey AE, Defor TE, Gooley TA, *et al.* Allogeneic hematopoietic cell transplantation for hematologic malignancy: relative risks and benefits of double umbilical cord blood. *Blood* 2010;116(22):4693–9.

7. Eapen M, Rubinstein P, Zhang MJ, Stevens C, Kurtzberg J, Scaradavou A, *et al.* Outcomes of transplantation of unrelated donor umbilical cord blood and bone marrow in children with acute leukaemia: a comparison study. *Lancet* 2007;369(9577):1947–54.

8. Rocha V, Cornish J, Sievers EL, Filipovich A, Locatelli F, Peters C, *et al.* Comparison of outcomes of unrelated bone marrow and umbilical cord blood transplants in children with acute leukemia. *Blood* 2001;97(10):2962–71.

9. Raiola AM, Dominietto A, di Grazia C, Lamparelli T, Gualandi F, Ibatici A, *et al.* Unmanipulated haploidentical transplants compared with other alternative donors and match sibling grafts. *Biol Blood Marrow Transplant* 2014;20(10):1573–9.

10. Anasetti C, Beatty PG, Storb R, Martin PJ, Mori M, Sanders JE, *et al.* Effect of HLA incompatibility on graft-*versus*-host disease, relapse, and survival after marrow transplantation for patients with leukemia or lymphoma. *Hum Immunol* 1990;29(2):79–91.

11. Beatty PG, Clift RA, Mickelson EM, Nisperos BB, Flournoy N, Martin PJ, *et al.* Marrow transplantation from related donors other than HLA-identical siblings. *N Engl J Med* 1985;313(13):765–71.

12. Ash RC, Horowitz MM, Gale RP, van Bekkum DW, Casper JT, Gordon-Smith EC, *et al.* Bone marrow transplantation from related donors other than HLA-identical siblings: effect of T cell depletion. *Bone Marrow Transplant* 1991;7(6):443–52.

13. Aversa F, Terenzi A, Tabilio A, Falzetti F, Carotti A, Ballanti S, et al. Full haplotype-mismatch hematopoietic stem-cell transplantation: a phase II study in patients with acute leukemia at high risk of relapse. *J Clin Oncol* 2005;23(15):3447–54.

14. Martelli MF, Di Ianni M, Ruggeri L, Falzetti F, Carotti A, Terenzi A, et al. HLA-haploidentical transplantation with regulatory and conventional T-cell adoptive immunotherapy prevents acute leukemia relapse. *Blood* 2014;124(4):638–44.

15. Wang Y, Liu DH, Liu KY, Xu LP, Zhang XH, Han W, et al. Long-term follow-up of haploidentical hematopoietic stem cell transplantation without in vitro T cell depletion for the treatment of leukemia: nine years of experience at a single center. *Cancer* 2013;119(5):978–85.

16. Rizzieri DA, Koh LP, Long GD, Gasparetto C, Sullivan KM, Horwitz M, et al. Partially match, nonmyeloablative allogeneic transplantation: clinical outcomes and immune reconstitution. *J Clin Oncol* 2007;25(6):690–7.

17. Kanda J, Long GD, Gasparetto C, Horwitz ME, Sullivan KM, Chute JP, et al. Reduced-intensity allogeneic transplantation using alemtuzumab from HLA-match related, unrelated, or haploidentical related donors for patients with hematologic malignancies. *Biol Blood Marrow Transplant* 2014;20(2):257–63.

18. Luznik L, O'Donnell PV, Symons HJ, Chen AR, Leffell MS, Zahurak M, et al. HLA-haploidentical bone marrow transplantation for hematologic malignancies using nonmyeloablative conditioning and high-dose, posttransplantation cyclophosphamide. *Biol Blood Marrow Transplant* 2008;14(6):641–50.

19. O'Donnell PV, Luznik L, Jones RJ, Vogelsang GB, Leffell MS, Phelps M, et al. Nonmyeloablative bone marrow transplantation from partially HLA-mismatch related donors using posttransplantation cyclophosphamide. *Biol Blood Marrow Transplant* 2002; 8(7):377–86.

20. Kanakry CG, Ganguly S, Zahurak M, Bolanos-Meade J, Thoburn C, Perkins B, et al. Aldehyde dehydrogenase expression drives human regulatory T cell resistance to posttransplantation cyclophosphamide. *Sci Transl Med* 2013;5(211):211ra157.

21. Ross D, Jones M, Komanduri K, Levy RB. Antigen and lymphopenia-driven donor T cells are differentially diminished by post-transplantation administration of cyclophosphamide after hematopoietic cell transplantation. *Biol Blood Marrow Transplant* 2013;19(10):1430–8.

22. Kasamon YL, Luznik L, Leffell MS, Kowalski J, Tsai HL, Bolanos-Meade J, et al. Nonmyeloablative HLA-haploidentical bone marrow transplantation with high-dose posttransplantation cyclophosphamide: effect of HLA disparity on outcome. *Biol Blood Marrow Transplant* 2010;16(4):482–9.

23. Castagna L, Crocchiolo R, Furst S, Bramanti S, El-Cheikh J, Sarina B, et al. Bone marrow compared with peripheral blood stem cells for haploidentical transplantation with a nonmyeloablative conditioning regimen and post-transplantation cyclophosphamide. *Biol Blood Marrow Transplant* 2014;20(5):724–9.

24. Raiola AM, Dominietto A, Ghiso A, Di Grazia C, Lamparelli T, Gualandi F, et al. Unmanipulated haploidentical bone marrow transplantation and posttransplantation cyclophosphamide for hematologic malignancies after myeloablative conditioning. *Biol Blood Marrow Transplant* 2013;19(1):117–22.

25. Raj K, Pagliuca A, Bradstock K, Noriega V, Potter V, Streetly M, et al. Peripheral blood hematopoietic stem cells for transplantation of hematological diseases from related, haploidentical donors after reduced-intensity conditioning. *Biol Blood Marrow Transplant* 2014;20(6):890–5.

26. Solomon SR, Sizemore CA, Sanacore M, Zhang X, Brown S, Holland HK, et al. Haploidentical transplantation using T cell replete peripheral blood stem cells and myeloablative conditioning in patients with high-risk hematologic malignancies who lack conventional donors is well tolerated and produces excellent relapse-free survival: results of a prospective phase II trial. *Biol Blood Marrow Transplant* 2012;18(12):1859–66.

27. Ciurea SO, Mulanovich V, Saliba RM, Bayraktar UD, Jiang Y, Bassett R, et al. Improved early outcomes using a T cell replete graft compared with T cell depleted haploidentical hematopoietic stem cell transplantation. *Biol Blood Marrow Transplant* 2012;18(12):1835–44.

28. Wagner JE, Eapen M, Carter SL, Haut PR, Peres E, Schultz KR, et al. No survival advantage after double umbilical cord blood (UCB) compared to single UCB transplant in children with hematological malignancy: results of the Blood and Marrow Transplant Clinical Trials Network (BMT CTN 0501) Randomized Trial. *ASH Annual Meeting Abstracts* 2012;120(21):359.

29. Hwang WY, Samuel M, Tan D, Koh LP, Lim W, Linn YC. A meta-analysis of unrelated donor umbilical cord blood transplantation *versus* unrelated donor bone marrow transplantation in adult and pediatric patients. *Biol Blood Marrow Transplant* 2007;13(4):444–53.

30. Eapen M, Rocha V, Sanz G, Scaradavou A, Zhang MJ, Arcese W, et al. Effect of graft source on unrelated donor haemopoietic stem-cell transplantation in adults with acute leukaemia: a retrospective analysis. *Lancet Oncol* 2010;11(7):653–60.

31. Rocha V, Labopin M, Ruggeri A, Blaise D, Rio B, Cornelissen JJ, et al. Outcomes after double cord blood transplantation compared to single cord blood transplantation in adults with acute leukemia given a reduced intensity conditioning regimen. *ASH Annual Meeting Abstracts* 2012;120(21):232.

32. Lindemans CA, Chiesa R, Amrolia PJ, Rao K, Nikolajeva O, de Wildt A, et al. Impact of thymoglobulin prior to pediatric unrelated umbilical cord blood transplantation on immune reconstitution and clinical outcome. *Blood* 2014;123(1):126–32.

33. Brunstein CG, Barker JN, Weisdorf DJ, DeFor TE, Miller JS, Blazar BR, et al. Umbilical cord blood transplantation after nonmyeloablative conditioning: impact on transplantation outcomes in 110 adults with hematologic disease. *Blood* 2007;110(8):3064–70.

34. Brunstein CG, Fuchs EJ, Carter SL, Karanes C, Costa LJ, Wu J, et al. Alternative donor transplantation after reduced intensity conditioning: results of parallel phase 2 trials using partially HLA-mismatch related bone marrow or unrelated double umbilical cord blood grafts. *Blood* 2011;118(2):282–8.

35. Szabolcs P, Cairo MS. Unrelated umbilical cord blood transplantation and immune reconstitution. *Semin Hematol* 2010;47(1):22–36.

36. Jacobson CA, Turki AT, McDonough SM, Stevenson KE, Kim HT, Kao G, *et al*. Immune reconstitution after double umbilical cord blood stem cell transplantation: comparison with unrelated peripheral blood stem cell transplantation. *Biol Blood Marrow Transplant* 2012;18(4):565–74.

37. Ruggeri A, Peffault de Latour R, Carmagnat M, Clave E, Douay C, Larghero J, *et al*. Outcomes, infections, and immune reconstitution after double cord blood transplantation in patients with high-risk hematological diseases. *Transpl Infect Dis* 2011;13(5):456–65.

38. Klein AK, Patel DD, Gooding ME, Sempowski GD, Chen BJ, Liu C, *et al*. T-cell recovery in adults and children following umbilical cord blood transplantation. *Biol Blood Marrow Transplant* 2001;7(8):454–66.

39. Komanduri KV, St John LS, de Lima M, McMannis J, Rosinski S, McNiece I, *et al*. Delayed immune reconstitution after cord blood transplantation is characterized by impaired thymopoiesis and late memory T-cell skewing. *Blood* 2007;110(13):4543–51.

40. Kanda J, Chiou LW, Szabolcs P, Sempowski GD, Rizzieri DA, Long GD, *et al*. Immune recovery in adult patients after myeloablative dual umbilical cord blood, match sibling, and match unrelated donor hematopoietic cell transplantation. *Biol Blood Marrow Transplant* 2012;18(11):1664–1676 e1.

41. Dominietto A, Raiola AM, Bruno B, Pende D, Meazza R, Gualandi F, *et al*. Fast immune recovery following unmanipulated haploidentical BMT with post-transplant high-dose cyclophosphamide as GvHD prophylaxis: a comparison with siblings, unrelated donors, cord blood (EBMT abstract). *Bone Marrow Transplant* 2012;47:S257–S258.

42. El-Cheikh J, Roberto C, Sabine F, Stefania B, Barbara S, Angela G, *et al*. Comparison of umbilical cord blood and haploidentical donor grafts in adults with high risk hematologic diseases after fludarabine cyclophosphamide and TBI 2Gy based reduced-intensity conditioning regimen stem cell transplantation. *Blood* 2013;122(21):3288.

43. González-Vicent M, Molina B, Andión M, Sevilla J, Ramirez M, Pérez A, *et al*. Allogeneic hematopoietic transplantation using haploidentical donor vs. unrelated cord blood donor in pediatric patients: a single-center retrospective study. *Euro J Haematol* 2011;87(1):46–53.

44. Mo XD, Zhao XY, Liu DH, Chen YH, Xu LP, Zhang XH, *et al*. Umbilical cord blood transplantation and unmanipulated haploidentical hematopoietic SCT for pediatric hematologic malignancies. *Bone Marrow Transplant* 2014;49(8):1070–5.

45. Huang XJ, Liu DH, Liu KY, Xu LP, Chen H, Han W. Donor lymphocyte infusion for the treatment of leukemia relapse after HLA-mismatch/ haploidentical T-cell-replete hematopoietic stem cell transplantation. *Haematologica* 2007;92(3):414–7.

46. Yan CH, Liu DH, Xu LP, Liu KY, Zhao T, Wang Y, *et al*. Modified donor lymphocyte infusion-associated acute graft-*versus*-host disease after haploidentical T-cell-replete hematopoietic stem cell transplantation: incidence and risk factors. *Clin Transplant* 2012;26(6):868–76.

47. Zeidan AM, Forde PM, Symons H, Chen A, Smith BD, Pratz K, *et al*. HLA-haploidentical donor lymphocyte infusions for patients with relapsed hematologic malignancies after related HLA-haploidentical bone marrow transplantation. *Biol Blood Marrow Transplant* 2014;20(3):314–8.

48. Roth JA, Bensink ME, O'Donnell PV, Fuchs EJ, Eapen M, Ramsey SD. Design of a cost-effectiveness analysis alongside a randomized trial of transplantation using umbilical cord blood *versus* HLA-haploidentical related bone marrow in advanced hematologic cancer. *J Comp Eff Res* 2014;3(2):135–44.

Chapter

62

Adoptive Cell Therapy for Cancer Using T-Cells Genetically Engineered to Express Chimeric Antigen Receptors

Sarwish Rafiq and Renier J. Brentjens

Introduction

Adoptive cell therapy with allogeneic hematopoietic cell transplant (allo-HCT) has a high rate of relapse in patients with leukemia. This failure is due in part to minimal beneficial graft-*versus* leukemia (GvL) effect. Immune cells that specifically recognize and respond to cancer cells can enhance the GvL effect. To achieve this, T-cells can be genetically engineered to recognize tumor cells with synthetic receptors termed chimeric antigen receptors (CARs). CAR T-cells have been demonstrated to have antitumor efficacy in preclinical models and in clinical trials, and represent a promising treatment strategy for cancer. This chapter will describe CARs and discuss the uses of CAR T-cell therapy.

Evolution of Chimeric Antigen Receptors (CARs)

Currently, there is no consensus for the optimal design of CARs. CARs consist of multiple functional domains (Figure 62.1). Each of these domains plays a vital role in the utility and effectiveness of the CAR T-cells.

The antigen-recognition domain is the extracellular part of the CAR and is most commonly composed of a linked variable heavy and light chain domain from a monoclonal antibody that form a single-chain variable fragment (scFv). A CAR can be created against any antigen for which a monoclonal antibody can be generated[1], in a human leukocyte antigen (HLA)-independent manner. This includes surface antigens such as proteins, carbohydrates, and glycolipids. More

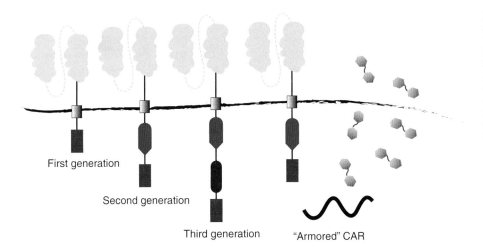

First generation

Second generation

Third generation

"Armored" CAR

Figure 62.1. Schematic representation of chimeric antigen receptors (CAR) and "Armored" CARs. First-generation CAR T-cells have the CD3ζ signaling domain. Second-generation CAR T-cells contain a costimulatory domain in addition to the CD3ζ domain. Third-generation CAR T-cells have multiple costimulatory domains in addition to the activation CD3ζ domain. "Armored" CAR T-cells are characterized by their ability to express proteins that protect them from the tumor microenvironment.

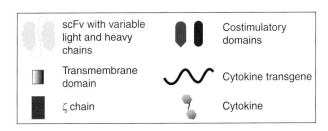

scFv with variable light and heavy chains

Costimulatory domains

Transmembrane domain

Cytokine transgene

ζ chain

Cytokine

recently, human phage display libraries allow for the generation of scFvs to virtually any target antigen, including intracellular antigen-derived peptides bound to HLA molecules, in an HLA-restricted manner akin to a T-cell receptor (TCR)[2].

The antigen-recognition domain is fused to the hinge and transmembrane domains, and subsequently the intracellular signaling domains. The hinge region gives flexibility to the antigen-binding domain, which is required for appropriate binding to target antigens[1]. The transmembrane region anchors the CAR to the cell membrane and may allow for dimerization of the signaling domains. The majority of CARs currently being studied have hinge and transmembrane domains derived from either CD8α or CD28, although others such as the FcR transmembrane domain have been utilized[3].

During normal T-cell activation, the TCR recognizes a peptide antigen in the context of an HLA molecule and then signals an activation pathway to the T-cell. One protein present in the TCR is CD3ζ, which contains immunoreceptor tyrosine-based activation motifs (ITAMs) that are phosphorylated upon TCR-mediated antigen recognition and initiate the "signal 1" pathway in T-cell activation. First-generation CARs contain a single cytoplasmic activation domain that is derived from the CD3ζ chain. T-cells modified to express first-generation CARs demonstrated antigen recognition and target cell lysis[4]. However, first-generation CAR T-cells exhibited limited antitumor efficacy and were often anergized or underwent apoptosis[5]. Furthermore, T-cells transduced with first-generation CARs did not have robust cytokine responses and did not proliferate upon repeated antigen exposure both in-vitro and in-vivo[6].

Second-generation CARs include the addition of a costimulatory "signal 2" signaling domain in addition to the CD3ζ activation domain. In natural T-cell activation, CD80 and CD86 on APCs form the B7 complex that binds to CD28 on T-cells to provide costimulation, or "signal 2". Costimulation is needed to ensure T-cell proliferation upon repeated antigen exposures, avoidance of anergy and apoptosis, as well as robust cytokine secretion[7]. In CARs, "signal 2" can be provided by a number of different costimulatory domains. CD28 and CD137 (4-1BB) are the most commonly used domains, although other costimulatory signals used include CD134 (OX-40), DNAX-activation protein 10 (DAP10), and CD27[1]. Importantly, inclusion of a costimulatory signaling domain results in increased persistence and proliferation of human and mouse CAR T-cells, enhanced antitumor efficacy, and production of cytokines such as IL-2 and IFN-γ[8–11]. The superior persistence of second-generation CAR T-cells has also been demonstrated in patients that were infused with a mixture of CD3ζ- or CD28/CD3ζ-containing CD19-targeted CAR T-cells for the treatment of non-Hodgkin lymphoma (NHL)[12]. Comprehensive studies comparing the different costimulatory domains to each other have yet to provide a definitive answer to the optimal signaling domain for CAR T-cells. CD28- or 4-1BB-containing CAR T-cells did not show differential effects in

preclinical *in-vivo* studies[13] and clinical trials with either have yielded promising results[14–16].

Third-generation CARs contain two costimulatory signaling domains in addition to the activating CD3ζ domain. These CAR T-cells are reported to have even greater potency in mouse models[13,17–19]. Whether third-generation CAR T-cells enhance antitumor efficacy of therapy compared to second-generation CAR T-cells in the clinical setting has not been directly studied.

Clinical Trials with CAR-Modified T-Cells in B-Cell Malignancies

CD19 is the most extensively investigated CAR T-cell target to date. It is expressed on a wide range of B-cells during development and on most B-cell malignancies. CD19-specific CAR T-cells were the first to mediate eradication of systemic tumors in mouse models[8]. This and other preclinical studies[1] paved the way to moving towards the first clinical trials in B-cell malignancies using autologous patient-derived CD19-targeted CAR T-cells.

CD19-Directed T-Cells for Acute Lymphocytic Leukemia

To date, the most promising clinical trial outcomes with CAR T-cell therapy have been in the treatment of patients with relapsed or refractory B-cell acute lymphoblastic leukemia (B-ALL) using CD19-targeted CAR T-cells.

The initial results of CD19-specific CAR T-cell treatment for relapsed B-ALL were reported by Memorial Sloan Kettering Cancer Center (MSKCC), where five patients were treated with autologous second-generation CD19-specific CAR T-cells [20]. The CAR contained an scFv derived from the SJ25C1 antibody hybridoma and utilized the CD28/CD3ζ signaling domains. All of the patients treated in this study achieved minimum residual disease negative complete remissions (MRD–CR)[21]. All patients also achieved a molecular remission, as assessed by deep-sequencing polymerase chain reaction. Four of these five patients underwent a standard of care allo-stem cell transplant (SCT). Updated reports on 32 B-ALL patients showed an overall CR rate of 91% and the majority of these patients also continuing on to an allo-SCT[14]. The MSKCC studies reported transient B-cell aplasias as well as other toxicities including high-grade fevers, hypotension, obtundation, and seizure-like activity. These symptoms were likely due to markedly elevated serum cytokine levels and, grouped together, are referred to as a cytokine release syndrome (CRS).

Confirmatory studies of CD19-targeted CAR T-cells in relapsed B-ALL patients have been reported by investigators at the Abramson Family Cancer Research Institute at the University of Pennsylvania (UPenn)[15]. Researchers initially described two pediatric patients with relapsed B-ALL treated with CD19-targeted CARs at the Children's Hospital of

Pennsylvania. The CD19-specific CAR contained an scFv domain from the anti-CD19 FMC63 antibody hybridoma and 4-1BB/CD3ζ signaling domains. Both patients achieved an MRD–CR but experienced toxicities including CRS and B-cell aplasia. One patient experienced disease relapse about 2 months after treatment. The relapsed tumor was found to be a CD19– tumor escape variant. An updated report of this study reported a 90% CR response rate in a total of 30 children and adults.

Additionally, the National Cancer Institute (NCI) performed a clinical trial using CD19-specific CAR T cells containing the CD28/CD3ζ costimulatory domain and a CD19-binding scFv derived from the FMC63 antibody hybridoma. A 70% CR rate was reported in 20 pediatric and young adult patients with relapsed or refractory B-ALL[22]. The toxicities reported in this study included B-cell aplasias, severe CRS in three patients, and reversible neurotoxicity in six patients.

Furthermore, researchers at the Fred Hutchinson Cancer Center (FHCRC) reported using CAR T cells with a FMC63-derived CD19-specific scFv and 4-1BB/CD3ζ signalling domains to achieve complete bone marrow remissions in 27 out of 29 patients with relapsed or refractory B-ALL[23]. The patients were treated with a defined subset of CD4+ and CD8+ central memory CAR T cells. Severe CRS was seen in 15 out of 30 patients and two patients died due to toxicities related to the CAR T cell infusion. One of the patients developed severe CRS that was unresponsive to treatment, while the other had irreversible neurotoxicity.

CD19-directed CAR T-cells for Treatment of Low-Grade B-Cell Malignancies

Clinical trials investigating CD19-specific CAR T-cells for the treatment of low-grade B-cell malignancies such as chronic lymphocytic leukemia (CLL) have been performed at a number of research institutes.

Investigators at MSKCC reported on the outcomes of treating eight patients with refractory or relapsed CLL with autologous CD19-specific CD28/CD3ζ CAR T-cells[20]. An initial cohort of patients did not receive prior conditioning and had no clinical response to the CD19-targeted CAR T-cells. In patients that received prior chemotherapy conditioning with cyclophosphamide, three out of the four evaluable patients experienced either stable disease or a significant reduction in lymphadenopathy. The study implicates the importance of preconditioning on the clinical outcomes of patients treated with CAR T-cells. Toxicities reported in this study include rigors, chills, and transient fevers after transfusion of T-cells but no overt evidence of a CRS.

Researchers at UPenn reported initial results of the treatment of 3 CLL patients with CD19-targeted, 41BB/CD3ζ-containing second-generation CAR-modified T-cells[24]. Of this initial cohort, two patients achieved long-lasting MRD– CRs and one patient had a partial response (PR). This report described toxicities with CAR T-cell therapy similar to the

flu-like symptoms associated with CRS. A follow-up study of additional CLL patients treated on this trial had an overall response rate of 57% with four out of 14 patients achieving complete recovery and four out of 14 achieving a partial recovery[25].

The NCI reported treating a patient with advanced follicular lymphoma with a second-generation CAR[26]. The patient had regression of lymphoma and persistent B-cell aplasia, indicating CAR T-cell function, and no acute toxicities related to treatment. In a subsequent report, four relapsed CLL patients were treated with CD19-specific CAR T-cells. All patients received nonmyeloablative-conditioning chemotherapy consisting of fludarabine and cyclophosphamide prior to CAR T-cell treatment. One patient achieved a CR and three patients achieved PRs[27]. Two of these patients experienced prolonged B-cell aplasias, again indicating persistence and function of infused CAR T-cells. Four patients with follicular lymphoma (FL) and one with splenic marginal zone lymphoma were also treated on this study and of these five patients, four achieved PRs. Four of the eight total patients in this study developed hypogammaglobulinemia due to B-cell aplasia and the majority of patients experienced CRS-like symptoms associated with elevated levels of cytokines such as interferon-γ (IFN- γ) and tumor necrosis factor (TNF). Recently, these authors have reported on outcomes of CD19-specific CAR T-cell treatment of 15 patients with advanced refractory diffuse large B-cell lymphoma (DLBCL) or indolent B-cell malignancies[28]. CRS toxicities reported after CD19-specific CAR T-cell infusion were similar to that seen in CLL and ALL with this treatment and included fever, hypotension, and delirium. Although one patient died suddenly on this study and was not evaluable, eight patients achieved CRs, four experienced PRs, and one had stable disease. The numerous remissions achieved in this study suggest that DLBCL may be more susceptible to CD19-directed CAR T-cell therapy than CLL.

Finally, researchers at the FHCRC recently reported the results from a phase I trial using CD19-specific CAR T cells in 32 adult patients with relapsed and/or refractory B-cell non-Hodgkin's lymphoma[29]. Patients were treated with a defined CD4+ and CD8+ central memory CAR T cell product and a 33% total CR rate was achieved. Severe CRS was reported in 13% of patients treated and grade ≥3 neurotoxicity in 28% of patients.

CD20-Directed T-Cells for Lymphoma

CD20 is another B-cell-specific antigen found on many B-cell malignancies. Investigators at the FHCRC reported on the clinical trial outcomes of patients with relapsed or refractory B-cell lymphoma or mantle cell lymphoma who were treated with autologous CD20-directed first-generation CAR T-cells. Patients received cytoreductive chemotherapy prior to multiple CAR T-cell infusions. Of the seven patients treated, minimal toxicities were noted and two patients maintained their previously established CRs, one achieved a PR, and four patients experienced stable disease[30]. In a follow-up study, three relapsed indolent B-cell or mantle cell lymphoma patients were treated with third-generation CD20-directed CAR T-cells containing CD3ζ activating domain and both CD28 and 4-1BB costimulatory domains[31]. Again, patients received cytoreductive chemotherapy prior to CAR T-cell infusion. Two out of the three patients treated remained progression free for over 12 months. Low levels of CAR T-cells were detected in the peripheral blood of these patients for up to 1 year after treatment. Adverse effects reported in this study included fevers and hypotension, similar to the symptoms observed in the CD19-specific CAR T-cell trials. B-cell aplasias were not observed. The modest results observed in both of these studies may be due to the method of gene transfer (electroporation instead of the more widely utilized retroviral gene transfer) and the prolonged *ex-vivo* cell expansion protocols required to achieve adequate numbers of CAR T-cell levels for therapy. The investigators at FHCRC aim to switch to a lentiviral method of gene transfer with a predicted shorter period of *ex-vivo* CAR T-cell expansion period in future studies[31].

The disparity in clinical outcomes between B-ALL and low-grade B-cell malignancies remains unexplained. However, multiple etiologies may be responsible. First, CLL patients may have increased tumor bulk at the time of CD19-targeted CAR T-cell infusion *versus* patients treated with relapsed B-ALL. Second, the tumor microenvironment may differ between B-ALL and CLL/low-grade lymphomas as the latter may inhibit CAR T-cell function with the presence of regulatory T-cells (Tregs), myeloid-derived suppressor cells (MDSC), tumor-associated macrophages (TAM), and/or inhibitory cytokines[32,33]. Third, CLL patients are known to have inherent T-cell defects[34,35], which may result in impaired T-cell effector functions of the autologous CAR T-cell product.

Future of CAR T-Cell Therapy

Alternative CAR Targets for Hematologic Malignancies

The restricted expression of antigens such as CD19 on normal and malignant B-cells has led to some clinical success of targeting this antigen with CAR T-cells. Alternative tumor-associated antigen (TAA) targets are required to apply CAR T-cell therapy to the treatment of a wider range of hematologic and solid tumor malignancies. A multitude of TAA-directed CARs have been explored for hematologic and solid malignancies and an exhaustive list can be found elsewhere[1]. Here, we will discuss clinical trial results utilizing CAR T-cell in a subset of malignancies. A complete list of open actively recruiting clinical trials in the United States with CAR T-cells is provided in Table 62.1.

A B-cell malignancy that may benefit from CAR T-cell therapy is multiple myeloma (MM). MM is a disease of malignant plasma B-cells and due to the late stage of the B-cell development in which the malignancy occurs, CD19 or CD20 are rarely expressed on these cells. Potential targets for CAR T-cell therapy include common MM markers such as CD138, CD38, or CD56. However, these markers are also widely expressed on normal tissues[36]. CAR T-cells responding to these markers on normal tissue could result in significant on-target, off-tumor toxicities. Clinical trial studies investigating CAR T-cells therapy of MM target antigens with more limited expression including the immunoglobulin kappa light chain (Igκ) and B-cell maturation antigen (BCMA). Given that B-cells express surface immunoglobulins with either kappa or lambda light chains in a clonally restricted manner, Igκ may represent a more selective antigen for MM. MM cells themselves are clonal and therefore may be targeted by CAR T-cells specific to the Ig light chain expressed by the malignant cells. Ongoing clinical trials at Baylor College of Medicine are investigating CAR T-cells with CD28/CD3ζ signaling domains against Igκ in patients with MM (NCT00881920), as well as NHL and CLL. The Lewis Y (LeY) carbohydrate antigen, related to the Lewis blood group antigen family, is another potential target for CAR T-cell treatment of MM[37]. BCMA is expressed on most cases of MM. Researchers at the NCI reported treating 12 patients with a BCMA-targeted CAR containing an scFv from the 11D5-3 scFv and CD28/CD3ζ signalling domains[38]. Four doses of CAR T cells were studied. At dose levels 3 and 4, two patients achieved PRs and one achieved a CR. Patients treated at the highest dose of cells experienced CRS. This trial is ongoing (NCT02215967) as well as two additional trials in MM utilizing BCMA-targeted CAR T cells (NCT02658929 and NCT02546167).

Acute myeloid leukemia (AML) is a non-B-cell hematologic malignancy in which CAR T-cell treatment could improve patient outcome. However, AML is a heterogeneous collection of cancers forming in cells of myeloid origin, and subsequently identification of suitable CAR targets is difficult. Furthermore, long-term targeting of all myeloid cells can be detrimental to patients, as they play a vital role in innate immunity to bacterial and viral pathogens. Lewis Y (LeY) antigen is overexpressed on AML cells and LeY-specific CAR T-cells were investigated for safety and clinical efficacy at the Peter MacCallum Cancer Centre in Australia[39]. Patients received preconditioning treatment with fludarabine-containing chemotherapy and were infused with CD28/CD3ζ containing second-generation LeY-specific CAR T-cells[39]. One patient achieved a transient cytogenetic remission, an additional patient experienced a transient reduction in blasts, and two patients had stable disease. Despite these modest antitumor responses, CAR T-cells were detected and activated *in-vivo* for up to 10 months after treatment. Significantly, to date this study has reported no significant infusion-related adverse events or on-target, off-tumor toxicities. Meanwhile, identification of other suitable targets for AML CAR T-cell therapy remain in preclinical studies and ideal targets remain largely elusive.

Table 62.1 Ongoing clinical trials in the United States utilizing CAR T-cells

Antigen	Disease	Sponsor
B-cell maturation antigen	Multiple myeloma	bluebird bio (NCT02658929), National Cancer Institute (NCI) (NCT02215967), University of Pennsylvania (NCT02546167)
CD19	CD19+ B-cell malignancies	Baylor College of Medicine (NCT02050347) (NCT01853631), City of Hope Medical Center (NCT02146924) Fred Hutchinson Cancer Research Center (NCT01865617), Juno Therapeutics Inc (NCT02631044) (NCT02535364), Kite Pharma, Inc. (NCT02348216) (NCT02614066) (NCT02625400) (NCT02926833), Memorial Sloan Kettering Cancer Center (NCT01860937) (NCT01430390) (NCT01044069), MD Anderson (NCT02529813), NCI (NCT02659943), Novartis Pharmaceuticals (NCT02445248), Seattle Children's Hospital (NCT02028455), University of Pennsylvania (NCT02030834) (NCT02030847) (NCT02640209) (NCT02624258)
CD22	CD22+ malignancies	NCI (NCT02315612), University of Pennsylvania (NCT02650414)
CD30	Lymphomas, Non-Hodgkin lymphoma, Hodgkin lymphoma	UNC Lineberger Comprehensive Cancer Center (NCT02663297) (NCT02690545)
CD123	Acute myeloid leukemia	City of Hope (NCT02159495)
CD171	Neuroblastoma	Seattle Children's Hospital (NCT02311621)
EGFRVIII	Glioma, glioblastoma, brain cancer	NCI (NCT01454596) University of Pennsylvania (NCT02209376) (NCT02666248),
GD-2	GD-2+ solid tumors, non-neuroblastoma, Sarcoma	Baylor College of Medicine (NCT02107963) (NCT01953900), NCI (NCT02107963)
Her2	Sarcoma, gliobastoma	Baylor College of Medicine (NCT00902044) (NCT02442297)
IL13Rα2	Malignant Glioma	City of Hope Medical Center (NCT02208362)
Kappa immunoglobulin	Lymphoma, myeloma, leukemia	Baylor College of Medicine (NCT00881920)
Mesothelin	Mesothelin+ tumors, breast cancer	Memorial Sloan Kettering Cancer Center (NCT02792114), NCI (NCT01583686), University of Pennsylvania (NCT02388828)
MUC16ecto	Epithelial Ovarian, Fallopian Tube or primary peritoneal cancer	Memorial Sloan Kettering Cancer Center (NCT02498912)
Prostate Specific Membrane Antigen	Castrate Metastatic Prostate Cancer	Memorial Sloan Kettering Cancer Center (NCT01140373)

From clinicaltrials.gov

Alternative CAR Targets for Solid Malignancies

CAR therapy in solid tumors is a new frontier for immunotherapy. There are a number of limitations that may hinder CAR T-cells in these malignancies. First, as with hematologic malignancies, TAA with limited expression on normal tissues are difficult to identify. Second, solid tumor structure lends itself to an immunosuppressive tumor microenvironment that may suppress CAR T-cell expansion and function *in-vivo*. Regulatory cells potentially found in this environment include MDSC, Tregs, and TAMs, all of which have been shown to suppress T-cell function[40,41]. Furthermore, regulatory receptors on T-cells such as programmed cell death 1 (PD-1) and cytotoxic T-lymphocyte-associated protein 4 (CTLA-4) may suppress T-cell function[40]. These combined issues may explain the, to date, relative paucity of clinically meaningful responses to CAR T-cell therapy for solid tumors.

CAR T-cell therapy has been investigated for the treatment of ovarian cancer with modest results[42]. The NCI treated

14 patients with metastatic ovarian cancer with CAR T-cells specific for α-folate receptor (FR) without preconditioning[42]. The FR-directed CAR is composed of an scFv derived from the MOv18 antibody hybridoma fused to the signaling domain of the Fc receptor γ chain. Patients safely tolerated FR-directed CAR T-cell infusions but no reduction in tumor burden was observed in any patients. Levels of CAR T-cells rapidly declined following infusion and FR-directed CAR T-cells labled with ^{111}In showed that T-cells did not localize to the tumor site in patients. The lack of clinical responses seen in this trial was hypothesized to be due to the absence of CAR T-cell trafficking and persistence.

More promising results were seen in high-risk neuroblastoma patients treated with G_{D2}-directed ganglioside (GD2) first-generation CAR T-cells at the Baylor College of Medicine[43]. Nineteen patients were treated in this study without preconditioning, eight that were in remission and 11 with active disease. No severe toxicities were associated with GD2-directed CAR T-cell infusion. Three out of the 11 patients with active neuroblastoma achieved long-term CRs, although one patient had bone marrow disease that relapsed after 6 weeks. The GD2-directed CAR T-cells had long-term persistence at low levels, which correlated with longer survival of patients. Low levels of persisting CAR T-cells were safely tolerated and may be the key to the success of this therapy in neuroblastoma.

Mesothelin is another attractive target for CAR T-cell therapy of solid tumors. It is an extracellular protein expressed on normal mesothelial cells and is overexpressed on a number of cancers[44]. Investigators at UPenn treated patients with pancreatic adenocarcinoma or malignant pleural mesothelioma with second-generation mesothelin-specific CAR T-cells containing an scFv derived from the murine monoclonal antibody SS1 and 4-1BB/CD3ζ signaling domains[44]. CAR expression was achieved with mRNA electroporation into autologous patient T-cells, resulting in transient expression of the CAR on the surface of T-cells. Transient CAR expression was hypothesized to decrease on-target, off-tumor toxicity. Patients were given multiple infusions of CAR T-cells and three out of four patients safely tolerated CAR T-cell therapy. One patient developed anaphylaxis and cardiac arrest shortly after the third infusion of CAR T-cells. Given that the scFv of this CAR was derived from a mouse antihuman mesothelin antibody, the authors of this study hypothesized that the anaphylaxis was a result of an antimouse/CAR immune response. Human anti-mouse antibodies were detected in the serum samples of this patient. However, all of the CD19-specific CAR T-cell trials reported to date utilize CARs derived from mouse antihuman monoclonal antibodies and adverse events such as these have not been observed elsewhere. The overall antitumor efficacy of the mesothelin-directed CAR T-cells was not reported, although the authors noted that one patient died from progressive disease.

Dual-Targeting CARs

TAA can be expressed on normal as well as malignant cells. A strategy to enhance the specificity of CAR is to target two separate antigens. One model of dual-targeting CARs utilizes T-cells coexpressing two CARs with different specificities. There are a number of preclinical studies in solid tumors of bispecific CAR T-cells, such as Her2 and IL-13Rα[45] and folate-binding protein and ERBB2[46]. These studies found that bispecific CAR T-cells specifically kill cancer cells and offset tumor antigen escape.

A second model of dual specific targeting CAR T-cells aims to specifically target cancer cells and spare normal tissues through the expression of two recognition receptors that split activation and costimulation signaling domains and are hypothesized to only activate T-cells when both receptors are bound[47]. Expression of split activation and costimulation CARs spare cells that express the antigen individually (normal tissues) and allow CAR T-cell lysis of targets that express both antigens (tumor tissues).

Additionally, supportive cells of the tumor microenvironment and cancer cells can be both targeted by combinatory targeting CAR T-cells. Targeting fibroblast activation protein-α (FAP) on cancer-associated fibroblasts found in tumor-associated stroma in addition to erphrin type-A receptor 2 (EphA2) found in lung cancer with CAR T-cells leads to enhanced antitumor efficacy[48]. Together, these approaches aim to overcome toxicities associated with CAR T-cell therapy and may also decrease the growth risk of tumor escape variants.

"Armored" CARs

CARs can be "armored" with a defense system in order to remain functional in the suppressive tumor microenvironment of malignancies such as CLL and solid tumors (Figure 62.2). "Armored" CAR T-cells may be protected from the suppressive cells and cytokines of the tumor microenvironment and may recruit endogenous immune effector cells to the site of the tumor. In addition, the "armored" CAR T-cells may modulate the patient's immune landscape to favor effective antitumor responses.

Several investigators have reported on "armored" tumor-specific T-cells genetically engineered to secrete the proinflammory cytokine IL-12[49–51]. IL-12 is a pleiotropic cytokine naturally secreted by dendritic cells, macrophages, and B-cells and stimulates growth, differentiation, and effector function of T-cells[50]. Modifying tumor-targeted CAR T-cells to express IL-12 allows for the cytokine to be secreted specifically at the tumor site. Localized delivery of IL-12 minimizes systemic levels of the cytokine, which have been highly toxic to patients when administered systemically[51]. Preclinical studies with first- and second-generation IL-12-secreting CAR T-cells mediated enhanced antitumor efficacy, persistence, and resistance to Treg-mediated suppression, as compared to control CAR T-cells[36,50]. Alternative models of IL-12 secreting tumor-targeted T-cells have demonstrated that IL-12 can also overcome microenvironment suppression by cells such as MDSC and TAM[49]. Given the toxicities associated with systemic IL-12 infusions, CAR T-cells secreting IL-12 could present a

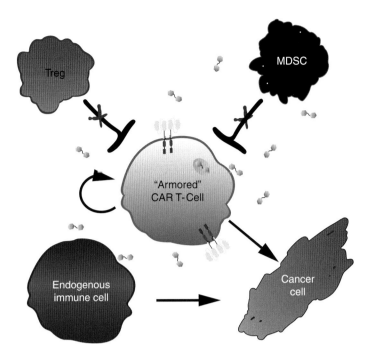

Figure 62.2. Possible mechanisms of action of "armored" CAR T-cells. Cytokines secreted by "armored" CAR T-cells act in an autocrine and paracrine manner to enhance CAR T-cell and endogenous immune cell function against cancer cells, as well as overcome immune suppression by regulatory T-cells (Treg) and myeloid-derived suppressor cells (MDSC).

safety risk, and awaits careful investigation of this approach in the clinical setting. A phase I clinical trial currently open at MSKCC that is utilizing IL-12 secreting CAR T cells that target MUC-16ecto in recurrent ovarian cancer (NCT02498912)[52].

The tumor microenvironment can be modulated in other ways. CAR T-cells can be engineered to express a variety of proteins including chemokines or immunostimulatory ligands. One report of CAR T-cells co-expressing ligands describes first-generation CAR T-cells targeted to prostate-specific membrane antigen (PMSA) and "armored" to co-express the costimulatory ligands CD80 and CD137 (4-1BBL)[53]. CD80 or 4-1BBL on the CAR T-cells stimulates CD28 or 4-1BB in an autocrine manner to provide costimulation to the T-cells without the need for APCs. The CD80/4-1BBL "armored" PMSA-directed CAR T-cells showed antigen-specific proliferation and elimination of established tumors in mice by both auto- and trans-costimulation of CAR T-cells, as compared to unarmored CAR T-cells.

"Armored" CAR T-cells may be necessary for successful immunotherapy in hematologic and solid tumor malignancies with hostile tumor microenvironments. The efficacy of "armored" CAR T-cells, although promising in the preclinical setting, awaits verification in clinical trials.

Controversies in the Field of CAR T-Cell Therapy

Optimal Design of Second-Generation CARs: CD28 or 4-1BB

The most extensive clinical studies with CAR T-cells have utilized second-generation CARs containing either CD28 or 4-1BB costimulatory domains. However, between these two designs, the ideal or superior costimulatory domain remains undefined. Whether one costimulatory domain results in longer-lasting CAR T-cells than the other is uncertain, although there is preliminary clinical evidence to suggest 4-1BB-containing CAR T-cells may have greater *in-vivo* persistence compared to CD28 containing CAR T-cells[15,21]. The role of CAR T-cell persistence and the relationship between persistence of CAR T-cells and their functional capacity over time are also unclear. Whereas persistence is important to tumor eradication, in some settings long-term CAR T-cell persistence and function may result in undesired on-target, off-tumor toxicity. Currently there are no clinical reports directly comparing CD28 to 4-1BB second-generation CAR T-cells in terms of efficacy or persistence/long-term CAR T-cell function. However, both CD28 and 4-1BB containing second-generation CAR T-cells have shown effective antitumor responses in clinical trials[15,21].

Preconditioning Regimes

Preparative preconditioning regimes prior to adoptive T-cell therapy were necessary in preclinical mouse models for successful CAR T-cell therapy in immune-competent mice[50,54]. Preconditioning of patients prior to CAR T-cell therapy appears to be essential for therapeutic response but the underlying mechanisms as well as optimal conditioning regimens remain undefined. Favorable patient outcomes were noted when CLL patients received chemotherapy conditioning prior to CAR T-cell therapy[1]. Individual research centers have differing preparatory protocols, timing of infusions, and some administer exogenous IL-2 to support the infused CAR T-cells. Despite variations across different treatment centers, the question of optimal preparative conditioning warrants further investigation with an aim to achieve the best possible patient outcomes with CAR T-cell therapy.

Target Antigen Selection: On-Target, Off-Tumor Responses

On-target, off-tumor responses are immune responses mediated by CAR T-cells that cause damage to normal tissues. This occurs when normal tissues express the antigen targeted by CAR T-cells. One example of on-target, off-tumor response is the prolonged B-cell aplasia and hypogammaglobulinemia seen with successful CD19-specific CAR T-cell therapy[20]. This is a manageable side effect that can be treated with infusions with γ-globulins. However, this treatment is expensive and leaves patients at a higher risk of infection. This on-target, off-tumor toxicity is unavoidable when using CD19 as a target for CAR T-cells.

On-target, off-tumor responses can be more severe with other CAR T-cells. Selection of TAAs is important and not all antigens are safe to target, even if the antigen has been successfully targeted with an antibody. An example of an unsafe target for CAR T-cell therapy is ERBB2[55]. The structure of the third-generation ERBB2-directed CAR was derived from the clinically approved antibody trastuzumab (Herceptin) and included both the CD28 and 4-1BB costimulatory domains along with CD3ζ activating domain. A metastatic colon cancer patient was treated with third-generation ERBB2-directed CAR T-cells and died shortly after treatment[55]. The authors of the study hypothesized the toxicity observed with ERBB2-directed CAR T-cell therapy was due to low levels of ERBB2 expression on many normal tissues, including lung epithelial cells. ERBB2 targeting serves as an example that not all on-target, off-tumor toxicities are as manageable as B-cell aplasia and further that safety of targeting a given antigen with a MAb does not translate into safety when the same antigen is targeted by a CAR.

Given the dangers involved with this therapy, a reliable method to eliminate CAR T-cells in the event of CAR T-cell toxicity needs to be established. High-dose steroids rapidly reverse CRS symptoms but the lymphotoxic effects can affect the clinical outcome of patients[14]. A suicide gene can be incorporated into the CAR design that rapidly eradicates CAR T-cells in the event of toxicity or severe side effects. A number of suicide genes have been clinically tested[20]. Clinical experience in allogeneic transplant patients treated with T-cells modified with the inducible caspase 9 (iCaspase-9) suicide gene demonstrates this is an effective option for rapidly and safely eliminating T-cells after injection with a cognate dimerizing agent in the event of graft-*versus*-host disease[56]. The expression of a nonfunctional, truncated version of the epidermal growth factor receptor (EGFRt) on the T-cell surface along with the CAR is another mechanism of eliminating CAR T-cells *in-vivo*[20]. CAR T-cells are eradicated after administration of the clinically available anti-EGFR antibody cetuximab via antibody-dependent cell-mediated cytoxicity or activation

of the complement cascade. CAR T-cells containing suicide genes have only recently been clinically applied in patients but will be required in future clinical studies using more potent "armored" CAR T-cells, as well as CAR T-cells targeted to novel antigens with enhanced potential for on-target off-tumor toxicity.

Management of CAR T-Cell Related Toxicities

CRS is a surge in inflammatory cytokines seen in some patients up to one month after CAR T-cell infusion. CRS is caused by large numbers of activated T-cells and has been correlated with intense antitumor response in CD19-targeted CAR T-cell trials at multiple centers[24,27,57]. Severe CRS has been associated with high levels of cytokines such as IFNγ, IL6, sgp130, and sIL6R[58]. Symptoms of CRS include hypotension and high fevers. Reversible neurologic complications such as delirium and seizure-like activity have also been reported[59]. CRS is manageable with high-dose steroids, vasopressors, and supportive care. IL-6 levels were seen to be key to the toxic response seen in patients[15], and the anti-IL-6R antibody tocilizumab has been used to dampen the effects of CRS. However, this treatment has been reported to not be effective in all cases of CRS[28]. Furthermore, there is concern that the treatment of CRS may decrease the antitumor effect of CAR T-cell therapy. In addition, the severity of CRS in patients has been correlated to increased tumor burden at the time of CAR T cell infusion[20,23]. Staging the level and symptoms of CRS may be key to balancing the management of this syndrome and the effective CAR T-cell response. A correlation has been found between the serum levels of the acute-phase reactant C-reactive protein (CRP) and CRS severity[14]. Therefore, levels of CRP may serve as a guideline to clinicians to determine if patients need closer monitoring in the ICU setting and predict whether pharmacologic intervention is needed.

Summary and Perspectives

CD19-targeted CAR T-cell therapy has proven to be effective in relapsed B-ALL patients. As illustrated in this chapter, CAR T-cell therapy has been less successful in other malignancies. The challenge now is to be able to expand this technology to other hematologic and solid malignancies.

One obstacle impeding application of CAR T-cell therapy to a wider range of cancers is target antigen selection, which is a challenge in many malignancies. The ideal target antigen is one that is only expressed by malignant cells. However, no entirely cancer-specific extracellular proteins have been described that are disease- and not patient-specific. CAR T-cell therapy against TAA results in on-target, off-tumor effects that can have moderate to severe toxicities in patients, including death. Therefore, antigen identification is vital. Recent preclinical success in determining more specific TAA by scFv phage display libraries or by dual-targeting of antigens may allow improved CAR target antigen selection.

Broad CAR T-cell therapy success may be dependent on optimal CAR design, preconditioning regimen, and management of toxicities. While it may be necessary to determine which costimulatory domain is ideal for antitumor activity and persistence of CAR T-cells, efficacy has been reported with both CD28 and 4-1BB containing second-generation CARs. Likewise, while preconditioning in general has been essential for effective CAR T-cell responses in B-cell leukemias, the various institutes conducting these studies use widely differing chemotherapy regimes, the consequences of which remain unknown. In addition, CRS has been noted in a subset of patients in most CAR T-cell trials. While CRP may serve as a marker for CRS, diagnosis, staging, treatment, and management of CRS without limiting CAR T-cell-mediated clinical

benefit has yet to be optimized and needs further clinical investigation.

Lastly, the immunosuppressive microenvironment may impede effective CAR T-cell therapy. Through modulation of the tumor microenvironment and recruitment of the endogenous immune system, "armored" CAR T-cells can overcome this suppression. However, "armored" CAR T-cells may carry increased risks to patient safety. Therefore, a safety switch is necessary before moving these cellular therapies into the clinic. CAR T-cells have been proven as an effective cellular therapy against cancer and through enhancement of design as well as identification of suitable and safe tumor targets has the potential to ultimately be a novel approach for therapy in a wide range of malignancies.

References

1. Sadelain M, Brentjens R, Riviere I. The basic principles of chimeric antigen receptor design. *Cancer Discovery.* 2013;3(4):388–98. PubMed PMID: 23550147. Pubmed Central PMCID: PMC3667586.

2. Dao T, Yan S, Veomett N, Pankov D, Zhou L, Korontsvit T, *et al.* Targeting the intracellular WT1 oncogene product with a therapeutic human antibody. *Science Translational Medicine.* 2013;5(176):176ra33. PubMed PMID: 23486779. Pubmed Central PMCID: PMC3963696.

3. Hudecek M, Lupo-Stanghellini MT, Kosasih PL, Sommermeyer D, Jensen MC, Rader C, *et al.* Receptor affinity and extracellular domain modifications affect tumor recognition by ROR1-specific chimeric antigen receptor T cells. *Clinical Cancer Research: An Official Journal of the American Association for Cancer Research.* 2013;19(12):3153–64. PubMed PMID: 23620405. Pubmed Central PMCID: PMC3804130.

4. Eshhar Z, Waks T, Gross G, Schindler DG. Specific activation and targeting of cytotoxic lymphocytes through chimeric single chains consisting of antibody-binding domains and the gamma or zeta subunits of the immunoglobulin and T-cell receptors. *Proceedings of the National Academy of Sciences of the United States of America.* 1993;90(2):720–4. PubMed PMID: 8421711. Pubmed Central PMCID: PMC45737.

5. Brocker T, Karjalainen K. Signals through T cell receptor-zeta chain alone are insufficient to prime resting T lymphocytes. *The Journal of Experimental Medicine.* 1995;181(5):1653–9. PubMed PMID: 7722445. Pubmed Central PMCID: PMC2192006.

6. Gong MC, Latouche JB, Krause A, Heston WD, Bander NH, Sadelain M. Cancer patient T cells genetically targeted to prostate-specific membrane antigen specifically lyse prostate cancer cells and release cytokines in response to prostate-specific membrane antigen. *Neoplasia.* 1999;1(2):123–7. PubMed PMID: 10933046. Pubmed Central PMCID: PMC1508130.

7. Maher J, Brentjens RJ, Gunset G, Riviere I, Sadelain M. Human T-lymphocyte cytotoxicity and proliferation directed by a single chimeric TCRzeta /CD28 receptor. *Nature Biotechnology.* 2002;20(1):70–5. PubMed PMID: 11753365.

8. Brentjens RJ, Latouche JB, Santos E, Marti F, Gong MC, Lyddane C, *et al.* Eradication of systemic B-cell tumors by genetically targeted human T lymphocytes co-stimulated by CD80 and interleukin-15. *Nature Medicine.* 2003;9(3):279–86. PubMed PMID: 12579196.

9. Kowolik CM, Topp MS, Gonzalez S, Pfeiffer T, Olivares S, Gonzalez N, *et al.* CD28 costimulation provided through a CD19-specific chimeric antigen receptor enhances in vivo persistence and antitumor efficacy of adoptively transferred T cells. *Cancer Research.* 2006;66(22):10995–1004. PubMed PMID: 17108138.

10. Finney HM, Akbar AN, Lawson AD. Activation of resting human primary T cells with chimeric receptors: costimulation from CD28, inducible costimulator, CD134, and CD137 in

series with signals from the TCR zeta chain. *Journal of Immunology.* 2004;172(1):104–13. PubMed PMID: 14688315.

11. Hombach A, Sent D, Schneider C, Heuser C, Koch D, Pohl C, *et al.* T-cell activation by recombinant receptors: CD28 costimulation is required for interleukin 2 secretion and receptor-mediated T-cell proliferation but does not affect receptor-mediated target cell lysis. *Cancer Research.* 2001;61(5):1976–82. PubMed PMID: 11280755.

12. Savoldo B, Ramos CA, Liu E, Mims MP, Keating MJ, Carrum G, *et al.* CD28 costimulation improves expansion and persistence of chimeric antigen receptor-modified T cells in lymphoma patients. *The Journal of Clinical Investigation.* 2011;121(5):1822–6. PubMed PMID: 21540550. Pubmed Central PMCID: PMC3083795.

13. Carpenito C, Milone MC, Hassan R, Simonet JC, Lakhal M, Suhoski MM, *et al.* Control of large, established tumor xenografts with genetically retargeted human T cells containing CD28 and CD137 domains. *Proceedings of the National Academy of Sciences of the United States of America.* 2009;106(9):3360–5. PubMed PMID: 19211796. Pubmed Central PMCID: PMC2651342.

14. Davila ML, Riviere I, Wang X, Bartido S, Park J, Curran K, *et al.* Efficacy and toxicity management of 19-28z CAR T cell therapy in B cell acute lymphoblastic leukemia. *Science Translational Medicine.* 2014;6(224):224ra25. PubMed PMID: 24553386.

15. Grupp SA, Kalos M, Barrett D, Aplenc R, Porter DL, Rheingold SR, *et al.*

Chimeric antigen receptor-modified T cells for acute lymphoid leukemia. *The New England Journal of Medicine*. 2013;368(16):1509–18. PubMed PMID: 23527958. Pubmed Central PMCID: PMC4058440.

16. Jackson HJ, Rafiq S, Brentjens RJ. Driving CAR T cells forward. *Nature Reviews Clinical Oncology*. 2016;13:370–83.

17. Zhong XS, Matsushita M, Plotkin J, Riviere I, Sadelain M. Chimeric antigen receptors combining 4-1BB and CD28 signaling domains augment PI3kinase/AKT/Bcl-XL activation and CD8+ T cell-mediated tumor eradication. *Molecular Therapy: The Journal of the American Society of Gene Therapy*. 2010;18(2):413–20. PubMed PMID: 19773745. Pubmed Central PMCID: PMC2839303.

18. Tammana S, Huang X, Wong M, Milone MC, Ma L, Levine BL, et al. 4-1BB and CD28 signaling plays a synergistic role in redirecting umbilical cord blood T cells against B-cell malignancies. *Human Gene Therapy*. 2010;21(1):75–86. PubMed PMID: 19719389. Pubmed Central PMCID: PMC2861957.

19. Wang J, Jensen M, Lin Y, Sui X, Chen E, Lindgren CG, et al. Optimizing adoptive polyclonal T cell immunotherapy of lymphomas, using a chimeric T cell receptor possessing CD28 and CD137 costimulatory domains. *Human Gene Therapy*. 2007;18(8):712–25. PubMed PMID: 17685852.

20. Brentjens RJ, Riviere I, Park JH, Davila ML, Wang X, Stefanski J, et al. Safety and persistence of adoptively transferred autologous CD19-targeted T cells in patients with relapsed or chemotherapy refractory B-cell leukemias. *Blood*. 2011;118(18):4817–28. PubMed PMID: 21849486. Pubmed Central PMCID: PMC3208293.

21. Brentjens RJ, Davila ML, Riviere I, Park J, Wang X, Cowell LG, et al. CD19-targeted T cells rapidly induce molecular remissions in adults with chemotherapy-refractory acute lymphoblastic leukemia. *Science Translational Medicine*. 2013;5(177):177ra38. PubMed PMID: 23515080. Pubmed Central PMCID: PMC3742551.

22. Lee DW, Kochenderfer JN, Stetler-Stevenson M, Cui YK, Delbrook C, Feldman SA, et al. T cells expressing CD19 chimeric antigen receptors for acute lymphoblastic leukaemia in children and young adults: a phase 1 dose-escalation trial. *Lancet*. 2015;385(9967): 517–28.

23. Turtle, CJ, Hanafi LA, Berger C, Gooley TA, Cherian S, Hudecek M, et al. CD19 CAR–T cells of defined CD4+ : CD8+ composition in adult B cell ALL patients. *Journal of Clinical Investigation*. 2016;126(6).

24. Porter DL, Levine BL, Kalos M, Bagg A, June CH. Chimeric antigen receptor-modified T cells in chronic lymphoid leukemia. *The New England Journal of Medicine*. 2011;365(8):725–33. PubMed PMID: 21830940. Pubmed Central PMCID: PMC3387277.

25. Porter DL, Hwang WT, Frey NV, Lacey SF, Shaw PA, Loren AW, et al. Chimeric antigen receptor T cells persist and induce sustained remissions in relapsed refractory chronic lymphocytic leukemia. *Science Translational Medicine*. 2015;7(303):303–39.

26. Kochenderfer JN, Wilson WH, Janik JE, Dudley ME, Stetler-Stevenson M, Feldman SA, et al. Eradication of B-lineage cells and regression of lymphoma in a patient treated with autologous T-cells genetically engineered to recognize CD19. *Blood*. 2010;116(20):4099–102. PubMed PMID: 20668228. Pubmed Central PMCID: PMC2993617.

27. Kochenderfer JN, Dudley ME, Feldman SA, Wilson WH, Spaner DE, Maric I, et al. B-cell depletion and remissions of malignancy along with cytokine-associated toxicity in a clinical trial of anti-CD19 chimeric-antigen-receptor-transduced T cells. *Blood*. 2012;119(12):2709–20. PubMed PMID: 22160384. Pubmed Central PMCID: PMC3327450.

28. Kochenderfer JN, Dudley ME, Kassim SH, Somerville RP, Carpenter RO, Stetler-Stevenson M, et al. Chemotherapy-refractory diffuse large B-cell lymphoma and indolent B-cell malignancies can be effectively treated with autologous T-cells expressing an anti-CD19 chimeric antigen receptor. *Journal of Clinical Oncology: Official Journal of the American Society of Clinical Oncology*. 2015;33(6): 540–9. PubMed PMID: 25154820.

29. Turtle, et al. Immunotherapy of non-Hodgkin's lymphoma with a defined ratio of CD8+ and CD4+ CD19-specific chimeric antigen receptor–modified T cells. *Science Translational Medicine*. 2016;8(355).

30. Till BG, Jensen MC, Wang J, Chen EY, Wood BL, Greisman HA, et al. Adoptive immunotherapy for indolent non-Hodgkin lymphoma and mantle cell lymphoma using genetically modified autologous CD20-specific T-cells. *Blood*. 2008;112(6):2261–71. PubMed PMID: 18509084. Pubmed Central PMCID: PMC2532803.

31. Till BG, Jensen MC, Wang J, Qian X, Gopal AK, Maloney DG, et al. CD20-specific adoptive immunotherapy for lymphoma using a chimeric antigen receptor with both CD28 and 4-1BB domains: pilot clinical trial results. *Blood*. 2012;119(17):3940–50. PubMed PMID: 22308288. Pubmed Central PMCID: PMC3350361.

32. Burger JA, Ghia P, Rosenwald A, Caligaris-Cappio F. The microenvironment in mature B-cell malignancies: a target for new treatment strategies. *Blood*. 2009;114(16):3367–75. PubMed PMID: 19636060.

33. Herishanu Y, Perez-Galan P, Liu D, Biancotto A, Pittaluga S, Vire B, et al. The lymph node microenvironment promotes B-cell receptor signaling, NF-kappaB activation, and tumor proliferation in chronic lymphocytic leukemia. *Blood*. 2011;117(2):563–74. PubMed PMID: 20940416. Pubmed Central PMCID: PMC3031480.

34. Christopoulos P, Pfeifer D, Bartholome K, Follo M, Timmer J, Fisch P, et al. Definition and characterization of the systemic T-cell dysregulation in untreated indolent B-cell lymphoma and very early CLL. *Blood*. 2011;117(14):3836–46. PubMed PMID: 21270444.

35. Riches JC, Davies JK, McClanahan F, Fatah R, Iqbal S, Agrawal S, et al. T-cells from CLL patients exhibit features of T-cell exhaustion but retain capacity for cytokine production. *Blood*. 2013;121(9):1612–21. PubMed PMID: 23247726. Pubmed Central PMCID: PMC3587324.

36. Davila ML, Bouhassira DC, Park JH, Curran KJ, Smith EL, Pegram HJ, et al. Chimeric antigen receptors for the adoptive T cell therapy of hematologic malignancies. *International Journal of Hematology*. 2014;99(4):361–71. PubMed PMID: 24311149.

37. Neeson P, Shin A, Tainton KM, Guru P, Prince HM, Harrison SJ, et al. Ex vivo culture of chimeric antigen receptor

T cells generates functional CD8+ T-cells with effector and central memory-like phenotype. *Gene Therapy*. 2010;17(9):1105–16. PubMed PMID: 20428216.

38. Ali SA, Shi V, Maric I, Wang M, Stroncek DF, Rose JJ, et al. T cells expressing an anti–B-cell maturation antigen chimeric antigen receptor cause remissions of multiple myeloma. *Blood*. 2016;128:1688–700.

39. Ritchie DS, Neeson PJ, Khot A, Peinert S, Tai T, Tainton K, et al. Persistence and efficacy of second generation CAR T cell against the LeY antigen in acute myeloid leukemia. *Molecular Therapy: The Journal of the American Society of Gene Therapy*. 2013;21(11):2122–9. PubMed PMID: 23831595. Pubmed Central PMCID: PMC3831035.

40. Gajewski TF, Schreiber H, Fu YX. Innate and adaptive immune cells in the tumor microenvironment. *Nature Immunology*. 2013;14(10):1014–22. PubMed PMID: 24048123. Pubmed Central PMCID: PMC4118725.

41. Lee JC, Hayman E, Pegram HJ, Santos E, Heller G, Sadelain M, et al. In vivo inhibition of human CD19-targeted effector T-cells by natural T regulatory cells in a xenotransplant murine model of B cell malignancy. *Cancer Research*. 2011;71(8):2871–81. PubMed PMID: 21487038. Pubmed Central PMCID: PMC3094720.

42. Kershaw MH, Westwood JA, Parker LL, Wang G, Eshhar Z, Mavroukakis SA, et al. A phase I study on adoptive immunotherapy using gene-modified T cells for ovarian cancer. *Clinical Cancer Research: An Official Journal of the American Association for Cancer Research*. 2006;12(20 Pt 1):6106–15. PubMed PMID: 17062687. Pubmed Central PMCID: PMC2154351.

43. Louis CU, Savoldo B, Dotti G, Pule M, Yvon E, Myers GD, et al. Antitumor activity and long-term fate of chimeric antigen receptor-positive T-cells in patients with neuroblastoma. *Blood*. 2011;118(23):6050–6. PubMed PMID: 21984804. Pubmed Central PMCID: PMC3234664.

44. Maus MV, Haas AR, Beatty GL, Albelda SM, Levine BL, Liu X, et al. T-cells expressing chimeric antigen receptors can cause anaphylaxis in humans. *Cancer Immunology Research*. 2013;1(1):26–31. PubMed PMID: 24777247.

45. Hegde M, Corder A, Chow KK, Mukherjee M, Ashoori A, Kew Y, et al. Combinational targeting offsets antigen escape and enhances effector functions of adoptively transferred T cells in glioblastoma. *Molecular Therapy: The Journal of the American Society of Gene Therapy*. 2013;21(11):2087–101. PubMed PMID: 23939024. Pubmed Central PMCID: PMC3831041.

46. Duong CP, Westwood JA, Berry LJ, Darcy PK, Kershaw MH. Enhancing the specificity of T-cell cultures for adoptive immunotherapy of cancer. *Immunotherapy*. 2011;3(1):33–48. PubMed PMID: 21174556.

47. Kloss CC, Condomines M, Cartellieri M, Bachmann M, Sadelain M. Combinatorial antigen recognition with balanced signaling promotes selective tumor eradication by engineered T-cells. *Nature Biotechnology*. 2013;31(1):71–5. PubMed PMID: 23242161.

48. Kakarla S, Chow K, Mata M, Shaffer DR, Song XT, Wu MF, et al. Antitumor effects of chimeric receptor engineered human T-cells directed to tumor stroma. *Molecular Therapy: The Journal of the American Society of Gene Therapy*. 2013;21(8):1611–20. PubMed PMID: 23732988. Pubmed Central PMCID: PMC3734659.

49. Chmielewski M, Hombach AA, Abken H. Of CARs and TRUCKs: chimeric antigen receptor (CAR) T cells engineered with an inducible cytokine to modulate the tumor stroma. *Immunological Reviews*. 2014;257(1):83–90. PubMed PMID: 24329791.

50. Pegram HJ, Lee JC, Hayman EG, Imperato GH, Tedder TF, Sadelain M, et al. Tumor-targeted T-cells modified to secrete IL-12 eradicate systemic tumors without need for prior conditioning. *Blood*. 2012;119(18):4133–41. PubMed PMID: 22354001. Pubmed Central PMCID: PMC3359735.

51. Leonard JP, Sherman ML, Fisher GL, Buchanan LJ, Larsen G, Atkins MB, et al. Effects of single-dose interleukin-12 exposure on interleukin-12-associated toxicity and interferon-gamma production. *Blood*. 1997;90(7):2541–8. PubMed PMID: 9326219.

52. Koneru M, O'Cearbhaill R, Pendharkar S, Spriggs DR, Brentjens RJ. A phase I clinical trial of adoptive T cell therapy using IL-12 secreting MUC-16ecto directed chimeric antigen receptors for recurrent ovarian cancer. *Journal of Translational Medicine*. 2015;13:102.

53. Stephan MT, Ponomarev V, Brentjens RJ, Chang AH, Dobrenkov KV, Heller G, et al. T cell-encoded CD80 and 4-1BBL induce auto- and transcostimulation, resulting in potent tumor rejection. *Nature Medicine*. 2007;13(12):1440–9. PubMed PMID: 18026115.

54. Davila ML, Kloss CC, Gunset G, Sadelain M. CD19 CAR-targeted T-cells induce long-term remission and B Cell Aplasia in an immunocompetent mouse model of B cell acute lymphoblastic leukemia. *PLoS one*. 2013;8(4):e61338. PubMed PMID: 23585892. Pubmed Central PMCID: PMC3621858.

55. Morgan RA, Yang JC, Kitano M, Dudley ME, Laurencot CM, Rosenberg SA. Case report of a serious adverse event following the administration of T-cells transduced with a chimeric antigen receptor recognizing ERBB2. *Molecular Therapy: The Journal of the American Society of Gene Therapy*. 2010;18(4):843–51. PubMed PMID: 20179677. Pubmed Central PMCID: PMC2862534.

56. Di Stasi A, Tey SK, Dotti G, Fujita Y, Kennedy-Nasser A, Martinez C, et al. Inducible apoptosis as a safety switch for adoptive cell therapy. *The New England Journal of Medicine*. 2011;365(18):1673–83. PubMed PMID: 22047558. Pubmed Central PMCID: PMC3236370.

57. Kalos M, Levine BL, Porter DL, Katz S, Grupp SA, Bagg A, et al. T cells with chimeric antigen receptors have potent antitumor effects and can establish memory in patients with advanced leukemia. *Science Translational Medicine*. 2011;3(95):95ra73. PubMed PMID: 21832238. Pubmed Central PMCID: PMC3393096.

58. Teachey DT, Lacey SF, Shaw PA, Melenhorst J, Maude SL, Frey N, et al. Identification of predictive biomarkers for cytokine release syndrome after chimeric antigen receptor T-cell therapy for acute lymphoblastic leukemia. *Cancer Discovery*. 2016; 10.1158/2159-8290.CD-16-0040.

59. Bonifant CL, Jackson HJ, Brentjens RJ, Curran KJ. Toxicity and management in CAR T-cell therapy. *Molecular Therapy: Oncolytics*. 2016;3:16011; doi:10.1038/mto.2016.11.

Chapter

63

NK Cells for Cancers

Dean A. Lee

Introduction to NK Cell Recognition and Killing of Targets

NK cells are lymphocytes of the innate immune system with cytotoxic and regulatory functions, which are critical mediators of immune responses against infections and malignancies[1]. NK cells are typically defined as CD56-expressing lymphocytes that lack a T-cell receptor (e.g., CD3-negative), comprising approximately 10% of all blood lymphocytes[2]. As members of the innate immune system, they express only germline-encoded receptors and lack the genetic recombination of receptors essential for T-, B-, and NKT-cell development. NK cells are highly heterogeneous, express a variegated array of activating and inhibitory receptors, and are triggered to kill target cells when the balance of activation and inhibition exceeds a preset threshold in favor of activation. Once triggered, NK cells mediate target cell killing through the release of cytolytic granules containing perforin and granzyme, or through activation of apoptosis by ligation of death receptors (Fas, DR4, DR5). In addition to these direct cytolytic mechanisms, NK cells also produce cytokines such as IFN-γ, which are important in initiating subsequent adaptive immune responses.

NK Cell Receptors

NK cells were initially identified in the 1970s on the basis of recognizing malignant targets without prior sensitization[3,4]. In addition to direct recognition of cell targets, they are also important mediators of antibody-dependent cell cytotoxicity (ADCC), wherein the low-affinity antibody receptor FcγRIIIa (CD16a) binds to the Fc portion of IgG antibodies resulting in a potent activation signal to the NK cell. Their importance in this regard will not be discussed further, as we will focus on the direct role of NK cells in the context of hematopoietic cell transplantation (HCT).

Inhibitory receptors on NK cells primarily recognize major histocompatibility complex (MHC) class I molecules on potential targets, preventing NK-mediated lysis of cells that express normal levels of self MHC. The primary inhibitory receptors are members of the killer immunoglobulin-like receptor (KIR) family, a highly diverse group of NK receptors with cytoplasmic tails containing either short activating (immunoreceptor tyrosine-based activating motif; ITAM) or long inhibitory

(immunoreceptor tyrosine-based inhibition motif; ITIM) domains. Fourteen KIR genes and two pseudogenes have been identified on chromosome 19q13.4 and are extremely polymorphic. The C-type lectin receptors in the NKG2 family are also polymorphic, and either recognize self through nonclassical MHC class I (e.g., human leukocyte antigen (HLA)-E recognized by NKG2A and NKG2C) or recognize danger signals such as stress-related ligands (e.g., MICA recognized by NKG2D). Other activating receptors include the family of natural cytotoxicity receptors (NKp30, NKp44, NKp46, and NKp80). NKG2A mediates an inhibitory signal, whereas NKG2C mediates an activation signal, both in response to HLA-E. NKG2A and NKG2C may function together as a rheostat for signaling depending on the peptides present in HLA-E.

Models of NK Cell Recognition

The "missing self" model for NK cell allorecognition was formed on the basis of numerous observations that MHC class I expression on-target cells correlated inversely with their susceptibility to NK cell lysis, and on data showing that rejection of bone marrow from β2m-deficient mice (which lack MHC class I expression) was fully mediated by NK cells in the recipient[5]. Subsequent murine studies dissecting the basis for "hybrid resistance" in bone marrow transplantation – which could not be explained by T-cell mechanisms – identified an essential role for NK cell recognition of self MHC class I as an inhibitory signal[6,7]. Exploitation of this property as a means for augmenting NK function against leukemia has been a major source of interest in using HLA haplotype matched donors for hematopoietic cell transplantation (haplo-HCT), but also has relevance for matched allogeneic HCT (allo-HCT) and even autologous HCT (auto-HCT) transplants, as will be discussed below.

However, "missing self" is an oversimplification of NK cell regulation, since a lack of MHC class I is not sufficient alone to induce NK cytotoxicity, nor is its presence always sufficient to prevent NK cytotoxicity[8]. The recognition that NK cell killing also requires engagement of activating receptors has led to the modified model of "altered self", which, in addition to the loss of MHC described by "missing self," includes activation signals delivered by the neo-expression of surface ligands and/or peptides that interfere with MHC recognition (e.g., HLA-E as described above). This further modification of the model provides an explanation for how NK cells can recognize virus-infected or transformed cells without inducing graft-*versus*-host disease (GvHD), since these activating ligands are not expressed on normal healthy tissues.

Models for Predicting NK Cell Alloreactivity in Humans

The 14 functionally expressed KIR genes are present or absent in many haplotype combinations such that most individuals lack one or more KIR genes. In addition to their haplotype variability, KIR genes are highly polymorphic, are variably expressed between NK cells, and functional reactivity is educated by interaction with the host HLA haplotypes (termed "licensing"). Thus, the functional repertoire available on NK cells varies greatly between individuals. Importantly, the allelic variations in KIR can be simplified into A and B haplotypes[9], with B haplotypes having greater numbers of activating KIR genes.

Inhibitory KIRs are specific for HLA isotypes on the basis of conserved amino acid residues at position 80. Approximately 60% of HLA-C alleles have the amino acid asparagine (N) at residue 80 – referred to as Group C1. This N80 residue confers binding of the HLA to KIR2DL2 and KIR2DL3. The other 40% of HLA-C alleles – referred to as Group C2 – have lysine (K) at residue 80 that confers binding to KIR2DL1. Similarly, about 30% of HLA-B alleles carry the supertypic serologic epitope HLA-Bw4, defined primarily by threonine (T) at residue 80 which confers binding to KIR3DL1. Thus, given both parental alleles and speaking strictly of the primary inhibitory KIRs that recognize MHC class I, it is possible for the HLA type of an individual to restrict inhibitory HLA interactions to as few as one (e.g., C2/C2 homozygous and Bw4–) or as many as three (C1/C2 heterozygous and Bw4+) inhibitory KIRs.

Licensing is the process by which NK cells possessing inhibitory KIRs "learn" to be most sensitive to the HLA that are expressed by the individual as "self." Although most individuals will have NK cells expressing all three major inhibitory KIRs, the NK cells which interact with the cognate ligand during development will be rendered the most active. For example, NK cells expressing KIR2DL1 that develop in an individual who is Group C2 homozygous will be "licensed" to recognize Group C2, and therefore more likely to recognize a cell as missing self when Group C2 is missing, whereas NK cells expressing KIR2DL2 will not interact with a ligand and will therefore be hypofunctional.

Predicting Missing Self

Missing Ligand Model

The simplest model for NK cell recognition of targets is the missing ligand model. In this model, NK cells bearing an inhibitory KIR interact with a cell missing the cognate HLA

ligand, and therefore are predicted to be less inhibited than their counterparts for which a cognate ligand is present. As mentioned above, it is possible for individuals to have as few as one or as many as three MHC alleles that mediate such inhibitory "self" signals. As such, only the patient's HLA type is required for predictions using this model. Individuals possessing HLA that inhibit all three groups of KIR would have the most inhibited NK cells, whereas individuals possessing only one group of inhibitory HLA alleles would only inhibit the NK cells expressing the matching KIR, and the rest would be less inhibited (Figure 63.1A). Importantly, this model can be applied to matched allo-transplant, autotransplant, and non-transplant settings because a mismatch between a donor and recipient is not implied. Also important is that this model ignores the effect of licensing.

Ligand–Ligand Mismatch Model

This model is not based on HLA mismatch *per se*, but mismatch of the broad HLA groups with respect to KIR recognition (Group C1, Group C2, and Bw4 mentioned above). Mismatch in the graft-*versus*-lymphoma (GvL) direction is defined in this model as a donor having a KIR-ligand HLA group that is missing in the recipient (e.g., Group C1/C2 heterozygous haploidentical donor for a Group C2 homozygous recipient) (Figure 63.1B). In this model, the presence of the most active licensed NK cells – and their potential for released inhibition by a ligand missing in the recipient – is assumed on the basis of donor and recipient HLA typing. This model is therefore only predictive in the setting of HLA-mismatched donors, and although it incorporates the concept of licensing, it ignores KIR genotype and assumes the presence of the inhibitory KIR (which may be incorrect ~10% of the time).

KIR–KIR-Ligand Mismatch Model

This model is a refinement of the Ligand–Ligand mismatch model, and requires HLA typing of the donor and recipient and KIR typing of the donor. A mismatch in this model is defined as the donor having an inhibitory KIR and the cognate HLA, but the cognate HLA is missing in the recipient (e.g., KIR2DL2+, Group C1/C2 heterozygous haploidentical donor for a Group C2 homozygous recipient) (Figure 63.1C). This model is the most stringent in predicting alloreactivity on the basis of licensed NK cells, but as for the Ligand–Ligand model, it only applies to mismatched transplants.

KIR–KIR Mismatch Model

In the KIR–KIR mismatch model, emphasis is placed on the differences in KIR genotype between the recipient and the donor. This model assumes some degree of immunologic pressure (immunoediting) placed on the cancer by the patient's own NK cells during carcinogenesis. Since KIR gene inheritance is widely variable, the presence of new KIR genes in the donor may result in new alloreactive interactions by NK cell subsets. Although the basis for benefit is primarily attributed to KIR-B donors in KIR A recipients, this model also

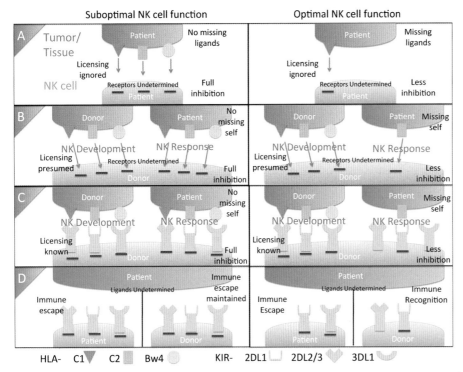

Figure 63.1. Models for predicting NK cell activity on the basis of "missing self". (**A**) **Missing Ligand model:** patient HLA is classified according to the number of KIR ligands present to provide inhibitory signals. The more ligands present, the more potential inhibition, and the fewer ligands present, the less inhibition. The model may be applied to matched and autologous transplant or nontransplant settings, but ignores licensing and does not assess for the presence of relevant KIR. (**B**) **Ligand–Ligand Mismatch model:** patient and donor HLA is classified according to the number of KIR ligands present to provide inhibitory signals, and optimal donors are considered those who have ligands that the patient is missing, resulting in less inhibition of the donor NK cells. The model only applies to mismatched transplants, and only presumes licensing occurs because it does not assess for the presence of relevant KIRs. (**C**) **KIR–KIR-Ligand Mismatch model:** patient and donor HLA is classified according to the number of KIR ligands present to provide inhibitory signals, and donor KIR genotype is determined. Optimal donors are considered those who have an inhibitory KIR and cognate ligand for which the patient is missing the ligand, resulting in less inhibition of the donor NK cells. The model only applies to mismatched transplants, and is the most stringent regarding licensing. (**D**) **KIR–KIR Mismatch model:** patient and donor KIR are determined, and optimal donors are considered those who have KIRs that the patient is missing. The model can be applied to matched or mismatched transplants, but does not assess the effect of HLA haplotype on licensing or inhibition.

allows for a benefit from donor KIR licensing in recipients who lack one of the major inhibitory KIR (Figure 63.1D).

Altered Self or Injured Self

Whereas a missing self-interaction leads to the release of NK cells from inhibition, it is not sufficient on its own to mediate NK cell activation. NKG2D recognition of stress ligands is relatively uniform across donors, but the inheritance of activating KIR is highly variable, and the relative composition of NKG2C+ *versus* NKG2A+ NK cells is highly variable across donors. Several models are proposed for predicting enhanced NK cell activation from activating receptor variability among donors.

Activating KIR Content

In this model, the number of activating KIRs inherited by an individual is determined by KIR genotyping. Current methods allow only for identifying that a KIR gene has been inherited, and do not allow discrimination between those who inherit one from those with two copies of a given gene. Specific activating KIRs may be more relevant to predicting outcomes

for certain malignancies, but the majority of reports stratify patients based on KIR content in groups (e.g., 0–1, 2–3, or 4+ activating KIR). The ligands have not been identified for most activating KIRs, although some bind to the same HLA group as defined above for inhibitory KIRs. This model does not take into account the effect of HLA haplotype on these activating KIRs, although a few small studies have taken this effect into consideration as independent endpoints showing benefit for donor-activating KIRs that bind recipient HLA[10].

KIR Haplotype

An alternative to quantifying the total number of activating KIRs is to stratify individuals into major haplotype groups. Approximately 50% of individuals fit into a relatively uniform group of genotypes which specifically lack *KIR2DL5*, *KIR2DS1*, *KIR2DS2*, *KIR2DS3*, *KIR2DS5*, and *KIR3DS1* genes and therefore possess few or no activating KIRs, referred to as "KIR A." The remainder of genotypes which each include at least one of these genes are designated "KIR-B." Broadly speaking, the KIR haplotype model can be thought of as a simplification of KIR content, with KIR-B representing individuals whose NK cells possess more activating receptors and therefore more potential for activation. However, some variants of this model have demonstrated a more profound effect for KIR-B genotypes that are defined by the genes on the centromeric end of the KIR locus compared to those on the telomeric end, suggesting that total activating KIR gene content may not be as important as specific activating KIRs.

NKG2A *versus* NKG2C

Donor-derived NK cells initially emerging from the allograft have an immature phenotype with low KIR expression and overexpression of NKG2A. By 6 to 9 months postengraftment, NK cells acquire phenotypic characteristics of mature cells[11], including a transition to expressing more NKG2C and less NKG2A[12]. Importantly, the maturation of NK cells expressing KIR and the transition to NKG2C may be enhanced by CMV reactivation[13–15].

NK Cells in Transplantation: Demonstrating Antitumor, Antiviral, and Anti-GvHD Effects in Clinical Trials

NK cells have antitumor effects, reduce GvHD, and mediate antiviral responses, each of which may impact the overall survival after HCT. Individually assessing each of these factors within each of the possible models and across all types of transplants has led to conflicting conclusions and confusion within the field. Nonetheless, data are accumulating in each of these settings that support a strong role for NK cells in disease-free survival after HCT, as listed in the Table 63.1.

Haplotype Matched HCT

As mentioned above, the Ligand–Ligand and KIR–KIR-ligand models predict potential benefit by manipulating NK cell licensing in an HLA-mismatched transplant setting. As such, all four predictive models for NK cell alloreactivity, and the predictive models for NK cell function can be applied to mismatched transplants. Thus, it is not surprising that the data are strongest for an NK cell effect in this setting. While prospective studies that select donors on this basis are not yet mature, retrospective studies have provided the proof-of-principle for this approach, demonstrating decreased leukemia relapse when donor:recipient pairs have a KIR–KIR-ligand mismatch. It is important to note that the impact of NK cells on transplant outcomes may differ across the approaches for GvHD prevention. The KIR–KIR-ligand model was superior to the Ligand–Ligand model in the T-cell-depleted setting[16], whereas the KIR–KIR and KIR A/B models were more predictive in the post-transplant cyclophosphamide setting[17].

Matched Allo-HCT, Including Cord Blood Transplants

Importantly, KIR mismatch is associated with increased risk of GvHD in cord blood transplants using reduced intensity conditioning regimens[18]. Missing ligand was also associated

with GvHD in matched allo-HCT, but was highly associated with the lack of T-cell depletion or ATG[19], suggesting that the NK cells were not directly responsible for GvHD but may play a role in providing T-cell help. Cord blood transplants may provide more opportunity to select for mismatch based on the Ligand–Ligand or KIR–KIR-ligand models because of acceptable levels of GvHD when mismatched for HLA.

Autologous HCT

Auto-HCT cannot benefit from prospective donor selection, but the benefits of missing ligand could be used for risk stratification, perhaps by identifying individuals with low benefit from autotransplant who could derive more benefit from an allo-HCT. In diseases where NK cell reconstitution predicts outcomes, augmenting post-transplant NK cell recovery may improve overall survival.

Future Research
Preclinical Models

Few preclinical studies assessing potential roles for NK cells in treating cancer incorporate HLA type and expression of cancer cell lines or KIR typing or licensing of the NK cells obtained from normal donors for *in-vitro* studies, making it difficult to translate the findings to clinical transplantation. In addition, murine NK cell biology and genetics vary greatly from humans, making murine studies of cancer difficult to extrapolate directly to human disease or the transplant setting. Moreover, murine xenograft models are typically NK cell deficient, if not completely lacking in NK cell function. In light of these problems, future research will need to clearly identify the HLA and KIR genotypes of research cell lines, and refined animal models will need to be developed, including outbred large animal models.

NK Cell Subsets

Recent approaches in high-dimension phenotyping have revealed great heterogeneity in NK cell subsets, suggesting there may be thousands of different types of NK cells based on differential inheritance patterns and variegated receptor expression[20]. Application of such methods to identify the unique subsets of NK cells that are primarily responsible for tumor recognition and control will enable better donor selection, graft manipulation, and cell engineering.

In addition, identifying Ligand–Ligand or KIR–KIR-Ligand mismatched family donors is possible for only a minority of patients, and KIR-B haplotypes are also present in a minority of donors, such that many patients may not have donors available with an "ideal" NK cell genotype. Future research must address methods for manipulating the receptor repertoire or KIR licensing in order to increase the "ideal" donor characteristics in otherwise suboptimal donor–recipient pairs.

Table 63.1 Transplant outcome benefits attributed to NK cells

Disease/context	Predictive factor	Benefit	Reference
Haplotransplant/mismatched			
AML, ALL, haplo-T-cell-depleted	Ligand–Ligand mismatch, any	AML – Survival[a] ALL – (NS)	Ruggeri et al. 2002[31]
AML/ALL/MDS/CML/ NHL/HD/MM MMUD	Ligand–Ligand mismatch	OS,[b] DFS[c]	Giebel et al. 2003[32]
Myeloid leukemias, MMUD	Ligand–Ligand mismatch	Relapse[a]	Beelen et al. 2005[33]
CML, MMUD	Ligand–Ligand mismatch	Relapse,[b] EFS[a]	Elmaagacli et al. 2005[34]
AML, haplo-T-cell-depleted	KIR–KIR-Ligand mismatch	AML Relapse,[c] EFS,[a] OS[a]	Ruggeri et al. 2007[16]
Myeloid or lymphoid leukemia, haplo-post-Tx Cy	KIR–KIR KIR A versus B	OS,[b] EFS[a] OS[a]	Symons et al. 2010[17]
Hematologic malignancies, MUD or haplo	Post-transplant NK cell activity	Relapse[a]	Lang et al. 2011[35]
CML, haplo-HCT	Missing Ligand Activating KIR–KIR Ligand	Relapse,[a] OS[a] Relapse[a]	Zhao et al. 2014[10]
ALL, haplo-T-cell-depleted	KIR A versus B	EFS[a]	Oevermann et al. 2014[36]
Hematologic malignancies, haplo-HCT	KIR A versus B	Relapse[b]	Michaelis et al. 2014[37]
Hematologic malignancies, haplo-HCT	KIR2DS1/KIR3DS1	NRM,[a] EFS,[a] Infection[b]	Mancusi, Blood. 2015 125(20):3173-82
Matched allo-transplant, including CBT			
AML/ALL/MDS/CML, MSD-HCT	NK cell dose in allograft	aGvHD,[a] cGvHD[b]	Yamasaki et al. 2003[38]
Acute leukemia, MSD-HCT	Presence of both 2DS1 and 2DS2	Relapse[a] OS – NS	Verheyden et al. 2005[39]
AML/MDS, MSD	Missing ligand	Relapse – NS DFS[a]	Hsu et al. 2005[40]
Unselected malignant and nonmalignant, MSD-HCT	NK cell dose in allograft	Engraftment[c] Infection[b] NRM[a]	Kim et al. 2005[41]
Hematologic malignancies, MUD HCT	Missing ligand	Relapse[b]	Hsu et al. 2006[42]
Myeloid, MUD-, or MMUD-HCT	Missing ligand	Relapse[a]	Miller et al. 2007[19]
AML, MUD-, or MSD-HCT (T-depleted)	NK cell recovery at day 30	AML – aGvHD[b] Relapse[c] NRM[b] OS[c] ALL– (NS)	Savani et al. 2007[43]
AML, ALL UCBT	Ligand–Ligand mismatch	DFS,[b] OS,[b] relapse[a]	Willemze et al. 2009[44]
AML, MUD-, or MMUD-HCT	Ligand–Ligand mismatch KIR A versus B	RFS[b] RFS[b]	Cooley et al. 2009[45]
AML, MUD-HCT	KIR A versus B	Relapse,[b] DFS[a]	Cooley et al. 2010[46]
Unselected malignant and nonmalignant, MUD-HCT	KIR A versus B	Bacterial infections[a]	Tomblyn et al. 2010[47]
Hematologic malignancies, UCBT	Post-transplant NK cell recovery	OS[a]	Yamamoto et al. 2013[48]
Autotransplant			
Solid tumors, Lymphoma	KIR–KIR-Ligand	Relapse,[a] EFS[a]	Leung et al. 2007[49]
Neuroblastoma	Missing ligand	PFS[a] OS[b]	Venstrom et al. 2009[50]

NS – not significant.
[a] $P \leq 0.05$.
[b] $P \leq 0.01$.
[c] $P \leq 0.001$.

The Role of NKG2C+ NK Cells in Leukemic Control

Similarly, the importance of generating NKG2C+ mature NK cells in post-transplant immune reconstitution has been associated with decreased leukemia relapse[13,14], but the mechanisms for leukemic control by these cells is not fully understood. Again, improved understanding of NK cell subsets will enable better transplant engineering.

Identify Best GvH Prophylaxis, Cytokines, and Conditioning to Promote NK Reconstitution

NK cell reconstitution and participation in GvL and GvHD responses are dependent on the conditioning regimen[18] and methods of GvHD prophylaxis. Particularly in the setting of haplo-HCT new approaches for graft manipulation such as αβTCR-depletion[21] and GvHD prevention with post-transplant cyclophosphamide[22] will need to be fully characterized for their effect on NK cell reconstitution and function. Even the selection of post-transplant immunosuppressants may need to be reconsidered across platforms with the aim of optimizing NK cell function[23].

Controversies

In-vivo *versus* Ex-vivo Expansion

Approaches to improving either functional or numeric NK cell reconstitution after HCT can be divided among those that promote *in-vivo* proliferation or maturation, such as cytokines or lymphodepletion, or those that rely on *ex-vivo* expansion, activation, or maturation systems. NK cells may be collected by apheresis, T-cell-depleted to avoid GvHD, and infused in the post-transplant setting to augment GvL, reduce GvHD, or reduce infectious complications[24–26]. Alternatively, *ex-vivo* propagation using feeder cells[27–30] may enable large doses of highly activated autologous or allogeneic NK cells to be infused. *Ex-vivo* approaches have the advantages of removing the NK cells from potentially suppressive tumor microenvironments, allow for selective manipulation of desirable subsets, and avoiding systemic or off-target effects. For instance, high-dose IL-2 is highly effective at activating NK cells, but concentrations necessary to achieve activation and proliferation *in-vivo* also cause systemic inflammatory symptoms and may promote Treg proliferation and function. New approaches using IL-12, IL-15, or IL-21 are currently under investigation. On the other hand, *ex-vivo* systems may take weeks for propagation and maturation, require complex and costly specialized facilities for cell manufacturing, and may be limited by replicative senescence. The best solutions may involve delivering *ex-vivo*-propagated cells to patients in combination with optimizing *in-vivo* proliferation and survival. A hybrid approach involving short-term culture in cytokines (to achieve a highly-active memory-like phenotype) followed by *in vivo* expansion (induced by lymphodepletion) appears promising.

Identifying and Applying the Most Predictive Models of NK Cell Alloreactivity

The six competing models mentioned above for predicting optimal donor–recipient pairs on the basis of KIR need to be systematically compared and contrasted in large cohorts across transplant platforms and donor sources. Unfortunately, no current models take into consideration the role of both inhibitory and activating KIR biology, such as considering HLA-specific activating KIR (e.g., KIR2DS1) as a confounding factor to KIR–KIR-ligand stratification. Inconsistency in the collection of donor KIR genotypes contributes to the lack of information on KIR-based effects in transplant research. Recent high-quality publications describing highly effective new platforms for HLA-haplotype mismatch transplant have not addressed the role of KIRs in this setting[22] because of the lack of donor KIR information. Priority for funding and for publication in high-quality journals should be given to research that adequately assesses the predictive power of each of the models. More importantly, transplant consortia and donor programs should begin collecting KIR genotype data on all donors prospectively to enable broad-based research across disease and donor types.

The Role of NK Cells in GvHD

NK cells have been strongly associated with suppressing GvHD in many preclinical murine models. One proposed mechanism is through elimination of recipient dendritic cells responsible for cross-presentation of recipient minor antigens to donor T-cells[31]. However, studies in human transplantation have shown conflicting results, with some showing increased GvHD, some decreased GvHD, and many showing no effect. Adoptive transfer of activated NK cells in both murine experiments and human trials have shown very little propensity for directly causing GvHD, although a recent report suggests that highly active NK cells may exacerbate subclinical GvHD if adoptively transferred post-transplant[26]. Controversy over the role that NK cells have in either promoting or protecting from GvHD will likely require the identification of temporal events in the genesis of GvHD, and may depend on all of the repertoire and activation variables described above for antitumor responses, in addition to the timing of adoptive transfer in relation to the transplanted stem cells.

References

1. Raulet DH, Guerra N. Oncogenic stress sensed by the immune system: role of natural killer cell receptors. *Nat Rev Immunol.* 2009;9(8):568–80. Epub 2009/07/25.

2. Almeida-Oliveira A, Smith-Carvalho M, Porto LC, Cardoso-Oliveira J, Ribeiro Ados S, Falcao RR, et al. Age-related changes in natural killer cell receptors from childhood through old age. *Hum Immunol.* 2011;72(4):319–29. Epub 2011/01/26.

3. Kiessling R, Klein E, Wigzell H. "Natural" killer cells in the mouse. I. Cytotoxic cells with specificity for mouse Moloney leukemia cells. Specificity and distribution according to genotype. *Eur J Immunol.* 1975;5(2):112–7. Epub 1975/02/01.

4. Herberman RB, Nunn ME, Lavrin DH. Natural cytotoxic reactivity of mouse lymphoid cells against syngeneic acid allogeneic tumors. I. Distribution of reactivity and specificity. *Int J Cancer.* 1975;16(2):216–29. Epub 1975/08/15.

5. Murphy WJ, Koh CY, Raziuddin A, Bennett M, Longo DL. Immunobiology of natural killer cells and bone marrow transplantation: merging of basic and preclinical studies. *Immunol Rev.* 2001;181:279–89. Epub 2001/08/22.

6. Ljunggren HG, Karre K. In search of the 'missing self': MHC molecules and NK cell recognition. *Immunol Today.* 1990;11(7):237–44.

7. Raulet DH, Correa I, Corral L, Dorfman J, Wu MF. Inhibitory effects of class I molecules on murine NK cells: speculations on function, specificity and self-tolerance. *Semi Immunol.* 1995;7(2):103–7. Epub 1995/04/01.

8. Farag SS, Caligiuri MA. Human natural killer cell development and biology. *Blood Rev.* 2006;20(3):123–37. Epub 2005/12/21.

9. Uhrberg M, Valiante NM, Shum BP, Shilling HG, Lienert-Weidenbach K, Corliss B, et al. Human diversity in killer cell inhibitory receptor genes. *Immunity.* 1997;7(6):753–63. Epub 1998/01/16.

10. Zhao XY, Chang YJ, Xu LP, Zhang XH, Liu KY, Li D, et al. HLA and KIR genotyping correlates with relapse after T-cell-replete haploidentical transplantation in chronic myeloid leukaemia patients. *Br J Cancer.* 2014;111(6):1080–8. Epub 2014/08/01.

11. Shilling HG, McQueen KL, Cheng NW, Shizuru JA, Negrin RS, Parham P. Reconstitution of NK cell receptor repertoire following HLA-matched hematopoietic cell transplantation. *Blood.* 2003;101(9):3730–40. Epub 2003/01/04.

12. Giebel S, Dziaczkowska J, Czerw T, Wojnar J, Krawczyk-Kulis M, Nowak I, et al. Sequential recovery of NK cell receptor repertoire after allogeneic hematopoietic SCT. *Bone Marrow Transplant.* 2010;45(6):1022–30. Epub 2010/02/02.

13. Beziat V, Liu LL, Malmberg JA, Ivarsson MA, Sohlberg E, Bjorklund AT, et al. NK cell responses to cytomegalovirus infection lead to stable imprints in the human KIR repertoire and involve activating KIRs. *Blood.* 2013;121(14):2678–88. Epub 2013/01/18.

14. Foley B, Cooley S, Verneris MR, Pitt M, Curtsinger J, Luo X, et al. Cytomegalovirus reactivation after allogeneic transplantation promotes a lasting increase in educated NKG2C+ natural killer cells with potent function. *Blood.* 2012;119(11):2665–74. Epub 2011/12/20.

15. Foley B, Cooley S, Verneris MR, Curtsinger J, Luo X, Waller EK, et al. Human cytomegalovirus (CMV)-induced memory-like NKG2C(+) NK cells are transplantable and expand in vivo in response to recipient CMV antigen. *J Immunol.* 2012;189(10):5082–8. Epub 2012/10/19.

16. Ruggeri L, Mancusi A, Capanni M, Urbani E, Carotti A, Aloisi T, et al. Donor natural killer cell allorecognition of missing self in haploidentical hematopoietic transplantation for acute myeloid leukemia: challenging its predictive value. *Blood.* 2007;110(1):433–40. Epub 2007/03/21.

17. Symons HJ, Leffell MS, Rossiter ND, Zahurak M, Jones RJ, Fuchs EJ. Improved survival with inhibitory killer immunoglobulin receptor (KIR) gene mismatches and KIR haplotype B donors after nonmyeloablative, HLA-haploidentical bone marrow transplantation. *Biol Blood Marrow Transplant.* 2010;16(4):533–42. Epub 2009/12/08.

18. Brunstein CG, Wagner JE, Weisdorf DJ, Cooley S, Noreen H, Barker JN, et al. Negative effect of KIR alloreactivity in recipients of umbilical cord blood transplant depends on transplantation conditioning intensity. *Blood.* 2009;113(22):5628–34. Epub 2009/03/31.

19. Miller JS, Cooley S, Parham P, Farag SS, Verneris MR, McQueen KL, et al. Missing KIR ligands are associated with less relapse and increased graft-*versus*-host disease (GVHD) following unrelated donor allogeneic HCT. *Blood.* 2007;109(11):5058–61.

20. Horowitz A, Strauss-Albee DM, Leipold M, Kubo J, Nemat-Gorgani N, Dogan OC, et al. Genetic and environmental determinants of human NK cell diversity revealed by mass cytometry. *Sci Transl Med.* 2013;5(208):208ra145. Epub 2013/10/25.

21. Bertaina A, Merli P, Rutella S, Pagliara D, Bernardo ME, Masetti R, et al. HLA-haploidentical stem cell transplantation after removal of alphabeta+ T and B cells in children with nonmalignant disorders. *Blood.* 2014;124(5):822–6. Epub 2014/05/30.

22. Kanakry CG, O'Donnell PV, Furlong T, de Lima MJ, Wei W, Medeot M, et al. Multi-institutional study of post-transplantation cyclophosphamide as single-agent graft-*versus*-host disease prophylaxis after allogeneic bone marrow transplantation using myeloablative busulfan and fludarabine conditioning. *J Clin Oncol.* 2014;32(31):3497–505. Epub 2014/10/01.

23. Derniame S, Perazzo J, Lee F, Domogala A, Escobedo-Cousin M, Alnabhan R, et al. Differential effects of mycophenolate mofetil and cyclosporine A on peripheral blood and cord blood natural killer cells activated with interleukin-2. *Cytotherapy.* 2014;16(10):1409–18.

24. Rubnitz JE, Inaba H, Ribeiro RC, Pounds S, Rooney B, Bell T, et al. NKAML: a pilot study to determine the safety and feasibility of haploidentical natural killer cell transplantation in childhood acute myeloid leukemia. *J Clin Oncol.* 2010;28(6):955–9. Epub 2010/01/21.

25. Choi I, Yoon SR, Park SY, Kim H, Jung SJ, Jang YJ, et al. Donor-derived natural killer cells infused after human leukocyte antigen-haploidentical hematopoietic cell transplantation: a dose-escalation study. *Biol Blood Marrow Transplant.* 2014;20(5):696–704. Epub 2014/02/15.

26. Shah NN, Baird K, Delbrook CP, Fleisher TA, Kohler ME, Rampertaap S, et al. Acute GVHD in patients receiving IL-15/4-1BBL activated NK cells following T cell depleted stem cell transplantation. *Blood.* 2015;125(5):784–92.

27. Fujisaki H, Kakuda H, Shimasaki N, Imai C, Ma J, Lockey T, et al. Expansion of highly cytotoxic human natural killer

cells for cancer cell therapy. *Cancer Res.* 2009;69(9):4010–7. Epub 2009/04/23.

28. Denman CJ, Senyukov VV, Somanchi SS, Phatarpekar PV, Kopp LM, Johnson JL, *et al.* Membrane-bound IL-21 promotes sustained ex vivo proliferation of human natural killer cells. *PLoS One.* 2012;7(1):e30264. Epub 2012/01/27.

29. Spanholtz J, Preijers F, Tordoir M, Trilsbeek C, Paardekooper J, de Witte T, *et al.* Clinical-grade generation of active NK cells from cord blood hematopoietic progenitor cells for immunotherapy using a closed-system culture process. *PLoS One.* 2011;6(6):e20740. Epub 2011/06/24.

30. Berg M, Lundqvist A, McCoy P, Jr., Samsel L, Fan Y, Tawab A, *et al.* Clinical-grade ex vivo-expanded human natural killer cells up-regulate activating receptors and death receptor ligands and have enhanced cytolytic activity against tumor cells. *Cytotherapy.* 2009;11(3):341–55. Epub 2009/03/25.

31. Ruggeri L, Capanni M, Urbani E, Perruccio K, Shlomchik WD, Tosti A, *et al.* Effectiveness of donor natural killer cell alloreactivity in mismatched hematopoietic transplants. *Science.* 2002;295(5562):2097–100.

32. Giebel S, Locatelli F, Lamparelli T, Velardi A, Davies S, Frumento G, *et al.* Survival advantage with KIR ligand incompatibility in hematopoietic stem cell transplantation from unrelated donors. *Blood.* 2003;102(3):814–9.

33. Beelen DW, Ottinger HD, Ferencik S, Elmaagacli AH, Peceny R, Trenschel R, *et al.* Genotypic inhibitory killer immunoglobulin-like receptor ligand incompatibility enhances the long-term antileukemic effect of unmodified allogeneic hematopoietic stem cell transplantation in patients with myeloid leukemias. *Blood.* 2005;105(6):2594–600. Epub 2004/11/13.

34. Elmaagacli AH, Ottinger H, Koldehoff M, Peceny R, Steckel NK, Trenschel R, *et al.* Reduced risk for molecular disease in patients with chronic myeloid leukemia after transplantation from a KIR-mismatched donor. *Transplantation.* 2005;79(12):1741–7. Epub 2005/06/24.

35. Lang P, Pfeiffer M, Teltschik HM, Schlegel P, Feuchtinger T, Ebinger M, *et al.* Natural killer cell activity influences outcome after T cell depleted stem cell transplantation from matched unrelated and haploidentical donors. *Best Pract Res Clin Haematol.* 2011;24(3):403–11. Epub 2011/09/20.

36. Oevermann L, Michaelis SU, Mezger M, Lang P, Toporski J, Bertaina A, *et al.* KIR B haplotype donors confer a reduced risk for relapse after haploidentical transplantation in children with ALL. *Blood.* 2014;124(17):2744–7. Epub 2014/08/15.

37. Michaelis SU, Mezger M, Bornhauser M, Trenschel R, Stuhler G, Federmann B, *et al.* KIR haplotype B donors but not KIR-ligand mismatch result in a reduced incidence of relapse after haploidentical transplantation using reduced intensity conditioning and CD3/CD19-depleted grafts. *Ann Hematol.* 2014;93(9):1579–86. Epub 2014/04/29.

38. Yamasaki S, Henzan H, Ohno Y, Yamanaka T, Iino T, Itou Y, *et al.* Influence of transplanted dose of CD56 + cells on development of graft-*versus*-host disease in patients receiving G-CSF-mobilized peripheral blood progenitor cells from HLA-identical sibling donors. *Bone Marrow Transplant.* 2003;32(5):505–10. Epub 2003/08/28.

39. Verheyden S, Schots R, Duquet W, Demanet C. A defined donor activating natural killer cell receptor genotype protects against leukemic relapse after related HLA-identical hematopoietic stem cell transplantation. *Leukemia.* 2005;19(8):1446–51. Epub 2005/06/24.

40. Hsu KC, Keever-Taylor CA, Wilton A, Pinto C, Heller G, Arkun K, *et al.* Improved outcome in HLA-identical sibling hematopoietic stem-cell transplantation for acute myelogenous leukemia predicted by KIR and HLA genotypes. *Blood.* 2005;105(12):4878–84.

41. Kim DH, Sohn SK, Lee NY, Baek JH, Kim JG, Won DI, *et al.* Transplantation with higher dose of natural killer cells associated with better outcomes in terms of non-relapse mortality and infectious events after allogeneic peripheral blood

stem cell transplantation from HLA-matched sibling donors. *Eur J Haematol.* 2005;75(4):299–308. Epub 2005/09/09.

42. Hsu KC, Gooley T, Malkki M, Pinto-Agnello C, Dupont B, Bignon JD, *et al.* KIR ligands and prediction of relapse after unrelated donor hematopoietic cell transplantation for hematologic malignancy. *Biol Blood Marrow Transplant.* 2006;12(8):828–36. Epub 2006/07/26.

43. Savani BN, Mielke S, Adams S, Uribe M, Rezvani K, Yong AS, *et al.* Rapid natural killer cell recovery determines outcome after T-cell-depleted HLA-identical stem cell transplantation in patients with myeloid leukemias but not with acute lymphoblastic leukemia. *Leukemia.* 2007;21(10):2145–52. Epub 2007/08/04.

44. Willemze R, Rodrigues CA, Labopin M, Sanz G, Michel G, Socie G, *et al.* KIR-ligand incompatibility in the graft-*versus*-host direction improves outcomes after umbilical cord blood transplantation for acute leukemia. *Leukemia.* 2009;23(3):492–500. Epub 2009/01/20.

45. Cooley S, Trachtenberg E, Bergemann TL, Saeteurn K, Klein J, Le CT, *et al.* Donors with group B KIR haplotypes improve relapse-free survival after unrelated hematopoietic cell transplantation for acute myelogenous leukemia. *Blood.* 2009;113(3):726–32. Epub 2008/10/24.

46. Cooley S, Weisdorf DJ, Guethlein LA, Klein JP, Wang T, Le CT, *et al.* Donor selection for natural killer cell receptor genes leads to superior survival after unrelated transplantation for acute myelogenous leukemia. *Blood.* 2010;116(14):2411–9. Epub 2010/06/29.

47. Tomblyn M, Young JA, Haagenson MD, Klein JP, Trachtenberg EA, Storek J, *et al.* Decreased infections in recipients of unrelated donor hematopoietic cell transplantation from donors with an activating KIR genotype. *Biol Blood Marrow Transplant.* 2010;16(8):1155–61. Epub 2010/03/04.

48. Yamamoto W, Ogusa E, Matsumoto K, Maruta A, Ishigatsubo Y, Kanamori H. Recovery of natural killer cells and

prognosis after cord blood transplantation. *Leuk Res.* 2013;37(11):1522–6. Epub 2013/10/08.

49. Leung W, Handgretinger R, Iyengar R, Turner V, Holladay MS, Hale GA. Inhibitory KIR-HLA receptor-ligand mismatch in autologous haematopoietic stem cell transplantation for solid tumour and lymphoma. *Br J Cancer.* 2007;97(4):539–42. Epub 2007/08/02.

50. Venstrom JM, Zheng J, Noor N, Danis KE, Yeh AW, Cheung IY, *et al.* KIR and HLA genotypes are associated with disease progression and survival following autologous hematopoietic stem cell transplantation for high-risk neuroblastoma. *Clin Cancer Res.* 2009;15(23):7330–4. Epub 2009/11/26.

Chapter

64

Immune Therapy with Cytotoxic T-Lymphocytes for Treatment of Infections

Michael D. Keller, Conrad Russell Y. Cruz, and Catherine M. Bollard

Introduction

In the period following hematopoietic cell transplantation (HCT), infections are a leading cause of morbidity and mortality[1–4]. Advances in prophylactic therapy have reduced the early burden of viral and fungal infections, therapeutic options for breakthrough infections are complicated by toxicities, and for many viral infections, there are no effective treatments[5–9]. It has been well established that T-cell reconstitution is the key factor in controlling viral infection following HCT, and factors that influence the speed of T-cell recovery also impact the risk of viral infection in this period (see Chapter 27) [2,3]. The use of donor lymphocyte infusions from the stem cell donor was discovered to be an effective salvage therapy for viral infections in HCT recipients prior to T-cell recovery, but risk of potentially severe graft-*versus*-host disease (G*v*HD) remains[10]. From this early work, the field of cytotoxic T-lymphocyte (CTL) immunotherapy has emerged as a safer method of expediting T-cell reconstitution against specific targets. The growth of CTL therapy has been dependent on several advances in immunobiology, including: (i) the knowledge of conserved T-cell epitopes for various pathogens[11–13], (ii) improvements in *ex-vivo* culture of T-cells and antigen-presenting cells[14–16], and (iii) rapid tests to evaluate the effector function and MHC-restriction of T-cells[17,18].

The trials utilizing antiviral CTLs represent the majority of studies to date; preclinical studies and early clinical trials of antifungal CTLs have also shown promise. Adoptive immunotherapy targeting tumor targets is also a burgeoning field, and has recently been reviewed[19]. Here, we will summarize the methodologies and results of trials with antipathogen CTL therapy, and will review recent preclinical advances that are instrumental in providing the framework for future CTL therapy-related clinical studies.

Methodologies of CTL Production

Ideally, CTL production requires the selection of pathogen-specific T-cells and the exclusion of alloreactive T-cells. This has been accomplished previously via three pathways: (1) direct selection of donor cells, (2) stimulation and *ex-vivo* culture of donor T-cells from peripheral blood mononuclear cells (PBMCs), or (3) genetic modification of T-cells to confer specific recognition of pathogen or pathogen-infected cells (Figure 64.1).

Direct selection relies on cell sorting of donor PBMCs, usually after a short stimulation with the antigen of interest [20]. This can be achieved via multimer selection (selecting for T-cells with a T-cell receptor (TCR) of known antigen specificity), or by column selection of interferon-γ-producing T-cells following a brief stimulation with an antigen of interest. Selection strategies have the advantages of very rapid manufacturing time and using existing GMP (good manufacturing practice)-compliant sorting technologies. However, this technique requires leukapheresis of donors in order to collect sufficient cells for clinical use. Additionally, it requires detectable pathogen-specific T-cells in the periphery, and thus would not be a viable option for manufacturing of CTLs from pathogen-naïve donors nor for pathogens that induce a poor memory response. Multimer selection has the disadvantage of selecting only CD8+ T-cells of a limited specificity and MHC-restriction, which could allow pathogen evasion and possibly impair CTL persistence[21]. Previous studies have suggested that residual binding of multimers may impact T-cell function *in-vitro*[22], though the recent development of reversible streptamer technology for selection bypasses this potential risk[23]. IFN-γ selection allows inclusion of polyclonal antigen-specific CD4+ and CD8+ T-cells, and allows selection of a wider range of antigen-specific cells in the final collected product.

Alternately, stimulation and *ex-vivo* culture permits expansion of single or multiple pathogen-specific CTLs. Culture has several advantages over cell selection, including generation of polyclonal CTLs, and expansion of cells to clinically useful volumes from a small volume of blood[24]. These advantages come at the expense of the culture and processing time required for CTL stimulation and expansion, which can vary from 10 days to >4 weeks, depending on the donor source. Loss of the ability of cells to self-renew and impaired persistence *in-vivo* has been a longstanding concern with the use of prolonged *ex-vivo* culture and expansion methods[25]. However, it should be noted that clinical trials utilizing virus-specific T-cells post-HCT have demonstrated prolonged persistence in spite of *ex-vivo* culture of the adoptively transferred T-cells[26]. Additionally, studies have demonstrated that

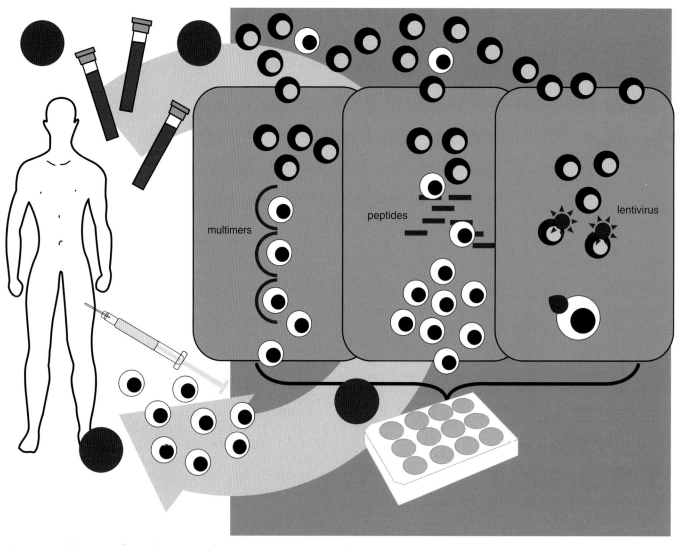

Figure 64.1. Schematic of antipathogen-specific CTL immunotherapy. Blood from various donors (autologous, allogeneic, umbilical cord blood) (1) is drawn, and peripheral blood mononuclear cells (2) are then subjected to different methods of generating T-cells. Cell *selection* utilizes either multimers displaying a pathogen-derived peptide in the setting of a type I HLA molecule, or column selection utilizing *ex-vivo* stimulation of T-cells with antigens followed by selection of IFN-γ· or CD154 expressing T-cells via antibody-coated immunomagnetic beads. *Ex-vivo* cell *expansion* culture utilizes stimulation of T-cells by antigen-displaying APCs, which can be produced via antigenic peptide pools, viral transduction, or nucleofection. A rapid protocol can produce CTL in 10–12 days from virus-seropositive donors after a single stimulation, whereas production of CTL derived from cord blood require three stimulations over a minimum of 28 days. Finally, *genetic modification* involves the transfer of high-affinity pathogen-specific T-cell receptors or chimeric antigen receptors to redirect specificity of T-cells. These cells are then expanded in culture (3) to sufficient numbers for subsequent clinical infusion (4).

ex-vivo culturing with pathogen-specific stimuli reduces alloreactivity *in-vitro*[13], likely due to cell death or outgrowth by pathogen-specific T-cells. Moreover, any residual alloreactivity detected in *ex-vivo* expanded virus-specific T-cell lines has been shown to be clinically insignificant[27]. Early trials of virus-specific CTL therapy depended on the use of virus-infected antigen-presenting cells, such as cytomegalovirus (CMV) lysates, CMV-infected fibroblasts, or EBV-lymphoblastoid cells lines as a stimulant for expansion of donor-derived memory T-cells[28–30]. Subsequent knowledge of dominant and highly conserved antigens such as CMV-pp65 and adenovirus hexon and penton have permitted the replacement of live viral stimulation with either 15-mer peptide pools spanning viral proteins or DNA plasmid-transduced antigen-presenting cells [31,32]. Newer methods to rapidly grow and manipulate antigen-presenting cells have also enabled the use of a wider population of donors and targeting of a greater number of pathogens in a single CTL culture[14,33]. Optimization of cytokine cocktails for CTL culture has also allowed improved yields and targeted cellular phenotypes. In the recent rapid CTL protocol, IL-4 and IL-7 have been shown to produce CD4+ T-cells with a predominantly Th1 phenotype, whereas IL-2 and IL-15 seem to favor NK proliferation at the expense of T-cells[32]. Finally, studies have shown that central memory T-cells, characterized by expression of CD62L and CD45RA have superior persistence *in-vivo* following adoptive transfer, and may be the ideal cell population for adoptive immunotherapy[34,35]. Consequently, studies using both selection and culture methods have demonstrated the presence of central memory T-cells in the resulting CTL products[23,32].

Modification of T-cells to redirect specificity involves the use of vectors to introduce the transgene – either a high-affinity T-cell receptor, or a chimeric antigen receptor. TCR gene transfer uses a high-affinity TCR clone (usually obtained from patients who demonstrate high specificity towards a particular antigen) that can provide immune protection against pathogens expressing the corresponding antigen. T-cell antigen specificity derived from a heterodimeric complex of two immunoglobulin-like proteins (α and β) that form part of the TCR complex[36], coupled with advances in viral-mediated gene transfer technology, allowed for the genetic modification of T-cells. This resulted in the cloning and subsequent transfer of the α and β genes of the TCR from such patients into recipient T-cells, bestowing upon them the high-affinity specificity characteristic of the original donor clone. The process described is the basis for the production of tumor-specific T-cells via TCR gene transfer[37]. Chimeric antigen receptors (CARs), on the other hand, are composed of an extracellular region that mediates antigen recognition (this region consists of a single-chain variable fragment of a monoclonal antibody recognizing a particular antigen) and an intracellular region that mediates signaling upon ligand binding (this region consists of the TCR zeta chain alone for first-generation CARs, the zeta chain and the signaling domain of the CD28 costimulatory molecule for second-generation CARs, and an additional signaling domain from another costimulatory molecule, e.g., 41BB, for third-generation CARs) [38]. The transfer of high-affinity TCRs to confer specificity against pathogens has been used to recognize CMV-infected cells[39], HPV-infected cells[40], hepatitis B-infected cells[41], hepatitis C-infected cells[42], tuberculosis-infected cells[43], SARS-infected cells[44], chlamydia-infected cells[45], and HIV-infected cells[46]. Currently, two major approaches have used chimeric antigen technology for generating pathogen-specific T-cells: for recognition of CD4 in HIV-infected cells [47–50] and for recognition of β-glucans in fungi[51]. These are discussed in the relevant sections below.

Clinical and Preclinical Studies of Antiviral CTLs

Cytomegalovirus

CMV was the first virus targeted in early CTL therapy trials, and remains a primary focus in many subsequent studies (Table 64.1). Cobbold *et al.* published the first clinical report in which CD8$^+$ CMV-specific CTLs were isolated via tetramer selection[52]. Complete or partial clinical responses were achieved in nine patients who received infusions,

though there were limited data on long-term persistence of infused CTLs.

CTL production utilizing *ex-vivo* cell culture has been the most common methodology to date, and accounts for the majority of patients treated in clinical trials of antipathogen adoptive immunotherapy (Table 64.1) over the past decade. Walter *et al.* and colleagues were among the first to show that stimulation of donor PBMC by CMV-extracts resulted in expansion of CMV-specific CTLs, which lost alloreactivity after several weeks of *ex-vivo* culture but retained antiviral activity[30]. With subsequent advances in cell culture methods, most recent CTL therapy trials have included CMV in multiviral CTL products, which are described below.

Several studies have utilized IFN-γ column selection (Gamma capture, Miltenyi) to produce CMV-CTLs. In a trial by Feuchtinger *et al.*, partial to complete responses were seen in 15 of 18 patients who were given a single dose of CMV-CTLs isolated by this method[53]. Peggs *et al.* also used IFN-γ selection to produce CMV-CTL, using either recombinant pp65 or an overlapping peptide pool of 15-mers covering the pp65 protein as stimulants[54]. They were successful in protecting seven patients who were prophylactically treated, while *in-vivo* expansion of CMV-CTLs was detected in 11 patients infused who had detectable CMV[54]. Schmitt *et al.* produced CMV-CTLs from HCT donors utilizing reversible streptamers with MHC-restricted pp65 peptides[23]. These products were used to successfully treat two patients who developed CMV reactivation during treatment of GvHD after HCT.

EBV

EBV-CTLs have been used for prevention and treatment of post-transplantation lymphoproliferative disease (PTLD) (see Chapter 22) as well as EBV+ lymphoma in several trials, most of which utilized cell culture for CTL manufacturing. Rooney *et al.* successfully used irradiated EBV-lymphoblastoid cells (EBV-LCL) to generate EBV-specific CTLs, which were effective as prophylaxis or treatment for EBV PTLD in 114 patients [26,29]. Of note, the first 26 patients received gene-marked CTLs, and follow-up studies showed persistence of the gene-marked cells for as long as 105 months following infusion (Table 64.1).

Several studies have used selection technology to produce EBV-CTLs. Uhlin *et al.* used HLA-A2-specific pentamers to produce EBV-CTLs from the haploidentical mother of a patient who underwent cord blood transplantation and subsequently developed EBV PTLD[55]. A complete clinical response was obtained following two doses of CTLs. Moosmann *et al.* treated six patients with EBV-induced PTLD with EBV-CTLs developed by IFN-γ selection, and achieved complete responses in the three patients with early disease, but no response in three patients with advanced, multiorgan disease [56]. Most recent targeting of EBV has been through use of either multiviral CTL products or third-party derived EBV-CTLs, both of which are described below.

Table 64.1 Previous clinical trials of virus-specific T-cell therapy

Study	Pathogen specificity	Setting	T-cell donor	Methodology	Patient accrual	Number of centers
Cobbold et al. 2005[111]	CMV	HCT	HCT donor or third party	Tetramer selection	9	1
Feuchtinger et al. 2010[53]	CMV	HCT	HCT donor or third party	IFN-γ column selection	18	1
Peggs et al. 2011[112]	CMV	HCT	HCT donor	IFN-γ column selection	18	1
Haque et al. 1998[85]	EBV	SOT	Autologous	EBV-LCL stimulation	3	1
Haque et al. 2001[75]	EBV	SOT	Third party	Irradiated EBV-LCL	1	1
Haque et al. 2002[76]	EBV	SOT	Third party	Irradiated EBV-LCL	8	1
Haque et al. 2007[77]	EBV	SOT	Third party	Irradiated EBV-LCL	33	1
Uhlin et al. 2010[113]	EBV	HCT	Related haploidentical donor	Multimer selection	1	1
Moosman et al. 2010[56]	EBV	HCT	HCT donor	IFN-γ column selection	6	1
Barker et al. 2010[78]	EBV	HCT	Third-party donor	EBV-LCL stimulation	2	1
Heslop et al. 2010[26]	EBV	HCT	HCT donor	Irradiated EBV-LCL stimulation	114	3
Basso et al. 2013[84]	EBV	HCT	Autologous	EBV-LCL stimulation	1	1
Qasim et al. 2011[114]	Adv	HCT	Third party	IFN-γ column selection	1	1
Feuchtinger et al. 2006[115]	Adv	HCT	HCT donor	IFN-γ column selection	9	1
Lieberman et al. 1997[66]	HIV	N/A	Autologous	CD8+ HIV-specific ex-vivo expanded	6	1
Mitsuyasu et al. 2000[68]	HIV	N/A	Autologous	CD4-ζ CAR transduction	24	1
Deeks et al. 2002[67]	HIV	N/A	Autologous	CD4-ζ CAR transduction	40	5
Tebas et al. 2013[69]	HIV	N/A	Autologous CD4-T-cells	Transduction with antisense gene to HIV env	17	1
Tebas et al. 2014[70]	HIV	N/A	Autologous CD4-enriched	CCR5 gene editing via ZFN	12	1
Balduzzi et al. 2011[116]	JCV	HCT	HCT donor	Pepmix-pulsed PBMC	1	1
Uhlin et al. 2012[117]	CMV/EBV/Adv	HCT	HCT donor or third-party	Pentamer selection	8	1
Perruccio et al. 2005[100]	CMV or Aspergillus	HCT	HCT donor	Stimulation of PBMC with CMV antigen or inactivated conidia	10	1
Leen et al. 2006[118]	CMV/EBV/Adv	HCT	HCT donor	Ad5f35pp65 transduced LCL	26	3
Mickelwaite et al. 2008[59]	CMV/Adv	HCT	HCT donor	Ad5f35pp65 transduced DC	12	1
Leen et al. 2009[58]	EBV/Adv	HCT	HCT donor	Ad5f35null transduced LCL	13	3
Leen et al. 2013[79]	CMV/EBV/Adv	HCT	Third-party donor	Ad5f35pp65 transduced LCL	47	8
Gerdemann et al. 2013[119]	CMV/EBV/Adv	HCT	HCT donor	Nucleofection of DCs	12	3
Blyth et al. 2013[62]	CMV or CMV/Adv	HCT	HCT donor	NLV-peptide pulsing or Ad5f35pp65 transduction of DCs	50	2

Table 64.1 (cont.)

Study	Pathogen specificity	Setting	T-cell donor	Methodology	Patient accrual	Number of centers
Papadopoulou et al. 2014 [64]	Adv, EBV, CMV, BKV, HHV6	HCT	HCT donor	Rapidly generated EBV, adenovirus, CMV, BK virus, HHV6-specific T-cells following stimulation with peptide mixes	11	1

CMV: cytomegalovirus; HCT: hematopoietic stem cell transplantation; EBV: Epstein–Barr virus; SOT: solid organ transplantation; EBV-LCL: Epstein–Barr virus–lymphoblastoid cell line; Adv: adenovirus; HIV: human immunodeficiency virus; JCV: JC virus; ZFN: Zinc-finger nuclease; CAR: chimeric antigen receptor; PBMC: peripheral blood mononuclear cells; DC: dendritic cells; BKV: BK virus; HHV6: human herpesvirus-6.

Adenovirus

Many studies have targeted adenovirus (Adv) through CTL production, predominantly in multiviral CTL products (below)[15,57–59]. A small number of clinical studies have exclusively targeted Adv by selection technology. Feuchtinger et al. successfully produced Adv-CTLs by IFN-γ selection for treatment of nine patients with drug-refractory Adv infections [60]. In-vivo CTL expansion was demonstrated in five of six patients tested, and four patients had clearance of disease.

Of note, in all studies utilizing cell selection, clinical benefit was seen in spite of very low cell doses ($<5 \times 10^4$ cells/kg in most studies)[60,61].

Multiviral CTL Trials

Some recent antiviral CTL therapy trials have sought to target multiple viruses, with CMV, EBV, and Adv being the main targets as the three leading causes of viral-associated mortality in the post-HCT period (Table 64.1) (see Chapter 24). The development of the clinical grade Adv vector Ad5f35pp65, which contains immunodominant CMV antigen pp65, permitted transduction of either donor-derived dendritic cells or EBV-LCL for use as antigen-presenting cells (APCs) for CTL culture. Leen et al. used this strategy to produce triviral (CMV, EBV, Adv-specific) CTLs, which were utilized in a dose-escalation trial to treat 26 patients[15]. No adverse effects were seen at doses ranging from 5×10^6 to 1×10^8 cells/m^2, and all patients were effectively protected against CMV, EBV, and Adv diseases. However, though EBV and CMV-specific CTLs showed persistence by IFN-γ ELISpot, Adv-specific CTLs were not detectable except in the setting of infection. A follow-up trial utilized Ad5f35-transduced EBV-LCL to produce EBV and Adv-specific CTLs, which were infused into 13 patients as prophylaxis or treatment of EBV and Adv following HCT [58]. Though the products provided effective protection against EBV and Adv in-vivo, Adv-specific CTLs were again not detectable except in the setting of Adv infection, suggesting that even at levels below the limits of detection by IFN-γ ELISpot, the Adv-specific CTLs provided protection and were able to undergo expansion in the setting of viral infection. Ad5f35pp65-transduced dendritic cells were similarly used by Micklethwaite et al. to produce CMV and Adv-specific CTLs,

which were clinically effective in 12 patients who received infusions following HCT[59]. Only two subsequent episodes of CMV reactivation occurred in the setting of administration of prednisone at levels as low as 0.5 mg/kg/day. Blyth et al. similarly treated 50 patients following HCT with triviral (CMV, EBV, Adv-specific) CTLs which were derived by a mix of methods: 10 were produced by pulsing donor DCs with the HLA-A2 restricted CMV peptide NLVPMVATV, and 40 were produced using Ad5f35pp65-transduced donor DCs[62]. Only 5 of the 50 patients developed CMV reactivations following CTL infusions, and 1 of these 5 required antiviral pharmacotherapy after being treated with steroids for acute GvHD.

Recent protocol advances have validated the use of 15-mer peptide pools encompassing immunodominant viral antigens in place of viral transduction of APC, thus removing the potential safety and regulatory barriers associated with use of viral vector[31]. The use of gas-permeable rapid-expansion (G-Rex) bioreactors has further simplified CTL culture[63]. Gerdemann et al. combined these two advances to develop a rapid protocol that yields CTLs at clinical volumes in 10–12 days, and provided effective antiviral protection in 10 patients who were infused following HCT[32]. A more recent study further modified this rapid protocol to produce 5-virus-specific CTLs targeting EBV, CMV, Adv, HHV6, and BK virus infections in a single T-cell product for patients following allogeneic HCT[64]. Papadopolou et al. produced 48 CTL lines from HCT donors, and found that 14 of the lines recognized all 5 of the component viral targets, while 35 (73%) recognized 3 or more viruses by IFN-γ ELISpot assay. Of note, 22 of the HCT donors were CMV seronegative, and lines produced from these donors predictably lacked CMV specificity. These lines were used to treat 11 patients following HCT. Three patients were treated prophylactically and remained free of viral infections. The remaining eight were treated for 18 viral reactivations, and all of them experienced partial or complete responses against CMV, EBV, Adv, and HHV6. Only one patient failed to clear BK virus, and study of the associated CTL line showed that the donor did not display BK reactivity.

Naik et al. recently reviewed the use of CTL therapy in patients with primary immunodeficiency disorders on previous and current trials[128]. Of 36 patients reviewed, CTL therapy resulted in complete or partial antiviral responses in

81% of patients. Notably, one patient with CTP synthase 1 deficiency who developed EBV-lymphoproliferative disease prior to transplantation was successfully treated with partially HLA-matched CTL from a third-party donor.

CTL Therapy for HIV Infection

The use of CTL therapy for treatment of HIV has drawn interest but only limited success to date, as has been recently reviewed [65]. Prior attempts to expand and reinfuse autologous HIV-specific CTLs met with only transient improvement in viral count[66]. A larger number of trials have focused on the use of genetically modified CTL to target HIV, either via transduction of a modified T-cell receptor or CARs. These trials have established safety of these approaches, but only limited antiviral efficacy[67,68]. The outgrowth of escape mutants with alterations to the target epitope remains a problem when using a single target. A more successful approach has been genetic modification of autologous T-cells to produce HIV resistance. One novel methodology was to introduce an antisense gene complementary to HIV *env* to T-cells via lentiviral transduction, which was administered to 17 patients without adverse events[69]. Tebas *et al.* demonstrated that though these CTLs persisted for only a mean of 5 weeks, they homed to gut associated lymphoid tissue, and exerted genetic pressure on HIV *env*. In two of eight patients who underwent antiviral treatment interruption, viral load remained undetectable for 4 and 14 weeks, suggesting that the modified CTLs have transient antiviral activity. In another study, CCR5-delta32 mutations were introduced to CD4-enriched T-cells through the use of a zinc finger nuclease[70]. These autologous CCR5-edited T-cells were subsequently infused to 12 patients, and remained detectable for up to 42 months. In six patients who underwent antiviral treatment interruption, decline in CD4+ T-cells was slower in modified than in nonmodified T-cells. That viremia did occur shortly after treatment interruption is not surprising as CXCR4-trophic HIV strains are well described. Most recently, dual gene editing of CXCR4 and CCR5 via zinc finger nucleases was successful in a T-cell line, and preclinical studies showed that these cells were highly resistant to HIV infection[71]. Whether this approach could prevent primary infection or augment existing infection in a meaningful way is yet to be seen.

CTL Therapy for Other Viruses

A small number of other viruses have been targeted via adoptive immunotherapy. The JCV is a ubiquitous polyoma virus which can cause progressive multifocal leukoencephalopathy (PML), a devastating neurologic disease, in patients who are profoundly immunocompromised, including recipients of HCT or solid organ transplants and patients with advanced HIV or primary immunodeficiency disorders. Balduzzi *et al.* described the use of donor-derived JCV-specific CTLs in a 14-year-old patient who developed PML in the setting of prolonged steroid treatment for GvHD following HCT[72]. These CTLs were manufactured using 15-mer peptide pools

encompassing the JC viral antigens VP1 and LT, and were cultured for 26 days. The patient received two doses of JCV-specific CTLs, and had a remarkable and sustained improvement, including clearance of JCV-DNA from the CSF and substantial improvements in his neurologic status.

The human papillomavirus (HPV) is not an uncommon late complication of HCT, particularly in patients treated for primary immunodeficiency disorders (see Chapter 53). HPV has also been evaluated in preclinical studies as a potential target for CTL therapy. Ramos *et al.* have described the use of peptide pools spanning the HPV E6 and E7 proteins to generate HPV-specific CTLs from patients with oropharyngeal or cervical cancer, many of which arise due to HPV16 infection [73]. The resulting CTLs showed specific activity against HPV E6 and E7, and also showed antitumor activity against the HPV16 cervical cancer cell line CaSki.

Human Parainfluenza Virus is also a frequent cause of respiratory tract infection in immunocompromised patients. A recent article suggested that Human Parainfluenza 3 (HPIV3) accounts for 40% of viral pneumonia in patients who have undergone hematopoietic stem cell transplantation[129], with mortality rates in adults varying from 22–76%[130]. A recent preclinical study suggested that HPIV3-specific CTLs can be produced by rapid *ex vivo* expansion using peptide pools spanning 4 of the 6 viral proteins[131]. These HPIV3-specific CTLs were predominantly CD4$^+$ T-cells, and were shown to be polyfunctional in vitro based on IFNg and TNFα production on viral peptide restimulation.

Adverse Events in Antigen-Specific CTL Therapy

Adverse events following administration of *ex-vivo* cultured CTL products in 381 infusions for 180 patients on 18 protocols were reviewed by the groups at Baylor College of Medicine [74]. Twenty-four mild adverse events were reported within 6 hours of infusion, with nausea and vomiting being most common, and 22 nonserious adverse events (fever, chills, nausea) occurred within 24 hours. No significant GvHD was attributable to CTL infusion. The only significant complications of CTL therapy have been rare reports of systemic inflammatory responses following EBV-CTL therapy in patients with bulky EBV+ lymphomas. Blyth *et al.* reported that seven cases of acute GvHD occurred following CTL infusion, though some were attributable to corticosteroid weaning prior to CTL infusion, and additionally the authors noted that the degree of HLA mismatch was greater in patients who received CTL therapy *versus* controls[62].

Novel Strategies for CTL Therapy
Third-Party CTL Use

Until recently, the selection or culture of antipathogen CTLs was dependent on the presence of pathogen-specific memory T-cells in donor blood. These protocols failed to help recipients of pathogen-naïve hematopoietic cell products, a population that has been well described to be at increased risk of viral infection following HCT.

One answer to this problem is the use of "off-the-shelf" CTLs derived from third-party donors. This approach has been successfully used in several studies. Haque *et al.* were the first to validate this strategy, and treated 8 patients in a phase 1 trial of partially matched EBV-CTLs for PTLD in the setting of solid organ transplantation[75,76], and subsequently 33 patients in a phase 2 trial using a similar approach[77]. The latter trial demonstrated a response rate of 64% at 5 weeks and 52% at 6 months, with outcomes correlating to the degree of HLA match between the CTL donor and recipient. This strategy has similarly been employed after HCT. Barker *et al.* successfully treated two patients with refractory EBV PTLD following cord blood transplantation (CBT) with third-party EBV-specific CTLs[78]. Leen *et al.* utilized a bank of 32 CTL lines with characterized activity against EBV, CMV, and Adv to identify matched lines for 50 patients with refractory viral infections. These infusions resulted in partial or complete antiviral responses in 74%, 78%, and 67% of those with CMV, Adv, and EBV, respectively[79]. This represents a dramatic improvement from the standard therapy response rate in eight patients for whom a matched line could not be found, who had a response rate of 13% and mortality rate of 75%. In spite of only partial HLA-matching (1–4 loci), only two patients developed grade I GvHD. The lower rate of response against EBV relative to CMV and Adv may be reflective of a greater breadth of immunodominant epitopes that differ by MHC types, which complicates the task of selecting the ideal third-party line with both antiviral activity and proper MHC-restriction.

Third-party CTL treatment has also been successful using selection methodology. Uhlin *et al.* used pentamer selection to produce antiviral CTL specific for CMV, EBV, or Adv from related third-party donors for six patients with refractory viral infections (four with CMV, and one each with EBV and Adv) [57]. Five of six patients had partial or complete responses. Notably, an infant with severe combined immunodeficiency was treated *prior* to CBT with CMV-CTL derived from her mother, with a 10-fold reduction in her CMV DNA level. Wg and Qasim *et al.* used IFN-γ selection to manufacture Adv-CTL from related third-party donors to treat two patients who underwent HCT and subsequently developed Adv viremia[80]. Though treatment successfully cleared the Adv infection in one patient, she developed grade III skin and liver GvHD[61]. Curiously, cytogenetic studies of liver tissue showed infiltration with T-cells from the original HCT donor but not from the CTL donor. The authors postulated that this was due to a "bystander" effect of CTLs on the HCT donor cells; however, such an effect has not been observed in larger trials utilizing third-party CTL therapy.

TCR Gene Transfer

Several studies have explored the possibility of transducing CTLs with a TCR with known viral specificity[81–83]. This offers a novel strategy to develop CTLs from pathogen-naïve donors, but imposes the additional regulatory requirements of transgenic technology. Additionally, the use of a single anti-viral TCR may risk antigenic escape by the pathogen. Nonetheless, a current trial of transgenic CTLs utilizing a retroviral vector with a CMV-specific TCR is ongoing in the United Kingdom (E. Morris *et al.*, MRC# G0701703).

CTL Manufacture from Pathogen-Naïve Donors

An important landmark in the field of adoptive immunotherapy has been the successful development of virus-specific CTLs from virus-naïve donors. Hanley *et al.* first demonstrated that CTLs could be produced from a 20% fraction from cord blood using donor-derived dendritic cells (DCs) and EBV-lymphoblastoid cell line (LCL) as APCs, and Ad5f35pp65 transduction as a source of CMV and Adv antigens[14]. The resulting cell lines had specific antiviral activity against CMV, EBV, and Adv in IFN-γ ELISpot analysis as well as Cr[51] cytotoxicity assays with no evidence of alloreactivity. Curiously, epitope mapping showed that the immunodominant epitopes recognized by cord blood-derived CTLs differed from CTLs manufactured from CMV and EBV seropositive adult donors, with the HLA-A2-restricted epitope NLVPMVATV notably absent in the cord blood derived lines. Despite this finding, CTLs manufactured from cord blood have been used successfully in 12 CBT recipients to date in the ongoing ACT-CAT trial (Safety, Toxicity, and MTD of One Intravenous IV Injection of Donor CTLs Specific for CMV and Adenovirus # NCT00880789).

Most recently, Hanley *et al.* have also successfully manufactured multiviral CTLs from CMV-naïve adult donors[33]. To do so, CMV-CTLs were produced from CD45RA+ naïve T-cells isolated via column selection, and stimulated by donor DCs pulsed with CMV 15-mer peptide pools. Preclinical data suggest that they have similar antiviral activity, and the current MUSTAT trial (Multivirus-Specific Cytotoxic T-Lymphocytes for the Prophylaxis and Treatment of EBV, CMV, and Adenovirus Infections Post-Allogeneic Stem Cell Transplant # NCT01945814) will seek to compare the clinical efficacy of CTLs derived from CMV-seropositive *versus* CMV-naïve donors.

Autologous CTL Production for Recipients of Solid Organ Transplant

In recipients of solid organ transplants, EBV PTLD is a significant long-term risk, and though Rituxan is effective in some cases, treatment often requires reduction of immunosuppression, which can potentially lead to graft rejection. The successful use of autologous EBV-CTLs has been described in several studies [84]. Haque *et al.* prophylactically treated three EBV-positive organ recipients with several infusions of autologous EBV-CTLs, which were successful in reducing EBV viral load without adverse reactions in spite of ongoing treatment with calcineurin inhibitors[85]. Basso *et al.* treated a heart transplant patient who had developed Hodgkin lymphoma-type PTLD 8 years after transplantation with autologous EBV-CTLs as an adjunctive treatment with chemotherapy[84]. Remission was obtained without alteration in the patient's immunosuppressive regimen (cyclosporine and everolimus), similar to that seen by Haque *et al.*[85]. This supports previous observations that calcineurin inhibitors impact proliferation, but do not notably affect cytotoxic function of T-cells[86].

Antifungal CTLs

Fungal infections are a well-described risk after allogeneic HCT (see Chapter 25). But these opportunistic infections are virtually unknown outside the immunocompromised setting. *Candida*, present as a commensal in the gastrointestinal tract, can cause mucocutaneous colonization of the skin and mouth, or severe life-threatening systemic infections. *Aspergillus*, a ubiquitous environmental mold, frequently causes invasive pulmonary infection, but has been documented to cause more widespread infection and neurologic disease[87]. Patients with congenital or acquired defects in neutrophils (including cancer patients with neutropenia as a result of therapy), and those receiving immunosuppressive therapy post-lung transplant and allogeneic HCT have the highest risks for opportunistic mycoses[88].

The importance of Th17 immunity in controlling *Candida* infections has been well demonstrated by forms of primary immunodeficiency such as Hyper-IgE syndrome and chronic mucocutaneous candidiasis as well as HIV infection[89,90]. The importance of T-cell immunity in defense against invasive aspergillosis and mucormycosis is less clear, while their ties to innate defense (most notably neutrophil function) are well established. Further a recent study evaluated patients with chronic granulomatous disease who have a high prevalence of IA and demonstrated that these patients have abundant *Aspergillus*-specific T-cells with increased IFN-γ production compared to healthy controls[91]. Despite these uncertainties, fungal infections may be a valid target for treatment via adoptive immunotherapy after HCT.

The adaptive immune response against invasive aspergillosis is believed to center on the CD4+ T-cell. Several preclinical studies have been successful in developing CTLs with activity against *Candida*, *Aspergillus*, and *Rhizopus* species (Table 64.2). Beck *et al.* successfully produced *Aspergillus*-specific CTLs by stimulation of PBMCs with antigens from *Aspergillus* extracts, followed by IFN-γ selection and culture[92]. The resulting population was predominantly CD4+ memory (CD45RO+) cells, but demonstrated IFN–γ production in response to several species of *Aspergillus* as well as *Penicillium*. The authors also showed that these T-cells enhanced hyphal damage by neutrophils and APCs *in-vitro*. Tramsen *et al.* similarly used IFN-γ selection following stimulation with cellular extracts from *Candida albicans*, *Aspergillus fumigatus*, and *Rhizopus oryzae* to produce multifungal-specific CTL lines, which were also almost exclusively CD4+ CD45RO+ HLA-DR+[93]. These lines displayed pathogen-specific activation markers (IFN-γ, CD154, TNF-α) and also enhanced oxidative activity of

neutrophils when co-incubated with antigen and APCs and tested via the 123-dihydrorhodamine assay. Khanna *et al.* described a novel selection method based on up-regulation of CD154 to produce multi-pathogen-specific T-cells against CMV, EBV, Adv, *Candida*, and *Aspergillus*[94]. Donor PBMCs were incubated with peptide libraries from CMV-pp65, EBV-LMP2, Adv-Hexon, *Candida* MP65, and a 15mer peptide from *Aspergillus* CRF1. Following 14 days of culture, the investigators showed pathogen-specific IFN-γ production, proliferation, and cytotoxicity *in-vitro*. Although these results are intriguing, there are limited data regarding the relative importance of MP65 and CRF1 in antifungal immunity[95,96]. Schmidt *et al.* expanded memory/effector Th1 cells following stimulation with Rhizopus extracts for T-cell therapy of mucormycosis. These cells demonstrated specificity not just against the original *R. oryzae* extract, but to other mucorales species as well[97]. Tramsen *et al.* generated *Candida*-specific T-cells following stimulation with cellular extracts of *Candida albicans*. These T-cells mediated hyphal damage *in-vitro*, and increased activity of neutrophils against hyphae[98]. Finally, a unique strategy was proposed by Kumaresan *et al.*, when they transduced T-cells with the β-glucan receptor dectin[51]. The carbohydrate β-glucan is found in most fungi[99], and so the investigators used its natural ligand, dectin-1, as a recognition receptor coupled to a chimeric CD28 and CD3-zeta transgene, to initiate signaling from T-cells upon ligation of the carbohydrates in fungi. The group showed the ability of T-cells (through an as yet unknown mechanism) to mediate damage to hyphae *in-vitro* and *in-vivo* following recognition of the cell wall[51].

Perruccio *et al.* developed CTLs via stimulation of donor PBMCs with inactivated conidia from *Aspergillus fumigatus*, followed by several weeks of culture, resulting in clonal CD4+ CTLs with anti-*Aspergillus* activity by IFN-γ ELISpot[100]. These donor T-cell clones specific for *Aspergillus* antigens were then infused in patients following HLA-haplotype mismatch transplant. Twenty-three patients developed invasive aspergillosis after transplant: 10 received anti-*Aspergillus* T-cells, while 13 did not. Of the 10 patients treated with T-cell therapy, nine cleared the infection. In contrast, of the 13 untreated patients, only seven cleared the infection. *Aspergillus*-specific T-cells were detected in high frequencies in the patients who received T-cell immunotherapy, while they were barely detectable in control subjects[100].

Again, these studies are intriguing but several key issues remain. First, a better understanding of the immunodominant T-cell targets for various fungal species is needed. Second, standardized, GMP-compliant fungal antigen sources are necessary to allow consistency and valid comparisons between future clinical trials.

Controversies Surrounding Cytotoxic T-Lymphocytes for Treatment of Infections

Although significant progress has been made, many important questions remain regarding ideal CTL production

Table 64.2 Preclinical studies of T-cell therapy against nonviral infections

Study	Pathogen specificity	Donor	Methodology
Beck et al. 2006[92]	Aspergillus	Healthy donors	IFN-γ selection after stimulation of PBMCs with Aspergillus extracts
Khanna et al. 2011[94]	Aspergillus, Candida, Rhizopus	Healthy donors	CD154 selection after stimulation of PBMCs with fungal extracts
Tramsen et al. 2013[93]	Aspergillus, Candida, Rhizopus	Healthy donors	IFN-γ selection after stimulation of PBMCs with fungal extracts
Kumaresan et al. 2014	Aspergillus (potentially other pathogens)	Healthy donors	Transduction of CTL with chimeric antigen receptor directed against B-glucans
Tramsen et al. 2009[120]	Aspergillus	Healthy donors	Expansion of anti-Aspergillus T-cell using Aspergillus extracts
Gaundar et al. 2012[121]	Aspergillus, Candida, Penicillium	Healthy donors	Expansion of fungus-specific T-cells using a lysate from A. fumigatus
Tramsen et al. 2007[98]	Candida	Healthy donors	IFN-γ capture of T-cells following stimulation with C. albicans cellular extract
Stuehler et al. 2011[122]	Candida and Aspergillus	Murine cells	Crf1-stimulated T-cells
Jolink et al. 2013[123]	Aspergillus	Healthy donors	CD137 selection following stimulation with Crf1 and catalase 1
Feng et al. 2000[124]	Tuberculosis	Murine cells	Transgenic TCR-transduced cells
Stemberger et al. 2014[125]	Listeria	Murine cells	MHC-streptamer-enriched antigen-specific T-cells
Bhardra et al. 2013[126]	Toxoplasma	Murine cells	Acutely infected animals
Polley et al. 2006[127]	Leishmania	Murine cells	(Proof-of-principle) – targeting of OVA-expressing parasites
Roan and Starnbach 2006[45]	Chlamydia	Murine cells	Transgenic TRC-transduced cells

methods and the relative clinical efficacy of the various T-cell products.

Is There an Antigen Limit?

As manufacture of CTLs expands to include more pathogens in a single culture, the possibility of antigenic competition between the different pathogen-specific T-cells has caused many to question the limits of CTL monocultures. This concern has certainly been validated in attempts to produce multivirus-specific CTLs from donors who are CMV-naïve, in which the resulting culture is dominated by memory-derived EBV and Adv-specific T-cells. Though the relative proportions of individual virus-specific CTLs decrease as the number of antigens increase, this has not seemed to impact the efficacy of these products in clinical trials. Recent studies have challenged the upper antigen limit of CTL monoculture, as Gerdemann et al. successfully produced CTLs specific for seven viruses (CMV, EBV, Adv, BK, HHV6, RSV, and influenza) utilizing peptide pools for 15 antigens, and demonstrated specific activity against all targeted viruses via IFN-γ ELISpot[32]. As additional preclinical studies attempt to add further pathogens

to monoculture, it remains to be seen whether an increased number of targets will increase the potential for alloreactivity and/or compromise specific CTL function or persistence in-vivo.

Are T-Cells Compatible with Immunosuppressive Medications?

The need for immunosuppressive medications is common in recipients of allogeneic HCT, and unfortunately the use of these drugs also suppresses CTL products. Most existing protocols require recipients to be receiving less than 0.5 mg/kg/day prednisone and at least 30 days out from any anti-T-cell serotherapy in order to receive a CTL infusion. Calcineurin inhibitors such as cyclosporine A, tacrolimus, or sirolimus would similarly impact the clinical benefits of CTLs at therapeutic doses.

One answer to this problem is to produce genetically modified CTLs that have resistance to immunosuppressive medications. Several exciting studies have successfully demonstrated the viability of this concept. De Angelis et al. produced EBV-specific CTLs with resistance to tacrolimus by knockdown of FKBP12 via a retrovirally transduced specific siRNA

[101]. Transduction of CTLs did not impact antiviral activity, and the cells showed activity in a mouse EBV-lymphoma model in the presence of tacrolimus. Brewin *et al.* similarly produced EBV-specific CTLs with resistance to both cyclosporine A and tacrolimus by direct mutation of calcineurin [102]. The mutation had no impact on the phenotype or antiviral activity of the CTLs *in-vitro*, and mutated cells showed a growth advantage in the presence of calcineurin inhibitors.

Though similarly modified cells have not been used clinically to date, they have great potential in treating both HCT and solid organ transplant recipients. Future extension of these studies could potentially facilitate production of CTLs with resistance to monoclonal biologic agents such as alemtuzumab.

What Are the Optimal Culture Conditions?

With the increasing use of virus-specific CTLs to prevent and treat viral infections in immune compromised patients, the major challenge centers on the optimal production method for generating the most efficacious CTL product. There has always been concern that multiple rounds of stimulation with antigen and prolonged culture may lead to T-cell exhaustion, and groups have attempted to decrease production time using newer bioreactors[103]. Infusing the "correct" subpopulation of T-cells is also another point of contention. Recently, a new population of "stem cell memory T-cells" has been putatively identified – which possess characteristics ideal for use in adoptive immunotherapy. These cells are believed to persist longer *in-vivo*, maintaining a pool of memory cells that can readily repopulate the antigen-specific effector population when needed[104].

Can T-Cells Be Used against Nonviral Pathogens?

The use of T-cells against nonviral targets has met with limited success so far with only one published clinical trial demonstrating the utility of fungus-specific CTLs. No trials thus far have evaluated T-cell therapies for bacterial and parasitic infections. Despite many studies evaluating the T-cell response *in-*

vitro, there remains no consensus regarding the importance of T-cells in defense against aspergillosis. Athymic nude mice do not have increased susceptibilities to aspergillosis[105], and there are currently no data showing susceptibilities to *Aspergillus* in SCID patients. Aspergillosis is considered an uncommon opportunistic infection in AIDS, despite the obvious deficiency in CD4+ T-cells[106]. There is currently conflicting evidence of T-cell activity against *Aspergillus* in the literature where we note that while some groups find T-cell responses in healthy donors, others – like us – could not. Their functions in protective immunity are still in debate, with the earlier model of harmful Th17 responses[107] being questioned by recent findings showing protection arising from Th17[108]. The main evidence supporting a protective role for T-cells stems from epidemiologic studies showing HCT patients at risk for *Aspergillus* late after neutrophil engraftment (when presumably only T-cells are deficient and the neutrophils have already repopulated)[109]. However, an important caveat to this observation is the concern that there may be undocumented deficiencies within the neutrophil compartment of these patients and neutrophils may not be fully functional for months after HCT[110].

Conclusion

Several hundred patients have received antipathogen CTLs, which have been established as a safe and highly effective therapy following allogeneic HCT. Further studies to identify preserved viral T-cell epitopes, probe the antigen limits in CTL monoculture, and test the clinical efficacy of immunosuppressive-resistant CTLs will further broaden the usefulness of this treatment strategy. As rapid advances in protocols and methods of manufacture broaden the availability of this therapy, in time CTL therapy may become the standard of care following allogeneic HCT.

Acknowledgments

This work was supported by the NICHD K12-HD-001399 award to M.D.K. and CPRIT R01 RP100469 and NCI P01 CA148600-02 awards to C.M.B.

References

1. Boeckh M, Leisenring W, Riddell SR, *et al.* Late cytomegalovirus disease and mortality in recipients of allogeneic hematopoietic stem cell transplants: importance of viral load and T cell immunity. *Blood.* 2003;101(2):407–414.

2. Brunstein CG, Weisdorf DJ, DeFor T, *et al.* Marked increased risk of Epstein–Barr virus-related complications with the addition of antithymocyte globulin to a nonmyeloablative conditioning prior to unrelated umbilical cord blood transplantation. *Blood.* 2006;108(8):2874–2880.

3. Myers GD, Krance RA, Weiss H, *et al.* Adenovirus infection rates in pediatric recipients of alternate donor allogeneic bone marrow transplants receiving either antithymocyte globulin (ATG) or alemtuzumab (Campath). *Bone Marrow Transplant.* 2005;36(11):1001–1008.

4. Neofytos D, Horn D, Anaissie E, *et al.* Epidemiology and outcome of invasive fungal infection in adult hematopoietic stem cell transplant recipients: analysis of Multicenter Prospective Antifungal Therapy (PATH) Alliance registry. *Clin Infect Dis.* 2009;48(3):265–273.

5. Avery R. Update in management of Ganciclovir-resistant cytomegalovirus infection. *Curr Opin Infect Dis.* 2008;21:433–437.

6. Biron KK. Antiviral drugs for cytomegalovirus diseases. *Antiviral Res.* 2006;71(2–3):154–163.

7. Nichols WG, Corey L, Gooley T, *et al.* Rising pp65 antigenemia during preemptive anticytomegalovirus

therapy after allogeneic hematopoietic stem cell transplantation: risk factors, correlation with DNA load, and outcomes. *Blood.* 2001;97(4):867–874.

8. Ljungman P, Deliliers GL, Platzbecker U, et al. Cidofovir for cytomegalovirus infection and disease in allogeneic stem cell transplant recipients. The Infectious Diseases Working Party of the European Group for Blood and Marrow Transplantation. *Blood.* 2001;97(2):388–392.

9. Kuehnle I, Huls MH, Liu Z, et al. CD20 monoclonal antibody (rituximab) for therapy of Epstein–Barr virus lymphoma after hemopoietic stem-cell transplantation. *Blood.* 2000;95(4):1502–1505.

10. Papadopoulos EB, Ladanyi M, Emanuel D, et al. Infusions of donor leukocytes to treat Epstein–Barr virus-associated lymphoproliferative disorders after allogeneic bone marrow transplantation. *N Engl J Med.* 1994;330(17):1185–1191.

11. Slezak SL, Bettinotti M, Selleri S, Adams S, Marincola FM, Stroncek DF. CMV pp65 and IE-1 T cell epitopes recognized by healthy subjects. *J Transl Med.* 2007;5:17.

12. Leen AM, Christin A, Khalil M, et al. Identification of hexon-specific CD4 and CD8 T cell epitopes for vaccine and immunotherapy. *J Virol.* 2008;82(1):546–554.

13. Bollard CM, Rooney CM, Heslop HE. T-cell therapy in the treatment of post-transplant lymphoproliferative disease. *Nat Rev Clin Oncol.* 2012;9(9):510–519.

14. Hanley PJ, Cruz CR, Savoldo B, et al. Functionally active virus-specific T cells that target CMV, adenovirus, and EBV can be expanded from naive T-cell populations in cord blood and will target a range of viral epitopes. *Blood.* 2009;114(9):1958–1967.

15. Leen AM, Myers GD, Sili U, et al. Monoculture-derived T lymphocytes specific for multiple viruses expand and produce clinically relevant effects in immunocompromised individuals. *Nat Med.* 2006;12(10):1160–1166.

16. Sili U, Huls MH, Davis AR, et al. Large-scale expansion of dendritic cell-primed polyclonal human cytotoxic T-lymphocyte lines using lymphoblastoid cell lines for adoptive immunotherapy. *J Immunother.* 2003;26(3):241–256.

17. Kern F, Faulhaber N, Frommel C, et al. Analysis of CD8 T cell reactivity to cytomegalovirus using protein-spanning pools of overlapping pentadecapeptides. *Eur J Immunol.* 2000;30(6):1676–1682.

18. Hanley PJ, Shaffer DR, Cruz CR, et al. Expansion of T cells targeting multiple antigens of cytomegalovirus, Epstein–Barr virus and adenovirus to provide broad antiviral specificity after stem cell transplantation. *Cytotherapy.* 2011;13(8):976–986.

19. Kalos M, June CH. Adoptive T cell transfer for cancer immunotherapy in the era of synthetic biology. *Immunity.* 2013;39(1):49–60.

20. Sellar RS, Peggs KS. The role of virus-specific adoptive T-cell therapy in hematopoietic transplantation. *Cytotherapy.* 2012;14(4):391–400.

21. Hansen SG, Powers CJ, Richards R, et al. Evasion of CD8+ T cells is critical for superinfection by cytomegalovirus. *Science.* 2010;328(5974):102–106.

22. Neudorfer J, Schmidt B, Huster KM, et al. Reversible HLA multimers (Streptamers) for the isolation of human cytotoxic T lymphocytes functionally active against tumor- and virus-derived antigens. *J Immunol Methods.* 2007;320(1–2):119–131.

23. Schmitt A, Tonn T, Busch DH, et al. Adoptive transfer and selective reconstitution of streptamer-selected cytomegalovirus-specific CD8+ T cells leads to virus clearance in patients after allogeneic peripheral blood stem cell transplantation. *Transfusion.* 2011;51(3):591–599.

24. Bollard CM, Kuehnle I, Leen A, Rooney CM, Heslop HE. Adoptive immunotherapy for posttransplantation viral infections. *Biol Blood Marrow Transplant.* 2004;10(3):143–155.

25. Gattinoni L, Klebanoff CA, Palmer DC, et al. Acquisition of full effector function in vitro paradoxically impairs the in vivo antitumor efficacy of adoptively transferred CD8+ T-cells. *J Clin Invest.* 2005;115(6):1616–1626.

26. Heslop HE, Slobod KS, Pule MA, et al. Long-term outcome of EBV-specific T-cell infusions to prevent or treat EBV-related lymphoproliferative disease in transplant recipients. *Blood.* 2010;115(5):925–935.

27. Melenhorst JJ, Leen AM, Bollard CM, et al. Allogeneic virus-specific T-cells with HLA alloreactivity do not produce GVHD in human subjects. *Blood.* 2010;116(22):4700–4702.

28. Peggs KS, Verfuerth S, Pizzey A, et al. Adoptive cellular therapy for early cytomegalovirus infection after allogeneic stem-cell transplantation with virus-specific T-cell lines. *The Lancet.* 2003;362(9393):1375–1377.

29. Rooney CM, Smith CA, Ng CY, et al. Infusion of cytotoxic T-cells for the prevention and treatment of Epstein–Barr virus-induced lymphoma in allogeneic transplant recipients. *Blood.* 1998;92(5):1549–1555.

30. Walter EA, Greenberg PD, Gilbert MJ, et al. Reconstitution of cellular immunity against cytomegalovirus in recipients of allogeneic bone marrow by transfer of T-cell clones from the donor. *N Engl J Med.* 1995;333(16):1038–1044.

31. Trivedi D, Williams RY, O'Reilly RJ, Koehne G. Generation of CMV-specific T lymphocytes using protein-spanning pools of pp65-derived overlapping pentadecapeptides for adoptive immunotherapy. *Blood.* 2005;105(7):2793–2801.

32. Gerdemann U, Keirnan JM, Katari UL, et al. Rapidly generated multivirus-specific cytotoxic T lymphocytes for the prophylaxis and treatment of viral infections. *Mol Ther.* 2012;20(8):1622–1632.

33. Hanley PJC, Melenhorst J, Scheinberg P, et al. Naïve T-cell-derived CTL recognize atypical epitopes of CMVpp65 with higher avidity than CMV-seropositive donor-derived CTL – a basis for treatment of post-transplant viral infection by adoptive transfer of T-cells from virus-naïve donors. ISCT 2013 Annual Meeting (Abstract); 2013.

34. Berger C, Jensen MC, Lansdorp PM, Gough M, Elliott C, Riddell SR. Adoptive transfer of effector CD8+ T-cells derived from central memory cells establishes persistent T cell memory in primates. *J Clin Invest.* 2008;118(1):294–305.

35. Willinger T, Freeman T, Hasegawa H, McMichael AJ, Callan MF. Molecular signatures distinguish human central memory from effector memory CD8 T cell subsets. *J Immunol.* 2005;175(9):5895–5903.

36. Janeway C. *Immunobiology: The Immune System in Health and Disease.* 6th ed. New York: Garland Science; 2005.

37. Leen AM, Rooney CM, Foster AE. Improving T cell therapy for cancer. *Ann Rev Immunol.* 2007;25:243–265.

38. Eshhar Z. Tumor-specific T-bodies: towards clinical application. *Cancer Immunol Immunother.* 1997;45(3–4):131–136.

39. Schub A, Schuster IG, Hammerschmidt W, Moosmann A. CMV-specific TCR-transgenic T cells for immunotherapy. *J Immunol.* 2009;183(10):6819–6830.

40. Scholten KB, Turksma AW, Ruizendaal JJ, *et al.* Generating HPV specific T helper cells for the treatment of HPV induced malignancies using TCR gene transfer. *J Transl Med.* 2011;9:147.

41. Gehring AJ, Xue SA, Ho ZZ, *et al.* Engineering virus-specific T-cells that target HBV infected hepatocytes and hepatocellular carcinoma cell lines. *J Hepatol.* 2011;55(1):103–110.

42. Zhang Y, Liu Y, Moxley KM, *et al.* Transduction of human T-cells with a novel T-cell receptor confers anti-HCV reactivity. *PLoS Pathogens.* 2010;6(7): e1001018.

43. Luo W, Zhang XB, Huang YT, *et al.* Development of genetically engineered CD4+ and CD8+ T cells expressing TCRs specific for a *M. tuberculosis* 38-kDa antigen. *J Mol Med (Berl).* 2011;89(9):903–913.

44. Oh HL, Chia A, Chang CX, *et al.* Engineering T-cells specific for a dominant severe acute respiratory syndrome coronavirus CD8 T cell epitope. *J Virol.* 2011;85(20):10464–10471.

45. Roan NR, Starnbach MN. Antigen-specific CD8+ T cells respond to *Chlamydia trachomatis* in the genital mucosa. *J Immunol.* 2006;177(11):7974–7979.

46. Ueno T, Fujiwara M, Tomiyama H, Onodera M, Takiguchi M. Reconstitution of anti-HIV effector functions of primary human CD8 T lymphocytes by transfer of HIV-specific alphabeta TCR genes. *Eur J Immunol.* 2004;34(12):3379–3388.

47. Masiero S, Del Vecchio C, Gavioli R, *et al.* T-cell engineering by a chimeric T-cell receptor with antibody-type specificity for the HIV-1 gp120. *Gene Ther.* 2005;12(4):299–310.

48. Sahu GK, Sango K, Selliah N, Ma Q, Skowron G, Junghans RP. Anti-HIV designer T-cells progressively eradicate a latently infected cell line by sequentially inducing HIV reactivation then killing the newly gp120-positive cells. *Virology.* 2013;446(1–2): 268–275.

49. Bitton N, Verrier F, Debre P, Gorochov G. Characterization of T cell-expressed chimeric receptors with antibody-type specificity for the CD4 binding site of HIV-1 gp120. *Eur J immunol.* 1998;28(12):4177–4187.

50. Joseph A, Zheng JH, Follenzi A, *et al.* Lentiviral vectors encoding human immunodeficiency virus type 1 (HIV-1)-specific T-cell receptor genes efficiently convert peripheral blood CD8 T lymphocytes into cytotoxic T lymphocytes with potent in-vitro and in vivo HIV-1-specific inhibitory activity. *J Virol.* 2008;82(6):3078–3089.

51. Kumaresan PR, Manuri PR, Albert ND, *et al.* Bioengineering T cells to target carbohydrate to treat opportunistic fungal infection. *Proc Natl Acad Sci USA.* 2014;111(29):10660–10665.

52. Cobbold M, Khan N, Pourgheysari B, *et al.* Adoptive transfer of cytomegalovirus-specific CTL to stem cell transplant patients after selection by HLA-peptide tetramers. *J Exp Med.* 2005;202(3):379–386.

53. Feuchtinger T, Opherk K, Bethge WA, *et al.* Adoptive transfer of pp65-specific T-cells for the treatment of chemorefractory cytomegalovirus disease or reactivation after haploidentical and matched unrelated stem cell transplantation. *Blood.* 2010;116(20):4360–4367.

54. Peggs KS, Thomson K, Samuel E, *et al.* Directly selected cytomegalovirus-reactive donor T-cells confer rapid and safe systemic reconstitution of virus-specific immunity following stem cell transplantation. *Clin Infect Dis.* 2011;52(1):49–57.

55. Uhlin M, Okas M, Gertow J, Uzunel M, Brismar TB, Mattsson J. A novel haplo-identical adoptive CTL therapy as a treatment for EBV-associated lymphoma after stem cell transplantation. *Cancer Immunol Immunother.* 2010;59(3):473–477.

56. Moosmann A, Bigalke I, Tischer J, *et al.* Effective and long-term control of EBV PTLD after transfer of peptide-selected T cells. *Blood.* 2010;115(14):2960–2970.

57. Uhlin M, Gertow J, Uzunel M, *et al.* Rapid salvage treatment with virus-specific T-cells for therapy-resistant disease. *Clin Infect Dis.* 2012;55(8):1064–1073.

58. Leen AM, Christin A, Myers GD, *et al.* Cytotoxic T lymphocyte therapy with donor T-cells prevents and treats adenovirus and Epstein–Barr virus infections after haploidentical and matched unrelated stem cell transplantation. *Blood.* 2009;114(19):4283–4292.

59. Micklethwaite KP, Clancy L, Sandher U, *et al.* Prophylactic infusion of cytomegalovirus-specific cytotoxic T lymphocytes stimulated with Ad5f35pp65 gene-modified dendritic cells after allogeneic hemopoietic stem cell transplantation. *Blood.* 2008;112(10):3974–3981.

60. Feuchtinger T, Matthes-Martin S, Richard C, *et al.* Safe adoptive transfer of virus-specific T-cell immunity for the treatment of systemic adenovirus infection after allogeneic stem cell transplantation. *Br J Haematol.* 2006;134(1):64–76.

61. Qasim W, Derniame S, Gilmour K, *et al.* Third-party virus-specific T-cells eradicate adenoviraemia but trigger bystander graft-*versus*-host disease. *Br J Haematol.* 2011;154(1):150–153.

62. Blyth E, Clancy L, Simms R, *et al.* Donor-derived CMV-specific T cells reduce the requirement for CMV-directed pharmacotherapy after allogeneic stem cell transplantation. *Blood.* 2013;121(18):3745–3758.

63. Vera JF, Brenner LJ, Gerdemann U, *et al.* Accelerated production of antigen-specific T-cells for preclinical and clinical applications using gas-permeable rapid expansion cultureware (G-Rex). *J Immunother.* 2010;33(3):305–315.

64. Papadopoulou A, Gerdemann U, Katari UL, *et al.* Activity of broad-spectrum T cells as treatment for Adv, EBV, CMV, BKV, and HHV6 infections after HSCT. *Sci Transl Med.* 2014;6(242):242ra283.

65. Lam S, Bollard C. T-cell therapies for HIV. *Immunotherapy.* 2013;5(4):407–414.

66. Lieberman J, Skolnik PR, Parkerson GR, 3rd, *et al.* Safety of autologous, ex vivo-expanded human immunodeficiency virus (HIV)-specific cytotoxic T-lymphocyte infusion in HIV-infected patients. *Blood.* 1997;90(6):2196–2206.

67. Deeks SG, Wagner B, Anton PA, *et al.* A phase II randomized study of HIV-specific T-cell gene therapy in subjects with undetectable plasma viremia on combination antiretroviral therapy. *Mol Ther.* 2002;5(6):788–797.

68. Mitsuyasu RT, Anton PA, Deeks SG, *et al.* Prolonged survival and tissue trafficking following adoptive transfer of CD4zeta gene-modified autologous CD4(+) and CD8(+) T-cells in human immunodeficiency virus-infected subjects. *Blood.* 2000;96(3):785–793.

69. Tebas P, Stein D, Binder-Scholl G, *et al.* Antiviral effects of autologous CD4 T-cells genetically modified with a conditionally replicating lentiviral vector expressing long antisense to HIV. *Blood.* 2013;121(9):1524–1533.

70. Tebas P, Stein D, Tang WW, *et al.* Gene editing of CCR5 in autologous CD4 T cells of persons infected with HIV. *New Engl J Med.* 2014;370(10):901–910.

71. Didigu CA, Wilen CB, Wang J, *et al.* Simultaneous zinc-finger nuclease editing of the HIV coreceptors ccr5 and cxcr4 protects CD4+ T-cells from HIV-1 infection. *Blood.* 2014;123(1):61–69.

72. Balduzzi A, Lucchini G, Hirsch HH, *et al.* Polyomavirus JC-targeted T-cell therapy for progressive multiple leukoencephalopathy in a hematopoietic cell transplantation recipient. *Bone Marrow Transplant.* 2011;46(7):987–992.

73. Ramos CA, Narala N, Vyas GM, *et al.* Human papillomavirus type 16 E6/E7-specific cytotoxic T lymphocytes for adoptive immunotherapy of HPV-associated malignancies. *J Immunother.* 2013;36(1):66–76.

74. Cruz CR, Hanley PJ, Liu H, *et al.* Adverse events following infusion of T cells for adoptive immunotherapy: a 10-year experience. *Cytotherapy.* 2010;12(6):743–749.

75. Haque T, Taylor C, Wilkie GM, *et al.* Complete regression of posttransplant lymphoproliferative disease using partially HLA-matched Epstein Barr virus-specific cytotoxic T-cells. *Transplantation.* 2001;72(8):1399–1402.

76. Haque T, Wilkie GM, Taylor C, *et al.* Treatment of Epstein–Barr-virus-positive post-transplantation lymphoproliferative disease with partly HLA-matched allogeneic cytotoxic T-cells. *Lancet.* 2002;360(9331):436–442.

77. Haque T, Wilkie GM, Jones MM, *et al.* Allogeneic cytotoxic T-cell therapy for EBV-positive posttransplantation lymphoproliferative disease: results of a phase 2 multicenter clinical trial. *Blood.* 2007;110(4):1123–1131.

78. Barker JN, Doubrovina E, Sauter C, *et al.* Successful treatment of EBV-associated posttransplantation lymphoma after cord blood transplantation using third-party EBV-specific cytotoxic T lymphocytes. *Blood.* 2010;116(23):5045–5049.

79. Leen AM, Bollard CM, Mendizabal AM, *et al.* Multicenter study of banked third-party virus-specific T cells to treat severe viral infections after hematopoietic stem cell transplantation. *Blood.* 2013;121(26):5113–5123.

80. Wy Ip W, Qasim W. Management of adenovirus in children after allogeneic hematopoietic stem cell transplantation. *Adv Hematol.* 2013;2013:176418.

81. Schub A, Schuster IG, Hammerschmidt W, Moosmann A. CMV-specific TCR-transgenic T-cells for immunotherapy. *J Immunol.* 2009;183(10):6819–6830.

82. Xue SA, Gao L, Ahmadi M, *et al.* Human MHC Class I-restricted high avidity CD4 T-cells generated by co-transfer of TCR and CD8 mediate efficient tumor rejection in vivo. *Oncoimmunology.* 2013;2(1):e22590.

83. Frumento G, Zheng Y, Aubert G, *et al.* Cord blood T cells retain early differentiation phenotype suitable for immunotherapy after TCR gene transfer to confer EBV specificity. *Am J Transplant.* 2013;13(1):45–55.

84. Basso S, Zecca M, Calafiore L, *et al.* Successful treatment of a classic Hodgkin lymphoma-type post-transplant lymphoproliferative disorder with tailored chemotherapy and Epstein–Barr virus-specific cytotoxic T lymphocytes in a pediatric heart transplant recipient. *Pediatr Transplant.* 2013;17(7):E168–173.

85. Haque T, Amlot PL, Helling N, *et al.* Reconstitution of EBV-specific T cell immunity in solid organ transplant recipients. *J Immunol.* 1998;160(12):6204–6209.

86. Savoldo B, Goss J, Liu Z, *et al.* Generation of autologous Epstein–Barr virus-specific cytotoxic T-cells for adoptive immunotherapy in solid organ transplant recipients. *Transplantation.* 2001;72(6):1078–1086.

87. Romani L. Immunity to fungal infections. *Nat Rev Immunol.* 2004;4(1):1–23.

88. Groll AH, McNeil Grist L. Current challenges in the diagnosis and management of invasive fungal infections: report from the 15th International Symposium on Infections in the Immunocompromised Host: Thessaloniki, Greece, 22–25 June 2008. *Int J Antimicrob Agents.* 2009;33(2):101–104.

89. Milner JD, Holland SM. The cup runneth over: lessons from the ever-expanding pool of primary immunodeficiency diseases. *Nat Rev Immunol.* 2013;13(9):635–648.

90. Kim CJ, McKinnon LR, Kovacs C, *et al.* Mucosal Th17 cell function is altered during HIV infection and is an independent predictor of systemic immune activation. *J Immunol.* 2013;191(5):2164–2173.

91. Cruz CR, Lam S, Hanley PJ, *et al.* Robust T cell responses to aspergillosis in chronic granulomatous disease: implications for immunotherapy. *Clin Exp Immunol.* 2013;174(1):89–96.

92. Beck O, Topp MS, Koehl U, *et al.* Generation of highly purified and functionally active human TH1 cells against *Aspergillus fumigatus. Blood.* 2006;107(6):2562–2569.

93. Tramsen L, Schmidt S, Boenig H, *et al.* Clinical-scale generation of multi-specific anti-fungal T cells targeting Candida, Aspergillus and mucormycetes. *Cytotherapy.* 2013;15(3):344–351.

94. Khanna N, Stuehler C, Conrad B, *et al.* Generation of a multipathogen-specific T-cell product for adoptive immunotherapy based on activation-dependent expression of CD154. *Blood.* 2011;118(4):1121–1131.

95. Gomez MJ, Maras B, Barca A, La Valle R, Barra D, Cassone A. Biochemical and immunological characterization of MP65, a major mannoprotein antigen of the opportunistic human pathogen *Candida albicans. Infect Immun.* 2000;68(2):694–701.

623

96. Jolink H, Meijssen IC, Hagedoorn RS, *et al.* Characterization of the T-cell-mediated immune response against the *Aspergillus fumigatus* proteins Crf1 and catalase 1 in healthy individuals. *J Infect Dis.* 2013;208(5):847–856.

97. Schmidt S, Tramsen L, Perkhofer S, *et al.* Characterization of the cellular immune responses to Rhizopus oryzae with potential impact on immunotherapeutic strategies in hematopoietic stem cell transplantation. *J Infect Dis.* 2012;206(1):135–139.

98. Tramsen L, Beck O, Schuster FR, *et al.* Generation and characterization of anti-Candida T-cells as potential immunotherapy in patients with Candida infection after allogeneic hematopoietic stem-cell transplant. *J Infect Dis.* 2007;196(3):485–492.

99. Goodridge HS, Wolf AJ, Underhill DM. Beta-glucan recognition by the innate immune system. *Immunol Rev.* 2009;230(1):38–50.

100. Perruccio K, Tosti A, Burchielli E, *et al.* Transferring functional immune responses to pathogens after haploidentical hematopoietic transplantation. *Blood.* 2005;106(13):4397–4406.

101. De Angelis B, Dotti G, Quintarelli C, *et al.* Generation of Epstein–Barr virus-specific cytotoxic T lymphocytes resistant to the immunosuppressive drug tacrolimus (FK506). *Blood.* 2009;114(23):4784–4791.

102. Brewin J, Mancao C, Straathof K, *et al.* Generation of EBV-specific cytotoxic T cells that are resistant to calcineurin inhibitors for the treatment of posttransplantation lymphoproliferative disease. *Blood.* 2009;114(23):4792–4803.

103. Vera JF, Brenner LJ, Gerdemann U, *et al.* Accelerated production of antigen-specific T-cells for preclinical and clinical applications using gas-permeable rapid expansion cultureware (G-Rex). *J Immunother.* 2010;33(3):305–315.

104. Gattinoni L, Lugli E, Ji Y, *et al.* A human memory T cell subset with stem cell-like properties. *Nat Med.* 2011;17(10):1290–1297.

105. Williams DM, Weiner MH, Drutz DJ. Immunologic studies of disseminated infection with Aspergillus fumigatus in the nude mouse. *J Infect Dis.* 1981;143(5):726–733.

106. Holding KJ, Dworkin MS, Wan PC, *et al.* Aspergillosis among people infected with human immunodeficiency virus: incidence and survival. Adult and Adolescent Spectrum of HIV Disease Project. *Clin Infect Dis.* 2000;31(5):1253–1257.

107. Zelante T, De Luca A, Bonifazi P, *et al.* IL-23 and the Th17 pathway promote inflammation and impair antifungal immune resistance. *Eur J Immunol.* 2007;37(10):2695–2706.

108. Werner JL, Gessner MA, Lilly LM, *et al.* Neutrophils produce interleukin 17A (IL-17A) in a dectin-1- and IL-23-dependent manner during invasive fungal infection. *Infect Immun.* 2011;79(10):3966–3977.

109. Marr KA, Carter RA, Boeckh M, Martin P, Corey L. Invasive aspergillosis in allogeneic stem cell transplant recipients: changes in epidemiology and risk factors. *Blood.* 2002;100(13):4358–4366.

110. Zimmerli W, Zarth A, Gratwohl A, Speck B. Neutrophil function and pyogenic infections in bone marrow transplant recipients. *Blood.* 1991;77(2):393–399.

111. Cobbold M, Khan N, Pourgheysari B, *et al.* Adoptive transfer of cytomegalovirus-specific CTL to stem cell transplant patients after selection by HLA-peptide tetramers. *J Exp Med.* 2005;202(3):379–386.

112. Peggs KS, Thomson K, Samuel E, *et al.* Directly selected cytomegalovirus-reactive donor T cells confer rapid and safe systemic reconstitution of virus-specific immunity following stem cell transplantation. *Clin Infect Dis.* 2011;52(1):49–57.

113. Uhlin M, Okas M, Gertow J, Uzunel M, Brismar TB, Mattsson J. A novel haplo-identical adoptive CTL therapy as a treatment for EBV-associated lymphoma after stem cell transplantation. *Cancer Immunol Immunother.* 2010;59(3):473–477.

114. Qasim W, Derniame S, Gilmour K, *et al.* Third-party virus-specific T-cells eradicate adenoviraemia but trigger bystander graft-*versus*-host disease. *Br J Haematol.* 2011;154(1):150–153.

115. Feuchtinger T, Matthes-Martin S, Richard C, *et al.* Safe adoptive transfer of virus-specific T-cell immunity for the treatment of systemic adenovirus infection after allogeneic stem cell transplantation. *Br J Haematol.* 2006;134(1):64–76.

116. Balduzzi A, Lucchini G, Hirsch HH, *et al.* Polyomavirus JC-targeted T-cell therapy for progressive multiple leukoencephalopathy in a hematopoietic cell transplantation recipient. *Bone Marrow Transplant.* 2011;46(7):987–992.

117. Uhlin M, Gertow J, Uzunel M, *et al.* Rapid salvage treatment with virus-specific T cells for therapy-resistant disease. *Clin Infect Dis.* 2012;55(8):1064–1073.

118. Leen AM, Myers GD, Sili U, *et al.* Monoculture-derived T lymphocytes specific for multiple viruses expand and produce clinically relevant effects in immunocompromised individuals. *Nat Med.* 2006;12(10):1160–1166.

119. Gerdemann U, Katari UL, Papadopoulou A, *et al.* Safety and clinical efficacy of rapidly-generated trivirus-directed T-cells as treatment for adenovirus, EBV, and CMV infections after allogeneic hematopoietic stem cell transplant. *Mol Ther.* 2013;21(11):2113–2121.

120. Tramsen L, Koehl U, Tonn T, *et al.* Clinical-scale generation of human anti-Aspergillus T-cells for adoptive immunotherapy. *Bone Marrow Transplant.* 2009;43(1):13–19.

121. Gaundar SS, Clancy L, Blyth E, Meyer W, Gottlieb DJ. Robust polyfunctional T-helper 1 responses to multiple fungal antigens from a cell population generated using an environmental strain of *Aspergillus fumigatus. Cytotherapy.* 2012;14(9):1119–1130.

122. Stuehler C, Khanna N, Bozza S, *et al.* Cross-protective TH1 immunity against *Aspergillus fumigatus* and *Candida albicans. Blood.* 2011;117(22):5881–5891.

123. Jolink H, Meijssen IC, Hagedoorn RS, *et al.* Characterization of the T-cell-mediated immune response against the *Aspergillus fumigatus* proteins Crf1 and catalase 1 in healthy individuals. *J Infect Dis.* 2013;208(5):847–856.

124. Feng CG, Britton WJ. CD4+ and CD8+ T cells mediate adoptive immunity to aerosol infection of *Mycobacterium bovis* bacillus Calmette-Guerin. *J Infect Dis.* 2000;181(5):1846–1849.

125. Stemberger C, Graef P, Odendahl M, *et al.* Lowest numbers of primary CD8(+) T cells can reconstitute protective immunity upon adoptive immunotherapy. *Blood.* 2014;124(4):628–637.

126. Bhadra R, Cobb DA, Khan IA. Donor CD8+ T cells prevent *Toxoplasma gondii* de-encystation but fail to rescue the exhausted endogenous CD8 + T cell population. *Infect Immun.* 2013;81(9):3414–3425.

127. Polley R, Stager S, Prickett S, *et al.* Adoptive immunotherapy against experimental visceral leishmaniasis with CD8+ T cells requires the presence of cognate antigen. *Infect Immun.* 2006;74(1):773–776.

128. Naik S, Nicholas SK, Martinez CA, *et al.*, Adoptive immunotherapy for primary immunodeficiency disorders with virus-specific T lymphocytes. *J Allergy Clin Immunol.* 2016;137(5):1498–505.

129. Henrickson KJ. Parainfluenza viruses. *Clin Microbiol Rev.* 2003;16(2):242–64.

130. Nichols WG, Corey L, Gooley T, *et al.* Parainfluenza virus infections after hematopoietic stem cell transplantation: risk factors, response to antiviral therapy, and effect on transplant outcome. *Blood.* 2001;98(3):573–8.

131. McLaughlin L, Lang H, Williams E, *et al.* Human parainfluenza virus-3 can be targeted by rapidly ex vivo expanded T lymphocytes. *Cytotherapy.* 2016;18(12): 1515–24.

Chapter

65

Strategies to Augment Graft-*versus*-Leukemia and -Lymphoma Effects

A. John Barrett

Introduction

It has long been realized that the curative effect of allogeneic hematopoietic cell transplant (allo-HCT) depends heavily on the immune control of the transplant recipient's malignancy by an allogeneic graft-*versus*-leukemia or *versus* lymphoma (GvL) effect (referred to hereafter as the GvL effect). GvL is mediated through both T-lymphocytes and natural killer (NK) cells and

their mechanisms of action are summarized in Figures 65.1 and 65.2 and reviewed in reference[1]. Hematologic diseases vary in their susceptibility to the GvL effect according to the type of malignancy, the degree to which the disease has progressed through pretransplant treatments, and the disease burden at the time of allo-HCT. In the last decade the field of HCT and Cell Therapy has made huge progress in HCT: improvements have

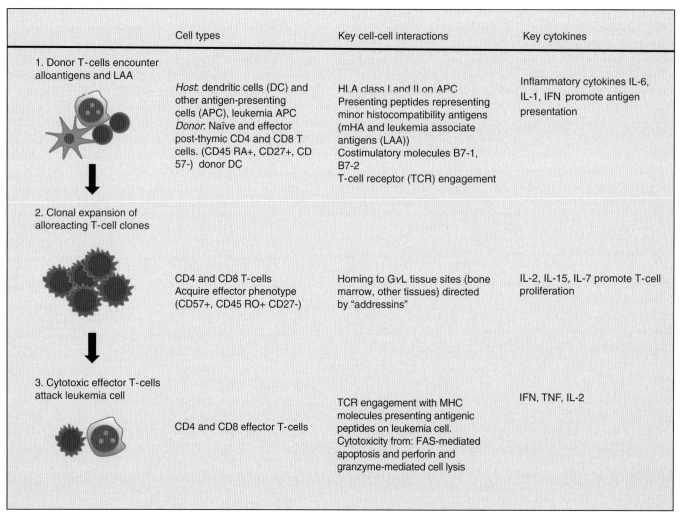

	Cell types	Key cell-cell interactions	Key cytokines
1. Donor T-cells encounter alloantigens and LAA	*Host:* dendritic cells (DC) and other antigen-presenting cells (APC), leukemia APC *Donor:* Naïve and effector post-thymic CD4 and CD8 T cells. (CD45 RA+, CD27+, CD 57-) donor DC	HLA class I and II on APC Presenting peptides representing minor histocompatibility antigens (mHA and leukemia associate antigens (LAA)) Costimulatory molecules B7-1, B7-2 T-cell receptor (TCR) engagement	Inflammatory cytokines IL-6, IL-1, IFN promote antigen presentation
2. Clonal expansion of alloreacting T-cell clones	CD4 and CD8 T-cells Acquire effector phenotype (CD57+, CD45 RO+ CD27-)	Homing to GvL tissue sites (bone marrow, other tissues) directed by "addressins"	IL-2, IL-15, IL-7 promote T-cell proliferation
3. Cytotoxic effector T-cells attack leukemia cell	CD4 and CD8 effector T-cells	TCR engagement with MHC molecules presenting antigenic peptides on leukemia cell. Cytotoxicity from: FAS-mediated apoptosis and perforin and granzyme-mediated cell lysis	IFN, TNF, IL-2

Figure 65.1. Mechanism of T-cell-mediated GvL.

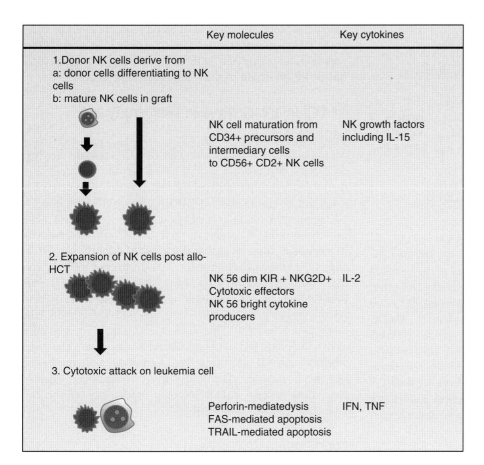

Figure 65.2. Mechanism of NK cell-mediated GvL.

reduced transplant-related mortality dramatically. This has permitted safe transplants for individuals up to 70 years of age. Unfortunately, leukemic relapse remains the unfinished business of allo-HCT whatever the graft source. Relapse rates even in early favorable-risk patients (e.g., acute myeloid leukemia in first remission) remain in the order of 20% and reach over 60% in transplants for advanced, late-stage high-risk disease (e.g., refractory leukemias). It is therefore reasonable to question whether we have reached the limits of the GvL potential of HCT from current transplant approaches. The recognition of transplant strategies to optimize GvL effects with new techniques to augment GvL show promise. Here we will consider the best ways to deliver transplants that maximize their "natural GvL" capacity and describe the strengths and limitations of recent developments that aim to specifically boost the GvL effect without potentiating or risking graft-*versus* host disease (GvHD)[1].

Choosing the Best Transplant Approach at the Ideal Time – Improve Disease-Free Survival without Increments in Treatment-Related Mortality: Is It Possible?

Results of large numbers of transplants from multiple centers provide reliable data about the GvL potential which can guide the selection of the optimum transplant approach to maximize

GvL. Because factors that increase the antitumor effect of the transplant (as identified by decreased post-transplant relapse rates) are frequently inversely linked with transplant-related mortality (TRM), it is important to describe effects which can augment GvL not only by their effect on relapse rates, but also in terms of disease-free survival (DFS) to account for the deleterious impact of a variety of strategies that reduce relapse rates while increasing the TRM.

Timing of Transplant: Why Is It Important?

The single most powerful factor affecting relapse is the state of the disease at the time of transplant (see Chapters 32 to 49). It is well known that the best outcomes and the lowest relapse rates are seen in patients transplanted early in the course of their disease. In most cases of acute leukemia, this means transplanting in first and not subsequent remission, in lymphomas after the first treatment failure, rather than after disease refractoriness to multiple agents has become established, and for myelodysplastic syndromes (MDS), transplantation before the marrow shows excess of blast cells. In the United States, a significant proportion of patients with high-risk acute leukemias (where HCT is indicated in first remission) are referred late, either in second or subsequent remission. It is salutary to note that simply selecting the optimum time for transplant could improve DFS by over 25% because of the considerably lower relapse rates of allo-HCT transplanted at the optimum moment.

Donor Compatibility

It is generally assumed that increasing disparity between donor and recipient in their human leukocyte antigen (HLA) antigens and the *minor* histocompatibility antigens (mHAs) presented by HLA class I and II molecules can increase GvL, albeit at the expense of increased GvHD and TRM (see Chapters 12 and 13). The higher relapse rates observed in transplants between identical twins compared with HLA-matched sibling donors attests to the importance of mHA disparity in GvL[2].

Identical Twin Donors: Should They Even Be Considered for Allograft?

Since identical twins share both HLA and mHA identity the only GvL effect in such HCT may be ascribed to the fact that the incoming donor immune system is not tolerized to the leukemia and it is reasonable to question whether there is any GvL effect from an identical twin transplant. Intriguing data from the Center for International Blood and Marrow Transplant (CIBMTR) showed that higher marrow cell doses (CD34+ cells $>3\times10^8$/kg) were associated with lower relapse rates in CML identical twin transplants, suggesting that there may be some ability to improve GvL effects even with identical twin donors. Identical twin HCT represents a special case where the higher relapse rate is offset by a very low TRM. Thus it is reasonable to perform identical twin transplants in patients with relatively low risk of relapse[3].

HLA-Matched Donors

Compared with HLA-matched sibling donors (MSD), match unrelated donors (MUD) differ from their recipients both in the degree of matching of HLA class I and II molecules and their mHAs (see Chapters 7 and 8). However, a recent large retrospective study failed to convincingly show a significant benefit in relapse rates for the outbred donor compared with the HLA-matched sibling[4].

HLA-Haplotype Mismatch Donors

It has also been assumed that HLA-haplotype mismatch HCT confers lower relapse rates than transplants from HLA-MSD. Unfortunately, there are no evaluable side-by-side comparisons between HLA-MSD and mismatched family donor transplants to clearly determine this assumption. It is notable that relapse of leukemia after HLA-haplotype mismatch HCT is frequently accompanied with a down-regulation (by the leukemia) of the mismatched HLA haplotype, cutting off the strong alloimmune reaction against the mismatched HLA haplotype [5]. Thus, somewhat surprisingly (with the important exception of identical twin transplant), definitive evidence for differences in the potency of GvL determined by HLA and mHA compatibility is lacking (see Chapter 59).

Graft Source and Relapse Rates

There is now a large body of data concerning relapse rates from the three main donor graft sources: bone marrow (BM), peripheral blood (PB), and cord blood (CB) reviewed in reference[5]. Relapse rates after CB transplants do show lower relapse rates compared with MUD-HCT[6]. Relapses after BM or PB grafts fail to show important differences[6].

NK Cell Alloreactivity: Can We Identify and Capture It?

An important factor mediating GvL in mismatch and matched HCT is the degree of compatibility between donor NK cells and their targets as characterized by matched or mismatch killer immunoglobulin receptor (KIR)/HLA groups (see Chapter 7). NK alloreactivity is controlled by other genes outside the MHC on chromosome 6 leading to diversity of NK alloreactivity independent from HLA-matching. KIR disparity in HLA-haplotype mismatch transplants, HLA-matched sibling, and matched unrelated HCT carries a potent GvL effect, at least in myeloid malignancies, resulting in significant differences in relapse probabilities between transplants with and without KIR incompatibility[7,8,9]. The problem is that these reports differ as to which KIR groups confer favorable effects on relapse and whether such NK GvL is restricted to myeloid malignancies or can also be detected after transplants for lymphoid malignancies. Thus a clear insight into the mechanism of the NK GvL effect remains undefined.

Conditioning Regimens

Apart from the role that conditioning plays in minimizing the disease burden thereby favoring effective control of malignancy from the GvL effect (see Chapter 27), conditioning regimens can influence the GvL effect through the degree of immunoablation they achieve, which in turn determines the time required to achieve full donor T-cell chimerism. There are both experimental and clinical data to support the greater efficacy of GvL when early donor T-cell chimerism is achieved[10].

CD34+ and CD3+ Cell Dose: Effect on Relapse Risk?

The quantity as well as the quality of immune cells transferred in the graft to the recipient affect the subsequent GvL potential of the transplant. Beyond the impact of CD34+ dose on engraftment potential (ascribed to a "veto" effect on recipient T-cells[11]), the dose of CD34+ cells affects both transplant outcome and relapse probability. We showed in T-cell-depleted (TCD) HLA-MSD HCT (myeloablative setting), all receiving the same T-cell dose of around 5×10^5 CD3+ cells/kg, that relapse risk was lower when greater than the median CD34+ cell dose of $>5\times10^6$ CD34+ cells/kg was achieved [12]. A large retrospective study from the CIBMTR also confirmed a favorable effect on relapse of CD34+ cell doses $>6\times10^6$/kg in unmanipulated HCT[13]. The basis for a GvL effect of CD34+ cell dose is unknown. Data supporting a favorable effect of T-cell dose are less clear. Peripheral blood grafts provide about 10-fold higher CD3+ cells than bone marrow grafts but while it is agreed that PB grafts confer more GvHD than bone marrow grafts, there is little impact of PB on reduced relapse rates[14].

Optimizing the Graft-*versus*-Host Prophylaxis in T-cell-Replete Allografts: Does It Affect GvL?

Numerous anecdotal reports associate immunosuppressive therapy (IST) with relapse, and conversely the occasional achievement of a remission when IST treatment is stopped (see Chapter 26). These observations support the assumption that the GvL alloresponse is equally susceptible to the effects of IST as GvH alloreacting T-cells. The duration as well as the type of IST may be critical in weakening the GvL effect, but without any clear knowledge of how long the GvL effect is required it is not possible to strategize optimal treatment approaches (see Chapter 12 and 13). Indeed the requirement for a prolonged GvL effect may vary with diseases. The very late relapses (up to 17 years post-allograft) seen in CML transplant recipients strongly suggest that GvL represents a permanent state of disease control, which if interrupted, may provoke a relapse[15].

In contrast, the very rare cases of relapse beyond 5 years from allo-HCT in acute leukemias suggest a shorter required time period for effective GvL. In an attempt to find a balance between effective GvHD control and functional GvL effects, several investigators have sought to minimize IST by reducing the dose of calcineurin inhibitors. Results in both adults and children suggest that lower target levels of cyclosporine achieve lower relapse rates without augmenting GvHD risks[16,17]. Therefore, more studies to determine the minimum safe use of calcineurin inhibitors for GvHD prophylaxis seem worthwhile (see Chapter 70).

Lastly the choice of IST may be important. Several agents that suppress GvHD have direct activity against hematologic malignancies: imatinib, a weak immune suppressor, can target Ph+ ALL and CML; sirolimus suppresses GvHD but has potential activity against B-cell lymphomas. Preliminary observations suggest that sirolimus could be used to advantage after allotransplants for NHL and ALL[18]. In the same way, the anti CD20+ monoclonal antibody rituximab is of interest because of its dual properties of targeting B-cell lymphomas as well as suppressing chronic GvHD[19] (see Chapter 19).

T-cell Depletion: How Does It Affect GvL?

Initial reports, mainly in CML, that TCD increases relapse have been a deterrent to the widespread application of this transplant approach despite the successful reduction in both acute and chronic GvHD (see Chapter 29). *In-vivo* TCD with monoclonal antibodies has, however, remained popular especially in older patients receiving reduced intensity conditioning (RIC) regimen because of the favorable low TRM[20]. Best outcomes require judicious dose and timing of antilymphocyte antibodies to steer between too much immunosuppression with consequent viral infections and increased relapse rates, and too little with consequent GvHD.

ATG and Relapse Risk

In a recent meta-analysis of outcomes from six reported studies in over 1500 patients, relapse mortality was not significantly increased by ATG and OS was improved because of a reduced TRM[21]. We can therefore conclude that *in-vivo* TCD is not deleterious to the GvL effect with ATG (although the correct or optimal dose of ATG remains a matter of debate) perhaps because effective GvHD prevention with IST offsets the potent adverse impact of steroids given to treat GvHD.

Ex-vivo T-cell Depletion

As a means to better control T-cell dose in the transplant, some groups have employed *ex-vivo* TCD using immunomagnetic beads coated with CD34+ antibody to positively select CD34+ cells or antilymphocyte antibodies to negatively select CD34+ cells. In the HLA-MSD-HCT myeloablative setting current TCD methods (where a small residual T-cell population is reinfused in the order of 10^5 CD3+ cells/kg) appear to favor improved OS because of reduced TRM and reduced risk of chronic GvHD in the absence of increased relapse, at least in acute leukemias[22]. Retrospective comparisons of *ex-vivo* TCD and unmanipulated related or unrelated HLA-matched HCT in AML in first remission from Memorial Sloane Kettering Cancer Center show no significant difference in relapse rates between the two approaches[23]. These promising data for *ex-vivo* TCD have set the scene for prospective studies comparing TCD and non-TCD approaches. The TCD has also been applied in HLA-haplotype mismatch HCT by the Perugia group where the benefit of minimizing GvHD offsets any potential increased risk of relapse (see Chapters 59 and 61). In this setting the role of alloreacting NK cells in minimizing relapse is apparent[24].

Moving Forward: GvL without Concurrent GvHD

Current approaches of TCD and GvHD prophylaxis suffer from the inability to selectively inactivate the GvHD alloreactions while conserving GvL. This limitation has stimulated attempts to use newer *in-vitro* or *in-vivo* selective TCD to target lymphocyte subsets which lack GvHD reactivity (summarized in Figure 65.3). Target T-cell subsets which are predominantly but not exclusively responsible for causing acute GvHD are CD8+ T-cells and naïve (nonantigen experienced post-thymic) T-cells. Based on the successful demonstration of naïve TCD in animals, clinical trials are now underway[25]. However, there are no data in humans to determine how much GvL alloreactions are preserved by these subset depletion strategies.

Antibodies against Single or Multiple Activation Markers of T-cells

A strategy with the potential to conserve GvL alloreacting cells while depleting the GvHD reactive cells is to activate the donor's T-cells by exposure to normal (nonmalignant)

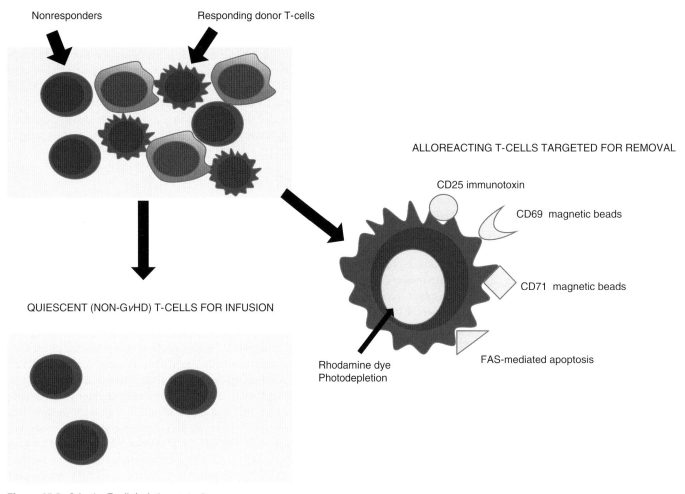

Figure 65.3. Selective T-cell-depletion strategies.

recipient antigen-presenting cells (APCs). In this method of selective allodepletion approach, alloreacting (GvHD reactive) T-cells are targeted by antibodies against single or multiple activation markers of T-cells such as *CD25*, *CD71*, *CD69*, and *FAS*. Purging techniques used include conjugation of a toxin to the antibody, or removal of antibody-coated cells by magnetic beads[26].

Photodepletion

An alternative selection approach (photoselection) relies upon a relatively increased uptake and retention of rhodamine dyes by activated T-cells. T-cells cultured with nonmalignant stimulator cells from the patient become activated and retain dye [26]. By exposing the culture to light, the activated cells are killed by free radical release from retained dye and purged from the cell mix. By excluding leukemia cells from the stimulators, nonactivated GvL reacting cells can be retained. Clinical trials have been performed using various selective allodepletion techniques in both HLA-matched and HLA-mismatched situations. The consensus is that alloresponses in HLA-matched individuals are not strong enough to power the level

of selectivity achieved by these relatively crude techniques. In contrast very promising results have been reported using photoselection in HLA-haplotype mismatch HCT[27,28]. Refer to Chapters 59 and 61 for further reading on selective alloreactive T-cell depletion.

Post-transplant Cyclophosphamide

Pioneered by the Johns Hopkins transplant group, Fuchs *et al.* have developed a highly effective strategy to block GvHD by eliminating donor T-cells and conserving regulatory T (Treg) cells in the early period of allostimulation[28,29]. The critical element is the careful timing of the dose of cyclophosphamide on days +3 and +4 post-transplant of unmanipulated marrow or peripheral blood. While powerful alloresponses are blocked, populations of T-cells that establish reactions to viruses and possibly naïve T-cell populations responsible for GvL reactions against leukemia/lymphoma-associated antigens (LAA) are spared together with Treg cells. Disappointingly, relapse remains a significant cause of treatment failure with this approach leaving open to question whether GvL reactivity is indeed conserved[29,30].

"Super Donor Lymphocyte Infusions": Increasing Susceptibility of Malignant Cells to T-Cell and NK Cell Attack

Preemptive DLI

The remarkable success of donor lymphocyte infusions (DLIs) when first used to treat post-transplant relapse in a series of CML patients initiated the almost universal use of DLI (when available) as an adjunct to any attempts at relapse treatment. It is now clear that DLI have their greatest impact on CML and some lymphomas, while their therapeutic impact on relapsed acute leukemias and MDS is modest. To optimize the effect of DLI, a number of investigators have explored the use of preemptive DLI, given usually within the first 3 months after HCT to boost the G*v*L effect and prevent relapse. Similar strategies combine molecular approaches to monitor early recurrence of disease with DLI. Preemptive DLI strategies and DLI are discussed further in Chapter 25 (also discussed prophylactic DLI) and Chapter 26 and are reviewed in reference[31]. Given the partial control of disease usually associated with DLI many investigators have sought to boost G*v*L either by increasing T-cell activation and cytotoxic potential with cytokines, or by increasing susceptibility of the leukemia or lymphoma cell to cytotoxic attack by T-cells or NK cells (reviewed in reference[32]).

Adding Another Agent to DLI

Several studies have explored the use of GM-CSF and interferon-α to increase antigen presentation by myeloid leukemia cells[33]. In the absence of controlled trials there is no clear evidence that these efforts increase the capacity of DLI to control leukemia. Most promising is the use of hypomethylating agents to increase presentation of tumor-specific antigens. For patients with MDS and AML, HCT trials using azacytidine are underway to evaluate this agent to boost G*v*L in the early post-transplant setting[34].

Enhancing G*v*L Effect with Lenalidomide?

The thalidomide derivative lenalidomide has several immune properties that could also enhance G*v*L. Firstly it promotes dendritic cell 1 (DC1) type APCs which elicit cytotoxic T-cells and secondly it enhances cytotoxic *Th1* cells. Lenalidomide and the proteasome inhibitor bortezomib have been used as a maintenance therapy after autologous HCT in patients with multiple myeloma (MM) (see Chapter 46) and these agents deserve exploration in the allo-HCT (see Chapters 19 and 48) setting for other lymphoid malignancies[35].

Vaccines in Allo-HCT: Opportunity and Limitation

Despite extensive animal studies, vaccines targeting leukemia have not been widely explored. Studies with influenza vaccine show that it is feasible to generate T-cell responses with vaccine, especially if the donor is first vaccinated and the recipient receives further boosting post-infusion of a graft containing the primed donor lymphocytes[36]. Vaccines against the unique idiotype M protein in MM have been explored by Kwak *et al.* In a small study, donors were vaccinated with the idiotype myeloma protein prior to bone marrow transplantation in 5 HLA-matched patients with MM. Patients showed transfer of idiotype-specific T-cells and three patients showed sustained responses[37]. Vaccines targeting common antigens expressed by leukemia such as WT1, PRAME, and Proteinase 3 are other possible approaches to boosting G*v*L. WT1 and PR1 vaccines have been reported to produce responses in myeloid leukemias and MDS but have not been evaluated in the post-transplant setting[38]. These studies emphasize that allo-HCT offers a unique opportunity to boost G*v*L by vaccination of the donor. However, concerns about the risks of administering leukemia antigens to the donor have generally restricted this approach.

T-Cell Therapy to Enhance G*v*L Effect: Which Antigens to Target?

It is a widely held perception that G*v*L can only be optimized if the G*v*L alloreaction is completely separated from the G*v*HD alloresponse. Indeed many transplanters refer to the separation of G*v*HD and G*v*L as the "holy grail" of allo-HCT. Table 65.1 lists the differences between G*v*HD and G*v*L that have been studied to engineer such transplants.

Targeting G*v*L through Specific Antigens: Minor Histocompatibility and Leukemia-Associated Antigens

Of the differences between G*v*HD and G*v*L reactions, the antigenic disparities between G*v*HD and G*v*L targets have attracted most interest since they offer the opportunity for precise targeting of G*v*L antigens by discrete T-cell clones via their antigen-specific T-cell receptors. Two major classes of antigens, mHA and LAA, are the focus of strategies to generate G*v*L-specific T-cells as illustrated in Figure 65.4.

Minor Histocompatibility Antigens as Targets for G*v*L

mHAs are self-peptides presented by HLA class I and II molecules on the cell surface (Table 65.2). Inherited polymorphisms of the amino acid sequence in proteins are commonplace and give rise to diversity in amino acid sequences of the peptides presented by HLA molecules. mHAs elicit a T-cell alloresponse if two conditions are satisfied; first the alleleic peptide sequence must be presented by class I or II HLA molecules and second the donor must not share the allele with the recipient so that the donor's T-cell receptors recognize the recipient allele as foreign and respond by clonal expansion. Many mHAs are derived from ubiquitous proteins found in

Table 65.1 Strategies to separate GvL from GvHD

Strategy	GvL conserved	GvHD suppressed	Comments
Cell-based approaches			
Deplete CD8	+	(+)	Modest separation
Deplete naïve cells	+	(+)	Under evaluation
Transfuse NK cells	+	−	NK cells do not cause GvHD
Tregs infusion	+?	(+)	Controls GvHD, may not block GvL
Selective T-cell depletion	+	(+)	Effective *in-vitro*, *in-vivo* unclear
T-cells with suicide gene	+	−	Abrogates GvHD after GvL effect
mHA-specific T-cells	++	−	Can *increase* GvL specifically
LAA-specific T-cells	++	−	Can *increase* GvL specifically
CAR cells	++	−	
Immune modulation			
Low-dose cyclosporine	+	(+)	Reduces relapse but stops GvHD
Lenalidomide	+	(+?)	Immune function enhancer
Vaccines	+	−	Potential to boost GvL specifically
Direct effect on the leukemia/lymphoma			
Azacytidine	+	−	Increases expression of LAA
Sirolimus (NHL)	+	−	Suppresses GvHD
Rituximab	+	−	Treats cGvHD

+ GvL conserved; ++ GvL enhanced; (+) reduced GvHD; − no GvHD/no impact on GvHD.

diverse tissues. Such mHAs represent targets for both GvHD and GvL reacting T-cells. GvL targets are less frequent; they are the mHA peptides derived from the breakdown of proteins unique to hematopoietic lineages. Nevertheless, it is estimated that there are many hundreds of mHAs that could elicit GvL-restricted responses. Since the first identification of HA-1, a hematopoiesis-restricted mHA, more have been described with restriction to B-cell lineages, myeloid lineages, or to hematopoietic lineages in general. Even HLA-matched donor–recipient pairs from the same family have hundreds of mHAs differences and the current list is still the tip of a large iceberg of unknown mHAs. Harnessing mHAs to generate GvL reacting T-cells has proved difficult in practice because only mHAs that have a balanced polymorphism have practical applicability[39,40]. By way of illustration, if a recipient possesses an mHA with an allele frequency of 50%, an HLA-matched related donor has a 25% chance of lacking the same allele since mHAs and HLA antigens are inherited separately. Thu, the probability in an HLA-matched related pair for the donor to make an alloreaction against the recipient's mHAs is 12.5%. HA1 represents an "ideal" antigen. Its frequency in northern European populations is about 40% but many other

mHAs are either too rare or too frequent to make the chance of finding a donor that recognizes an mHA antigen as foreign. While the situation is mitigated by selecting favorable mHA mismatches from a list of unrelated donors, the only alternative is to work on a case by case basis to identify mHAs that are specific for a particular donor–recipient pair. Indeed Bleakley *et al.* have used this approach to identify new mHAs with GvL potential in a series of HLA-matched donor–recipient pairs. Using dendritic cells (DCs) as APC from the patient they elicited multiple clones of mHA reacting T-cells from the donor. Nonspecific alloreacting cells which also recognized recipient fibroblasts were excluded. Leukemia-specific clones were further selected by their ability to recognize the recipient's leukemia cells. GvL reactivity was demonstrated by the ability of the chosen T-cell clones to eliminate the leukemia in an immunodeficient mouse model[41]. In a few patients, donor mHA-specific T-cells have been given post-allo-HCT with evidence of leukemia control. While this approach is proof-of-principle the strategy is constrained by the "boutique" nature of its expensive high technology approach that restricts it to academic centers. Furthermore without a comprehensive knowledge of the tissue expression of novel mHAs,

Table 65.2 Minor histocompatibility antigens with GvL potential

mHA	HLA restriction	Percent disparity matched sibling donor[a]	Percent disparity unrelated donor[a]
HA-1	A*0201; A*0206	6.4	11.6
LRH-1	B*0702	4.9	7.5
ACC-2	B*4403	3.6	6.7
HEATR 1	B*0801	3.1	5.6
ACC-1	A*2402	2.8	5.2
ACC-6	B*4402; B*4403	2.3	5.9
HA-2	A*0201	1.8	2.5
SP110	A*0301	1.6	2.5
LBLY75-1K	DRB1*1301	1.2	2.4
HA-1	B*60; B*40012	<1	<1
ACC1	A*2402	<1	<1
CD19	DQ, A1*05; B1*02	10.4	15.9
HB-1	B*4402; B*4403	3.9	6.8
HB1	B*4402; B*4403	1.2	1.3

Origin: alleles of diverse normal intracellular proteins of the hematopoietic lineage.
Antigenicity: powerful for donors lacking the recipient's alleleic peptide sequence.
[a] Probability of having an HLA-matched donor recognizing the antigen.

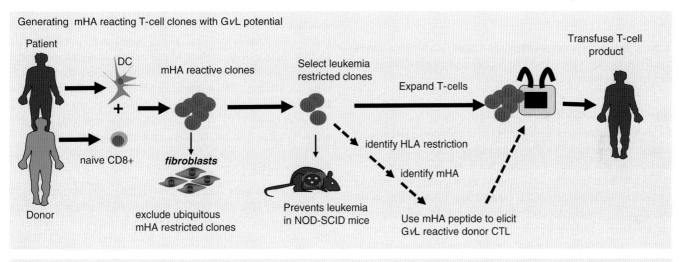

Generating mHA reacting T-cell clones with GvL potential

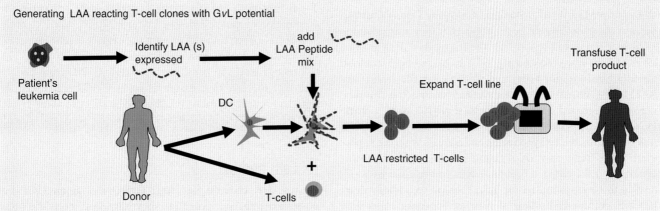

Generating LAA reacting T-cell clones with GvL potential

Figure 65.4. Strategies to generate GvL reacting T-cells with mHA or LAA.

633

Table 65.3 Common LAA with GvL potential

	AML	CML	ALL	CLL
WT1	+	+	+	−
Proteinase 3	+	+	−	−
PRAME	+	+	+	−
RHAMM	+	+	+	+
Aurora A Kinase	+	+	+	−
MAGE A3	+	+	−	+
MP11	−	−	−	+
HAGE	+	+	−	−
BCR/ABL	−	+	Ph+	−
NyEso1	−	+	−	+
BMI-1	−	+	−	−
Telomerase	+	+	+	+
Fibromodulin	−	−	−	+
Syntaxin	−	−	−	+

Ph+: Philadelphia chromosome-positive leukemias.
Origin: overexpressed or aberrantly expressed proteins, many known tumor-specific antigens.
Antigenicity: variable avidity, epitopes vary according to HLA type.

there is a risk of unwanted and potentially dangerous cross-reactivity of the mHA-specific T-cells and normal tissues as described by Warren *et al.*[42].

Leukemia-Associated Antigens

As an alternative to targeting mHAs, other investigators have sought to generate T-cells recognizing LAA (Table 65.3). Improvements in culture techniques used to develop virus-specific T-cells from healthy donors have paved the way for generating high-potency CTL recognizing LAA. Nagai *et al.*, for example, sought to elicit high-avidity CTL recognizing a single tumor antigen epitope (Aurora Kinase) and subsequently sequenced and cloned the TCR to transduce into T-cells to generate highly potent T-cell lines targeting a specific LAA epitope[43]. By incorporating a *Sleeping Beauty* transposon into the gene cassette bearing the TCR they subverted the T-cell machinery to present only the transduced TCR heterodimer. T-cells lines recognizing WT1 have also been made in this way but have not been used in clinical trials (see Chapter 23). The limitation of this strategy is that the immune response is focused on a single epitope restricted by a single HLA class I molecule (usually HLA-A-0201 or HLA-A-2401). This constrains the cell product to individuals with the appropriate HLA type and risks tumor escape through down-regulation of the targeted protein. Furthermore, the regulatory hurdles to be surmounted for gene therapy technology deter the early commercialization of such an approach. Also such

manipulated T-cells carry a risk of cross-reactivity with healthy tissues[44]. To avoid these constraints, and modeled upon successful adoptive therapy with multivirus-specific T-cells, we have explored the generation of multileukemia antigen-specific T-cells[45,46]. Peptide libraries from up to five leukemia antigens are incubated with DCs and used to induce multi-LAA-specific CD4+ and CD8+ T-cells. Such T-cell lines can be generated from any donor and have antileukemia activity. Clinical trials to treat or prevent relapse after HCT with infusions of multi-LAA-specific T-cells are now underway (NCT02203903).

Improving T-Cell Function through Gene Modification

CAR T-Cells and BiTE Cells

The arming of cytotoxic lymphocytes with a chimeric antigen receptor (CAR) bearing an immunoglobulin molecule by gene transfer creates a cytotoxic cell which has superior binding through its antibody to the target, activating the T-cell to exert cytotoxic damage to the malignant cell target. Results are extremely promising (see Chapter 62), but the approach is limited by the lack of truly leukemia-specific surface molecules leading to indiscriminate targeting of normal cells bearing the same surface antigen. Thus CAR cells directed against CD20+ cells on acute lymphocytic leukemia (ALL) cells also eliminate nonmalignant B-cells. At present myeloid malignancies lack suitable target surface molecules. A variant of this approach which avoids the complication of gene insertion are bi-antigen-specific T (BiTE) cells (see Chapter 33). A bispecific antibody attaches to surface antigens on the malignant cells and captures T-cells through the surface expressed CD3 molecule bringing the cytotoxic potential of the T-cell to bear on the malignant cell target[47,48].

Suicide Gene Transduction

Techniques to eliminate GvHD reacting cells by inserting a suicide gene into the grafted lymphocyte fraction permits a "safe" form of GvHD which can be abrogated by administering the suicide agent. Two systems have been explored. Initial approaches inserted viral tyrosine kinase tyrosine into the T-cell inoculum rendering the grafted T-cells susceptible to elimination by ganciclovir (see Chapter 29)[49]. More recently, T-cells have been transduced with the caspase 9 gene rendering the transduced cells sensitive to a caspase 9 activator[50]. This technology works in principle to separate GvHD from GvL by virtue of the fact that it suffices for a GvHD reaction to be initiated in order for the GvL effect to be effective while GvHD can be abolished immediately afterwards with the suicide agent.

NK Cells and GvL

Because NK cells do not exert GvHD in human HCT but possess strong GvL potential, they have long been the focus of cell therapy strategies. The opportunity to select a donor with KIR groups permitting alloreactivity against the recipient HLA groups should make it possible to generate G*v*L reactive NK cells to use after transplant to enhance G*v*L. A detailed account of NK cell therapy is given in Chapter 63 and is reviewed in reference[9].

Other T-Cell Subsets

Several cytotoxic cell types have G*v*L potential through non-HLA restricted targeting. NKT cells are CD3+ T-cells with non-HLA restricted NK-like cytotoxicity generated by incubation of T-cells with high doses of interleukin-2[51]. Interest in gamma-delta T-cells has been stimulated by several observations that high frequencies of these cells post-HCT confer a lower relapse incidence in ALL transplant recipients. Gamma-delta T-cells can be generated by exposure to biphosphonates (drugs used to increase bone mineralization) to create sufficient cell numbers for infusion[52]. Currently there has been no substantial application of these cell types in the allo-transplant setting.

Controversies and Future Directions

While this chapter outlines some very promising areas of development in ways to control and enhance the G*v*L effects, the absence of solid data in these new areas of research means that controversies abound as to the best approach to use.

Is It Possible to Design a Transplant Approach that Improves on Current Relapse Rates?

While there are ongoing efforts to refine the conditioning regimen and post-allo-HCT prophylaxis it would seem that the limits have been reached. Rather, more promising avenues of research appear to favor ways to co-opt the donor's immune system with specific therapies aimed at boosting G*v*L beyond its natural limits.

T-Cells or NK Cells?

The field of G*v*L is somewhat dichotomized between proponents of NK-mediated *versus* T-cell-mediated G*v*L. In favor of NK-based strategies are the large impacts on relapse seen in various genetic disparities between donor and recipient KIR ligands and their recipient targets. Against a central role for NK-mediated G*v*L is the possibility that the effect is restricted to myeloid malignancies. Furthermore, the failure of NK infusions so far to impact disease post-HCT reduces enthusiasm for relying on NK cells to deliver reliable G*v*L. In contrast, the well-defined role of T-cells in G*v*HD and G*v*L places T-cells in a stronger position to be developed to enhance G*v*L.

Does Selective T-Cell Depletion Spare G*v*L?

Whether the donor T-cell alloresponse to major and minor histocompatibility antigens is eliminated (*in-vitro* or *in-vivo*) to prevent G*v*HD, the preservation of G*v*L T-cell reactivity relies upon the persistence of leukemia recognizing T-cells that were not activated by recipient antigen presentation. Such antigens would include antigens overexpressed or uniquely expressed by the leukemia including LAA and some mHA. However, we do not know if such residual G*v*L reacting cells would suffice to initiate effective G*v*L reactions. Hence, selective depletion may be best considered as a means to avoid the need for G*v*HD prophylaxis, thus serving as a platform to infuse potent leukemia-reacting lymphocytes with enhanced G*v*L properties.

Does DLI Offer Any Substantial GvL Effect for Malignancies Other Than CML?

While DLI served us well in achieving dramatic second remissions and prolonged survivals when used to treat relapsed CML, the benefit of DLI for acute leukemias boosted by cytokines or judicious timing after chemotherapy has been minimal. It can be reasonably asked whether there is any role for the time-honored approach of giving unmodified DLI for relapse in these situations. Rather, the dismal outcomes for patients who relapse after HCT should be seen as an opportunity to explore new treatments. Sadly, while relapse is the single most important cause of treatment failure after HCT, there is a paucity of clinical trials exploring novel strategies to treat the problem.

What Is the Future for Genetically Transduced T-cells?

Genetic modification of cells for human therapy incurs a huge burden of regulatory control not only on the manufacture of the cell product but on the long-term outcome for the recipient. For example, the FDA requires 15 years of follow-up for recipients of genetically modified T-cells. Such controls are disincentives for commercialization of such T-cell therapies. The dramatic successes reported with CAR-modified T-cells have nevertheless sparked much enthusiasm for such T-cell therapeutics with huge investment by pharmaceutical companies. Evidence of broadened success of genetically modified T-cell therapies, whether by CAR modifications, T-cell receptor insertion, or ways to enhance cytotoxicity, may overcome the natural reluctance of corporate entities to embrace cell therapy. Depending on therapeutic success or failure, the next decade will establish the trajectory of T-cell therapy as a realistically funded, widely used treatment approach to prevent and treat relapse pre-or post-HCT.

Acknowledgment

This work was supported by the Intramural Research Program of the NIH.

References

1. Barrett AJ. Understanding and harnessing the graft-*versus*-leukaemia effect. *Br J Haematol.* 2008;142(6):877–88.

2. Gale RP, Horowitz MM, Ash RC, Champlin RE, Goldman JM, Rimm AA, Ringdén O, Stone JA, Bortin MM. Identical-twin bone marrow transplants for leukemia. *Ann Intern Med.* 1994;120(8):646–52.

3. Barrett AJ, Ringdén O, Zhang MJ, Bashey A, Cahn JY, Cairo MS, Gale RP, Gratwohl A, Locatelli F, Martino R, Schultz KR, Tiberghien P. Effect of nucleated marrow cell dose on relapse and survival in identical twin bone marrow transplants for leukemia. *Blood.* 2000;95(11):3323–7.

4. Ringdén O, Pavletic SZ, Anasetti C, Barrett AJ, Wang T, Wang D, Antin JH, Di Bartolomeo P, Bolwell BJ, Bredeson C, Cairo MS, Gale RP, Gupta V, Hahn T, Hale GA, Halter J, Jagasia M, Litzow MR, Locatelli F, Marks DI, McCarthy PL, Cowan MJ, Petersdorf EW, Russell JA, Schiller GJ, Schouten H, Spellman S. The graft-*versus*-leukemia effect using matched unrelated donors is not superior to HLA-identical siblings for hematopoietic stem cell transplantation. *Blood.* 2009;113(13):3110–8.

5. Vago L, Toffalori C, Ciceri F, Fleischhauer K. Genomic loss of mismatched human leukocyte antigen and leukemia immune escape from haploidentical graft-*versus*-leukemia. *Semin Oncol.* 2012;39(6):707–15.

6. Weisdorf D, Which donor or graft source should you choose for the strongest GVL? Is there really any difference. *Best Pract Res Clin Haematol* 2013; 26: 293–6.

7. Pegram HJ, Ritchie DS, Smyth MJ, Wiernik A, Prince HM, Darcy PK, Kershaw MH. Alloreactive natural killer cells in hematopoietic stem cell transplantation. *Leuk Res.* 2011;35(1):14–21.

8. Moretta L, Locatelli F, Pende D, Marcenaro E, Mingari MC, Moretta A. Killer Ig-like receptor-mediated control of natural killer cell alloreactivity in haploidentical hematopoietic stem cell transplantation. *Blood.* 2011;117(3):764–71.

9. Davies JO, Stringaris K, Barrett JA, Rezvani K. Opportunities and limitations of natural killer cells as adoptive therapy for malignant disease. *Cytotherapy.* 2014;May 20. [Epub of print]

10. Reshef R, Hexner EO, Frey NV, Stadtmauer EA, Luger SM, Mangan JK, Gill SI, Vassilev P, Lafferty KA, Smith J, Van Deerlin VM, Mick R4, Porter DL. Early donor chimerism levels predict relapse and survival after allogeneic stem-cell transplantation with reduced intensity conditioning. *Biol Blood Marrow Transplant.* 2014; Jul 9. [Epub ahead of print]

11. Reisner Y, Gur H, Reich-Zeliger S, Martelli MF, Bachar-Lustig E. Hematopoietic stem cell transplantation across major genetic barriers: tolerance induction by megadose CD34 cells and other veto cells. *Ann N Y Acad Sci.* 2005;1044:70–83.

12. Singh AK, Savani BN, Albert PS, Barrett AJ. Efficacy of CD34+ stem cell dose in patients undergoing allogeneic peripheral blood stem cell transplantation after total body irradiation.*Biol Blood Marrow Transplant.* 2007;13(3):339–44.

13. Ringdén O, Barrett AJ, Zhang MJ, Loberiza FR, Bolwell BJ, Cairo MS, Gale RP, Hale GA, Litzow MR, Martino R, Russell JA, Tiberghien P, Urbano-Ispizua A, Horowitz MM. Decreased treatment failure in recipients of HLA-identical bone marrow or peripheral blood stem cell transplants with high CD34 cell doses. *Br J Haematol.* 2003;121(6):874–85.

14. Chang YJ, Weng CL, Sun LX, Zhao YT. Allogeneic bone marrow transplantation compared to peripheral blood stem cell transplantation for the treatment of hematologic malignancies: a meta-analysis based on time-to-event data from randomized controlled trials. *Ann Hematol.* 2012;91(3):427–37.

15. Norkin M, Uberti JP, Schiffer CA. Very late recurrences of leukemia: why does leukemia awake after many years of dormancy? *Leuk Res.* 2011;35(2):139–44.

16. Bacigalupo A, Vitale V, Corvo R, Barra S, Lamparelli T, Gualandi F, Mordini N, Berisso G, Bregante S, Raiola AM, Van Lint MT, Frassoni F. The combined effect of total body irradiation (TBI) and cyclosporin A (CyA) on the risk of relapse in patients with acute myeloid leukaemia undergoing allogeneic bone marrow transplantation. *Br J Haematol.* 2000;108:99–104.

17. Locatelli F, Zecca M, Rondelli R, Bonetti F, Dini G, Prete A, Messina C, Uderzo C, Ripaldi M, Porta F, Giorgiani G, Giraldi E, Pession A. Graft *versus* host disease prophylaxis with low-dose cyclosporine-A reduces the risk of relapse in children with acute leukemia given HLA-identical sibling bone marrow transplantation: results of a randomized trial. *Blood.* 2000;95:1572–9.

18. Pulsipher MA, Langholz B, Wall DA, Schultz KR, Bunin N, Carroll WL, Raetz E, Gardner S, Gastier-Foster JM, Howrie D, Goyal RK, Douglas JG, Borowitz M, Barnes Y, Teachey DT, Taylor C, Grupp SA. The addition of sirolimus to tacrolimus/methotrexate GVHD prophylaxis in children with ALL: a phase 3 Children's Oncology Group/Pediatric Blood and Marrow Transplant Consortium trial. *Blood.* 2014;123(13):2017–25.

19. Khouri IF, Lee MS, Saliba RM, Andersson B, Anderlini P, Couriel D, Hosing C, Giralt S, Korbling M, McMannis J, Keating MJ, Champlin RE. Nonablative allogeneic stem cell transplantation for chronic lymphocytic leukemia: impact of rituximab on immunomodulation and survival. *Exp Hematol.* 2004;32(1):28–35.

20. Champlin RE, Passweg JR, Zhang MJ, Rowlings PA, Pelz CJ, Atkinson KA, Barrett AJ, Cahn JY, Drobyski WR, Gale RP, Goldman JM, Gratwohl A, Gordon-Smith EC, Henslee-Downey PJ, Herzig RH, Klein JP, Marmont AM, O'Reilly RJ, Ringdén O, Slavin S, Sobocinski KA, Speck B, Weiner RS, Horowitz MM.T-cell depletion of bone marrow transplants for leukemia from donors other than HLA-identical siblings: advantage of T-cell antibodies with narrow specificities. *Blood.* 2000;95(12):3996–4003.

21. Sheng Z, Ma H, Pang W, Niu S, Xu J. In vivo T-cell depletion with antithymocyte globulins improves overall survival after myeloablative allogeneic stem cell transplantation in patients with hematologic disorders. *Acta Haematol.* 2013;129(3):146–53. doi: 10.1159/000343604. Epub 2012 Nov 30.

22. Devine SM, Carter S, Soiffer RJ, Pasquini MC, Hari PM, Stein A, Lazarus HM, Linker C, Stadtmauer EA, Alyea EP, Keever-Taylor CA, O'Reilly RJ. Low-risk of chronic graft *versus* host disease and relapse associated with

T-cell depleted peripheral blood stem cell transplantation for acute myeloid leukemia in first remission: results of the Blood and Marrow Transplant Clinical Trials Network (BMT CTN) Protocol 0303. *Biol Blood Marrow Transplant*. 2011;17:1343–1351.

23. Bayraktar UD, de Lima M, Saliba RM, Maloy M, Castro-Malaspina HR, Chen J, Rondon G, Chiattone A, Jakubowski AA, Boulad F, Kernan NA, O'Reilly RJ, Champlin RE, Giralt S, Andersson BS, Papadopoulos EB.Ex vivo T cell-depleted *versus* unmodified allografts in patients with acute myeloid leukemia in first complete remission. *Biol Blood Marrow Transplant*. 2013;19(6):898–903.

24. Aversa F, Martelli MF, Velardi A. Haploidentical hematopoietic stem cell transplantation with a megadose T-cell-depleted graft: harnessing natural and adaptive immunity. *Semin Oncol*. 2012;39(6):643–52.

25. Bleakley M, Heimfeld S, Jones LA, Turtle C, Krause D, Riddell SR, Shlomchik W. Engineering human peripheral blood stem cell grafts that are depleted of naïve T cells and retain functional pathogen-specific memory T cells. *Biol Blood Marrow Transplant*. 2014;20(5):705–16.

26. Mielke S, Solomon SR, Barrett AJ. Selective depletion strategies in allogeneic stem cell transplantation. *Cytotherapy*. 2005;7(2):109–15.

27. Bastien JP, Roy J, Roy DC.Donor selective T-cell depletion for haplotype-mismatched allogeneic stem cell transplantation. *Semin Oncol*. 2012;39(6):674–82.

28. Amrolia PJ, Muccioli-Casadei G, Huls H, Adams S, Durett A, Gee A, Yvon E, Weiss H, Cobbold M, Gaspar HB, Rooney C, Kuehnle I, Ghetie V, Schindler J, Krance R, Heslop HE, Veys P, Vitetta E, Brenner MK. Adoptive immunotherapy with allodepleted donor T-cells improves immune reconstitution after haploidentical stem cell transplantation. *Blood*. 2006;108(6):1797–808.

29. Fuchs EJ. Human leukocyte antigen-haploidentical stem cell transplantation using T-cell-replete bone marrow grafts. *Curr Opin Hematol*. 2012;19:440–7.

30. Kanakry CG, Ganguly S, Zahurak M, Bolaños-Meade J, Thoburn C, Perkins

B, Fuchs EJ, Jones RJ, Hess AD, Luznik L. Aldehyde dehydrogenase expression drives human regulatory T cell resistance toposttransplantation cyclophosphamide. *Sci Transl Med*. 2013;5(211):211ra157.

31. Baron F, Beguin Y. Preemptive cellular immunotherapy after T-cell-depleted allogeneic hematopoietic stem cell transplantation. *Biol Blood Marrow Transplant*. 2002;8:351–9.

32. Chang YJ, Huang XJ.Donor lymphocyte infusions for relapse after allogeneic transplantation: when, if and for whom? *Blood Rev*. 2013;27:55–62.

33. Kolb HJ, Rank A, Chen X, Woiciechowsky A, Roskrow M, Schmid C, Tischer J, Ledderose G.In-vivo generation of leukaemia-derived dendritic cells. *Best Pract Res Clin Haematol*. 2004;17:439–51.

34. Martino M, Fedele R, Moscato T, Ronco F.Optimizing outcomes following allogeneic hematopoietic progenitor cell transplantation in AML: the role of hypomethylating agents. *Curr Cancer Drug Targets*. 2013;13:661–9.

35. Joks M, Jurczyszyn A, Machaczka M, Skotnicki AB, Komarnicki M. The roles of consolidation and maintenance therapy with novel agents after autologous stem cell transplantation in patients with multiple myeloma. *Eur J Haematol*. 2015;94(2):109–14.

36. Neelapu SS, Munshi NC, Jagannath S, Watson TM, Pennington R, Reynolds C, Barlogie B, Kwak LW.Tumor antigen immunization of sibling stem cell transplant donors in multiple myeloma. *Bone Marrow Transplant*. 2005;36:315–23.

37. Weng J, Cha SC, Matsueda S, Alatrash G, Popescu MS, Yi Q, Molldrem JJ, Wang M, Neelapu SS, Kwak LW. Targeting human B-cell malignancies through Ig light chain-specific cytotoxic T lymphocytes. *Clin Cancer Res*. 2011;17(18):5945–52.

38. Rezvani K, Barrett AJ. Characterizing and optimizing immune responses to leukaemia antigens after allogeneic stem cell transplantation. *Best Pract Res Clin Haematol*. 2008;21:437–53.

39. Falkenburg JH, Willemze R.Minor histocompatibility antigens as targets of cellular immunotherapy in leukaemia. *Best Pract Res Clin Haematol*. 2004;17:415–25.

40. Riddell SR, Bleakley M, Nishida T, Berger C, Warren EH. Adoptive transfer of allogeneic antigen-specific T cells. *Biol Blood Marrow Transplant*. 2006;12 (Suppl 1):9–12

41. Bleakley M, Otterud BE, Richardt JL, Mollerup AD, Hudecek M, Nishida T, Chaney CN, Warren EH, Leppert MF, Riddell SR. Leukemia-associated minor histocompatibility antigen discovery using T-cell clones isolated by in vitro stimulation of naive CD8+ T cells. *Blood*. 2010;115(23):4923–33.

42. Warren EH, Fujii N, Akatsuka Y, Chaney CN, Mito JK, Loeb KR, Gooley TA, Brown ML, Koo KK, Rosinski KV, Ogawa S, Matsubara A, Appelbaum FR, Riddell SR. Therapy of relapsed leukemia after allogeneic hematopoietic cell transplantation with T cells specific for minor histocompatibility antigens. *Blood*. 2010;115(19):3869–78.

43. Nagai K, Ochi T, Fujiwara H, An J, Shirakata T, Mineno J, Kuzushima K, Shiku H, Melenhorst JJ, Gostick E, Price DA, Ishii E, Yasukawa M. Aurora kinase A-specific T-cell receptor gene transfer redirects T lymphocytes to display effective antileukemia reactivity. *Blood*. 2012;119:368–76.

44. Linette GP, Stadtmauer EA, Maus MV, Rapoport AP, Levine BL, Emery L, Litzky L, Bagg A, Carreno BM, Cimino PJ, Binder-Scholl GK, Smethurst DP, Gerry AB, Pumphrey NJ, Bennett AD, Brewer JE, Dukes J, Harper J, Tayton-Martin HK, Jakobsen BK, Hassan NJ, Kalos M, June CH. Cardiovascular toxicity and titin cross-reactivity of affinity-enhanced T cells in myeloma and melanoma. *Blood*. 2013;122(6):863–71.

45. Weber G, Gerdemann U, Caruana I, Savoldo B, Hensel NF, Rabin KR, Shpall EJ, Melenhorst JJ, Leen AM, Barrett AJ, Bollard CM. Generation of multi-leukemia antigen-specific T cells to enhance the graft-*versus*-leukemia effect after allogeneic stem cell transplant. *Leukemia*. 2013;27:1538–47.

46. Weber G, Caruana I, Rouce RH, Barrett AJ, Gerdemann U, Leen AM, Rabin KR, Bollard CM.Generation of tumor antigen-specific T cell lines from pediatric patients with acute lymphoblastic leukemia–implications for immunotherapy. *Clin Cancer Res*. 2013;19:5079–91.

47. Duong CP, Yong CS, Kershaw MH, Slaney CY, Darcy PK. Cancer

immunotherapy utilizing gene-modified T cells: From the bench to the clinic.*Mol Immunol.* 2015;67(2 Pt A):46–57.

48. Hoffman LM, Gore L. Blinatumomab, a bi-specific anti-CD19/CD3 BiTE(®) antibody for the treatment of acute lymphoblastic leukemia: perspectives and current pediatric applications. *Front Oncol.* 2014; 4:63.

49. Oliveira G, Greco R, Lupo-Stanghellini MT, Vago L, Bonini C. Use of TK-cells in haploidentical hematopoietic stem cell transplantation. *Curr Opin Hematol.* 2012;19:427–33.

50. Tey SK, Dotti G, Rooney CM, Heslop HE, Brenner MK. Inducible caspase 9 suicide gene to improve the safety of allodepleted T cells after haploidentical stem cell transplantation. *Biol Blood Marrow Transplant.* 2007;13:913–24.

51. Karadimitris A, Chaidos A. The role of invariant NKT cells in allogeneic hematopoietic stem cell transplantation. *Crit Rev Immunol.* 2012;32:157–71.

52. Locatelli F, Merli P, Rutella S. At the bedside: innate immunity as an immunotherapy tool for hematological malignancies. *J Leuk Biol.* 2013;94:1141–57.

Chapter

66

Expanded Umbilical Cord Cells: Benefits and Limitations

Rohtesh S. Mehta, Katayoun Rezvani, and Elizabeth J. Shpall

Introduction

Cord blood (CB) is an attractive donor source for patients who lack an human leukocyte antigen (HLA)-matched peripheral blood (PB) or bone marrow (BM) graft for an allogeneic (allo) hematopoietic cell transplant (HCT). The probability of finding an HLA-matched PB or BM donor is only about 40% and is lower for patients of non-Caucasian origin[1]. Since the first human umbilical cord blood transplant (CBT), which took place in 1988[2], the number of CBTs has been increasing gradually, especially for younger patients. From 2002 through 2011, the preferred donor sources were PB and BM; CB was used in only 3–6% of allo-HCTs in patients >20 years old and about 20% of allo-HCTs in patients <20 years old. However, in 2010–11, the corresponding numbers for CBT were 12% and 43%, respectively[1]. Improved transplantation procedures and increasing awareness of CB biology and its distinctive benefits are among the reasons for the surge in CBT.

Advantages and Disadvantages of CBT

Among alternative donor transplantation procedures, CBT holds several unique advantages, including ease of collection, negligible risk of infection transmission, ready availability, lack of donor attrition, better tolerability of a greater degree of HLA mismatch, and yet lower incidence of graft-*versus*-host disease (GvHD) among alternative donor sources[3–8]. The rapidity of procuring HLA-typed cryopreserved CB units is exceedingly beneficial for patients in urgent need of allograft. However, CBT is associated with a higher risk of graft rejection, delayed engraftment, and immune reconstitution which can lead to an increased risk of infection, relapse, or nonrelapse mortality (NRM)[9,10]. These adverse effects are partly explained by the low total number of nucleated cells (TNCs) and CD34+ cell doses available for CBT, which are only about 5–10% of the doses available in PB or BM allografts. The cell dose is directly proportional to transplant outcome in CBT. Patients receiving less than 1.7×10^5 CD34+ cells/kg experience delayed engraftment and a higher rate of treatment-related mortality (TRM)[7]. The minimum recommended TNC dose is $2.5–3 \times 10^7$/kg for 5–6/6 HLA-matched CBT; a higher dose is needed for additional mismatches. In CBT trials using a "myeloablative" conditioning (MAC) regimen,

the median CD34+ cell dose ranged from 0.9×10^5/kg to 1.2×10^5/kg, which produced neutrophil and platelet engraftment at a median of 22–27 days and 40–90 days, respectively. The corresponding engraftment times for BM transplant are about 18–22 days and 25–40 days[11–15].

Two strategies to increase the cell dose are[1] to use double-unit CBT (dCBT) and[2] to use *ex-vivo* expansion of CB progenitor cells. Although the use of dCBT is safe and circumvents the limitation of low cell dose[16], it does not yield the "more rapid" engraftment seen with PB and BM allotransplants. *Ex-vivo* expansion of CB provides an excellent platform because there are far more colony-forming unit–granulocyte-macrophages (CFU-GMs) in CB than in adult PB and about the same number as in BM[17,18]. Further, the primitive subpopulation of CB progenitor cells, as defined by their CD34+CD38− immunophenotype, has greater proliferative ability than BM progenitor cells[19,20].

Low cell doses have traditionally also prohibited the successful use of adoptive cellular immunotherapies that have been effectively employed with other types of allo-grafts to manage infection or disease relapse[21–24]. *Ex-vivo* engineering not only allows expansion of hematopoietic progenitor cells but also creates an array of research opportunities in antivirus and antitumor adoptive immunotherapies, GvHD prevention (see Chapter 12), and homing augmentation (discussed later in the chapter).

Ex-vivo Expansion of CB Progenitor Cells

A variety of *ex-vivo* expansion techniques have been explored, varying from the choice of primary cell population of interest (CD34+, CD133+, or mononuclear cells), type of device used for purification, selection of culture medium, presence or absence of stromal support, and culture duration. Further, the cytokines used range from any combination of stem cell factor (SCF), granulocyte colony-stimulating factor (G-CSF), GM colony-stimulating factor (GM-CSF), Fms-like tyrosine kinase 3 ligand (FLT3-L), interleukin (IL)-3, IL-6, IL-11, megakaryocyte growth and differentiation factor, and thrombopoietin (TPO)[25–33]. The timing of thawing of CB in relation to the time of transplant and the proportion of the graft used for expansion have also varied considerably in trials.

Static Culture Method with Cytokines

One of the earliest trials used the "static culture" technique, whereby CD34+ cells were purified from CB mononuclear cells with the Isolex 300-i device (Nexell, Irvine, CA) and anti-CD34 antibody. This process yielded only 30–45% of the initial thawed CD34+ cells. Purified CD34+ cells were then cultured in medium containing SCF, G-CSF, and megakaryocyte growth and differentiation factor for 10 days, which resulted in a median expansion of 4-fold. Yet, the median CD34+ dose available for infusion in adult patients was only 0.89×10^5/kg (median TNC count, 0.79×10^7/kg); this outcome was attributed to the initial significant cell loss resulting from the selection technique. The median time to neutrophil or platelet engraftments depended on the study stratum and cohort (range 26–31 days and 73–126 days, respectively), without any statistical differences. Further, the rate of acute or chronic GvHD in adults was 80% and 90%, respectively, despite no detectable T-cells in the CD34+-expanded population[34].

Continuous Perfusion Method

An automated continuous perfusion culture device, such as the Aastrom Replicell bioreactor, continuously perfuses the culture system with cytokines and maintains optimal culture conditions based on a computer-generated system that continuously monitors the biologic and physiologic environment. In a clinical trial using this system, CB samples were thawed on day 0, a majority of which was infused unmanipulated on the same day (median TNC count, 2.05×10^7/kg), but a small fraction (TNC count, $1-2 \times 10^8$) was used for expansion and infused on day 12 for a "boost." The culture medium was supplemented with cytokines, including PIXY321 (a fusion protein of IL-3 and GM-CSF), FLT3-L, and erythropoietin. This resulted in an increased TNC count by a median of 2.4-fold, and CD34+ expansion was variable and feeble (median 0.5-fold; range 0.09- to 2.45-fold). The median dose of expanded cells infused was 2.05×10^7/kg, and the median time to neutrophil or platelet engraftment was 22 and 71 days, respectively. Three out of 22 patients failed to achieve engraftment, and 2 died prior to engraftment. Moderate or severe acute GvHD occurred in eight patients (36%). Of note, the study included mostly pediatric patients (median age 4.5 years; median weight 17 kg)[35].

This study raised concerns about the potential loss of early progenitor cells (EPCs) because CD34+ cells differentiate into mature cells during *ex-vivo* expansion, leading to an increased TNC count[36]. Thus, methods to block the *in-vitro* differentiation of CD34+ cells in an attempt to expand the number of EPCs have been explored.

Early Progenitor Cell Differentiation Blockers

Copper Chelators

The role of copper in the proliferation and differentiation of progenitor cells is well defined. Techniques incorporating copper chelators in the culture medium have been developed to block early progenitor cell (EPC) differentiation[37]. A preclinical study showed that the addition of a polyamine copper chelator, tetraethylenepentamine, to culture medium with FLT3-L, IL-6, TPO, and SCF inhibited the differentiation of EPCs (CD34+CD38−, or CD34+Lin−) without affecting the proliferation of mature committed cells (CD34+Lin+). In a preliminary study, 3 weeks of culturing purified CD133+ cells resulted in substantial expansion of CD34+ cells (89-fold), CD34+CD38− cells (30-fold), and CFU unit cells (172-fold). Transplantation of *ex-vivo*-expanded cells in NOD-SCID mice resulted in significantly superior engraftment compared with transplantation with unexpanded cells[38].

Clinical Studies of Expansion of CB Progenitor Cells: StemEx® (Copper Chelation-Based)-Based Expansion?

On the basis of encouraging preclinical results, a phase 1–2 study was conducted at the MD Anderson Cancer Center. A fraction of single-unit cryopreserved CB samples was thawed on day −20, from which enriched CD133+ cells were cultured in bags using tetraethylenepentamine (TEPA) and the cytokine cocktail described for the previous study. Overall, an average expansion of TNCs and CD34+ cells of 219-fold and 6-fold, respectively, was observed after 3 weeks of culturing. The expanded cells were infused into the patients 24 hours following the infusion of the unmanipulated CB fraction. The median number of TNCs infused was 2.23×10^7/kg (range 1.12×10^7/kg to 5.63×10^7/kg). The median time to neutrophil or platelet engraftment was 30 and 48 days, respectively, which is similar to the times for historical recipients of unmanipulated single CB units[39]. A subsequent large prospective multinational trial conducted using this technique reported faster neutrophil engraftment (21 *versus* 28 days; $P < 0.0001$) and an improved overall survival at 100 days (84.2% *versus* 74.6%; 95% CI 0.5 (0.26–0.95); $P = 0.035$)) without any differences in acute or chronic GvHD compared with controls from the Center for International Blood and Marrow Transplant Research (CIBMTR) and Eurocord registries[40]. This methodology holds the promise of increasing the number of CBT being performed while potentially reducing its short-term morbidity and mortality.

Nicotinamide

Nicotinamide (NAM), a form of vitamin B3, has an important role in the adhesion, migration, proliferation, and differentiation of embryonic stem cells and primary nonhematopoietic cells[41]. In a preclinical study, culturing with CD34+-selected CB cells supported by SCF, TPO, IL-6, and FLT3-L with or without NAM resulted in an CD34+ expansion of about 40-fold in both treatment groups. However, the EPCs (CD34+Lin− cells) expanded to a notably greater degree in NAM-treated cells, which also exhibited enhanced migratory potential in response to CXCL12. Transplantation of carboxy-fluorescein diacetate succinimidyl ester (CFSE)-labeled cells into irradiated NOD/SCID mice showed a 3-fold increased number of CD34+CFSE+ cells with BM homing potential and about a 7-fold increase in engraftment potential compared with untreated cells[42].

Clinical Study with Expansion of CB Progenitor Cells: Addition of Nicotinamide?

In a phase 1 trial, NAM-treated cord was co-infused with an unmanipulated cord in 11 adults with hematologic malignancies. The time to neutrophil engraftment (13 versus 25 days), but not the platelet engraftment, was significantly shorter than the institutional historical controls[43].

Notch Signaling

The instrumental role of Notch signaling in the early development and differentiation of many invertebrate systems led to the discovery of TAN1, the human Notch homolog in CD34+ BM cells[44]. Later, constitutive Notch signaling was shown to establish immortalized, cytokine-dependent cell lines. In that study, primitive mouse BM cells were transduced with a retrovirus expressing the intracellular domain of Notch1 and a green fluorescent protein (GFP). After 2 days, GFP+ cells were isolated and cultured in liquid culture medium with SCF, IL-6, IL-11, and FLT3-L, where the cells continued to proliferate undifferentiated without any stromal support for over 8 months. Notably, the cells retained their ability to differentiate ex-vivo or in-vivo into either myeloid cells in the presence of GM-CSF or lymphoid cells in the presence of SCF, IL-3, and IL-7[45].

In subsequent studies, CD34+-selected CB cells were transduced with an engineered Notch ligand (Delta1$^{ext-IgG}$) and cultured for 16 days in serum-free medium with IL-3, IL-6, TPO, SCF, and FLT3-L, which led to an average expansion of CD34+ cells of 222-fold, as compared to 68-fold expansion for cells cultured with control immunoglobulin G. Infusion of the expanded cells into NOD-SCID mice showed a substantially superior in-vivo repopulating ability (compared with control mice) that resulted in both myeloid and lymphoid human cell engraftment. Further, human cell engraftment, defined as $\geq$0.5% human CD45+ cells in the BM, was observed as early as 10 days after the transplant in all mice receiving Delta1$^{ext-IgG}$-cultured cells.

Clinical Study with Expansion of CB Progenitor Cells Notch-Mediated Expansion?

A phase I study is ongoing in patients with acute leukemia who are undergoing MAC dCBT, in which one ex-vivo expanded unit is infused 4 hours after the infusion of an unmanipulated unit. In the preliminary analysis (n=10), the median time to neutrophil engraftment was 16 days. No infusion-related toxicities were noted; primary graft rejection occurred in one patient. All evaluable patients developed grade 2 acute GvHD,

except one who had grade 3 acute GvHD. There was no extensive chronic GvHD, while limited chronic GvHD was noted in three patients. At a median follow-up of 354 days, 70% of the patients were in complete remission with sustained engraftment. Interestingly, two patients had long-term persistence of the expanded cells, until day 180 and day 240. However, the expanded cells did not persist beyond 1 year, after which the unexpanded CB unit completely contributed to engraftment[46].

Mesenchymal Stem Cell-Supported Expansion Techniques

An entirely distinct technique of ex-vivo expansion focuses on simulating the in-vivo environment of EPC growth thereby circumventing any manipulations to the EPC differentiation pathway. Mesenchymal stem cells (MSCs) form a BM "niche" for hematopoiesis by producing cytokines and other proteins that regulate cell proliferation and homing. Ex-vivo coculturing of MSCs promotes the growth of hematopoietic stem cells [47]. Although purified CD34+ or CD133+ cells can be supported in cultures without MSC support and with the help of cytokines alone, the purification process itself can result in a significant upfront loss of cell numbers. The median recovery of the target cells in the previously described studies was about 35% (range 4–70%). Therefore, even after significant expansion with cytokine-supported cultures, the ultimate cell dose may not be satisfactory. In this regard, coculture with MSC is advantageous because this approach does not require initial purification of CD34+ or CD133+ cells[48].

MSCs can be obtained from the BM harvest of an HLA haploidentical family member. However, it takes a long time to generate the final product for the transplant because of obvious logistic difficulties. The availability of clinical grade "off-the-shelf" MSC precursor cells, such as Mesoblast (Mesoblast Limited, Melbourne, Australia), has significantly shortened this process (see Chapter 68)[49].

Landmark Study: Mesenchymal Stem Cell-Supported Expansion

In a landmark study with 31 patients that used this technique, one unit was expanded ex-vivo for 2 weeks and infused concurrently with the unexpanded unit. The culture resulted in 12.2-, 30.1-, and 17.5-fold increases in the TNC, CD34+, and colony-forming unit-C populations, respectively, producing final median doses of 5.84×10^7/kg, 0.97×10^6/kg, and 3×10^6/kg, respectively. There were no notable differences in the expansion achieved from family member-derived or "off-the-shelf" MSC. The median time to neutrophil or platelet engraftment was 15 and 42 days, respectively; these values were significantly shorter than the CIBMTR control times. The rates of grade II–IV acute GvHD (42%), grade III–IV acute GvHD (13%), and chronic GvHD (45%) were similar to the CIBMTR control times[50].

Role of *Ex-vivo* Expansion in Adoptive Immunotherapy

The effect of the notably improved engraftments seen with some of the novel techniques described above on long-term immune reconstitution is unknown. Moreover, disease relapse, infection, and GvHD are still the leading causes of mortality in all types of transplants[1]. To counter these adverse outcomes, adoptive immunotherapy has been employed in other types of transplants (see Chapter 64) except for CBT, primarily due to the low cell counts in CBT. The implementation of *ex-vivo* expansion has now introduced these therapies to CBT as well.

Cord Blood Virus-Specific Cytotoxic T-Lymphocytes: CB for Viral Infections?

The delayed immune reconstitution and the naivety of the CB immune system create the risk of critical infection after CBT. Among viruses, cytomegalovirus (CMV), Epstein–Barr virus (EBV), and adenovirus are the most commonly encountered infections[51]. The use of donor PB-derived virus-specific cytotoxic T-lymphocytes (CTLs) in the PB allo-HCT setting[21–24] is relatively straightforward as these infections are almost universal and generation of virus-specific CTLs requires relatively straightforward expansion of the memory T-lymphocytes. However, CB mandates the priming of naïve T-cells to specific infections followed by their *ex-vivo* expansion[52–54].

Initial preclinical studies concentrated on the generation of single virus-specific CTLs, such as CTLs against EBV[54] or CMV[53]. However, multivirus-specific CTLs possessing activity against EBV, CMV, and adenovirus have been created and are currently being tested in a clinical trial[52]. In this study, the *ex-vivo* expansion was performed with only 20% of the CB graft in the setting of a single CBT. Preliminary results (n=8) showed this method to be safe and effective for expanding virus-specific CTLs *in-vivo*. None of the eight patients who received CB-derived CTLs developed acute toxicity or grade II or higher acute GvHD. More strikingly, the CTLs were able to clear reactivated CMV infection within weeks of infusion in most of the patients without the use of conventional treatment. Similarly, all patients with high EBV loads and almost every patient with adenovirus infection were able to clear the viruses[55].

Cord Blood Donor Lymphocyte Infusion: CB for Relapse Disease?

The use of donor lymphocyte infusion (DLI) to treat relapse or persistent disease after an allo-HCT dates back to over a decade[56]. With *ex-vivo* expansion using anti-CD3/CD28 magnetic enrichment techniques and culture with IL-2, CB T-cells can now be expanded by a median of 100-fold while maintaining their polyclonal T-cell receptor diversity[57]. This advancement has allowed CB-donor DLI to proceed to a phase 1 clinical trial (ClinicalTrials.gov:NCT01630564).

Cord Blood Leukemia-Specific Cytotoxic T-Lymphocytes: Better than PB CTL?

In general, leukemia cells are poorly immunogenic and possess an immunosuppressive profile. However, by virtue of uncertain mechanisms, CB T-cells may recognize tumor cells better than PB T-cells[58]. Several techniques to generate leukemia-specific CTL have been reported, which are described elsewhere.

With the use of one of those methods, adenovirus-transduced CD40L+ CB T-cells demonstrated *in-vivo* leukemia-specific cytotoxicity in a mouse model with no evidence of GvHD[59]. A different method targeted tumor-associated antigens, a large number of which have been identified[60]. One study reported the generation of multitumor-associated antigen-specific CTLs carrying activity against WT1, NE, Pr3, MAGE-A3, and PRAME from PB as well as CB. In contrast to PB-derived CTLs, which were primarily reactive against a particular antigen, CB-derived CTLs did not target a particular antigen. CB-derived CTLs could thus be used clinically against a broad range of myeloid malignancies[61].

One of the major breakthroughs in the field of adoptive immunotherapy was the introduction of chimeric receptor antigen (CAR) T-cells, which are created by gene transfer using a lentiviral or retroviral vector. Since the first reported case of its use in 1990, CAR T-cell therapy has evolved considerably[62–68]. Most recently, CD19-specific CAR T-cells were created with a novel nonvirus-based gene transfer technique, known as the *Sleeping Beauty*. In this method, T-cells are electroporated to simultaneously introduce two DNA plasmids consisting of a transposon (CD19RCD28) and a transposase. This technique is currently under investigation in a clinical trial[69,70].

Combined Antitumor and Antivirus Immunotherapy

Taking the genetically modified T-cell approach one step further, single-product CD19-CAR T-cells have been created that not only possess an antitumor effect but also are active against EBV, CMV, and adenovirus[71].

Cord Blood Natural Killer Cell Antitumor Immunotherapy

Natural killer (NK) cells are another enticing candidate for adoptive immunotherapy due to their multiple potential advantages over T-cells[72,73]. *Ex-vivo* expansion of CB NK cells not only increases their numbers but also results in their activation. Several approaches have been conceived to expand CB NK cells *ex-vivo*.

One technique is a two-step process of isolating and expanding CD34+ cells for 2 weeks and then expanding and differentiating NK cells for 5 weeks. Although this process resulted in the generation of functional human NK cells in excess of four log from freshly collected CB samples[74], it is a technically tedious and lengthy procedure. Another method involves positively selecting CD56+CD3− NK cells from CB mononuclear cells and culturing them in IL-2-containing medium for 2 weeks. This approach led to a median expansion of 92-fold, increased expression of activating receptor NKp44, no change in killer cell immunoglobulin-like receptor expression, and enhanced *in-vivo* antileukemia activity in a NOD-SCID-IL2Rγ^{null} mouse model[75]. In a novel technique using a GP500 gas-permeable bioreactor and a feeder layer of irradiated artificial antigen-presenting cells, a mean expansion of 1848-fold of NK cells from fresh CB and a mean expansion of 2389-fold from frozen CB samples were reported. The expanded NK cells demonstrated significant *in-vivo* cytotoxicity against a multiple myeloma target in a mouse model[76].

Clinical Studies: Cord Blood NK Cells for Cancer

Two phase 1–2 clinical trials are evaluating the safety and efficacy of prophylactic CB NK infusion in the setting of CBT for patients with chronic lymphocytic leukemia (ClinicalTrials.gov: NCT01619761) and in conjunction with autologous HCT for patients with multiple myeloma (ClinicalTrials.gov:NCT01729091).

Role of *Ex-vivo* Expansion in Preventing GvHD

Although the risk of severe acute or chronic GvHD is significantly lower with CBT than with transplants using alternative donor grafts, GvHD remains one of the leading causes of TRM. Naturally occurring regulatory T-cells (Treg cells) can inhibit alloreactive T-cells, reduce the risk of GvHD and graft rejection, improve immune reconstitution, and prevent opportunistic infections without restricting the graft-*versus*-leukemia effect of the graft[77]. Despite these impressive roles, the clinical use of Treg cells for transplantation has been implemented rather slowly due to the very low number of Treg cells in circulation and the risk of low purity of extraction, which can lead to the presence of activated conventional T-cells which can actually trigger GvHD. CB offers certain advantages over PB for Treg cell immunotherapy. First, there is a paucity of memory T-cells in CB compared with in PB, which reduces contamination by conventional T-cells. Second, Treg cells represent a marginally higher proportion of TNCs in CB (approximately 5%) and their purification is noted to be superior to that of PB.

Various protocols have been formulated to purify CB Treg cells *ex-vivo*. A study that used two-step magnetic separation to extract CB Treg cells *ex-vivo* resulted in a roughly 100-fold expansion[78]. Another method of coculturing, which purified Treg cells with engineered artificial antigen-presenting cells, yielded a Treg cell expansion of >1250-fold with significant *in-vivo* suppression of GvHD in a xenogenic

GvHD lethality model[79]. A recent study from the MD Anderson Cancer Center demonstrated the feasibility of using clinically relevant "off-the-shelf" *ex-vivo*-expanded Treg cells from third-party cryopreserved CB samples. Infusion of the purified *ex-vivo*-expanded Treg cells followed by infusion of allogeneic PB mononuclear cells the next day prevented GvHD and prolonged survival in irradiated NOD-SCID IL-2Rγ^{null} mice[80].

Clinical Studies: Infusion of Tregs to Prevent GvHD but at What Cost?

A "first-in-human" single-center, phase 1 dose-escalating trial revealed the feasibility, safety, and effectiveness of using *ex-vivo*–expanded Treg cells from partially HLA-matched third-party cryopreserved CB samples in 23 patients with hematologic malignancies who were undergoing CBT[81]. However, an update of the study reported increased cumulative density of viral reactivations within the first 30 days of infusion as compared with the historical controls but no difference in the rate of fungal infection, NRM, or PFS. These results suggested heightened immune suppression with Treg cell infusion that may raise the risk of viral reactivation[82]. An ongoing phase 1 study is evaluating further dose escalations (from 1×10^5 to 3000×10^5 Treg cells/kg body weight); the findings will shed more light on this issue (Clinicaltrial.gov; NCT00602693).

Role of *Ex-vivo* Expansion in Enhancing Homing

Apart from boosting the cell dose for a transplant and permitting the use of adoptive immunotherapies, *ex-vivo* expansion allows for research involving augmentation of the homing capacity of CB progenitor cells and consequent engraftment. This approach is being tested in clinical trials using different techniques.

Ex-vivo Fucosylation of CB CD34+ Cells and Clinical Implications

Successful homing of graft is a multistep process and includes interactions between adhesion molecule receptors (E- or P-selectins) on vascular endothelial cells and selectin ligands on hematopoietic cells. One of the major shortcomings of CBT is deficient homing to BM, which is attributed to poor fucosylation of the selectin ligands, such as P-selectin glycoprotein ligand 1[83]. A recent study at the MD Anderson Cancer Center showed that compared with unmanipulated human CB CD34+ cells, human CB CD34+ cells treated with fucosyltransferase (FT)-VI and GDP-fucose improved their homing capacity, resulting in faster and significantly higher rates of engraftment in mouse models[84]. A later study suggested that although both FT-VI and FT-VII have similar potential to fucosylate CB CD34+ cells, FT-VII was also able to fucosylate T- and B-lymphocytes. This ability may play a crucial role in promoting the graft-*versus*-leukemia effect while minimizing GvHD[85]. A clinical trial involving infusion of one unmanipulated CB unit and one *ex-vivo* fucosylated CB unit is currently assessing the efficacy of this approach in improving clinical endpoints (ClinicalTrials.gov Identifier: NCT01471067).

Ex-vivo CB Cells Treatment with Prostaglandin E2 Analogs

Ex-vivo pulse treatment by prostaglandin E2 (PGE2) stimulates the growth and homing potential of multilineage progenitor cells. This stimulation has been postulated to be mediated via up-regulation of the apoptosis-inhibiting protein *Survivin*, proliferation genes such as cyclin D1 (leading to selective stimulation and self-renewal capabilities of primitive hematopoietic stem cells), and up-regulation of the chemokine receptor CXCR4[86].

A phase 1 clinical trial recently evaluated the safety and efficacy of a PGE2 derivative (dmPGE2) in the dCBT setting involving *ex-vivo* treatment of one of the CB units. The study included two separate cohorts: the smaller unit was incubated with dmPGE2 in 6 of the 9 patients in cohort 1, while the larger unit underwent *ex-vivo* treatment prior to the infusion in all 12 patients in cohort 2 and the remaining 3 patients in cohort 1. The median time to neutrophil engraftment was 24 days and 17.5 days in cohorts 1 and 2, respectively. The corresponding times for platelet engraftments were 72.5 and 43 days. Two of the nine patients in cohort 1 experienced graft failure, while no graft failure occurred in the second cohort. In addition, the second cohort demonstrated sustained engraftment from PGE2-treated CB in some patients for up to 27 months. Additional studies are ongoing[87].

Ex-vivo CB Cells Treatment with DPP-IV Inhibitor

Dipeptidyl peptidase-4 (DPP-IV)/CD26 is a membrane-bound peptidase that inhibits the migratory potential of CD34+ cells by cleaving CXCL12/SDF-1α (stromal cell-derived factor 1) at its N-terminal[88]. An active form of DPP-IV/CD26 is present on a small subset of CB CD34+ cells. Inhibition of DPP-IV activity using a specific inhibitor (Diprotin-A) significantly increased the homing capacity of CD34+/CD26+ cells[88] as well as long-term engraftment of Sca-1+lin⁻ BM donor cells in mouse models[89]. The role of an oral DPP-IV inhibitor, sitagliptin, is currently under investigation in a phase 2 study (Clinicaltrials.gov, NCT00862719).

Current Challenges of *Ex-vivo* Expansion

Some earlier studies raised the apprehension that *ex-vivo* expansion may increase the number of "low quality" hematopoietic progenitor cells that are capable of short-term reconstitution, resulting in faster but nonsustained engraftment that could ultimately lead to graft failure. This is implied even

in the most recent studies using novel techniques in which *in-vivo* persistence of the expanded CB was observed for only a few patients and was eventually lost, at which time the unexpanded CB provided complete engraftment. However, the use of dCBT ensures short-term rapid engraftment from the expanded CB and long-term engraftment from the unexpanded CB, thus providing a dependable mechanism to prevent graft rejection. Significant progress in the field of *ex-vivo* expansion could be achieved by increasing the number of "high-quality" BM-repopulating EPCs capable of providing durable engraftment.

Another area for improvement is shortening the duration required for *ex-vivo* expansion. Currently, even the most advanced techniques require at least 10–14 days of culture before the final product is ready. This extended time delays transplantation, which is undesirable for patients in urgent need of a transplant. Further, although the results on engraftment noted in some recent studies are highly encouraging, the effects on immune reconstitution and long-term clinical outcomes are not yet known. Finally, there is a risk of graft contamination by any kind of *ex-vivo* graft manipulation. However, these procedures are conducted in good manufacturing practice-grade laboratories by trained professionals, so the risk is theoretical. Moreover, to date all of the clinical studies have shown these techniques to be safe. The economics of these novel procedures will become an important part of the decision-making process once any of these methods get approval for routine practice (see Chapter 61).

Summary and Future Directions

CB is an attractive alternative donor source for patients lacking a suitable HLA-identical donor. It is readily available, is well tolerated, and results in less GvHD compared with transplants using BM or PB despite a greater degree of HLA mismatch. However, the low cell dose in CB grafts contributes to adverse outcomes such as graft rejection, delayed engraftment, and poor immune reconstitution, creating the risks of disease relapse and infection.

The advent of *ex-vivo* expansion, in conjunction with better understanding of CB biology and its management, has resulted in a remarkable surge in the number of CBTs performed over the past decade. The techniques for *ex-vivo* expansion have advanced impressively: methods range from "static culture" to continuous perfusion; a variety of cytokines and culture media are available; specific, isolated subpopulation of CB cells (CD34+ or CD133+ cells, T-lymphocytes, or NK cells) can be expanded; and EPCs specifically may be expanded by blocking their *ex-vivo* differentiation by using copper chelators or NAM or by targeting *Notch* signaling and the use of stromal cells to simulate *in-vivo* growth environment for CB progenitor cells *ex-vivo*. Many of the recent studies have shown substantially enhanced CB engraftment in clinical trials that approach those observed with transplants using alternative donor material.

Ex-vivo expansion not only increases the cell dose for a transplant but also opens doors for a host of fascinating graft engineering studies. It has permitted the generation and clinical use of multiple virus-specific and leukemia-specific CTLs to prevent or combat viral infection and disease relapse, respectively. *Ex-vivo*-expanded Treg cell infusions are being tested in clinical trials as a G*v*HD prophylaxis. Further, studies are ongoing to augment the homing potential of CB progenitor cells using *ex-vivo* fucosylation, prostaglandin E2 analogs, and DPP-IV inhibitors.

Despite the recent dramatic innovations, the field of *ex-vivo* expansion is still in a state of infancy. An ideal *ex-vivo* expansion process will be concise, be reproducible across laboratories, lead to the largest possible expansion of "high-quality"

hematopoietic progenitor cells, produce the final product quickly, and ultimately improve the clinical outcomes.

Acknowledgments

The authors would like to thank Nina D. Shah, Chitra M. Hosing, Betul Oran, Amanda L. Olson, Uday R. Popat, Amin M. Alousi, Simrit Parmar, Partow Kebriaei, Laurence J.N. Cooper, Priti Tewari, Joshua Kellner, and Ian K. Mc Niece at the Department of Stem Cell Transplantation and Cellular Therapy, UT MD Anderson Cancer Center, Houston, TX, and Catherine M. Bollard and Patrick J. Hanley at the Children's National Hospital System and The George Washington University, Washington, DC.

References

1. Pasquini M, Wang Z. Current use and outcome of hematopoietic stem cell transplantation: CIBMTR Summary Slides, 2013. Available at: http://www.cibmtr.org.

2. Gluckman E, Broxmeyer HA, Auerbach AD, Friedman HS, Douglas GW, Devergie A, et al. Hematopoietic reconstitution in a patient with Fanconi's anemia by means of umbilical-cord blood from an HLA-identical sibling. *The New England Journal of Medicine.* 1989;321(17):1174–8.

3. Gluckman E, Rocha V, Boyer-Chammard A, Locatelli F, Arcese W, Pasquini R, et al. Outcome of cord-blood transplantation from related and unrelated donors. Eurocord Transplant Group and the European Blood and Marrow Transplantation Group. *The New England Journal of Medicine.* 1997;337(6):373–81.

4. Kurtzberg J, Laughlin M, Graham ML, Smith C, Olson JF, Halperin EC, et al. Placental blood as a source of hematopoietic stem cells for transplantation into unrelated recipients. *The New England Journal of Medicine.* 1996;335(3):157–66.

5. Kurtzberg J, Prasad VK, Carter SL, Wagner JE, Baxter-Lowe LA, Wall D, et al. Results of the Cord Blood Transplantation Study (COBLT): clinical outcomes of unrelated donor umbilical cord blood transplantation in pediatric patients with hematologic malignancies. *Blood.* 2008;112(10):4318–27.

6. Rubinstein P, Carrier C, Scaradavou A, Kurtzberg J, Adamson J, Migliaccio AR,

et al. Outcomes among 562 recipients of placental-blood transplants from unrelated donors. *The New England Journal of Medicine.* 1998;339(22):1565–77.

7. Wagner JE, Barker JN, DeFor TE, Baker KS, Blazar BR, Eide C, et al. Transplantation of unrelated donor umbilical cord blood in 102 patients with malignant and nonmalignant diseases: influence of CD34 cell dose and HLA disparity on treatment-related mortality and survival. *Blood.* 2002;100(5):1611–8.

8. Wagner JE, Rosenthal J, Sweetman R, Shu XO, Davies SM, Ramsay NK, et al. Successful transplantation of HLA-matched and HLA-mismatched umbilical cord blood from unrelated donors: analysis of engraftment and acute graft-*versus*-host disease. *Blood.* 1996;88(3):795–802.

9. Eapen M, Rocha V, Sanz G, Scaradavou A, Zhang MJ, Arcese W, et al. Effect of graft source on unrelated donor haemopoietic stem-cell transplantation in adults with acute leukaemia: a retrospective analysis. *The Lancet Oncology.* 2010;11(7):653–60.

10. Jacobson CA, Turki AT, McDonough SM, Stevenson KE, Kim HT, Kao G, et al. Immune reconstitution after double umbilical cord blood stem cell transplantation: comparison with unrelated peripheral blood stem cell transplantation. *Biology of Blood and Marrow Transplantation: Journal of the American Society for Blood and Marrow Transplantation.* 2012;18(4):565–74.

11. Laughlin MJ, Barker J, Bambach B, Koc ON, Rizzieri DA, Wagner JE, et al. Hematopoietic engraftment and survival in adult recipients of

umbilical-cord blood from unrelated donors. *The New England Journal of Medicine.* 2001;344(24):1815–22.

12. Ooi J, Takahashi S, Tomonari A, Tsukada N, Konuma T, Kato S, et al. Unrelated cord blood transplantation after myeloablative conditioning in adults with acute myelogenous leukemia. *Biology of Blood and Marrow Transplantation: Journal of the American Society for Blood and Marrow Transplantation.* 2008;14(12):1341–7.

13. Arcese W, Rocha V, Labopin M, Sanz G, Iori AP, de Lima M, et al. Unrelated cord blood transplants in adults with hematologic malignancies. *Haematologica.* 2006;91(2):223–30.

14. van Heeckeren WJ, Fanning LR, Meyerson HJ, Fu P, Lazarus HM, Cooper BW, et al. Influence of human leucocyte antigen disparity and graft lymphocytes on allogeneic engraftment and survival after umbilical cord blood transplant in adults. *British Journal of Haematology.* 2007;139(3):464–74.

15. Sato A, Ooi J, Takahashi S, Tsukada N, Kato S, Kawakita T, et al. Unrelated cord blood transplantation after myeloablative conditioning in adults with advanced myelodysplastic syndromes. *Bone Marrow Transplantation.* 2011;46(2):257–61.

16. Barker JN, Weisdorf DJ, DeFor TE, Blazar BR, McGlave PB, Miller JS, et al. Transplantation of 2 partially HLA-matched umbilical cord blood units to enhance engraftment in adults with hematologic malignancy. *Blood.* 2005;105(3):1343–7.

17. Broxmeyer HE, Douglas GW, Hangoc G, Cooper S, Bard J, English D, et al. Human umbilical cord blood as a

potential source of transplantable hematopoietic stem/progenitor cells. *Proceedings of the National Academy of Sciences of the United States of America.* 1989;86(10):3828–32.

18. Broxmeyer HE, Gluckman E, Auerbach A, Douglas GW, Friedman H, Cooper S, *et al*. Human umbilical cord blood: a clinically useful source of transplantable hematopoietic stem/progenitor cells. *International Journal of Cell Cloning.* 1990;8 Suppl 1:76–89; discussion 91.

19. Hao QL, Shah AJ, Thiemann FT, Smogorzewska EM, Crooks GM. A functional comparison of CD34 + CD38- cells in cord blood and bone marrow. *Blood.* 1995;86(10):3745–53.

20. Cardoso AA, Li ML, Batard P, Hatzfeld A, Brown EL, Levesque JP, *et al*. Release from quiescence of CD34+ CD38- human umbilical cord blood cells reveals their potentiality to engraft adults. *Proceedings of the National Academy of Sciences of the United States of America.* 1993;90(18):8707–11.

21. Doubrovina E, Oflaz-Sozmen B, Prockop SE, Kernan NA, Abramson S, Teruya-Feldstein J, *et al*. Adoptive immunotherapy with unselected or EBV-specific T cells for biopsy-proven EBV+ lymphomas after allogeneic hematopoietic cell transplantation. *Blood.* 2012;119(11):2644–56.

22. Leen AM, Myers GD, Sili U, Huls MH, Weiss H, Leung KS, *et al*. Monoculture-derived T lymphocytes specific for multiple viruses expand and produce clinically relevant effects in immunocompromised individuals. *Nature Medicine.* 2006;12(10):1160–6.

23. Heslop HE, Slobod KS, Pule MA, Hale GA, Rousseau A, Smith CA, *et al*. Long-term outcome of EBV-specific T-cell infusions to prevent or treat EBV-related lymphoproliferative disease in transplant recipients. *Blood.* 2010;115(5):925–35.

24. Peggs KS, Thomson K, Samuel E, Dyer G, Armoogum J, Chakraverty R, *et al*. Directly selected cytomegalovirus-reactive donor T cells confer rapid and safe systemic reconstitution of virus-specific immunity following stem cell transplantation. *Clinical Infectious Diseases: An Official Publication of the Infectious Diseases Society of America.* 2011;52(1):49–57.

25. Lazzari L, Lucchi S, Porretti L, Montemurro T, Giordano R, Lopa R,

et al. Comparison of different serum-free media for ex vivo expansion of HPCs from cord blood using thrombopoietin, Flt-3 ligand, IL-6, and IL-11. *Transfusion.* 2001;41(5):718–9.

26. Lazzari L, Lucchi S, Rebulla P, Porretti L, Puglisi G, Lecchi L, *et al*. Long-term expansion and maintenance of cord blood haematopoietic stem cells using thrombopoietin, Flt3-ligand, interleukin (IL)-6 and IL-11 in a serum-free and stroma-free culture system. *British Journal of Haematology.* 2001;112(2):397–404.

27. McNiece I, Jones R, Cagnoni P, Bearman S, Nieto Y, Shpall EJ. Ex-vivo expansion of hematopoietic progenitor cells: preliminary results in breast cancer. *Hematology and Cell Therapy.* 1999;41(2):82–6.

28. McNiece I, Kubegov D, Kerzic P, Shpall EJ, Gross S. Increased expansion and differentiation of cord blood products using a two-step expansion culture. *Experimental Hematology.* 2000;28(10):1181–6.

29. Mohamed AA, Ibrahim AM, El-Masry MW, Mansour IM, Khroshied MA, Gouda HM, *et al*. Ex vivo expansion of stem cells: defining optimum conditions using various cytokines. *Laboratory Hematology: Official Publication of the International Society for Laboratory Hematology.* 2006;12(2):86–93.

30. Piacibello W, Sanavio F, Garetto L, Severino A, Dane A, Gammaitoni L, *et al*. Differential growth factor requirement of primitive cord blood hematopoietic stem cell for self-renewal and amplification vs proliferation and differentiation. *Leukemia.* 1998;12(5):718–27.

31. Purdy MH, Hogan CJ, Hami L, McNiece I, Franklin W, Jones RB, *et al*. Large volume ex vivo expansion of CD34-positive hematopoietic progenitor cells for transplantation. *Journal of Hematotherapy.* 1995;4(6):515–25.

32. Yao CL, Chu IM, Hsieh TB, Hwang SM. A systematic strategy to optimize ex vivo expansion medium for human hematopoietic stem cells derived from umbilical cord blood mononuclear cells. *Experimental Hematology.* 2004;32(8):720–7.

33. Yao CL, Feng YH, Lin XZ, Chu IM, Hsieh TB, Hwang SM. Characterization

of serum-free ex vivo-expanded hematopoietic stem cells derived from human umbilical cord blood CD133(+) cells. *Stem Cells and Development.* 2006;15(1):70–8.

34. Shpall EJ, Quinones R, Giller R, Zeng C, Baron AE, Jones RB, *et al*. Transplantation of ex vivo expanded cord blood. *Biology of Blood and Marrow Transplantation: Journal of the American Society for Blood and Marrow Transplantation.* 2002;8(7):368–76.

35. Jaroscak J, Goltry K, Smith A, Waters-Pick B, Martin PL, Driscoll TA, *et al*. Augmentation of umbilical cord blood (UCB) transplantation with ex vivo-expanded UCB cells: results of a phase 1 trial using the AastromReplicell System. *Blood.* 2003;101(12):5061–7.

36. Koller MR, Palsson MA, Manchel I, Palsson BO. Long-term culture-initiating cell expansion is dependent on frequent medium exchange combined with stromal and other accessory cell effects. *Blood.* 1995;86(5):1784–93.

37. Peled T, Landau E, Mandel J, Glukhman E, Goudsmid NR, Nagler A, *et al*. Linear polyamine copper chelator tetraethylenepentamine augments long-term ex vivo expansion of cord blood-derived CD34+ cells and increases their engraftment potential in NOD/SCID mice. *Experimental Hematology.* 2004;32(6):547–55.

38. Peled T, Mandel J, Goudsmid RN, Landor C, Hasson N, Harati D, *et al*. Pre-clinical development of cord blood-derived progenitor cell graft expanded ex vivo with cytokines and the polyamine copper chelator tetraethylenepentamine. *Cytotherapy.* 2004;6(4):344–55.

39. de Lima M, McMannis J, Gee A, Komanduri K, Couriel D, Andersson BS, *et al*. Transplantation of ex vivo expanded cord blood cells using the copper chelator tetraethylenepentamine: a phase I/II clinical trial. *Bone Marrow Transplantation.* 2008;41(9):771–8.

40. Stiff PJ, Montesinos P, Peled T, Landau E, Rosenheimer N, Mandel J, *et al*. StemEx®(copper chelation based) ex vivo expanded umbilical cord blood stem cell transplantation (UCBT) accelerates engraftment and improves 100 day survival in myeloablated patients compared to a registry cohort undergoing double unit UCBT: results

of a multicenter study of 101 patients with hematologic malignancies. *Blood* 2013;122(21):295.

41. Peled T, Shoham H, Aschengrau D, Yackoubov D, Frei G, Rosenheimer GN, et al. Nicotinamide, a SIRT1 inhibitor, inhibits differentiation and facilitates expansion of hematopoietic progenitor cells with enhanced bone marrow homing and engraftment. *Experimental Hematology.* 2012;40(4):342–55 e1.

42. Peled T, Adi S, Peleg I, Rosenheimer NG, Daniely Y, Nagler A, et al. Nicotinamide modulates ex-vivo expansion of cord blood derived CD34 + cells cultured with cytokines and promotes their homing and engraftment in SCID mice. *Blood.* 2006;108(Abstract 725):Oral Session, ASH December 12, 2006.

43. Horwitz ME, Chao NJ, Rizzieri DA, Long GD, Sullivan KM, Gasparetto C, et al. Umbilical cord blood expansion with nicotinamide provides long-term multilineage engraftment. *The Journal of Clinical Investigation.* 2014;124(7):3121–8.

44. Milner LA, Kopan R, Martin DI, Bernstein ID. A human homologue of the Drosophila developmental gene, Notch, is expressed in CD34+ hematopoietic precursors. *Blood.* 1994;83(8):2057–62.

45. Varnum-Finney B, Xu L, Brashem-Stein C, Nourigat C, Flowers D, Bakkour S, et al. Pluripotent, cytokine-dependent, hematopoietic stem cells are immortalized by constitutive Notch1 signaling. *Nature Medicine.* 2000;6(11):1278–81.

46. Delaney C, Heimfeld S, Brashem-Stein C, Voorhies H, Manger RL, Bernstein ID. Notch-mediated expansion of human cord blood progenitor cells capable of rapid myeloid reconstitution. *Nature Medicine.* 2010;16(2):232–6.

47. Deans RJ, Moseley AB. Mesenchymal stem cells: biology and potential clinical uses. *Experimental Hematology.* 2000;28(8):875–84.

48. Robinson SN, Simmons PJ, Yang H, Alousi AM, Marcos de Lima J, Shpall EJ. Mesenchymal stem cells in ex vivo cord blood expansion. *Best Practice & Research Clinical Haematology.* 2011;24(1):83–92.

49. Simmons PJ, Torok-Storb B. Identification of stromal cell precursors in human bone marrow by a novel monoclonal antibody, STRO-1. *Blood.* 1991;78(1):55–62.

50. de Lima M, McNiece I, Robinson SN, Munsell M, Eapen M, Horowitz M, et al. Cord-blood engraftment with ex vivo mesenchymal-cell coculture. *The New England Journal of Medicine.* 2012;367(24):2305–15.

51. Ruggeri A, Peffault de Latour R, Carmagnat M, Clave E, Douay C, Larghero J, et al. Outcomes, infections, and immune reconstitution after double cord blood transplantation in patients with high-risk hematological diseases. *Transplant Infectious Disease: An Official Journal of the Transplantation Society.* 2011;13(5):456–65.

52. Hanley PJ, Cruz CR, Savoldo B, Leen AM, Stanojevic M, Khalil M, et al. Functionally active virus-specific T cells that target CMV, adenovirus, and EBV can be expanded from naive T-cell populations in cord blood and will target a range of viral epitopes. *Blood.* 2009;114(9):1958–67.

53. Park KD, Marti L, Kurtzberg J, Szabolcs P. In vitro priming and expansion of cytomegalovirus-specific Th1 and Tc1 T cells from naive cord blood lymphocytes. *Blood.* 2006;108(5):1770–3.

54. Sun Q, Burton RL, Pollok KE, Emanuel DJ, Lucas KG. CD4(+) Epstein–Barr virus-specific cytotoxic T-lymphocytes from human umbilical cord blood. *Cellular Immunology.* 1999;195(2):81–8.

55. Hanley P, Leen A, Gee AP, Leung K, Martinez C, Krance RA, et al. Multi-virus-specific T-cell therapy for patients after hematopoietic stem cell and cord blood transplantation. *Blood.* 2013;122(21):140.

56. Chang YJ, Huang XJ. Donor lymphocyte infusions for relapse after allogeneic transplantation: when, if and for whom? *Blood Reviews.* 2013;27(1):55–62.

57. Parmar S, Robinson SN, Komanduri K, St John L, Decker W, Xing D, et al. Ex vivo expanded umbilical cord blood T cells maintain naive phenotype and TCR diversity. *Cytotherapy.* 2006;8(2):149–57.

58. Ramsay AG, Xing D, Decker WK, Burks JK, Wierda WG, Gribben JG, et al. Compared to adult peripheral blood t cells, cord blood T cells show enhanced immunological recognition of chronic lymphocytic leukemia tumor cells. *Blood.* 2008;112(Abstract 2333).

59. Decker WK, Shah N, Xing D, Lapushin R, Li S, Robinson SN, et al. Generation of functional CLL-specific cord blood CTL using CD40-ligated CLL APC. *PLoS One.* 2012;7(12):e51390.

60. Anguille S, Van Tendeloo VF, Berneman ZN. Leukemia-associated antigens and their relevance to the immunotherapy of acute myeloid leukemia. *Leukemia.* 2012;26(10):2186–96.

61. Weber G, Gerdemann U, Caruana I, Savoldo B, Hensel NF, Rabin KR, et al. Generation of multi-leukemia antigen-specific T cells to enhance the graft-*versus*-leukemia effect after allogeneic stem cell transplant. *Leukemia.* 2013;27(7):1538–47.

62. Rosenberg SA, Aebersold P, Cornetta K, Kasid A, Morgan RA, Moen R, et al. Gene transfer into human – immunotherapy of patients with advanced melanoma, using tumor-infiltrating lymphocytes modified by retroviral gene transduction. *The New England Journal of Medicine.* 1990;323(9):570–8.

63. Till BG, Jensen MC, Wang J, Chen EY, Wood BL, Greisman HA, et al. Adoptive immunotherapy for indolent non-Hodgkin lymphoma and mantle cell lymphoma using genetically modified autologous CD20-specific T cells. *Blood.* 2008;112(6):2261–71.

64. Birkholz K, Hombach A, Krug C, Reuter S, Kershaw M, Kampgen E, et al. Transfer of mRNA encoding recombinant immunoreceptors reprograms CD4+ and CD8+ T cells for use in the adoptive immunotherapy of cancer. *Gene Therapy.* 2009;16(5):596–604.

65. Savoldo B, Ramos CA, Liu E, Mims MP, Keating MJ, Carrum G, et al. CD28 costimulation improves expansion and persistence of chimeric antigen receptor-modified T cells in lymphoma patients. *The Journal of Clinical Investigation.* 2011;121(5):1822–6.

66. Hosing C, Kebriaei P, Wierda W, Jena B, Cooper LJ, Shpall E. CARs in chronic lymphocytic leukemia – ready to drive. *Current Hematologic Malignancy Reports.* 2013;8(1):60–70.

67. Kohn DB, Sadelain M, Glorioso JC. Occurrence of leukaemia following

gene therapy of X-linked SCID. *Nature Reviews Cancer*. 2003;3(7):477–88.

68. Scholler J, Brady TL, Binder-Scholl G, Hwang WT, Plesa G, Hege KM, et al. Decade-long safety and function of retroviral-modified chimeric antigen receptor T cells. *Science Translational Medicine*. 2012;4(132):132ra53.

69. Kebriaei P, Huls H, Singh H, Olivares S, Figliola M, Kumar PR, et al. First clinical trials employing Sleeping Beauty gene transfer system and artificial antigen presenting cells to generate and infuse T cells expressing CD19-specific chimeric antigen receptor. *Blood*. 2013;122(21):166.

70. Huls MH, Figliola MJ, Dawson MJ, Olivares S, Kebriaei P, Shpall EJ, et al. Clinical application of Sleeping Beauty and artificial antigen presenting cells to genetically modify T cells from peripheral and umbilical cord blood. *Journal of Visualized Experiments*. 2013 (72):e50070.

71. Micklethwaite KP, Savoldo B, Hanley PJ, Leen AM, Demmler-Harrison GJ, Cooper LJ, et al. Derivation of human T lymphocytes from cord blood and peripheral blood with antiviral and antileukemic specificity from a single culture as protection against infection and relapse after stem cell transplantation. *Blood*. 2010;115(13):2695–703.

72. Baron F, Petersdorf EW, Gooley T, Sandmaier BM, Malkki M, Chauncey TR, et al. What is the role for donor natural killer cells after nonmyeloablative conditioning? *Biology of Blood and Marrow Transplantation: Journal of the American Society for Blood and Marrow Transplantation*. 2009;15(5):580–8.

73. Ruggeri L, Capanni M, Urbani E, Perruccio K, Shlomchik WD, Tosti A, et al. Effectiveness of donor natural killer cell alloreactivity in mismatched hematopoietic transplants. *Science*. 2002;295(5562):2097–100.

74. Spanholtz J, Tordoir M, Eissens D, Preijers F, van der Meer A, Joosten I, et al. High log-scale expansion of functional human natural killer cells from umbilical cord blood CD34-positive cells for adoptive cancer immunotherapy. *PLoS One*. 2010;5(2):e9221.

75. Xing D, Ramsay AG, Gribben JG, Decker WK, Burks JK, Munsell M, et al. Cord blood natural killer cells exhibit impaired lytic immunological synapse formation that is reversed with IL-2 exvivo expansion. *Journal of Immunotherapy*. 2010;33(7):684–96.

76. Shah N, Martin-Antonio B, Yang H, Ku S, Lee DA, Cooper LJ, et al. Antigen presenting cell-mediated expansion of human umbilical cord blood yields log-scale expansion of natural killer cells with anti-myeloma activity. *PLoS One*. 2013;8(10):e76781.

77. Di Ianni M, Falzetti F, Carotti A, Terenzi A, Castellino F, Bonifacio E, et al. Tregs prevent GVHD and promote immune reconstitution in HLA-haploidentical transplantation. *Blood*. 2011;117(14):3921–8.

78. Godfrey WR, Spoden DJ, Ge YG, Baker SR, Liu B, Levine BL, et al. Cord blood CD4(+)CD25(+)-derived T regulatory cell lines express FoxP3 protein and manifest potent suppressor function. *Blood*. 2005;105(2):750–8.

79. Hippen KL, Harker-Murray P, Porter SB, Merkel SC, Londer A, Taylor DK, et al. Umbilical cord blood regulatory T-cell expansion and functional effects of tumor necrosis factor receptor family members OX40 and 4-1BB expressed on artificial antigen-presenting cells. *Blood*. 2008;112(7):2847–57.

80. Parmar S, Liu X, Tung SS, Robinson SN, Rodriguez G, Cooper LJ, et al. Third-party umbilical cord blood-derived regulatory T cells prevent xenogenic graft-*versus*-host disease. *Cytotherapy*. 2014;16(1):90–100.

81. Brunstein CG, Miller JS, Cao Q, McKenna DH, Hippen KL, Curtsinger J, et al. Infusion of ex vivo expanded T regulatory cells in adults transplanted with umbilical cord blood: safety profile and detection kinetics. *Blood*. 2011;117(3):1061–70.

82. Brunstein CG, Blazar BR, Miller JS, Cao Q, Hippen KL, McKenna DH, et al. Adoptive transfer of umbilical cord blood-derived regulatory T cells and early viral reactivation. *Biology of Blood and Marrow Transplantation: Journal of the American Society for Blood and Marrow Transplantation*. 2013;19(8):1271–3.

83. Xia L, McDaniel JM, Yago T, Doeden A, McEver RP. Surface fucosylation of human cord blood cells augments binding to P-selectin and E-selectin and enhances engraftment in bone marrow. *Blood*. 2004;104(10):3091–6.

84. Robinson SN, Simmons PJ, Thomas MW, Brouard N, Javni JA, Trilok S, et al. Ex vivo fucosylation improves human cord blood engraftment in NOD-SCID IL-2Rgamma(null) mice. *Experimental Hematology*. 2012;40(6):445–56.

85. Robinson SN, Thomas MW, Simmons PJ, Lu J, Yang H, Parmar S, et al. Fucosylation with fucosyltransferase VI or fucosyltransferase VII improves cord blood engraftment. *Cytotherapy*. 2014;16(1):84–9.

86. Hoggatt J, Singh P, Sampath J, Pelus LM. Prostaglandin E2 enhances hematopoietic stem cell homing, survival, and proliferation. *Blood*. 2009;113(22):5444–55.

87. Cutler C, Multani P, Robbins D, Kim HT, Le T, Hoggatt J, et al. Prostaglandin-modulated umbilical cord blood hematopoietic stem cell transplantation. *Blood*. 2013;122(17):3074–81.

88. Christopherson KW, 2nd, Hangoc G, Broxmeyer HE. Cell surface peptidase CD26/dipeptidylpeptidase IV regulates CXCL12/stromal cell-derived factor-1 alpha-mediated chemotaxis of human cord blood CD34+ progenitor cells. *Journal of Immunology*. 2002;169(12):7000–8.

89. Christopherson KW, 2nd, Hangoc G, Mantel CR, Broxmeyer HE. Modulation of hematopoietic stem cell homing and engraftment by CD26. *Science*. 2004;305(5686):1000–3.

Gene Therapy in Hematopoietic Cell Transplants

67

Hua Fung and Stanton L. Gerson

Introduction

Gene therapy represents a new promising genetic treatment for many genetic or acquired hematologic disorders. Basically, gene therapy involves the introduction of a functional gene to replace a mutated gene or a therapeutic gene to provide treatment. In many cases, patient's blood cells are removed and hematopoietic stem cells or T-cells are carefully purified by antibody selection. The therapeutic genes placed within a genetically modified vector, typically viral, are delivered by receptor binding and internalization into target cells. These gene-modified cells are then reinfused back into the patient. Since this method modifies cells outside the patient's body, it is called *ex-vivo* gene therapy. In the other approach, called *in-vivo* gene therapy, direct injection of therapeutic gene-containing vectors into the patient results in varying degrees of gene transfer and is less cell-selective (Figure 67.1). Once inside the target cell, the gene becomes expressed either after DNA insertion or from an

episome, producing therapeutic protein for treatment. If the gene-modified cells are long-lived and able to expand inside the body, as is a property of hematopoietic stem cells (HSC), a single-gene therapy may be sufficient to provide a lifelong therapeutic effect. Indeed, current gene therapy technologies have reached the point that single-gene hematologic deficiency diseases can be permanently corrected, for example, X-linked severe combined immunodeficiency (X-SCID)[1,2] and adenosine deaminase deficiency severe combined immunodeficiency (ADA-SCID)[3].

Gene therapy has come a long way from the mid-1980s when the first experiment of stem cell gene transfer was successful. However, several serious obstacles appeared that have slowed the clinical advancement of this technology. First, the difficulty in delivering a modified gene into HSC because of their lack of cell surface receptors and quiescent state[4]. Second, the early X-SCID gene therapy was interrupted because 20% of patients developed malignancy (T-lymphoid leukemia)

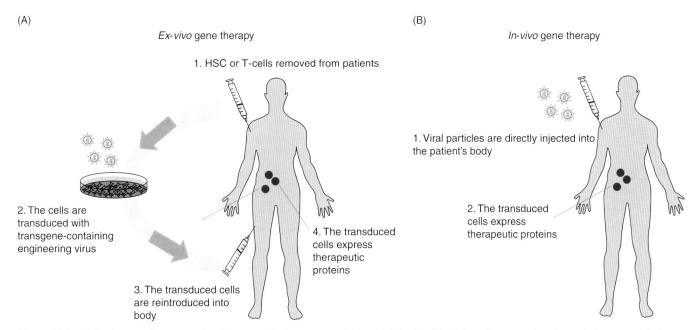

(A)   *Ex-vivo* gene therapy

1. HSC or T-cells removed from patients

2. The cells are transduced with transgene-containing engineering virus

3. The transduced cells are reintroduced into body

4. The transduced cells express therapeutic proteins

(B)   *In-vivo* gene therapy

1. Viral particles are directly injected into the patient's body

2. The transduced cells express therapeutic proteins

Figure 67.1. (A) *Ex-vivo* gene therapy involves four steps: (1) take out patient's blood (HSC or T-cells); (2) the cells are transduced outside the patient's body by engineering virus that contains a transgene; (3) the transduced cells are infused back into the patient's body; (4) inside body, the transduced cell starts to produce therapeutic proteins. (B) *In-vivo* gene therapy is done by directly injecting viral particles into the patient's body.

649

from insertional mutagenesis within 3–6 years of gene therapy. The retroviral vectors contained powerful enhancer elements within the long terminal repeats (LTRs), which transcriptionally activated lymphocyte proliferative signals from nearby *LMO2* proto-oncogenes[5]. Today, after almost three decades, these issues have been gradually addressed. With an array of cytokines and improved lentiviral vectors, the *ex-vivo* HSC transduction rate in humans can reach 50–80%[6,7]. In addition, introduction of a myeloablative conditioning regimen that directly damages endogenous stem cells to advantage homing and engraftment of the donor stem cells, using drugs such as busulfan, melphalan, and 1,3-bis-(2-chloroethyl)-1-nitrosourea (BCNU) prior to stem cell infusion, is an effective method to increase stem cell niche-homing and engraftment rates to 1–2 copies of gene marking/cell[6,7]. High stem cell engraftment rates are critical for the gene therapy of chronic granulomatous disease, X-linked adrenoleukodystrophy, and metachromatic leukodystrophy[6–9]. Moreover, the safer so-called self-inactivating (SIN) new-generation viral vectors have been developed, in which viral LTR enhancers were completely removed. Using these vectors, not a single case of therapy-related malignancy has been found in several clinical trials, some of which have run for as long as 7–8 years[6,7]. Gene therapy is no longer just a theory because some trials have achieved sustained clinical correction (that is, phenotypic correction of the genetic defect) for as long as 12 years. Gene therapy has thus undergone a new renaissance.

Gene Therapy Targeted Cells
Hematopoietic Stem Cells (HSCs)

HSCs have been traditionally used as the cell of choice for gene therapy. There are several reasons for using HSCs. First, many blood disorders are hematopoietic diseases and therefore gene-corrected HSCs are obviously the first candidate for replacement. Second, HSCs are a long-lived and self-renewing population and therefore may reduce or eliminate the need for repeated administrations of the gene therapy. Technically HSCs are readily removed from the body via the circulating blood or bone marrow or collected from umbilical cord blood. They are also easily identified and manipulated in the laboratory and can be returned to patients by infusion. Third, engineered HSCs are able to home to the marrow, become quiescent, and differentiate into many types of blood cells such as T- and B-lymphocytes, red blood cells, natural killer cells, monocytes, macrophages, granulocytes, eosinophils, basophils, and megakaryocytes. Thus gene transduction of HSCs provides the possibility to correct defects in all hematopoietic lineages. Finally, HSCs or their progeny migrate to a number of different tissues, including liver, spleen, lung, brain, and lymph nodes. These may be strategic locations for localized delivery of therapeutic agents for disorders unrelated to the blood system, such as liver diseases and metabolic disorders such as Gaucher's disease.

Non-stem Cells

HSC progeny have limited replication capacity and are short lived except perhaps for the lymphocyte series. For some gene-deficient diseases involving T cells (such as SCID and HIV), using the HSC as a T-cell precursor creates the opportunity to provide gene therapy to a specific lineage. The underlying mechanism is still not very clear but memory T-cells are long-lived. Within the memory T-cell compartment, at least three subsets have been identified: T memory stem cells, T central memory cells, and effector memory T-cells[10]. T memory stem cells and T central memory cells can quickly expand to large numbers of effector T-cells when they are reactivated[11]. In fact, T-cell gene therapy has been shown to be very effective in some cancer gene therapy. Effector T-cells are "executioners" in cell-mediated immunity, having a capacity to directly eradicate diseased cells. However, cancer cells in general make themselves "invisible" to T-cells. For this reason researchers modified T-cells by adding new gene-encoding receptors, so-called chimeric antigen receptors (CARs), that recognize antigens presented by cancer cells that can invoke a strong immune reaction, such as CD19 of B-cell lymphocytic leukemia[11,12]. Once the CAR-modified T-cells are transfused into patients' bodies, they become very active specifically towards cancer cells. In recent clinical trials anti-CD19 CAR T-cells almost completely eliminated all cancer cells in two patients with end-stage B-cell chronic lymphocytic leukemia (CLL)[11,12].

Compared to HSC, one advantage of using gene modified T-cells to therapeutically alter only the T-lymphoid lineage is to leave undisturbed a normal functional hematopoietic system. However, this is also a limitation of T-cells in gene therapy. For example, when using T-cells to correct X-SCID, although T-cells recover to near normal level, the other types would not be affected. In this setting, B-cells are not corrected, and the longevity of gene transfer suffers from the limited expansion of the T-cell population. Thus, the patient may remain on immunoglobulin replacement therapy and natural killer cell (B-cell derived) deficiency may be persistent.

Retroviral Vectors in Gene Therapy

Retroviral vectors can be genetically modified to contain the gene of interest. Viral preparations can be purified and stored. The vector system efficiently inserts reverse transcribed viral DNA into the host genome, which is preferred in gene therapy designed to establish long-term expression of the transgene. The most commonly used retroviral vectors are γ-retroviral and lentiviral vectors. The most commonly used lentiviral vectors are HIV-1 based, and other lentiviral vector backbones are derived from simian immunodeficiency virus (SIV) or foamy viruses. Lentiviral vectors have at least three advantages over γ-retroviral vectors. First, the lentiviral vector preintegration complex is able to cross the nuclear membrane of the host cell even in the absence of mitosis, and therefore it is able to transduce nondivided cells such as HSCs[13]. Second, the lentiviral vector preintegration complex is more stable and stays longer prior to integration, which would give more chances for integration[14]. Finally, γ-retroviral vector prefer to integrate near gene transcription start sites, whereas lentiviral vector integration is more evenly distributed[15]. Moreover, γ-retroviral vector integration more closely aligns to gene transcription regulatory regions such as CpG <Define?> islands, mammalian conserved noncoding sequences, and conserved transcriptional factor binding sites, suggesting that γ-retroviral vector integrations have a greater chance of altering the regulatory mechanisms of nearby genes, thus altering their expression, than lentiviral vectors[15]. Lentiviral vectors have thus emerged as an important advance for safer gene therapy in hematologic disorders with minimal likelihood of insertional gene expression altering mutagenesis.

Transplantation Conditioning

To increase stem or T-cell engraftment, a myeloablative therapy prior to transplantation is often applied[16]. Full myeloablative conditioning would result in the obliteration of nearly all stages of the hematopoietic cells over a period of several days. At the end of this period, the bone marrow is profoundly hypocellular, with an intact stroma containing a few residual plasma cells and macrophages. This environment is ideal for infused genetically modified cell homeostatic expansion. In addition, supporting cytokines and some genetic modifications could confer on infused cells a homing, engraftment, and expansion growth advantage; both of them would significantly increase homeostatic expansion[17]. A controversial point for using myeloablative conditioning is that HSCs are vital cells for human life and aging[18]. A relatively limited number (10000–30000) of long-term repopulating HSCs exist in humans[19]. Losing the long-term repopulating HSCs may impair hematopoiesis unless the genetically altered HSCs fully engraft. In this sense the myeloablative therapy needs to be tempered with the lifelong outlook for the recipient. Therefore this treatment must be applied extremely carefully and the overall clinical benefit should be assessed in each individual case.

Nevertheless, an excellent engraftment environment alone is still insufficient for a successful transplantation. Early efforts in CAR gene therapy provide a useful case study. The principle of CAR cancer therapy was established 25 years ago, but all early gene therapies were unsuccessful [17]. Initially, it was thought that effector T-cells were superior because they secreted high levels of effector cytokines and were proficient killers of tumor targets in-vitro. However, transferring large numbers of effector T-cells proved to be ineffective[17]. We now know they are terminally differentiated cells, with limited replicative capacity insufficient to kill advanced cancers[17]. Moreover the heterogeneity and potential variable of polyclonal unselected cells could affect the efficacy of eliminating cancer. The success of CAR

therapy was not evident until a subset of highly replicative T-cells including naïve T-cells was discovered[20], consisting of central memory T-cells[21], Th17 cells[22], and T stem memory cells[23]. Conversely, some regulatory T-cells will block an antitumor response of transferred lymphocytes[24]. With these considerations in mind, transferring a few highly replicative T-cells has been demonstrated to be sufficient to eradicate end-stage cancers because of outstanding in-vivo expansion (>1000 times) [11]. Thus, a successful transplantation is not dependent on how many bulky T-cells infused but whether these cells are able to expand inside the body. This may also be applied to HSC-based gene therapy; many efforts have failed simply because modified cells could not expand. Like lymphocytes, only a small fraction of HSCs are long-term repopulating HSCs[19]. Therefore, how to define and select those highly replicative HSCs for transplantation will be a key factor for successful HSC gene therapy.

Gene Therapy Successes

There have been many successful gene therapies for hematologic diseases in recent years. Here we have just selected two of them as examples. X-SCID is a single gene-deficient disease caused by mutations in the interleukin-2 receptor gene, γIL2RG[25]. Lacking functional γIL2RG causes absence of T-cells and natural killer cells and poorly functional B-cells. X-SCID is a fatal disease. Patients often die within the first 2 years of life without medical interventions[25]. During 1999–2006, 20 X-SCID children were treated in two gene therapy trials [1,2]. Because patients lacked an HLA-identical donor, all 20 were given a single γ-retroviral vector-mediated gene therapy, in which a wild γIL2RG gene was delivered into patients' T-cells. Five to twelve years after the gene transfer procedure, 17 of the 20 treated participants are alive and display nearly full correction of the T-cell deficiency by genetically modified T-cells[1,2].

Wiskott–Aldrich syndrome (WAS) is another single-gene disorder due to mutations in WAS protein (WASp) gene[26]. The WASp codes a protein called WASP, which activates actin polymerization in almost all blood cells. Congenital deficiency in WASp is associated with microthrombocytopenia, recurrent infections, eczema, a high incidence of autoimmunity, and lymphoreticular malignancy (lymphoma and leukemia)[26]. Replacement gene therapy with a normal WASp offers the only hope of cure. In 2010 three patients in the United States were given gene therapy following busulfan conditioning and γ-retroviral vector WASp modified autologous HSC, with high degrees of engraftment – gene marking of 26%, 5%, and 4% of neutrophils, respectively. In two of the patients the long-term gene marking was 1.1% and 0.03% of neutrophils. Gene-marked neutrophils have sustained full correction of oxidase activity for 34 and 11 months, respectively, with full or partial resolution of infection in those two patients[27].

Gene Therapy for Hematologic Cancers

Gene therapy for cancer treatment has been widely exploited. A book published in 2014 details the new developments in this field[28]. Here we have selected two significant developments. One of the most creative approaches is CAR for B-cell lymphocytic leukemia, in which patients' T-cells were modified to target their own cancers[11]. The human immune system attacks foreign invaders such as viruses, bacteria, and parasitic worms very efficiently, but it doesn't always recognize cancer cells because cancer cells uniformly express self antigens and usually develop several mechanisms to induce T-cell tolerance. There is a strongly expressed antigen CD19 on the cell surface of all types of B-cells including B-lymphocytic malignancies. However, CD19 is also present on normal B-cells. In order to attack CD19 leukemia cells, a patient's own normal CD4 and CD8 T-cells are isolated from the blood and genetically engineered to express the B-cell CD19 antigen as the T-receptor (CD19-CAR) via a lentiviral vector. The resultant CD19-CAR consists of a single-chain variable fragment (scFv) of a CD19-specific antibody as an extracellular CD19 antigen-binding moiety, a linker (Hinge) and transmembrane domain, and an intracellular signaling CD3ζ domain (Figure 67.2).

The CD19-CAR-modified T-cells were then given as a single-dose reinfused into the patient. The engineered T-cells recognize CD19-cancer cells. This recognition triggers an immune response that activates T-cells, which causes T-cell proliferation. The activated CD8 (killer) T-cells can directly kill CD19 cells by releasing cytotoxins such as perforin and granulysin[29], while activated CD4 (helper) T-cells release cytokines that enhance the cytotoxic function of macrophages and killer T-cells. Importantly, the CAR is designed to recognize CD19 in a simple antigen–antibody interaction, which is independent of the major histocompatibility complex (MHC) that determines an antigen "self" or "nonself"[11]. This design not only directly kills all types of CD19 cells very efficiently, but also avoids mechanisms that cancer cells use to escape immunorecognition, including down-regulation of the MHC, reduction of costimulatory molecules, induction of suppressive cytokines, and recruitment of regulatory T-cells[30].

The success of recent trials is largely due to two important improvements[11]. First, a T-cell-specific costimulatory 4-1BB was added into the CAR signaling domains (second-generation CAR, see Figure 67.2). This modification enhances CAR signaling strength and persistence, subsequently increasing cytotoxicity. Second, a subset of T-cells with strong replicative capacity were carefully selected for the transplantation, which is probably the decisive factor to ensure a sustained and strong immune response[11,17]. The initial clinical trial reported in 2011 from the University of Pennsylvania focused on three advanced, chemotherapy-resistant CLL patients. The transplantation induced a dramatic tumor-killing response (tumor lysis syndrome), which started at day 14 post-transplantation with fevers, rigors, diaphoresis, anorexia, nausea, and diarrhea. A large amount of cancer cells was rapidly destroyed and by

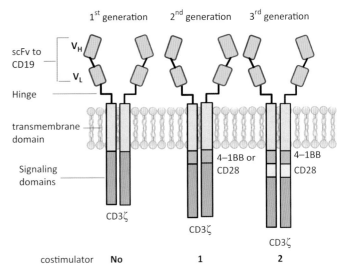

Figure 67.2. Structure of chimeric antigen receptors (CARs). First-generation CARs are 3-fragment fusion proteins with a single-chain fragment antibody (scFv) containing the heavy (V_H) and light chain (V_L) variable regions specific to a TAA, a CD8 transmembrane domain, and a T-cell receptor cytoplasmic signaling domain CD3ζ. Second-generation CARs are the successful versions used in a 2011 clinical trial, in which a costimulator 4-1BB or CD28 was added. Third-generation CARs have the addition of two tandem costimulators (two of CD28, 4-1BB, OX40, CD27, and inducible T-cell costimulatory (CD278)). CARs usually form a dimer.

day 23, no CLL cells could be detected in the bone marrow[11]. CD19-CAR T-cells trafficked to the bone marrow, expanded, and persisted in the blood for at least 6 months in all three patients[11], indicating an excellent result for the transplantation. This immunotherapy induced a complete, durable remission in two of the patients lasting over 4 years to date and a partial response in the third. There were three major side effects. First, as a trade off, the normal B-cells were attacked by CD19-CAR T-cells; B-cell aplasia was common and the patients were usually given immunoglobulin supplements. Second, cytokine release syndrome can occur because of an immune response, resulting in activated T-cells and release of large amounts of cytokines by macrophage cells, which can induce fever, hypotension, hypoxia, and neurologic changes. Severe cytokine release syndrome has been treated with tocilizumab, an IL-6 receptor-blocking antibody. The last side effect is tumor lysis syndrome, which can result in end-organ damage to lung and kidney. The triumph of the pioneer trial has inspired numerous clinical studies with CD19-CAR T-cells to CD19 positive CLL, acute lymphocytic leukemia (ALL), B-cell non-Hodgkin lymphoma, and myeloma. Impressive clinical results of CD19-CAR T-cell-treated ALL trials have been recently published by the National Cancer Institute[31] and Memorial Sloan Kettering Cancer Center[32]. In addition to CD19, other antigens such as CD20, CD22, CD30, and CD33 have also been tested for their potential as therapeutic targets for hematologic malignancies[30].

Another creative strategy is to enhance the conventional chemotherapy by protecting the marrow through gene

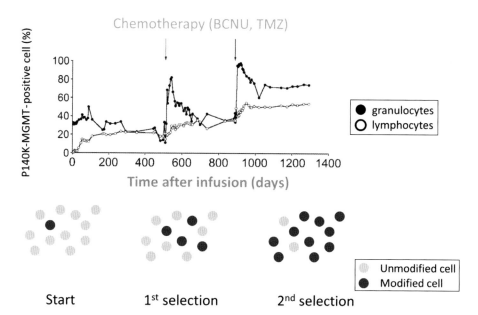

Figure 67.3. An example of P140K-MGMT in-vivo selection in a monkey. The P140K-MGMT-modified cell numbers continued to increase after each chemotherapy session (selective pressures). Modified from Beard B. *JCI* 120/2345 (2010).

transfer. This method will also provide a selection method for the transduced HSCs over time. Chemotherapy has a limited therapeutic window due to its severe toxic effect to bone marrow cells and its leukemogenesis potential. Since the main lethal effect of certain alkylating chemotherapy treatments is DNA damage, especially O^6-methylguanine, a number of investigators have pursued a strong chemoresistant DNA repair gene, a mutant (P140K) of O^6-methylguanine-DNA methyltransferase (MGMT). This gene produces an MGMT protein capable of DNA repair but resistant to a known inhibitor, O^6-benzylguanine. When introduced into HSC by a γ-retroviral vector, the P140KMGMT gene confers resistance to temozolomide and BCNU, both used in the treatment of glioma. In two ongoing trials, this gene transduction into HSCs is being used early in the course of treatment of glioma. Over time, the goals are to improve tolerance to these chemotherapy agents, allow dose escalation, and improve the treatment response to more cycles of chemotherapy. In one recent phase 1 clinical trial, it was demonstrated that intensification of chemotherapy was feasible, and there was a clear improvement in therapy outcome and patient survival in a small study [33,34]. A similar result was also observed in our ongoing clinical trial with a lentiviral vector produced by Lentigen (reported at the American Society of Hematology 2014 Annual Meeting). As noted below, use of P140KMGMT to select HSCs transduced with another gene is now an emerging technology.

New Technologies Used in Gene Therapy
In-vivo Selection and MGMT Selective Method
The question of whether stem cell gene therapy can cure a disease is largely reliant on whether corrected cells can ultimately functionally replace the deficient cells. An interesting finding in the early successful gene therapy of X-SCID and ADA-SCID is that a low (0.1–1%) engraftment rate is sufficient

for long-term correction, and the single most important factor is that the corrected transgene confers a selective *in-vivo* survival advantage[35]. By contrast, a main reason for poor response to gene therapy is that the gene-corrected cells have no or weak selective advantage that does not provide a clinically meaningful benefit. Therefore, the *in-vivo* selection process is a key element in the success of clinical gene therapy.

In fact, the gene-corrected cells in the majority of current known hematologic genetic diseases have no *in-vivo* selection advantage[35]. To overcome this problem, a second *selectable* gene was used to coexpress with the corrected gene introduced into the cell, which turned nonselectable corrected cells into selectable cells[35]. The selectable gene can be cloned into a vector along with the corrected gene driven by a single or separate promoter. Initial experiments have identified several selectable genes including those for multidrug-resistant proteins dihydrofolate reductase and MGMT[35]. However, MGMT shows the most promising results in experiments in large animals and humans. MGMT encodes an important DNA repair enzyme O^6-methylguanine-DNA-methyltransferase, which confers resistance to the cytotoxicity of alkylating chemotherapy agents such as BCNU and temozolomide (TMZ)[36]. Studies found that P140K-MGMT has a more than l0-fold stronger resistance effect[37]. Therefore, P140K-MGMT-expressed cells can be selected after BCNU and TMZ exposure (Figure 67.3). Recent clinical trials have clearly demonstrated that P140K-MGMT protected the gene-modified cells from TMZ-induced toxicity[33]. This strategy has also been used in an HIV gene therapy mouse model[38]. Successful gene therapy with good gene marking levels (~30%) are dependent on three factors: high HSC transduction rate, high engraft rate, and *in-vivo* selection[35]. However, a recent trial indicates that with excellent transduction rates (80–90%) and excellent engraft rates (gene copy marking/genome >0.5), two factors would be sufficient to achieve a sustained gene

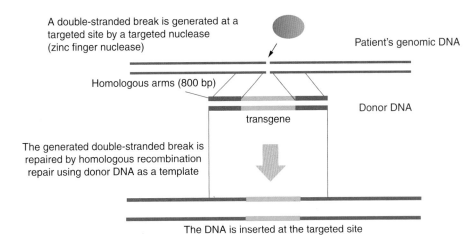

A double-stranded break is generated at a targeted site by a targeted nuclease (zinc finger nuclease)

Patient's genomic DNA

Homologous arms (800 bp)

Donor DNA

transgene

The generated double-stranded break is repaired by homologous recombination repair using donor DNA as a template

The DNA is inserted at the targeted site

Figure 67.4. Targeted transgene insertion. A targeted nuclease such as zinc finger nuclease first generates a double-stranded break (DSB). Then the DSB is repaired by homologous recombination repair using a donor DNA with a transgene inserted within two homologous arms. When the repair is finished, the transgene will be inserted at the targeted site.

correction even without an *in-vivo* selection mechnism[7]. Nevertheless, even with low transduction rates and engraftment rates, MGMT-mediated *in-vivo* selection for the HSC population certainly will be a valuable tool for successful gene therapy.

Overcoming Genotoxicity by Targeted-Insertion Gene Therapy

To achieve a sustained gene correction, many gene therapies have used integrated viral vectors such as γ-retroviral or lentiviral vectors. However, the viral insertion causes mutagenesis. In the past, gene therapies for X-SCID[39], WAS[40], and chronic granulomatous disease[41] have indicated that activation of proto-oncogenes upon γ-retroviral insertion in their vicinity is associated with the development of lymphoproliferative, myelodysplastic syndromes and lymphoid leukemia.

More recently, improved lentiviral vectors have added many safe features to gene therapy protocols. These include no preference for integration near promoters, removal of viral promoter/enhancer, and production of self-inactivating sequences or so-called suicide genes that would selectively kill genetically altered cells. However, in experimental models, an association of gene therapy lentiviral vector insertion-induced clonal dominance[9] with the development of murine leukemia[42] has been reported. Thus, wherever DNA insertion is possible a risk of insertional mutagenesis remains, and documenting of clonal evolution and insertion sites will remain important. Furthermore, determining whether a therapy-related cancer is related to lentiviral vector insertions within gene regions remains a priority for safety[15]. To date, the US Food and Drug Administration has not approved single-gene therapy in the United States. The review boards are appropriately conservative about the risk of exogenous gene insertion.

One way to reduce this risk is to select preferred sites of DNA insertion. Recently developed gene-targeting and gene-editing technologies could make this possible. Gene editing is a genetic engineering technique that allows the insertion of DNA at a desired location[43]. It starts with artificially engineered

nucleases, such as zinc finger nucleases, which can create a double-stranded break (DSB) at a targeted DNA sequence anywhere in the human genome. The DSBs would then be repaired by homologous recombination (HR) repair or non-homologous end-joining repair. However, if the zinc finger nucleases are co-transfected with another plasmid (donor DNA plasmid), in which a desired DNA such as a transgene has been inserted within a sequence (homologous arms) that is homologous to the flanking sequences of the DSB, use of this DNA as a template by HR would lead to insertion at a targeted location (Figure 67.4). Using zinc finger nuclease it has been well demonstrated that a DNA (up to 9.6 kb)[44] can be inserted precisely into a selected location on the human genome. There are several known safe harbors in the human genome. For example, the *PPP1R12C* gene on chromosome 19 (*AAVS1* locus) where frequently integrated by adeno-associated virus (AAV), but AAV infection is not associated with any known pathophysiology[45]. Recently, studies have successfully inserted several genes into the *AAVS1* site of human cells, including stem cells, using zinc finger nuclease gene targeting methods[44,46]. However, the gene correction rate of gene editing is still very low (~1%)[47]. Fortunately, gene targeting is a fast-growing field. Many new technologies have developed in recent years. The newly discovered transcription activator-like effector nuclease (TALEN)[48] and RNA-guided endonuclease, the clustered, regularly interspaced, short palindromic repeats (CRISPR)[49] technology, have shown great promise. TALEN and CRISPR are both much easier and faster than the zinc finger nuclease technique. These new gene-targeted technologies together may one day finally solve the retroviral insertion mutagenesis safety problems.

Conclusions

The field of gene therapy for hematologic diseases remains one of the most exciting areas of research for new therapeutics. The ongoing advances and continuous evolution, largely focused on medical need and safety, are coupled with continued breakthroughs in genetic modification technology. The possibility of using induced pluripotent stem cells to derive the desired precursor population and newer CRISPR approaches to gene modification suggest that gene therapy will remain at the interface of experimentation and clinical investigation for the next decade and beyond.

References

1. Hacein-Bey-Abina S, Hauer J, Lim A, Picard C, Wang GP, Berry CC, et al. Efficacy of gene therapy for X-linked severe combined immunodeficiency. *N Engl J Med*. 2010;363(4):355–64.

2. Zhang L, Thrasher AJ, Gaspar HB. Current progress on gene therapy for primary immunodeficiencies. *Gene Ther*. 2013;20(10):963–9.

3. Candotti F, Shaw KL, Muul L, Carbonaro D, Sokolic R, Choi C, et al. Gene therapy for adenosine deaminase-deficient severe combined immune deficiency: clinical comparison of retroviral vectors and treatment plans. *Blood*. 2012;120(18):3635–46.

4. Vollweiler JL, Zielske SP, Reese JS, Gerson SL. Hematopoietic stem cell gene therapy: progress toward therapeutic targets. *Bone Marrow Transplant*. 2003;32(1):1–7.

5. Howe SJ, Mansour MR, Schwarzwaelder K, Bartholomae C, Hubank M, Kempski H, et al. Insertional mutagenesis combined with acquired somatic mutations causes leukemogenesis following gene therapy of SCID-X1 patients. *J Clin Invest*. 2008;118(9):3143–50.

6. Aiuti A, Biasco L, Scaramuzza S, Ferrua F, Cicalese MP, Baricordi C, et al. Lentiviral hematopoietic stem cell gene therapy in patients with Wiskott-Aldrich syndrome. *Science*. 2013;341(6148):1233151.

7. Biffi A, Montini E, Lorioli L, Cesani M, Fumagalli F, Plati T, et al. Lentiviral hematopoietic stem cell gene therapy benefits metachromatic leukodystrophy. *Science*. 2013;341(6148):1233158.

8. Grez M, Reichenbach J, Schwable J, Seger R, Dinauer MC, Thrasher AJ. Gene therapy of chronic granulomatous disease: the engraftment dilemma. *Mol Ther*. 2011;19(1):28–35.

9. Cartier N, Hacein-Bey-Abina S, Bartholomae CC, Veres G, Schmidt M, Kutschera I, et al. Hematopoietic stem cell gene therapy with a lentiviral vector in X-linked adrenoleukodystrophy. *Science*. 2009;326(5954):818–23.

10. Gattinoni L, Restifo NP. Moving T memory stem cells to the clinic. *Blood*. 2013;121(4):567–8.

11. Porter DL, Levine BL, Kalos M, Bagg A, June CH. Chimeric antigen receptor-modified T cells in chronic lymphoid leukemia. *N Engl J Med*. 2011;365(8):725–33.

12. Kalos M, Levine BL, Porter DL, Katz S, Grupp SA, Bagg A, et al. T cells with chimeric antigen receptors have potent antitumor effects and can establish memory in patients with advanced leukemia. *Sci Transl Med*. 2011;3(95):95ra73.

13. Cooray S, Howe SJ, Thrasher AJ. Retrovirus and lentivirus vector design and methods of cell conditioning. *Methods Enzymol*. 2012;507:29–57.

14. Naldini L, Blomer U, Gage FH, Trono D, Verma IM. Efficient transfer, integration, and sustained long-term expression of the transgene in adult rat brains injected with a lentiviral vector. *Proc Natl Acad Sci U S A*. 1996;93(21):11382–8.

15. Cattoglio C, Pellin D, Rizzi E, Maruggi G, Corti G, Miselli F, et al. High-definition mapping of retroviral integration sites identifies active regulatory elements in human multipotent hematopoietic progenitors. *Blood*. 2010;116(25):5507–17.

16. Gyurkocza B, Sandmaier BM. Conditioning regimens for hematopoietic cell transplantation: one size does not fit all. *Blood*. 2014;124(3):344–53.

17. Barrett DM, Singh N, Porter DL, Grupp SA, June CH. Chimeric antigen receptor therapy for cancer. *Annu Rev Med*. 2014;65:333–47.

18. Kenyon J, Fu P, Lingas K, Thomas E, Saurastri A, Santos Guasch G, et al. Humans accumulate microsatellite instability with acquired loss of MLH1 protein in hematopoietic stem and progenitor cells as a function of age. *Blood*. 2012;120(16):3229–36.

19. Abkowitz JL, Catlin SN, McCallie MT, Guttorp P. Evidence that the number of hematopoietic stem cells per animal is conserved in mammals. *Blood*. 2002;100(7):2665–7.

20. Hinrichs CS, Borman ZA, Cassard L, Gattinoni L, Spolski R, Yu Z, et al. Adoptively transferred effector cells derived from naive rather than central memory CD8+ T cells mediate superior antitumor immunity. *Proc Natl Acad Sci U S A*. 2009;106(41):17469–74.

21. Berger C, Jensen MC, Lansdorp PM, Gough M, Elliott C, Riddell SR. Adoptive transfer of effector CD8+ T cells derived from central memory cells establishes persistent T cell memory in primates. *J Clin Invest*. 2008;118(1):294–305.

22. Paulos CM, Carpenito C, Plesa G, Suhoski MM, Varela-Rohena A, Golovina TN, et al. The inducible costimulator (ICOS) is critical for the development of human T(H)17 cells. *Sci Transl Med*. 2010;2(55):55ra78.

23. Gattinoni L, Lugli E, Ji Y, Pos Z, Paulos CM, Quigley MF, et al. A human memory T cell subset with stem cell-like properties. *Nat Med*. 2011;17(10):1290–7.

24. Lee JC, Hayman E, Pegram HJ, Santos E, Heller G, Sadelain M, et al. In vivo inhibition of human CD19-targeted effector T cells by natural T regulatory cells in a xenotransplant murine model of B cell malignancy. *Cancer Res*. 2011;71(8):2871–81.

25. Cavazzana-Calvo M, Fischer A, Hacein-Bey-Abina S, Aiuti A. Gene therapy for primary immunodeficiencies: Part 1. *Curr Opin Immunol*. 2012;24(5):580–4.

26. Aiuti A, Bacchetta R, Seger R, Villa A, Cavazzana-Calvo M. Gene therapy for primary immunodeficiencies: Part 2. *Curr Opin Immunol*. 2012;24(5):585–91.

27. Kang EM, Choi U, Theobald N, Linton G, Long Priel DA, Kuhns D, et al. Retrovirus gene therapy for X-linked chronic granulomatous disease can achieve stable long-term correction of oxidase activity in peripheral blood neutrophils. *Blood*. 2010;115(4):783–91.

28. Lattime EC, Gerson SL. *Gene therapy of cancer: translational approaches from preclinical studies to clinical implementation*. 3rd ed. San Diego, CA: Academic Press; 2014.

29. Ma LL, Spurrell JC, Wang JF, Neely GG, Epelman S, Krensky AM, et al. CD8 T cell-mediated killing of Cryptococcus neoformans requires granulysin and is dependent on CD4 T cells and IL-15. *J Immunol.* 2002;169(10):5787–95.

30. Han EQ, Li XL, Wang CR, Li TF, Han SY. Chimeric antigen receptor-engineered T cells for cancer immunotherapy: progress and challenges. *J Hematol Oncol.* 2013;6:47.

31. Brentjens RJ, Davila ML, Riviere I, Park J, Wang X, Cowell LG, et al. CD19-targeted T cells rapidly induce molecular remissions in adults with chemotherapy-refractory acute lymphoblastic leukemia. *Sci Transl Med.* 2013;5(177):177ra38.

32. Davila ML, Riviere I, Wang X, Bartido S, Park J, Curran K, et al. Efficacy and toxicity management of 19–28z CAR T cell therapy in B cell acute lymphoblastic leukemia. *Sci Transl Med.* 2014;6(224):224ra25.

33. Adair JE, Beard BC, Trobridge GD, Neff T, Rockhill JK, Silbergeld DL, et al. Extended survival of glioblastoma patients after chemoprotective HSC gene therapy. *Sci Transl Med.* 2012;4(133):133ra57.

34. Adair JE, Johnston SK, Mrugala MM, Beard BC, Guyman LA, Baldock AL, et al. Gene therapy enhances chemotherapy tolerance and efficacy in glioblastoma patients. *J Clin Invest.* 2014;124(9):4082–92.

35. Neff T, Beard BC, Kiem HP. Survival of the fittest: in vivo selection and stem cell gene therapy. *Blood.* 2006;107(5):1751–60.

36. Zielske SP, Gerson SL. Lentiviral transduction of P140K MGMT into human CD34(+) hematopoietic progenitors at low multiplicity of infection confers significant resistance to BG/BCNU and allows selection in vitro. *Mol Ther.* 2002;5(4):381–7.

37. Davis BM, Roth JC, Liu L, Xu-Welliver M, Pegg AE, Gerson SL. Characterization of the P140K, PVP(138–140)MLK, and G156A O6-methylguanine-DNA methyltransferase mutants: implications for drug resistance gene therapy. *Hum Gene Ther.* 1999;10(17):2769–78.

38. Chung J, Scherer LJ, Gu A, Gardner AM, Torres-Coronado M, Epps EW, et al. Optimized lentiviral vectors for HIV gene therapy: multiplexed expression of small RNAs and inclusion of MGMT(P140K) drug resistance gene. *Mol Ther.* 2014;22(5):952–63.

39. Knight S, Zhang F, Mueller-Kuller U, Bokhoven M, Gupta A, Broughton T, et al. Safer, silencing-resistant lentiviral vectors: optimization of the ubiquitous chromatin-opening element through elimination of aberrant splicing. *J Virol.* 2012;86(17):9088–95.

40. Deichmann A, Brugman MH, Bartholomae CC, Schwarzwaelder K, Verstegen MM, Howe SJ, et al. Insertion sites in engrafted cells cluster within a limited repertoire of genomic areas after gammaretroviral vector gene therapy. *Mol Ther.* 2011;19(11):2031–9.

41. Gaussin A, Modlich U, Bauche C, Niederlander NJ, Schambach A, Duros C, et al. CTF/NF1 transcription factors act as potent genetic insulators for integrating gene transfer vectors. *Gene Ther.* 2012;19(1):15–24.

42. Heckl D, Schwarzer A, Haemmerle R, Steinemann D, Rudolph C, Skawran B, et al. Lentiviral vector induced insertional haploinsufficiency of Ebf1 causes murine leukemia. *Mol Ther.* 2012;20(6):1187–95.

43. Gaj T, Gersbach CA, Barbas CF, 3rd. ZFN, TALEN, and CRISPR/Cas-based methods for genome engineering. *Trends Biotechnol.* 2013 Jul;31(7):397–405.

44. Fung H, Weinstock DM. Repair at single targeted DNA double-strand breaks in pluripotent and differentiated human cells. *PLoS One.* 2011;6(5): e20514.

45. Smith JR, Maguire S, Davis LA, Alexander M, Yang F, Chandran S, et al. Robust, persistent transgene expression in human embryonic stem cells is achieved with AAVS1-targeted integration. *Stem Cells.* 2008;26(2):496–504.

46. DeKelver RC, Choi VM, Moehle EA, Paschon DE, Hockemeyer D, Meijsing SH, et al. Functional genomics, proteomics, and regulatory DNA analysis in isogenic settings using zinc finger nuclease-driven transgenesis into a safe harbor locus in the human genome. *Genome Res.* 2010;20(8):1133–42.

47. Urnov FD, Miller JC, Lee YL, Beausejour CM, Rock JM, Augustus S, et al. Highly efficient endogenous human gene correction using designed zinc-finger nucleases. *Nature.* 2005;435(7042):646–51.

48. Reyon D, Tsai SQ, Khayter C, Foden JA, Sander JD, Joung JK. FLASH assembly of TALENs for high-throughput genome editing. *Nat Biotechnol.* 2012;30(5):460–5.

49. Sander JD, Joung JK. CRISPR-Cas systems for editing, regulating and targeting genomes. *Nat Biotechnol.* 2014;32(4):347–55.

Chapter

68

Regenerative Medicine: The Future?

Kerry Atkinson

Historical Perspective

Prehistory

The earliest concept of regenerative medicine appears to have occurred in 800 BC pre-Athenian Greek mythology and was later reiterated in the Greek tragedy written by Aeschylus in 500 BC called *Prometheus Bound*. Prometheus was a Titan (a Greek deity) who sided with Zeus and the ascending Olympian gods in the vast cosmological struggle against Cronus and the other Titans. Prometheus was therefore on the conquering side of the cataclysmic war of the Greek gods, the Titanomachy, in which Zeus and the Olympian gods ultimately defeated Cronus and the other Titans.

The Prometheus myth first appeared in the late 8th Century BC Greek epic poet Hesiod's *Theogony*. At the Mekone, a sacrificial meal marking the "settling of accounts" between mortals and immortals, Prometheus played a trick on Zeus, the King of the Gods. He presented two sacrificial offerings to the Olympian: a selection of beef placed inside an ox's stomach (nourishment hidden inside a displeasing exterior), and a bull's bones wrapped completely in "glistening fat" (something inedible hidden inside a pleasing exterior). Zeus chose the latter, setting a precedent for future sacrifices: henceforth, humans would keep that meat for themselves and burn the bones wrapped in fat as an offering to the gods.

This angered Zeus, who hid fire from humans in retribution. Prometheus, however, stole fire back in a giant fennel-stalk and restored it to humanity. This further enraged Zeus. As punishment, Zeus had Prometheus chained to a rock where his liver was eaten daily by an eagle, only to have it regenerate at night, due to his immortality. Each day the eagle would eat Prometheus' liver. Each night his liver would regenerate. Years later, the Greek hero Heracles (Hercules) slayed the eagle and freed Prometheus from his chains.

It is interesting that the liver is one of the few human organs that can self-regenerate to a significant extent.

Developments in the 20th Century

The term "Regenerative Medicine" was first used in a 1992 article on hospital administration by Leland Kaiser. Kaiser's paper closed with a series of short paragraphs on future technologies that would impact hospitals. One such paragraph had "Regenerative Medicine" as a bold print title and went on to

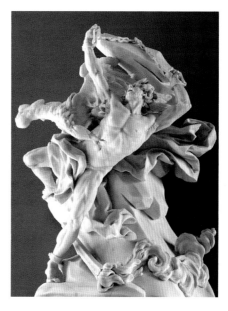

Figure 68.1. The eagle eating the liver of Prometheus in 800 BC (painted by Theodoor Rombouts, 1597–1637). This image, reproduced here from Wikimedia Commons, is in the public domain. PD 1923.

state "A new branch of medicine will develop that attempts to change the course of chronic disease and in many instances will regenerate tired and failing organ systems"[1].

In 2006, the US National Institutes of Health defined regenerative medicine as "the process of creating living, functional tissues to repair or replace tissue or organ function lost due to age, disease, damage, or congenital defects". More specifically, regenerative medicine has developed as a branch of translational research involving stem cells and their progeny and often involving tissue engineering technology and the use scaffolds. It deals with the "process of replacing, engineering or regenerating human cells, tissues or organs to restore or establish normal function"[1]. Regenerative medicine also includes the possibility of growing tissues and organs in the laboratory and safely implanting them when the body cannot heal itself. If a regenerated organ's cells could be derived from the patient's own tissue or cells, this would potentially solve the problem of the shortage of organs available for donation, and the problem of organ transplant rejection.

The Hematopoietic Stem Cell

Progress was slow in regenerative medicine after the description of the regeneration of Prometheus' liver and it was not until 2760 years later when McCulloch and Till[2] in

Canada described hematopoietic stem cells that further progress was made. Their discovery led directly to human bone marrow transplantation in the late 1960s as a therapy of last resort for leukemia that was refractory to conventional chemotherapy. Dr Don Thomas pioneered this technique and was awarded the Nobel Prize in Medicine in 1990. Bone marrow transplantation (and subsequently transplantation of mobilized peripheral blood stem and progenitor cells and cord blood transplantation – known collectively as hematopoietic stem cell (HSC) transplantation) initially utilized myeloablative chemotherapy or chemotherapy and total body irradiation to eradicate the patient's leukemia. In so doing, the recipient's own marrow was eradicated and the transplanted donor HSCs enabled regeneration of a new hematopoietic and immune system of donor origin in the recipient[3,4]. It was subsequently discovered that a major contributing component to the cure of such leukemias was the graft-*versus*-leukemia effect mediated by donor T-cells in the HSC inoculum[5].

HSC transplantation has been part of clinical practice for over 40 years and represents the most prominent example, indeed the only current example, of mainstream regenerative medicine in the clinic.

The Mesenchymal Stem Cell

The next discovery relevant to the development of regenerative medicine was made in 1974 by Dr Friedenstein and his colleagues in Russia[6]. They discovered another stem cell in the bone marrow that could give rise to at least some of the skeletal tissues of the body such as the bones, cartilage, tendon, muscles, and fat. They measured the number of cells that they were able to grow in the laboratory by using the clonal growth in agar of cells that resembled fibroblasts and such colonies were called colony-forming unit-fibroblast (CFU-F). The stem cell is known as the mesenchymal stem cell and its progeny are known as mesenchymal stromal cells (MSCs) or mesenchymal progenitor cells.

Organ-Specific Stem Cells

Organ-specific stem cells have been identified in the gastrointestinal tract[7], skeletal muscle[8], skin[9], central nervous system[10], endometrium[11], heart[12], and liver[13].

The Human Embryonic Stem Cell

The next major breakthrough that contributed to this new form of medicine was the discovery of the human embryonic stem cell (ESC) by James Thomson at the University of Wisconsin in 1998[14]. This was an exponential leap in the potential development of the field of regenerative medicine because all the tissues of the body could be derived from such cells. There were two prime areas of concern. On an ethical level, human ESCs could only be obtained by destroying a living human embryo, as the process involved enucleating the

contents of the fertilized egg at the four-cell stage of growth. In medical terms, the concern was that mice injected with ESCs developed teratomas: tumors consisting of tissues from each of the three germ layers – the ectoderm, the endoderm, and the mesoderm. Indeed this capacity became the recognized test of the ESC's pluripotent ability – that is to say, the ability to differentiate into cells or tissues of each of the three germ layers.

The Human Induced Pluripotent Stem Cell

Relief on the ethical side occurred when Dr Shinya Yamanaka's group in Japan described the ability to derive pluripotent stem cells by injecting normal mature cells with four genes – Klf4, c-Myc, Oct-3/4, and Sox-2[15]. Thus, these cells could be derived in the laboratory without the need to utilize living human embryos and were much more acceptable than ESCs to many people – both in the scientific community and in the general public. These cells were known as induced pluripotent stem cells (iPSCs).

The problem was not solved yet, however, since some of the genes used by Dr Yamanaka and his colleagues initially were known oncogenes (e.g., c-Myc) and integration of the injected genes into the nucleus resulted in their random integration into the genome, which could lead to the activation of other endogenous oncogenes if the injected gene integrated next to one of these. Furthermore, differentiation protocols had to be designed to drive iPSCs down the desired differentiation pathway for therapeutic use – be it to neurons or cardiomyocytes or retinal epithelial cells or any other type of cell required by the patient.

In 2013 researchers successfully reprogramed adult cells in a living animal for the first time, creating stem cells that have the ability to grow into any tissue found in the body. Until then these cells had only ever been created in Petri dishes in the laboratory after being removed from the animal. However, researchers at the Spanish National Cancer Research Centre in Madrid, Spain, were able to create these cells in the bodies of living mice[16].

Scaffolds Using Decellularized Human Organs
Biologic Scaffolds

In June 2008, at the Hospital Clínic de Barcelona, Professor Paolo Macchiarini and his team, of the University of Barcelona, performed the first tissue-engineered tracheal transplantation. Adult stem cells were extracted from the patient's bone marrow, grown into a large population, and matured into cartilage cells, or chondrocytes, using an adaptive method originally devised for treating osteoarthritis. The team then seeded the newly grown chondrocytes, as well as epithelial cells, into a decellularized (free of donor cells) tracheal segment that was donated from a 51-year-old transplant donor who had died of cerebral hemorrhage. After 4 days of seeding, the graft was used to replace the patient's left main bronchus. After 1 month, a biopsy elicited local bleeding, indicating that the blood vessels had already grown back successfully[17].

In 2012, Professor Paolo Macchiarini and his team improved upon the 2008 implant by transplanting a laboratory-made trachea seeded with the patient's own cells, and in 2013 his group bioengineered a rat esophagus[18]. In the United States, Anthony Atala's group has been involved in similar bioengineering and is employing three-dimensional printing to help generate individual body organs[19].

Synthetic Scaffolds

A large number of materials have been used to provide synthetic scaffolds for cells prior to their implantation into the recipient. A commonly used synthetic material is polylactic acid (PLA). This is a polyester which degrades within the human body to form lactic acid, a naturally occurring chemical which is easily removed from the body. Similar materials are polyglycolic acid (PGA) and polycaprolactone (PCL): their degradation mechanism is similar to that of PLA, but they exhibit respectively a faster and a slower rate of degradation compared to PLA.

Clinical Results

Bone Marrow Hematopoietic Stem Cells

The Hematopoietic and Immune Systems

There are minimal data to suggest that bone marrow HSCs play a major role in the regeneration of any tissues other than the hematopoietic and immune systems after HSC transplantation. They perform the latter magnificently although hematopoietic cell recovery is faster than some cells of the adaptive immune system, specifically functional T- and B-lymphocytes. Furthermore, mobilized peripheral blood stem and progenitor cell transplantation produces faster recovery than bone marrow transplantation, which, in turn, produces faster recovery than cord blood transplantation, at least in adults. It is still astonishing that 40 years after a brother has received an HLA-identical transplant from a sister that metaphases of cells from his hematopoietic and immune system cells continue to show only an XX karyotype (and vice versa (i.e., XY) with brother to sister transplants).

In stark contrast to this, the marrow stromal cells of the host remain, indicating their significant resistance to very high-dose chemoradiation or chemotherapy.

Acute Myocardial Infarction

In the past a number of investigators have suggested that adult bone marrow (BM) cells may enable cardiac regeneration after acute myocardial infarction, suggesting that marrow serves as a reservoir for cardiac precursor cells. A detailed study investigating the role of murine marrow HSCs in mice given a myocardial infarction negated this. Balsam and colleagues[20] studied the ability of c-kit-enriched BM cells, Lin- c-kit+ BM cells, and c-kit+ Thy1.1lo Lin- Sca-1+ long-term reconstituting hematopoietic stem cells to regenerate myocardium in a model of myocardial infarction. Cells were isolated from transgenic mice expressing green fluorescent protein (GFP) and injected directly into ischemic myocardium of wild-type mice. Abundant GFP+ cells were detected in the myocardium after 10 days, but by 30 days, few cells were detectable. These GFP+ cells did not express cardiac tissue-specific markers, but rather, most of them expressed the hematopoietic marker CD45 and myeloid marker Gr-1. The role of circulating cells in the repair of ischemic myocardium using GFP+-GFP- parabiotic mice was investigated in the same study: again, no evidence of myocardial regeneration from blood-borne partner-derived cells was found. The data suggested that even in the microenvironment of the injured heart, c-kit-enriched BM cells, Lin-c-kit+ BM cells, and c-kit+ Thy1.1lo Lin- Sca-1+ long-term reconstituting hematopoietic stem cells adopt only traditional hematopoietic fates.

Corneal Ulceration

A study was conducted to evaluate the therapeutic effects of topically applied bone marrow (BM) cells and CD117-positive hematopoietic stem (CD117+) cells on alkali-induced corneal ulcers in mice[21]. Bone marrow cells and CD117+ cells were isolated from syngeneic mice and labeled with an intracellular cell tracer. Defined corneal wounds were produced in 89 eyes of syngeneic mice and allowed to partially heal *in-vivo* for 6 hours. The alkali-burned eyes were enucleated 6 hours post-injury and randomly divided into three groups. The control group (33 eyes) was incubated with medium only. The treatment groups received either BM cells (30 eyes) or CD117+ cells (26 eyes) suspended in medium. The re-epithelialization process of corneal defects was qualitatively and quantitatively assessed and statistically analyzed. The corneas were examined by histologic and immunohistochemical methods. We found that the re-epithelialization of corneal wounds in both treatment groups was significantly accelerated as compared to the control group. During the follow-up period (85 hours), the corneal transparency was comparable in all groups. Morphologic investigations of corneas from control and treatment groups showed no evident differences in the phenotype of the regenerated epithelium. Additionally, corneas in the treatment groups were devoid of donor-derived BM cells and CD117+ cells, respectively. This study provided evidence that topical application of BM cells or CD117+ cells can be used to reconstruct corneal surfaces. Because neither BM cells nor CD117+ cells were integrated into the corneal epithelium, it was suggested that soluble factors could be responsible for the positive effect of BM cells and CD117+ cells on corneal wound healing.

Skeletal Muscle

It had previously been shown that bone marrow cells contribute to skeletal muscle regeneration, but the nature of marrow cell(s) involved in this process was unknown. Abedi *et al.*[22] used an immunocompetent and an immunocompromised model of bone marrow transplantation to characterize the type of marrow cells participating in regenerating skeletal muscle fibers in mice. Animals were transplanted with different populations of marrow cells from GFP transgenic mice and the presence of GFP+ muscle fibers were evaluated in the cardiotoxin-injured tibialis anterior muscles. GFP+ muscle fibers were found mostly in animals that received either CD45–, lineage–, c-kit+, Sca-1+, or Flk-2+ populations of marrow cells, suggesting that HSC or more differentiated hematopoietic cells rather than mesenchymal cells are responsible for the formation of GFP+ muscle fibers. A Mac-1 positive population of marrow cells was also associated with the emergence of GFP+ skeletal muscle fibers. However, most of this activity was limited to either Mac-1+, Sca+, or Mac-1+ c-kit+ cells with long-term hematopoietic repopulation capabilities, indicating a hematopoietic stem cell phenotype for these cells

Mobilized Peripheral Blood Stem and Progenitor Cells

Acute Myocardial Infarction

Investigators hypothesized that mobilized peripheral blood hematopoietic cells would accelerate recovery from acute myocardial infarction and gave granulocyte colony-stimulating factor (G-CSF) to patients who had had an acute myocardial infarction: in fact this had an adverse impact on the infarct, presumably because even greater numbers of neutrophils were attracted to the already inflamed myocardium by the administration of G-CSF[23].

Another study prospectively randomized 27 patients with myocardial infarction who underwent coronary stenting into three groups: G-CSF-mobilized peripheral blood hematopoietic cells (n=10), G-CSF alone (n=10), and a control group (n=7) [24]. Changes in left ventricular systolic function and perfusion were assessed after 6 months. Seven patients from the cell infusion group, three from the G-CSF group, and one from the control group had been assessed at the time of the report. G-CSF injection and intracoronary infusion of the mobilized PBHC did not aggravate inflammation and ischemia during the periprocedural period. Exercise capacity, myocardial perfusion, and systolic function improved significantly in patients who received cell infusion. However, an unexpectedly high rate of in-stent restenosis at initial coronary artery lesion in patients who received G-CSF was noted, and enrollment was therefore stopped.

The Presence of Donor Hematopoietic Stem Cells in Organs Other Than the Hematopoietic and Immune Systems

It is worth noting, however, that a minor degree of donor cell chimerism has been documented in organs other than the hematopoietic and immune systems. For example, Körbling et al.[25] performed biopsy specimens from the liver, gastrointestinal tract, and skin from 12 patients who had undergone transplantation of hematopoietic stem cells from peripheral blood (11 patients) or bone marrow (1 patient). Six female patients had received transplants from a male donor. Five had received a sex-matched transplant, and one had received an autologous transplant. Hematopoietic stem cell engraftment

was verified by cytogenetic analysis or restriction-fragment-length polymorphism analysis. The biopsies were studied for the presence of donor-derived epithelial cells or hepatocytes with the use of fluorescence in situ hybridization of interphase nuclei and immunohistochemical staining for cytokeratin, CD45 (leukocyte common antigen), and a hepatocyte-specific antigen. All six recipients of sex-mismatched transplants showed evidence of complete hematopoietic donor chimerism. XY-positive epithelial cells or hepatocytes accounted for 0 to 7% of the cells in histologic sections of the biopsy specimens. These cells were detected in liver tissue as early as day 13 and in skin tissue as late as day 354 after the transplantation of peripheral-blood stem cells.

Although present in these tissues, the numbers detected were too small to hypothesize that they could have played any role in regeneration of these organs.

Cord Blood Hematopoietic Stem Cells

There are many articles in the scientific literature suggesting that cord blood cells play a role in regeneration of a number of tissues. However, the majority of these reports refer to cord blood cells or cord blood stem cells, without indicating whether the population responsible for the regenerative effects are hematopoietic stem cells, mesenchymal cells, endothelial cells, or other cell types. While cord blood is a proven and useful source of CD34+ hematopoietic stem cells for HSC transplantation, mesenchymal cells are only found in first trimester cord blood and not in cord blood taken after delivery of a normal term pregnancy. Their possible role in the regeneration of tissues other than the hematopoietic system will not be further discussed.

Other Cells of the Hematopoietic and Immune Systems

T-Cells and HIV Infection

In June 2014 the USA biotechnology company Calimmune was given approval to continue with the second cohort of subjects with HIV. This phase 1/2 clinical trial focuses on CCR5, a chemokine receptor that plays a key role in enabling HIV to infect cells. Blocking CCR5 may provide the cells with a protective shield against HIV, which in turn would help retain immune system functionality. In the first phase of this study four HIV-positive participants were infused with their own blood stem cells as well as mature T cells that had been modified to carry a gene that blocks production of CCR5. The hope is that those stem cells will then create a new blood system that is resistant to HIV.

The Role of Mesenchymal Cells in Regenerative Medicine

The Biology of Mesenchymal Stem Cells

Mesenchymal cells are the cells currently employed in most attempts at tissue and organ regeneration using cellular therapy (for organs other than the hematopoietic and immune systems). Mesenchymal cells were first described in the bone marrow by Friedenstein *et al.*[6]. The identity of cells that establish the hematopoietic microenvironment in human bone marrow, and of clonogenic skeletal progenitors found in bone marrow stroma, remained elusive until Sacchetti *et al.* demonstrated that MCAM/CD146-expressing subendothelial cells in human marrow stroma were capable of transferring, upon transplantation, the hematopoietic microenvironment to heterotopic sites *in-vivo* in mice, coincident with the establishment of identical subendothelial cells within the miniature bone organ that was established by the transplantation of these cells[26]. Establishment of subendothelial stromal cells in developing a heterotopic bone marrow *in-vivo* was found to occur via specific, dynamic interactions with developing bone marrow sinusoids. Subendothelial stromal cells residing on the sinusoidal wall were found to be major producers of Angiopoietin-1, a pivotal molecule of the HSC niche involved in vascular remodeling. These data revealed the functional relationships between establishment of a hematopoietic microenvironment *in-vivo*, establishment of skeletal progenitors in BM sinusoids, and angiogenesis. These investigators showed that mesenchymal stem cells could both self-renew and could differentiate in mice into osteoblasts to form bone, which was subsequently colonized by the recipient mouse's hematopoietic cells.

The direct relationship between mesenchymal cells and hematopoietic stem cells was further amplified by the work of Mendez-Ferrer *et al.*[27]. They demonstrated that mesenchymal stem cells, identified using nestin expression, constituted an essential HSC niche component. Nestin+ mesenchymal stem cells contained all the CFU-F activity and could be propagated as nonadherent "mensspheres" that could self-renew and expand in serial transplantations. Nestin+ mesenchymal stem cells were found to be spatially associated with HSCs and adrenergic nerve fibers, and to highly express HSC maintenance genes. These genes, and others triggering osteoblastic differentiation, were selectively downregulated during enforced HSC mobilization or beta-3 adrenoreceptor activation. Whereas parathormone administration doubled the number of bone marrow nestin+ cells and favored their osteoblastic differentiation, *in-vivo* nestin+ cell depletion rapidly reduced HSC content in the bone marrow. Purified HSCs homed to an area near nestin+ mesenchymal stem cells in the bone marrow of lethally irradiated mice, whereas *in-vivo* nestin+ cell depletion significantly reduced bone marrow homing of hematopoietic progenitors. These results confirmed the unprecedented partnership between the two distinct somatic stem cell types described previously by Sacchetti's group and indicated a unique niche in the bone marrow made of heterotypic stem cell pairs.

Mesenchymal stem cells exist in small numbers in marrow at a frequency of between 1 in 10^4 and 1 in 10^5 of nucleated marrow cells. This makes it difficult to obtain sufficient numbers for clinical application. Their progeny, however,

known as mesenchymal stromal cells (MSCs), can be grown in large numbers because of their ability to expand *ex-vivo* by adherence to plastic and can be used for both basic research and clinical application. The abbreviation MSC in this chapter refers to mesenchymal *stromal* cells and not to mesenchymal stem cells.

Clinical use of the findings of the Sacchetti and Mendez-Ferrer groups was made by de Lima and colleagues who used a monolayer of mesenchymal stromal cells on which to expand the HSCs from a cord blood unit for clinical transplantation. Patients were transplanted with one unmanipulated cord unit and one unit of the cord blood cells incubated on the MSC monolayer[28]. Transplantation of cord blood cells expanded with mesenchymal stromal cells appeared to be safe and effective. Expanded cord blood in combination with unmanipulated cord blood significantly improved engraftment, compared to unmanipulated cord blood only.

The Biology of Mesenchymal Stromal Cells

The cell surface phenotype of mesenchymal stromal cells is characteristic but not unique – for example, fibroblasts express many of the same antigens. Human MSCs express CD73, CD105, CD29, CD44, CD49d, CD90, CD146, CD166, and HLA class I. Upon incubation with interferon-γ, they can be induced to express MHC class II antigens.

MSCs are pericytes – they wrap around the endothelium of capillaries[29,30]. They can, therefore, be isolated from every vascularized tissue or organ. While all MSCs are pericytes, not all pericytes are MSCs: in arterioles, arteries, and veins smooth muscle cells also cover the endothelium, allowing these vessels to contract.

MSCs have two characteristics that are advantageous for their use in the clinic. Firstly, there appears to be no need for tissue-matching between the MSC donor and the MSC recipient. In mice we have shown this in a murine model of allergic asthma in which Balb/c mice (H2^d) sensitized to house dust mite received two-haplotype-mismatched MSCs from

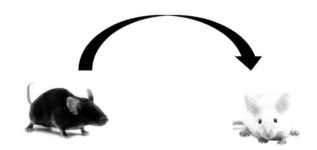

Donor-derived MSCs
- C57BL/6 male mice
- MHC haplotype: **H2^b**

Animal model of asthma
- BALB/c female mice
- MHC haplotype: **H2^d**

Figure 68.2. An example of an allogeneic transplantation model of allergic murine asthma: MSCs from C57BL/6 mice were able to dramatically improve pulmonary function in Balb/c mice sensitized to the house dust mite despite the cells being transplanted across a two-haplotype-mismatched barrier.

Table 68.1. Mechanisms by which MSCs appear to mediate therapeutic benefit

1. Differentiation into mesodermal lineage[45]

2. Paracrine secretion of immunomodulatory molecules to down-regulate excessive inflammation (Lee *et al*. Cell Stem Cell 2009)

3. Induction of tolerance by inducing T-cell apoptosis and increasing Treg cells to produce immune tolerance (Akiyama *et al*. Cell Stem Cell 2012)

4. Transfer of MSC-derived mitochondria to damaged target cells (Islam *et al*. Nature Medicine 2012)

5. Stimulate the abundance and lineage commitment of endogenous organ-specific stem cells[56]

6. Gene replacement?

C57BL/6 mice (H2^b), with marked improvement in pulmonary function (K Dhuang, PhD thesis, in preparation). This was also illustrated in one of the first descriptions of the use of MSCs in the clinic: Le Blanc *et al*. infused third-party haploidentical (parental) MSCs into a recipient of an allogeneic transplant recipient with severe graft-*versus*-host disease refractory to conventional treatment[31].

Since then MSCs from unrelated volunteers have been widely used in almost all clinical trials with MSCs (see for example reference[32]).

This characteristic enables the manufacture and cryopreservation of MSCs so that they are available as an "off-the-shelf" product for any acute or chronic clinical setting when needed. They thus appear to be the nucleated cell equivalent of Rhesus-negative Group O red blood cells.

Secondly, MSCs injected intravenously preferentially home to at least some sites of inflammation. For example, intravenously injected murine MSCs preferentially homed to a small skin incision on one side of the abdomen after their passage through the lungs.

In addition to their apparent ability to evade the immune surveillance of the recipient's immune system, MSCs are actively suppressive of T-cell, B-cell, NK cell, and dendritic cell function[33,34]. This may be one of the mechanisms by which MSCs avoid rejection by the recipient's immune system.

As indicated above, MSCs used for laboratory and clinical investigations need to be expanded in *ex-vivo* culture to obtain sufficient cell numbers to work with. While some changes have been described with increasing passage number, we have found murine MSCs at passage 10 still able to suppress T-cell alloreactivity *in-vitro*, maintain hematopoietic stem cells *in-vitro*, improve cardiac function after acute myocardial infarction *in-vivo* and improve pulmonary function in allergic asthma *in-vivo*.

A number of different mechanisms have been described by which MSCs appear to mediate their therapeutic effects *in-vivo*. These are listed in Table 68.1.

One further area of discussion is the source of MSCs used: two questions are relevant: firstly, do MSCs derived from

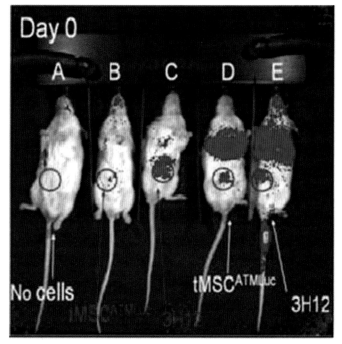

Figure 68.3. Murine MSCs injected intravenously via the tail vein homed preferentially to a small cutaneous wound on the right underside of the recipient mouse after their passage through the lungs. Murine MSCs transgenic for the luciferase gene were imaged by their photon emission capability (best seen in mice D and E). Mouse A was a control and received no MSCs.

different organs or tissues differ in their biologic characteristics? Secondly, are MSCs from a specific and healthy source better, worse, or the same in terms of their ability to mediate a therapeutic benefit in the corresponding diseased target organ or tissue? I am unaware of any such comparisons to answer the second question. However, while many biologic characteristics are shared between MSCs from different sources, there are differences in gene expression between MSCs from different sources, both in the mouse and in humans. A study we conducted compared murine MSCs from bone marrow, heart, and kidney. The cell surface antigen display was virtually identical in MSCs from each source, although the intensity of expression differed. The ability of MSCs from bone marrow was the most suppressive of T-cell alloproliferation in a mixed leukocyte reaction, while renal MSCs were moderately immunosuppressive and cardiac MSCs showed very little immune suppression capability (Figures 68.4 and 68.5)[35]. Gene expression was quite different between the three different populations and the genes overexpressed in canonical pathways varied according to the MSC source (Table 68.2). Similarly, when we compared MSCs from normal human adult bone marrow with MSCs isolated from term placenta, the MSCs from each source were similar in their cell surface antigen display, mesodermal differentiation ability *in-vitro*, and capacity to inhibit T-cell alloproliferation *in-vitro*[36], but again differed in their gene expression profile (N. Matigian *et al*., unpublished data).

Morphologically, MSCs derived from human placenta were heterogeneous in size but homogeneous in appearance: they

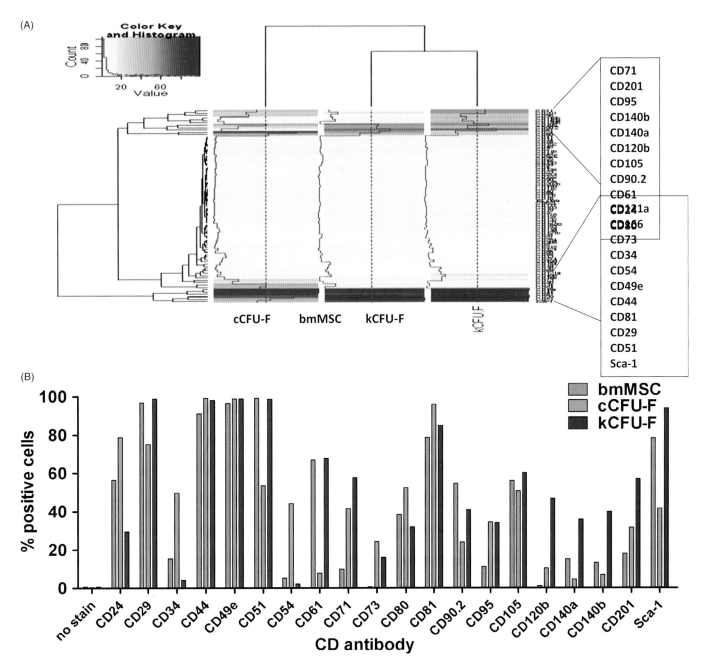

Figure 68.4. CD cell surface epitope expression of murine bone marrow/bone MSCs, cardiac CFU-Fs, and kidney CFU-F populations[35].

had a large dense nucleus and much cytoplasm with many vacuoles present.

Clinical Results

The Role of Mesenchymal Stromal Cells in Regenerative Medicine

The Hematopoietic and Immune Systems

Expansion of Hematopoietic Cells on a Monolayer of Human Mesenchymal Stromal Cells

The expansion of human cord blood hematopoietic stem cells on a monolayer of human mesenchymal stromal cells has been

outlined above. This finding is of considerable significance since cord blood transplantation in adults (as opposed to children) is markedly hampered by slow hematopoietic engraftment in adults because of the low number of CD34+ cells present in cord blood units. Overcoming this slow engraftment rate would make cord blood safer and thus more readily accessible to adults requiring an HSC transplant for whom no living HLA-matched related or unrelated donors are available.

Graft-*versus*-Host Disease

Katarina Le Blanc's description of the therapeutic effect of haploidentical MSCs in a patient with treatment-refractory graft-*versus*-host disease following an HSC transplant from an unrelated donor was one of the first and most startling indications of the potential therapeutic value of these cells[31]. A phase 2 multicenter study suggested that they did indeed have therapeutic value in this setting[32]. The therapeutic effect seems to be most marked in children. Human allogeneic bone marrow-derived MSCs have been granted marketing approval in Canada and New Zealand for severe acute GvHD following allogeneic HSC transplantation in children.

Wound Repair

MSCs play a critical role in wound healing[37]. Several studies have been published which demonstrated their clinical usefulness[38]. They reported that the direct application of autologous bone marrow-derived MSCs (BM-MSCs) in patients with chronic wounds could achieve wound closure and tissue reconstruction. They observed that the direct injection of fresh whole BM into the edges of the wound followed by topical application of cultured MSCs managed to completely close chronic ulcers in three patients in whom conventional treatment had failed. Furthermore, remarkable results can be achieved in the treatment of chronic wounds by combining BM-MSCs with tissue engineering. A trial was performed on five patients with acute or chronic wounds which were treated with autologous BM-MSCs applied with a fibrin spray as a cell delivery system. Biopsies of these wounds revealed that the MSCs migrated to the wound and stimulated elastin expression, thus improving the structure of the extracellular matrix [39]. In a similar study a collagen sponge was used to administer autologous BM-MSCs to 20 patients with chronic wounds. The results showed that the MSC-impregnated collagen compound enhanced wound healing in 18 of 20 patients and accelerated tissue regeneration[40].

Limb Ischemia and Foot Ulcers

Lu *et al.* found that BM-MSC therapy appeared to be better tolerated and more effective than BM mononuclear cells for

Table 68.2 Over-representation of genes involved in cellular processes and canonical pathways in the three murine MSC-like cell populations using Ingenuity Pathway Analysis

Cell population	Over-representation of genes involved in cellular processes and canonical pathways
Bone marrow MSCs	Cell cycle Genetic disorders *Cell-mediated immunity* *Connective tissue disorders* Gene expression
Cardiac CFU-Fs	Skeletal and muscular development Nervous system development and function Tissue development *Cardiovascular system development and function* Organ development Developmental disorders Lymphoid tissue structure and function Skeletal and muscular development
Kidney CFU-Fs	*Renal/urologic system development and function* Organ development Tissue development Infection mechanism

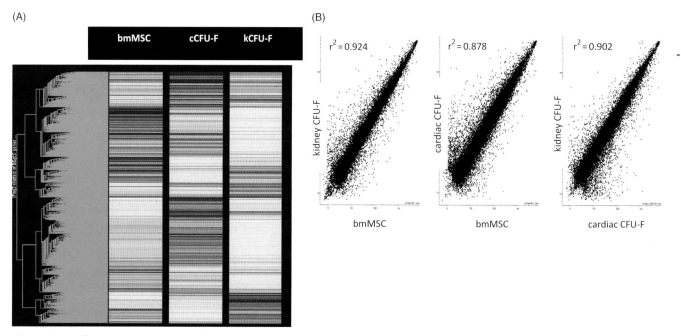

Figure 68.5. Differential gene expression profiles of murine bone marrow/bone MSCs, cardiac CFU-Fs and kidney CFU-F populations[35]. (A) Gene tree. (B) Pearson's correlation coefficients.

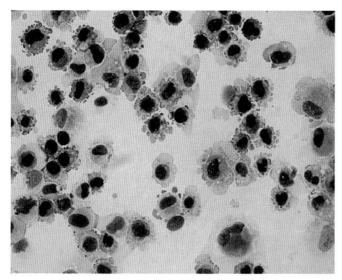

Figure 68.6. A comparison of size, CD cell surface markers, and mesodermal differentiation of human bone marrow-derived MSCs and human placenta-derived MSCs[36].

increasing lower limb perfusion and promoting foot ulcer healing in diabetic patients with critical limb ischemia[41]. In 2012, Lee *et al.* published a study in which they applied several intramuscular ASC injections in 15 critical limb ischemia patients. The authors observed clinical improvement in 66.7% of cases, with patients exhibiting a significant decrease in the pain rating scale and improved claudication walking distance[42].

Perianal Fistulae

In 2008, García-Olmo *et al.* used MSCs derived from adipose tissue for treating perianal fistulae[43]. Cells were obtained by liposuction and a subsequent expansion process. They were then administered according to a protocol which involved infusion of the cells into the target lesion along with fibrin glue. The results obtained compared the MSCs plus fibrin glue application to fibrin glue alone. The MSCs were effective at inducing healing in complex perianal fistulas. Unfortunately, a low proportion of the stem cell-treated patients with closure after the procedure remained free of recurrence after more than 3 years of follow-up.

Rectovaginal Fistulae

The same group published in 2010 the first results of using allogeneic MSCs derived by liposuction to treat rectovaginal fistulae associated with Crohn's disease. Although the fistulae remained open, considerable improvement was noted[44].

Musculoskeletal Disorders
Nonunion Bone Fractures

de Steiger *et al.* reported the use of autologous bone marrow-derived MSCs to treat bone fractures that had failed to unite using conventional orthopedic treatment[45]. At the time of

surgery, the *ex-vivo* expanded cells were implanted onto a hydroxyl apatite/tricalcium phosphate matrix and placed in the nonunion site. Eight of 11 patients united at a mean time of 24 weeks. One patient appeared to be uniting, union in one was uncertain, and failure to unite occurred in one patient.

Critical Bone Defects

Quarto *et al.* published a report in which three patients underwent successful treatments with *ex-vivo* expanded autologous bone marrow-derived MSCs that were seeded on macroporous hydroxyapatite scaffolds. Each patient was immobilized in an external fixator and osteointegration was achieved in each patient by the second postoperative month[46].

Craniofacial Defects

Craniofacial defects encompass cranial defects, cleft palate-related deformities, and mandibular defects. The traditional treatment for cranial bone repair has involved using autologous bone grafts, derived from scapula, ribs, fibula, or iliac crest. However, access to these tissues is limited and often associated with secondary site morbidity. Two human clinical trials examined the efficacy of MSCs to repair cranial defects. These studies used autologous MSCs combined with collagen-coated scaffolds for adults[47], or MSCs combined with hydroxyapatite and polylactic polymer scaffolds in child patients[48]. Both trials reported promising outcomes, with gross general morphology and CT imaging revealing bone formation at the transplant site and an accompanying reduction in defect size in patients with alveolar cleft defects and general cranial defects.

Spinal Fusion

Gan and colleagues demonstrated the efficacy of using enriched preparations of autologous bone marrow-derived MSCs combined with tricalcium phosphate for posterior spinal fusion in 41 patients. Long-term follow-up indicated that 95% of cases exhibited good spinal fusion at 34 months following treatment, with only minor adverse effects in four patients relating to inflammation of their wounds, which resolved with standard therapy[49].

Osteoarthritis

By 2012, 21 studies of the use of intra-articular MSCs to repair the cartilage defect in subjects with osteoarthritis had been reported, with those with the largest number of evaluable patients reporting generally favorable results. A randomized double-blind trial sponsored by Osiris Therapeutics Inc. involved 55 patients who received either 50 million or 150 million bone allogeneic marrow-derived MSCs into an affected joint. Patients reported significantly reduced pain and MRI scans showed a decrease in degenerative bone changes[50].

Nejadnik compared 36 patients given autologous MSCs with 36 given autologous chondrocytes. Those receiving MSCs reported improvement in physical function[51].

Cartilage Injuries

Cartilaginous injuries can arise from either traumatic injury or disease. In human studies, the favored scaffold for cartilage repair appears to be collagen based, which is more flexible and resorbable, unlike the osteoinductive hydroxyapatite/tricalcium phosphate ceramic scaffolds preferred for long bone fracture repair. Several case studies reported that all the patients that received autologous MSC therapy demonstrated substantial improvement in their symptoms and showed evidence of cartilage repair and the ability to resume their sporting and daily activities. The progress of the patients was followed for up to 5 years, with no evidence of adverse effects from the MSC therapy[52,53].

Tendinopathies

Our group has explored the use of allogeneic placenta-derived MSCs in subjects with Achilles tendinopathy refractory to conventional treatment including surgery and exercise programs. There were no serious adverse events related to the administration of the MSCs and, although designed as a phase 1 safety, feasibility, and dose escalation trial, the therapeutic response has been impressive (M. Young, unpublished data).

Cardiac Disease
Ischemic Cardiomyopathy/Chronic Heart Failure

Accumulating data support the use of bone marrow (BM)-derived MSCs in animal models (e.g., pigs) to restore cardiac function and tissue perfusion in chronic cardiac injury. Based on results obtained in pigs. At the time of writing. Da Silva and Hare are conducting phase 1/2 clinical trials to address the safety, cell type, cell dose, delivery technique, and efficacy of MSCs in patients with ischemic cardiomyopathy/chronic heart failure. MSCs for these trials were isolated from harvested BM and then processed and expanded for intracardiac injection. The BM-MSCs in use for the clinical trials were of clinical grade, having been processed successfully in an FDA-approved cGMP facility[54]. Hare's group has conducted four clinical trials comprising 107 patients. All trials revealed safety and a reduction in myocardial infarct size and improvement in functional parameters such as the 6-minute walk time and the Minnesota Living with Heart Failure Score[55]. Interestingly, injection of bone marrow-derived cells into the heart stimulates endogenous cardiomyocytes and promotes cardiac repair[56].

Lung Disease
Chronic Obstructive Pulmonary Disease (COPD)

Osiris Therapeutics Inc. sponsored a trial in which subjects with severe COPD received four infusions of allogeneic unrelated bone marrow-derived MSCs. This trial demonstrated that MSCs were safe in this setting.

Idiopathic Pulmonary Fibrosis

Our group has been involved in a phase 1 trial of allogeneic placenta-derived MSCs in subjects with idiopathic pulmonary fibrosis. This disease occurs in the 3rd to 5th decades and is universally fatal without lung transplantation. There were no adverse events associated with administration of the MSCs and pulmonary function and CT scan results remained stable throughout the 6-month follow-up period[57]. The rationale for this trial was the beneficial effect that MSCs have on a bleomycin-induced model of pulmonary fibrosis in mice.

Autoimmune Diseases
Systemic Lupus Erythematosus

Several small uncontrolled case series have been reported in subjects with systemic lupus erythematosus with promising results[58,59]. Multicenter randomized, controlled clinical trials are needed to confirm these results.

Multiple Sclerosis

Yamout *et al.* explored the safety of bone marrow-derived MSCs in subjects with multiple sclerosis[60]. They injected *ex-vivo* expanded autologous MSCs intrathecally in 10 patients with advanced multiple sclerosis. Patients were assessed at 3, 6, and 12 months. Assessment at 3–6 months revealed Expanded Disability Scale Score (EDSS) improvement in 5/7, stabilization in 1/7, and worsening in 1/7 patients. Magnetic resonance imaging at 3 months revealed new or enlarging lesions in 5/7 and gadolinium-enhancing lesions in 3/7 patients. Vision and low contrast sensitivity testing at 3 months showed improvement in 5/6 and worsening in 1/6 patients. Early results suggested clinical, but not radiologic, efficacy and evidence of safety with no serious adverse events.

Other Conditions

As of September 2014, 420 clinical trials were listed on ClinicalTrials.gov with a search for "mesenchymal stem cells." In addition to those described above, the use of MSCs in other conditions included the following:

Musculoskeletal disorders. Anterior cruciate ligament repair, degenerative disc disease, osteoporotic bone fractures, alveolar bone loss, osteogenesis imperfecta, bone cysts, facioscapulohumeral dystrophy, periodontitis, osteonecrosis of the femoral head, leg length inequality, rotator cuff tear, foot and ankle fusion procedures, after meniscectomy.
Cardiac disorders. Acute myocardial infarction, dilated cardiomyopathy, congestive cardiac failure.
Nervous system disorders. Ischemic stroke, parkinsonism, amyotrophic lateral sclerosis, autism, anoxic and hypoxic brain injury, Alzheimer's disease, hereditary ataxia, retinitis pigmentosa, cerebellar ataxia, Duchenne muscular dystrophy, dementia, tauopathies, delirium, cognitive disorders, hereditary retinal dystrophy, optic nerve disease.
Autoimmune disorders. Sjögren syndrome, type 1 diabetes mellitus, type 2 diabetes mellitus, rheumatoid arthritis, primary biliary cirrhosis, ulcerative colitis, Crohn's disease, systemic sclerosis (scleroderma), ankylosing spondylitis.

Hepatic disorders. Hepatic cirrhosis, Wilson's disease.

Bowel diseases. Inflammatory bowel disease: ulcerative colitis and Crohn's disease.

Pulmonary disorders. Acute respiratory distress syndrome, emphysema, bronchopulmonary dysplasia, asthma, pulmonary arterial hypertension, postoperative air leaks after lung resection.

Renal disease. Cisplatin-induced acute renal failure in patients with solid organ cancers, chronic renal disease, occlusive vascular disease of the kidney.

Ischemic disorders other than AMI and stroke. Limb ischemia due to Buerger disease, diabetic foot ulcers, erectile dysfunction.

Skin diseases. Epidermolysis bullosa, burns, cutaneous photoaging.

Eye diseases. Limbus insufficiency syndrome, glaucoma.

Infectious diseases. HIV, neutropenic enterocolitis, septic shock with severe neutropenia.

Solid organ transplantation. Renal transplant rejection, obliterative bronchiolitis after lung transplantation.

Hematopoietic stem cell transplantation. Marrow graft failure after HSC transplantation, co-transplantation with allogeneic HSC transplantation, expansion of cord blood cells.

Miscellaneous disorders. Vocal cord scarring, aplastic anemia, hemophilia, familial hypercholesterolemia, urinary incontinence in women, fecal incontinence, male infertility, prostate cancer, premature ovarian failure, breast reconstruction, endometrial receptivity, aging frailty, with chemotherapy for ovarian cancer, sarcoma and small intestine neoplasms, generation of dendritic cells from cord blood stem cells.

This list contains a total of 87 different clinical settings.

The Role of Other Adult Somatic Cells in Regenerative Medicine

Cardiac Cells

Capricor Therapeutics has completed a phase I clinical study using autologous cardiac cells obtained by myocardial biopsy and grown as cardiospheres prior to their injection directly into the coronary artery of patients who had had an acute myocardial infarction. A total of 31 patients 18 years or older with a recent myocardial infarction ($\leq$4 weeks) were enrolled in the trial. These patients had documented left ventricular dysfunction with ejection fraction (EF) between 25–45%. The trial demonstrated significantly reduced infarct (scar) size and increased healthy heart muscle. The study challenged long-standing convention that cardiac scarring is permanent and that healthy heart muscle cannot be restored and provided early evidence for cardiac regeneration. The study also demonstrated improved regional function and trends pointing towards the reversal of adverse cardiac remodeling[61,62].

The company has now initiated a similar study using allogeneic cardiospheres.

The Role of Organ-Specific Stem or Progenitor Cells in Regenerative Medicine

Skeletal Myoblasts

Skeletal myoblasts have been used to treat subjects with severe ischemic heart disease. However, one serious adverse event was the development of ventricular arrhythmias in some of the subjects into whose myocardium the skeletal myoblasts were injected[63].

Neural Stem Cells

The biotechnology company Stem Cells Inc. has completed two phase 1 clinical trials using the company's proprietary neural cell product called HuCNS-SC. One trial recruited subjects with neuronal ceroid lipofuscinosis (Batten disease): this trial showed the cells to be safe. Three of six subjects are alive at 5 years after transplantation. The second trial was performed in subjects with the rare disorder Pelizaeus–Merzbacher disease, a fatal myelination disorder in children: magnetic resonance imaging showed evidence of donor-derived myelin and modest gains in neurologic function. Two phase 1/2 trials are in progress: one in subjects with thoracic spinal cord injury and the other in age-related macular degeneration.

HuCNS-SC is a highly purified composition of adult human neural stem cells. HuCNS-SC cells are based on work done in 1999 by the company[64]. Scientists at the company were the first to identify cell surface markers for the human neural stem cell and developed monoclonal antibodies against these markers in order to isolate a highly purified, expandable population of neural stem cells from human brain tissue[65]. Prepared under controlled conditions and processed to cGMP standards, the HuCNS-SC cells are purified, expanded in culture, cryopreserved, and then stored, ready to be transplanted.

These human neural stem cells are currently in clinical development for spinal cord injury and for Pelizaeus–Merzbacher disease, a fatal myelination disorder in children.

The Role of Cells Derived from Embryonic Stem Cells in Regenerative Medicine

Spinal Cord Injury

Geron Corporation Inc. in the United States treated five subjects with spinal cord injury using oligodendrocyte progenitor cells derived from human ESCs. The trial was stopped for strategic reasons, but follow-up studies on the five patients has shown no serious side effects due to administration of the cells and in four of the five patients MRI scans have shown that the size of the injury site in the spinal cord had decreased. Asterias Biotherapeutics acquired all the cell therapy assets of

Geron in 2013 and in 2014 has been funded by the California Institute of Regenerative Medicine (CIRM) to initiate a phase 1 trial using up to 10 times the number of cells used in the Geron trial. Additionally it will focus on spinal cord injuries arising in the neck between the 5th and 7th cervical vertebra: such people are paraplegic (CIRM press release, August 2014).

Type 1 Diabetes Mellitus

In August 2014 ViaCyte Inc. obtained approval from the USA Food and Drug Administration to start a phase 1/2 clinical trial for treatment for type 1 diabetes using its VC-01 product. The VC-01 therapy is the combination of PEC-01 cells, a proprietary pancreatic endoderm cell product derived through directed differentiation of an inexhaustible human embryonic stem cell line, and its Encaptra drug delivery system, a proprietary immune-protecting and retrievable encapsulation medical device. This combination of cells and device is a thin plastic pouch containing an immature form of pancreatic cells that, when implanted under the skin, are designed to mature and become insulin-producing and other cells needed to regulate blood glucose levels. These cells are able to sense when blood glucose is high, and then secrete insulin to restore it to a healthy level. In effect this is designed to mimic the glucose-regulating functions of the pancreas, which, in people with type 1 diabetes mellitus, no longer works (CIRM press release, August 2014).

HIV

In June 2014 the USA biotechnology company Calimmune was given approval to continue with the second cohort of subjects with HIV. This phase 1/2 clinical trial focuses on CCR5, a chemokine receptor that plays a key role in enabling HIV to infect cells. Blocking CCR5 may provide the cells with a protective shield against HIV, which in turn would help retain immune system functionality. In the first phase of this study four HIV-positive participants were infused with their own blood stem cells as well as mature T-cells that had been modified to carry a gene that blocks production of CCR5. The hope is that those stem cells will then create a new blood system that is resistant to HIV (CIRM press release, June 2014).

Age-Related Macular Degeneration

Humayun *et al.* have received funding from CIRM to initiate a clinical trial of retinal pigment epithelial cells derived from human ESCs and grown on a scaffold that will be implanted into the eye of subjects with age-related macular degeneration (CIRM press release, December 2013).

The Role of Cells Derived from Induced Pluripotent Stem Cells in Regenerative Medicine

Age-Related Macular Dystrophy

A new study in Japan is the first clinical trial on humans using induced pluripotent stem cells (iPSCs). The phase I study will test the safety and feasibility of using autologous iPSCs taken from adult patients to treat blindness due to age-related macular degeneration (RIKEN press release, July 2013).

The study is led by Dr Masayo Takahashi of the Laboratory for Retinal Regeneration, RIKEN Center for Developmental Biology, and conducted in collaboration with the Institute for Biomedical Research and Innovation with support from the Kobe City Medical Centre General Hospital; the study began recruiting patients on August 1 2014.

The protocol for this study involves the establishment of autologous iPSCs from each of the research participants, which will then be differentiated into retinal pigment epithelial (RPE) cells using a novel technology that allows these epithelial cells to be transplanted in monolayer cell sheets without the use of synthetic scaffolds or matrices. The cell sheets will be shaped into 1.3×3 mm grafts and transplanted into the affected site of a single eye, following excision of the damaged RPE and neovascular tissues.

Transplant sites will be monitored closely for functional integration and potential adverse reactions for an initial intensive observation period of 1 year, and subsequent follow-up observation for 3 years.

Current Good Manufacturing Practice

Current Good Manufacturing Practices (cGMP) are practices required in order to conform to guidelines recommended by therapeutic regulatory agencies that control the authorization and licensing for manufacture and sale of food, drug products, and active pharmaceutical products. These guidelines provide minimum requirements that a pharmaceutical or a food product manufacturer must meet to ensure that the products are of high quality and do not pose any risk to the consumer or public.

In Australia, the Therapeutic Goods Authority (TGA) regulates therapeutic drugs, cells, and tissues, and medical devices that are used in humans. Cells that are expanded *ex-vivo* are mandated by the TGA to be manufactured using the principles of cGMP for phase II, III, and IV clinical trials. However, since we were utilizing a cellular product that had not been administered previously to humans, namely placenta-derived MSCs, we elected to manufacture our MSCs for phase I clinical trials using cGMP principles to maximize the safeness of the cells as well as the safety of the cell manufacturing staff and the reputation of our institution. This process was time-consuming, laborious, and expensive, but we considered it appropriate. A key component to cGMP manufacturing is the standard operating procedures and protocols used in the manufacture of the cells. Our Quality Assurance Program developed over 2000 documents to cover this. Steps in the manufacturing procedure to isolate MSCs from term placenta are shown in Figures 68.7–68.11. In order to be used for clinical trials the isolated MSCs at the end of each passage must fulfil the following criteria: viability >70% by Trypan blue dye exclusion, negative Gram stain, sterility on 14-day microbial culture, negative *Mycoplasma* test, negative 16s rRNA test, purity >85% CD73+/CD105+ and <1% CD45+, endotoxin level <2 EU/mL, and a normal karyotype.

Three weeks before the planned administration of the manufactured MSCs, a test vial corresponding to each bag or vial intended for clinical trial use is thawed. To be used in a clinical trial, the MSCs must fulfil the following criteria: viability >70% by Trypan blue dye exclusion, sterility on 14-day microbial culture, negative *Mycoplasma* test, and negative 16s rRNA test.

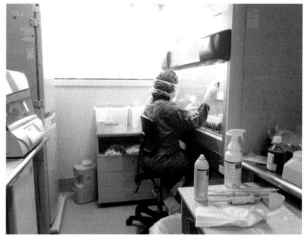

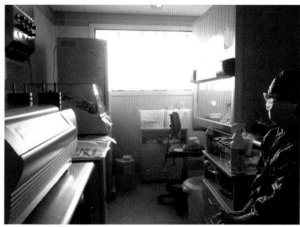

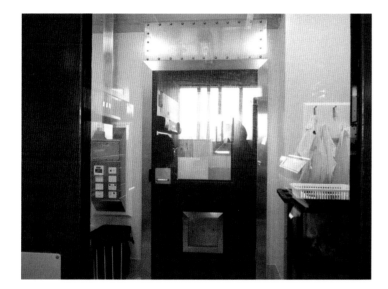

Figure 68.7. A Giemsa-stained cytospin preparation showing the morphology of human placenta-derived MSCs in suspension x400 (Brooke *et al.*, 2008).

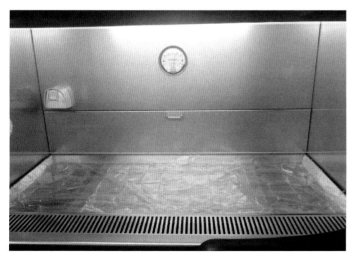

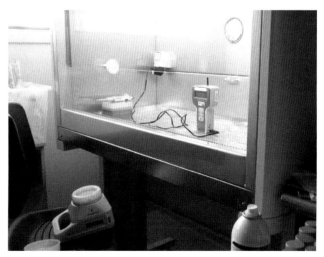

Figure 68.8. The Good Manufacturing Process (GMP). The anteroom where reagents are stocked and the clean room where the MSC isolation took place.

Conclusions

It is likely that regenerative medicine will have an impact on all areas of medicine over the next two to three decades. It seems unlikely that hematopoietic stem cells will play a role in this, apart from the essential role in regeneration of the hemato- poietic and immune systems after the chemotherapy or che- moradiation used immediately pretransplant.

At present the main cells involved in clinical trials in the regenerative medicine area are mesenchymal stromal cells. As of September 2014, 420 trials with mesenchymal cells were registered with ClinicalTrials.gov.

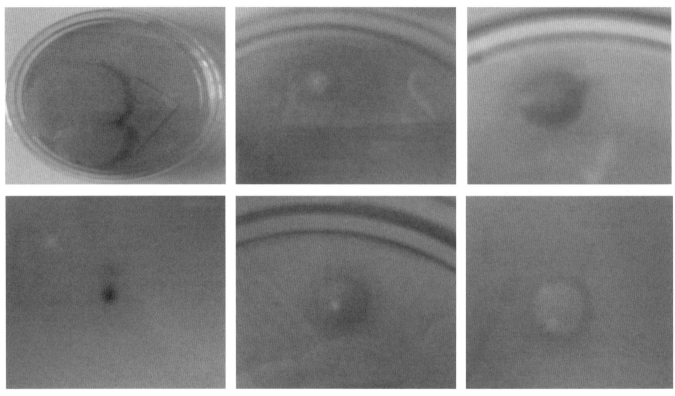

Figure 68.9. The Good Manufacturing Process (GMP). The environmental monitoring process. Culture dishes are placed in the biohazard hood to monitor air-borne microbes (left photograph) and the temperature in the hood is monitored (right photograph).

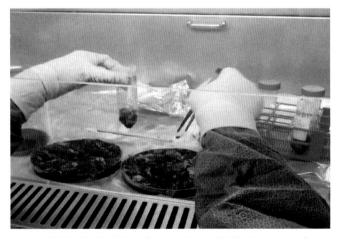

Figure 68.10. The Good Manufacturing Process (GMP). Finger swabs from the MSC production scientists are routinely monitored.

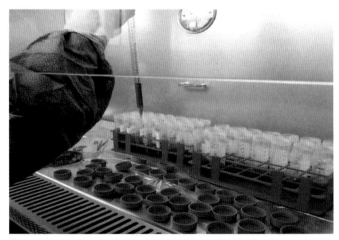

Figure 68.11. The Good Manufacturing Process (GMP). The placenta is received from the operating room where the elective Caesarian section took place and where it was double-bagged. It is removed from the container in which the bags had been placed. It is then cut up using scissors and scalpels into smaller and smaller pieces followed by a collagenase digest. This day is termed day 0 of the MSC isolation and *ex-vivo* expansion process.

The differentiated progeny of embryonic stem cells may play a role in regenerative medicine, but there remain ethical concerns of destroying a human embryo in order to obtain them, as well as their teratoma generation potential, should some of the cells administered have not differentiated and some ESCs are inadvertently coadministered. However, four trials in the United States in which progeny derived from human ESCs have already started or are approved to start: they are in the fields of severe spinal cord injury, type 1 diabetes mellitus, HIV, and age-related macular degeneration.

The differentiated progeny of induced pluripotent stem cells are also likely to play an important role in regenerative medicine since the ethical concern about destruction of a living human embryo does not apply to them. The teratoma risk, however, does also apply to iPSCs and maximizing the safety of their differentiated progeny before their administration will be required. Possible approaches include the inclusion of a suicide gene in the infused cells, so that they can be switched off and destroyed should a tumor occur. It should be emphasized that the teratoma occurring in animals in receipt of ESCs or iPSCs are not malignant tumors – they are teratomas, not teratocarcinomas. Although they would usually be amenable to

surgical excision should they occur, they could develop at sites where surgery is hazardous, for example in the spinal cord. The first clinical trial in the world was due to start recruiting subjects in August 2014 in Japan. The targeted disease is age-related macular regeneration.

Organ-specific stem cells and their differentiated progeny are also likely to play a significant role in regenerative medicine.

For treatment of some diseases by stem cells or their differentiated progeny, scaffolds to hold the cells at the specific disease site will be necessary. In some cases these will be decellularized human organs or tissues. In other cases they will be synthetic scaffolds.

In parallel with the use of stem cells and their differentiated progeny or of somatic cells for regenerative medicine, a completely different approach is already well underway: the use of bionic organs. The bionic ear made by the Australian company Cochlear has been a dramatic clinical treatment for deaf people. Work on a bionic eye and bionic limbs are underway.

Medicine in the 21st century will be as different as medicine in the 20th century was to that of the 19th century.

References

1. L.R. Kaiser. The future of multihospital systems. *Topics in Health Care Financing* 1992; 18: 32–45.

2. E.A. McCulloch and J.E. Till. The radiation sensitivity of normal mouse bone marrow cells, determined by quantitative marrow transplantation into irradiated mice. *Radiation Research* 1960; 13: 115–25.

3. J. Storek and R.P. Witherspoon. Immunological reconstitution after hematopoietic stem cell transplantation. In: Atkinson K., Champlin R., Ritz, J., Fibbe W., Ljungman P. and Brenner, M.K. eds. *Clinical Bone Marrow and Blood Stem Cell Transplantation*. Cambridge, Cambridge University Press, 2004: 194–226.

4. H.J. Kolb, K. Atkinson and M. Reinhold. Cellular therapy. In: *The BMT Data Book Including Cellular Therapy*. Cambridge, Cambridge University Press, 2013: 209–33.

5. P.L. Weiden, N. Flournoy, E.D. Thomas *et al*. Antileukemic effect of graft-*versus*-host disease in human recipients of allogeneic-marrow grafts. *N Engl J Med*. 1979; 300:1068–73.

6. A.J. Friedenstein, R.K. Chailakhyan, N.V. Latsinik *et al*. Stromal cells responsible for transferring the

microenvironment of the hemopoietic tissues. Cloning in vitro and retransplantation in vivo. *Transplantation*. 1974; 17: 331–40.

7. N. Barker, M. van de Wetering and H. Clevers. The intestinal stem cell. *Genes Dev*. 2008; 22:1856–64.

8. J.C.J. Chen and D.J. Goldhamer. Skeletal muscle stem cells. *Reprod Biol Endocrinol*. 2003; 1: 101–19.

9. C. Blanpain and E. Fuchs. Epidermal stem cells of the skin. *Annu Rev Cell Dev Biol* 2006; 22: 339–73.

10. N. Uchida, D.W. Buck, S. He *et al*. Direct isolation of human central nervous system stem cells. *Proc Nat Acad Sci*. 2000; 97: 14720–5.

11. C.E. Garget and H. Masuda. Adult stem cells in the endometrium. *Mol Hum Reprod*. 2010; 16: 818–34.

12. A.P. Beltrami, L. Barlucchi, D. Torella *et al*. Adult cardiac stem cells are multipotent and support myocardial regeneration. *Cell* 2003; 114: 763–76.

13. A. Myajima, M. Tanaka and T. Itoh. Stem/progenitor cells in liver development, homeostasis, regeneration, and reprogramming. *Cell Stem Cell* 2014; 14: 561–74.

14. J.A. Thomson, J. Itskovitz-Eldor, S. Sander *et al*. Embryonic stem cell lines

derived from human blastocysts. *Science*; 1998; 282: 1145–7.

15. K. Takahashi, K. Tanabe, M. Ohnuki *et al*. Induction of pluripotent stem cells from adult human fibroblasts by defined factors. *Cell* 2007; 131: 861–72.

16. M. Abad, L. Mosteiro, C. Pantoja *et al*. Reprogramming in vivo produces teratomas and iPS cells with totipotency features. *Nature* 2013; 502, 340–5.

17. P. Macchiarini, P. Jungebluth, T. Go *et al*. Clinical transplantation of a tissue-engineered airway. *Lancet*; 2008: 372, 2023–30.

18. S. Sjöqvist, P. Jungebluth, M.L. Lim *et al*. Experimental orthotopic transplantation of a tissue-engineered oesophagus in rats. *Nature Communications* 2014, 5: 3562.

19. A. Atala and S.V. Murphy. 3D bioprinting of tissues and organs. *Nat Biotechnol*. 2014; 32: 773–85.

20. L.B. Balsam, A.J. Wagers, J.L. Chistenson. Haematopoietic stem cells adopt mature haematopoietic fates in ischaemic myocardium. *Nature* 2004; 428: 668–73.

21. S. Saadettin, M. Ulf, N. Schilling *et al*. Bone marrow cells and CD117-positive haematopoietic stem cells promote corneal wound healing. *Acta Ophthalmologica* 2012; e367–e373.

22. M. Abedi, B.M. Foster, K.D. Wood *et al.* Haematopoietic stem cells participate in muscle regeneration. *Br J Haematol.* 2007; 138: 792–801.

23. J.C. Kovacic, P. Macdonald, M.P. Feneley *et al.* Safety and efficacy of consecutive cycles of granulocyte-colony stimulating factor, and an intracoronary CD133+ cell infusion in patients with chronic refractory ischemic heart disease: The G-CSF in Angina patients with IHD to stimulate Neovascularization (GAIN I) trial. *Am Heart J* 2008; 156: 954–63.

24. H.-J. Kang, H.-S. Kim, S.-Y. Zhang *et al.* Effects of intracoronary infusion of peripheral blood stem-cells mobilised with granulocyte-colony stimulating factor on left ventricular systolic function and restenosis after coronary stenting in myocardial infarction: the MAGIC cell randomised clinical trial. *Lancet* 2004; 363: 751–56.

25. M. Körbling, R.L. Katz, A. Khanna *et al.* Hepatocytes and epithelial cells of donor origin in recipients of peripheral-blood stem cells. *N Engl J Med.* 2002; 346: 738–46.

26. B. Sacchetti, A. Funari, S. Michienzi *et al.* Self-renewing osteoprogenitors in bone marrow sinusoids can organize a hematopoietic microenvironment. *Cell* 2007; 131: 324–36.

27. S. Mendez-Ferrer, T.V. Michurina, F. Ferraro *et al.* Mesenchymal and haematopoietic stem cells form a unique bone marrow niche. *Nature* 2010; 466: 829–34.

28. M. de Lima, I. McNiece, S.N. Robinson *et al.* Cord-blood engraftment with ex-vivo mesenchymal-cell coculture. *N Engl J Med.* 2012; 367: 2305–15.

29. M. Crisan, S. Yap, L. Casteilla *et al.* A perivascular origin for mesenchymal stem cells in multiple human organs. *Cell Stem Cell* 2008; 3: 301–13.

30. L. Da Silva Meireles, A.I. Caplan, N.B. Nardi *et al.* In search of the in vivo identity of mesenchymal stem cells. *Stem Cells.* 2008; 26: 2287–99.

31. K. Le Blanc, I. Rasmusson, B. Sundberg *et al.* Treatment of severe acute graft-*versus*-host disease with third party haploidentical mesenchymal stem cells. *Lancet* 2004; 363: 1439–41.

32. K. Le Blanc, F. Frassoni, L. Ball *et al.* Mesenchymal stem cells for treatment of steroid-resistant, severe, acute graft-*versus*-host disease: a phase II study. *Lancet* 2008; 371: 1579–86.

33. K. Le Blanc and O. Ringden. Immunobiology of human mesenchymal stem cells and future use in hematopoietic stem cell transplantation. *Biol Blood Marrow Transplant.* 2005; 11: 321–34.

34. N.G. Singer and A.I. Caplan. Mesenchymal stem cells: mechanisms of inflammation. *Annu Rev Pathol Mech Dis.* 2011; 6: 457–78.

35. R. Pelekanos, L.I. Gongora, T. Doan *et al.* Comprehensive genotype/phenotype analysis of renal and cardiac MSC-like populations supports strong congruence with bone marrow MSC despite maintenance of distinct identities. *Stem Cell Res.* 2012; 5: 58–73.

36. S. Barlow, G. Brooke, K. Chatterjee *et al.* Comparison of human placenta- and bone marrow-derived multipotent mesenchymal stem cells. *Stem Cells Dev* 2008; 17: 1095–108.

37. S. Maxson, E.A. Lopez, D. Yoo *et al.* Concise Review: Role of mesenchymal stem cells in wound repair. *Stem Cells Transl Med.* 2012; 1: 142–9.

38. E.V. Badivas, M. Abedi, J. Butmarc *et al.* Participation of bone marrow derived cells in cutaneous wound healing. *J Cell Physiol.* 2003; 196: 245–50.

39. V. Falanga, S. Iwamoto, M. Chartier *et al.* Autologous bone marrow-derived cultured mesenchymal stem cells delivered in a fibrin spray accelerate healing in murine and human cutaneous wounds. *Tissue Eng.* 2007; 13: 1299–312.

40. T. Yoshikawa, H. Mitsuno, I. Nonaka *et al.* Wound therapy by marrow mesenchymal cell transplantation. *Plast Reconstr Surg.* 2008; 121: 860–77.

41. D. Lu, B. Chen and Z. Liang. Comparison of bone marrow mesenchymal stem cells with bone marrow-derived mononuclear cells for treatment of diabetic critical limb ischemia and foot ulcer: a double-blind, randomized, controlled trial. *Diabetes Res Clin Pract.* 2011; 92: 26–36.

42. H.C. Lee, S.G. An, H.W. Lee *et al.* Safety and effect of adipose tissue-derived stem cell implantation in patients with critical limb ischemia: a pilot study. *Circ J.* 2012; 76: 1750–60.

43. D. Garcia-Olmo, M. Garcia-Arranz and D. Herreros. Expanded adipose-derived stem cells for the treatment of complex perianal fistula including Crohn's disease. *Expert Opin Biol Ther.* 2008; 8: 1417–23.

44. D. García-Olmo, D. Herreros, P. De-La-Quintana *et al.* Adipose-derived stem cells in Crohn's rectovaginal fistula. *Case Rep Med.* 2010: 961758.

45. R. de Steiger, R Ferrugia, M. Richardson *et al.* OR14: A safety study of autologous mesenchymal precursor cells in the management of non-union of tibial and fibular fractures. *J Bone Joint Surg Br.* 2010; 92: 203–4.

46. R. Quarto, M. Mastrogiacomo, R. Cancedda *et al.* Repair of large bone defects with the use of autologous bone marrow stromal cells. *N Engl J Med.* 2001; 344: 385–6.

47. M. Gimbel, R.K. Ashley, M. Sisodia *et al.* Repair of alveolar cleft defects: reduced morbidity with bone marrow stem cells in a resorbable matrix. *J Craniofac Surg.* 2007; 18: 895–901.

48. F. Velardi, P.R. Amante, M. Caniglia *et al.* Osteogenesis induced by autologous bone marrow cells transplant in the pediatric skull. *Childs Nerv Syst.* 2006; 22: 1158–66.

49. Y. Gan, K. Dai, P. Zhang *et al.* The clinical use of enriched bone marrow stem cells combined with porous beta-tricalcium phosphate in posterior spinal fusion. *Biomaterials* 2008; 29: 3973–82.

50. C.T. Vangsness, T.D. David, W.G. David *et al.* A randomized clinical trial using mesenchymal stem cells for meniscus regeneration and osteoarthritis. http://www.aaos.org/Education/anmeet/education/Sports_Medicine_Arthoroscopy_Abstracts.pdf 2012.

51. H. Nejadnik, J.H. Hui, E.P. Feng Choong *et al.* Autologous bone marrow-derived mesenchymal stem cells *versus* autologous chondrocyte implantation: an observational cohort study. *Am J Sports Med.* 2010; 38: 1110–16.

52. S. Wakitani, M. Nawata, K. Tensho *et al.* Repair of articular cartilage defects in the patello-femoral joint with autologous bone marrow mesenchymal cell transplantation: three case reports involving nine defects in five knees. *J Tissue Eng Regener Med* 2007; 1: 74–9.

53. R. Kuroda, K. Ishida, T. Matsumoto *et al.* Treatment of a full-thickness articular cartilage defect in the femoral condyle of an athlete with autologous bone-marrow stromal cells. *Osteoarthritis Cartilage* 2007; 15: 226–31.

54. J.S. Da Silva and J.M. Hare. Cell-based therapies for myocardial repair: emerging role for bone marrow-derived mesenchymal stem cells (MSCs) in the treatment of the chronically injured heart. *Methods Mol Biol.* 2013; 1037: 145–63.

55. A.W. Heldman, D.L. DiFede, J.E. Fishman *et al.* Transendocardial mesenchymal stem cells and mononuclear bone marrow cells for ischemic cardiomyopathy: the TAC-HFT randomized trial. *JAMA.* 2014; 311: 62–73.

56. F.S. Loffredo, M.L. Steinhauser, J. Gannon *et al.* Bone marrow-derived cell therapy stimulates endogenous cardiomyocyte progenitors and promotes cardiac repair. *Cell Stem Cell* 2011; 8: 389–98.

57. D.C. Chambers, D. Enever, N. Ilic *et al.* Safety of mesenchymal stromal cell therapy for idiopathic pulmonary fibrosis. *Respirology.* In press.

58. L. Sun, D. Wang, J. Liang *et al.* Umbilical cord mesenchymal stem cell transplantation in severe and refractory systemic lupus erythematosus. *Arthritis Rheum.* 2010; 62: 2467–75.

59. J. Liang, H. Zhang and B. Hua. Allogeneic mesenchymal stem cells transplantation in refractory systemic lupus erythematosus: a pilot clinical study. *Ann Rheum Dis.* 2010; 69: 1423–9.

60. B. Yamout, R. Hourani, H. Salti *et al.* Bone marrow mesenchymal stem cell transplantation in patients with multiple sclerosis: a pilot study. *J Neuroimmunol.* 2010; 227: 185–9.

61. R.R. Makkar, R.R. Smith, K. Cheng *et al.* Intracoronary cardiosphere-derived cells for heart regeneration after myocardial infarction (CADUCEUS): a prospective, randomised phase I trial. *Lancet.* 2012; 379: 895–904.

62. K. Malliaras, R.R. Makkar, R.R. Smith *et al.* Intracoronary cardiosphere-derived cells after myocardial infarction: evidence of therapeutic regeneration in the final 1-year results of the CADUCEUS trial (CArdiosphere-Derived aUtologous stem CElls to reverse ventricUlar dySfunction). *J Am Coll Cardiol.* 2014; 63: 110–22.

63. P. Menache. Skeletal myoblasts and cardiac repair. *J Mol Cell Cardiol.* 2008; 45: 545–53.

64. N. Uchida, D.W. Buck, S. He *et al.* Direct isolation of human central nervous system stem cells. *Proc Nat Acad Sci USA.* 2000; 97: 14720–5.

65. A. Tsukamoto, N. Uchida, A. Capela *et al.* Clinical transplantation of human neural stem cells. *Stem Cell Res Ther.* 2013; 4: 102–13.

Chapter

69

Statistics: Do We Understand the Results of Our Analyses?

Binod Dhakal and Parameswaran Hari

Introduction

In blood and bone marrow transplants clinical decision-making is often based on limited high-level evidence. Prospective clinical trials are rare except in the multicenter network setting and practice change difficult to effect. Clinicians are prone to biases and often misjudge statistical significance in their search for definitive answers to clinical questions. In this chapter, we describe the common statistical issues in the analysis and interpretation of transplant studies with a special emphasis on the common pitfalls.

The typical outcomes of interest are events occurring post-transplant such as death, relapse or disease progression, graft failure, graft-*versus*-host disease (GvHD), and infection. Summarizing these outcomes or comparing these outcomes between defined groups is the essence of most studies.

Proper Handling of Time: Concepts of Truncation and Censoring

Outcomes of interest occur at random times post-transplant and sometimes do not occur during the observation period. Subjects in whom the event of interest has not occurred prior to the time of last observation are considered "right censored" (since the unobserved event is potentially to the right of the censoring time). Truncation is an adjustment needed to account for the sampling bias resulting when only those individuals whose lifetimes lie within a certain interval can be observed. For example, clinicians often want to compare survival after GvHD. If the analysis were to simply consider time of transplant as the start time, subjects at risk at any given point in time thereafter would include those alive after GvHD and not the total numbers of subjects alive. In this simplistic approach, subjects are not included in the denominator unless they experienced GvHD. Since all subjects begin in the non-GvHD arm and do not move into the GvHD arm until random times post-transplant, data in the GvHD arm are considered left truncated. Thus we need to adjust for the bias resulting from the condition that subjects in the GvHD arm must live for a certain period (without GvHD) until they get GvHD and experience the outcome of interest (death after GvHD).

Guarantee Time Bias

Another relatively common error resulting from improper handling of time in transplant studies is called guarantee time bias. This bias arises from comparing outcomes between subjects with or without a post-transplant condition such as GvHD, complete remission, etc. Any analysis between groups defined by a classifying event occurring sometime during follow-up but timed from enrollment or study therapy is prone to this type of bias[1]. In transplant analyses comparing survival among groups which developed GvHD *versus* no GvHD, bone marrow recovery *versus* no bone marrow recovery, complete response *versus* no complete response, etc. are prone to this error. The problem arises because the grouping event (GvHD, complete response etc.) is not known at the time of transplant. There are acceptable methods of performing such analyses such as incorporating the grouping event as a time-dependent covariate in Cox models, landmark analysis.

Competing Risk Data and Survival Data

Transplant outcomes can be classified into two types based on how they need to be analyzed. Survival data such as mortality (survival) and treatment failure (combined endpoint of death or relapse) are typically summarized by a Kaplan–Meier curve. Subjects either experience the event of interest or are censored at the time of last observation. Competing risk data, on the other hand, are outcomes where the occurrence of one event precludes the occurrence of another, e.g., death in remission and relapse (where the latter precludes the former and vice versa). Such data are appropriately summarized using the cumulative incidence function to account for competing risk (Table 69.1). Cumulative incidence curves take into account the fact that persons at risk for the event of interest (e.g., relapse) can be eliminated from experiencing that risk by competing events (nonrelapse death). If a Kaplan–Meir estimate of relapse is obtained, deaths in remission would typically be treated as censored observations resulting in an overestimate of relapse risk.

Comparing Post-transplant Outcomes

The most common analyses in transplants involve comparing subgroups based on subject- (age, performance state, etc.),

Table 69.1 Competing risks in transplants

Outcome	Competing risks
Relapse	Death in remission
Progression	Death without progression
Acute GvHD	Death without acute GvHD, relapse, second transplant
Bone marrow recovery	Death without bone marrow recovery
Death from disease of interest	Death due to any other cause

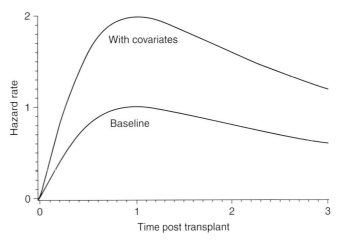

Figure 69.1 Relationship between hazard rates.

disease- (remission state, white blood count (WBC), etc.), or transplant (conditioning regimen, graft dose, etc.)-related variables known at the time of transplant. When the defining variable is based on a post-transplant event (e.g., GvHD or bone marrow recovery), special consideration is required.

Unadjusted Comparisons

These are crude comparisons which assume that baseline prognostic factors are balanced between comparison groups and there are no confounding factors affecting outcomes differentially between the groups of interest. Unadjusted comparisons may be carried out by three approaches[2]. The first involves events that occur shortly after transplant such as bone marrow recovery. In this situation, we may choose an interval in advance. Subjects who experience the event in this window (e.g. platelets >50×10E+9/L at day 30) are considered a *success* and subjects on-study for interval but do not experience the event are a *failure*. The second approach compares survival (or disease-free survival) or cumulative incidence curves (e.g., relapse or death in remission at fixed points). Estimated probabilities are computed using either the Kaplan–Meier or cumulative incidence curves. A third approach compares the entire survival experience for subjects in the groups by comparing hazard rates using the (weighted) log-rank test[3].

Adjusted Comparisons and the Cox Proportional Hazards Model

Regression models or multivariate analyses are used to address confounding and imbalance of baseline risks between groups. The aim of multivariate analysis is to interrogate the relationship between the outcome variable and other variables considered simultaneously in a mathematical model.

Regression models such as the Cox proportional hazard model can be used to determine subject-, disease-, and transplant-related variables which may influence one or more outcomes post-transplant. These models are also used to adjust for imbalances in baseline risk between groups of subjects making possible comparisons between treatments. The Cox proportional hazard model uses the hazard rate to model

timing of events. The hazard rate is defined as the chance of the event of interest occurring in the next instant of time for a subject yet to experience the event. The Cox model assumes that the hazard rate for a given subject can be factored into a baseline hazard rate (common to all subjects) and a parametric function of the covariates which describe the subject characteristics[4]. Figure 69.1 shows the relationship between hazard rates for a single binary covariate based on the Cox model. These curves are hump-shaped typical of the hazard rate plot for treatment failure post-transplant.

For results of the Cox model to be valid the model assumptions must be correct. The most important assumption is the proportional hazard assumption which states that the effects of the risk factors are constant over time. There are different ways of adjusting the Cox model when there is clear violation of proportional hazard assumption. One way is to divide the post-transplant interval into distinct time intervals so that within each interval the proportionality assumption holds. A second way is to stratify the Cox model on the nonproportional covariate[5].

The Cox model can be used to analyze both survival data and competing risk data. For the competing risk data it models cause-specific hazard defined as the rate at which subjects at risk to experience the event of interest as well as the competing event experience the event of interest[6]. Pseudo-value regression is another approach to analyze competing risk data. This method allows to directly model the cumulative incidence function at a fixed time point as well compare the entire cumulative incidence curve. It is critical to define the aim of the analysis as the results of the cause-specific Cox model and pseudo-value regression for competing risk data could be quite different[7].

Common Errors in Analyses of Transplant Studies

Examples of common errors in analyses of transplant data include:

1. Mis-specification of the time of origin (start time) resulting in biased estimates of the outcome probabilities of interest. For example, comparing transplant in first complete remission with transplant in second complete remission starting with time of transplant as origin. This ignores the additional time pretransplant subjects need to have lived before achieving 2nd remission. Another issue in this example is that persons who died without transplant after relapsing (either before/after reaching 2nd remission) are ignored.

2. Mis-identifying the at-risk population (using the wrong denominator): the denominator of an estimated probability must include all subjects at risk. For example, a study comparing planned double (tandem) transplants *versus* single transplants should include all subjects intended to receive a second transplant whether or not it was done.

3. Comparing outcomes between subjects with or without a condition developing only post-transplant. For example, a direct comparison of survival in subjects achieving a complete response *versus* those not achieving a complete response.

4. Misinterpreting time-dependent covariates (such as engraftment and GvHD) which vary over time as time-fixed covariates (such as age and KPS) known at time of transplant. When the effect of time-fixed covariates on outcome is mediated through time-dependent covariates and both are included in the analysis, further confounding can occur, for example, comparing subjects with chronic GvHD to subjects without chronic GvHD. In this situation estimates in the chronic GvHD cohort will be biased by the implicit assumption all subjects are at risk for GvHD. In reality some subjects die before experiencing GvHD.

5. Misinterpreting time varying fixed effects which occur when the effects of a fixed covariate on outcome change over time. This effect should be distinguished from time-dependent covariates. For example, the effect of a defined short interval of maintenance therapy post-transplant on long-term survival could change depending on when maintenance therapy is stopped.

Interpreting Results

Overinterpreting Statistical Significance for Clinical Decision-Making

The *P*-value can be thought of as the probability that any observed difference between two groups resulted from chance alone. When the concept of *P*-value was introduced in the 1920s by R. A. Fisher it was intended to judge whether the evidence was significant and worthy of second look as part of a fluid, nonnumerical process that combined data and knowledge to lead to scientific conclusions[8]. Unfortunately it is common among clinicians to rely heavily on a published *P*-value <0.05 for clinical decision-making or to judge the effect of a study intervention solely by the *P*-value. Some

Table 69.2 Common misconceptions regarding *P*-values[14]

All of the following are false:
1. If *P*=0.05 the null hypothesis has only a 5% chance of being true
2. A nonsignificant difference (*P*≥0.05) means there is no difference between the groups
3. A statistically significant finding is clinically important
4. Studies with *P*-values on opposite sides of 0.05 are conflicting
5. Studies with same *P*-value provide the same evidence against the null hypothesis
A scientific conclusion or treatment policy should be based on whether or not the *P*-value is significant

common misinterpretations of the *P*-value are summarized in Table 69.2. The first misconception is the most pervasive. The *P*-value is broadly described as the probability of the observed result plus more extreme results if the null hypothesis were true.

For example, the probability of observing five consecutive heads in a coin flipping experiment is 3.125% (or 1/32). This corresponds to a one-sided *P*=0.03 or a two-sided *P*=0.06 (since we are also interested in the other extreme of all tails). This does not automatically lead to the conclusion that the coin is not a fair coin, or that it has only a 3% or 6% chance of being a fair coin. The probability simply indicates that a result of five consecutive heads (and more extreme results) could be observed at least 6% of the time.

In interpreting published data for clinical decision-making it is best to be skeptical about the *P*-value. The *P*-value does not make statements about reality. In fact, the magnitude of an observed effect is better appreciated through the confidence interval since it incorporates both the size and imprecision in effect estimated by the data. In other words, the better question when comparing treatments should be, how much of an effect is there? Bayesian statisticians have argued for the use of Bayes factor (likelihood ratio) as an evidentiary measure especially in clinical decision-making (Table 69.3).

Statistical tests are best interpreted in the context of biologic plausibility and scientific knowledge. In clinical medicine, a positive diagnostic test does not mean someone has a disease. Similarly a significant *P*-value does not always confirm a research hypothesis especially when it is at odds with biologic plausibility. Bayesian approaches and prior probabilities need to be incorporated in clinical decision-making[9].

Misinterpreting the Hazard Ratio

Hazard ratios are used to express the effects of interventions in time-to-event or survival analyses. Cox models generate a hazard ratio (HR) and confidence interval. HR is a ratio of the hazard rate in the study group *versus* controls.

A hazard is the rate at which events happen. The probability of an event happening in a short time interval is the length of time multiplied by the hazard. The hazard rate is calculated as the probability that if the event of interest has not already occurred it will occur in the next time interval divided by the

Table 69.3 Evidentiary properties of Bayes factor *versus* P-value

Evidential property	P-value	Bayes factor
Information about effect size	No	Yes
Uses only observed data?	No	Yes
Explicit alternative hypothesis?	No	Yes
Positive evidence?	No	Yes
Sensitivity to stopping rules?	Yes	No
Easily combined across experiments?	No	Yes
Part of a formal system of inference?	No	Yes

length of that interval. The time interval is made very brief such that the hazard rate represents an instantaneous rate. Although the hazard rate may vary with time the assumption in Cox proportional hazard models for survival analyses is that the hazard in one group is a constant proportion of the hazard in the other. This proportion is the hazard ratio. For example in a study where progression-free survival is the endpoint the hazard ratio indicates the relative likelihood of the events of interest (such as death or progression) in treated *versus* control subjects at any given time point.

A common pitfall when interpreting hazard rates is to infer time effects. For example, if the hazard rate for mortality in a study group is 0.5, a common misconception is the assumption that median survival was doubled in the study group or that subjects in the control group were twice as likely to die by a certain number of years. In reality a hazard rate of 0.5 means only that a study group subject who is still alive at a certain time point has one-half the chance of dying at the next point in time compared with someone in the control group. In other

words, time effects should not be inferred from the hazard rate. Changes in hazard rate only affect the risk of the outcome and should be described alongside a measure of time to understand the size of the treatment effect[10].

Limitations of Published Data

There is emerging evidence that false findings may be in the majority or even the vast majority of publications[11–13]. Bias in research has been defined as the combination of factors in the design, data, analysis, and presentation that tends to produce false research findings. Ioannidis *et al.* proposed:

1. Published findings are less likely to be true in fields where study populations are small and where the effect size is small. This is mainly a function of decreasing power and positive predictive value.
2. Flexible designs, definitions, and outcomes and greater numbers of relationships tested tend to produce research findings less likely to be true.

The transplant field exhibits all of the above issues. Trials typically have few subjects and complex relationships between prognostic variables. Many transplant practices produce small incremental benefits difficult to prove statistically but which may be important clinically. Networking of investigators, large collaborative studies, randomized trial designs, and networked data collection are critical to progress. The Blood and Marrow Transplant Clinical Trials Network (BMT CTN) is a network of US transplant centers and a data coordinating center at the Center for International Blood and Marrow Transplant Research (CIBMTR). It has been highly successful in moving the transplant field to an era of collaborative randomized clinical trials with more than 7500 subjects enrolled in prospective studies.

References

1. Giobbie-Hurder A, Gelber RD, Regan MM. Challenges of guarantee-time bias. *J Clin Oncol.* 2013;31(23):2963–9.
2. Klein JP, Rizzo JD, Zhang MJ, Keiding N. Statistical methods for the analysis and presentation of the results of bone marrow transplants. Part I: unadjusted analysis. *Bone Marrow Transplant.* 2001;28(10):909–15.
3. Tarone RE, Ware JH. On distribution-free tests for equality for survival distributions. *Biometrika.* 1977;64:156–160.
4. Hahn T, McCarthy PL, Carreras J, Zhang MJ, Lazarus HM, Laport GG, *et al.* Simplified validated prognostic model for progression-free survival after autologous transplantation for hodgkin lymphoma. *Biol Blood Marrow Transplant.* 2013;19(12):1740–4.
5. Klein JP, Rizzo JD, Zhang MJ, Keiding N. Statistical methods for the analysis and presentation of the results of bone marrow transplants. Part 2: Regression modeling. *Bone Marrow Transplant.* 2001;28(11):1001–11.
6. Logan BR, Zhang MJ, Klein JP. Regression models for hazard rates *versus* cumulative incidence probabilities in hematopoietic cell transplantation data. *Biol Blood Marrow Transplant.* 2006;12(1 Suppl 1):107–12.
7. Klein JP, Andersen PK. Regression modeling of competing risks data based on pseudovalues of the cumulative incidence function. *Biometrics.* 2005;61(1):223–9.
8. Goodman SN. Of P-values and Bayes: a modest proposal. *Epidemiology.* 2001;12(3):295–7.
9. Goodman SN. Toward evidence-based medical statistics. 1: The P value fallacy. *Ann Intern Med.* 1999;130(12):995–1004.
10. Uno H, Claggett B, Tian L, Inoue E, Gallo P, Miyata T, *et al.* Moving beyond the hazard ratio in quantifying the between-group difference in survival analysis. *J Clin Oncol.* 2014;32(22):2380–5.
11. Colhoun HM, McKeigue PM, Davey Smith G. Problems of reporting genetic associations with complex outcomes. *Lancet.* 2003;361(9360):865–72.
12. Ioannidis JP. Microarrays and molecular research: noise discovery? *Lancet.* 2005;365(9458):454–5.
13. Ioannidis JP. Genetic associations: false or true? *Trends Mol Med.* 2003;9(4):135–8.
14. Goodman, S. A dirty dozen: twelve P-value misconceptions. *Sem Hematol.* 2008;45(3):135–14.

Pharmacologic Controversies in Hematopoietic Cell Transplants

Elizabeth C. DiMaggio and Helen Leather

Pretransplant Pharmacologic Controversies

Conditioning Regimens

Controversy #1: What Is the Optimal Melphalan Dose for Plasma Cell Myeloma Subjects with Renal Insufficiency?

Approximately 20%[1] to 50%[2,3] of newly diagnosed multiple myeloma patients present with renal impairment, with 9% requiring dialysis[2]. Contributing factors leading to kidney injury include proximal tubular damage via monoclonal light chains, increased uric acid or calcium, use of nephrotoxic medications, dehydration, infection, cast nephropathy, and less commonly, amyloid deposit or plasma cell infiltration[4,5]. High-dose chemotherapy (HDC) with hematopoietic cell support is both a standard of care, and a vital component, in the treatment of eligible patients with multiple myeloma. The management of HDC in multiple myeloma patients with renal impairment poses a challenge to clinicians. One approach is to reduce the dose of HDC to compensate for anticipated reduced clearance, e.g., reducing the standard melphalan dose of $200\,\text{mg/m}^2$ to $140\,\text{mg/m}^2$ in patients with renal insufficiency[5–7]. To date, there are at least 15 case reports, retrospective analyses, and prospective studies addressing the use of melphalan given alone or concomitantly with other conditioning therapy in patients with renal insufficiency (including patients on hemodialysis) for the treatment of various solid tumors and hematologic malignancies[1–3,5,6,8–17]. Various definitions of renal impairment or renal failure have been applied including a serum creatinine of $>176.8\,\text{mmol/L}$ ($>2\,\text{mg/dL}$), estimated CrCL of ≤ 60 mL/min, or dialysis dependent with melphalan doses ranging from $50\,\text{mg/m}^2$ to $200\,\text{mg/m}^2$. Unfortunately, the data supporting dose reductions in renal impairment are limited and contradictory at best (Table 70.1). The majority of the data confirm the feasibility of melphalan use over a range of doses from $50\,\text{mg/m}^2$ to $200\,\text{mg/m}^2$ in patients with renal insufficiency, failure, or dialysis dependence[3,9,10,12–15]. With regard to adverse reactions, neither Tricot et al.[8] nor Parikh et al.[5] noted significant toxicities when using melphalan $200\,\text{mg/m}^2$ in

patients with CrCL <40 mL/min (including five on dialysis) or patients with a serum Cr $>2\,\text{mg/dL}$ prior to autologous HCT, respectively. Contrary to these findings, other groups have reported comparable event-free survival (EFS) and overall survival (OS) but with less toxicity when using doses of melphalan less than $200\,\text{mg/m}^2$ (range $100\,\text{mg/m}^2$ to $180\,\text{mg/m}^2$) in patients with serum Cr >2, CrCL ≤ 60 mL/min, or on hemodialysis[1,2,6,11] (Table 70.1). At lower melphalan doses, patients were observed to have less mucositis, pulmonary, cardiac, neurologic, and dermatologic complications, shorter hospitalization periods, and less intravenous antibiotic use.

Practice Points

Collectively, the above data do not strongly support or oppose melphalan dose reduction in patients with renal insufficiency. A truly scientific and definitive answer on the role of reduced dose melphalan conditioning cannot be made due to a lack of controlled randomized data. Contrasting study designs, differing patient populations, small sample sizes, and varying definitions of renal insufficiency or failure make it impossible to draw direct comparisons and make definitive conclusions. Current review of the topic and guidelines from the International Myeloma Working Group support the role of lower dose melphalan ($100–140\,\text{mg/m}^2$) in patients with renal impairment and those who are dialysis dependent without compromising efficacy[4,7].

Controversy#2: What is the Optimal Seizure Prophylaxis When Administering Busulfan in a Conditioning Regimen?

Busulfan was first established in HCT conditioning regimens in the 1980s[18,19]. It readily distributes into the cerebrospinal fluid at concentrations similar to that of plasma resulting in central nervous system (CNS) toxicities, namely seizures, which have been reported in up to 10% of the adult and 7.5% of the pediatric population when administered without preventive anticonvulsants[20–24]. Since first reported, premedication with seizure prophylaxis is recommended prior to initiation of busulfan and should continue for at least 24 hours following the last busulfan dose[25,26]. Unfortunately options are limited as many anticonvulsants can cause significant side

Table 70.1 Melphalan dosing in MM patients with renal insufficiency

Reference	n	Conditioning	Inclusion/definition of RI or RF	Dialysis	Toxicity	NRM	TRM	CR	PFS	EFS	OS
Kergueris et al. 1994 [17]	6	Mel 140mg/m² – single agent	CrCL ≤20 mL/min/1.73 m² (n=3)	0 patients on dialysis	Mucositis in patients with severe renal insufficiency	NR	NR	NR	NR	NR	NR
	8	Mel 140mg/m² – plus radiation									
	2	Mel 140mg/m² – plus busulfan									
	4	Mel 140mg/m² – in BEAM									
Tricot et al. 1996[8]	20	Mel 200mg/m²ᵃ divided equally on 2 consecutive days (day −3 and −2)	CrCL ≤40 mL/min (n=6)	5 patients were on dialysis	Longer fever durations and hospitalizations in renal failure patients	NR	NR	NR	NR	NR	NR
Badros et al. 2001 [1]	60ᵃ	Mel 200mg/m²ᵃ divided equally and infused over 20 min on 2 consecutive days (day −3 and −2)	SCr >2mg/dL or patients on dialysis (n=81)	38 patients were on dialysis at time for first auto-HCT (n=27 Mel 200; n=11 Mel 140); dialysis performed before Mel and again 24–48h after stem cell infusion	Mucositis 93% Complications: Pulmonary 57% Cardiac 21% Neurologic 36%	NR	7%	35%	NR	Overall 48% (3-year)	Overall 55% (3-year)
	21ᵃ	Mel 140mg/m²ᵃ given as a single infusion day −2			Mucositis 67% Complications: Pulmonary 17% Cardiac 0% Neurologic 37%	NR	5%	33%	NR		
Lee et al. 2004[11]	32	Mel 200mg/m² infused on day −2	RF on maintenance dialysis at time of auto-HCT (n=59)	32 patients on dialysis; dialysis performed 24–36h after Mel before stem cell infusion		NR	12%ᵇ (6 mo)	46%	NR	24% (5-year)	36% (5-year)
	27	Mel 140mg/m² infused on day −2									
Knudsen et al. 2005 [3]	16	Mel 200mg/m²	CrCL <60mL/min (n=29)	8 patients were on dialysis	Antibiotics (days) 13 (median 4–34) Fever (days) 4 (median 0–21) Hospitalization (days) 22 (median 15–47)	NR	17%	NR	NR	25 months	NR
	10	Mel 140mg/m²			Antibiotics (days) 10 (median 0–17) Fever (days) 4 (median 0–4) Hospitalization (days) 19 (median 19–21)						
	3	Mel 200mg/m² divided equally on 2 consecutive days			Antibiotics (days) 25 (median 7–65) Fever (days) 16 (median 0–36) Hospitalization (days) 39 (median 18–73)						

Table 70.1 (cont.)

Reference	n	Conditioning	Inclusion/ definition of RI or RF	Dialysis	Toxicity	NRM	TRM	CR	PFS	EFS	OS
Raab et al. 2006[2]	17	Mel 100mg/m² (dialysis pts)	End-stage RF on maint. dialysis (n=17)	17 patients on dialysis	Antibiotics (days) 10 (median 0–22) Fever (days) 3 (median 0–20) Hospitalization (days) 19 (median 13–63)	NR	6%	NR	NR	23.4 months (P=0.71)	35.6 months (P=0.44)
	17	Mel 200mg/m² (SCr within NL limits)			Antibiotics (days) 6 (median 0–10) Fever (days) 2 (median 0–9) Hospitalization (days) 17 (median 13–22)		6%			18.3 months	52.3 months
Parikh et al. 2009 [5]	33	Mel 200mg/m²ᵃ divided equally on 2 consecutive days (day −4 and −3)	SCr ≥2mg/dL for >1 month pre-auto-HCT (n=46)	10 patients on dialysis		0% 100 d	NR	22%	36% (3 yr)	NR	64% (3-year)
	9	Mel 180mg/m²ᵃ divided equally on 2 consecutive days (day −4 and −3)				15% 100d for Mel 180+140					
	4	Mel 140mg/m²ᵃ divided equally on 2 consecutive days (day −4 and −3)									
Abidi et al. 2012[6]	3	Mel 140mg/m²	CrCL <60mL/ min (n=15)	NR	OM Grade 2 (n=1) OM Grade 3 (n=1) OM Grade 1 (n=1) OM Grade 3 (n=1) OM Grade 2 (n=1) OM Grade 3 (n=4) OM Grade 4 (n=2) Other: death due to multiorgan failure (n=1) Other: CHF, interstitial pneumonitis, bullous dermatitis (n=1)	NR	NR	NR	NR	NR	NR
	3	Mel 160mg/m²									
	6	Mel 180mg/m²									
	3	Mel 200mg/m²									

Abbreviations: auto-HCT, autologous hematopoietic cell transplant; BEAM, BCNU, etoposide, cytarabine, melphalan; CHF, congestive heart failure; CR, complete remission; CrCL, creatinine clearance; EFS, event-free survival; IV, intravenous; maint, maintenance; Mel, melphalan; NL, normal; NR, not reportec; NRM, nonrelapse mortality; OM, oral mucositis; OS, overall survival; PFS, progression-free survival; pts, patients; RF, renal failure; RI, renal insufficiency; SCr, serum creatinine; TRM, transplant-related mortality.

ᵃ According to patient tolerance and response to first auto-HCT, a second auto-HCT was planned after 3–6 months with a dose of melphalan at 140mg/m² (n=7) or 200mg/m² (n=24).

ᵇ TRM after first auto-HCT; 23 patients went on to receive a second auto-HCT.

effects, drug interactions, and have long half-lives which require a long lead time to attain therapeutic concentrations. The goal is to select optimal prophylaxis that avoids or minimizes these concerns while providing adequate protection against neurotoxicity.

In the initial pharmacokinetic studies of busulfan, phenytoin was most commonly the antiepileptic of choice. A drug interaction between both drugs was discovered, such that concomitant administration yields higher busulfan clearance due to glutathione-S-transferase induction[21]. Variation in levels can be avoided with busulfan drug monitoring and therapeutic dose adjustments. An effective inducer of the hepatic cytochrome P450 enzyme system, phenytoin, may also alter the concentrations of supportive medications. Lastly, in dosing phenytoin, it is prudent to give a loading dose to obtain rapid therapeutic concentrations and weight-based dosing is the standard of care in the field of neurology.

More appealing are medications with fewer drug interactions and shorter half-lives, such as benzodiazepines (clonazepam, lorazepam) or levetiracetam. Benzodiazepines may cause sedation, weakness, or respiratory depression, but do provide additive antiemetic properties, produce few drug interactions, and have favorable pharmacokinetic profiles, all without the need for drug monitoring[24,27]. Both toxicity and drug interactions of levetiracetam are minimal, also without the need for therapeutic drug monitoring[24]. Finally, lorazepam and levetiracetam are available in intravenous formulation thus facilitating rapid therapeutic levels. The summary of the literature supporting the outlined options is detailed in Table 70.2. While the majority of these analyses are represented by the pediatric population, and the prophylaxis dosing and administration differs from study to study, the overall incidence of seizures is low (0–4%) with the exception of the sole case report[20,23,24,27–29,31,32].

Practice Points

As there have not been any direct comparisons between antiepileptic agents, it is not possible to conclude superiority of one versus another. All agents are associated with success in case reports/case series/small studies and are appropriate options. Each center should choose their preferred agent.

Controversy #3: What is the Best Way to Dose Conditioning Regimens/Drugs: Ideal, Adjusted, or Actual Body Weight?

More than one-third of adults in the United States are obese and as such the likelihood of HCT recipients being obese is high[33]. In the "myeloablative" HCT setting, chemotherapy is typically dosed to levels very close to those where significant or fatal side effects occur. For patients who are obese, where dosing is based on actual body weight, the concern is dosing for "fat weight" might result in significant toxicity; moreover there is a contrary concern that dosing on a lower adjusted

body weight in obese individuals will result in "under dosing" and lower efficacy/relapse. Recently there have been several reviews/position papers on dosing chemotherapy in obese individuals, and their overall recommendations are:

a. The American Society of Clinical Oncology evaluated the published literature (small observational studies, case reports, and pharmacokinetic studies) from 1996 to 2010 largely in breast, ovarian, colon, and lung cancer patients [24]. They found that a significant number of patients (up to 40%), received doses of chemotherapy not based on actual body weight, rather alternative lower doses. Their recommendations included[34]:

   a. Actual body weight (ABW) should be used when dosing chemotherapy, regardless of obesity

      i. No evidence that toxicity, either short-term or long-term, is increased with this strategy

      ii. No significant differences in myelosuppression are observed when ABW dosing is used

   b. Where dose-reduction strategies are employed such as for renal or hepatic impairment, resumption of full-weight-based dosing be implemented as soon as safely possible

      i. There are no data supporting greater dose reductions in obese versus nonobese populations

   c. Fixed-dose cytotoxic chemotherapy is rarely justified

   d. BSA (body surface area) calculations can be performed using any of the standard formulas (e.g., Mosteller, DuBois and Dubois, Haycock, Gehan and George, Boyd)

b. The American Society for Blood and Marrow Transplantation Practice Guideline Committee specifically evaluated HCT literature between 1946 and June 2012, as these patients were not well studied in the ASCO guideline, to develop a position statement on conditioning chemotherapy dosing in obese HCT recipients[35]. Their findings concluded[35]:

   a. There was insufficient information to make Level I or II evidence-based conclusions on chemotherapy dosing in obese HCT patients as a consequence of small series; lack of information on key variables such as weight, height, and BMI; retrospective studies; and use of PK-guided dosing adjustments

   b. Individual recommendations according to preparative agent were provided and supported by the committee and are outlined in Table 70.3.

Lastly, Weiss and colleagues performed a review of the literature on obesity and HCT[36]. They made a number of recommendations for future studies, that were similarly echoed by Bubalo and colleagues and included: use adjusted ideal body weight for dose calculation for research studies of HCT with curative intent; evaluate PK and PD of chemotherapeutic agents relative to weight and quantitative measurements of total and compartmental adipose tissue masses; and integrate

Table 70.2 Summary of studies investigating busulfan seizure prophylaxis

Citation	n	Age, years (range)	Preparative regimen	Busulfan dose	Seizure prophylaxis	Seizure prophylaxis dose	Started before Bu	Ended after Bu	Seizure incidence	Adverse effects	Comments
Vassal et al. 1990[20]	27	1–17	Bu alone BuCy BuMel BuCyMel BuCyTiot	600mg/m²	Clonazepam	0.1mg/kg/day CIVI	NR	NR	0%	NR	
Chan et al. 2002[24]	29	0.5–19	TiotBuCy BuCy	40mg/m² PO or 0.8mg/kg IV q6h×12 doses 1mg/kg PO q6h×16 doses	Lorazepam	0.02–0.05mg/kg IV or PO q6h	30 min pre-ea. Bu dose	24h	0%	Drowsiness; muscle twitch; sedation; weakness	
Bubalo et al. 2008[28]	46	22–75	BuMel BuMelTiot BuCy BuFluTBI	1mg/kg/dose PO×12–16 doses or IV 3.2mg/kg/day×1–2 days	Clonazepam plus levetiracetam	0.5mg PO BID 250–500mg PO BID	24h	24h	0%	Sedation; confusion	
Caselli et al. 2008[31]	16	1–17	BuMel BuMelCy BuCy	1mg/kg q6h PO for 4 days (n=13) 1.2mg/kg q6h IV for 4 days (n=3)	Lorazepam	0.1mg/kg/day CIVI	12h	24h	0%	Drowsiness	
Hamidieh et al. 2010[23]	30	1.08–15	NR	Disease dependent: 0.2–5mg/kg/day PO q6h for 4 days	Lorazepam	0.5mg/kg q6h PO	30 min pre-ea. Bu dose	72h	0%	Sedation; agitation; excitement; headache; dizziness; hallucination; urinary incontinence	PK studies done; no change in Bu clearance observed
Soni et al. 2012[27]	28 25	0.4–21 0.8–23	NR	NR	Levetiracetam Fosphenytoin	10mg/kg/dose q12h IV 15mg/kg LD followed by maint to a daily trough of 10–20µg/mL starting 24h post	6–12h 6–12h	24–48h 24–48h	0% 4%	None None	
Diaz-Carrasco et al. 2013[30]	33	15–69	BuMel BuCy FluBu BuCyFlu TiotFluBu	3.2mg/kg q24h (for 2–4 days)	Clonazepam	1mg q8h IV	12h	24h	0%	NR	Lorazepam 1mg q day prescribed as hypnotic in 63.6%
Yazal Erdem et al. 2014[32]	1	16	BuCy	3.2mg/kg/day IV for 4 days	Levetiracetam plus valproic acid	25–40mg/kg/day 26mg/kg/day	NR	NR	100%	NR	Pt with history of epilepsy
Caselli et al. 2014[29]	954	1.3–19	NR	Dose not reported; all oral form	Lorazepam Carbamazepine	0.03–0.06mg/kg/day IV 0.02–0.05mg/kg q6h PO 10–15mg/kg/day	24h 24h–5 days	NR NR	0.5% total	NR	13 seizures total but only 5 thought to be Bu-related

Abbreviations: Bu, busulfan; CIVI, continuous intravenous infusion; Cy, cyclophosphamide; Flu, fludarabine; LD, loading dose; Mel, melphalan; NR, not reported; TBI, total body irradiation; Tiot, thiotepa.

Table 70.3 Dosing recommendations for HCT conditioning agents in the obese individual[35]

Agent	Suggested dosing	Additional information
Alemtuzumab	Flat dosing in adults based upon regimen selected	Addition of this agent to conditioning regimens continues to evolve and there are currently no data on dose adjustments for obese individuals
Busulfan	Dose on ABW25 in adults (obese and nonobese) receiving per kilogram dosing or BSA based on TBW for m^2 dosing. All regimens >12mg/kg PO equivalent are recommended to have PK targeting as appropriate for the disease state. Regimens using doses >12mg/kg PO equivalent do not have sufficient information to recommend routine PK monitoring at this time. Pediatric patients should be dosed upon TBW with similar monitoring guidelines	PK monitoring has reduced SOS/VOD from an occurrence rate of approximately 20% to <5% AUC/C_{ss} targeting varies by regimen For BuCy regimens the MTD is 16mg/kg PO equivalent over 4 days for adults For Bu/Flu and BuFlu-alemtuzumab MTD based upon daily AUC have been determined Dosing with other combinations of agents is still being determined
Carboplatin	Dose adults on BSA based on TBW	No current literature consensus for dosing carboplatin based on AUC for HCT regimens or adjustments on dosing during HCT for obese individuals
Carmustine	Dose adults on BSA based on TBW unless >120% IBW then dose on BSA based on ABW25	Pulmonary toxicity >50% at 600mg/m^2 with multiple agent regimens. MTD of 1200mg/m^2 as single agent with 9.5% pulmonary toxicity
Clofarabine	Dose adults and children on BSA based on TBW	Addition of this agent to conditioning regimens continues to evolve and there are currently no data on dose adjustments for obese individuals
Cyclophosphamide	Dose on the lesser of TBW or IBW for Cy200. For Cy120 dosing can be either IBW or TBW until >120% IBW then dose based on ABW25. The former method is preferred for adults and the latter is preferred in pediatrics	
Cytarabine	Dose adults and children on BSA based on TBW	Cytarabine dosing generally lower than dose used in leukemia consolidation regimens
Etoposide	Dose adults on ABW25 for mg/kg dosing and BSA based on TBW for BSA based dosing	DLT of mucositis
Fludarabine	Dose adults on BSA based on TBW	Risk factors and effects of chemotherapy on post-treatment leukoencephalopathy still being studied for conditioning regimen doses above 125mg/m^2
Melphalan	Dose adults on BSA based on TBW	DLT of mucositis. Adjustments for age and renal function are still not standardized
Pentostatin	Dose adults on BSA based on TBW	Addition of this agent to conditioning regimens continues to evolve and there are currently no data on dose adjustments for obese individuals
Thiotepa	Dose adults on BSA based on TBW unless >120% IBW then dose on BSA based on ABW40	Multi-agent MTD is 500–750mg/m^2, single-agent MTD is 900mg/m^2
Antithymocyte globulin – equine	Dose on mg/kg based on TBW	Addition of this agent to conditioning regimens continues to evolve and there are currently no data on dose adjustments for obese individuals
Antithymocyte globulin – rabbit	Dose on mg/kg based on TBW	Addition of this agent to conditioning regimens continues to evolve and there are currently no data on dose adjustments for obese individuals

ABW25 indicates IBW +0.25(TBW-IBW); ABW40, IBW þ .4(TBW-IBW); AUC, area under the curve; Bu, busulfan; BMI, body mass index; BSA, body surface area; Css, concentration at steady-state; Cy, cyclophosphamide; Cy120, cyclophosphamide 120mg/kg; Cy200, cyclophosphamide 200mg/kg; DLT, dose-limiting toxicity; Flu, fludarabine; IBW, ideal body weight; MTD, maximum tolerated dose; PK, pharmacokinetics; PO, oral; SOS, sinusoidal obstruction syndrome; TBW, total body weight; VOD, veno-occlusive disease.

dose-escalation studies with curative intent and include PK, PD, biomarkers, and assessment of adipose tissue mass; evaluate relative to patient outcomes. If these recommendations are followed it might be possible to make definitive recommendations in the future.

Practice Points

With the disparity in recommendations between ASCO and ASBMT, it would be prudent for HCT practitioners to follow the ASBMT recommendations, specifically as they evaluated HCT studies where significantly higher doses of chemotherapy are administered.

Post-transplant Pharmacologic Controversies

Graft-*versus*-Host Disease

Controversy#1: What Are Optimal Serum Concentrations When Tacrolimus Is Combined with Sirolimus?

Historically, target serum concentrations for single-agent tacrolimus and sirolimus have been 5–20 ng/mL and 3–12 ng/mL, respectively. However HCT centers tend to adopt their own "normal range" and the optimal target levels when both immunosuppressants are utilized is not clearly defined.

Over the last decade a number of smaller studies have investigated the addition of sirolimus to calcineurin-immunosuppressive regimens in an attempt to remove the need for methotrexate from graft-*versus*-host disease (GvHD) prophylaxis due to its toxicity. Most of the research on this approach was performed by the Dana-Farber Group in both HLA-matched related donor (MRD) and HLA-matched unrelated donor (MUD) allogeneic HCT patients where GvHD prophylaxis with sirolimus and tacrolimus (starting day −3; target serum concentrations of 3–12 ng/mL and 5–10 ng/mL, respectively) was associated with low rates of acute and chronic GvHD and nonrelapse mortality (NRM), with high rates of relapse-free survival (RFS) and OS[37,38].

The results from these studies served as the basis for the large Bone Marrow Transplant Clinical Trials Network (BMT CTN) randomized, multicenter, phase 3 trial of 304 HLA MRD HCT recipients comparing the combination of sirolimus-tacrolimus to methotrexate-tacrolimus as GvHD prophylaxis[39]. Patients were conditioned with either cyclophosphamide/total body irradiation (TBI) or etoposide/TBI. GvHD prophylaxis consisted of sirolimus and tacrolimus starting on day −3 with target serum concentrations of 3–12 ng/mL and 5–10 ng/mL, respectively. In the comparator group, tacrolimus was given identically and the methotrexate (Mtx) was given as 15 mg/m^2 IV on day +1 and 10 mg/m^2 per day intravenously on days +3, +6, and +11. Rates of acute

GvHD were similar between both the sirolimus and the methotrexate group, lending support to the role of non-Mtx-based GvHD prophylaxis regimens. The Mtx-based regimen resulted in a significantly longer time to both neutrophil and platelet engraftment. There was no difference in the incidence of veno-occlusive disease (VOD) and thrombotic microangiopathy (TMA) between both groups. These results support the role of tacrolimus-sirolimus as GvHD prophylaxis as an alternative to methotrexate-based regimens (see Chapters 12 and 13).

Other HCT groups have also evaluated tacrolimus-sirolimus regimens and demonstrated different results. Rodriguez and colleagues demonstrated higher rates of acute GvHD and TMA in HLA MRD HCT recipients (Table 70.4)[40]. There were differences in the preparative regimens they used (fludarabine-melphalan (n=46); TBI-etoposide (n=28); and busulfan cyclophosphamide (n=11)), and they demonstrated an association between preparative regimen and the occurrence of TMA (7% *versus* 25% *versus* 55%, respectively; $P<0.005$). There was no relationship between TMA and immunosuppression levels. Pidala and colleagues conducted a prospective, randomized study comparing combination sirolimus-tacrolimus to standard methotrexate-tacrolimus GvHD prophylaxis in HLA MUD or MRD-HCTs[41]. Their immunosuppression targets varied from the previous studies such that when given in combination, the target tacrolimus and sirolimus levels were 3–7 ng/mL and 5–14 ng/mL, respectively. In earlier work by Pidala and colleagues, when these two agents were given concurrently, these levels were considered standard targets to reduce risk of TMA[42]. Interestingly, toxicity was similar among both groups as no difference was found in the time to both neutrophil ($P=0.57$) and platelet ($P=0.6$) engraftment, mucositis ($P=0.12$), VOD incidence ($P=0.56$), or TMA incidence ($P=0.48$). However, rates of grade II–IV acute GvHD were significantly lower in the sirolimus-tacrolimus group (43% *versus* 89%, $P<0.001$) largely due to differences in grade II GvHD. Regardless, survival and relapse outcomes did not differ among the study groups as well.

Practice Points

There are no data available directly comparing outcomes if different tacrolimus-sirolimus concentrations are targeted, thus it is not possible to determine the optimal goals. The largest trial from the BMT CTN targeted levels of 3–12 ng/mL for sirolimus and 5–10 ng/mL for tacrolimus with comparable GvHD rates and low toxicity and should be the current standard.

Controversy #2: Should Mycophenolate Mofetil (MMF) Levels be Monitored in HCT Candidates?

As a prodrug, esterases quickly hydrolyze MMF to the active component, mycophenolic acid (MPA), which blocks inosine monophosphate dehydrogenase. MPA has a high affinity for albumin with up to 99% protein bound with only the free MPA being pharmacologically active[43]. Low albumin has been

Table 70.4 Combination sirolimus and tacrolimus for GvHD prophylaxis

Citation	n	Median age yr (range)	HCT type	Donor	PB versus BM	Preparative regimen	GvHD prophylaxis and dose	CI start day	Target level (ng/mL)	Acute GvHD	Chronic GvHD	VOD	TMA	Relapse	Outcomes (DFS, EFS, NRM, OS)
Phase 3															
Cutler et al. 2014 [39]	304	45 (19–59) 43 (13–58)	MA	MRD	PB	Cy/TBI VP16/TBI	Group 1: SIR‡ /TAC℗ n=151 Group 2: TAC℗/MTX¶ n=153	−3/−3 −3 (TAC)	5–10 TAC 3–12 SIR 5–10 TAC	26% II–IV (P=0.48) 34% II–IV	53% 45% (P=0.06)	11% (VOD+ TMA+ endothelial injury) 5%		28% 29% (P=0.8)	DFS: 53%/OS: 59% DFS: 54%/OS: 63% (P=0.77, P=0.36)
Phase 2															
Cutler et al. 2004 [37]	30	42 (19–54)	MA	MRD	PB	Cy/TBI	SIR‡/TAC ℗	−3/−3	5–10 TAC 3–12 SIR	10% II–IV (100 days)	39%	10%	13%	NR	NRM: 6% (1 yr) RFS: 71% (1 yr) OS: 67% (1 yr)
Cutler et al. 2007 [38]	83	53 (18–59) 44 (22–54)	MA	MRD (n=53) MUD	PB	Cy/TBI	SIR‡/TAC℗	−3/−3	5–10 TAC 3–12 SIR	18.9% II–IV 23.3% II–IV	58.3% 59.3%	9.4% 6.7%	9.4% 3.3%	17% 13.3%	NRM: 5.7% (100 day) OS 1 yr/2 yr: 77.4%/ 69.8% NRM: 3.3% (100 day) OS 1 yr/2 yr: 76.7%/ 76.7%
Rodriguez 2010 [40]	85	48 (10–67)	RIC MA	MSD	PB BM	Flu/Mel VP16/TBI Bu/Cy	SIR‡/TAC℗	−3/−3	5–10 TAC 3–12 SIR	40% II–IV	51%	2%	19%	34% (2 yr)	NRM: 10.2 (2 yr) OS: 66% (2 yr) DFS: 58% (2 yr)
Pidala et al. 2012 [41]	74	49 (25–68) 48 (23–69)	NR	MSD (n=35) MUD	PB	Flu/Bu Pento/Bu Flu/Mel	Group 1: SIR♭ /TAC℗ n=37 Group 2: TAC ℗/Mtx¶ n=37	−1/−3 −3 (TAC)	3–7 TAC 5–14 SIR 5–15 TAC	43% II–IV (P<0.001, a) 14% III–IV (P=0.71, b) 89% II–IV (a) 11% (b)	53% 70% (P=0.68)	5.4% 2.7% (P=0.56)	24.3% 18.9% (P=0.57)	18% 31% (2 yr, P=0.09)	NRM: 28%/OS: 61% NRM: 8%/OS: 69% (2 yr, P=0.025)(2 yr, P=0.66)
Shayani 2013 [65]	177	46 (10–70)	RIC MA	MSD (n=82) MUD	PB BM	Flu/Mel Cy/TBI VP16/TBI Bu/Cy	SIR‡ /TAC℗	−3/−3	5–10 TAC 3–12 SIR	50.5% II–IV	71.3%	NR	17%/ 22%*	31.1% (2 yr)	NRM: 15.8 (2 yr) OS: 59.9% (2 yr) EFS: 51.7% (2 yr)

Abbreviations: BM, bone marrow; Bu, busulfan; CI, calcineurin inhibitor; CIVI, continuous intravenous infusion; Cy, cyclophosphamide; DFS, disease-free-survival; EFS, event-free survival; flu, fludarabine; GvHD, graft-versus-host disease; HCT, hematopoietic cell transplantation; MA, myeloablative; Md, median; Mel, melphalan; MRD, matched related donor; MSD, matched sibling donor; Mtx, methotrexate; MUD, matched unrelated donor; n, number; NR, not reported; NRM, nonrelapse mortality; OS, overall survival; PB, peripheral blood; Pento, pentostatin; RFS, relapse-free survival; RIC, reduced intensity conditioning; SIR, sirolimus; TAC, tacrolimus; TBI, total body irradiation; TMA, thrombotic microangiopathy; VOD, veno-occlusive disease; VP-16, etoposide; yr(s), year(s).
Notes: * Definite TMA in 17% of patients and probable TMA in 22% of patients (probable due to missing a test value); ℗ TAC: 0.02 mg/kg per day CIVI; ¶ Mtx: 15 mg/m² on day 1, 10 mg/m² on days 3, 6, 11; ♭ Sir: 9 mg oral loading dose followed by maintenance; ‡ Sir: 12 mg oral loading dose followed by daily doses of 4 mg with the 4 mg dose adjusted to reach target level.

shown to correspond with rapid clearance of total MPA. Clearance is also increased by concomitant cyclosporine administration and decreased in patients with either renal or hepatic impairment[44]. The aforementioned, plus weight-based dosing, contribute to variability noted in MPA plasma concentrations[45]. While monitoring MMF levels has been studied in solid organ transplantation, it is not well established in the allogeneic HCT population. Several factors likely contribute to inconsistent practices including both the variation and inconvenience in methods of measurement (trough, steady-state plasma concentrations (Css), area-under-the-plasma concentration curve (AUC), or as Bayesian estimates of AUC); as well as determining which component of the metabolized MMF to measure, namely the unbound, total MPA product, or both. Finally, clinical outcomes reported in the literature are not consistent and the relevance of Css levels, trough levels, and unbound and free MPA is unclear.

An early study by Giaccone et al.[46] examined the association of both total and unbound MPA with donor chimerism, graft rejection, acute GvHD, and relapse in 85 adult (age 17–70 years) NMA HLA-matched MUD-HCT recipients. Patients with a total MPA Css less than 3 µg/mL were at an increased risk for low (<50%) donor CD3 cell chimerism; and those below 2.5 µg/mL, at risk for graft rejection. A positive association was also observed with free MPA Css and chimerism. These associations were not reported with trough (total MPA or free MPA) concentrations, and measurement of this level was deemed clinically meaningless. No significant associations were seen with any MPA measurements and either relapse or GvHD. McDermott and colleagues analyzed Css total MPA, Css free MPA, and total MPA trough concentrations in 308 related and unrelated HCT recipients for associations in graft rejection, day 28 donor T-cell chimerism, acute GvHD, relapse, nonrelapse mortality (NRM), cytomegalovirus (CMV) reactivation, and OS[45]. In contrast to Giacconne et al.'s study, a relationship between total MPA Css and donor T-cell chimerism was not detected. In those receiving an unrelated graft, an association was seen with low MPA Css and grades III to IV acute GvHD and NRM. No clinical outcomes were associated with trough levels. Measuring MPA AUCs in HCT recipients of both MRD and MUD has also been explored. In a small prospective study of 15 patients, Royer et al. observed that patients with lower total MPA AUCs exhibited more GvHD [47]. Recently, the association between MPA trough levels and outcomes in double-unit cord blood transplants (dCBT) was assessed[48]. No association was detected between mean week 1 and 2 trough levels and incidence of grade II to IV acute GvHD, day 100 neutrophil engraftment, platelet engraftment, nor duration of total parenteral nutrition (TPN) (used to assess gastrointestinal toxicity). Only an increased risk for grade III and IV acute GvHD was associated with low trough levels.

Practice Points

Although it would be ideal to establish a simple monitoring strategy for MPA that resembles that observed with calcineurin inhibitors, benefit has not been documented consistently in all HCT subtypes (MRD and MUD) and validated using all measurement strategies. Steady-state levels appear to correlate to outcomes better than a trough level or AUC measurement; however, numerous blood draws are necessary to gather and calculate the pharmacokinetic data, a task that is both laborious and inconvenient to the patient. As a consequence, it would seem that there is not sufficient evidence to support the routine monitoring of MMF levels at this time.

Controversy#3: How Should Hypomagnesemia Caused by Calcineurin Inhibitors Be Managed?

Calcineurin inhibitors have been reported to cause many adverse effects including nephrotoxicity, electrolyte disturbances/metabolic toxicity, neurotoxicity, increased infections, and hypertension; all requiring frequent monitoring and intervention[49–51]. In particular, electrolyte changes include magnesium wasting, which can eventually result in seizures, altered mental status, or cardiac arrhythmias[49]. Though unclear, it is surmised that magnesium reabsorption is blocked at sites in the more distal tubules by calcineurin inhibitors[49–51]. Consequently, levels have been observed to drop within the first 3 weeks following HCT, and loss is maintained throughout tacrolimus or cyclosporine therapy, thus precipitating the need for concomitant supplementation [49]. If mild and asymptomatic, oral supplementation may be warranted assuming the patient can tolerate it (no signs and symptoms of nausea or vomiting) and has good gastrointestinal absorption without diarrhea. More acute cases require parenteral replacement[49,52].

Practice Points

Table 70.5 serves as a general guideline, although currently there is no literature recommending or comparing replacement

Table 70.5 Guideline for magnesium replacement

Grade	Measurement (ng/dL)	Replacement	Comment
0	Within normal limits	No replacement	
1	<Lower limit of normal − 1.2	No replacement necessary or Oral supplementation with magnesium gluconate 500–1000 mg orally three times daily	May cause diarrhea
2	<1.2−0.9	Magnesium sulfate 4 g IV weekly	Cardiac monitoring may be necessary
3	<0.9−0.7	Frequent IV infusions of magnesium sulfate 4–8 g daily or every other day	
4	<0.7		

Note: Adapted from reference [51].

strategies in the HCT population, and each institution must adopt their own monitoring, prevention, and treatment algorithms based on its severity.

What Are the Major Pharmacokinetic Drug Interactions Relevant to GvHD Prophylaxis Medications?

Pharmacologic complications are highly prevalent in HCT due to the number of medications required to ensure success. A recent study examining potential drug interactions in allogeneic or autologous HCT recipients reported average number of administered medications during a single hospital stay was 31.8 + 4.96[53]. This number of medications means that the likelihood of a drug interaction is high. All drug interactions are important, but those impacting the preparative regimen and the post-transplant immune suppression are most important owing to their role in a successful outcome. Drug interactions, both reported and theoretical, for tacrolimus are outlined in Table 70.6, for cyclosporine in Table 70.7, and

for sirolimus in Table 70.8. All members of the HCT team should be aware of the potential for drug interactions and adjust the doses of medications, or choose an alternative agent where possible.

Controversy#4: How Long Antifungal Prophylaxis Should be Administered in the Absence of GvHD?

The use of antifungal agents as prophylaxis against yeasts and mold infections in IICT recipients is commonplace and supported by a wide body of evidence[54–62]. Over the last two decades we have learned that: fluconazole prophylaxis is better than placebo[59–62]; itraconazole has improved efficacy over itraconazole, although at the cost of increased toxicity and lower tolerability[60,61]; micafungin is more effective than fluconazole although hampered by being an intravenous drug [63]; posaconazole is similar in efficacy to fluconazole in preventing all fungal infections, although superior in preventing proven/probable invasive aspergillosis in allogeneic HCT patients with GvHD[55]; and lastly voriconazole treatment is

Table 70.6 Clinically relevant pharmacokinetic drug interactions with tacrolimus

Drug	Data type	Proposed mechanism of interaction by drug	Clinical effect (potential or actual)	Recommended action
Amiodarone	Case report	CYP3A4 inhibition	No PK parameters reported Prolonged QTc interval	Monitor cardiac function.
Antivirals				
Adefovir	PK study	CYP3A4 inhibition CYP2C9 inhibition	$\leftrightarrow$ Tacrolimus PK parameters	Not a clinically significant interaction; can be safely coadministered.
Boceprevir	PK study	CYP3A4 inhibition	$\uparrow$ Tacrolimus AUC$_{inf}$ 15.8-fold $\uparrow$ Tacrolimus C$_{max}$ 9.75-fold $\downarrow$ Tacrolimus CL 18-fold $\uparrow$ Tacrolimus t½ 2-fold $\leftrightarrow$ Bocepravir PK	Dose reduction of tacrolimus and also extension of the dosing interval
Emtricitabine/tenofovir	PK study	Not reported	$\leftrightarrow$ AUC$_\tau$, C$_{max}$, and C$_\tau$	Not a clinically relevant interaction; can be safely coadministered
Oseltamivir	PK study	Not reported	$\leftrightarrow$ Tacrolimus C$_{max}$, AUC, T$_{max}$ $\uparrow$ Tacrolimus C$_{min}$ 13%	Not a clinically relevant interaction
Telaprevir	Theoretical	CYP3A4 inhibition	$\uparrow$ Tacrolimus [ ]	Monitor tacrolimus blood levels and dosemodify accordingly
Azole antifungals				
Fluconazole Itraconazole Posaconazole Voriconazole	Case reports; PK study	CYP3A4 inhibition	$\uparrow$ Tacrolimus C$_{min}$ → $\uparrow$ toxicity[a] See fluconazole, itraconazole, posaconazole, and voriconazole drug-interaction tables	Monitor levels. $\downarrow$ Tacrolimus doses as follows: by 40% for fluconazole; by 50–60% for itraconazole; 66% for voriconazole (reduce starting tacrolimus dose to 33% of the regular dose at the start of voriconazole), by 75–80% for posaconazole (reduce the starting tacrolimus dose to 33% of the regular dose at the start of posaconazole)

Table 70.6 (*cont.*)

Drug	Data type	Proposed mechanism of interaction by drug	Clinical effect (potential or actual)	Recommended action
Calcium channel blockers				
Amlodipine	Case report; PK study	CYP3A5 inhibition in intestine	↓ Tacrolimus CL/F 2.2-fold in CYP3A5 expressers ↓ Amlodipine AUC in both expressers and nonexpressers of CYP3A5	Monitor tacrolimus concentrations
Diltiazem	*In-vitro* Case report	CYP3A5*3 inhibition	↑ Tacrolimus AUC 26–177% ↑ C_{min} [ ] tacrolimus → ↑ toxicity	Monitor levels. ↓ Tacrolimus dose Drug interaction most profound in CYP3A5 expressers
Verapamil	*In-vitro*	CYP3A4 inhibition	↑ Exposure → toxicity	Monitor levels. ↓ Tacrolimus dose
Chloramphenicol	Case report	CYP3A4 inhibition	↑ Tacrolimus AUC 7.5-fold → toxicity	Monitor levels. ↓ Tacrolimus dose
Everolimus	PK study	Not reported	↓ Tacrolimus bioavailability	Monitor levels. ↑ Tacrolimus dose
Imatinib mesylate	Hypothesis	CYP3A4 inhibition	Unknown, anticipate ↑ [ ] tacrolimus	Monitor levels
Macrolide antibiotics				
Clarithromycin Erythromycin	Case reports *In-vitro*; case reports	CYP3A4 inhibition	↑ Tacrolimus C_{min} 2-fold →↑ toxicity ↑ Tacrolimus C_{min} 6-fold → ↑ toxicity	Monitor levels. ↓ Tacrolimus dose Monitor levels. ↓ Tacrolimus dose
Protease inhibitors				
Atazanavir	Case report	Weak CYP3A4 inhibition	↓ Tacrolimus [ ]	Monitor levels and ↑ Tacrolimus dose accordingly; the opposite interaction to other PIs experienced.
Darunavir, fosamprenavir, indinavir, lopinavir, nelfinavir, saquinavir, tipranivir	Theoretical	CYP34 inhibition	↑ Tacrolimus [ ]	Monitor levels. ↓ Tacrolimus dose
Ritonavir	Case report	CYP3A4 inhibition	↑ Tacrolimus [ ]	Monitor levels. ↓ Tacrolimus dose
Phenobarbital	*In-vitro*; case reports	CYP3A4 induction	↓ Tacrolimus [ ] → GvHD	Monitor levels. ↑ Tacrolimus dose
Phenytoin	Case report	CYP3A4 induction	↓ Tacrolimus [ ] → GvHD	Monitor levels. ↑ Tacrolimus dose
Ranolazine	Case report	CYP3A4 inhibition P-gp pump inhibition	↑ Tacrolimus [ ]	Monitor levels. ↓ Tacrolimus dose; authors suggest a 70% ↓ in dose
Rifampin	Healthy volunteers	CYP3A4 induction	↓ Tacrolimus AUC_{po} 68% ↓ Tacrolimus AUC_{iv} 35% ↓ F_{PO} 51%	Monitor levels. ↑ Tacrolimus dose
St John's wort	Case report	CYP3A4 induction ↑ P-gp transporter expression	↓ Tacrolimus [ ] → GvHD	Monitor levels. ↑ Tacrolimus dose
Theophylline	Case report	CYP3A4 inhibition	↑ Exposure → toxicity	Monitor levels. ↓ Tacrolimus dose

[ ] = concentration; ↑ = increased; → = leads to; ↓ = decreased; ↔ = no change; AUC = area under the curve; C_{min} = trough concentration; F = bioavailability; GvHD = graft-*versus*-host disease; P-gp = P-glycoprotein; PK = pharmacokinetic; CYP3A4 = cytochrome P450 3A4 isoenzyme.
[a] Drug interaction occurs when both agents administered orally and where fluconazole dose is >200mg/day.

Table 70.7 Clinically relevant pharmacokinetic drug interactions with cyclosporine

Drug	Data type	Proposed mechanism of interaction by drug	Clinical effect (potential or actual)	Recommended action
Antivirals				
Bocepravir	PK study	CYP3A4 inhibition	↑ Cyclosporine AUC_{inf} 2.7-fold ↓ Cyclosporine C_{max} 1–89-fold ↑ Cyclosporine $t\frac{1}{2}$ 25% ↓ Cyclosporine CL 2 fold	The magnitude of increase is thought to be outside a clinically meaningful interaction. Monitor cyclosporine levels and adjust accordingly
Oseltamivir	PK study	Not applicable	↔ Cyclosporine C_{max}, AUC, T_{max}	Can be safely coadministered
Telaprevir	Theoretical	CYP3A4 inhibition	↑ Cyclosporine [ ]	Monitor cyclosporine blood levels and dose modify accordingly
Argatroban	Case report	CYP3A4 induction	↓ Cyclosporine [ ]	Monitor cyclosporine blood levels and dosemodify accordingly
Azole antifungals				
Fluconazole Itraconazole Posaconazole Voriconazole	Case reports; PK studies	CYP3A4 inhibition	↑ Cyclosporine C_{min} → ↑ toxicity See other azole interaction Appendices	Monitor levels. ↓ Cyclosporine dose Monitor levels. ↓ Cyclosporine dose Monitor levels. ↓ Cyclosporine dose
Calcium channel blockers[a] (diltiazem, verapamil)	PK studies; case reports	CYP3A4 inhibition	↑ Cyclosporine C_{min} → ↑ toxicity ↓ Cyclosporine CL 50–70%	Monitor levels. ↓ Cyclosporine dose
Carbamazepine	Case report	CYP3A4 induction	↓ Cyclosporine [ ] → GvHD	Monitor cyclosporine levels. ↑ Cyclosporine dose Change to nonenzyme inducing antiepileptic
Chlorpamphenicol	Case report	Unknown	↑ Cyclosporine C_{min} → ↑ toxicity	Monitor cyclosporine levels. ↓ Cyclosporine dose
Colchicine	PK study	Unknown	↑ Colchicine C_{max} 224% ↑ Colchicine $AUC_{0-\infty}$ 215% ↓ Colchicine CL 72%	Reduce the colchicine dose by ≥50% when coadministering with cyclosporine
Efavirenz	Case report	CYP3A4 induction	↓ Cyclosporine C_{min} by 30%	Increase cyclosporine dose; monitor levels
Etoposide	PK study	↓ Clearance via P-glycoprotein mechanism	↑ Etoposide AUC 59% ↓ Etoposide CL 35% ↑ Etoposide $t\frac{1}{2}$ → > toxicity	Cyclosporine has been used to overcome P-glycoprotein resistance
Everolimus	PK study; case reports	P-gp transport inhibition by cyclosporine	↑ Everolimus [ ]	Monitor for signs of everolimus toxicity
Fluoroquinolones Norfloxacin[b]	Case report	CYP3A4 inhibition	↑ Cyclosporine C_{min} → ↑ toxicity	Monitor cyclosporine levels. ↓ Cyclosporine dose (~43%) ** *conflicting data* **
Grapefruit juice	PK study	CYP3A4 inhibition	↑ Cyclosporine AUC 186% ↑ Cyclosporine C_{max} 150% ↓ Cyclosporine CL 43%	Monitor cyclosporine levels

Table 70.7 *(cont.)*

Drug	Data type	Proposed mechanism of interaction by drug	Clinical effect (potential or actual)	Recommended action
HMG-CoA reductase inhibitor				
Simvastatin	Case report	CYP3A4 inhibition	↑ Cyclosporine [ ]	Monitor cyclosporine levels; monitor for rhabdomyolysis
Imatinib mesylate	Hypothesis	CYP3A4 inhibition	Unknown, anticipate ↑ [ ] Cyclosporine	Monitor cyclosporine levels
Macrolide antibiotics				
Clarithromycin Erythromycin	Case reports Case reports	CYP3A4 inhibition CYP3A4 inhibition	↑ Cyclosporine C_{min} 26–33% ↑ Cyclosporine C_{min} 4.7-fold → toxicity	Monitor cyclosporine levels. ↓ Cyclosporine dose Monitor Cyclosporine levels. ↓ Cyclosporine dose by 50%
Mycophenolate mofetil (MMF)	PK studies	Attenuates enterohepatic recirculation of MPAG/MPA	↓ MPA AUC ↑ MMF C_{min} 2-fold when cyclosporine discontinued	Monitor patient for side effects of MMF
Phenytoin	PK studies; case reports	CYP3A4 induction	↓ Cyclosporine C_{min} ↓ Cyclosporine AUC 50% → ↑ toxicity	Monitor cyclosporine levels. ↑ Cyclosporine dose
Protease inhibitors				
Darunavir, fosamprenavir, indinavir, lopinavir, nelfinavir, saquinavir, tipranivir	Theoretical	CYP34 inhibition	↑ Cyclosporine [ ]	Monitor levels. ↓ Cyclosporine dose
Raltegravir	Case report	Effect on UGT1A1	↔ Cyclosporine [ ]	Can be safely coadministered without interaction
Rifampin	Healthy volunteers	CYP3A4 induction	↓ Cyclosporine AUC_{IV} 28% ↓ Cyclosporine AUC_{PO} 73% ↓ Cyclosporine F 63%	Avoid if possible ↑ Cyclosporine doses according to levels
Sirolimus oral liquid	Healthy volunteers	CYP3A4 inhibition of sirolimus; inhibition P-glycoprotein transport	↑ Sirolimus C_{max} 116%[c] ↑ Sirolimus AUC 230%[c] ↑ Sirolimus C_{max} 37%[d] ↑ Sirolimus AUC 80%[d]	Administer sirolimus 4 hours after administration of cyclosporine. Monitor tacrolimus levels if necessary
Sirolimus tablets	Healthy volunteers		↑ Sirolimus C_{max} 512%[c] ↑ Sirolimus AUC 148%[c] ↑ Sirolimus C_{max} 33%[d] ↑ Sirolimus AUC 33%[d]	Administer sirolimus 4 hours after administration of cyclosporine Monitor tacrolimus levels if necessary
Sildenafil	PK study	CYP3A4 inhibition	↑ Sildenafil C_{max} 44% ↑ Sildenafil AUC 90% ↑ t½ (elimination)	Start sildenafil at 25 mg to avoid profound hypotension May need to adjust antihypertensives if coprescribed
St John's wort	Case reports	Hypericin: P-gp Hyperforin : CYP3A4 and CYP2B6 intestinal and hepatic induction	↓ Cyclosporine C_{min} → GvHD	Avoid

[ ] = concentration; ↑ = increased; → = leads to; ↓ = decreased; AUC = area under the curve; C_{min} = trough concentration; CL = clearance; F = bioavailability; GvHD = graft-*versus*-host disease; PK = pharmacokinetic; CYP3A4 = cytochrome P450 3A4 isoenzyme. MPA = mycophenolic acid.

[a] Nifedipine does not increase cyclosporine levels and can be used safely.

[b] Ciprofloxacin[52] and levofloxacin[53] have been studied and no clinically significant interaction exists.

[c] Pharmacokinetic changes to sirolimus when administered simultaneously with cyclosporine dose.

[d] Pharmacokinetic changes to sirolimus when administered 4 hours after cyclosporine dose.

Table 70.8 Clinically relevant pharmacokinetic drug interactions with sirolimus

Drug	Data type	Proposed mechanism of interaction by drug	Effect (potential or actual)	Recommended action
Amiodarone	Case report	CYP3A4 inhibition of sirolimus; inhibition P-glycoprotein transport	↑ Sirolimus [ ] → ↑ toxicity	Monitor sirolimus levels. ↓ Sirolimus dose
Azole antifungals				
Fluconazole	Theoretical	CYP3A4 inhibition	↑ Sirolimus [ ]	Monitor levels. ↓ Sirolimus dose
Itraconazole	Case reports	CYP3A4 inhibition	↑ Sirolimus [ ] → ↑ toxicity	Monitor levels. ↓ Sirolimus dose
Ketoconazole	PK study	CYP3A4 inhibition	↑ Sirolimus C_{max} 4.3-fold	Monitor levels. ↓ Sirolimus dose
Posaconazole	Case reports	CYP3A4 inhibition	↑ Sirolimus AUC 10.9-fold	Monitor levels. ↓ Sirolimus dose
Voriconazole	PK study	CYP3A4 inhibition	↑ Sirolimus C_{max} 572% ↑ Sirolimus AUC 788% ↑ Sirolimus [ ] → ↑ toxicity	Monitor levels. ↓ Sirolimus dose
Bosentan	Theoretical	Impaired absorption and elimination via gut CYP3A4	↓ Sirolimus [ ]	Monitor sirolimus levels
Calcineurin inhibitors				
Cyclosporine Oral liquid		CYP3A4 inhibition of sirolimus; inhibition P-glycoprotein transport	↑ Sirolimus [ ] → ↑ toxicity	Administer sirolimus 4 hours after administration of cyclosporine Monitor sirolimus concentrations If cyclosporine is discontinued do not forget to increase sirolimus doses
Tacrolimus Tablets	Solid organ transplant patients		↔ Sirolimus or tacrolimus concentrations	Monitor tacrolimus levels if necessary.
Calcium channel blockers[a]				
Diltiazem	PK studies Case reports	CYP3A4 inhibition	↑ Sirolimus C_{max} 1.4-fold ↑ Sirolimus T_{max} 1.3-fold ↑ Sirolimus AUC 1.6-fold ↔ Sirolimus on diltiazem PK	Monitor sirolimus levels and adjust dose accordingly
Nicardipine	Not reported	CYP3A4 inhibition	↑ Sirolimus [ ]	Monitor sirolimus levels and adjust dose accordingly
Verapamil	PK study	CYP3A4 inhibition P-glycoprotein inhibition	↑ Sirolimus C_{max} 2.3-fold ↑ Sirolimus AUC 2.2-fold ↔ Sirolimus T_{max} ↑ Verapamil C_{max} 1.5-fold ↑ Verapamil AUC 1.5-fold	Monitor sirolimus levels and adjust dose accordingly
Carbamazepine	Theoretical	CYP3A4 induction	↓ Sirolimus [ ]	Monitor sirolimus levels and adjust dose accordingly
Fosphenytoin	See phenytoin			
Grapefruit juice	Theoretical	CYP3A4 inhibition	↑ Sirolimus [ ]	Avoid concomitant use
Imatinib	Theoretical	CYP3A4 inhibition	↑ Sirolimus [ ]	Monitor sirolimus levels, and adjust accordingly
Macrolide antibiotics				
Clarithromycin	Case report	CYP3A4 inhibition of sirolimus; inhibition P-glycoprotein transport	↑ Sirolimus [ ] 9-fold → ↑ toxicity	Monitor sirolimus levels. ↓ Sirolimus dose Coadministration not recommended

Table 70.8 (cont.)

Drug	Data type	Proposed mechanism of interaction by drug	Effect (potential or actual)	Recommended action
Erythromycin	PK study	CYP3A4 inhibition of sirolimus Inhibition P-gp transport	↑ Sirolimus C_{max} 4.4-fold ↑ Sirolimus AUC 4.2-fold ↑ Erythromycin C_{max} 1.6-fold ↑ Erythromycin AUC 1.7-fold	Monitor sirolimus levels. ↓ sirolimus doses based on levels
Nevirapine	Theoretical	CYP3A4 induction	↓ Sirolimus [ ]	Monitor sirolimus levels, and adjust accordingly
Nilotinib	Theoretical	CYP3A4 inhibition	↑ Sirolimus [ ]	Monitor sirolimus levels, and adjust accordingly
Phenytoin	Case reports	CYP3A4 induction	↓ Sirolimus [ ] → ↓ efficacy ↓ Sirolimus AUC	Monitor sirolimus levels. ↑ Sirolimus dose
Rifabutin	Theoretical	CYP3A4 induction P-glycoprotein induction	↓ Sirolimus AUC ↓ Sirolimus C_{max}	Avoid if possible – use an alternative ↑ Sirolimus doses according to levels
Rifampin	PK study	CYP3A4 induction P-glycoprotein induction	↑ Sirolimus CL 5.5-fold ↓ Sirolimus AUC 82% ↓ Sirolimus C_{max} 71%	Avoid if possible. Use an alternative ↑ Sirolimus doses according to levels
St John's wort (*Hypericum perforatum*)	Case report	CYP3A4 induction	↓ Sirolimus [ ] → GvHD	Avoid
Telaprevir	Theoretical	CYP3A4 inhibition P-gp pump inhibition	↑ Sirolimus [ ]	Monitor sirolimus levels; monitor renal function
Troleandomycin	Theoretical	Inhibition of gut CYP3A4	↑ Sirolimus [ ]	Monitor sirolimus levels

Sirolimus is a substrate for cytochrome P450 3A4 and P-glycoprotein. Coadministration of drugs that are inducers of either of these pathways will result in a reduction in blood levels of sirolimus and coadministration of drugs that are inhibitors of either of these pathways will result in an increase in the blood levels of sirolimus.

[ ] = concentration; ↑ = increased; → = leads to; ↓ = decreased; AUC = area under the curve; C_{min} = trough concentration; C_{max} = maximum serum concentration; CL = clearance; F = bioavailability; GvHD = graft-*versus*-host disease; LD = loading dose; P-gp = P-glycoprotein; PK = pharmacokinetic; CYP3A4 = cytochrome P450 3A4 isoenzyme.

associated with a trend to fewer invasive fungal infections including *Aspergillus* infections yet no difference in RFS and OS[57].

For low-risk HCT patients, namely those undergoing autologous HCT or allogeneic HCT with an anticipated duration of neutropenia of 14 days or less, prophylaxis strategies should be directed towards *Candida* species. Consensus guidelines recommend administration of fluconazole (doses ≥200 mg/day) starting with conditioning or just following completion of conditioning (if azoles other than fluconazole are being used, there is a concern for drug interactions between voriconazole/posaconazole/ itraconazole and chemotherapy, and as such they should only be started once the chemotherapy has been eliminated, which is generally 5 half-lives of the cytotoxic)[64]. What is not clear is the optimal discontinuation time for fluconazole. Two large randomized trials have been conducted comparing fluconazole to placebo, one where fluconazole was discontinued once the ANC was >1000/microliter[62] and the other from the Fred Hutchinson Cancer Center where fluconazole prophylaxis was continued until day +75

post-transplant[59,60]. In the latter, prolonged administration of fluconazole to day +75 was associated with significantly better survival compared to placebo, a lower rate of invasive candidiasis, and lower *Candida*-related mortality among placebo recipients[59]. In addition fluconazole recipients appeared to have lower acute GvHD rates. Based on this study some centers may choose to administer prophylaxis until day +100, although the mechanism by which fluconazole prophylaxis improved overall survival and lowered GvHD rates is unknown. With this in mind, many centers choose to stop azole prophylaxis in patients without GvHD/steroid use upon neutrophil count recovery. Factors likely to contribute to earlier discontinuation include the potential for drug interactions between azoles and immunosuppressive medications, the patient pill burden, adverse effects, and economic considerations.

For high-risk patients undergoing allogeneic HCT with an anticipated duration of neutropenia of >14 days, GvHD necessitating steroids, or extensive chronic GvHD mold-active prophylaxis is required. Several studies have been conducted with mold-active azoles and echinocandins in high-risk allo-geneic HCT patients[55,56,57,60,61,63]. Itraconazole prophylaxis has been shown to be effective but bioavailability and tolerance concerns are limitations. Amphotericin preparations are also active and several studies have shown efficacy, but toxicity and the need for parenteral administration have made this suboptimal to administer over the prolonged risk period. Several trials have tested lipid amphotericin B as adjunctive treatment with promising results and one randomized prophylaxis trial found that repeated inhalations of liposomal amphotericin B resulted in a protective effect with a reduction in invasive aspergillosis in patients treated for acute myelogenous leukemia. This has not yet been evaluated in HCT patients.

In recent years invasive aspergillosis prophylaxis studies have focused on the mold-active azoles, posaconazole and voriconazole. Posaconazole prophylaxis was found to be associated with a trend to fewer invasive fungal infections (IFI) of all types and fewer cases of invasive aspergillosis (IAs) in HCT patients with GvHD receiving corticosteroids. However, it is important to note that the benefit was confined to the subgroup of patients with positive galactomannan testing (GM) at the start of the study drug. Two large randomized trials examined voriconazole prophylaxis in HCT patients. In one trial voriconazole was compared to fluconazole[57]. Both voriconazole and fluconazole were well tolerated and had similar rates of survival free of IFI at 6 months. Risk factors for IFIs were GvHD, older age, and an underlying disease of AML. In the subgroup of patients transplanted for AML, there were fewer IFIs and better fungal-free survival with voriconazole than with fluconazole prophylaxis. In another trial, voriconazole was compared with itraconazole[56]. There were similar rates of IFIs and survival, but voriconazole was better tolerated than itraconazole.

Prophylaxis with mold-active agents is typically initiated with conditioning (provided no interaction) or the day of HCT. The optimal duration of antimold prophylaxis is not known. The overarching principle is that it should cover the interval of risk. Most mold infections historically occurred during the first 100 days after transplant. Thus, the largest clinical trials of *Aspergillus* prophylaxis used 100 days as the duration of study drug[57]. However, patients with ongoing active GvHD after 100 days or who otherwise have persistent severe T-cell immunodeficiency (the major host defense responsible for protection) are at continuing risk and several observational studies suggest an increase in late mold infections beyond 100 days. Such patients should be considered for continued antimold prophylaxis until immune recovery. Peripheral blood lymphocyte or CD4+ cell counts have been used as markers of cell-mediated immune competence in other situations, but there is a dearth of studies documenting how useful they are after HCT. Functional assays of T-cell function are needed to provide better indicators of the interval at risk.

The decision to continue mold-active prophylaxis is complex, as the treatments used are associated with well-known side effects that may impact quality of life, drug interactions with immunosuppressants, and the acquisition cost, which is a burden that impacts patients directly with large copays. Furthermore we now practice in the era of novel diagnostics such as galactomannan and PCR assays, which can be used to prompt evaluation with CT scans, bronchoscopic evaluation when indicated, and early initiation of presumptive antifungal therapy. This strategy of screening with early therapy when IA is suspected is sometimes often referred to as "preemptive" therapy. Several trials have evaluated this approach with promising results and this has been advocated by some experts as a viable alternative to universal prophylaxis for mold IFIs. Therefore the opposing opinion is that it might be feasible to discontinue the mold-active agent upon hematopoietic reconstitution, and monitor the patient regularly with routine galactomannan assays through day +100 (or longer when GvHD is present or long-term corticosteroids are being used), only initiating preemptive treatment in patients who have a positive galactomannan assay result.

Practice Points

1. There is considerably varied literature on the need to modify the dose of melphalan in HCT candidates. A review of the topic and current guidelines from the International Myeloma Working Group support the role of lower dose melphalan (100–140 mg/m^2) in patients with renal impairment and those who are dialysis dependent without compromising efficacy.

2. Seizure prophylaxis in patients conditioned with busulfan includes phenytoin, lorazepam, clonazepam, or levetiracetam. Due to a lack of comparative studies, no one agent can be deemed superior over the other, and as all have demonstrated activity in small studies, the choice will be center dependent.

3. There is insufficient literature to support definitive dosing recommendations in HCT candidates. With the paucity of controlled data, the guidelines recently published should be followed. Patients undergoing HCT are already receiving doses of chemotherapy that are close to the lethal toxicity and as such these patients should be managed differently than dosing of standard chemotherapy in obese individuals.

4. The optimal levels of sirolimus and tacrolimus are 3–12 ng/mL and 5–10 ng/mL, respectfully. This should be the current standard as supported by data from the recent large BMT CTN phase 3 trial.

5. There is insufficient evidence to support routine monitoring of MMF levels in adult HCT patients at this time.

6. There is no literature comparing magnesium replacement strategies in the HCT population and each institution must adopt their own monitoring, prevention, and treatment algorithms based on its severity.

7. Drug interactions in the HCT population are common owing to the number of necessary medications to make the

procedure a success. All members of the clinical team should be aware of these interactions, and dose modify accordingly.

8. The value of prophylaxis in HCT is unequivocal, what is not clear is the optimal duration of the prophylaxis strategy. The literature support the continuation of fluconazole in low-risk patients through day +75 post-HCT, and the use of voriconazole through day 100 where antimold activity is required. However in the "real world" treatment is often abbreviated with both agents being discontinued upon hematopoietic reconstitution in the absence of active GvHD. Provided a preemptive monitoring strategy is in place, the latter approach appears to be feasible for molds.

References

1. Badros A, Barlogie B, Siegel E, *et al.* Results of autologous stem cell transplant in multiple myeloma patients with renal failure. *Br J Haematol.* 2001;114(4):822–9.

2. Raab MS, Breitkreutz I, Hundemer M, *et al.* The outcome of autologous stem cell transplantation in patients with plasma cell disorders and dialysis-dependent renal failure. *Haematologica.* 2006;91(11):1555–8.

3. Knudsen LM, Nielsen B, Gimsing P, Geisler C. Autologous stem cell transplantation in multiple myeloma: outcome in patients with renal failure. *Eur J Haematol.* 2005;75:27–33.

4. Dimopoulos MA, Terpos E, Chanan-Khan A, *et al.* Renal impairment in patients with multiple myeloma: a consensus statement on behalf of the International Myeloma Working Group. *J Clin Oncol.* 2010;28(33):4976–84.

5. Parikh GC, Amjad AI, Saliba RM, *et al.* Autologous hematopoietic stem cell transplantation may reverse renal failure in patients with multiple myeloma. *Biol Blood Marrow Transplant.* 2009;15(7):812–6.

6. Abidi MH, Agarwal R, Ayash L, *et al.* Melphalan 180 mg/m^2 can be safely administered as conditioning regimen before an autologous stem cell transplantation (ASCT) in multiple myeloma patients with creatinine clearance 60 mL/min/1.73 m^2 or lower with use of palifermin for cytoprotection: results of a phase I trial. *Biol Blood Marrow Transplant.* 2012;18(9):1455–61.

7. Bodge MN, Reddy S, Thompson MS, Savani BN. Preparative regimen dosing for hematopoietic stem cell transplantation in patients with chronic kidney disease: analysis of the literature and recommendations. *Biol Blood Marrow Transplant.* 2014;20(7):908–19.

8. Tricot G, Alberts DS, Johnson C, *et al.* Safety of autotransplants with high-dose melphalan in renal failure: a pharmacokinetic and toxicity study. *Clin Cancer Res.* 1996;2(6):947–52.

9. Tosi P, Zamagni E, Ronconi S, *et al.* Safety of autologous hematopoietic stem cell transplantation in patients with multiple myeloma and chronic renal failure. *Leukemia.* 2000;14:1310–13.

10. Hamaki T, Katori H, Kami M, *et al.* Successful allogeneic blood stem cell transplantation for aplastic anemia in a patient with renal insufficiency requiring dialysis. *Bone Marrow Transplant.* 2002;30:195–8.

11. Lee CK, Zangari M, Barlogie B, *et al.* Dialysis-dependent renal failure in patients with myeloma can be reversed by high-dose myeloablative therapy and autotransplant. *Bone Marrow Transplant.* 2004;33(8):823–8.

12. Termuhlen AM, Grovas A, Klopfenstein K, *et al.* Autologous hematopoietic stem cell transplant with melphalan and thiotepa is safe and feasible in pediatric patients with low normalized glomerular filtration rate. *Pediatr Transplant.* 2006;10:830–4.

13. de Souza JA, Saliba RM, Patah P, *et al.* Moderate renal function impairment does not affect outcomes of reduced-intensity conditioning with fludarabine and melphalan for allogeneic hematopoietic stem cell transplantation. *Biol Blood Marrow Transplant.* 2009;15:1094–9.

14. Tendas A, Cupelli L, Dentamaro T, *et al.* Feasibility of a dose-adjusted fludarabine-melphalan conditioning prior autologous stem cell transplantation in a dialysis-dependent patient with mantle cell lymphoma. *Ann Hematol.* 2009;88:285–6.

15. Choi HS, Kim SY, Lee JH, *et al.* Successful allogeneic stem-cell transplantation in a patient with myelodysplastic syndrome with hemodialysis-dependent end-stage renal disease. *Transplantation.* 2011;92: e28–e29.

16. van Besien K, Schouten V, Parsad S, *et al.* Allogeneic stem cell transplant in renal failure: engraftment and prolonged survival, but high incidence of neurologic toxicity. *Leuk Lymphoma.* 2012;53:158–9.

17. Kergueris MF, *et al.* Pharmacokinetics of high-dose melphalan in adults: influence of renal function. *Anticancer Res.* 1994;14:2379–82.

18. Santos GW, Tutschka PJ, Brookmeyer R, *et al.* Marrow transplantation for acute nonlymphocytic leukemia after treatment with busulfan and cyclophosphamide. *N Engl J Med.* 1983;309(22):1347–53.

19. Tutschka PJ, Copelan EA, Klein JP. Bone marrow transplantation for leukemia following a new busulfan and cyclophosphamide regimen. *Blood.* 1987;70(5):1382–8.

20. Vassal G, Deroussent A, Hartmann O, *et al.* Dose-dependent neurotoxicity of high-dose busulfan in children: a clinical and pharmacological study. *Cancer Res.* 1990;50(19):6203–7.

21. Hassan M, Oberg G, Björkholm M, Wallin I, Lindgren M. Influence of prophylactic anticonvulsant therapy on high-dose busulphan kinetics. *Cancer Chemother Pharmacol.* 1993;33(3):181–6.

22. Sureda A, Pérez de Oteyza J, García Laraña J, Odriozola J. High-dose busulfan and seizures. *Ann Intern Med.* 1989;111(6):543–4.

23. Hamidieh AA, Hamedani R, Hadjibabaie M, *et al.* Oral lorazepam prevents seizure during high-dose busulfan in children undergoing hematopoietic stem cell transplantation: a prospective study. *Pediatr Hematol Oncol.* 2010;27(7):529–33.

24. Chan KW, Mullen CA, Worth LL, *et al.* Lorazepam for seizure prophylaxis during high-dose busulfan administration. *Bone Marrow Transplant.* 2002;29(12):963–5.

25. Eberly AL, Anderson GD, Bubalo JS, McCune JS. Optimal prevention of seizures induced by high-dose busulfan. *Pharmacotherapy.* 2008;28(12):1502–10.

26. Grigg AP, Shepherd JD, Phillips GL. Busulphan and phenytoin. *Ann Intern Med.* 1989;111(12):1049–50.

27. Soni S, Skeens M, Termuhlen AM, *et al.* Levetiracetam for busulfan-induced seizure prophylaxis in children undergoing hematopoietic stem cell transplantation. *Pediatr Blood Cancer.* 2012;59(4):762–4.

28. Bubalo JS, Kovascovics TJ, Meyers G, *et al.* Clonazepam and levetiracetam for prevention of busulfan-induced seizures: a singer-center experience [abstract]. *Biol Blood Marrow Transplant* 2008;14(2 suppl 2):Abstract 467.

29. Caselli D, Rosati A, Faraci M, *et al.* Bone Marrow Transplantation Working Group of the Associazione Italiana Ematologia Oncologia Pediatrica. Risk of seizures in children receiving busulphan-containing regimens for stem cell transplantation. *Biol Blood Marrow Transplant.* 2014;20(2):282–5.

30. Diaz-Carrasco MS, Olmos R, Blanquer M, *et al.* Clonazepam for seizure prophylaxis in adult patients treated with high dose busulfan. *Int J Clin Pharm.* 2013;35(3):339–43.

31. Caselli D, Ziino O, Bartoli A, *et al.* Continuous intravenous infusion of lorazepam as seizure prophylaxis in children treated with high-dose busulfan. *Bone Marrow Transplant.* 2008;42(2):135–6.

32. Yazal Erdem A, Azık F, Tavil B, *et al.* Busulfan triggers epileptic seizures under levetiracetam and valproic acid therapy. *Pediatr Transplant.* 2014;18(4):412–3.

33. Ogden CL, Carroll MD, Kit BK, Flegal KM. Prevalence of childhood and adult obesity in the United States, 2011–2012. *JAMA.* 2014;311(8):806–14.

34. Griggs JJ, Mangu PB, Anderson H, *et al.* Appropriate chemotherapy dosing for obese adult patients with cancer: American Society of Clinical Oncology Clinical Practice Guideline. *J Clin Oncol.* 2012;30:1553–61.

35. Bubalo J, Carpenter PA, Majhail N, *et al.* Conditioning chemotherapy dose adjustment in obese patients: A review and position statement by the American Society for Blood and Marrow Transplantation Practice Guideline Committee. *Biol Blood Marrow Transplant.* 2014;20: 600–16.

36. Weiss BM, Vogl DT, Berger NA, Stadtmauer EA, Lazarus HM. Trimming the fat: obesity and hematopoietic cell transplantation. *Bone Marrow Transplant.* 2013;48: 1152–60.

37. Cutler C, Kim HT, Hochberg E, *et al.* Sirolimus and tacrolimus without methotrexate as graft-*versus*-host disease prophylaxis after matched related donor peripheral blood stem cell transplantation. *Biol Blood Marrow Transplant.* 2004;10(5):328–36.

38. Cutler C, Li S, Ho VT, *et al.* Extended follow-up of methotrexate-free immunosuppression using sirolimus and tacrolimus in related and unrelated donor peripheral blood stem cell transplantation. *Blood.* 2007;109(7):3108–14.

39. Cutler C, Logan B, Nakamura R, *et al.* Tacrolimus/sirolimus vs tacrolimus/ methotrexate as GVHD prophylaxis after matched, related donor allogeneic HCT. *Blood.* 2014;124(8):1372–7.

40. Rodriguez R, Nakamura R, Palmer JM, *et al.* A phase II pilot study of tacrolimus/sirolimus GVHD prophylaxis for sibling donor hematopoietic stem cell transplantation using 3 conditioning regimens. *Blood.* 2010;115(5):1098–105.

41. Pidala J, Kim J, Jim H, *et al.* A randomized phase II study to evaluate tacrolimus in combination with sirolimus or methotrexate after allogeneic hematopoietic cell transplantation. *Haematologica.* 2012:97(12):1882–9.

42. Pidala J, Tomblyn M, Nishihori T, *et al.* Sirolimus demonstrates activity in the primary therapy of acute graft-*versus*-host disease without systemic glucocorticoids. *Haematologica.* 2011;96(9):1351–6.

43. Li H, Mager DE, Sandmaier BM, *et al.* Population pharmacokinetics and dose optimization of mycophenolic acid in HCT recipients receiving oral mycophenolate mofetil. *J Clin Pharmacol.* 2013;53(4):393–402.

44. Kim H, Long-Boyle J, Rydholm N, *et al.* Population pharmacokinetics of unbound mycophenolic acid in pediatric and young adult patients undergoing allogeneic hematopoietic cell transplantation. *J Clin Pharmacol.* 2012;52(11):1665–75.

45. McDermott CL, Sandmaier BM, Storer B, *et al.* Nonrelapse mortality and mycophenolic acid exposure in nonmyeloablative hematopoietic cell transplantation. *Biol Blood Marrow Transplant.* 2013;19(8):1159–66.

46. Giaccone L, McCune JS, Maris MB, *et al.* Pharmacodynamics of mycophenolate mofetil after nonmyeloablative conditioning and unrelated donor hematopoietic cell transplantation. *Blood.* 2005;106:4381–8.

47. Royer B, Larosa F, Legrand F, *et al.* Pharmacokinetics of mycophenolic acid administered 3 times daily after hematopoietic stem cell transplantation with reduced-intensity regimen. *Biol Blood Marrow Transplant.* 2009;15(9):1134–9.

48. Harnicar S, Ponce DM, Hilden P, *et al.* Intensified mycophenolate mofetil dosing and higher mycophenolic acid trough levels reduce severe acute graft-*versus*-host disease after double-unit cord blood transplantation. *Biol Blood Marrow Transplant.* 2015;21(5):920–5.

49. Aisa Y, Mori T, Nakazato T, *et al.* Effects of immunosuppressive agents on magnesium metabolism early after allogeneic hematopoietic stem cell transplantation. *Transplantation.* 2005;80(8):1046–50.

50. Woo M, Przepiorka D, Ippoliti C, *et al.* Toxicities of tacrolimus and cyclosporin A after allogeneic blood stem cell transplantation. *Bone Marrow Transplant.* 1997;20(12):1095–8.

51. Saif MW. Management of hypomagnesemia in cancer patients receiving chemotherapy. *J Support Oncol.* 2008;6(5):243–8.

52. Atsmon J, Dolev E. Drug-induced hypomagnesaemia : scope and management. *Drug Saf.* 2005;28(9):763–88.

53. Gholaminezhad S, Hadjibabaie M, Gholami K, *et al.* Pattern and associated factors of potential drug-drug interactions in both pre- and early post-

hematopoietic stem cell transplantation stages at a referral center in the Middle East. *Ann Hematol.* 2014;93(11):1913–22.

54. Cornely OA, Maertens J, Winston DJ, *et al.* Posaconazole *versus* fluconazole or itraconazole prophylaxis in patients with neutropenia. *N Engl J Med.* 2007;356:348–59.

55. Ullmann AJ, Lipton JH, Vesole DH, *et al.* Posaconazole or fluconazole for prophylaxis in severe graft-*versus*-host disease. *N Engl J Med.* 2007;356:335–47.

56. Marks DI, Pagliuca A, Kibbler CC, *et al.* Voriconazole *versus* itraconazole for antifungal prophylaxis following allogeneic hematopoietic stem-cell transplantation. *Br J Haematol.* 2011;155:318–27.

57. Wingard JR, Carter SL, Walsh TJ, *et al.* Randomized, double-blind trial of fluconazole *versus* voriconazole for prevention of invasive fungal infection after allogeneic hematopoietic cell transplantation. *Blood.* 2010;116(24):5111–18.

58. Slavin MA, Osborne B, Adams R, *et al.* Efficacy and safety of fluconazole prophylaxis for fungal infections after marrow transplantation – a prospective, randomized, double-blind study. *J Infect Dis.* 1995;171:1545–52.

59. Marr KA, Seidel K, Slavin MA, *et al.* Prolonged fluconazole prophylaxis is associated with persistent protection against candidiasis-related death in allogeneic marrow transplant recipients: long-term follow-up of a randomized, placebo-controlled trial. *Blood.* 2006;96:2055–61.

60. Marr KA, Crippa F, Leisenring W, *et al.* Itraconazole *versus* fluconazole for prevention of fungal infections in patients receiving allogeneic stem cell transplants. *Blood.* 2004;103:1527–33.

61. Winston DJ, Maziarz RT, Chandrasekar PH, *et al.* Intravenous and oral itraconazole *versus* intravenous and oral fluconazole for long-term antifungal prophylaxis in allogeneic hematopoietic stem-cell transplant recipients. A multicenter, randomized trial. *Ann Intern Med.* 2003;138(9):705–13.

62. Goodman JL, Winston DJ, Greenfield RA, *et al.* A controlled trial of fluconazole to prevent fungal infections in patients undergoing bone marrow transplantation. *N Engl J Med.* 1992;326(13):845–51.

63. van Burik JA, Ratanatharathorn V, Stepan DE, *et al.* Micafungin *versus* fluconazole for prophylaxis against invasive fungal infections during neutropenia in patients undergoing hematopoietic stem cell transplantation. *Clin Infect Dis.* 2004;39(10):1407–16.

64. Tomblyn M, Chiller T, Einsele H, *et al.* Guidelines for preventing infectious complications among hematopoietic cell transplantation recipients: A global perspective. *Biol Blood Marrow Transplant.* 2009;15:1143–238.

65. Shayani S, Palmer J, Stiller T, *et al.* Thrombotic microangiopathy associated with sirolimus levels following allogeneic hematopoietic cell transplantation with tacrolimus/sirolimus-based GVHD prophylaxis. *Biol Blood Marrow Transplant.* 2013;19(2):298–304.

Chapter

71

Quality of Life: Can We Really Make a Difference?

Nandita Khera and Navneet S. Majhail

Introduction

The World Health Organization (WHO) defines quality of life (QoL) as an "individual's perception of their position in life in the context of the culture and value systems in which they live and in relation to their goals, expectations, standards and concerns"[1]. Health-related QoL is a broad, multidimensional concept that includes physical, social, role, and psychologic function as impacted by a disease or treatment. Given the increase in patient survival achieved with current strategies for hematopoietic cell transplantation (HCT), QoL has emerged as a significant medical outcome measure and an important focus for researchers and healthcare providers. Multiple cross-sectional and longitudinal studies evaluating QoL in HCT recipients have contributed to our current understanding about the trajectory of QoL starting from HCT to as long as 20 years after HCT. These studies have demonstrated early impairment in QoL, followed by eventual recovery in greater than 60% of patients between 1 to 4 years after the HCT. This chapter provides an overview of the current literature on the trajectory of quality of life after HCT, with a specific focus on measurement and predictors of QoL. We will conclude by describing interventions to help improve QoL, exploring the lacunae in the state of our current knowledge and outlining research priorities in the area. While related issues such as employment/financial toxicity, sexuality, and impact on caregiver are important to QoL in HCT survivors, detailed discussion about these topics is beyond the scope of this chapter.

Impact of HCT on QoL

Multiple medical complications after HCT can negatively impact a patient's performance of daily activities, return to work, interpersonal and family relationships, and sense of personal well-being, thus making QoL an important clinical outcome. Studies show that full recovery after HCT is a 3- to 5-year process and that the trajectory of QoL is influenced by transplant type (autologous *versus* allogeneic), phase (early *versus* late), and complications (e.g., chronic graft-*versus*-host disease (G*v*HD))[2]. Impairments can begin prior to HCT due to the underlying diagnosis and treatments. A majority of patients report high global QoL despite many symptoms and

limitations in activity[2]. Most longitudinal studies suggest that overall QoL declines rapidly after HCT, reaches a nadir around 30 days after allogeneic HCT and 10–14 days after autologous HCT, then begins to improve with a fluctuating trajectory to return close to baseline between 3 months to 1 year after HCT. Lee *et al.* have reported that autologous patients start their recovery sooner than allogeneic HCT recipients with a detectable difference at 6 months post-HCT although the rates at 1 year were comparable for both groups [3]. While continued long-term impairments may be seen in all domains of QoL for allogeneic HCT survivors, they are mainly evident in physical functioning, role functioning, and overall QoL for the autologous HCT survivors[4]. A recent study showed similar QoL outcomes in patients transplanted more than 20 years ago for thalassemia as compared to the general population[5].

In addition to medical complications, HCT recipients are at risk for sexual dysfunction, occupational disability, economic burden, negative body image, and difficulties with social reintegration which have an adverse impact on QoL[6–9]. However, some positive sequelae including improved self-esteem, perception of a new meaning in life, redirected life priorities, increased compassion, improved social, marital and family relationships, and heightened spirituality have also been reported after HCT[10]. While studies in other areas have shown the potential of QoL to be a prognostic indicator for survival, it is not yet validated in the case of HCT.

Although QoL research in pediatric HCT recipients has lagged behind adults, considerable progress has been made in recent years[11]. Somewhat similar to the adults, QoL in childhood HCT survivors improves over a 4- to 12-month period post-HCT and no differences can be found between autologous and allogeneic survivors more than 3 years from HCT. In addition to more intensive treatment and pre-HCT cognitive, behavioral, and social functioning, family variables are important predictors for QoL in pediatric HCT patients [12]. A recent report from the Children's Oncology Group comparing QoL between 5-year survivors of childhood AML treated with chemotherapy with or without autologous or allogeneic HCT reported similar QoL scores among treatment groups and decreased QoL in those with more self-reported health conditions or cancer-related pain[13].

Table 71.1 Instruments used in QoL assessments in HCT

Generic	Cancer specific	HCT specific
- Medical Outcomes Study Short form-36 (SF-36)[10,31,49] - Medical Outcomes Study Short Form-12 (SF-12)[29,50] - Patient-Reported Outcomes Measurement Information System (PROMIS)[36] - Hospital and Anxiety Depression Scale (HADS)[53]	- Functional Assessment of Cancer Therapy – General (FACT-G)[26] - European Organization for the Research and Treatment of Cancer Quality of Life Questionnaire (EORTC-QLQ C30)[7] - Cancer Rehabilitation Evaluation System – Short Form (CARES-SF)[51] - Cancer Rehabilitation Evaluation System (CARES) [54]	- Functional Assessment of Cancer Therapy–Bone Marrow Transplant Module (FACT-BMT)[25,31] - City of Hope/Stanford Long- term BMT Survivor Index (COH-QoL)[17] - Chronic GvHD Symptom Scale[33,52]

Measurement of QoL in HCT

Instruments for Assessment

There is enormous heterogeneity in the measures used for assessment of QoL in HCT patients. While generic measures such as EORTC-QLQ 30 or SF-36 may be useful for comparing HCT patients with other groups, they are less sensitive to HCT-specific effects. HCT-specific measures are more helpful especially in clinical trials to capture disease and treatment-related distress. Thus, it is important to consider the objective or purpose for obtaining the information, when selecting among the various different measures. Table 71.1 summarizes the instruments that have been used in HCT literature. Various modalities have been used to administer these instruments including by computer, mail, or telephone interview.

Issues in QoL Assessment in HCT

Response Shift

Response shift refers to a change in the meaning of one's self-evaluation of QoL as a result of a change in the medical condition of the patient[14]. In HCT, this phenomenon may help patients cope and enable them to experience good QoL, especially good psychologic function, despite the medical complications of HCT[15]. Hence, patients' perception of their QoL may improve over time on long-term follow-up after transplantation.

Proxy Responder

When patients are unable to provide information about their QoL, family or friends who are termed as proxy responders may be used. In pediatric cases, proxy responders usually are parents of the young child.

Clinically Meaningful Change

Clinically meaningful change in the area of QoL is challenging to define since there is a multitude of QoL instruments available, each with different units of measurement[16]. Also, it may be different based on perspective (patient *versus* clinician). Factors to consider in defining clinically meaningful change include the severity of the baseline QoL, the precision of the measurement instrument, and the direction of change.

Anchor-based methods and distribution-based methods have been used to identify clinically meaningful change. Whereas anchor-based methods include cross-sectional approaches and longitudinal approaches, distribution-based methods include those based on statistical significance, sample variability, and measurement precision. Use of multiple methods is recommended because both approaches have advantages and limitations.

Attrition Due to Mortality and Loss to Follow-up

Missing data due to death or loss of follow-up is commonly seen in studies evaluating longitudinal QoL after HCT and can range from 20 to 65% at 1 year after HCT[2,17,18]. It is felt that the QoL in general, is poorer for people who do not have complete data due to death, relapse, or study drop out. Studies have used various methods to address this issue including statistical modeling to estimate and control for attrition, supplementing with pattern mixture models, or reporting dichotomous outcomes for different subgroups[3,17,19].

Predictors of QoL after HCT

Patient Characteristics

Older age, female sex, advanced disease, lower educational level, lower pre-HCT functioning level, and lower household income have been shown to be predictors of poorer QoL and higher distress after HCT (Table 71.2)[17,20–22]. Other factors affecting QoL after HCT include level of social support, coping styles, and personality[2,23,24].

Transplant Characteristics

Conditioning

The studies comparing QoL after myeloablative *versus* reduced intensity transplants have been mostly observational and have indicated comparable QoL between the two groups.[25,26]

Graft Type

There are few data available about QoL after alternative donor transplants. Liu *et al.* recently reported a higher proportion of patients in the umbilical cord blood transplant group (as

Table 71.2 Predictors of QoL in HCT recipients

Patient factors
- Age
- Gender
- Race and ethnicity
- Education level
- Household income
- Pre-HCT functional level
- Social support
- Coping styles and personality
- Marital status

Disease factors
- Diagnosis
- Disease status at transplant
- Pre-HCT treatment

Transplant factors
- Previous HCT
- Occurrence of post-transplant complications
- Chronic graft-*versus*-host disease

opposed to matched sibling donor transplants) who were alive for more than 1 year, did not suffer from chronic GvHD, and returned to work[27]. Results from QoL data analysis, which was done as a substudy of the Blood and Marrow Transplant Clinical Trials Network (BMT CTN) 0201 study comparing peripheral blood *versus* bone marrow as an unrelated donor graft source, is awaited.

Post-transplant Factors

The presence of late effects has been reported to be associated with lower physical functioning, overall perception of health status as poor, and a lower likelihood of returning to work/ school in both autologous and allogeneic HCT recipients [28,29]. Chronic GvHD is a late complication itself as well as predisposing to a host of other problems. It occurs in 30–70% of HCT patients with a median time of onset between 4 and 6 months after HCT, though 5–10% of cases can be diagnosed 1 year after HCT[30]. While it was known that it is a predictor of poor QoL, studies from the Chronic GvHD Consortium in the last few years have provided valuable information about the patient-reported outcomes in patients with this complication. In one of their earlier studies, the group showed that chronic GvHD severity as per National Institutes of Health (NIH) criteria was independently associated with QoL, adjusting for age[31]. Patients with moderate and severe chronic GvHD had physical functioning comparable to that of patients with systemic sclerosis, systemic lupus erythematosus, and multiple sclerosis, and greater impairment compared with common chronic conditions including diabetes, hypertension, and chronic lung disease[31]. It was also reported that overlap type of chronic GvHD was associated not only with poorer overall survival but also greater functional impairment, and higher symptom burden[32]. More recently, they have shown that despite higher physical and functional limitations,

older patients with moderate or severe chronic GvHD have preserved QoL and similar overall survival and nonrelapse mortality when compared to younger patients[33].

Interventions to Improve QoL

The first step in improving QoL is providing information about QoL to patients to help them with decision-making about HCT. A cross-sectional survey study to assess HCT physician attitudes about QoL identified the scope for increasing the proportion of the physicians who would use QoL results to modify practice if the results were more understandable[34]. The next step is screening for problems in QoL at different phases of the HCT. The increasing emphasis on incorporating "Patient-reported outcomes (PRO)" into clinical practice has led to development of simple tools such as NCCN distress thermometer to screen for distress in HCT patients [35]. Wood *et al.* have recently demonstrated the feasibility of frequent collection of electronic PROs in the early post-HCT period[36].

Most providers would acknowledge that interventions to improve QoL are an integral part of the post-HCT care. Indeed, the guidelines for screening and preventive care practices for survivors of HCT recommend periodic evaluations for psychosocial complications as well as assessment of caregiver psychologic adjustment after HCT[37]. However, it is increasingly becoming clearer that interventions to improve QoL are relevant throughout the HCT continuum (Table 71.3).

Several interventions can help improve QoL after HCT, similar to what has been reported in cancer literature, although only a few have actually been studied in HCT. These include pharmacotherapy to treat pain, anxiety, and depression, exercise programs, cognitive restructuring, mindfulness-based practices for developing positive emotions, more effective partner support, group acceptance in support groups, sharing experiences through verbal, artistic or written expression, and giving back. Most of these interventions can be categorized into three broad categories used so far to help enhance QoL in HCT recipients.

Exercise

A Cochrane review showed that exercise in cancer patients may have beneficial effects on overall QoL and certain specific domains including cancer-specific concerns, body image/self-esteem, emotional well-being, sexuality, sleep disturbance, social functioning, anxiety, fatigue, and pain[38]. In the arena of HCT, Wiskemann *et al.* reviewed multiple studies reporting the benefits of exercise interventions in attenuating a range of physical and psychosocial problems associated with HCT and improving the QoL[39]. Table 71.4 summarizes exercise trials in HCT. It is important to note that the positive effects of exercise may vary significantly as a function of the underlying disease; the type of HCT; the nature, intensity, and duration of the exercise program; and the fitness and lifestyle of the patient.

Table 71.3 Interventions to improve QoL through the continuum of HCT

Intervention	Pre-HCT	HCT	Post-HCT
Education			
Information about the risks and benefits of HCT especially in regards to QoL	✓		
Enhancing knowledge of post-HCT outcomes and follow-up care			✓
Screening			
Screen patients for psychosocial health needs	✓	✓	✓
Psychopharmacologic interventions			
Medications to treat anxiety, depression, and other mental health problems	✓	✓	✓
Health promotion interventions			
Exercise programs (supervised *versus* home based)	✓	✓	✓
Provider monitoring of health behaviors	✓	✓	✓
Logistical and financial assistance			
Financial planning/supplemental grants	✓	✓	✓
Connect patients to psychosocial health services (social work/ psychology/psychiatry)	✓	✓	✓
Patient navigation resources to help with coordination of care	✓	✓	✓
Behavioral interventions			
Counseling and psychotherapy (including teaching coping skills)	✓	✓	✓
Cognitive rehabilitation and behavioral strategies	✓	✓	✓
Stress management/relaxation techniques	✓	✓	✓
Support groups	✓	✓	✓
Management of late complications that impact QoL (e.g., sexual dysfunction, chronic GvHD, pain issues)			✓

Table 71.4 Summary of studies assessing the impact of exercise in HCT

Study	Study characteristics	Type of transplants	Intervention	Results
Wiskemann et al.[55]	Multicenter randomized controlled trial	Allogeneic HCT (n=105)	Partly self-administered exercise intervention	Improvement in fatigue, physical fitness/ functioning global distress in exercise group
Dimeo et al. [56]	Single center	Conventional chemotherapy (n=45) and autologous HCT (n=21)	Daily exercise on treadmill	Reduced treatment-related loss of physical performance
Jarden et al. [57]	Single-center randomized controlled trial	Allogeneic HCT (n=42)	Multimodal intervention(with exercise, relaxation training, and psycho-education)	No statistically significant effect on QoL, fatigue, psychologic well-being, or on physical activity levels, but longitudinal trends favored the intervention group
DeFor et al. [58]	Single-center randomized controlled trial	Allogeneic HCT (n=100)	Structured walking regimen (daily treadmill walking)	Smaller (not statistically significant) decline in KPS in the exercise group than in the control group; statistically significant only in the subset of older and less fit patients receiving nonmyeloablative conditioning. Higher scores for physical and emotional well-being in exercise group in this subset *also*

Table 71.4 (*cont.*)

Study	Study characteristics	Type of transplants	Intervention	Results
Wilson *et al.* [59]	Single center, pilot study	Autologous HCT (n=13) Allogeneic HCT (n=4)	Home-based aerobic exercise programs	Improved scores of aerobic fitness, fatigue severity, and physical well-being
Baumann *et al.* [60]	Single-center randomized controlled trial	Autologous HCT (n=18) Allogeneic HCT (n=46)	Exercise therapy (aerobic endurance training and an "ADL-training") twice a day	Significant differences in favor of the exercise group regarding strength, endurance, lung function, and quality of life
Knols *et al.* [61]	Two-center randomized controlled trial	Autologous HCT (n=80) Allogeneic HCT (n=51)	Supervised exercise program, incorporating both endurance and resistive strength exercises	Improved physical performance measures though no statistically significant change in QoL
Hayes *et al.* [54]	Single-center randomized controlled trial	Autologous HCT (n=12)	3-month, moderate-intensity, mixed-type exercise program	Statistically significant improvements in overall QoL and endorsed problems and average severity of problems in both the physical and psychosocial domains were observed for the exercise group but not the control group, following the 3-month recovery period
Jacobsen *et al.* [49]	Multicenter randomized trial through the BMT CTN	Autologous HCT (n=358) Allogeneic HCT (n=351)	Patients randomized to 4 interventions: self-directed exercise, self-administered stress management, both, or neither	At day 100, no difference in QoL, treatment distress, sleep quality, pain and nausea between exercise and no exercise groups

Psychosocial Interventions

Psychosocial interventions such as cognitive behavioral therapy (CBT) have been shown to reduce emotional distress and improve mood and QoL in cancer patients, although there are various methodologic issues in combining the studies[40]. In HCT, very few studies have assessed the impact of such interventions specifically on QoL. Two of these studies have shown the impact of hypnosis training or relaxation and imagery training in reducing pain[41,42]. DuHamel *et al.* showed the efficacy of telephone-administered CBT intervention in reducing illness-related post-traumatic stress disorder symptoms, general distress, and depressive symptoms in 89 HCT survivors[43]. Recently, a study of 110 breast cancer patients scheduled to receive an autologous HCT reported the effectiveness of a comprehensive coping strategy program with significant improvement in overall QoL, health and functioning, and socioeconomic and psychologic/spiritual well-being[44]. A pilot study evaluating the impact of Mindfulness-Based Resilience Training in solid organ and stem cell transplant recipients showed clinically significant improvements in stress, depression, anxiety, and sleep (Cynthia Stonnington, personal communication).

Educational Interventions

While no information is available on the impact of pre-HCT education on QoL of HCT patients, there are some data in cancer patients. A brief orientation program in newly diagnosed cancer patients showed lower state anxiety, lower overall distress, and fewer patients reporting depressive symptoms in the intervention group[45]. Most transplant centers provide standard educational materials on the post-HCT course to the patient as well as caregivers both before and at multiple time points after HCT. A recent qualitative study sought to describe the perspective of patients about education related to QoL after HCT. The focus group participants in the study noted the profound impact of post-HCT complications on QoL and their sense of recovery. They felt that the timing, content, and format of education regarding HCT should be flexible and more tailored to individual patients[46].

Educational efforts in the post-HCT phase are being studied currently. Empowering the patients by providing education about treatment exposures and follow-up care to help improve the overall health and well-being of survivors using individualized survivorship care plans is the main goal of an ongoing study for HCT recipients (Navneet Majhail, personal communication). Investigators are also studying the use of internet-based programs for enhancing survivorship outcomes including QoL after HCT by providing tailored educational opportunities to HCT survivors[47].

Combining various approaches may help better manage psychosocial issues and foster improved QoL[48]. The BMT CTN 0902 randomized study recently reported the impact of combining 15-minute exercise training with stress management using paced abdominal breathing, progressive muscle relaxation with guided imagery, and coping self-statements on physical and mental functioning of 711 HCT recipients at 100 days after HCT[49]. No differences were observed between the groups in physical and mental functioning scores or overall survival, hospitalization days until day +100 and in other patient-reported outcomes, including treatment-related distress, sleep quality, pain, and nausea. Various possible explanations for inability to detect benefit from the interventions were put forth by the study investigators including use of lower intensity training sessions, measuring the outcomes too early, and self-reported measures not being sensitive enough to detect the difference. The study also emphasized the importance of factors such as timing of intervention around HCT, targeting specific at-risk groups, and more intensive and personalized intervention that may result in better outcomes.

Controversies

Although a variety of cross-sectional and longitudinal studies have provided us with the depth and breadth of research on the trajectory of psychosocial recovery after HCT and predictors of QoL, there continue to be several areas of controversy and important gaps still exist in the literature. There is a need to better evaluate the impact of the advances in techniques of HCT in the last decade, e.g., the impact of reduced intensity/nonmyeloablative transplants, alternative donor sources, and newer GvHD prophylaxis regimens on the post-HCT QoL. It is also not clear as to what impact the comorbidities or more extensive pre-HCT treatments may have on the survivor's health and functional status and their risk for poor psychosocial outcomes including financial hardship after HCT. There needs to be a paradigm shift in QoL research with studies incorporating all domains (physiologic, psychosocial, and economic) while trying to design interventions to address post-HCT QoL. An ideal intervention would have the potential for widespread dissemination in the setting of fragmented post-HCT care, be relatively inexpensive, and be easy to administer without using too many resources. With the present literature, it is not clear which patient might benefit from which intervention. More research is needed to determine if certain demographic, disease, or HCT-related characteristics would predict whether a patient is likely to benefit more from one specific type of intervention than another. Many interventions presently being investigated are complex and require expertise and resources to implement. As research in this area matures, emphasis will need to be placed on taking interventions to the clinic so that they can be applied in the "real world scenario." Last, but not least, the costs and resource needs for implementing specific interventions will have to be considered as part of clinical trials. With the increasing focus on the needs of survivors, the time seems to be ripe for continuing efforts to not only have the HCT survivors live, but also to "live well."

References

1. The World Health Organization Quality of Life Assessment (WHOQOL): position paper from the World Health Organization. *Soc Sci Med.* 1995;41:1403–9.

2. Syrjala KL, Langer SL, Abrams JR, Storer B, Sanders JE, Flowers ME *et al.* Recovery and long-term function after hematopoietic cell transplantation for leukemia or lymphoma. *JAMA* 2004;291(19):2335–43.

3. Lee SJ, Fairclough D, Parsons SK, Soiffer RJ, Fisher DC, Schlossman RL *et al.* Recovery after stem-cell transplantation for hematologic diseases. *J Clin Oncol.* 2001;19(1):242–52.

4. Pidala J, Anasetti C, Jim H. Quality of life after allogeneic hematopoietic cell transplantation. *Blood.* 2009;114(1):7–19.

5. La Nasa G, Caocci G, Efficace F, Dessì C, Vacca A, Piras E *et al.* Long-term health-related quality of life evaluated more than 20 years after hematopoietic stem cell transplantation for thalassemia. *Blood.* 2013;122(13):2262–70.

6. Mosher CE, Redd WH, Rini CM, Burkhalter JE, DuHamel KN. Physical, psychological, and social sequelae following hematopoietic stem cell transplantation: a review of the literature. *Psycho-Oncology.* 2009;18(2):113–27.

7. Hensel M, Egerer G, Schneeweiss A, Goldschmidt H, Ho AD. Quality of life and rehabilitation in social and professional life after autologous stem cell transplantation. *Ann Oncol.* 2002;13(2):209–17.

8. Hamilton JG, Wu LM, Austin JE, Valdimarsdottir H, Basmajian K, Vu A *et al.* Economic survivorship stress is associated with poor health-related quality of life among distressed survivors of hematopoietic stem cell transplantation. *Psycho-Oncology.* 2013;22(4):911–21.

9. Kirchhoff AC, Leisenring W, Syrjala KL. Prospective predictors of return to work in the 5 years after hematopoietic cell transplantation. *J Cancer Surviv.* 2010;4(1):33–44.

10. Andrykowski MA, Bishop MM, Hahn EA, Cella DF, Beaumont JL, Brady MJ et al. Long-term health-related quality of life, growth, and spiritual well-being after hematopoietic stem-cell transplantation. *J Clin Oncol.* 2005;23(3):599–608.

11. Parsons SK, Phipps S, Sung L, Baker KS, Pulsipher MA, Ness KK. NCI, NHLBI/PBMTC First International Conference on Late Effects after Pediatric Hematopoietic Cell Transplantation: Health-Related Quality of Life, Functional, and Neurocognitive Outcomes. *Biol Blood Marrow Transplant.* 2012;18(2):162–71.

12. Clarke SA, Eiser C, Skinner R. Health-related quality of life in survivors of BMT for paediatric malignancy: a systematic review of the literature. *Bone Marrow Transplant.* 2008;42(2):73–82.

13. Schultz KA, Chen L, Chen Z, Kawashima T, Oeffinger KC, Woods WG *et al.* Health conditions and quality of life in survivors of childhood acute myeloid leukemia comparing post remission chemotherapy to BMT: a report from the children's oncology group. *Pediatr Blood Cancer.* 2014;61(4):729–36.

14. Jansen SJ, Stiggelbout AM, Nooij MA, Noordijk EM, Kievit J. Response shift in quality of life measurement in early-stage breast cancer patients undergoing radiotherapy. *Qual Life Res.* 2000;9(6):603–15.

15. Beeken RJ, Eiser C, Dalley C. Health-related quality of life in haematopoietic stem cell transplant survivors: a qualitative study on the role of psychosocial variables and response shifts. *Qual Life Res.* 2011;20(2):153–60.

16. Crosby R, Kolotkin R, Williams G. Defining clinically meaningful change in health related quality of life. *Value in Health.* 2001;4(2):177–7.

17. Wong FL, Francisco L, Togawa K, Bosworth A, Gonzales M, Hanby C et al. Long-term recovery after hematopoietic cell transplantation: predictors of quality-of-life concerns. *Blood.* 2010 115(12):2508–19.

18. McQuellon RP, Russell GB, Rambo TD, Craven BL, Radford J, Perry JJ et al. Quality of life and psychological distress of bone marrow transplant recipients: the 'time trajectory' to recovery over the first year. *Bone Marrow Transplant.* 1998;21(5):477–86.

19. Jacobs SR, Small BJ, Booth-Jones M, Jacobsen PB, Fields KK. Changes in cognitive functioning in the year after hematopoietic stem cell transplantation. *Cancer.* 2007;110(7):1560–7.

20. Andrykowski MA, Greiner CB, Altmaier EM, Burish TG, Antin JH, Gingrich R et al. Quality of life following bone marrow transplantation: findings from a multicentre study. *Br J Cancer.* 1995;71(6):1322–9.

21. Heinonen H, Volin L, Uutela A, Zevon M, Barrick C, Ruutu T. Gender-associated differences in the quality of life after allogeneic BMT. *Bone Marrow Transplant.* 2001;28(5):503–9.

22. Sun CL, Francisco L, Baker KS, Weisdorf DJ, Forman SJ, Bhatia S. Adverse psychological outcomes in long-term survivors of hematopoietic cell transplantation: a report from the Bone Marrow Transplant Survivor Study (BMTSS). *Blood.* 2011;118(17):4723–31.

23. Herzberg PY, Lee SJ, Heussner P, Mumm FH, Hilgendorf I, von Harsdorf S et al. Personality influences quality-of-life assessments in adult patients after allogeneic hematopoietic SCT: results from a joint evaluation of the prospective German Multicenter Validation Trial and the Fred Hutchinson Cancer Research Center. *Bone Marrow Transplant.* 2013;48(1):129–34.

24. Jenks Kettmann JD, Altmaier EM. Social support and depression among bone marrow transplant patients. *J Health Psychol.* 2008;13(1):39–46.

25. Diez-Campelo M, Perez-Simon JA, Gonzalez-Porras JR, Garcia-Cecilia JM, Salinero M, Caballero MD et al. Quality of life assessment in patients undergoing reduced intensity conditioning allogeneic as compared to autologous transplantation: results of a prospective study. *Bone Marrow Transplant.* 2004;34(8):729–38.

26. Bevans MF, Marden S, Leidy NK, Soeken K, Cusack G, Rivera P et al. Health-related quality of life in patients receiving reduced-intensity conditioning allogeneic hematopoietic stem cell transplantation. *Bone Marrow Transplant.* 2006;38(2):101–9.

27. Liu Hl, Sun Zm, Geng Lq, Wang Xb, Ding Ky, Tong J et al. Similar survival, but better quality of life after myeloablative transplantation using unrelated cord blood vs matched sibling donors in adults with hematologic malignancies. *Bone Marrow Transplant* 2014;49(8):1063–9.

28. Majhail NS, Ness KK, Burns LJ, Sun C-L, Carter A, Francisco L et al. Late effects in survivors of Hodgkin and non-Hodgkin lymphoma treated with autologous hematopoietic cell transplantation: a report from the Bone Marrow Transplant Survivor Study. *Biol Blood Marrow Transplant.* 2007;13(10):1153–9.

29. Khera N, Storer B, Flowers ME, Carpenter PA, Inamoto Y, Sandmaier BM et al. Nonmalignant late effects and compromised functional status in survivors of hematopoietic cell transplantation. *J Clin Oncol.* 2012;30(1):71–7.

30. Flowers ME, Parker PM, Johnston LJ, Matos AV, Storer B, Bensinger WI et al. Comparison of chronic graft-*versus*-host disease after transplantation of peripheral blood stem cells *versus* bone marrow in allogeneic recipients: long-term follow-up of a randomized trial. *Blood.* 2002;100(2):415–9.

31. Pidala J, Kurland B, Chai X, Majhail N, Weisdorf DJ, Pavletic S et al. Patient-reported quality of life is associated with severity of chronic graft-*versus*-host disease as measured by NIH criteria: report on baseline data from the Chronic GVHD Consortium. *Blood.* 2011;117(17):4651–7.

32. Pidala J, Vogelsang G, Martin P, Chai X, Storer B, Pavletic S et al. Overlap subtype of chronic graft-*versus*-host disease is associated with an adverse prognosis, functional impairment, and inferior patient-reported outcomes: a Chronic Graft-*versus*-Host Disease Consortium study. *Haematologica.* 2012;97(3):451–8.

33. El-Jawahri A, Pidala J, Inamoto Y, Chai X, Khera N, Wood WA et al. Impact of age on quality of life, functional status and survival in patients with chronic graft-versus-host disease. *Biol Blood Marrow Transplant.* 2014;20(9):1341–8.

34. Lee SJ, Joffe S, Kim HT, Socie G, Gilman AL, Wingard JR et al. Physicians' attitudes about quality-of-life issues in hematopoietic stem cell transplantation. *Blood.* 2004;104(7):2194–200.

35. Ransom S, Jacobsen PB, Booth-Jones M. Validation of the Distress Thermometer with bone marrow transplant patients. *Psycho-Oncology.* 2006;15(7):604–12.

36. Wood WA, Deal AM, Abernethy A, Basch E, Battaglini C, Kim YH et al. Feasibility of frequent patient-reported outcome surveillance in patients undergoing hematopoietic cell transplantation. *Biol Blood Marrow Transplant.* 2013;19(3):450–9.

37. Majhail NS, Rizzo JD, Lee SJ, Aljurf M, Atsuta Y, Bonfim C et al. Recommended screening and preventive practices for long-term survivors after hematopoietic cell transplantation. *Biol Blood Marrow Transplant.* 2012;18(3):348–71.

38. Mishra SI SR, Geigle PM, Berlanstein DR, Topaloglu O, Gotay CC, Snyder C. Exercise interventions on health-related quality of life for cancer survivors. *Cochrane Database Syst Rev.* 2012;8:CD008465.

39. Wiskemann J, Huber G. Physical exercise as adjuvant therapy for patients undergoing hematopoietic stem cell transplantation. *Bone Marrow Transplant.* 2007;41(4):321–9.

40. Jacobsen PB, Jim HS. Psychosocial interventions for anxiety and depression in adult cancer patients:

achievements and challenges. *CA Cancer J Clin.* 2008;58(4):214–30.

41. Syrjala KL, Cummings C, Donaldson GW. Hypnosis or cognitive behavioral training for the reduction of pain and nausea during cancer treatment: a controlled clinical trial. *Pain.* 1992;48(2):137–46.

42. Syrjala KL, Donaldson GW, Davis MW, Kippes ME, Carr JE. Relaxation and imagery and cognitive-behavioral training reduce pain during cancer treatment: a controlled clinical trial. *Pain.* 1995;63(2):189–98.

43. DuHamel KN, Mosher CE, Winkel G, Labay LE, Rini C, Meschian YM *et al.* Randomized clinical trial of telephone-administered cognitive-behavioral therapy to reduce post-traumatic stress disorder and distress symptoms after hematopoietic stem-cell transplantation. *J Clin Oncol.* 2010;28(23):3754–61.

44. Gaston-Johansson F, Fall-Dickson JM, Nanda JP, Sarenmalm EK, Browall M, Goldstein N. Long-term effect of the self-management comprehensive coping strategy program on quality of life in patients with breast cancer treated with high-dose chemotherapy. *Psycho-Oncology.* 2013;22(3):530–9.

45. McQuellon RP, Wells M, Hoffman S, Craven B, Russell G, Cruz J *et al.* Reducing distress in cancer patients with an orientation program. *Psycho-Oncology.* 1998;7(3):207–17.

46. Jim HS, Quinn GP, Gwede CK, Cases MG, Barata A, Cessna J *et al.* Patient education in allogeneic hematopoietic cell transplant: what patients wish they had known about quality of life. *Bone Marrow Transplant.* 2014;49(2):299–303.

47. Syrjala KL, Stover AC, Yi JC, Artherholt SB, Romano EM, Schoch G *et al.* Development and implementation of an Internet-based survivorship care program for cancer survivors treated with hematopoietic stem cell transplantation. *J Cancer Surviv.* 2011;5(3):292–304.

48. Jacobsen PB, Phillips KM, Jim HS, Small BJ, Faul LA, Meade CD *et al.* Effects of self-directed stress management training and home-based exercise on quality of life in cancer patients receiving chemotherapy: a randomized controlled trial. *Psycho-Oncology.* 2013;22(6):1229–35.

49. Jacobsen PB, Le-Rademacher J, Jim H, Syrjala K, Wingard JR, Logan B *et al.* Exercise and stress management training prior to hematopoietic cell transplantation: blood and marrow transplant clinical trials network (BMT CTN) 0902. *Biol Blood Marrow Transplant.* 2014;20(10):1530–6.

50. Lee SJ, Kim HT, Ho VT, Cutler C, Alyea EP, Soiffer RJ *et al.* Quality of life associated with acute and chronic graft-*versus*-host disease. *Bone Marrow Transplant.* 2006; 38(4):305–10.

51. Hjermstad MJ, Evensen SA, Kvaløy SO, Loge JH, Fayers PM, Kaasa S. The CARES-SF used for prospective assessment of health-related quality of life after stem cell transplantation. *Psycho-Oncology.* 2003;12(8):803–13.

52. Lee SJ, Cook EF, Soiffer R, Antin JH. Development and validation of a scale to measure symptoms of chronic graft-*versus*-host disease. *Biol Blood Marrow Transplant.* 2002;8(8):444–52.

53. Hjermstad MJ, Loge JH, Evensen SA, Kvaloy SO, Fayers PM, Kaasa S. The course of anxiety and depression during the first year after allogeneic or autologous stem cell transplantation. *Bone Marrow Transplant.* 1999;24(11):1219–28.

54. Hayes S, Davies PS, Parker T, Bashford J, Newman B. Quality of life changes following peripheral blood stem cell transplantation and participation in a mixed-type, moderate-intensity, exercise program. *Bone Marrow Transplant.* 2004;33(5):553–8.

55. Wiskemann J, Dreger P, Schwerdtfeger R, Bondong A, Huber G, Kleindienst N *et al.* Effects of a partly self-administered exercise program before, during, and after allogeneic stem cell transplantation. *Blood* 2011;117(9):2604–13.

56. Dimeo F, Schwartz S, Fietz T, Wanjura T, Boning D, Thiel E. Effects of endurance training on the physical performance of patients with hematological malignancies during chemotherapy. *Support Care Cancer.* 2003;11(10):623–8.

57. Jarden M, Baadsgaard MT, Hovgaard DJ, Boesen E, Adamsen L. A randomized trial on the effect of a multimodal intervention on physical capacity, functional performance and quality of life in adult patients undergoing allogeneic SCT. *Bone Marrow Transplant.* 2009;43(9):725–37.

58. DeFor TE, Burns LJ, Gold EM, Weisdorf DJ. A randomized trial of the effect of a walking regimen on the functional status of 100 adult allogeneic donor hematopoietic cell transplant patients. *Biol Blood Marrow Transplant.* 2007;13(8):948–55.

59. Wilson RW, Jacobsen PB, Fields KK. Pilot study of a home-based aerobic exercise program for sedentary cancer survivors treated with hematopoietic stem cell transplantation. *Bone Marrow Transplant.* 2005;35(7):721–7.

60. Baumann FT, Kraut L, Schule K, Bloch W, Fauser AA. A controlled randomized study examining the effects of exercise therapy on patients undergoing haematopoietic stem cell transplantation. *Bone Marrow Transplant.* 2009;45(2):355–62.

61. Knols RH, de Bruin ED, Uebelhart D, Aufdemkampe G, Schanz U, Stenner-Liewen F *et al.* Effects of an outpatient physical exercise program on hematopoietic stem-cell transplantation recipients: a randomized clinical trial. *Bone Marrow Transplant.* 2011;46(9):1245–55.

Epilogue

Armand Keating

In this book, you will have read of the many concepts, successes, and challenges that many of us encounter with hematopoietic cell transplantation (HCT). Our approach in this text has been to be more enquiring than didactic, and we hope that it will serve as an invitation to you to contribute your knowledge and expertise to improve this field further.

There is little doubt that the field is expanding and continues to be a highly active area of investigation. This applies not only to the increasing number of studies attempting to address the numerous complications facing HCT but also continues with expanding the indications for transplant, as for example in using genetically modified cells to treat rare, fatal, single-gene disorders such as lysosomal storage diseases. Indeed, if these successes continue, we can expect many more protocols with engineered hematopoietic and other cells in the near future.

As with many fields in medicine that are evolving, it has been interesting to note changes in the deployment of technology. A case in point is the noticeable reduction in the use of cord blood grafts in favor of hematopoietic cells from HLA haplotype mismatch donors. It remains to be seen whether or not this trend will continue.

A major challenge remains graft-*versus*-host disease (GvHD), and while the final chapter on the role of mesenchymal stromal cells (MSCs) in managing steroid-resistant acute GvHD has not yet been written, it will be prudent of us to keep an eye (or two) open for effective therapy with small molecules. Nonetheless, it has been disappointing that more cell therapy trials have not been undertaken in chronic GvHD, especially with MSCs. A multipronged approach to tackle this particularly challenging complication is very much in order. As you will have read, however, genomic and other approaches to GvHD prevention are likely to provide the most effective strategies.

As we review our successes with HCT, we would be wise to not overlook the long-term complications that the therapy engenders. This applies not only to the well-documented increase in second malignancies but also to the considerably more prevalent cardiovascular complications that only now are being recognized. We can speculate that the entire transplantation process is associated with a powerful inflammatory response, and here too, we could look perhaps to post-transplant cell therapy to mitigate the risks. As we now know, these late complications are not confined to allo-transplant but also apply to autologous HCT, albeit to a lesser extent.

There is considerable excitement with the highly promising results with immune-oncology, notably CAR T-cell and checkpoint inhibitor therapy (as much in the stock market as in the clinic, it would seem). It is unlikely that these treatments will supplant HCT, and if they do, then that will be all to the good, but in many cases they may simply serve as the oft-quoted "bridge to transplant." These developments will bring with them new challenges and potential complications.

It is evident that HCT is in a vibrant state but continues to require much work. We need to address, as best we can, the workforce shortage in the coming decade that many predict will be serious. As well as disseminating the basics and subtleties of HCT that I hope you will have found are covered in this text, I offer this challenge to you: please inspire your trainees to enter this field, to contribute their ingenuity and energy to the science and practice of HCT, and thereby ensure that more of our patients are cured and will go about their daily lives without serious complications.

Index

transplant *versus* non-transplant therapy, 53–4
allograft rejection. *See* graft failure
amphotericin B, 152, 155
anemia, 120, *See also* severe aplastic anemia (SAA); sickle cell disease (SCD)
aplastic, 3
anidulafungin, 154
antibiotics
  infection treatment in recipients, 136–7
    controversies, 137
  prophylaxis, 134–6
    patient requirements, 135–6
    post-engraftment infections, 136
    quinolone, 131–4
  resistance, 136–7
antifungal agents, 152–4
  combination therapy, 157
  controversies, 156–7
  cytotoxic T-lymphocyte immunotherapy, 618–23
  empiric antifungal therapy, 155
  invasive aspergillosis treatment, 156
  invasive candidiasis treatment, 155–6
  prophylaxis, 154–5
anti-T-cell antibodies. *See* antithymocyte globulin (ATG); conditioning regimens; T-cell depletion (TCD)
antithymocyte globulin (ATG), 106–7, 109
  ATG-Fresenius, 274
  dose and serum levels, 275–6
  GvHD prophylaxis, 164
  immune reconstitution impact, 285
  myeloablative conditioning, 274
  myelodysplastic syndromes, 332
  reduced intensity conditioning, 275
  relapse risk relationship, 629
aplastic anemia, 3
  severe. *See* severe aplastic anemia (SAA)
arthritis, 536
aspergillosis, 152, 618, *See also* fungal infections
  combination therapy, 157
  invasive aspergillosis treatment, 156
    comparative evidence of efficacy, 156
  prevention, 693
at-risk population identification, 676

Atgam, 274
atorvastatin, 108
autoimmune diseases, 531
  allo-HCT, 532
  arthritis, 536
  auto-HCT, 531–5
    controversies, 538–9
    efficacy variation, 539–41
    ex vivo graft selection, 538
    expertise requirement, 533
    funding issues, 533
    patient selection, 532–3
    peripheral blood mobilization, 538
    rationale, 531–2
    response predictor assessment, 543–4
    technique, 532
    timing, 532–3
  conditioning regimens, 538–9
  connective tissue diseases, 535–6
  future directions, 534, 545
  inflammatory bowel disease, 537
  mortality rates, 541
  neurological diseases, 536–7
  outcome measurements, 541
  post-transplant complications, 541–3
    fertility impact, 542
    immunocompromise, 541–2
    secondary autoimmune disease, 542
    secondary malignancies, 542
  regenerative medicine, 666
  transplant activity, 532–3
  type 1 diabetes, 537–8, 540
Autologous Bone Marrow Transplant Registry (ABMTR), 4
autologous HCT, 55–6, 97, *See also specific conditions*
  conditioning regimens, 249–50
  hematopoietic progenitor cell source, 17
  immune reconstitution, 198
  older patient selection, 54–6
  relapse prevention, 203–4
  tumor cell removal, 97
azacitidine
  maintenance therapy, 204–5
    controversies, 208
  myelodysplastic syndromes, 328
  relapse management, 232, 332
azoles, 153, *See also* antifungal agents

bacterial infections, 131
  at the time of HCT, 47
  carbapenem-resistant *Klebsiella pneumoniae*, 134

epidemiology in recipients, 132
  changes over time, 131
  pre-transplant evaluation, 44
  prophylaxis, 134–6
    patient requirements, 135–6
    post-engraftment infections, 136
    quinolone, 131–4
  treatment, 136–7
    controversies, 137
basiliximab, 113, 562
Batten disease, 667
B-cell recovery, 197
BCR/ABL positive ALL, 216–17, *See also* Philadelphia chromosome-positive ALL
beclomethasone, 113
Berlin Patient, 554
beta-thalassemia major
  allo-HCT, 514–16, 520
    adult patients, 520
    current experience, 515
    early experience, 514–15
    iron overload issue, 521
    mixed chimerism following, 519
    outcomes, 515, 517
    risk class-based approach, 514
    second transplant, 520
  conditioning regimens, 513–14, 520
  donor selection, 516–20
    alternative related donors, 516
    cord blood transplant, 518
    haplotype mismatched family donors, 516–18
    unrelated donors, 518–19
  future directions, 521
  historical perspective, 513
  post-transplant monitoring, 519–20
  transplant-related complications, 519
    graft failure or rejection, 519
    GvHD, 519
bi-antigen specific T-cells (BITE), 634
bias in research, 677
BIO5192, 88
biological scaffolds, 658–9
biomarkers, 32
  GvHD, 173
    treatment guidance, 114–16
  transplant candidacy assessment, 55
BK-virus, 147, 150
blast crisis, 341
blinatumomab, 304, 312
blood group incompatibilities, 123, *See also* ABO blood group incompatibility; Rh

blood group incompatibility
  definitions, 123
  transfusion strategies, 126–7
blood transfusion, 126
  with ABO blood group mismatch, 126–7
  with Rh blood group mismatch, 127
bone defects, 665
bone fractures, non-union, 665
bone loss, 190
  prevention, 190
bone marrow failure (BMF)
  Fanconi anemia, 507
  syndromes, 501
bone marrow fibrosis, 355
bone marrow niche, 79, 81
  endosteal niche, 79–80
  perivascular niche, 81
  signaling pathways, 81
bone marrow transplantation
  ABO blood group incompatibility complications, 124
  history, 1–6, 97
  HLA-mismatched transplant, 562–4
  RBC reduction, 124
  second allogeneic HCT, 236
  severe aplastic anemia, 502
  tumor cell removal, 97
  versus peripheral blood cell grafts, 59, 346
bortezomib
  GvHD prevention, 107–8
  immunoglobulin light chain amyloidosis, 482
  maintenance therapy, 450, 461–2, 472
    cytogenetic risk implications, 462
    second primary malignancy association, 462
    with thalidomide, 462
  mantle cell lymphoma, 409
  multiple myeloma, 446–7, 449
bosutinib, 340
brentuximab vedotin (BV), 368–9
brincidofovir, 142–4
bronchoscopy, 183
Burkitt lymphoma (BL), 423
  HIV-associated, 552
busulfan, 18, 448, *See also* conditioning regimens
  beta-thalassemia major, 513
  HLA-mismatched transplant, 562
  neuroblastoma, 493
  optimal seizure prophylaxis, 678–82

natural killer (NK) cells, 602
  alloreactivity mechanism, 628
  alloreactivity prediction
      models, 603–5, 607
    altered or injured self, 604–5
    KIR–KIR mismatch model,
        603
    KIR–KIR-ligand mismatch
        model, 603
    ligand–ligand mismatch
        model, 603
    missing ligand model, 603
    missing self, 603–4
    NKG2A *versus* NKG2C, 605
  cell recognition models, 602–3
  controversies, 606–7
    in vivo versus ex vivo
        expansion, 604–7
    role in GvHD, 607
  cord blood NK cell anti-tumor
      immunotherapy, 642
  donor lymphocyte infusion
      augmentation, 228
  future research, 605–7
    leukemic control, 607
    NK cell reconstitution
        promotion, 607
    NK cell subsets, 605
    preclinical studies, 605
  graft rejection prevention in
      HLA-mismatched
      transplants, 560
  graft-*versus*-leukemia effect
      enhancement, 634–5
  receptors, 602–4
  recovery, 196–7
  transplantation and, 604–5
    auto-HCT, 605
    cord blood transplants, 605
    haplotype matched HCT,
        604–5
    matched allo-HCT, 605
    outcome benefits, 606
neural stem cells, 667
neuroblastoma, 491
  allo-HCT, 494–5
  antibody therapy following
      HCT, 495–6
  auto-HCT, 491–4
    candidates for, 491
    conditioning regimens,
        492–3
    graft purging, 493–4
    historical perspective, 491–2
    prior lymphodepletion, 496
    tandem/sequential HCT,
        492–3
  cellular therapy, 496
  controversies, 497
  future directions, 497
  minimal residual disease, 494
neurological diseases, 536–7
  regenerative medicine, 666
neuromyelitis optica (NMO),
    537, 540

neuronal ceroid lipofuscinosis,
    667
neutrophil recovery, 196
nicotinamide, 640
  cord blood progenitor cell
      expansion, 641
nilotinib, 339, 341
non-Hodgkin lymphoma (NHL).
    See also diffuse large
      B-cell lymphoma; HIV-
      associated lymphoma;
      primary CNS lymphoma
      (PCNSL); secondary CNS
      lymphoma (CNSL)
  age effect on auto-HCT
      outcome, 54–6
  donor lymphocyte infusion,
      227
  HCT-specific comorbidity
      index use, 28
nonmyeloablative conditioning
    (NMC), 19, 250, *See also*
      conditioning regimens
  diffuse large B-cell lymphoma,
      422
  HLA-mismatched transplant,
      563
  sickle cell disease, 526
Notch signaling, 641
  cord blood progenitor cell
      expansion, 641

ocular complications, 191
older patients. *See also* age
  acute myeloid leukemia,
      optimal conditioning
      regimen, 253–4
  age as a selection criterion,
      30–1
  allo-transplant
    candidate selection, 53–5
    outcomes, 52–3
  comorbidities, 23
  disease relapse risk, 53
  epidemiological trends, 51
  mantle cell lymphoma, 403–4
    maintenance therapy, 405–7
  severe aplastic anemia, 503
  transplant tolerance, 54
on-target, off-tumor responses,
    598
organ-specific complications, 184
organ-specific stem cells, 658
osteoarthritis, 665
osteoporosis, 190

pancytopenia, 501
panobinostat, 205
papovaviruses, 145–6
parainfluenza viruses (PIV), 145
paroxysmal nocturnal
      hemoglobinuria (PNH),
      504
passenger lymphocyte syndrome
    (PLS), 125

ABO mismatch, delayed
      hemolysis and, 125
  Rh mismatch, 127–8
Pegfilgrastim, 82–3
Pelizaeus–Merzbacher disease,
    667
penicillin prophylaxis, 136
pentostatin, 108
performance status (PS), 29
  transplant tolerance
      relationship, 54
peri-anal fistulae, 665
peripheral blood cell grafts
  ABO blood group
      incompatibility
      complications, 124
    antibody removal, 124
    HLA-mismatched transplants,
        563–4
    red blood cell removal, 124
    second allo-HCT, 236
    T-cell depletion requirement,
        271
    versus bone marrow grafts, 59,
        346
peripheral blood stem cells
    (PBSCs), 79, *See also*
      peripheral blood cell
      grafts
  mobilization, 79, 81–5
    autoimmune diseases, 538
    controversies, 85–7
    failure, 79
    G-CSF, 82, 85–6
    G-CSF plus chemotherapy
        (G/C), 84–5
    GM-CSF, 83
    novel agents, 81–7
    pegylated G-CSF, 82–3
    physical exercise, 89
    Plerixafor, 84–6
    stem cell factor (SCF), 84
peripheral T-cell lymphomas
    (PTCL), 428
  allo-HCT, 431–2
    first-line treatment, 431–2
    relapsed/refractory disease,
        432
    studies, 432
  auto-HCT, 429–31
    clinical trials, 430
    first-line treatment, 429–30
    relapsed/refractory disease,
        430–1
  chemotherapy, 428–9
    CHOP regimen, 428
    etoposide addition, 428
  conditioning regimens, 429–30
  subtypes, 428
  transplant-related
      controversies, 432
perivascular niche, 81
pharmacological controversies
  antifungal prophylaxis
      duration, 687–94

drug interactions in GvHD
      prophylaxis, 687
  post-transplant, 681–93
    calcineurin inhibitor-
        induced
        hypomagnesemia
        management, 686–7
    mycophenolate mofetil
        monitoring, 684–6
    optimal serum levels for
        combined tacrolimus and
        sirolimus, 684
  pretransplant conditioning
      regimens, 678–84
    dosing, 681–4
    melphalan optimal dose,
        678
    optimal seizure prophylaxis
        with busulfan, 678–81
Philadelphia chromosome-
      positive ALL, 292, 309
  conditioning regimen, 311–12
  cord blood *versus* HLA-
      haplotype matched donor
      HCT, 310–11
  need for allo-HCT, 309
  tyrosine kinase inhibitor
      therapy, 309–10
phlebotomy, 189
physical examination, 45
physical exercise. *See* exercise
pidilizumab, 421
plasma cell disorders, 14, *See also*
      immunoglobulin light
      chain amyloidosis (AL);
      multiple myeloma (MM);
      plasma cell myeloma
  donor lymphocyte infusion,
      227
plasma cell leukemia (PCL),
    471
plasma cell myeloma. *See also*
      multiple myeloma (MM)
  allo-HCT, 468
    controversies, 473
    early history, 468
    future directions, 473
    graft-*versus*-myeloma
        (GvM) effect, 470
    maintenance therapy, 472
    relapse treatment, 471–3
    response measurement, 472
    risk assessment and, 470–1
    upfront, 468–70
  conditioning regimens, 247
    melphalan optimal dose,
        678
  minimal residual disease
      detection techniques, 463
    studies, 464
pleiotrophin (PTN), 81
Plerixafor, 84–5
  allogeneic setting, 86
  cost, 86–7
  versus chemotherapy, 85